Orthopaedic Physical Therapy

Third Edition

Robert A. Donatelli, PhD, PT, OCS

Physiotherapy Associates
Alpharetta, Georgia
National Director of Sports Rehabilitation
Physiotherapy Associates
Memphis, Tennessee
Orthopaedic Track Chair
Rocky Mountain University
Provo, Utah

Michael J. Wooden, MS, PT, OCS

Physiotherapy Associates
Lilburn, Georgia
National Director of Clinical Research
Physiotherapy Associates
Memphis, Tennessee
Instructor, Division of Physical Therapy
Department of Rehabilitation Medicine
Emory University
Atlanta, Georgia

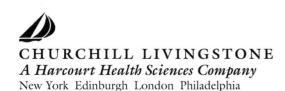

CHURCHILL LIVINGSTONE
A Harcourt Health Sciences Company
New York Edinburgh London Philadelphia

CHURCHILL LIVINGSTONE

A Harcourt Health Sciences Company

The Curtis Center
Independence Square West
Philadelphia, Pennsylvania 19106

Library of Congress Cataloging-in-Publication Data

Orthopaedic physical therapy / [edited by] Robert A. Donatelli, Michael J. Wooden—
3rd ed.
    p. ; cm.
  Includes bibliographical references and index.
  ISBN 0-443-07993-5
  1. Orthopedics. 2. Physical therapy. I. Donatelli, Robert. II. Wooden, Michael J.
  [DNLM: 1. Orthopedic Procedures—methods. 2. Musculoskeletal Diseases—therapy.
  3. Physical Therapy—methods. WE 168 O769 2001]
  RD736.P47 O79 2001
  616.7'0652—dc21

                                                                    00-046611

Acquisitions Editor: Andrew Allen
Senior Editorial Assistant: Suzanne Hontscharik
Production Manager: Donna L. Morrissey

ORTHOPAEDIC PHYSICAL THERAPY   ISBN 0-443-07993-5

Printed in the United States of America

Last digit is the print number: 9   8   7   6   5   4   3   2   1

To my most prized possession, Rachel Marie Donatelli

      R.A.D.

To Mary Lee for her love, understanding, and patience, patience, patience
To Gena, the real *writer in the family*
And to Trevor and Alec, my all-stars

      M.J.W.

Contributors

Jill Binkley, B.Sc.P.T., M.Sc.P.T.
Assistant Professor, School of Rehabilitation Sciences, McMaster University, Hamilton, Ontario, Canada; Physical Therapist, Appalachian Physical Therapy, Dahlonega, Georgia

Turner A. Blackburn, Jr., M.Ed., P.T.
Adjunct Assistant Professor, Department of Orthopaedics, Tulane University School of Medicine, Tulane University; Director, Tulane Institute of Sports Medicine, Tulane University Hospital and Clinic, New Orleans, Louisiana

Richard W. Bohannon, B.S., M.S., Ed.D.
Professor, Department of Physical Therapy, School of Allied Health, University of Connecticut, Storrs, Connecticut; Senior Scientist, Institute of Outcomes Research and Evaluation, Hartford, Connecticut

William G. Boissonnault, P.T., M.Sc., D.P.T.
Assistant Professor, Physical Therapy Program, University of Wisconsin–Madison, Madison, Wisconsin; Instructor, Krannert School of Physical Therapy, University of Indianapolis, Indianapolis, Indiana; Clinical Assistant Professor, College of Allied Health Sciences, University of Tennessee, Memphis, Tennessee; Adjunct Faculty, University of St. Augustine for Health Sciences, St. Augustine, Florida

Jean M. Bryan, Ph.D., M.P.T., O.C.S.
Professor, U.S. Army-Baylor University Graduate Program in Physical Therapy, San Antonio, Texas

Brenda Lipscomb Burgess, B.S., P.T., C.H.T.
Chief Hand Therapist, Progressive Sports Medicine and Physical Therapy, Decatur, Georgia

Robert A. Donatelli, Ph.D., P.T., O.C.S.
Physiotherapy Associates, Alpharetta, Georgia; National Director of Sports Rehabilitation, Physiotherapy Associates, Memphis, Tennessee; Orthopaedic Track Chair, Rocky Mountain University, Provo, Utah

Peter I. Edgelow, M.A., P.T.
Consultant to Kaiser Physical Therapy Residency Program in Advanced Orthopaedic Manual Therapy; Codirector, Physiotherapy Associates, Hayward Physical Therapy, Hayward, California

Robert L. Elvey, B.App.Sc., Grad. Dip. Manip. Ther.
Senior Lecturer, Curkin University; Physiotherapy Consultant, Southcare Physiotherapy, Perth, Western Australia

Mary L. Engles, M.S., P.T., O.C.S., M.T.C.
Former Adjunct Professor, 1986–96, Physical Therapist Assistant Program, Mesa College, San Diego, California; private practice, Sports Arena Physical Therapy, San Diego, California; chairperson, San Diego District, California Chapter, APTA, San Diego, California

Juan C. Garbalosa, Ph.D.
Assistant Professor, University of Hartford, West Hartford, Connecticut; Clinical Researcher, New Britain General Hospital, New Britain, Connecticut

Blanca Zita Gonzalez-King, B.S., P.T., C.H.T.
Private Consultant, Atlanta, Georgia; Clinical Instructor, Advance Rehabilitation Services, Marietta, Georgia

Gary W. Gray, B.S., A.T.C.
Director and Owner, Gary Gray Physical Therapy, Adrian, Michigan

Bruce A. Greenfield, M.M.Sc., P.T., O.C.S.
Instructor, Division of Physical Therapy, Department of Rehabilitation Medicine, Emory University, Atlanta, Georgia

Toby M. Hall, M.Sc., Post Grad. Dip. Manip. Ther.
Adjunct Senior Teaching Fellow, Curtin University; Director, Manual Concepts, Perth, Western Australia

William B. Haynes, M.D.
Orthopaedic Surgery and Sports Medicine, The Hughston Clinic, P.C., Alpharetta, Georgia

Stephanie Hoffman, M.S., P.T.
American Physical Therapy Association Member, La Jolla, California

Scot Irwin, D.P.T., M.A., B.A.
Associate Professor, North Georgia College and State University; Director, North Georgia Physical Therapy Faculty Practice, Dahlonega, Georgia

Steven C. Janos, M.S., P.T.
Assistant Professor, Department of Physical Therapy, University of Central Florida College of Health and Public Affairs, Orlando, Florida

Gregory S. Johnson, B.S., P.T.
Associate Instructor, Physical Therapy Schools, University of St. Augustine, Touro College, Long Island; Codirector, Institute of Physical Art Continuing Education Institute, Steamboat Springs, Colorado

Richard B. Johnston, III, M.D.
Clinical Instructor, Emory University; Partner, The Hughston Clinic, P.C., Atlanta, Georgia

Lee A. Kelley, M.D.
Piedmont Hospital, Sheperd Spinal Center, Atlanta, Georgia

Steven L. Kraus, P.T., O.C.S., M.T.C.
Clinical Assistant Professor, Division of Physical Therapy, Department of Rehabilitation Medicine, Emory University School of Medicine, Atlanta, Georgia

Shirley Kushner, M.Sc.P.T., B.Sc.P.T., B.P.E.
Family Lecturer, Department of Family Medicine, Faculty of Medicine, McGill University; Hertzl Family Practice Centre, Jewish General Hospital; Head Physiotherapist and Director, Physiotherapy Kushner, Montreal, Quebec, Canada

Leland C. McCluskey, M.D.
Staff Physician, Hughston Clinic, Columbus, Georgia

David A. McCune, M.Phty. St., P.T., O.C.S., A.T.C., F.A.A.O.M.P.T.
Adjunct Faculty, Upstate Medical University, Syracuse, New York

Monique Ronayne Peterson, B.S., P.T., O.C.S.
Research Advisor, Mount Saint Mary's College, Physical Therapy Program; Teaching Assistant, Orthopedic Class, Mount Saint Mary's College, Los Angeles, California

Robert M. Poole, P.T., M.Ed., A.T.C.
Corporate Director, Human Performance and Rehabilitation Center, Atlanta, Georgia

David C. Reid, B.P.T., M.D., M.Ch.(orth.), F.R.C.S.(C)
Professor, Department of Surgery, Faculty of Medicine; Honorary Professor, Physical Education Faculty; Adjunct Professor, Faculty of Rehabilitation Medicine, University of Alberta, Edmonton, Alberta, Canada

David Paul Rouben, M.D.
Visiting Professor, Orthopaedic Surgery, Western Galilee Medical Center, Techniow University, Haifa, Israel; Active Orthopaedic Surgeon, Jewish Hospital, Caritas Hospital, Norton Southwest Hospital, Louisville, Kentucky

David A. Schiff, M.D.
Peachtree Orthopaedic Clinic, Atlanta, Georgia

Lynn Snyder-Mackler, Sc.D., P.T.
Associate Professor, Department of Physical Therapy, University of Delaware, Newark, Delaware; Associate Research Professor, Department of Orthopedic Surgery, Thomas Jefferson University, Philadelphia, Pennsylvania

Robert B. Sprague, P.T., Ph.D., G.D.A.M.T.
Professor of Physical Therapy, Ithaca College, Ithaca, New York; Faculty, Maitland-Australian Physiotherapy Seminars, Cutchogue, New York; Burke Physical Therapy, Jacksonville, New York

Rick K. St. Pierre, M.D.
Director, Atlanta Center for Athletes; Director, Sports-Medicine Specialists; Medical Director, North Atlanta Orthopaedic Surgery Center; Fellow of the International College of Surgeons; Former Team Physician for the Atlanta Ruckus Professional Soccer Team and the Atlanta Glory Professional Basketball Team, Atlanta, Georgia

Steven A. Stratton, Ph.D., P.T., A.T.C.
Clinical Associate Professor, University Health Science Center of San Antonio School of Medicine, Physical Medicine and Rehabilitation Residency Program, San Antonio, Texas

Robert W. Sydenham, B.Sc., Dip.P.T., M.C.P.A., M.A.P.T.A., R.P.T., F.C.A.M.T.
Fellow, The Canadian Academy of Orthopaedic Manipulative Therapists; Director, URSA Foundation, Edmonds, Washington; Clinical Director, Lifemark Health Facility, Edmonton, Alberta, Canada

Dorie Syen, M.S., O.T.R./L., C.H.T.
Guest Lecturer, Emory University, Atlanta, Georgia; Brenau University, Gainesville, Georgia; Certified Hand Therapist, Atlanta Medical Center, Atlanta, Georgia

David Tiberio, Ph.D.
Associate Professor, Department of Physical Therapy, University of Connecticut, Storrs, Connecticut

Randy Walker, Ph.D., P.T.
Director, School of Rehabilitation Professions, and UC Foundation Associate Professor, Phyiscal Therapy Program, University of Tennessee at Chattanooga, Chattanooga, Tennessee

Ellen Wetherbee, M.S., P.T., O.C.S.
Academic Coordinator of Clinical Education, University of Hartford, West Hartford, Connecticut; Physical Therapist, Connal Physical Therapy, Windsor, Connecticut

Robbin Wickham, M.S., P.T.
Doctoral Fellow, Human Performance Laboratory, Ball State University, Muncie, Indiana

Joseph S. Wilkes, M.D.
Clinical Associate Professor, Orthopaedics, Emory University; Active Staff Member, Piedmont Hospital; Specialty Consulting, Crawford Long Hospital, Atlanta, Georgia; Active Staff Member, Fayette Community Hospital, Fayetteville, Georgia

Allyn L. Woerman, M.M.Sc., P.T.
Manager and Owner, Adult Rehabilitation Therapies, Lakewood, Washington

Michael J. Wooden, M.S., P.T., O.C.S.
Physiotherapy Associates, Lilburn, Georgia; National Director of Clinical Research, Physiotherapy Associates, Memphis, Tennessee; Instructor, Division of Physical Therapy, Department of Rehabilitation Medicine, Emory University, Atlanta, Georgia

Foreword

Donatelli and Wooden's *Orthopaedic Physical Therapy,* third edition, arrives at a time when the art and science of clinical practice is evolving at breakneck speed. Case management, primary care, differential diagnosis, consultation, and patient triage responsibilities are becoming the norm, as opposed to the exception, for the Orthopaedic Physical Therapist. At a time when pressures to increase productivity are prevalent, the American Physical Therapy Association has appropriately set very high standards of practice. Looking to the year 2020, the American Physical Therapy Association has established the vision of doctors of physical therapy providing physical therapy services. Orthopaedic Physical Therapy practitioners must rise to the occasion if we are to meet these challenges and continue to be cost-effective and efficacious members of the health care team.

Donatelli and Wooden have provided us with a wealth of information designed to enhance our clinical decision-making and technical skills. By assembling this group of experts from the Orthopaedic Physical Therapy clinical and research communities, and from the orthopaedic surgery and physical medicine communities, the editors have given readers access to the latest evidence related to the management of patients with musculoskeletal disorders. Donatelli and Wooden have assembled an eclectic group of experienced practitioners who expose the readers to multiple approaches of care for simple and complicated musculoskeletal conditions. A therapist would need to attend continuing education courses for years to be exposed to the ideas packed into this textbook.

Following a basic sciences foundation in the first section of the book, practical patient examination and intervention schemes are presented, first for the upper, then the lower quarter regions of the body. Excellent photographs and illustrations provide readers with a detailed understanding of anatomy, biomechanics, and orthopaedic pathology. The photographs illustrating examination and treatment techniques provide the detail necessary for readers to advance their observation, palpation, and manual therapy skills. Most importantly, the chapters are written in such a fashion that readers are allowed to join the experts in making difficult clinical decisions. The authors share the wisdom they have accumulated over the years through discussion, newly added patient cases, and updated reference lists. This "mentoring" will be invaluable to the physical therapy student, as well as to both the novice and the expert practitioner. New chapters in this edition include information on the science of muscle strengthening, foot orthotic therapy, and functional outcome measures for the orthopaedic patient.

The surgical information provided also sets this book apart from other similar textbooks. An understanding of the most current surgical approaches will not only enhance patient care directly but will also facilitate communication between therapists and physicians, which will then indirectly enhance the health care delivery to this patient population. The editors have recruited several new authors who, as orthopaedic surgeons, bring their expertise to the various descriptions of the latest surgical techniques. This textbook provides a strong link between the Orthopaedic Physical Therapist and the surgeon, with the patient being the ultimate winner.

I congratulate the editors and contributors for the update of this valuable clinical resource. The student and the experienced Orthopaedic Physical Therapist stand to greatly benefit by absorbing the wealth of information contained in this textbook. Donatelli and Wooden have made a significant contribution to the physical therapy profession's drive for clinical excellence and accountability.

William Boissonnault, P.T., D.P.T., M.Sc.
Assistant Professor, Program in Physical Therapy
Department of Surgery
University of Wisconsin, Madison
President, Orthopaedic Section
American Physical Therapy Association

Preface

We are pleased and proud to present the third edition of *Orthopaedic Physical Therapy*. We have expanded and updated this volume to meet our goal as set forth in previous editions: to present the current state of orthopaedic physical therapy practice as it has been influenced by research, advanced education, and specialization. The book is written for the physical therapy student, the general physical therapy practitioner, and the physical therapist specializing in orthopaedics. It will also be a valuable reference for allopathic and osteopathic physicians, podiatrists, and non-medical practitioners who treat orthopaedic dysfunction.

As before, this edition is divided into four main sections. The first section, Fundamental Principles, discusses the responses of body tissues and systems to trauma as well as immobilization and movement, and builds the foundation for safe and effective treatment. Previous chapters on *Tissue Response* and *Exercise Treatment for the Rehabilitated Patient* have been revised to include updated reference lists. A new chapter covering the *Theory and Practice of Muscle Strengthening in Orthopaedic Physical Therapy* will further guide the therapist in exercise prescription.

The Upper Quarter and Lower Quarter sections emphasize treatment of the individual, not just the site of the dysfunction. Because dysfunction syndromes often develop as a result of abnormal posture or movement patterns, the entire region must be evaluated. Within each of these sections, the relationships and interdependence of anatomy, mechanics, and kinesiology are discussed. Posture and gait are reviewed with emphasis on the interrelationship of structures during movement. Also presented are specific pathologies and dysfunction syndromes for each region. These include reviews of anatomy, local tissue responses to pathology and overuse, and physical therapy evaluation and treatment. Case studies and references for all chapters have been updated. Surgical options for restoring normal movement are discussed in detail. Chapters covering *New Advances in Lumbar Spine Surgery, Surgical Treatment of the Hip, Surgery of the Knee,* and *Reconstructive Surgery of the Foot and Ankle* have been substantially revised by new contributors, all orthopaedic surgeons. *Foot Orthotics: An Overview of Rationale, Assessment, and Fabrications,* has been added to provide the clinician with additional lower extremity treatment options.

The fourth section, Special Considerations, presents unique applications for orthopaedic physical therapy theory and practice. Of particular note is the new chapter dealing with *Measurement of Functional Status, Progress, and Outcome in Orthopaedic Clinical Practice.* Orthopaedic pathologies often encountered in the patient with neurologic dysfunction are presented, including implications, evaluation, and treatment. The section also contains a chapter on evaluation and treatment of soft tissue restrictions, which includes many helpful technical illustrations. Finally, the section concludes with another new chapter, *Evaluation and Treatment of Neural Tissue Pain Disorders.*

We have many people to thank for the evolution of the third edition. We could not have accomplished this without the unconditional support of the administration, clinicians, and office staffs of Physiotherapy Associates (and its parent company, the Stryker Corporation) whose reputation in the medical community fills us with pride, and with whom we have grown so much professionally. Similarly, we are grateful to our fellow faculty members at Emory University and Rocky Mountain University of Health Professions who have given us wonderful opportunities to learn, and to the many students we have had the absolute privilege to teach.

The expertise of so many people behind the scenes has contributed to this book's production. We are grateful to Andrew Allen for backing us (and pushing us!) all the way on this project, to Peg Waltner for keeping our shoulders to the wheel, and to Peggy Gordon for the finishing touches. Thanks also to Carol Binns for assistance with manuscript preparation.

We are indebted, of course, to our contributors for their thorough, insightful, and timely chapters. Because of their efforts we are confident this book will greatly enhance patient care.

Finally, we are grateful and fortunate to have wonderful families, whose love, patience, and encouragement are our greatest motivators.

Robert A. Donatelli, Ph.D., P.T., O.C.S.
Michael J. Wooden, M.S., P.T., O.C.S.

Contents

Section III
The Lower Quarter

Section IV
Special Considerations

CHAPTER 1
Tissue Response

Mary Engles

■ Normal Tissue

Muscle

In studying the human body and its response to its environment, we naturally proceed from the normal to the abnormal. Normal body tissues are grouped into four categories according to similarities of function and structure. In orthopaedic physical therapy we are most concerned with three of these: muscle; connective tissue (including bone, tendon, ligament, and fascia); and nerve. The fourth category, epithelium, is left to other specialists. Let us have a brief look at the normal structure and function of each of these tissues before moving on to examine the tissue-specific responses to mechanical stress, immobilization, and remobilization.

■ Normal Tissue

Muscle

Muscle is the tissue type that most completely expresses cell contractility.[1] It is a composite structure consisting of muscle cells or fibers and the connective tissue network that transmits the pull of the muscle cells.[1,2] The sarcomere, the basic contractile unit that makes up most of the muscle cell, is composed of actin and myosin.[1] These contractile proteins are arranged in a specific pattern, which gives muscle tissue its characteristic striated appearance. Sarcomeres are further arranged in parallel to form myofibrils (muscle fibers or cells), which in turn are arranged in bundles to form fascicles and finally a whole muscle (Fig. 1–1). Muscle fibers are cylindrical, with a diameter ranging from about 10 μm to about 100 μm— less than the diameter of a human hair.[3] This diameter is a major determinant of muscle fiber strength and is an index of changes in the level of use of the fiber. Muscle fiber length is likewise variable and has a profound influence on fiber contraction velocity and fiber excursion.[3] Other properties of muscle—morphology, metabolism,

physiology, and histochemistry—cause muscle fibers to be "typed." The metabolic classification into slow-oxidative (SO), fast oxidative-glycolytic (FOG), and fast-glycolytic is considered by many to be the most useful.[3] These characteristics reflect not only the contractile properties of the muscle fiber but also its response to exercise and immobilization. Chapter 2 of this book and other works describe the response of muscle to exercise.[4–6] The noncontractile element of the muscle, the connective tissue, is manifest at every level of muscle organization. Thin sheets of connective tissue surround each muscle fiber, becoming thicker as they surround each fascicle and finally enveloping the exterior of the muscle itself (Fig. 1–2). These delicate sheets of tissue provide a mechanical framework for contraction and a conduit for blood vessels and nerve fibers to reach the interior of the muscle. At either end of the muscle, collagen fibers extend beyond the muscle itself and blend with the connective tissue that forms the tendon, fascia, or aponeurosis, which anchors the muscle to its bony endpoint.

With the advent of electron microscopy in the early 1950s, the exact arrangement of the actin and myosin filaments within the sarcomere was discovered (Fig. 1–1). By comparing micrographs of muscle in the relaxed and contracted states, H.E. Huxley and coworkers in 1954 developed the "sliding filament" theory, which immediately gained widespread acceptance.[1] The manner in which this sliding occurs has been the subject of much study. When the muscle is relaxed, the lateral projections of the myosin filaments, formed by the tail-to-tail and spiral arrangement of the large myosin molecules,[7] lie close to their parent filament, whereas in contraction they project to contact the adjacent actin strands. Actin strands have a groove along their length due to their helical structure. A regulatory protein, tropomyosin, fits into this groove, which is also punctated at intervals by the protein troponin. Troponin is actually responsible for initiating

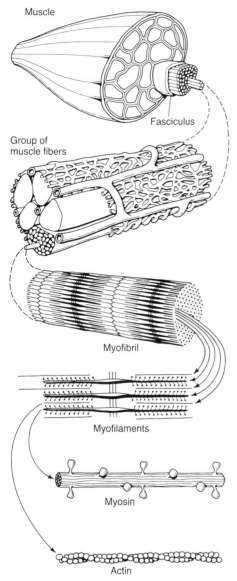

Muscle

Fasciculus

Group of
muscle fibers

Myofibril

Myofilaments

Myosin

Actin

Figure 1–1. Levels of organization within a skeletal muscle. (From Warwick et al.,[2] with permission.)

continued, actin filaments may overlap each other in the middle of the A band, and the Z bands may meet the ends of the myosin filaments. As the length of the sarcomere changes, so does the amount of overlap between actin and myosin. Since the number of possible cross-links between the two depends on the amount of overlap, it might be expected that a muscle would generate different tensions if it were made to contract at different lengths without being allowed to shorten.[2,6] Measurements confirm this expectation (Fig. 1–4).

The three types of muscle contraction—concentric, isometric, and eccentric—can be correlated with the behavior of the fine structure of the contractile mechanism of actin and myosin. In concentric contraction, in which a muscle shortens under a constant load to perform positive external work, actin and myosin cross-bridges are active in causing mutual sliding of the filaments. In isometric contraction, cross-bridges are made and broken repeatedly to maintain a constant muscle length under an external load. In eccentric contraction, a muscle generates tension while it is being actively lengthened by an external load. The precise behavior of the filaments has not been established in this type of contraction, but it is probable that cross-bridges are active in the usual manner while the actin and myosin are sliding apart.[2,8]

One often neglected structure also present in the muscle fiber environment is the satellite cell. This cell, located beneath the basal lamina, is a distinct entity with its own nucleus. While it plays no known role in normal muscle cell function, it has a crucial role in the ability of the muscle fiber to recover from injury. The satellite cell

muscle fiber contraction in the presence of calcium.[3] So, whereas the myosin-containing filament generates tension during muscle contraction, actin seems to regulate tension generation.[3]

In contracted muscle the actin filaments slide, in relation to the myosin, toward the center of the sarcomere, bringing the attached Z bands (Z stands for *zwitter*, the German word for "between") closer together, thus shortening the whole contractile unit (Fig. 1–3). This and many other observations indicate that muscle contraction may be caused by the successive making and breaking of cross-connections between thick myosin, those portions containing the projections, and thin actin filaments in a cyclical fashion, pulling the actin between the myosin toward the center of the sarcomere.[2] If contraction is

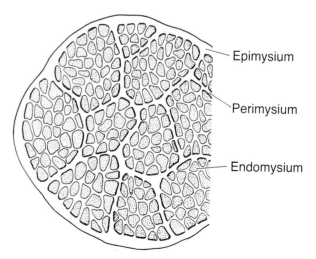

Epimysium

Perimysium

Endomysium

Figure 1–2. Striated muscle in cross section showing its connective tissue components and organization into bundles of muscle fibers. Epimysium encloses the entire muscle, perimysium surrounds each bundle of fibers, and endomysium lies between individual muscle fibers. (From Ham and Cormack,[1] with permission.)

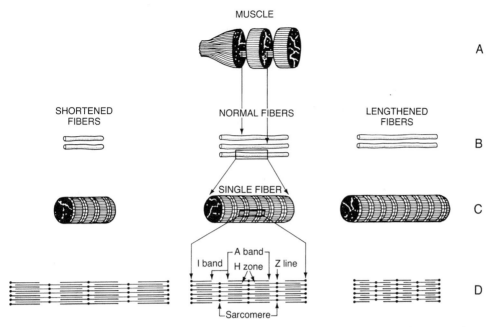

Figure 1–3. The structure of normal muscle (center) and the changes that occur when a muscle is in a shortened (left) or a lengthened position (right). (A) Skeletal muscle; (B) single muscle fibers; (C) myofibrils; (D) actin and myosin myofilaments. Note the increased and decreased sarcomere length in the shortened and lengthened fibers, respectively. (From Gossman et al.,[7] with permission.)

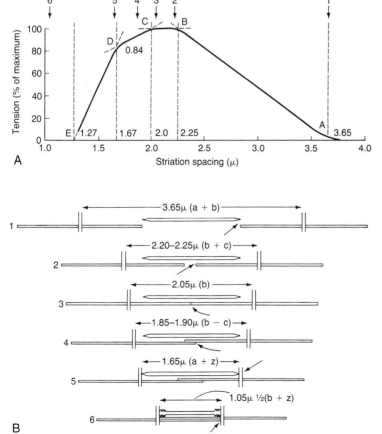

Figure 1–4. (A, B) Composite diagram showing the relationship of sarcomere length to the length–tension curve. a = 1.60 m; b = 2.05 m; c = 0.015 to 2.0 μm; z = 0.05 m. (From Gordon et al.,[50] with permission.)

is able to differentiate into a myofibroblast and form a new muscle fiber.[9] This regenerative process will be discussed later in the section on "Remobilization."

The last factor to be considered in the basic understanding of muscle structure and function is its innervation. Connections between nerves and muscles are very specific. Efferent, or motor, nerves supply each muscle via numerous axons. It has been shown that during growth and development, nerves unerringly project to the appropriate primitive muscle mass before any muscle fibers have been formed. This occurs even if the location of the appropriate muscle mass has been surgically altered.[10] One axon may supply one or many muscle fibers by means of branching. As the nerves contact the muscle fiber during growth and development, the synaptic neurotransmitter receptor sites begin to cluster around the site of contact.[11] The ratio of muscle fibers to axons in a muscle determines the fineness of the motion capabilities of that muscle. A single motor neuron and its axons together with all the muscle fibers it innervates are called a motor unit.[2,12] When stimulated, the fibers belonging to a single motor unit contract either completely or not at all—the "all or none" law. The force of contraction can vary because of circumstances such as the physiologic state of the fibers and the length–tension relationship. Within any one motor unit, all the fibers can be either red or white but not both.[1]

Sensory nerves also supply muscles, signaling the degree of contraction to the central nervous system (CNS). Information from muscle spindles and other sensory receptors provides awareness of the position and rate of movement of our body parts. These sensory organs can be classified under the broad category of mechanoreceptors because they respond to mechanical deformation or stimulation. Another category of receptors, called nociceptors, signals painful events, either mechanical or chemical, to the CNS. Nociceptors are more abundant in skin, connective tissue, and blood vessels than in the muscle belly itself.[12,13] Recent investigation of the long controverted phenomenon of trigger points indicates that intrafusal muscle fibers also have an innervation from the sympathetic nervous system.[14]

Connective Tissue

Connective tissue is found nearly everywhere in the body. It functions as a fibrous container for softer tissues, as a mechanical force transducer, as a chemical barrier, and as a highway for blood vessels and nerves (Fig. 1–5). Connective tissue is generally classified as loose or dense, regular or irregular, depending on the arrangement and quantity of collagen fibers within it (Fig. 1–6). Tendons and ligaments are considered to be dense connective tissue. Structurally, dense connective tissue is 80 percent

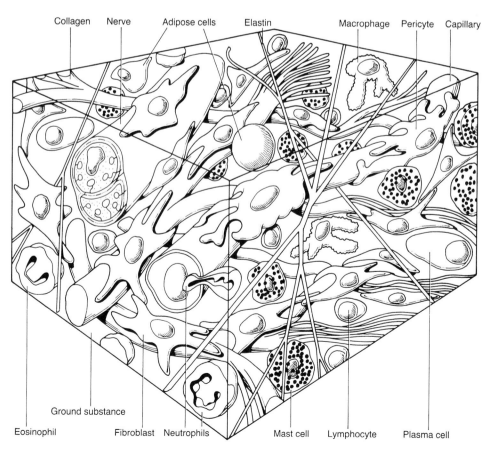

Collagen   Nerve   Adipose cells   Elastin   Macrophage   Pericyte   Capillary

Ground substance

Eosinophil   Fibroblast   Neutrophils   Mast cell   Lymphocyte   Plasma cell

Figure 1–5. A diagrammatic reconstruction of loose connective tissue showing the characteristic cell types, fibers, and intercellular spaces. (From Warwick et al.,[2] with permission.)

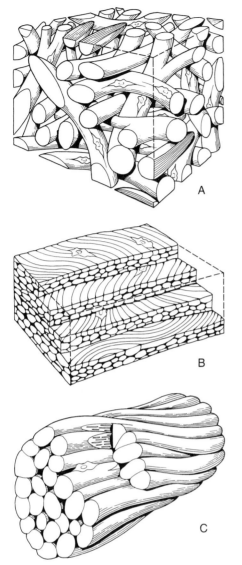

Figure 1–6. Three arrangements of collagen fibers. (A) Dense, irregular connective tissue; (B) a ligament; (C) a tendon. (From Warwick et al.,[2] with permission.)

water, 20 percent collagen fibers, and 2 percent cells and glycosaminoglycans (GAG).[1] Collagen represents 80 percent of the dry weight of connective tissue and is the only tensile-resistant protein in ligaments, tendon, and joint capsule.[15] The tensile strength of collagen has been estimated at 50 to 125 N/mm,[2] depending on the specimen tested.[16] Some studies of human collagen report loads at failure of 91 kilograms/force (kgf) for plantar fascia and 40 kgf for anterior cruciate ligament.[17,18] Clinically speaking, a dense, regular connective tissue structure such as a tendon is very strong. Tendon compliance studies indicate that tendons strain approximately 3 percent at maximum muscle tetany.[19,20] The tenoperiosteal junction is about five times stiffer than the musculotendinous junction. A tendon usually avulses from its bony attachment rather than tearing within its substance. The other

major components of connective tissue are water and GAG. They impart very important biomechanical properties to the tissue. GAG is a large, feather-like molecule with great affinity for water. This affinity greatly increases its space-occupying capabilities.[15,21,22] Water and GAG create a gel-like material that acts as both a lubricant and a spacer between the collagen fibers and imparts important physical and mechanical properties to the composite. Having an adequate tissue matrix between the collagen fibers decreases friction and maintains the interfiber distance necessary for the normal sliding movement that occurs between fibers.[15,22,23]

Collagen and GAG are produced by fibroblasts, the cells of connective tissue (Fig. 1–7). A collagen precursor molecule is assembled within the fibroblast and then secreted as tropocollagen.[1,24] Tropocollagen is then assembled in series via intermolecular bonds, or cross-links, to form collagen fibrils. The unique one-quarter overlap of this formation gives collagen its characteristic banded appearance.[1,25] The collagen continues to aggregate into bundles as needed by means of strong chemical bonds or intramolecular cross-links, finally forming a whole structure such as a tendon or a ligament (Fig. 1–8). Individual bundles have a wavy appearance, which permits small physiologic deformities to occur without placing the tissue under any stress.[25] Some recent studies indicate that not all connective tissue structures have identical ultrastructure or biochemistry.[26] Amiel et al.[27] and Frank et al.[28] identified histologic and biochemical differences between Achilles and patellar tendons and between different ligaments of the knee. Lyon et al.[26] reported differences in the cellular components of the medial collateral ligament (MCL) and the anterior cruciate ligament (ACL) of the knee. Using rabbits because of the similarity of their healing response in the MCL and ACL to that of humans, they demonstrated that while the MCL contained abundant spindle-shaped fibroblasts interspersed throughout the collagen fiber bundles, the cells of the ACL were ovoid, arranged in columns, and not in direct contact with the collagen matrix. The cellular organelles of these ovoid cells had an appearance somewhere between those of fibroblasts and chondrocytes. Remembering the limited healing capacity of fibrocartilage and articular cartilage, one might apply this concept to the drastic disparity in healing capacity between the human MCL and ACL. Other differences in tissue architecture were also noted between these two ligaments in the collagen fiber bundle arrangement and the crimp waveform alignment.

Physiologically, collagen is a rather sluggish substance.[21] In most forms, it is quite inert and has a slow turnover rate.[25] As fibers mature, the cross-links increase in strength. Attempts to modify the structure or alignment of collagen must therefore be prolonged and must be made early after injury or immobilization.[29] As collagen ages, more intermolecular cross-links form, and existing bonds become stronger.[15,25,30] The tissue thus becomes less extensible and more brittle. GAG has a more rapid

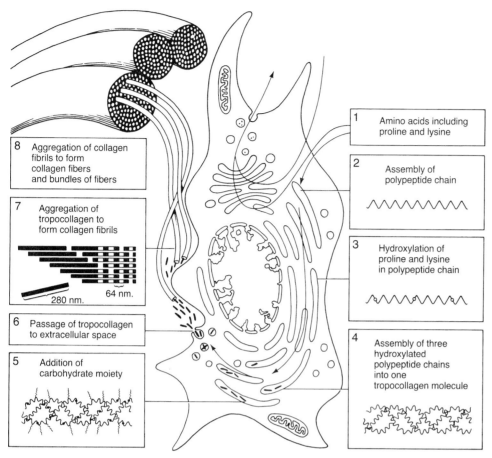

8 Aggregation of collagen fibrils to form collagen fibers and bundles of fibers

7 Aggregation of tropocollagen to form collagen fibrils

280 nm.   64 nm.

6 Passage of tropocollagen to extracellular space

5 Addition of carbohydrate moiety

1 Amino acids including proline and lysine

2 Assembly of polypeptide chain

3 Hydroxylation of proline and lysine in polypeptide chain

4 Assembly of three hydroxylated polypeptide chains into one tropocollagen molecule

Figure 1–7. The major steps in collagen synthesis by fibroblasts in connective tissue. (From Warwick et al.,[2] with permission.)

turnover rate and more active metabolism than collagen and thus appears to be more easily influenced by changes in the mechanical or chemical environment.[22,24]

Connective tissue does have abundant afferent innervation.[13,31] Although incapable of active movement, connective tissue does lengthen passively in response to internally or externally applied forces. These changes in length and tension are reported to the CNS by the different sensory receptors found within the tendons, ligaments, and articular capsule surrounding a joint. Wyke[32] classified these into four categories by size, structure, location, and function (Table 1–1). This rich supply of nerve endings, coupled with the muscle spindle endings, allows the CNS to monitor constantly the internal state of a particular joint. Type I, II, and III mechanoreceptors, via static and dynamic input, signal joint position, intra-articular pressure changes, and the direction, amplitude, and velocity of joint movements. Type II receptors are structurally contained in a thick, multilayered connective tissue capsule, which is subject to the same changes during immobi-

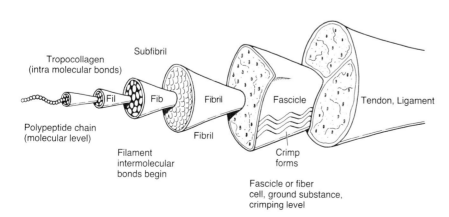

Tropocollagen (intra molecular bonds)

Subfibril

Fil   Fib   Fibril   Fascicle   Tendon, Ligament

Polypeptide chain (molecular level)

Filament intermolecular bonds begin

Fibril

Crimp forms

Fascicle or fiber cell, ground substance, crimping level

Figure 1–8. Organization of a tendon from tropocollagen to filament (Fil), fibril (Fib), fascicle, and whole tendon. Note the presence of crimping or waveforms at the fascicle level. (Redrawn from Betsch and Bauer,[25] with permission.)

□□□□□ □ □   □

Table 1–1. Classification of Articular Receptor Systems

Type	Morphology	Behavior
I	Fibrous capsule of joint (mainly superficial layers)	Static and dynamic receptors, low-threshold, slow adapting
II	Fibrous capsule of joint (mainly deeper layers) Articular fat pads	Dynamic mechanoreceptors, high-threshold, rapidly adapting
III	Joint ligaments	Dynamic mechanoreceptors, high-threshold, very slowly adapting
IV	Fibrous capsule Articular fat pads Ligaments Blood vessel walls	Pain receptors, high-threshold, nonadapting

(Modified from Wyke,[13] with permission.)

lization that affect other connective tissue structures. Type III mechanoreceptors are the homologues of the Golgi tendon organ. Functionally, the articular mechanoreceptors influence muscle tone, specifically the resistance of muscle to passive stretch.[33] Wyke[32] stated that type I and II mechanoreceptors synapse with fusimotor (γ) motoneurons via internuncial neurons. Type III receptors, being similar to Golgi tendon organs, can totally inhibit the excitability of the γ-motoneuron in nearby muscles when they are strongly stimulated. deAndrade et al.[34] demonstrated this inhibitory effect on the quadriceps muscle with an experimentally produced joint effusion. We see this clinically as the quadriceps "lag" after a knee injury or surgical procedure.

Freeman and Wyke[33] investigated the electromyographic (EMG) and stretch reflex responses of the tenotomized gastrocnemius muscle of the cat to passive ankle motion. When the ligaments and capsule were intact, the EMG activity and myotatic response of the muscle increased during passive ankle dorsiflexion, indicating facilitation. In contrast, the responses of the antagonistic tibialis anterior decreased. Local anesthesia of the ankle joint abolished these responses. Direct stimulation of the posterior joint capsule by means of gradual compression showed a progressive increase in the EMG activity of the gastrocnemius. This activity gradually returned to baseline with sustained gentle compression. Freeman and Wyke[33] concluded that mechanoreceptors provide valuable afferent pathways that influence muscle tone indirectly through mechanical stimulation of joint structures.

Peripheral Nerves

Peripheral nerves, like muscle, have both specialized cell components and a supporting connective tissue network[1,34] (Fig. 1–9). The fine structure of nerve fibers, or axons, follows the basic structure of a cell. The long processes of these nerve cells become the fibers that make

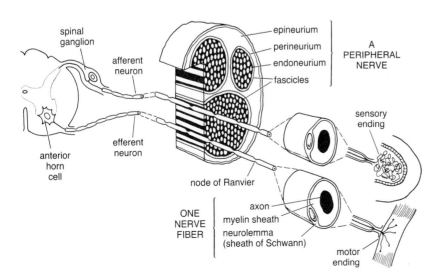

Figure 1–9. Organization of a peripheral nerve and its different parts. (From Ham and Cormack,[1] with permission.)

up the peripheral nerve.[1,2] Although organized in a bundled manner similar to that of muscle and connective structures, nerve fibers are unique in being surrounded by the fine cytoplasmic sheath called the neurolemma or sheath of Schwann[1] (Fig. 1–10). Some nerve fibers have a thick layer of myelin between the nerve and the neurolemma (myelinated fibers), whereas others do not (nonmyelinated fibers).[34] The myelin sheath is probably formed by the Schwann cell wrapping itself successively around the axon, gradually squeezing its own cytoplasm toward its nucleus so that its cell membranes fuse with each other. Unmyelinated fibers are merely invaginated into the Schwann cell rather than being wrapped in layers. Junctures between adjacent Schwann cells, down the length of an axon, form indentations called nodes of Ranvier.[1,2] These seem to facilitate conduction of impulses. Other functions attributed to the Schwann cell include collagen formation, transport of materials in the cell, transport of metabolites, protection of the nodal region from deformation, and maintenance of the ionic milieu.[34]

The connective tissue component of peripheral nerves consists of tubular sheaths, which encase successively the nerve fibers (endoneurium), the fascicles (perineurium), and the whole nerve (epineurium)[2] (Fig. 1–9). This is similar to the arrangement of muscle fibers into whole muscles. The connective tissue surrounding nerves serves not only as a mechanical protector but as a chemical one as well. It acts as a diffusion barrier, maintains internal pressure for axoplasm flow, provides uniform tensile strength, and maintains the conductile properties of the nerve.[34] Thickenings caused by an increase in connective tissue are observed along the course of the axon where nerves cross bones or occur near joints.

Within the nerve fascicles are different kinds of nerve fibers: sensory, motor, and sympathetic. These vary in quantity and arrangement.[2,34] As the nerve proceeds to its final destination, these components repeatedly unite and divide, forming plexi. Nerves have the same wavy pattern seen in connective tissue, even after removal of all the connective components of the nerve[34] (Fig. 1–11). As with connective tissue, this waviness disappears when gentle traction is applied.

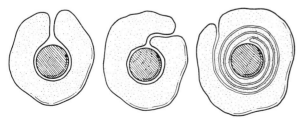

Figure 1–10. Early stages of the formation of a myelin sheath by a Schwann cell of the peripheral nervous system. (From Ham and Cormack,[1] with permission.)

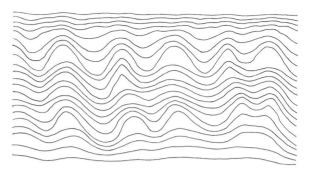

Figure 1–11. Drawing from a high-power photomicrograph of a longitudinal section of a small peripheral nerve, showing the snake-like appearance typical of such sections. (From Ham and Cormack,[1] with permission.)

Bone

Bone is essentially a highly vascular, constantly changing, mineralized connective tissue that is about 40 percent organic material (Fig. 1–12). Bone can be thought of as a passive system made up of collagen, stiffened by an extremely dense filling of calcium phosphate (Ca^{++}–P) (reordered to form hydroxyapatite) interspersed with small amounts of water, amorphous proteins, and cells. Or it can be seen as consisting most importantly of cells embedded in an amorphous, fibrous organic matrix permeated by inorganic bone salts.[1,22] The model we choose in considering the tissue we call bone depends on which of its functions we focus on: its function as the rigid support system for the body or the mineral reservoir.[1,22] Structurally, bone is similar to other forms of connective tissue in its main constituents but differs in both the quantity of the different components and the exact type of each component. Bone has a mineralized ground substance, whereas other connective tissues contain larger amounts of water and GAG. Bone receives a greater nutritional supply via its own blood vessels than do other connective tissues, which are largely avascular. Bone also has more cells per unit area than the other connective tissues. Because of this greater vascularity and cellularity, bone is capable of more rapid change, including healing and remodeling, than the other connective tissues.

The fine structure of bone varies widely with the age, location, and natural history of the tissue. Its collagen fiber framework varies from an almost random network of bundles to a highly organized system of parallel-fibered sheets or helical bundles. The inorganic matrix may exist as irregular dense masses with scattered bone cells, or it may be arranged as a series of thin sheets (lamellae) in a variety of patterns. Both types often develop as minute cylindrical masses (osteons), each with a central vascular canal. For our purposes, we can classify bone by the organization of its collagen fibers or by its general microstructure (Table 1–2).

It is difficult to understand bone as a tissue without some knowledge of its formation. The collagen of bone

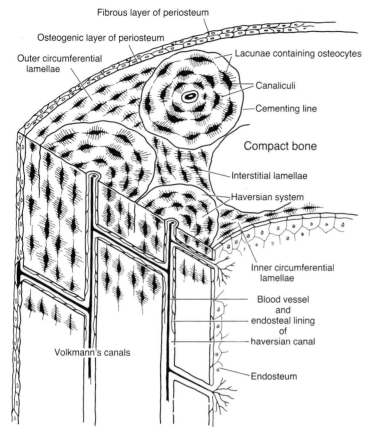

Fibrous layer of periosteum

Osteogenic layer of periosteum

Outer circumferential lamellae

Lacunae containing osteocytes

Canaliculi

Cementing line

Compact bone

Interstitial lamellae

Haversian system

Inner circumferential lamellae

Blood vessel and endosteal lining of haversian canal

Volkmann's canals

Endosteum

Figure 1–12. Appearance in cross section and longitudinal section of the components of the structure of the cortex of a long bone. In an actual bone, there would be many more Haversian systems than shown here. (From Ham and Cormack,[1] with permission.)

is produced in the same manner as that of ligament and tendon but by a different type of cell, the osteoblast. Collagen is laid down and then aggregates to form three distinct forms of bone: woven bone, lamellar bone, and parallel-fibered bone.[35] The collagen in woven bone is very fine and oriented almost randomly, like that of the skin. Woven bone contains many osteocytes and blood vessels. The spaces around the vessels are extensive, in contrast to those of lamellar bone.[35] The bone cells, called osteocytes, are contained within mineralized cavities (lacunae) and connect via fine processes through channels (canaliculi) with each other and with neighboring blood vessels.

Woven bone, or primary bone, is often replaced by lamellar bone during fetal growth and fracture repair. The collagen of lamellar bone is more precisely arranged than that of woven bone. The collagen and its ground substance are laid down in parallel sheets, with much less ground substance between the layers. The fibers are aligned within the plane of the lamella and are all oriented in the same direction. Within one lamella, however, there may be different domains of parallel-oriented fibers, similar to the arrangement of collagen in ligaments. Bundles of collagen may branch and are much thicker than those in woven bone. Parallel-fibered bone is structurally intermediate between woven bone and lamellar bone. It is highly calcified, but the collagen fiber bundles are less randomly arranged than those in woven bone. Parallel-fibered bone is found in particular bones in particular situations.[35]

Lamellar bone also exists in a separate form called a Haversian system, or osteon. Bone around a blood vessel is gradually eroded by bone-destroying cells, the osteoclasts, leaving a central cavity. Bone is then deposited on the inner surface of this cavity in concentric lamellae (Fig. 1–13). In cross section, the end result looks like an onion, with discernible cylindrical layers. Bone modeling and remodeling within this system occur via bone deposi-

□□□□□□ □ □ □

Table 1–2. Classification of Bone

Organization of collagen fibers
 Woven-fibered bone (coarse-bundled bone) has an irregular collagen network, includes embryonic bone, occurs in isolated patches in adults, is also formed during fracture repair
 Parallel-fibered bone includes all forms of lamellar bone and primary nonlamellar osteons
General microstructure
 Nonlamellar bone includes early woven-fibered bone and primary osteons
 Lamellar bone: almost all mature bone

(Modified from Warwick et al.,[2] with permission.)

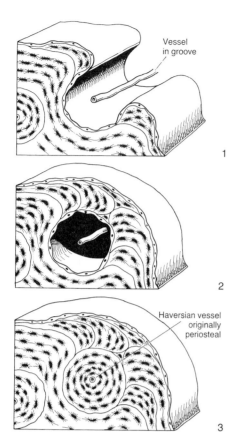

Figure 1–13. A representation of how the longitudinal grooves on the exterior of a growing bone shaft form tunnels and finally the Haversian system. (From Ham and Cormack,[1] with permission.)

tion and resorption, mediated by osteoblasts and osteoclasts, respectively.

The next higher order of structure is the mechanically important distinction between compact and cancellous bone. Cancellous bone is a framework of united bone spicules or trabeculae. During fetal development, a layer of osteoblasts forms deep to the outer dense sheath of connective tissue, the periosteum, which surrounds a whole bone. These osteoblasts deposit layers of bone, again called lamellae, beneath the periosteum. Near the time of birth, some locations of primary cancellous bone become compact bone. The trabeculae thicken by the addition of concentric lamellae around osteocytes and by rearrangement of the trabeculae into Haversian systems (Fig. 1–13). With the formation of many of these Haversian systems, the cancellous bone becomes compact bone. Osteoclasts remove bone centrally around the interior blood vessel of the Haversian system. Changes in bone occur in the same way during immobilization and remobilization.

All bones have an outer shell of compact, or cortical, bone and an inner mass of cancellous, or trabecular, bone. In some instances, the trabecular bone may be replaced by the medullary cavity or by an air space. Compact bone

is further distinguished from cancellous bone by the amount of mineralized tissue per total bone tissue volume. Compact bone is 5 to 30 percent porous, or nonmineralized, whereas cancellous bone is 30 to 90 percent porous.[23,35,36] The mineralized portion of cancellous bone appears as a three-dimensional latticework of trabeculae such as that seen in the head and neck of the femur (Fig. 1–14). Dense portions of cancellous bone also appear as plates such as those found in the pubis and lateral angle of the scapula. Other examples of dense portions of cancellous bone are the epiphyseal plates and the patellae.[35]

Mechanically, the trabecular bone structure is designed to provide support along the shaft of a long bone, thus resisting tension and bending. Plate structure gives more support near articular surfaces, which are subjected to compression and shear stresses. The collagen fibrils, which are evident in the trabecular and plate portions of cancellous bone, are usually aligned to present optimum resistance to the loads placed on the particular area. In areas subject to tension, collagen fibers are arranged parallel to the tensile load.[15] This orientation can be readily seen where tendons and ligaments attach to a bone and in areas subjected to tension under a bending load, such as the head and neck of the femur.[23]

The strength of bone is directly correlated with its degree of mineralization and with the number and organization of its osteons.[23] Demineralized bone has only 5 to 10 percent of the strength of mineralized bone.[35] The strength and strain of bone decrease as the number of osteons increases because of the relative weakness of the cement lines between them. Indeed, areas of bonding between osteons provide for more elastic and viscoelastic deformation.[22,37] The three types of osteons have different

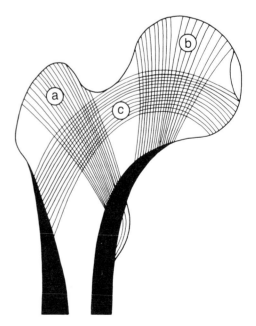

Figure 1–14. The trabeculae of the head and neck of the femur. (a) Lateral bundle; (b) medial bundle; (c) arcuate bundle. (From Rydell,[140] with permission.)

□□□□□ □ □ □

Table 1-3. Mechanical Stresses in Cancellous and Cortical Bone

Cancellous	Cortical
Compression	
Trabeculae are aligned according to compressive stresses. Greatest strain is available in lateromedial direction.	Longitudinal sections are strongest, then transverse, tangential, and radial. Ultimate compressive strength is greater than ultimate tensile strength. Strain is greatest in transverse section. Ultimate compressive strain is greater than ultimate tensile strain.
Tension	
Ultimate tensile strain is less than ultimate compressive strain. Ultimate strength is less than in cortical bone.	Longitudinal sections are strongest by eight times. Ultimate tensile strain is less than ultimate compressive strain.
Shear	
Trabeculae may be aligned according to direction of principal shear stress.	Longitudinal sections loaded perpendicularly are twice as strong as transverse sections loaded in parallel.

(Modified from Reigger,[22] with permission.)

tolerances for compression and elastic deformation, depending on the organization of the collagen fibers in each.[22] Compressive strength is greatest in type I and least in type III. Since collagen fibers resist tension along their axes, a longitudinal or steeply spiraling arrangement shows the greatest tensile strength, whereas a transverse arrangement (type I) has greater compressive strength.[22] See Table 1-3 for a summary of the differences between compact and cancellous bone. Because most whole bones are a combination of these two types of bony tissue, the strength of whole bone is greater than that of either tissue type alone.

Innervation of bone is supplied through finely distributed nerves within the periosteum, especially that of the articular extremities of the long bones, the vertebrae, and the larger flat bones. Fine myelinated and unmyelinated nerve fibers also accompany blood vessels into the interior of bones. These are nociceptors, which signal pain due to mechanical and chemical irritation.

■ Response to Mechanical Stress

The three principal mechanical loads or stresses are tension, compression, and shear. The mechanical response of a material to such a stress can be measured and plotted on a load–deformation (stress–strain) curve[23] (Fig. 1–15). Biologic tissue responds to mechanical stress by deforming according to specific mechanical and physical principles. The mechanical properties of biologic tissue containing large amounts of collagen are elasticity, viscoelasticity, and plasticity.[16,21,38–40] The physical properties are stress relaxation, creep, and hysteresis. These properties are defined in this section. Tissue with large amounts of collagen, such as bone and connective tissue, has also been found to respond to mechanical deformation by generating electrical polarity.[22,37,41] This is called the piezoelectric effect and is a characteristic of some substances with regular repeating molecular patterns such as collagen. Mechanical stress further triggers firing of different mechanoreceptors found in muscle, tendon, ligament, and joint capsule.[31–33,39] Intense mechanical deformation can also trigger the nociceptors found in these tissues.[31,39]

Clinically, when an outside force or load is applied, bone, muscle, ligament, and nerve respond by gradually

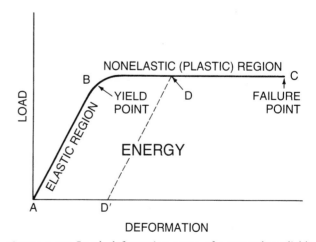

Figure 1–15. Load–deformation curve of a somewhat pliable material. The amount of permanent deformation that will occur if the structure is loaded to point D and then unloaded is represented by the distance between A and D′ (A–B, elastic region; B–C, plastic region). (From Frankel and Nordin,[23] with permission.)

lengthening. Because of their differences in collagen content, fiber arrangement, and inorganic components, these different tissues respond in slightly different ways. Individual collagen fibers deform very little. Instead, the unique arrangement of collagen into bundles of varying sizes and directional alignment within a tissue permits the different forms of tissue to have both strength and stiffness in varying amounts. The presence of a gel-like matrix allows the collagen bundles to move to align themselves along lines of stress application. Bone, muscle connective tissue, and nerve also respond differently, depending on the speed, duration, and magnitude of the applied load. The maximum stiffness for a tissue occurs along the lines of stress application if the load is applied slowly enough to permit time for collagen bundle realignment. The alignment of collagen fibers along lines of normal stress is lost during immobilization and is gradually regained through therapeutic stress application. The composition and amount of connective tissue matrix present are important factors in this time-dependent realignment phenomenon. Changes take place within connective tissue during immobilization that retard the realignment process.

Tissue-Specific Response to Mechanical Loading

Connective Tissue

Since tendons and ligaments are most often subjected to tension stress, this stress–strain curve has been well studied in connective tissue structures. Specific regions have been identified on the curve that correspond to specific material and clinical behavior (Fig. 1–16). Connective tissue responds to mechanical stress in a time-dependent

or viscoelastic manner.[16,21,25,38] Viscoelasticity is a mechanical property of materials that describes the tendency of a substance—in this instance, connective tissue—to deform at a certain rate, regardless of the speed of the externally applied force. When the deforming force is removed, the original shape of the tissue returns at a tissue-specific rate.[13,35] In engineering, this slow, predictable rate of deformation is also known as "creep" (Fig. 1–17). If the rate of load application is increased, other mechanical responses change to maintain a constant rate of deformation. Thus, a rapidly applied load will produce less deformation before failure than a slowly applied load. If the amount of deformation does not exceed the elastic range, the structure can return to its normal or original shape after the load is removed. If loading is continued into the plastic range, passing the yield point, the outermost fibers of the material will begin to tear (fail). Failure is thought to be a function of breaking of intermolecular cross-links rather than rupture of the chains of the collagen molecule.[42] If loading persists, that structure ultimately fails. An example of a load persisting until failure occurs, but where little deformation takes place, is an injury in an individual who starts a rapid acceleration sports activity without warming up. During sports activity, a large load is often applied rapidly to a connective tissue structure that has not been previously loaded in this way. Thus, the stress perceived by the tissue is high, and the failure point is reached quickly before much tissue elongation has had time to take place. This is often seen clinically as a midsubstance ligamentous tear.[43] A load of equal magnitude applied more slowly results in failure at the bone–ligament junction, where the connective tissue structure is weaker as it blends into the bone.[43,44]

Repeated loading, or cyclic loading, shows a change in mechanical response beginning with the first cycle and stabilizing after the sixth cycle.[37] Changes reflect an increased compliance (softening) of the tissue, an increased early stiffness, and a decreased load to failure.[25,45] The softening of the tissue in the first cycle and subsequent cycles reflects a release of energy from the tissue, called hysteresis, which is perhaps caused by internal friction (Fig. 1–17C). Increased tissue temperature has been recorded during repeated loading; hence, the term warm-up to describe repeated stretching before sports activities is particularly appropriate. Clinical experience also points to more connective tissue injuries occurring later in sports activities when ligaments and the joint capsule are warmed, more compliant, and less resistant to higher loads, and when muscles are fatigued.[46] Connective structures thus take less time to reach their yield and failure points. This warming of the tissue can also be induced therapeutically by the external application of heat.[40,47]

If a tissue is held under a constant external load and at a constant length, force relaxation occurs[15] (Fig. 1–17A). Although the external load on the tissue and the length of the tissue remain the same—for example, in a cylinder cast—the internal stress perceived by the tissue decreases.

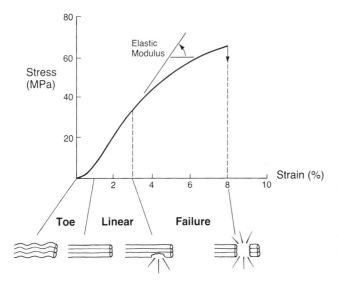

Figure 1–16. Typical normalized stress–strain curve for collagen. The curve provides mechanical parameters that are independent of tissue dimensions. (From Butler et al.,[38] with permission.)

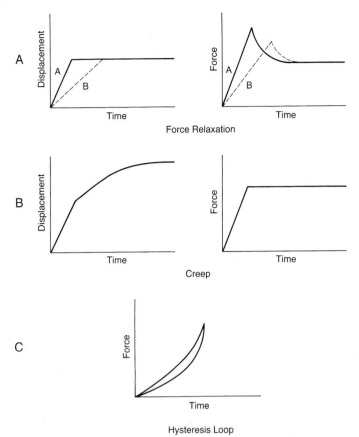

Force Relaxation

Creep

Hysteresis Loop

Figure 1–17. (A–C) Physical properties of collagen. (A) Initial loading; (B) subsequent loading. (From Butler et al.,[38] with permission.)

Thus, when the cylinder cast is removed, the tissue remains at its new length instead of immediately returning to its former length. The actual ultrastructural changes occurring during force relaxation have not been investigated, but we can surmise that collagen fibers are realigning along the lines of stress and that ground substance is perhaps also being redistributed. These mechanical properties of collagen-bearing tissues are important parameters for the rehabilitation process and for mobilization procedures. No specific or simple failure point can be stated for connective structures, as the specific mechanical behavior of a ligament or tendon depends on its individual cross section, length, and rate of loading in any situation. In general, connective tissue structures can tolerate 1.5 percent strain without any increase in stress; 1.5 to 3 percent is within physiologic limits; and 3 percent or greater begins to cause some mechanical failure.[45,47,48]

Bone

As might be expected, bone is considerably stiffer (deformation resistant) than muscle, connective tissue, or nerve because of its inorganic matrix. Because the collagen component of bone is embedded in this hard, mineralized matrix, it is not capable of rapid change in response to force application. As Wolff's law states, bone does respond to the forces placed on it, but it requires more time, often weeks or months, to manifest this change. Bone strength also varies according to the direction of stress. It is nonuniform in construction, and it is strongest where it is most often exposed to loading, as are the more mobile forms of connective tissue. It is strongest in compression (the opposite of the nonossified connective tissues) and weakest in shear.[22] The weakness of bone in shear and its slow physiologic response to mechanical forces are important properties to remember when applying mobilization techniques on or over bones that may be weakened from immobilizational osteoporosis or fracture healing. Recent studies by Wilson et al., using animal models, indicate that a manually applied compressive strain in excess of $-1,000\ \mu$ strain with an abnormal strain distribution within a bone could potentially stimulate osteogenesis within that bone. Levered bending was the technique that produced the greatest mean peak strains and greatest peak strains in vivo.[49]

Muscle

Muscle responds to mechanical stress by lengthening passively and by changing its ability to generate tension. These changes have been well represented by the passive length–tension curve[6] and the active isometric length–tension curve.[50] The development of passive tension in the muscle in response to length change is thought to be a result of both the tension-resisting capacity of the connective tissue of the muscle and the presence of a large structural protein within the myofibril aptly named titin.[51,52] Titin connects the thick myosin filaments end to end, thus passively supporting the sarcomere and stabilizing the myosin lattice.[51,52] Changes in tension-generating ability are thought to be a result of both the elastic response of the connective tissue that surrounds the muscle and the change in position of the actin and myosin. Electron microscopy has shown that the active tension-generating capacity of actin and myosin filaments has a small tolerance for length variations (Fig. 1–4). Because different muscles have different fiber bundle arrangements, each muscle has its own optimum isometric length–tension position.[2,6] The combination of connective tissue response and active length–tension response partially explains why different muscles generate their maximum tensions at slightly different joint angles.

Nerve

The mechanical responses of nerves to length changes appear to have been given little study. There is considerable clinical evidence that nerves have more tolerance for tension than for compression before physiologic injury occurs. A study on the mechanical behavior of the sciatic nerve during the straight leg raising test was conducted by Fahrni in 1966.[53] He found that the straight leg could be elevated 30 to 40 degrees before all the slack was taken up in the peripheral portions of the sciatic nerve. Nothing was reported on the microscopic mechanical events. Sunderland[29] reported that nerves can be stretched to some extent without damage. This may be because of the zigzag course of nerve fibers within a nerve. These waves are merely straightened out when a nerve is stretched to a certain point.

■ Trauma and Inflammation

Non-Tissue-Specific Response

Biologic tissue experiences mechanical trauma in the form of tension, compression, or shearing forces.[54] Muscle, nerve, connective tissue, and bone resist these mechanical stressors to differing degrees, depending on the specific components of the tissue, the physiologic state of the tissue, and the magnitude, velocity, and direction of the force. Whatever the trauma, once mechanical damage has occurred, the initial biologic response is a generalized non-tissue-specific inflammatory process (Table 1–4).

The initial stages of the inflammatory process are characterized by vascular changes.[24,54,55] The extent of these changes depends on the vascularity of the involved tissue; connective tissue has a smaller response than bone or muscle. Immediately after the injury, there is a brief period of vasoconstriction, lasting for 5 to 10 minutes.[54] Vessel walls become lined with leukocytes, erythrocytes,

□ □ □ □ □ □   □   □

Table 1–4. Inflammatory Process

Reaction phase
   1–3 days
   Vasodilation
   Edema
   Cell migration
   Debris removal
Repair phase
   48 hours–6 weeks
   Fibroplasia
   Wound closure
   Collagen content with random alignment
   Regeneration of small vessels
Remodeling phase
   3 weeks–12 months
   Reduction in wound size
   Increased wound strength
   Realignment of collagen
   Reduction of abnormal cross-links

and platelets.[24] Vasoconstriction is followed by active vasodilation of all local blood vessels and increased blood flow. The small venules increase in permeability, allowing plasma to leak through into the site of injury. Edema, or swelling, then becomes apparent at the injury site. A highly cellular environment develops, with active migration of leukocytes for "clean-up" of the damaged area.[56]

Once the debris has been removed by the leukocytes, the acute inflammatory process is completed and repair can begin.[55] Fibrocytes appear, possibly attracted by an electrical field within the wound area created by local hypoxia.[57] Proliferation of collagen produced by the fibroblasts begins to close any gap or defect in the tissue. A significant amount of collagen is present by the fourth or fifth day after injury and continues to increase for up to 6 weeks.[55] During this time, the injury site has very little tensile strength.[30] Immobilization is often needed to ensure an anatomically aligned repair.

In the absence of normal stress, the arrangement of collagen is random. Some ability to resist tension begins to develop at about the second week.[29,55] Collagen synthesis has been briefly described in the section on "Normal Tissue" and illustrated in Figure 1–7. To review, the collagen molecule is a triple helical structure manufactured by the fibroblast. In its initial molecular form, it is called tropocollagen.[1,24] The three chains making up the triple helix of tropocollagen are bonded by hydrogen bonds. Later, stronger chemical bonds form between the three chains. Outside the fibroblast, the tropocollagen units unite with each other in longer chains by overlapping their ends by one-quarter. This is the "quarter-stagger array," which gives collagen its unique banded appearance. Fibroblasts also produce the glycoproteins and GAG necessary for the ground substance of collagen.

Once a sufficient amount of collagen has been produced, the number of fibroblasts in the wound decreases. This marks the end of the proliferative or fibroplastic phase and the beginning of the maturation phase of wound healing. During the maturation phase, pronounced changes occur in the bulk, form, and strength of the scar tissue.[24] At the beginning of the phase, collagen is randomly oriented and the intermolecular bonds are weak. This appears to be the optimum time for applying gentle mobilization forces to reorient the collagen in a functional direction and to break any bonds that may have formed in an abnormal pattern.[15,23] As tension across a wound site increases, reorientation of collagen fiber bundles and collagen phagocytosis also increase.[58] Remodeling may continue for years, although more slowly. Even after 40 weeks, normal organization and concentration of collagen are not yet present.[55,57]

It is important to remember that wound healing is a continuum. Inflammation, fibroplasia, and remodeling may overlap each other slightly in time. Judgment is required when mobilizing an injury that may still be undergoing fibroplasia, as overzealous movement may stimulate further collagen production and thicken the scar formation.[55,57]

Tissue-Specific Responses

Bone

Bone has a more specialized reaction to injury than do the soft connective tissues. Since there is soft tissue (periosteum) around the bone, which may be torn in an injury, the same non-tissue-specific response does occur in this area. Since bone contains large quantities of specialized osteocytes, rather than fibroblasts, repair of the bone involves actual bone tissue rather than scar tissue.

Any trauma that fractures a bone results in the development of a callus (i.e., new tissue that forms around and between the ends of the fracture line or fragments). Within the first few days after a fracture, osteogenic cells begin to proliferate in the deep periosteum close to the fracture site, much as in the proliferative phase of connective tissue healing. Eventually, these cells form a collar around the fracture and begin to differentiate. The cells closest to a new blood supply become osteoblasts and form new bony trabeculae in this region. Cells farther away from a blood supply, in the more superficial parts of the collar of callus, become chondrocytes. As a result, cartilage develops in this outer part of the collar of callus. The callus becomes a three-layered structure consisting of an outer proliferating portion, a middle cartilaginous layer, and an inner area of new bony trabeculae (Fig. 1–18). Growth of the collar of callus continues until the two sides of the fragment meet and fuse. The callus also undergoes a remodeling phase, as do the soft tissues. Cartilage is eventually replaced with bone as the intercellular substance deposited between the chondrocytes be-

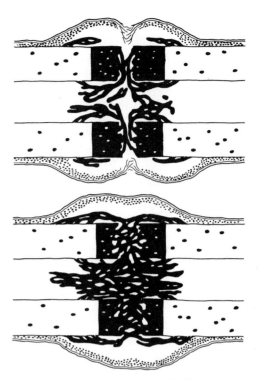

Figure 1–18. Process by which periosteal collars form, approach one another, and fuse in the repair of a fracture. Living bone is depicted in light gray, dead portions in dark gray, and new bone in black. (From Ham and Cormack,[1] with permission.)

comes calcified and the cells die. The trabeculae of bone that have formed close to the original fragments become firmly cemented to them and eventually to each other, thus bridging the fracture. The matrix of dead bone is gradually removed by osteoclasts. Osteoblasts move into the spaces opened by removal of dead bone and deposit new living bone. By replacing the cartilage of the callus with bone and converting cancellous bone into compact bone, the callus is gradually remodeled. Eventually the original line of the bone may be so well restored by this process that the fracture is almost undetectable by radiography or palpation.[1]

Nerve

Nerve also has a tissue-specific response to trauma because of its special tissue components and capabilities for repair. There is still the generalized inflammatory response and fibroplasia of the connective tissue component of the peripheral nerve. This results in interference with function for periods ranging from a few days to several weeks. Sensory nerves are affected more easily than motor nerves, and peripheral fibers are affected before inner fibers. Second-degree injuries result from pressure over a longer period of time and lead to axon death, especially distal to the injury.[1,24] Complete severance of a nerve produces anatomic and metabolic changes both proximal and distal to the point of injury. The generalized traumatic response of the nerve includes degeneration of the myelin sheath, with subsequent removal of debris by macrophages. New cytoplasm is synthesized, fibroblasts proliferate to bridge any defect created by the injury, and Schwann cells increase in number to restore the myelin sheath.[1,24] The Schwann cells grow in cords across the gap in the traumatized nerve. These cords provide guidance for any growing axons. The area of the damaged nerve may be enlarged due to fibroplasia for up to 3 weeks after injury. The severed axon degenerates both proximal and distal to the injury in the process called Wallerian degeneration. The degree of injury then dictates how much degeneration and how long the fibroplasia lasts. The axon then undergoes enlargement and budding. Excessive scar formation can deter the course of the growing axon buds to their target organs. Whether the axon reaches its proper destination at the distal end depends on the amount of scar tissue that has grown over the gap in the injured nerve.

Muscle

Muscle injuries represent one of the most common traumas in sports medicine. Muscles are also frequently injured in vehicular and industrial accidents via blunt trauma, laceration, or strain.[59] Blunt trauma represents a compression injury resulting in intramuscular bleeding and disruption of muscle fibers.[51] Trauma produces a laceration, whereas stretching may produce a strain or tear of muscle tissue components. Muscle spasm, whether neurologic from the ensuing pain or physiologic from the resulting fluid and cellular proliferation of the inflammatory response, may occur. This spasm limits the range of motion of the nearby joints. The amount of limitation may indicate the severity of the injury. A severe muscle contusion may result in myositis ossificans (i.e., the formation of bone tissue within the muscle). Caution must be used in mobilizing and exercising a severely contused muscle, as repeated trauma seems to stimulate the ossification process.[60]

Excessive tension may also injure a muscle; this is called a muscle strain. This strain may tear collagen fibers as well as muscle tissue itself if the failure point for that tissue is reached. The generalized inflammatory response of acute inflammation, repair, and remodeling occurs. Since muscle tissue has a limited potential for regeneration, any defect is usually filled with connective tissue scar. Some contractile function and thus strength may be lost, depending on the size of the defect.

■ Immobilization

The effects of immobilization have been well studied in bone, connective tissue, and muscle and to a much lesser extent in nerve.[15,61–70] The general consequence of immobilization is loss first of tissue substrate and later of the most basic tissue components. In connective tissue, the arrangement of collagen fiber also becomes random.

The net result of these physiologic changes is always a loss of the basic function of the tissue in question. The amount of loss depends on the degree of loss of tissue components. In bone, support and mineral reservoir capacities are diminished; in muscle, strength is compromised; in connective tissue, extensibility and tension resistance are reduced; and in nerve, sensitivity of some of the connective tissue-encapsulated receptors is reduced.

Bone

Bone accretion and absorption are maintained in equilibrium by weightbearing and muscular contraction.[61,71–75] Within 10 to 15 days of immobilization, the rate of bone turnover changes. Some sources report an initial increase in bone formation and absorption, with an eventual predominance of bone resorption by the 15th day.[61,71–74,76] The mineral content of the bone is also diminished, as reflected by increased excretion of urinary calcium. Increased excretion of hydroxyproline, an amino acid involved in collagen cross-linking, indicates destruction of the organic as well as the inorganic components of bone.[61] Loss of bone density is further evidenced by a disruption of the normal trabecular pattern, both in number and in arrangement.[77,78]

Localized loss of bone, such as that present in the distal fragment of a fractured long bone, is detectable on radiography when it constitutes a loss of 2 percent of total body calcium. This osteoporosis is most pronounced in the cancellous bone of the metaphysis and epiphysis, especially beneath the joint cartilage. True osteoporosis, a decrease in the total mass of the bony skeleton, is not detectable on radiography until 40 to 50 percent of the mineral content of the skeleton has been lost. The mechanical properties of bone also change with the loss of its organic and inorganic components. The hardness of bone steadily decreases with the duration of immobilization. By 12 weeks, it is reduced to 55 to 60 percent of normal.[61] The elastic resistance also declines, and the bone becomes more brittle and thus more easily fractured. Most of these losses are recoverable in a comparable period of time if immobilization lasts for 4 weeks or less. Components lost during an immobilization period of 12 weeks are also recoverable but require a longer recovery period.

The causes of osteoporosis have been associated with a change in blood flow during immobilization and a lack of normal mechanical stimulation.[61,71] Geiser and Trueta's study[71] of immobilized rabbits showed a decrease in filling of osseous blood vessels after 4 to 5 days. For the next 4 to 6 weeks, bone became hypervascular, and both bone formation and absorption increased. This was followed by a period of hypovascularity during which all activity declined. Cancellous bone showed only a network of thin, atrophic trabeculae. It was postulated that lack of muscle contraction reduced the suction effect on venous outflow and thus deprived distal areas of new blood.[71,72] The piezo-electric effect, thought to be important in maintaining normal bone activity, would also be lost in proportion to the loss of muscular activity.[73] Burr et al.[75] found that intracast muscle stimulation with implanted electrodes significantly altered the bone turnover rate in rabbit limbs immobilized for 17 days. Oscillating beds, which provide full weightbearing and thus muscle contraction, when used for brief periods, reduced urinary calcium loss by 50 percent.[61] Supine exercises and quiet sitting did not have the same effect.[61] Demineralization was less responsive to weightbearing if the subject was paralyzed, although paraplegics who used crutches for at least 1 hour per day seemed to be able to prevent the development of osteoporosis.[61]

Muscle

Changes with immobilization in muscle have been well investigated. Cooper's classic article[62] reported on ultrastructural changes in muscle from the limbs of cats immobilized for 2 to 22 weeks in plaster casts. Changes began appearing within 2 weeks, manifesting as a decrease in fiber size caused by loss of myofibrils. Sarcomere elements lost their normal configuration and alignment. The mitochondria decreased in size and number. As degeneration progressed, debris from the breakdown of these cellular elements accumulated as myelin figures and lipid droplets. In some fibers, all the myofilaments degenerated and the fibers shrank. Cell and basement membranes enfolded deeply and later became fragmented or separated from each other. As degeneration progressed, rows of nuclei appeared, forewarning of impending nuclear degeneration. Total nuclear degeneration left only a mass of chromatin. Adjacent to degenerating cells, macrophages increased in number. A fibrofatty infiltrate and connective tissue accumulated in the degenerating muscle. Wet weight of the muscles decreased 25 percent, and total weight decreased 32 percent. As muscle weight decreased, the ability to generate tension also decreased in even larger percentage. Muscle contraction and relaxation times increased, perhaps because of the development of cross-links between filaments, which were not allowed to move normally.[62]

Other studies affirm the concept that immobilization in the shortened position generates more unfavorable ultrastructural,[15,65] functional,[15,79–81] and biochemical changes than immobilization in either the resting or the lengthened position.[82] More recently, Appell,[59] in a review of changes in muscle after immobilization, stated that slow muscles with predominantly oxidative metabolism seem most affected. He surmised that this may be due in part to a complete loss of mitochondrial function during the first few days of nonuse and a decline in oxygen perfusion. Lieber et al.[83] also found a differential response in the dog quadriceps when it was immobilized for 10 weeks. Fiber atrophy was greatest in the vastus medialis and least in the rectus femoris. The authors concluded that postural muscles, muscles crossing only one joint,

and muscles with predominantly type I fibers were most susceptible to fiber atrophy. Other studies point to the same conclusion of differential atrophy among muscle fiber types.[64,79–85] Circumferential measurements have been found to be a misleading indicator of the extent of muscle fiber atrophy. Sargeant et al.[86] found that needle biopsy specimens taken from subjects with unilateral thigh wasting showed a 40 percent difference in mean fiber area despite only a 12 percent difference in fat-free thigh volume. Also noted was a 5 percent difference in midthigh circumference versus a 22 to 33 percent difference in quadriceps cross-sectional area. MacDougall et al.[87,88] showed similar results in a study of normal human elbows immobilized for 5 weeks. Further studies on the effects of aging in rats show an increased ratio of connective tissue to muscle with increasing age.[89]

The greatest loss of muscle mass occurs early in the immobilization period, evidently during the first 5 days. Lindboe and Platou[65] stated that in humans, muscle fiber size is decreased by 14 to 17 percent after 72 hours of immobilization.

Neural elements such as muscle spindles, motor nerves, and motor end plates appeared unaffected. Tabary et al.[63] found that muscle immobilized in a shortened position for 4 weeks lost 40 percent of its original sarcomeres and required an equal length of time for recovery. In this same study, muscles immobilized in a lengthened position gained 20 percent more sarcomeres and sustained no changes in the normal length–tension curve. Individual sarcomeres were found to have a decreased length, although total fiber length increased. There was no change in the response to resistance to passive tension. Muscles immobilized in the shortened position showed the opposite reaction: Sarcomeres were reduced in number but showed either no change or an increase in length. Fiber length increased, and there was an increase in resistance to passive tension. Muscles immobilized in the shortened position did lose weight more rapidly than those casted at resting length. Slow fibers appeared to be lost first.

Other researchers confirm the findings of Cooper[62] and provide clinical relevance to his research.[63–65] Booth,[64] in his review of the biochemical effects of immobilization on muscle, stated that there are lower levels of resting glycogen and ATP and more rapid depletion of ATP during exercise beginning as early as the sixth hour after immobilization. He noted that there is also an increase in lactate during work and a decreased ability to oxidize fatty acids. Lipman et al.[90] and Nicholson et al.[91] noted that when muscle contractile activity declines, even normal muscle shows decreased use of insulin and decreased glycogen synthesis. Muscle from the forearms of healthy humans at bed rest for 3 days shows a decreased ability of insulin to stimulate glucose uptake.

Changes in strength parameters have been investigated in animals and humans. MacDougall et al.[87] found a 35 percent decrease in elbow extension stength in human

□□□□□ □ □ □

Table 1–5. Biochemical Observations on Fibrous Connective Tissue from Immobilized Joints

	Results of Immobilization
Collagen	Mass reduced by about 10% Increased turnover Increased degradation rate Increased synthesis rate Increased reducible collagen cross-links
Glycosaminoglycans (GAG)	Total GAG reduced 20% Hyaluronic acid reduced 40% Sulfated GAG reduced 20%
Water content	Reduced 3–4%

(Modified from Akeson et al.,[68] with permission.)

volunteers after 5 weeks of immobilization. Berg et al.[92] reported a 22 percent decrease in maximum concentric peak torque and a 16 percent decrease in angle-specific torque for human lower limb muscles immobilized for 4 weeks. Several other authors reported decreases in the maximum twitch and tetanic force output per whole muscle and per unit cross-sectional area.[79,81,82,84] Again, decrements were greater when the muscle was immobilized in a shortened position. Other motor unit abnormalities reported include slowed contraction time,[62,93] increased recruitment of high-threshold motor units, decreased maximum firing rate, and lowered membrane resting potential.[94]

Another recently emphasized structural change in immobilized muscle is an increase in the intramuscular connective tissue or collagen content,[95–98] although not all authors agree.[99] Jozsa et al.[98] also found an increase in intramuscular capillary density. The greatest loss of muscle mass occurs early in the immobilization period, evidently during the first 5 days. Lindboe and Platou[65] stated that in humans, muscle fiber size is decreased by 14 to 17 percent after 72 hours of immobilization.

Connective Tissue

Akeson and associates[15,66–68] have been studying the effects of immobilization on connective tissue for three decades. In 1980, they presented the results of a study of the effects of immobilization on rabbit knee joints and formulated some theories on the pathomechanics of joint contracture. They found changes both in the collagen fibers of the connective tissue around the immobilized joints and in the intercellular substance of GAG and water (Table 1–5). In the intercellular substance, water content was decreased by 3 to 4 percent, and the connective tissue appeared "woody" rather than smooth and glistening.

An even greater decrease in concentration, 20 percent, was seen in the GAG portion of the intercellular substance. In contrast, total collagen remained unchanged. The authors theorized that this loss of water and GAG, while total collagen remained the same, would decrease the space between collagen fibers in the connective tissue and thus alter free movement between the fibers. This lack of free movement would tend to make the tissue less elastic, less plastic, and more brittle. Further, in the absence of normal stress during the immobilization period, collagen fibers would be laid down in a random pattern and cross-links might form in undesirable locations, inhibiting normal gliding movement (Fig. 1–19). Since the loss of intercellular substance would bring fibers closer together, cross-links might form more easily.

In support of the findings of Akeson et al. on the loss of connective tissue elasticity with immobilization, LaVigne and Watkins[69] reported that joints immobilized at 90 degrees for 0 to 64 days required increasing amounts of force to be moved through the normal range of motion. Capsular structures also failed at lower loads than control joints. Changes in the force required for motion and in the load at failure were evident only after 16 days of immobilization (Tables 1–6 and 1–7).

Ligaments immobilized for 8 weeks showed a decrease in maximum load to failure, a decrease in energy absorbed at failure, and an increase in extensibility.[100]

Although some joint stiffness can be attributed to gross adhesions and the formation of random cross-links within the collagen network, ligaments are affected somewhat differently. The random deposition of collagen characteristic of a stress-deprived tissue actually reduces the ability of a ligament to resist tensile forces. Further, weakness at the insertional site secondary to bone resorption further compromises the strength of the bone–ligament–

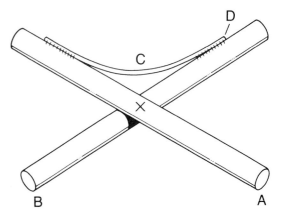

Figure 1–19. An idealized model demonstrating the interaction of collagen cross-links at the molecular level. A and B represent preexisting fibers, C represents the newly synthesized fibril, D represents the cross-links created as the fibril becomes incorporated into the fiber, and X represents the nodal point at which adjacent fibers are normally freely movable past each other. (From Akeson et al.,[15] with permission.)

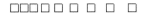

Table 1–6. Gross and Microscopic Changes in Synovial Joints Observed after Prolonged Immobilization

Tissue	Results of Immobilization
Synovium	Proliferation of fibrofatty connective tissue into the joint space
Cartilage	Adherence of fibrofatty connective tissue to cartilage surfaces Loss of cartilage thickness Pressure necrosis at points of contact when compression has been applied
Ligament	Disorganization of the parallel arrays of fibrils and cells
Ligament insertion site	Destruction of ligament fibers attaching to bone
Bone	Generalized osteoporosis of cancellous and cortical bone

(Modified from Akeson et al.,[68] with permission.)

bone complex.[101] Dehne and Torp[100] found that ligaments immobilized for 8 weeks showed a decrease in maximum load to failure, a decrease in energy absorbed at failure, and an increase in extensibility. Several recent studies point to an increase in intramuscular connective tissue, especially if the limb is concomitantly deprived of normal levels of oxygen.[97] Thus, both articular and muscular components conspire to render an immobilized limb stiff and weak.

The clinical implications of tissue immobilization are many. Bone that has undergone local osteoporosis after fracture or immobilization is less able to bear weight or withstand normal forces of compression, tension, and shear. Caution must be exercised when applying manual techniques to a joint that has been immobilized or is near a fracture site, particularly the small joints of the fingers. The phalanges are small, and the therapist's hands can easily grasp both the dorsal and palmar surfaces of the phalanx. Often, patients with the common problem of adhesive capsulitis are older and may have a combined osteoporosis of age and immobilization. Again, care must be taken to grade compression forces within the patient's pain tolerance and mechanical force absorption capabilities. As no studies are available on the forces applied during specific mobilization maneuvers or manual therapy techniques, the grading of forces applied to joints or over osteoporotic bone is still a matter of therapeutic judgment.

Muscles that have been immobilized will be weak because of loss of the intercellular constituents that are necessary for muscle contraction and because of decreased storage of energy-producing substrates. Muscles may also be tight if immobilized in a shortened position because the number of sarcomere will be reduced and intramuscular connective tissue may have formed abnormal cross-links. Since slow twitch fibers appear to be lost first, fatigue and low endurance will be most evident in postural activities and activities requiring sustained contraction. As muscle fatigues, its ability to absorb shock and protect neighboring joints is compromised. In short, muscle that has been immobilized or injured does not have the same contractile capacity as normal muscle, and therapeutic regimes must be altered and progressed accordingly.

Connective tissue likewise is compromised in strength, stiffness, and deformability after immobilization. This situation may be used to therapeutic advantage when stretching abnormal connective tissue or scar tissue, or it may limit the amount of stress that can be placed on an injured joint capsule, ligament, or tendon. A thorough knowledge of the time frame of connective tissue healing, the stress–strain curve, viscoelastic tissue behavior, and the extent of soft tissue injury is absolutely essential to the

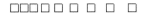

Table 1–7. Biomechanical Observations on Structures from 12-Week-Immobilized Joints

Tissue	Results of Immobilization
Joint composite	Range of motion on an arthrograph indicates that the force required for the first flexion–extension cycle is increased more than 12-fold.
Ligament	Stress–strain diagrams of collateral ligaments show increased deformation with a standard load (i.e., greater compliance). Tensile failure tests of collateral and cruciate ligaments show failure at a lower load, as well as lower energy-absorbing capacity of the immobilized bone–ligament complex (to about one-third of control values).

(Modified from Akeson et al.,[68] with permission.)

ability to exercise good therapeutic judgment in remobilization.

Nerve

Current investigations have revealed few structural changes in neural elements subjected to immobilization.[62] The dynamic function of muscle spindles, articular mechanoreceptors, motor efferents, and sensory afferents is difficult to assess experimentally, yet empirical data suggest a reflex effect on muscle atrophy secondary to joint damage or limb immobilization. In the late 1800s, Charcot[102] observed that paralysis and atrophy were more pronounced in the extensor muscle groups of the knee, hip, shoulder, and elbow after joint injury. Early experiments with dorsal rhizotomy showed reduced muscle wasting in cases of experimentally produced arthritis but no change in the muscle atrophy that accompanied joint immobilization.[103] Stokes and other authors did not feel that pain was the sole factor responsible in either case. Reflex quadriceps inhibition after invasive joint procedures[104] or experimentally produced joint effusion[105] has been recorded via integrated rectified EMG. Even a small joint effusion or an increase in intra-articular pressure can cause quadriceps muscle inhibition,[34,103,105] especially of the oblique fibers of the vastus medialis.[106] It seems that the less the periarticular tissue is disturbed during an invasive procedure, the less severe is the inhibition.[107]

Joint angle is also important in the reduction of reflex inhibition.[103] Even in the absence of a joint effusion, quadriceps contractions are inhibited less after arthrotomy and meniscectomy when the knee joint is positioned in slight flexion rather than full extension postoperatively.[103] This may be partially explained by variations in intra-articular pressure with joint angle or by dynamic reflexogenic activity. The Ruffini endings found at the insertions of ligaments fire more often at the extremes of range of motion to inhibit muscle contraction. Suppression of the H-reflex, which normally elicits muscle contraction, is also seen with an increase in intra-articular pressure.[103] Johansson et al.[108] found that the muscle spindles were highly sensitive to the low-threshold mechanoreceptors in the knee joint ligaments, thus increasing the resistance of the muscles to stretching and influencing effective joint stability. Further inhibition of extensor musculature can also be accomplished by facilitation of the flexor withdrawal response secondary to pain.

■ Remobilization

Mobilization of musculoskeletal injuries has changed greatly in some clinical practices in recent years.[109–114] The advent of the concept and technology of continuous passive movement in the late 1970s and early 1980s brought new dimensions to the prevention of deformity and limited movement after injury and to the promotion of healing of articular cartilage and connective tissue.[111–119] Modern surgery, antibiotics, and the use of cast bracing and intracast electrical stimulation have decreased the immobility period once thought necessary for adequate healing.[64] Physicians, physical therapists, and patients are requesting early mobilization of injuries within acceptable constraints of adequate healing and stability. Prevention rather than treatment of the sequelae of musculoskeletal injury and prolonged immobilization would be the ideal. Until this comes to pass, however, therapists will have to be prepared to evaluate and treat muscles, joints, ligaments, and tendons that have undergone the changes inherent in the inflammatory and immobilization processes.

Muscle, Bone, and Connective Tissue

Many studies are available on the response of muscle to mobilization. Most of these studies concentrate on the effects of exercise in normal subjects.[4, 5] This topic is treated at length in Chapter 2. For purposes of comparison, muscle regeneration begins within 3 to 5 days of the start of a reconditioning program after injury.[51,62] Within the first week, muscle weight increases. Some fibers may complete regeneration of their contractile elements by 1 to 3 days.[62] One week after release from immobilization, muscle fibers of cats immobilized for various lengths of time showed intense regenerative activity, although there was no evidence of mitosis. Fibers began to return to normal via endomysial proliferation. The sarcoplasm started to show evidence of fibrils, which then formed myofibrils. Mitochondria increased in number, and contractile proteins were added. Sarcomeres began forming randomly within a cell, and fiber regeneration also proceeded randomly in terms of geographic distribution. Sarcomeres were initially longer than normal, and A bands were not aligned in register until later in the regenerative process. As regeneration proceeded, sarcomere size and alignment became normal. Thick and thin filaments became better defined. Normal contraction and relaxation times were regained within the first week after release from immobilization.[62] Muscle weight was not quite normal by 6 weeks, but several authors reported normal weight and ultrastructure by 3 months.[120,121] Cooper[62] estimated that linear regeneration took place at the rate of 1 to 1.5 mm/day. Although structural recovery is rapid,[95] recently immobilized muscle may still be vulnerable to exercise-induced fiber damage for the first 14 to 28 days of vigorous recovery activities.[86]

Recent studies point to a protective effect of preimmobilization training for some muscles. Preconditioned rat hindlimb muscles lost a smaller percentage of slow oxidative fibers than did nonhypertrophied, age-matched controls[122] and showed less decrease in collagen synthesis and less formation of collagen cross-links.[99] Similar to their susceptibility to immobilizational atrophy, slow oxidative fibers (type II) recover less quickly during remobilization and seem to require the stimulus of an aerobic training program.[123]

Recovery in muscle takes place at a faster rate and begins substantially sooner after immobilization or trauma than in bone or connective tissue, most likely because of the superior vascular supply of muscle tissue.[62] Muscle immobilized for 4 weeks required an equal amount of time for recovery, as did bone immobilized for the same period of time.[61,63] Bone immobilized for longer periods of time, however, required proportionately longer periods for complete recovery. Connective tissue is the slowest of the tissues under consideration to return to normal after immobilization or injury. This may be because of its slow turnover rate, poor vascularity, or both. Ligaments that have been injured begin to regain tensile strength at about the fifth week after injury, depending on the severity of the injury.[124] A healing ligament may have about 50 percent of its normal strength by 6 months after injury, 80 percent after 1 year, and 100 percent only after 1 to 3 years, depending on the types of stresses placed on it and the prevention of repeated injury.[125] Thus, stressing a connective tissue structure during remobilization is important for full recovery, but it must be properly graded to avoid reinjury. Patients with ligament injuries or reconstructions need to be cautioned about returning gradually to preinjury activities. Since few studies are available on the exact stresses that functional and sports activities place on connective tissue structures, this is again a matter of clinical judgment. Because healing ligaments have a poor nerve supply, the protective effect of muscular contraction, mediated by the mechanoreceptors, is lost,[126] and pain cannot provide a guide to the appropriateness of any particular activity. Joint surfaces are also vulnerable to injury with a sudden increase in functional load.[127-131] Since the effects of periodic short immobilizations appear to be cumulative, it is important to avoid overstressing a recently mobilized limb to avoid reinjury and another period of immobilization.[130]

Studies are available on the response of articular cartilage injuries, total joint replacements, tendon lacerations, tendon transplants, and soft tissue injuries to intermittent and continuous movement.[111-115, 117-119] All of these studies reported an enhanced rate of healing, earlier recovery of normal range of motion, and improved strength over immobilized controls. Several researchers found that regular exercise and stress had the beneficial effect of increasing the mass of ligaments and tendons and rendering them stiffer and able to tolerate heavier loads at failure while preventing the accumulation of intramuscular connective tissue.[132] Biomechanical changes in reconditioned ligaments showed an increase in stress at the yield point, a longer plastic region of deformation, and an increase in maximum load capacity and energy at failure.[124,133,134] Early mobilization of healing tendon repairs decreased adhesion formation and thus increased mobility.[135] Strength was also enhanced compared with the immobilized controls.[136] Microscopic examination showed an increase in the size of collagen fibrils.[137]

Collagen is known to align along lines of stress application, especially during healing or reconditioning after immobilization.[58,134,139] Again, early during the repair phase of the healing process or soon after immobilization is the optimum time to begin any reconditioning program for connective tissue structures, involving either continuous passive movement, graded active exercise, manually applied passive movement, or supervised functional activity. Therapeutic intervention can be more effective when collagen is immature and intermolecular bonds are weak. Specific procedures that concentrate directly on the tissue structures involved would certainly be preferable to general activities, especially at the beginning of a program. When procedures are more specific, forces can be continually controlled and modified according to the response of the tissue and the patient. Without knowledge of the normal structure of the tissues we are dealing with; of the changes in these tissues with injury, immobilization, healing, and remobilization; and of the response of these tissues to the mechanical forces placed on them during physical therapy procedures, treatment is at best minimally therapeutic.

■ References

1. Ham AW, Cormack DH: Histology. 8th Ed. JB Lippincott, Philadelphia, 1979
2. Warwick R, Williams PL, Dyson H, et al: Gray's Anatomy. 37th Ed. Churchill Livingstone, Edinburgh, 1989
3. Lieber RL: Skeletal Muscle Structure and Function. Williams & Wilkins, Baltimore, 1992
4. Astrand P-O: Textbook of Work Physiology, Physiological Basis of Exercise. McGraw-Hill, New York, 1977
5. Gollnick P, Armstrong RB, Saubert CW IV, et al: Enzyme activity and fiber composition in skeletal muscle of untrained and trained men. J Appl Physiol 33:312, 1972
6. Soderberg GL: Kinesiology: Application to Pathological Motion. Williams & Wilkins, Baltimore, 1986
7. Gossman MR, Sahrman SA, Rose S: Review of length associated changes in muscle. Phys Ther 62:1800, 1982
8. Squire J: The Structural Basis of Muscular Contraction. Plenum Press, New York, 1981
9. Peachey LD, Franzini-Armstrong C: Structure and Function of Membrane Systems of Skeletal Mucle Cells. pp. 23–73. In Peachey LD (ed): Handbook of Physiology. American Physiological Society, Betheseda, MD, 1983
10. Landmesser LT: The generation of neuromuscular activity. Ann Rev Neurosci 3:279–302, 1980
11. Poo MM: Rapid lateral diffusion of functional A Ch receptors in embryonic muscle cell membrane. Nature 295:332–334, 1982
12. Brodahl A: Neurological Anatomy in Relation to Clinical Medicine. 3rd Ed. Oxford University Press, New York, 1981
13. Wyke B: The neurology of joints. Ann R Coll Surg 41:25, 1967
14. McNulty WH, Gevirtz RN, Hubbard DR, et al: Needle electromyographic evaluation of trigger point response to a

psychophysiological stressor. Psychophys 31(3):313–316, 1994

15. Akeson WH, Ameil D, Woo SL-Y: Immobility effects of synovial joints: the pathomechanics of joint contracture. Biorheology 17:95, 1980

16. Viidik A: On the rheology and morphology of soft collagenous tissue. J Anat 105:184, 1969

17. Van Brocklin JD, Ellis DG: A study of the mechanical behavior of toe extensor tendons under applied stress. Arch Phys Med 46:369, 1965

18. Kennedy JC, Hawkins RJ, Willis RB, et al: Tension studies of human knee ligaments. J Bone Joint Surg 58(A):350, 1976

19. Lieber RL, Brown CG, Trestik CL: Model of muscle–tendon interaction during frog semitendinosis fixed-end contractions. J Biomech 25:421, 1992

20. Lieber RL, Leonard ME, Brown CE, et al: Frog semitendinosus tendon load-strain and stress-strain properties during passive loading. Am J Physiol 261:C86–C92, 1991

21. Donatelli R, Owens-Burkhardt H: Effects of immobilization on the extensibility of periarticular connective tissue. J Orthop Sports Phys Ther 3:67, 1981

22. Reigger CL: Mechanical properties of bone. p. 3. In Davies GJ, Gould JA (eds): Orthopedic and Sports Physical Therapy. 2nd Ed. CV Mosby, St. Louis, 1985, and Reigger-Krugh CL: Bone. In Malone TR, McPoil TG, Nitz AJ (eds): Orthopedic and Sports Physical Therapy. 3rd Ed., CV Mosby, St. Louis, 1997

23. Frankel VH, Nordin M: Basic Biomechanics of the Skeletal System. Lea & Febiger, Philadelphia, 1980

24. Bryant WM: Wound Healing, Clinical Symposia. Vol. 29:3. CIBA Pharmaceutical, Summit, NJ, 1977

25. Betsch DF, Bauer E: Structure and mechanical properties of rat tail tendon. Biorheology 17:84, 1980

26. Lyon RM, Akeson WH, Amiel D, et al: Ultrastructural difference between the cells of the medial collateral ligament and the anterior cruciate ligament. Clin Orthop 272:279, 1991

27. Amiel D, Frank C, Harwood F, et al: Tendons and ligaments: a morphological and biomechanical comparison. J Orthop Res 1:257, 1984

28. Frank C, Amiel D, Woo SL-Y, et al: Normal ligament properties and ligament healing. Clin Orthop 196:15, 1985

29. Sunderland S: Nerves and Nerve Injuries. 2nd Ed. Churchill Livingstone, New York, 1978

30. Arem AJ, Madden JW: Effects of stress on healing wounds. 1. Intermittent noncyclical tension. J Surg Res 20:93, 1976

31. Rowinski M: Afferent neurobiology of the joint. p. 50. In Davies GJ, Gould JA (eds): Orthopedic and Sports Physical Therapy. CV Mosby, St. Louis, 1985

32. Wyke B: Articular neurology: a review. Physiotherapy 58:94, 1972

33. Freeman MAR, Wyke B: Articular reflexes at the ankle joint: an electromyographic study of normal and abnormal influences of ankle joint mechanoreceptors upon reflex activity in the leg muscles. Br J Surg 54:12, 1967

34. deAndrade JR, Grant CSJ, Dixon A: Joint distension and reflex muscle inhibition in the knee. J Bone Joint Surg 47(A):313, 1965

35. Currey J: The Mechanical Adaptations of Bones. Princeton University Press, Princeton, NJ, 1984

36. Ackerman LV, Spjut HF, Abell MR: Bones and Joints by 24 Authors. International Academy of Pathology Monograph #17. Williams & Wilkins, Baltimore, 1976

37. Bassett CAL: Electrical effects in bone. Sci Am 18:213, 1965

38. Butler DL, Grood ES, Noyes FR, et al: Biomechanics of ligaments and tendons. Exerc Sport Sci Rev 6:126, 1979

39. Zachezewski JE: Flexibility for the runner: specific program considerations. Top Acute Care Trauma Rehabil 10:9, 1986

40. Sapega AA, Quadenfeld TC, Moyer RA, et al: Biophysical factors in range of motion exercise. Phys Sports Med 9:57, 1981

41. Fukuda E: Mechanical deformation and electrical polarization in biological substances. Biorheology 5:199, 1968

42. Hirsch G: Tensile properties during tendon healing. Acta Orthop Scand, suppl. 153:1, 1974

43. Crowninshield RD, Pope MH: Strength and failure characteristics of rat medial collateral ligament. J Trauma 16:99, 1969

44. Noyes FR, DeLucas JL, Torvik PJ: Biomechanics of anterior cruciate ligament failure: an analysis of strain-rate sensitivity and mechanics of failure in primates. J Bone Joint Surg 56(A):236, 1974

45. Rigby BJ, Herai N, Spikes JD, et al: Mechanical properties of rat tail tendon. J Gen Physiol 43:265, 1959

46. Weismann MS, Pope MH, Johnson RJ: Cyclic loading in knee ligament injuries. Am J Sports Med 8:1, 1980

47. Lehmann JF, Masock ASJ, Warren CG, et al: Effect of therapeutic temperatures on tendon extensibility. Arch Phys Med Rehabil 51:481, 1970

48. Welsh RP, MacNab I, Riley V, et al: Biomechanical studies of rabbit tendon. Clin Orthop 81:171, 1971

49. Wilson AW, Davies HM, Edwards GA, et al: Can some physical therapy and manual techniques generate potentially osteogenic levels of strain within mammalian bone? Phys Ther JAPTA 79:931, 1999

50. Gordon AM, Huxley AF, Jilian FT: The variation in isometric tension with sarcomere length in vertebrate muscle fibers. J Physiol 184:185, 1966

51. Magid A, Law DJ: Myofibrils bear most of the resting tension in frog skeletal muscle. Science 230:1280–1282, 1985

52. Horowits R, Podolsky RJ: The positional stability of thick filaments in activated skeletal muscle depends on sarcomere length: evidence for the role of titin filaments. J Cell Biol 105:2217–2223, 1987

53. Fahrni WH: Observations on straight leg raising with special reference to nerve root adhesions. Can J Surg 9:44, 1966

54. Zarins B: Soft tissue injury and repair: biomechanical aspects. Int J Sports Med 3:9, 1982

55. Kellett J: Acute soft tissue injuries: a review of the literature. Med Sci Sports Exerc 18:5, 1986

56. Wilkerson GB: Inflammation in connective tissue: etiology and management. Athl Train Winter 298, 1985

57. van der Meulen JCH: Present state of knowledge on processes of healing in collagen structures. Int J Sports Med 3:4, 1982

58. McGaw WT: The effect of tension on collagen remodelling by fibroblasts: a stereological ultrastructural study. Connect Tissue Res 14:229, 1986

59. Appell HJ: Muscular atrophy following immobilization. A review. Sports Med 10:42, 1990

60. Turek SL: Orthopaedics: Principles and Their Application. 4th Ed. JB Lippincott, Philadelphia, 1984

61. Steinberg FU: The Immobilized Patient: Functional Pathology and Management. Plenum, New York, 1980

62. Cooper RR: Alterations during immobilization and regeneration of skeletal muscle in cats. J Bone Joint Surg 54(A):919, 1972

63. Tabary JC, Tabary C, Tardieu C, et al: Physiological and structural changes in the cat soleus muscle due to immobilization at different lengths by plaster casts. J Physiol 224:231, 1972

64. Booth FW: Physiologic and biochemical effects of immobilization on muscle. Clin Orthop 219:15, 1987

65. Lindboe CF, Platou CS: Effects of immobilization of short duration on the muscle fibre size. Clin Physiol 4:183, 1984

66. Akeson WH: An experimental study of joint stiffness. J Bone Joint Surg 43(A):1022, 1961

67. Akeson WH, Ameil D, LaViolette D: The connective tissue response to immobility: a study of the chondroitin 4- and 6-sulfate and dermatin sulfate changes in periarticular connective tissue of control and immobilized knees of dogs. Clin Orthop 51:183, 1967

68. Akeson WH, Ameil D, LaViolette D: The connective tissue response to immobility: an accelerated aging response. Exp Gerontol 3:239, 1968

69. LaVigne AB, Watkins RP: Preliminary results on immobilization-induced stiffness of monkey knee joints and posterior capsule. In Perspectives in Biomedical Engineering. Proceedings of a symposium, Biological Engineering Society, University of Strathclyde, Glasgow, June 1972. University Park Press, Baltimore, 1973

70. Noyes FR, Torvik PJ, Hyde WB, et al: Biomechanics of ligament failure II: an analysis of immobilization, exercise and reconditioning effects in primates. J Bone Joint Surg 56(A):1406, 1974

71. Geiser M, Trueta J: Muscle action, bone rarefication and bone formation. J Bone Joint Surg 40(B):282, 1958

72. Little K, De Valderama JF: Some mechanisms involved in the osteoporotic process. Gerontologia 14:109, 1968

73. Hardt AB: Early metabolic responses of bone to immobilization. J Bone Joint Surg 54(A):119, 1972

74. Hulth A, Olerud S: Disease of the extremities: II. A microangiographic study in the rabbit. Acta Chir Scand 120:338, 1961

75. Burr D, Frederickson R, Pavlinch C, et al: Intracast muscle stimulation prevents bone and cartilage deterioration in cast-immobilized rabbits. Clin Orthop 189:264, 1984

76. van der Wiel HE, Lips P, Nauta J, et al: Biochemical parameters of bone turnover during 10 days of bed rest and subsequent mobilization (abstract). Bone Miner 13:123, 1991

77. Li XJ, Jee WS, Chow SY, et al: Adaptations of cancellous bone to aging and immobilization in the rat: a single photon absorptiometry and histiomorphometry study (abstract). Anat Rec 227:12, 1990

78. Tuukkanen J, Wallmark B, Jalovaara P, et al: Changes induced in growing rat bone by immobilization and remobilization. Bone 12:113, 1991

79. Witzmann FA, Kim DH, Fitts RH: Effect of hindlimb immobilization on the fatigability of skeletal muscle (abstract). J Appl Physiol 54:1242, 1983

80. Witzmann FA, Kim DH, Fitts RH: Hind-limb immobilization: length-tension and contractile properties of skeletal muscle (abstract). J Appl Physiol 53:335, 1982

81. Simard CP, Spector SA, Edgerton VR: Contractile properties of rat hind limb muscles immobilized at different lengths (abstract). Exp Neurol 77:467, 1982

82. Robinson GA, Enoka RM, Stuart DG: Immobilization-induced changes in motor unit force and fatigability in the cat. Muscle Nerve 14:563, 1991

83. Lieber RL, Friden JO, Hargens AR, et al: Differential response of the dog quadriceps muscle to external skeletal fixation of the knee. Muscle Nerve 11:193, 1988

84. Mayer RF, Burke RE, Toop J, et al: The effect of long term immobilization on the motor unit population of the cat medial gastrocnemius muscle (abstract). Neuroscience 6:725, 1981

85. Kasper CE, White TP, Maxwell LC: Running during recovery from hindlimb suspension induces transient muscle injury (abstract). J Appl Physiol 68:533, 1990

86. Sargeant AJ, Davies CT, Edwards RH, et al: Functional and structural changes after disuse of human muscles. Clin Sci Mol Med 52:337, 1977

87. MacDougall JD, Ward GR, Sale DG, et al: Biochemical adaptations of human skeletal muscle to heavy resistance training and immobilization (abstract). J Appl Physiol 43:700, 1977

88. MacDougall JD, Elder GCB, Sale DG, et al: Effects of strength training and immobilization on human muscle fibers (abstract). Eur J Appl Physiol 43:25, 1980

89. Boreham CA, Watt PW, Williams PE, et al: Effects of ageing and chronic dietary restriction on the morphology of fast and slow muscles of the rat. J Anat 157:111, 1988

90. Lipman RL, Raskin P, Love T, et al: Glucose intolerance during decreased physical activity in man. Diabetes 21:101, 1972

91. Nicholson WF, Watson PA, Booth FA: Glucose uptake and glycogen synthesis in muscles from immobilized limbs (abstract). J Appl Physiol 56:431, 1984

92. Berg HE, Didley GA, Haggmark T, et al: Effects of lower limb unloading on skeletal muscle mass and function in humans (abstract). J Appl Physiol 70:1882, 1991

93. Duchateau J, Hainaut K: Effects of immobilization on contractile properties, recruitment and firing rates of human motor units. J Physiol 422:55, 1990

94. Zemkova H, Teisinger J, Almon RR, et al: Immobilization atrophy and membrane properties in rat skeletal muscle fibers (abstract). Eur J Physiol 416:126, 1990

95. Lieber RL, McKee-Woodburn T, Gershuni DH: Recovery of the dog quadriceps after 10 weeks of immobilization followed by 4 weeks of remobilization. J Orthop Res 7:408, 1989

96. Williams PE: Effect of intermittant stretch on immobilized muscle. Ann Rheum Dis 47:1014, 1988

97. Jozsa L, Reffy A, Demel S, et al: Quantitative alterations of intramuscular connective tissue in calf muscles of the rat during combined hypoxia and hypokinesia. Acta Physiol Hung 73:393, 1989

98. Jozsa L, Kannus P, Thoring J, et al: The effect of tenotomy and of immobilization on intramuscular connective tissue. A morphometric and microscopic study in rat calf muscles. J Bone Joint Surg 72(B):293, 1990

99. Karpakka J, Vaannanen K, Oravas S, et al: The effects of preimmobilization training and immobilization on collagen synthesis in rat skeletal muscle. Int J Sports Med 11:484, 1990

100. Dehne E, Torp RP: Treatment of joint injuries by immediate mobilization. Based on the spinal adaptation concept. Clin Orthop 77:218, 1971

101. Akeson WH, Amiel D, Abel MF, et al: Effects of immobilization on joints. Clin Orthop 219:33, 1987

102. Charcot JM: Clinical Lectures on the Diseases of the Nervous System. The New Syndenham Society, London, 1889

103. Young A, Stokes M, Iles JF: Effects of joint pathology on muscle. Clin Orthop 219:23, 1987

104. Stokes M, Young A: The contribution of reflex inhibition to arthrogenous muscle weakness. Clin Sci 67:7, 1984

105. Ekholm J, Eklund G, Skoglund S: On the reflex effects from the knee joint of the cat. Acta Physiol Scand 50:176, 1960

106. Iles JF, Stokes M, Young A: Reflex actions of knee joint afferents during contraction of the human quadriceps. Clin Physiol 10:489, 1990

107. Zimny ML: Mechanoreceptors in articular tissues (abstract). Am J Anat 182:16, 1988

108. Johansson J, Sjolander P, Sojka P: Receptors in the knee joint ligaments and their role in the biomechanics of the joint (abstract). Crit Rev Biomed Eng 18:341, 1991

109. Perry J: Contractures: a historical approach. Clin Orthop 219:8, 1987

110. Nicholas JA, Friedman MJ: Sprains and dislocations of joints and related structures. In Denton JR (ed): Orthopedics, Goldsmith Practice of Surgery 2:1. Harper & Row, Philadelphia, 1984

111. Salter RB, Simmonds DF, Malcolm BW, et al: The biological effect of continuous passive motion on the healing of full thickness defects in articular cartilage. J Bone Joint Surg 62(A):1232, 1980

112. Salter RB, Hamilton HW: Clinical application of basic research on continuous passive motion for disorders and injuries of joints: a preliminary report of a feasibility study. J Orthop Res 1:325, 1984

113. Coutts RD, Kaita J, Barr R, et al: The role of continuous passive movement in the postoperative rehabilitation of the total knee patient. Orthop Trans 6:277, 1982

114. Hamilton HW: Five years experience with continuous passive motion (CPM). J Bone Joint Surg 64(B):259, 1982

115. O'Driscoll SW, Kumar A, Salter RB: The effect of continuous passive motion on the clearance of a hemarthrosis. Clin Orthop 176:305, 1983

116. Salter RB: Motion vs rest: why immobilize joints? Presidential address to the Canadian Orthopedic Association. J Bone Joint Surg 64(B):251, 1982

117. Salter RB, Bell RS: The effect of continuous passive motion on the healing of partial thickness lacerations of the patellar tendon in the rabbit. Orthop Trans 5:209, 1981

118. Salter RB, Harris DJ, Bogoch E: Further studies on continuous passive motion (abstract). Orthop Trans 212:292, 1978

119. Salter RB, Minister RR: The effect of continuous passive motion on a semitendinosus tenodesis in the rabbit knee. Orthop Trans 6:292, 1982

120. Lash JW, Holtzer H, Swift H: Regeneration of mature skeletal muscle. Anat Rec 128:679, 1957

121. LeGros Clark WE: An experimental study of regeneration of mammalian striped muscle. J Anat 80:24, 1946

122. Ianuzzo CD, Blank S, Crassweller A, et al: Effect of hindlimb immobilization and recovery on compensatory hypertrophied rat plantaris muscle. Mol Cell Biochem 90:57, 1989

123. McNulty AL, Otto AJ, Kasper CE, et al: Effect of recovery mode following hind limb suspension on soleus muscle compensation in the rat. Int J Sports Med 13:6, 1992

124. Frank G, Woo SL-Y, Amiel D, et al: Medial collateral ligament healing. A multidisciplinary assessment in rabbits. Am J Sports Med 11:379, 1983

125. Tipton CM, James SL, Mergner W, et al: Influence of exercise on strength of medial collateral knee ligaments of dogs. Am J Physiol 218:894, 1970

126. Johansson H, Sjolander P, Sojka P: Receptors in the knee joint, ligaments and their role in the biomechanics of the joint. Crit Rev Biomed Eng 18:341, 1991

127. Tipton CM, Matthes RD, Maynard JA, et al: The influence of physical activity on ligaments and tendons. Med Sci Sports 7:165, 1975

128. Videman T: Connective tissue and immobilization: key factors in musculoskeletal degeneration? Clin Orthop 221:26, 1987

129. Videman T: Experimental osteoarthritis in the rabbit: comparison of different periods of repeated immobilization. Acta Orthop Scand 53:339, 1982

130. Videman T, Michelsson J-E: Inhibition of development of experimental osteoarthritis by distraction during immobilization. Int Res Comm Syst Ed Sci 5:139, 1977

131. Shimizu T, Videman T, Shimazaki K, et al: Experimental study on the repair of full thickness articular cartilage defects. J Orthop Res 5:187, 1987

132. Williams PE, Catanese T, Lucey EG, et al: The importance of stretch and contractile activity in the prevention of connective tissue accumulation in muscle. J Anat 158:109, 1988

133. Clayton ML, Weir GJ: Experimental investigation of ligament healing. Am J Surg 98:373, 1959

134. Viidik A: Tensile strength properties of Achilles tendon systems in trained and untrained rabbits. Acta Orthop Scand 40:261, 1969

135. Evans EB, Eggers GWN, Butler JK, et al: Experimental immobilization and remobilization of rat knee joints. J Bone Joint Surg 42(A):737, 1960

136. Gelberman R, Woo SL-Y, Lothringer K, et al: Effects of early intermittent passive mobilization on healing canine flexor tendons. J Hand Surg 7:170, 1982

137. Woo SL-Y, Gomez MA, Young-Kyun W, et al: Mechanical properties of tendons and ligaments II: the relationship of immobilization and exercise on tissue remodeling. Biorheology 19:397, 1982

138. Evans P: The healing process at a cellular level: a review. Physiotherapy 66:256, 1974

139. Cohen RE, Hooley CJ, McCrum NG: Viscoelastic creep of collagenous tissue. J Biomech 9:175, 1976

140. Rydell N: Biomechanics of the hip joint. Clin Orthop 92:6, 1973 Systems

CHAPTER 2

Exercise Treatment for the Rehabilitated Patient: Cardiopulmonary and Peripheral Responses

Scot Irwin

Rehabilitation services provided after an injury or surgery often fail to include a fitness training program for patients after they have completed the rehabilitation of their injury. Several stages are involved in completing this part of a rehabilitation program. Once the injured extremity or spine has achieved an acceptable level of function, program goals should be adjusted to achieve a state of fitness equivalent to that of the preinjured state.

This chapter discusses the completion of rehabilitation through exercise training. Exercise training requires the therapist to adhere to some basic principles of exercise physiology, including (1) designing a specific exercise program using an appropriate exercise mode to achieve the desired results, (2) recognizing the innate genetic limitations of each individual and thus the amount of improvement that can be expected, (3) developing cardiovascular conditioning by long-duration, continuous exercise of large muscle groups, and (4) increasing strength and power with high-intensity, short-duration bursts of activity.

These are principles, not laws. Each of these principles continues to be rigorously investigated, but for now, they are considered solid standards of exercise that can be followed with reasonable confidence. These principles are affected by several external variables that can influence the conditioning program and thus the desired outcomes. These variables include, but are not limited to, age, initial state of fitness, sex, temperature, altitude, medications, and individual motivation.

The purpose of this chapter is to highlight the principles, evaluation methods, and desired effects of exercise training programs used to complete the rehabilitation process after an injury. To achieve this purpose, the chapter is divided into four sections covering the effects of bed rest and deconditioning, the evaluation of cardiovascular condition, the principles of exercise prescription, and the effects of training.

Bed Rest and Deconditioning

Most extremity injuries, especially lower extremity injuries, are accompanied by a reduction in activity. Severe injuries, such as fractures and ligamentous tears, often result in short periods of complete bed rest and prolonged periods of inactivity.

The detrimental effects of bed rest have been thoroughly chronicled, especially in studies on the effects of weightlessness.[1] The effects of bed rest vary according to duration,[2-4] prior state of conditioning,[5] and the activity conducted during bed rest[2] (e.g., isometric or isotonic exercises, bathroom privileges). The time course of some of these changes is presented in Table 2–1.[2-5]

Many of the effects of bed rest occur within 3 days or less (Table 2–1). These changes are primarily attributed to changes in plasma volume, fluids and electrolytes, and venous compliance. With prolonged bed rest, the detrimental effects become more numerous and severe. They include losses in body weight, calcium, muscle strength, and maximum oxygen consumption. Some additional detrimental effects of bed rest include constipation, atelectasis, orthostatic hypotension, and osteoporosis.[6] However, some authors have demonstrated a significant increase in forced vital capacity and total lung capacity after bed rest of 11 to 12 days.[7] These data have been challenged by other researchers, who found no significant changes in static volumes after bed rest.[2]

There are numerous and sometimes conflicting reports on the effects of isometric and isotonic exercises used to reduce the detrimental effects of prolonged inactivity.[2,8] A summary of the effects of bed rest of 7 to 14 days on young male patients can also be found in Table 2–1.

Knowledge of the detrimental effects of bed rest will influence the treatment program chosen. The reader should not equate decreased activity with bed rest, for

□□□□□ □ □ □

Table 2-1. Effects of Bed Rest on Young Male Patients

Effect	1 Hr/Day Isotonic	7–14 Days No Exercise	1 Hr/Day Isometric
Changes in body composition	Increases fat loss Decreases lean loss Total weight loss is determined by diet	Loss of lean and fat mass	Total body weight loss may actually be greater
Plasma volume loss	Reduces loss to 7–8%	Plasma volume decreases by 300–500 ml (12–13%)	Reduces loss to 11%
VO_2	Decreases loss by about one-third (8–5%)	10–12%[a]	Decreases loss to about 4–5%
Glucose tolerance	Reduces glucose intolerance	Glucose tolerance worsens	Reduces glucose intolerance
Plasma calcium[b]	Reduces loss to 4%	11% loss continues steadily over 36 weeks	Reduces loss to 7%

Abbreviation: VO_2, maximum oxygen consumption.
[a]Depends on initial state of fitness. Men's rate of loss is less than women's.
[b]See references 2–5.

even modest activity such as sitting in a chair or performing mild isotonic or isometric exercise can reduce the detrimental effects of bed rest.[2] Normalization from the effects of bed rest can be achieved in only 7 days with an exercise conditioning program,[8] but many of the losses are reversible with resumption of normal activities.[8] The less time persons are subjected to bed rest or reduced activity, the less time it takes to return to their previous state of fitness.

Individuals at higher fitness levels, as determined by their maximum oxygen consumption (trained athletes), may lose a greater percentage of their maximum oxygen consumption during periods of inactivity than the average sedentary individual. They usually require a rigorous training program to regain the same relative state of fitness.[5] The higher the state of conditioning required, the greater the need for an individualized exercise prescription. The rehabilitation process is not complete simply because normal joint motion and muscular strength have returned. An individual, especially an athlete, should retrain the muscles, joints, and cardiopulmonary system to their premorbid state before resuming athletic endeavors. Untrained individuals may cause themselves further injury and achieve suboptimal performances.

■ Evaluation

Each individual should have a specifically designed exercise prescription based on a thorough evaluation of his or her maximum physical work capacity, neuromusculoskeletal limitations, and functional goals.

Physical work capacity can best be evaluated by performing an exercise test. This test can be as simple as a 12-minute walk or as sophisticated as a symptom-limited maximum thallium treadmill test. The choice of testing

method should match the mode of exercise to be prescribed and should be as sophisticated as the individual's age, cardiac risk factors, sex, and additional medical problems require. For example, if the mode of training will be biking, the exercise test should be performed on a bike. If the patient plans to participate in activities that require maximum cardiovascular performance, a symptom-limited maximum exercise test should be performed. Generally, if the patient is a male older than 35 years, he should be thoroughly screened by his physician before beginning an exercise program.[9] If he is younger than 35 years but has multiple risk factors for heart disease or any history of cardiac involvement (murmurs), he should also be cleared by his physician before initiating an exercise training program.[9]

A multitude of testing and evaluation modes are available. General guidelines for exercise testing can be found in the American College of Sports Medicine guidelines for testing and training.[9] Perhaps more important than the choice of testing methods is the interpretation of the test. A thorough discussion of exercise test interpretations is outside the scope of this chapter. For an in-depth discussion of this topic, see Astrand's *Textbook of Work Physiology*[10] and Ellestad's *Stress Testing*.[11]

A typical symptom-limited maximum exercise test completed on a 40-year-old man is depicted in Figures 2–1 and 2–2. This test was performed on a treadmill using a Bruce protocol.[12] Although this protocol is not ideal for exercise prescription, it is commonly used in exercise testing laboratories throughout the United States, especially for ruling out coronary disease. It is strongly recommended that any patient who is going to begin a walking, walk-jog, or higher-intensity exercise program have a symptom-limited maximum exercise test. If the patient is older than 35 years, this test should be completed in a formal exercise testing laboratory with the

TREADMILL TEST WORKSHEET
Clayton General Hospital

Name _____ Hosp. No _____ Date 1/12/87 Age 40

Sex M Weight 212 Height 6' 0" Diagnosis 0 _____

Reason for test Fitness Program _____ Protocol _____

ECG Interpretation Normal _____

Time 9:00 A.M. Medications None _____

Time last dose None _____ Time last cigarette None _____ Time last meal 6:00 P.M.

Physician: _____

_____

TEST RESULTS

Minutes Completed 7' 52" _____ Limiting Factors Leg fatigue, S.O.B. _____

Resting Heart rate 78 _____ Max. Heart rate 176 _____ Resting BP 108/78 _____

Max. BP 190/86 _____ BP Response normadaptive _____

_____

Chest Pain 0 _____

_____

Summary ST Segment Changes negative test to HR 176 _____

_____

Heart Sounds normal _____ Arrhythmias rare PVC's post exercise _____

Physical Work Capacity Fair-Good FAI 25% below predicted for a sedentary male _____

Remarks/Recommendations _____

_____

Figure 2–1. Treadmill test interpretation. (FAI, functional aerobic impairment; PVC, premature ventricular contraction; SOB, shortness of breath)

STAGE	MPH	GRADE	MINUTE	HR	BP	ARRHYTHMIAS	SYMPTOMS
PRE-EX							
SUPINE			1	76	110/70	0	0
SUPINE			2	78	118/78	0	0
BREATH-HOLD			1	66	102/70	0	0
HYPERVENT.			1	78	120/76	0	0
SITTING			1	78	130/70	0	0
STANDING			1	84	140/80	0	0
MPH	%	SEC.					
1.7	10		1	100	144/80	0	0
			2	110	150/78	0	0
			3	110	150/78	0	0
2.5	12		1	126	156/84	0	0
			2	136	166/84	0	0
			3	144	170/80	0	0
3.4	14	52"	1	160	186/86	0	S.O.B., leg pain
			2	176	190/86	0	
			3				
			1				
			2				
			3				
			1				
			2				
			3				
IMMEDIATE POST-EX.							
SUPINE			1	175	174/76	Rare PVC	
			2	160	156/70		
			3	140	148/72	xx	
			4	114	144/72	x	
			5	96	136/70		
			6	88	130/88		
			7	88	136/78		
			8				
			9				
			10				

Figure 2–2. Treadmill test worksheet.

appropriate personnel present. A study by Cahalin et al.[13] demonstrates the safety of this type of testing when completed independently by specially trained physical therapists. There are several alternative exercise test protocols that may more appropriately fit the needs of the patient or the program to be developed (Fig. 2–3).

A symptom-limited maximum exercise test gives us the following vital information: (1) actual symptom-limited maximum heart rate, (2) presence or absence of the normal cardiopulmonary responses to exercise, (3) presence or absence of electrocardiographic (ECG) abnormalities, (4) limiting symptoms, and (5) predicted physical work capacity.[12]

Despite attempts to formulate exercise prescriptions based directly on the treadmill exercise test,[15] I can state that, clinically, direct translation from a test to an exercise prescription is rarely possible. These tests should be considered as part of the patient's evaluation and as a screening process to rule out potentially dangerous pathologies. An exercise test can also be used to measure the extent of patient progress. Some protocols (Balke and Froelicher protocols) will enhance the therapist's ability to detect

improvements because they have smaller incremental increases at each stage of the test (Fig. 2–3).

Alternative forms of testing include biking and arm ergometry. The format for these tests is quite different. The treadmill test is a continuous test, whereas most arm or bike tests are intermittent. Participants are allowed to rest or pedal against lower resistance between 2- to 4-minute bouts of progressively higher-intensity exercise. Bike testing generally does not produce as high a cardiopulmonary response as treadmill testing because leg muscle fatigue occurs before the maximum cardiopulmonary level is attained. If your clinic does not have access to an exercise testing laboratory, simpler submaximal tests can be completed. A 6-minute walk test can be a useful evaluation, especially for people who have severe exercise intolerance. To complete this test, simply mark off a known distance and ask the patient to walk as far as he or she can in 6 minutes. Record the patient's resting and peak heart rates and blood pressures and any symptoms noted, and measure the distance the patient walked. The patient is allowed to stop and rest anytime during the 6 minutes and may resume the walk after each rest; the time, though,

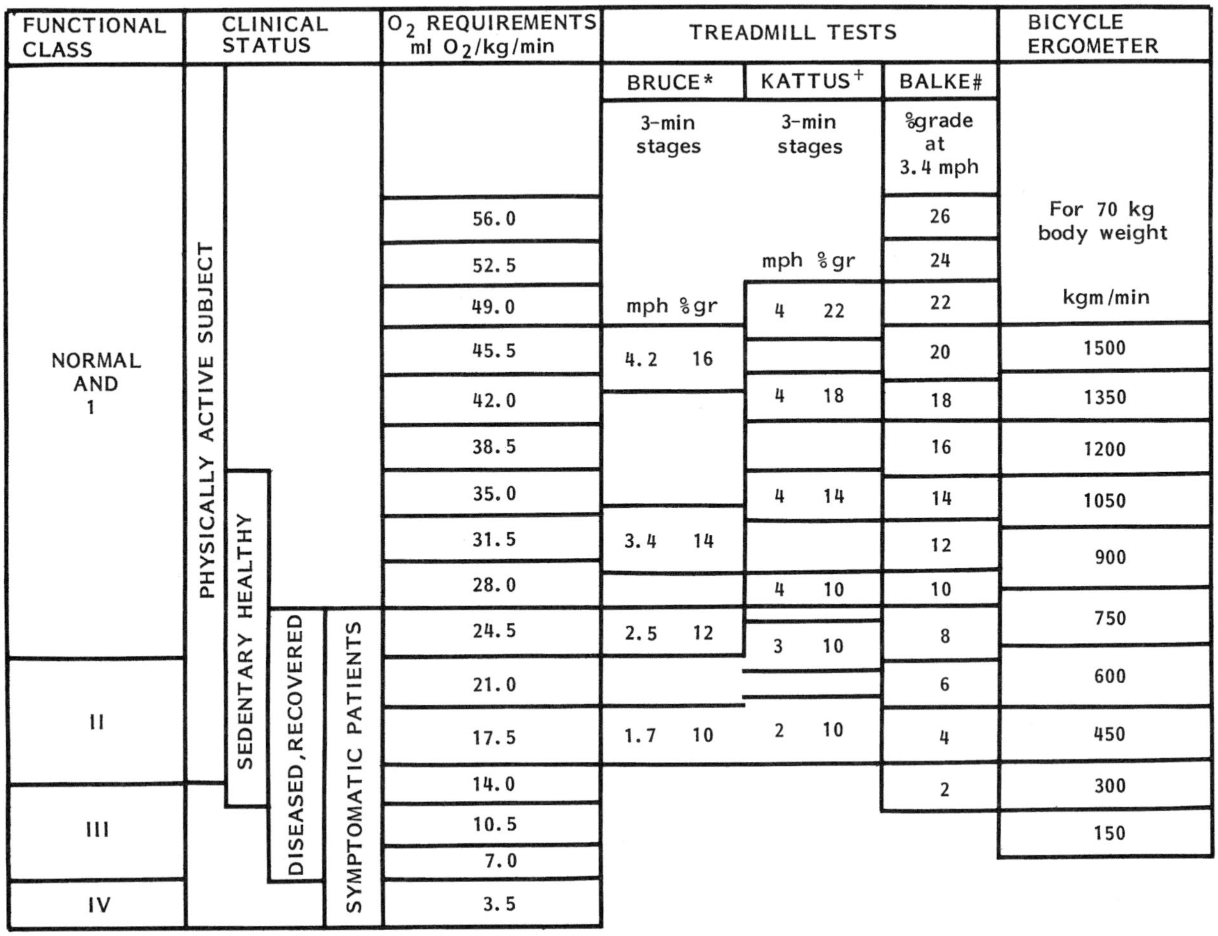

FUNCTIONAL CLASS	CLINICAL STATUS	O₂ REQUIREMENTS ml O₂/kg/min	TREADMILL TESTS BRUCE* 3-min stages (mph %gr)		KATTUS⁺ 3-min stages (mph %gr)		BALKE# %grade at 3.4 mph	BICYCLE ERGOMETER For 70 kg body weight kgm/min
NORMAL AND 1	PHYSICALLY ACTIVE SUBJECT	56.0					26	
		52.5					24	
		49.0			4	22	22	
		45.5	4.2	16			20	1500
		42.0			4	18	18	1350
		38.5					16	1200
		35.0			4	14	14	1050
	SEDENTARY HEALTHY	31.5	3.4	14			12	900
		28.0			4	10	10	
	DISEASED, RECOVERED / SYMPTOMATIC PATIENTS	24.5	2.5	12	3	10	8	750
II		21.0					6	600
		17.5	1.7	10	2	10	4	450
		14.0					2	300
III		10.5						150
		7.0						
IV		3.5						

Figure 2–3. Classification and oxygen requirements for different workloads on treadmill and bicycle ergometers. (gr, grade.) (Modified from Fortuin and Weiss,[14] with permission.)

is continuous. Rest periods are part of the 6 minutes. This information can be used as a baseline for exercise prescription and repeated to assess improvement.

Before an individualized exercise prescription is developed, a thorough neuromusculoskeletal evaluation should be completed, including a posture analysis with special attention to the strength, flexibility, and symmetry of the individual to be trained. For example, a patient who is going to start a walking or walk-jogging program should have a careful evaluation of lower extremity strength, range of movement, and gait, especially foot and ankle biomechanics (see Chapter 1). A posture analysis and an individualized muscle test are necessities. Elaboration of this part of the evaluation can be found in the work of Kendall and Kendall-McCreary.[16]

Any joint, strength, or postural asymmetries should be corrected before initiating, or as a part of, the patient's conditioning program. From my clinical experience, this will reduce subsequent complaints of pain and encourage continued exercise compliance. Routine reassessment of the program's intensity should also include a quick musculoskeletal screen to ensure that no detrimental changes have occurred as a result of training. Common clinical findings with walking and walk-jogging programs include shin splints, runner's hip, tightening of the hamstrings, knee pain, Achilles tendinitis, and calf pain. In some cases, a change in training mode is required. Biking and swimming are good alternatives, but reassessment and testing are required.

■ Principles of Exercise Prescription

We live in a society that is health conscious. Wellness is not a notion but a reality, but the forms of exercise that are sold by educated and uneducated individuals at all levels may not be the answer. In fact, the incidence of exercise-related injury has increased dramatically in recent years. A generalized exercise prescription, based on the idea that what is good for the instructor is good for all, may well be the reason.

An individualized exercise prescription requires more than that. An individualized exercise prescription must be based on a thorough evaluation and must take into consideration the mode, intensity, frequency, and duration of the exercise.

Selecting the mode of exercise is easy but is often poorly done. The mode of exercise should be chosen by approximating the individual's actual athletic endeavors as closely as possible. It should include methods of training that incorporate strengthening, improvement in flexibility, and endurance training. Emphasis on one of these three areas should be encouraged if the evaluation findings have identified a specific area of weakness. The mode of exercise should be specific. The principle of the specificity of exercise cannot be overstated. If an individual is

unable to train by performing the actual activity he or she wants to participate in, a mode of training that closely imitates that activity should be chosen. For example, a person suffering from a loss of physical work capacity because of prolonged bed rest or restricted activity needs a mode of exercise that most closely approaches his or her daily activities. This is usually best achieved by walking. However, a football star needs a program that incorporates modes of training to improve strength, flexibility, and endurance for repeated bouts of short-duration, high-intensity exercise; walking is not the best choice.

Once the mode or modes of exercise have been chosen, the next part of the exercise prescription is to decide the intensity of the exercise. Often at this point in a chapter about exercise prescription, the reader is exposed to a series of formulas and graphs. The formulas depict a reasonable but generally wide and unindividualized range of exercise target heart rates based on age. This information is available in almost any textbook on exercise physiology, so a brief summary will suffice here.

Heart rate is linearly related to oxygen consumption, especially between 40 and 90 percent of maximum effort. Cardiovascular fitness training is believed to occur best somewhere between 60 and 90 percent of an individual's maximum heart rate. This heart rate is predictable from the formula of 220 minus the person's age. The training heart rate can thus be computed by obtaining a maximum predicted heart rate (220 − age) and multiplying it by a fixed percentage. This formula uses the individual's resting heart rate, training percentage, and maximum heart rate to obtain a training heart rate. For example, a 30-year-old man with a resting heart rate of 60 would need to achieve a training heart rate of 151 to be training at a 70 percent intensity $(190 - 60)(.70) + 60$[17] (190 is 220 minus the man's age). All these formulas and numbers are entirely accurate and can even be used with a normal, relatively active, well-motivated, healthy population of people younger than 30 years. Exercise prescription for the rest of us is not that easy and should be carefully individualized to take into consideration each patient's current state of fitness, presence of disease (especially cardiopulmonary diseases), age, sex, altitude, temperature, and motivation.

In my clinical experience, these formulas are often not applicable. People recovering from injuries, bed rest, heart attacks, or surgery cannot and will not adhere to these generalized heart rate formulas. There are several reasons for this, including, but not limited to, medication, age, prior exercise habits, side effects of surgery, and motivation. So how does one determine an appropriate, useful intensity for an individual's exercise prescription? One of the best methods is to evaluate the person's response to the exercise program. This can be achieved by having the person carry out the program with you. I have found that many people, even after bypass surgery or a heart attack, can exercise continuously for 30 minutes at very low intensities. This is an excellent initial duration. The intensity is then increased according to the individual's response. For example, a patient returning to noncompetitive basketball after a foot injury needs endurance training. The patient is instructed to walk, beginning at 2.5 mph for 30 minutes. The therapist continuously assesses the patient's response to this intensity and adjusts the speed up or down accordingly. Maximal comfortable walking speed for most men is about 4.0–4.2 mph. Beyond this speed, most patients are more comfortable jogging. The intensity is then adjusted according to the needs of the patient. The desired outcome is an individual who can return to recreational basketball with a decreased risk of repeating his injury and a higher level of satisfaction.

There are two other ways to increase intensity using a treadmill. One is to maintain the speed and steepen the grade. I have found this to be effective before moving a patient to a jogging program. The maximum grade used is 5 percent. Steeper grades at high speeds tend to cause injuries, shin splints, calf pain, and knee pain. Another method for increasing intensity is to have the person jog at the same pace used for walking. This can even be done at low speeds of 3.6 to 4.0 mph. Jogging will increase the intensity of the exercise even though the speed may not have changed. Have the patient begin jogging at a low speed. After the patient can comfortably walk at a rate of 3.6 to 4.0 mph on a 1–3 percent grade for 30 to 45 minutes, he or she may begin a walk-jog program consisting of a 1-minute jog followed by a 5-minute walk at 3.6 to 4.0 mph on a level surface. The jogging duration is then gradually increased to a 5-minute jog alternating with a 10-minute walk, for a total of 30 to 45 minutes, on a level surface. Continuation of this process will result in the patient's eventually achieving an intensity that can be sustained without injury. In general, using a grade with jogging is not recommended, as this seems to enhance the risk of injury, especially in people older than 40 years. This gradual process of intensity changes from walking to jogging may require several weeks or months, depending upon the age and relative state of fitness of the individual prior to initiation of the program.

By integrating continuous musculoskeletal evaluation with a progressive method of assessing intensity, each person can achieve an exercise prescription with an appropriate mode, duration, and intensity for his or her personal needs. Frequency is determined by the individual's response to training and the individual's goals. When training patients to improve their cardiovascular fitness, I use a frequency of four to five times a week as a minimum. Often with low-level programs (1.5–2.5 mph), I will have a patient exercise twice a day four to five times a week. This requires the patient to carry out the greater part of the program at home. The therapist must therefore teach the patient about walking surfaces, shoes, and climate. Each of these variables can affect compliance and the incidence of injuries. Once a person has achieved an acceptable level of training, the frequency can be reduced to two to four times per week, although compliance can

easily fail at this juncture. People tend not to comply if too much time elapses between exercise days. Lifelong training may be as frequent as daily, although, again, the incidence of illness and injury will often make this impossible.

So, how does an exercise prescription evolve? For improving aerobic capacity, the mode is specific, and the intensity is individualized and intimately related to the duration of exercise. Finally, the frequency is determined by the goals of exercise: maintenance, improved fitness, or lifelong training. With these concepts in mind, the clinician should be able to complete the rehabilitation of an injured person regardless of age, sex, state of fitness, or type of injury.

■ Effects of Exercise Training

A chapter on exercise training would be incomplete without some discussion of the potential benefits of exercise. However, an in-depth analysis could encompass an entire textbook. Thus, this part of the chapter presentes a condensed version of the specific effects of an exercise training program using the principles already described.

The effects of exercise training fit nicely into two broad categories: central (cardiovascular) and peripheral effects. Each of these categories contributes to the net effect, which is an improvement in maximum oxygen consumption and physical work capacity.

The central or cardiovascular effects of exercise conditioning are well documented. An untrained individual can expect to achieve a 10 to 20 percent increase in maximum oxygen consumption over 3 to 6 months of training.

The primary central training effects are an increase in stroke volume, an increase in maximum cardiac output, a decrease in resting heart rate, and a decrease in heart rate and blood pressure at a given workload. These effects may require a minimum of 6 months of training or longer to achieve. In other words, at a workload of 4 mph, a person before training may exhibit a heart rate of 120 beats per minute and blood pressure of 170/80 mmHg, whereas after training the heart rate and blood pressure at this same workload will be significantly lower. The amount of improvement depends on several variables, including, but not limited to, the state of fitness of the individual before beginning exercise, the intensity and duration of training, the age of the individual, and the presence or absence of any systemic pathology. Those individuals who are most deconditioned before initiating an exercise program tend to have the greatest percentage improvement compared with more fit individuals. Low-intensity training programs, in which heart rates do not exceed 60 percent of maximum, may not produce the expected central training effects that higher levels of exercise training will achieve. The effects of training on elderly men and women appear to be very similar despite the somewhat lower intensities in the elderly.[18–23] Cardiopulmonary patients with severe ventricular dysfunction or advanced obstructive or restrictive lung disease may not demonstrate the same central training effects, and thus increases in their maximum oxygen-carrying capacity, but functional improvements can be dramatic. For an in-depth review of the effects of training on cardiopulmonary patients, see the work by Blessey.[24] Patients with coronary artery disease may never demonstrate improvement in stroke volume, although a small number of studies have demonstrated improvement after 12 months of training or more.[25]

The peripheral effects of training are more numerous and perhaps more rapidly attained. The initial effects of training are created peripherally. These effects include an increase in arterial oxygen extraction at the tissue level—the arteriovenous oxygen difference (A-Vo$_2$ difference)—the ability to withstand higher levels of lactic acid accumulation, increased concentrations of oxidative enzymes, increased numbers of mitochondria, increased muscle capillary density, and increased lean body mass. There is also a decrease in fat body mass.

These changes often account for most of the effects of exercise because they occur within the first 3 to 6 months of training.

■ Summary

The general state of fitness of most adults in the United States is perhaps fair at best. After an injury, bed rest, and prolonged inactivity, this condition may be significantly worsened. This chapter has reviewed (1) the causes of loss of fitness (in particular, bed rest); (2) methods for evaluating the condition of the individual through musculoskeletal screening and exercise stress testing; (3) the characteristics of a unique method for producing an individualized exercise prescription; and (4) the effects that exercise training should have on an individual's general state of fitness. Clinically, physical therapists should try to incorporate some form of exercise training into most of their patient care programs. This is especially important for individuals who are returning to vigorous recreational or athletic activities and for therapists who wish to complete the rehabilitation process.

■ References

1. Convertino VA: Exercise and adaptation to microgravity. pp. 815–843. In Fregley MJ, Blatteis CM (eds): Handbook of Physiology: Adaptation to the Environment, Section 4: Part 3: The Gravitational Environment. Oxford University Press, New York, 1995
2. Greenleaf JE, Kozolowski S: Physiological consequences of reduced activity during bed rest. Exerc Sport Sci Rev 10: 84, 1982
3. Downey JA, Myers SJ, Erwin GG, et al: The Physiological Basis of Rehabilitation Medicine. 2nd Ed. pp. 448–454. Butterworth-Heinemann, Boston, 1994
4. Winslow EH: Cardiovascular consequences of bed rest. Rev Cardiol 14:236, 1985
5. Saltin B, Blomquist CG, Mitchell JH, et al: Response to exercise after bed rest and after training. Circulation 38(Suppl 5):1, 1968
6. Brody LT: Mobility impairment. pp. 87–111. In Hall CM, Brody LT (eds): Therapeutic Exercise. Lippincott Williams & Wilkins, New York, 1998
7. Beckett WS, Vroman DN, Thompson-Gorman S, et al: Effect of prolonged bed rest on lung volume in normal individuals. J Appl Physiol 61:919, 1986
8. DeBusk RF, Convertino VA, Hung J, et al: Exercise conditioning in middle-aged men after 10 days of bed rest. Circulation 68:245, 1983
9. American College of Sports Medicine: Guidelines for Graded Exercise Testing and Exercise Prescription. 4th Ed. Lea & Febiger, Philadelphia, 1997
10. Astrand R: Textbook of Work Physiology. 4th Ed. McGraw-Hill, New York, 1993
11. Ellestad MH: Stress Testing: Principles and Practices. 3rd Ed. Williams & Wilkins, Baltimore, 1986
12. Bruce RA: Maximal oxygen uptake and normographic assessment of functional aerobic impairment in cardiovascular disease. Am Heart J 85:346, 1973
13. Cahalin LP, Blessey RL, Kummer D, et al: The safety of exercise testing performed independently by physical therapists. J Cardiopulmonary Rehabil 7:269, 1987
14. Fortuin N, Weiss JL: Exercise stress testing. Circulation 56(Suppl 5):699, 1977
15. Foster C, Lembarger K, Thomson N, et al: Functional translation of exercise responses from graded exercise testing to exercise training. Am Heart J 112:1309, 1986
16. Kendall FP, Kendall-McCreary E: Muscle function in relation to posture. In Muscle Testing and Function. 3rd Ed. Williams & Wilkins, Baltimore, 1983
17. Karvonen MJ, Kentola E, Mustola O: The effect of training on heart rate: a longitudinal study. Ann Med Exp Fenn 35: 307, 1957
18. Thomas SG, Cummingham DA, Rechnitzer PA: Determinants of the training response in elderly men. Med Sci Sports Exerc 17:667, 1985
19. Despres JP, Bouchard C, Tremblay A: Effects of aerobic training on fat distribution in male subjects. Med Sci Sports Exerc 17:113, 1985
20. Savage MP, Petratis MM, Thompson WH: Exercise training effects on serum lipids of prepubescent boys and adult men. Med Sci Sports Exerc 18:197, 1986
21. Gossard P, Haskell WL, Taylor BC, et al: Effects of low- and high-intensity home based exercise training on functional capacity in healthy middle-aged men. Am J Cardiol 57:446, 1985
22. Posner JD, Gorman BS, Klein HS: Exercise capacity in the elderly. Am J Cardiol 57:52C, 1986
23. Krisha AM, Boyles C, Cauley JA: A randomized exercise trial in older women: increased activity over two years and the factors associated with compliance. Med Sci Sports Exerc 18:557, 1986
24. Blessey R: The beneficial effects of aerobic exercise for patients with coronary artery disease. In Irwin S, Techlin JS (eds): Cardiopulmonary Physical Therapy. 3rd Ed. CV Mosby, St. Louis, 1995
25. Hagberg JM, Ehsani AA, Holloazy JO: Effect of 12 months of exercise training on stroke volume in patients with coronary artery disease. Circulation 67:1194, 1983

CHAPTER 3

Theory and Practice of Muscle Strengthening in Orthopaedic Physical Therapy

Robbin Wickham and Lynn Snyder-Mackler

Muscle strengthening is a core focus of orthopaedic physical therapy practice. This chapter will address issues of muscle physiology, skeletal muscle force generation, muscle fatigue, tissue healing, immobilization, and physiologic changes in training to provide the theoretical basis for muscle strengthening in training and rehabilitation. Case presentations will be used to illustrate how the science can inform practice.

Muscle Physiology

Contraction of a skeletal muscle cell is the result of a five-step process. An action potential arrives at the sarcolemma, and the intracellular calcium (Ca^{2+}) concentration rises. Ca^{2+} ions bind to troponin, a regulatory protein associated with tropomyosin, causing a change in the orientation of the troponin/tropomysin complex (Fig. 3–1). This change in conformation allows cross-bridges to form between the actin and myosin filaments. Once the stimulus is removed, the Ca^{2+} dissociates from the troponin, actin returns to its resting state, and further cross-bridge formation is disallowed. This five-step process is called the contraction-relaxation cycle.[1] We will now take a closer look at the mechanisms involved in this process.

Contraction of a muscle under voluntary control begins with an impulse generated in the motor cortex of the brain. The impulse is carried from the central nervous system to the muscle via a peripheral nerve that synapses at the sarcolemma of an individual muscle cell. Generation of an action potential changes the permeability of the cell membrane, and sodium and calcium ions from the extracellular fluid flow into the cell. The influx of extracellular Ca^{2+} by itself is insufficient to cause the conformational change in troponin/tropomysin complex. However, the increased intracellular Ca^{2+} concentration

stimulates the sarcoplasmic reticulum (SR) to release its stored Ca^{2+}. Calcium ions from the SR increase the cytosolic concentration of Ca^{2+} to more than 1 μM. At cytosolic Ca^{2+} concentrations greater than 1 μM, the Ca^{2+} binding sites on troponin are fully occupied, increasing the space occupied by this complex.[2] Steric hindrance causes rotation of the tropomyosin and actin filaments, leading to exposure of the cross-bridge binding site, and the cross-bridge on the myosin filament binds to the actin filament. Rotation of the cross-bridge head from a 90 degree angle to a 45 degree angle shortens the sarcomere (Fig. 3–2). Cross-bridge cycling continues until no further action potentials are received.[1] Throughout the action potential, the SR is actively resequestering Ca^{2+}. In the absence of a new action potential, the rate of Ca^{2+} uptake exceeds the rate of release, returning the cytosolic Ca^{2+} concentration to the resting level.[2] Actin resumes its resting conformation with the cross-bridge binding site blocked, and the skeletal muscle cell returns to the relaxed state.

The different types of muscle contraction have different adenosine triphosphate (ATP) requirements. During a concentric contraction, many cross-bridges are formed, dissociated, and reformed at the next available cross-bridge site on the actin filament. Each cycle, cross-bridge binding and dissociation, requires energy input of one ATP. At low loads, the rate of fiber shortening is high and cross-bridge cycling is rapid. ATP expenditure is consequently high. As the load is increased, the rate of muscle shortening decreases, with subsequently decreased ATP hydrolysis because the rate of cross-bridge cycling is decreased. If the load is further increased to the point where the muscle is unable to generate a force sufficient to overcome the load, no shortening occurs and the muscle contracts isometrically. ATP is still needed because the cross-bridges cycle but return to the same binding site during each cycle. An eccentric contraction requires no ATP expenditure because the cross-bridge remains in a

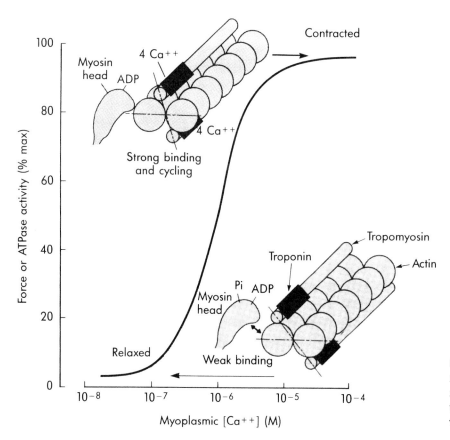

Figure 3–1. Ca^{2+} ions bind to troponin, a regulatory protein associated with tropomyosin, causing a change in the orientation of the actin filament. (From Murphy,[1] with permission.)

high-energy state during dissociation and therefore can bind to the actin filament again without further energy input.[2]

Muscle requires a constant supply of ATP for contraction. ATP promotes dissociation of the actin-myosin cross-bridge (actomyosin complex). Energy from the hydrolysis of ATP activates the dissociated cross-bridge, and another actomyosin complex can be formed. ATP also provides the energy for active resequestering of Ca^{2+} from the cytosol by the SR via the Ca^{2+}-ATPase pump. In the absence of ATP, rigor mortis ensues because the intracellular Ca^{2+} concentration remains elevated and the cross-bridge is held in a fixed position on the actin filament.[1,2]

Although ATP is the energy currency for all mammalian cells, other compounds including reduced nicotinamide adenine dinucleotide (NADH) and flavin adenine dinucleotide ($FADH_2$) serve as energy vouchers that can be converted to ATP under aerobic conditions. At rest, mammalian cells have minimal energy requirements and intracellular ATP concentrations are high. A high ATP concentration inactivates the enzyme pathways of energy production to conserve resources for times of need. At the onset of exercise the muscles use intracellular ATP stores as the initial energy source, but the cell can only store enough ATP for the first 2–3 seconds of exercise.[3] The cells need a way to replenish ATP rapidly if further work is to be performed. One method of replenishing ATP from adenosine diphosphate (ADP) is via the phosphagen (phosphocreatine) system. Phosphocreatine do-

nates a high-energy phosphate group to ADP to regenerate ATP. Direct phosphorylation from phosphocreatine supplies energy for only 10–20 seconds.[4]

Decreased intracellular ATP activates the enzymes involved in glycolysis, the rapid energy production system. With intense exercise the circulatory system is unable to supply sufficient oxygen to meet the needs of the cell. Glycolysis can, however, produce two ATP and two lactate molecules from one glucose molecule under fully anaerobic conditions.[5] Skeletal muscle is unable to use lactate for further energy production, and it is removed via the circulation to the liver. There it is reconverted to glucose or goes to the heart, where it can be used directly in energy production. Anaerobic glycolysis is a very inefficient means of supplying ATP and provides energy for only 1–3 minutes.

Mammalian cells have an alternate system for generating ATP from glucose when oxygen is plentiful. Glucose undergoes glycolysis, with a net production of two ATP, two molecules of pyruvate, and one NADH. Pyruvate enters the tricarboxylic acid (TCA) cycle (also called the Krebs cycle or the citric acid cycle). During the TCA cycle each molecule of pyruvate yields four NADH, one $FADH_2$, and one guanosine triphosphate (GTP) (an energy equivalent of ATP). Thus, one molecule of glucose gives two GTP, eight NADH, and two $FADH_2$ from the TCA cycle.[6] NADH and $FADH_2$ must undergo further processing to be converted to the usable energy currency ATP.

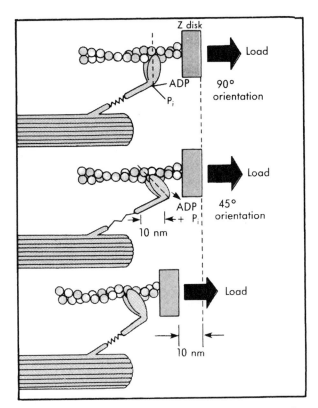

Figure 3–2. Sarcomere shortening as conformation of cross-bridge changes. (From Murphy,[1] with permission.)

NADH and FADH$_2$ transfer two electrons to a series of cytochromes within the mitochondrial inner membrane, which are alternately oxidized and reduced. Oxygen serves as the final electron acceptor in the electron transport or respiratory chain. Electron transfer is accompanied by release of hydrogen ions (H$^+$). The hydrogen ion concentration increases in the mitochondrial matrix, creating a proton gradient. ATP is produced by pumping the protons across the inner membrane when oxygen is present. During oxidative phosphorylation, 2.5 ATP are generated for every NADH molecule, transferring electrons to the respiratory chain, and 1.5 ATP are produced from oxidation of FADH$_2$. Under aerobic conditions, one molecule of glucose will yield 2 ATP, 2 GTP, 22.5 ATP from NADH, and 3 ATP from FADH$_2$, for a total of approximately 30 ATP equivalents.[7] Aerobic oxidation is a much more efficient mechanism for generating energy in a metabolically active cell.

Fats or triglycerides consist of a glycerol backbone and three fatty acid side chains. Triglycerides are a compact energy store yielding 9 kcal/g (compared to 4 kcal/g in carbohydrates). Accumulation of triglycerides in adipose cells functions as energy storage during time of plenty (postprandial). Cells cannot use fats directly to form ATP. The fats must first be hydrolyzed to the constituent parts. Glycerol, after a series of chemical reactions, is converted to pyruvate for use in energy production, as outlined earlier. Fatty acids undergo further degradation via the consecutive removal of two carbon fragments in a process called beta oxidation. Each round of beta oxidation yields one molecule of acetyl coenzyme A (acetyl CoA), NADH, and FADH$_2$. Acetyl CoA enters the critic acid cycle, and NADH and FADH$_2$ are oxidized in the electron transport chain. Naturally occurring fatty acids have an even number of carbons. Sixteen- and 18-carbon chains are most common in biological systems. Palmitic acid, a 16 carbon fatty acid, goes through seven cycles of beta oxidation, yielding eight acetyl CoA, seven NADH, and seven FADH$_2$. Each acetyl CoA yields the equivalent of 10 ATP in the citric acid cycle. Thus, the total ATP yield for the complete oxidation of one molecule of palmitic acid is 108 ATP. Two ATP were put into the system to activate the fatty acid before beta oxidation could occur, so the net ATP yield is 106 (compared to 30 ATP per glucose molecule).[8]

Carbohydrates and fats serve as the primary energy substrates. Ingested protein is used to maintain muscle protein, but it can be used in energy production under extreme starvation conditions. The conversion of protein to ATP is beyond the scope of this book, and the reader is referred to physiology or molecular biology books for further details.

The relative amount of carbohydrate usage compared to fat utilization depends on the intensity and length of exercise. At rest the body uses slightly more fatty acids to fuel metabolic processes than carbohydrates. Substrate use changes as the activity level increases. Dietary intake determines in part which fuels will be used. During light to moderate activity, fats and carbohydrates each generate half of the energy needed by the body. Carbohydrate utilization rises precipitously during exercise about the ventilatory threshold where the Krebs cycle is saturated and glycolysis again plays a primary role in energy generation for exercise. Carbohydrate is the only substrate that can be used in glycolysis. Substrate utilization also depends on the duration of the activity. For the first 20 minutes of activity, carbohydrates supply most of the energy needs. With prolonged moderate-intensity exercise, fat becomes the primary energy source as glucose and glycogen stores are depleted.[4]

■ Skeletal Muscle Force Generation

The force that an individual muscle can generate is modulated over a wide range. (Think of holding an egg versus gripping a baseball bat.) Grading of force can be accomplished by rate coding or recruitment of motor units. Rate coding refers to increasing or decreasing the frequency of motor neuron discharge, thus changing the firing rate of the muscle fibers within the motor unit.[9] The components of a motor unit are the alpha motor neuron and the muscle fibers it innervates. A muscle has thousands of motor units. Within a single motor unit the fiber type is constant. Different motor units within a single muscle have different types of fiber, and the proportion of the three fiber types in the muscle depends on the muscle's function. Individual fibers in a motor unit cannot functions independently. Therefore, an action potential that causes one fiber to fire causes all the fibers within that motor unit to fire (the all-or-none phenomenon).

Skeletal muscle fibers are classified into three groups based on the energy production system, contents of the cytoplasm, structural characteristics, and ability to generate tension. Type I fibers (slow oxidative, SO) rely on aerobic pathways for energy production. Consequently, oxidative enzyme concentrations, mitochondria content, capillary density, and myoglobin concentration are high. Because these cells generate more ATP per oxidized glucose molecule, the amount of intracellular glycogen, the storage form of glucose, is low.[10] As seen in Figure 3–3, type I fibers take longer to reach peak force and the twitch lasts longer. Despite a longer twitch, peak force output is low.[9] Neural impulses to slow fibers are delivered in long trains of low-frequency pulses.[11] High oxidative capacity, low-force output, and low-frequency neural input bestow fatigue resistance on the type I fibers.

Type IIb fibers, fast glycolytic or fast fatigue (FF) fibers, have a large cross-sectional area (CSA) composed primarily of contractile proteins. These fibers rely predominantly on anaerobic glycolysis for energy production. Because oxygen utilization is minimal, the number of mitochondria, capillary density, and myoglobin concentration is low. Glycolytic enzyme levels are high, as are glycogen stores.[10] These fibers are capable of generating large forces quickly (time to peak force is fast, and twitch duration is short), but they fatigue rapidly.[9] Nerves supplying type IIb fibers generate short bursts of high-frequency impulses.[11]

Type IIa fibers use both aerobic and anaerobic energy production systems and are identified as fast oxidative-glycolytic (FOG) or fast, fatigue-resistant (FR) fibers. Type IIa fibers represent an intermediate fiber type; consequently, oxidative and glycolytic enzymes are present in moderate amounts. Myoglobin, mitochondria, and capillary density are also found in moderate amounts. Glycogen stores are high to provide substrate for the less efficient glycolytic system. These FR fibers are capable of generating large forces.[10] The action potential following short, high-frequency bursts of stimulation resembles that of the type IIa fibers.[9,11]

Generally speaking, the FF motor units in a particular muscle generate more force than the FR fibers, which is still greater than the force production of the slow fibers. This does not hold true when one compares force output across different muscles within the same organism.[9]

The proportion of different fiber types in a muscle is determined in part by genetic predisposition, the type of activity performed, and the neural input. Buller et al.[12] demonstrated the influence of neural input on muscle by switching the nerves supplying a slow muscle (the soleus) and a fast muscle (medial gastrocnemius). Upon reinnervation, the fast muscle took on properties of its new innervation and became slower, while the slow muscle became faster. Continuous stimulation has been shown to promote the conversion of fast glycolytic fibers to SO fibers.[13] The ability to convert a fatigable skeletal muscle into a less fatiguable muscle has been exploited as a treatment for heart failure. In dynamic cardiomyoplasty, the latissimus dorsi (a relatively fatigable muscle) is conditioned via electrical stimulation to assume characteristics of cardiac muscle (the ultimate fatigue-resistant muscle) to augment left ventricular ejection.[14,15] Stimulation programs to promote the conversion of SO fibers to fast glycolytic (FF) fibers have not yet been elucidated.

Training techniques also influence the proportion of muscle fibers in a muscle. Training may develop the fibers best suited to perform a certain task while minimizing the development of other fibers. This has the effect of making the percentage of the developed fiber type greater on cross-sectional area while not changing the absolute number of each fiber type.

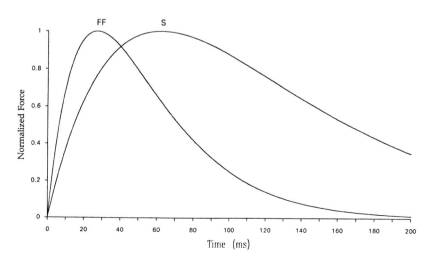

Figure

Figure 3–3. Model twitches of fast fatigable (FF) and slow (S) motor units. (From Clamann,[9] with permission.)

The strength of a motor unit depends on the fiber type, the number of fibers, and the force per unit area (specific tension). Contraction strength is variable, with a twitch contraction being on average only one-fifth as strong as a tetanic contraction. Rate coding, or increasing the frequency of stimulation of a motor unit, accounts for a fivefold increase in force production (average range = 2–15).[9] The muscle responds to the need for greater force by recruiting more motor units. Recruitment order is a function of motor unit size, activation threshold, and maximum force capability. Small, low-threshold motor units with low strength capacity are recruited first.[16, 17] This pattern of recruitment provides incremental increases in force production by the muscle (proportional control). For maximal force output, the largest motor units with high thresholds must be recruited and activated at a high rate.

Muscle Fatigue

Muscle fatigue is defined as the decreased ability to generate force following prior activity. Fatigue can be caused by decreased central nervous system (CNS) drive or by changes in local physiologic parameters. Decreased CNS drive (central activation) is found in neuromuscular diseases[18] and may be a factor in aged muscle,[18, 19] but there is significant controversy about the role that central activation failure (also called reflex inhibition) plays in healthy individuals or those without nervous system disease.[20]

The effect of fatigue on muscle activation acutely (within a series of contractions) and over time (recovery) is important to the development of scientifically based training and rehabilitation regimens because training programs use more than one contraction. While fatigue certainly plays a role in designing the number of repetitions, sets, and rest intervals in strength training programs, in many cases weakness is mischaracterized by patients and therapists as fatigue.[21] In the case of weak muscle, a very small amount of muscle fatigue may result in an inability to complete an activity. Fatigue will be implicated as the cause of the inability to perform the activity, while weakness is the real culprit.

Tissue Healing

Following an injury, regardless of the origin (trauma, bacterial infection, surgery, etc.), the damaged tissue undergoes a typical physiologic response.[22] The first 24–72 hours, the inflammatory stage, are characterized by redness, swelling, warmth, pain, and loss of function. The goal of the inflammatory phase is to "put out the fire," thus preventing injury to the surrounding tissues. The immediate response is arteriolar vasoconstriction to minimize blood loss. Injury to the tissue stimulates release of chemical messengers including prostaglandins, histamine,

thromboxanes, and bradykinin. These chemical messengers cause local vasodilation and increase vascular permeability. Vasodilation decreases the rate of blood flow through the vessel (think of the effect of opening and closing a nozzle on a water hose), allowing blood cells, especially leukocytes, to move toward the vessel wall (margination). Increased permeability results from contraction of the capillary endothelial cells, creating space between adjacent cells. Blood cells and large plasma proteins can leave the vessel through these spaces and collect in the interstitial space, creating an osmotic gradient. Water is attracted to the hyperosmotic area, and edema results. While edema formation is an undesirable outcome, the increased capillary permeability brings leukocytes (neutrophils, monocytes, and lymphocytes) and platelets to the area. Neutrophils are drawn to the injury site by chemotaxis. Monocytes convert to macrophages upon arrival at the injured tissue. Neutrophils and macrophages remove bacteria and cellular debris by phagocytosis. Lymphocytes tag invading bacteria for destruction by the immune system. Platelets deposit a fibrin mesh, forming a blood clot to prevent further bleeding.

The inflammatory process is a vital part of the healing response, so anti-inflammatory medications are contraindicated in the first 24–48 hours following injury. The goals of rehabilitation during the inflammatory phase are to decrease pain caused by irritating chemical agents (histamine, bradykinin, and prostaglandins), decrease swelling, and promote range of motion. Cold modalities are used not only for their analgesic effects, but also to decrease the metabolic rate of the surrounding healthy tissue to minimize hypoxic injury from the reduced blood supply to these tissues.

Repair and regeneration of the injured tissue characterizes the second phase of tissue healing. Tissue repair depends on resolution of inflammation, elimination of dead tissue, restoration of the blood supply, and formation of scar tissue. Certain tissues (epidermis, bone, and ciliated epithelial) can heal with native tissue in a process called tissue regeneration. Scar tissue is formed by fibroblasts that deposit a collagen and ground substance connective matrix. Decreased oxygen and elevated metabolic activity in the injured area stimulate the formation of capillary buds from healthy vessels in nearby tissues. The new capillaries interconnect to form a capillary bed supplying nutrients and removing waste from the healing tissue.

Anti-inflammatory medications are useful during this phase, as a prolonged inflammatory response delays healing. Rehabilitation during the repair phase is focused on restoring range of motion and applying controlled stress to the newly formed tissue to promote alignment of the collagen fibers and minimize adhesions. Because the collagen fibers are weak, it is important not to overstress the tissue and disrupt the fragile collagen scar.

Tissue healing is completed when the scar matures and remodels to its final form. Mature scar tissue is fibrous and inelastic and has no vascular supply. The scar is integrated into the injured tissue and the collagen fibers become thicker, increasing tensile strength, although never to the strength of the original tissue. The goals of rehabilitation during the maturation phase are to increase strength and neuromuscular control, with return to everyday activities and recreational pursuits.

Immobilization

Muscle

Immobilization has a profound and devastating effect on skeletal muscle, with atrophy noted after 1–2 weeks. Numerous experiments have demonstrated decreases in muscle weight[23] and CSA[24–26] following immobilization. Heslinga et al.[27] found an increased rate of atrophy in fast twitch fibers compared to slow twitch fibers. Immobilization in a shortened position has the further consequence of decreasing the number of series sarcomeres, with subsequent loss of muscle length.[28–30] Other structural changes observed following immobilization include a 50 percent decrease in muscle/tendon contact area with degenerative changes at the myotendinous junction,[31] formation of capillary fenestrae,[32] mitochondrial swelling with myofibrillar damage,[33] and deposition of connective tissue within the muscle.[32] Metabolic changes also occur during periods of immobilization. Protein synthesis is reduced secondary to decreased protein translation.[34] Immobilization promotes insulin resistance in muscle, leading to decreased glycogen stores when glucose is not transported into the cell and glycogen synthase enzyme activity is reduced.[35] The number of Na, K-ATPase pumps in the sarcolemma is decreased,[26] serum creatine kinase levels are elevated,[33] the inorganic phosphate/phosphocreatine ratio (Pi/PCr) is elevated,[25] succinate dehydrogenase activity is decreased,[36] and cytoplasm antioxidant enzyme activity is increased in response to the formation of peroxide radicals and superoxides during muscle degeneration.[37] These structural and metabolic changes lead to strength deficits of 50 percent.[25,26] Following immobilization, human subjects were unable to achieve maximum contraction during a burst superimposition test (a short burst of high-intensity electrical stimulation superimposed on a volitional contraction), indicating a central activating deficit.[25]

Bone

Immobilization is associated with reduced bone mass, osteopenia, and osteoporosis, with a subsequent increased risk of fracture when normal mechanical stress is applied to the weakened bone. Absence of stress on the bone leads to decreased osteoblast activity,[38] while osteoclast activity remains constant. Bone mineral loss does not resolve immediately upon return of normal stresses.

Houde et al.[39] reported decreased bone mineralization 5 weeks after remobilization of the hand and wrist following cast immobilization. Bone growth is regulated locally by many factors, including insulin-like growth factor 1 (IFG-1). Decreased expression of IGF-1 or membrane receptor resistance may play a role in the reduction of bone growth. Bikle and colleagues[40] found increased IGF-1 expression during immobilization, implicating a membrane receptor defect as the causative factor in cessation of bone growth.

Connective Tissues

Immobilization adversely affects musculoskeletal tissues other than muscle and bone. Tissues under reduced stress undergo physiologic and structural changes resulting in decreased load-bearing capacity. Collagen content is reduced in ligaments,[41,42] tendons,[42] and menisci[43] because these tissues become catabolic with disuse. The newly forming collagen is deposited in a haphazard pattern with low tensile strength.[44] Changes in the composition of the connective tissue matrix are also observed. Immobilized ligaments have less fibronectin,[41] menisci[45] and articular cartilage[46] show reduced aggregating proteoglycans (aggrecans), and water content is increased. Alterations in the matrix reduce tensile stiffness, with reduction of the capacity to resist deforming forces. Articular cartilage becomes thinner in the absence of normal joint stress.[47] Joint capsule adhesions formed during immobilization cause decreased range of motion (ROM) and joint volume with increased intracapsular pressure.[48]

Physiologic Changes of Training

Endurance Training

Physical activity induces changes in muscle composition, depending on the type of exercise performed. Low-load, high-repetition exercise promotes endurance gains by increasing mitochondrial density in muscle.[49] The advantages of increased mitochondrial density are greater efficiency of energy production, use of fatty acids as an energy substrate, and decreased use of muscle glycogen. Concomitant with the increase in mitochondria per unit area, the activity of enzymes associated with aerobic energy production increases.[50,51] Prolonged low-intensity exercise also stimulates capillary growth so that the oxygen diffusion distance remains low as the muscle enlarges.

The percentage of the different muscle fiber types changes with low-intensity exercise. Fast glycolytic (IIb) fibers decreased during a 12-week training program, while the percentage of type IIa fibers increased. Maximum muscle force, as measured by 1 repetition maximum (RM), was unchanged with training at low loads.[52] This outcome was not unexpected, as low-load exercise does not activate the high-threshold motor units, a requirement for strength gains to be realized.

Strength Training

Skeletal muscle changes are more pronounced with heavy resistance exercise. Within a few weeks of starting a resistance training program, changes in the myosin heavy chain (MHC) isoform (one of three polypeptide chains in the myosin filament) are observed.[53] The MHC isoform has a high degree of correlation with the muscle fiber type. The total quantity of contractile proteins increases, leading to muscle hypertrophy and an increase in the CSA of the muscle fiber. Increased amino acid uptake is stimulated by tension on myofilament.[54] High-intensity resistance training of the thigh musculature led to increases in maximal force output. A significant decrease in type IIb fibers was observed in as little as 2 weeks (four training sessions), with a concomitant decrease in MHC IIb content. Type IIa MHC protein increased at the same time.[55] The shift to a greater percentage of type IIa muscle fibers increases the oxidative capacity. Concomitant increases in capillary density and citrate synthase activity further support an increased oxidative state.[56] The fate of type I fibers during heavy resistance training is not clear. Some studies show increases in type I fibers,[57-59] while others demonstrate no change in the relative percentage of type I fibers.[60-62]

Heavy resistance training activates the high- and low-threshold motor units. Muscle CSA increases of 4.5–19.3 percent are observed in the first few months of training.[62-64] Without question, high-resistance strength training leads to increased muscle CSA. Whether this increase results from muscle hypertrophy, an increase in the radial diameter of fibers within the muscle, or hyperplasia, an increase in the number of fibers, is not fully known. Proponents of the hyperplasia theory point to increased numbers of muscle fibers in body builders[65,66] and the small fiber diameter in the hypertrophied deltoid muscle of wheelchair athletes.[67] A mechanism proposed for the increased fiber number states that a muscle fiber has a predetermined maximum volume and that cell growth exceeding that volume causes the fiber to split into two daughter cells.[68] The majority of the scientific studies, however, do not support the role of hyperplasia in muscle enlargement but rather report an increase in fiber CSA during high-resistance strength training. Kraemer et al.[52] and Pyka et al.[57] found increases in type I and IIa fiber CSA. Other studies showed an increase in type IIa with a decrease in type IIb muscle fibers subsequent to resistance training.[62] Muscle hypertrophy occurs via an increase in the size and number of myofibrils.[69] Actin and myosin content within the cell increases, along with the number of series sarcomeres. The accumulation of contractile proteins is accomplished by an increase in protein synthesis, a decrease in protein degradation, or both.[65,69]

Other physiologic changes result from resistance training. The type IIa fibers show increased oxidative enzyme activity.[70] The enzymes of anaerobic glycolysis, phosphofructokinase, and lactate dehydrogenase are unchanged.[71-73]

Glycogen, phosphocreatine, and ATP stores are not increased as the muscle fibers are able to generate sufficient ATP via oxidative phosphorylation.[72] The capacity to supply the cell with nutrients and oxygen is enhanced by increased capillarity[60] and increased myoglobin concentration. Reports of decreased capillary and myoglobin density[65] can be explained by the dilution effect of greater hypertrophy compared to capillary ingrowth or mitochondrial expression.

Strength Training in the Elderly

Muscle mass and bone mineral density (BMD) decrease with age. Muscle atrophy, or sarcopenia, is greatest in the type II fibers[74] and is associated with a decreased ability to perform activities of daily living including stair climbing, sit-to-stand transfers, and balance deficits. Muscle strength declines 15 percent per decade between 50 and 70 years of age and 30 percent per decade thereafter.[75,76] In the early 1980s, it was felt that elderly persons could not make strength gains based on the outcome of a study by Aniansson et al.[77] in which low-intensity training led to very modest strength gains. Recently, high-intensity resistance programs (three sets of eight repetitions at 80 percent 1 RM in three sessions per week) have been implemented with elderly subjects. Strength gains of 200 percent with increases in type I and type II fibers have been reported.[78] Strength gains have even been observed in the oldest elderly (>87 years) at intensities of 80 percent of 1 RM. More importantly, these strength gains were accompanied by increased walking speed, improved stair climbing, better balance, and an overall increase in movement throughout the day.[79]

Resistance training has the added benefit of reducing the loss of bone density that accompanies aging. Loss of bone density, osteoporosis, leads to significant morbidity in the form of hip fractures. Hip fracture is the number one predictor of inability to return to independent living. Osteogenesis, or new bone growth, results from applying stress to the bone. Resistance training at 80 percent of 1 RM in the elderly leads to increased BMD[80] or at least prevents the loss in BMD that has become a standard part of growing older.[81]

■ Strengthening

Strength refers to the ability of a muscle to generate force and depends on muscle CSA, length, fiber type distribution, and velocity of movement.[82] As described earlier, muscle CSA reflects the myofibril content of the muscle. Larger muscles have more myofibrils and are therefore able to generate more force. The length of the muscle fiber also influences force development according to Starling's law. Simply stated, muscle has an optimum length at which it is capable of generating the greatest force (length–tension curve). When the muscle is shortened (active insufficiency), myosin filaments collide with the Z disks and actin filaments overlap, preventing further shortening. If the muscle is stretched beyond its optimal length, the myosin-actin overlap is reduced and some of the cross-bridges are unable to bind during cross-bridge cycling. Lengthening beyond the optimal length leads to passive insufficiency. Muscles with a higher percentage of type II fibers are generally able to generate greater force than muscles with high type I content. Finally, during concentric contraction, the muscle is able to generate greater force at lower speeds compared to higher speeds. Previously, isokinetic testing within the first 12 weeks following ACL reconstruction using a patellar tendon graft was conducted at a rate of 180–300 degrees per second to decrease the tensile forces on the patellar tendon and patella. During eccentric contractions, the opposite holds true and the muscle is able to generate greater force at high speeds.

DeLorme[83] introduced strength training with weights in the early 1940s. He demonstrated that strength gains could be maximized with low-repetition, high-resistance programs. Further work showed that maximum strength gains occur when a load with resistance greater than 66 percent of 1 RM is lifted 10 times.[84,85] For continued strength gains, the load must be progressively increased. Failure to increase the resistance progressively results in less muscle activation, as fewer motor units are recruited to lift the unchanging load. Presently, weight lifting is a component of the training program of all athletes. Sports-specific resistance training increases strength, power, and endurance, enhancing the athlete's performance.

At different times of the year the goals of a strength training program change, reflecting the different training seasons (preseason, in-season, postseason, off-season). Strength and conditioning specialists are experts in developing periodized strength training programs to accomplish the goals of each season. While a complete discourse on the methods of periodized program design is beyond the scope of this book, it is helpful for the rehabilitation specialist to understand the basic tenets of periodization. A periodized program has three cycles. The macrocycle lasts throughout the entire training period (usually a year for a competitive athlete). The macrocycle is divided into blocks of time, mesocycles, each with specific goals and objectives. For a competitive athlete, mesocycles usually correspond to the preseason, in-season, postseason, and off-season periods. The daily workouts for 1 to 2 weeks make up the microcycle.[86] Several variables can be manipulated to facilitate goal achievement including exercises, order, volume, intensity, and rest between sets and exercises. The exercises are chosen to mimic the movement patterns of the sport. The order of exercise progresses from lifts or drills involving large muscle groups or multiple joints to lifts specific for the small muscle groups. The volume (sets and repetitions) can be changed to create heavy and light lifting days. Intensity, or the RM used

during lifts, depends on the goals. To increase strength, the weight chosen is usually less than 6 RM, while 20 RM may be used to increase endurance. Rest between sets and exercise is also manipulated to vary the intensity of the total workout.[87]

Periodization applies equally to the injured patient. A program for ACL reconstruction is described to demonstrate the use of a periodized program. The astute reader will note the resemblance of the periodized program to a criterion-based rehabilitation program previously described by Manal and Snyder-Mackler.[88] The macrocycle encompasses the time from injury until return to play. Mesocycles may include the preoperative phase, the early postoperative phase (days 1–7), the mid-postoperative phase (weeks 2–4), the late postoperative phase (weeks 5–12), and the return to activity phase (weeks 13–26) (Table 3–1).

■ Electrical Stimulation for Strengthening

Neuromuscular electrical stimulation (NMES) can also be used to increase muscular strength.[89] Electrically elicited muscular contraction, when used properly, can be more effective than volitional exercise during periods of decreased volitional control or reduced willingness to recruit the desired musculature. Evidence for effectiveness is strong.[89,90] There is a clear dose–response relationship between electrically elicited force and strengthening. Guidelines suggest a current intensity sufficient to elicit 50 percent of the volitional isometric force of the targeted musculature is the minimum dose for strength gains to be realized.[91] The intensity of stimulation needed to produce the necessary force of contraction can be uncomfortable for the patient, and the therapist must be willing and able to carry out the treatment at therapeutic intensities. The therapist must also have a method to measure the force output (dose) in order to determine if therapeutic levels are being reached.

■ Neural Adaptation

Early strength gains observed during resistance training programs cannot be explained by muscle changes, as contractile protein content and muscle CSA are unchanged. Increased strength in the absence of muscle hypertrophy is attributed to neural adaptation with training. As previously noted, force output is increased by recruiting more motor units or by increasing the rate of firing of the active motor units. Strength gains can also be achieved by coordinating firing of the synergists to the prime mover or inhibiting antagonist contraction.

Electromyography (EMG) is used to study the rate of action potentials and force output. The area under the curve, the integrated EMG (I-EMG), indicates the total

□□□□□ □ □ □

Table 3–1. Periodized ACL Program

	Goals	Microcycle (Sample Treatment)
	Full knee extension	Quad sets, straight leg raise (3 ×3 10)
Mesocycle	Quadriceps activation	NMES ×3 10 min
Preoperative	Decrease effusion	Ice, elevation, compression ×3 10 min
	ROM 0–90 degrees	Wall slides ×3 5 min
Early postoperative (days 1–7)	Quadriceps contraction	Patellar mobilizations—superior, inferior, and diagonals ×3 5 min
	Ambulating without crutches	Gait training—knee extension at heel strike
	Flexion within 10 degrees[a]	Cycling ×3 10 min
		Tibiofemoral mobilization with rotation (grade III/IV)
Mid-postoperative (weeks 2–4)	Full knee extension[a]	Prone hangs (with weights) ×3 10 min
		Superior patella glide ×3 5 min
	Quadriceps strength >.50%	Isokinetic intervals at 180 degrees per second, 360 degrees per second (2 ×3 10)
		NMES ×3 10 min
		Wall squats (3 ×3 10)
	Stairs—foot over foot	Step-ups and step-downs with a 6- to 8-inch block (3 ×3 10)
	Full ROM[a]	Prone quad stretch (5 ×3 45 sec)
Late postoperative (weeks 5–12)	Quadriceps strength >.80%	Standing terminal knee extensions (3 ×3 10)
		Leg press (3 ×3 10)
		Single leg cycling ×3 10 min
		Squats (3 ×3 10)
	Coordinate muscle firing	Perturbation training (3 ×3 1 min each exercise)
	Normal gait	Treadmill ×3 10 min
	Quadriceps strength >.95%	Increase intensity of exercises (3 ×3 20)
	Hop test >.85%	Agility drills ×3 10 min
Return to activity (weeks 13–26)		Treadmill running ×3 10 min
		Sport-specific perturbation training ×3 15 min

[a]Comparable to that of the uninvolved limb.

force output during a contraction. Surface EMG studies on the prime movers demonstrate the correlation between increases in strength and increases in the I-EMG[92]; thus, strength training improves activation of the prime mover by recruiting more motor units and increasing the firing rate. Furthermore, training one limb leads to increased strength in the contralateral limb, indicating a crossover effect in central processing.[93]

Synchronicity of muscle firing can also be evaluated using EMG. Strength training promotes synchronized firing of motor units during short, maximal contractions.[94] The role that synchronized firing plays in strength gains is unclear because asynchronous motor unit firing leads to greater force output during submaximal contraction.[95]

Prime mover activation can be easily studied by surface EMG. Changes in firing rate or motor unit recruitment in synergist muscles are more difficult to measure, but strength gains certainly suggest greater activation of synergist muscles. Increased activation with training im-

plies an inability to activate the muscle maximally in untrained persons. Sale[95] reviewed motor unit activation studies and concluded that untrained subjects were able to activate the muscles tested maximally. He postulated that the complex multijoint movements involved in weight lifting may result in central activation inhibition not observed in simple, single joint test motions.

Co-contraction of antagonist muscles is apparent during the initial performance of any task. (Remember the first time you tried to ice skate.) Antagonist co-contraction limits motor unit activation in agonist muscles. Antagonist inhibition as a result of training would be represented as increased prime mover strength.

Motor learning, or the integration of movement patterns in the motor cortex, also plays a role in the strength gains observed early in training. Research has shown that strength gains achieved through one type of muscle contraction have little carryover to other ranges. Multiangle isometrics are therefore used to strengthen muscles surrounding a painful joint. Dynamic muscle contractions exhibit a similar specificity for training. Higbie et al.[96] found that subjects trained with eccentric isokinetic exercise were stronger on eccentric testing, while those trained concentrically had greater strength on concentric testing.

Central and periperal neural adaptation, while not technically strengthening the muscle, is inextricably linked to strengthening paradigms and programs. The therapist needs to exploit neural adaptation for therapeutic benefit.

CASE STUDIES

CASE STUDY 1

A 19-year-old collegiate athlete originally dislocated her shoulder playing lacrosse in May. She underwent arthroscopic Bankart repair and rehabilitation. She was deemed adequately rehabilitated to return to playing field hockey in September because her shoulder would not be put in a compromised position by the demands of the sport. At the completion of her field hockey season in November, she asked to participate in two weekend lacrosse tournaments. Her surgeon was concerned about whether her shoulder was strong enough to withstand the rigors of lacrosse and referred her to a physical therapist for consultation.

Physical examination revealed excellent active and passive ROM, with no pain on any active or resisted motions. Strength and proprioceptive testing also revealed no abnormalities in any testing below 90 degrees of flexion or abduction. Above 90 degrees, however, there were significant strength and control deficits. Based on the evaluation, the athlete was not cleared to participate in the lacrosse tournaments. Instead, rehabilitation was reinstituted to prepare her for the upcoming lacrosse season in February.

This case illustrates the principles of motor learning, neural adaptation, and specificity of exercise. Rehabilitation focused on exercises that were progressively more challenging in elevated ROM. Abduction and posterior rotator cuff strengthening exercises were instituted above 90 degrees, with the shoulder moving into external rotation. A manually resisted D2 flexion (proprioceptive neuromuscular facilitatio [PNF]) pattern was used, beginning at 90 degrees of flexion and moving to full flexion. Rhythmic stabilization exercise was begun in the supine position and progressed to the sitting position, again in elevated ROM. Plyometric external rotation was begun in the supine position and progressed to the sitting position, and finally to standing. A weight-training program modified for her stabilization surgery was instituted,[97] and within 1 month, functional progression of lacrosse activities (throwing, catching, and cradling) was instituted. Return to play in February was uneventful.

CASE STUDY 2

A 24-year-old professional football running back who tore his ACL and medial meniscus in training camp was referred 4 days postinjury and 2 days after ACL reconstruction and medial meniscal repair. The patient was wearing a postoperative knee immobilizing orthosis and was non-weightbearing using axillary crutches. The orthosis and postoperative dressing were removed. His knee looked just as one would expect at this time after injury and surgery. Arthroscopy portals, the meniscal repair incision, the tibial incision, and the patellar tendon graft site incision were all visualized. His knee was swollen and a bit warm, but he had no real pain. He was a bit tentative about moving his knee at first but responded well to encouragement.

The first goal was to restore full extension equal to that on the opposite side in the first week. The patient had approximately 4 cm of hyperextension, as measured by a supine heel-height measurement on his left knee.[98] An electromechanical dynamometer was used in the CPM (continuous passive motion) mode and got his motion easily to 0–95 within 10 minutes. He was taught to perform active wall-slide exercises to maintain this newly acquired ROM. He was then able to bike on a stationary cycle and to maintain 60 RPMs for several minutes.

The patient demonstrated excellent quadriceps control with a small lag that was attributed to his effusion. He began our NMES protocol with his knee flexed to 60 degrees.[88] Two 3 by 5 inch self-adhesive electrodes were placed over the medial quadriceps distally and the proximal quadriceps laterally. A 2500-Hz alternating current with a 50 percent duty cycle at 75 bursts per second was delivered for 10 seconds with a 50-second rest period. His maximum voluntary isometric contraction torque was approximately 75 ft/lb, but electrically elicited forces of nearly 100 ft/lb were elicited by the end of the 10 contractions. Gait training without crutches, with his brace locked in full extension, was performed. He was able to negotiate stairs and walk comfortably on level surfaces before the end of the session. The only other typical postoperative concern in a person operated on acutely with a meniscal repair is scarring. The patient had had several previous surgeries but did not appear to develop a keloid scar. His incision healing was monitored, and scar mobility was addressed after the stitches were removed.

Physical therapy included the interventions begun on the first day. Stair climbing, upper body weight training, and left (uninvolved) leg weight training were begun on the second visit. Running on a mini-trampoline was also begun on visit two. He began squatting with free weights equal to his body weight at his first bilateral weight training exercise on week 4. The patient was seen for 10 visits over 4 weeks, and his care was transferred to the team's training staff when they returned from training camp. The patient had full extension and nearly full flexion. His quadriceps weakness was minimal, with only a 20 percent strength deficit, and therefore NMES was discontinued. His incisions were well healed. He had some graft-site pain that was resolving. He returned to play the following spring.

Summary

Strength training is essential for countering the muscle weakness that occurs with injury, disuse, and aging. Morphologic and physiologic characteristics of muscle can provide information that can be used to design more effective training regimens, especially for patients with muscle weakness. This chapter has endeavored to provide a systematic assessment of the physiologic response of muscle to repetitive contraction under conditions that occur during exercise (rest, fatigue, and recovery) in vivo and to examine its relationship to existing and proposed strength training programs for rehabilitation and training.

References

1. Murphy RA: Contractile mechanisms of muscle cells. p. 269. In Berne RM, Levy MN (eds): Physiology. 4th Ed. CV Mosby, St. Louis, 1998

2. Murphy RA: Skeletal muscle physiology. p. 282. In Berne RM, Levy MN (eds): Physiology. 4th Ed. CV Mosby, St. Louis, 1998

3. McArdle WD, Katch FI, Katch VL: Energy transfer in the body. p. 32. In Essentials of Exercise Physiology. Lea & Febiger, Philadelphia, 1994

4. Whitney EN, Rolfes SR: Fitness: physical activity, nutrients, and body adaptations. p. 509. In Understanding Nutrition. 7th Ed. West, Minneapolis, 1995

5. Stryer L: Glycolysis. p. 483. In Biochemistry. 4th Ed. WH Freeman, New York, 1995

6. Stryer L: Citric acid cycle. p. 509. In Biochemistry. 4th Ed. WH Freeman, New York, 1995

7. Stryer L: Oxidative phosphorylation. p. 529. In Biochemistry. 4th Ed. WH Freeman, New York, 1995

8. Stryer L: Fatty acid metabolism. p. 603. In Biochemistry. 4th Ed. WH Freeman, New York, 1995

9. Clamann HP: Motor unit recruitment and the gradation of muscle force. Phys Ther 73:830, 1993

10. Rose SJ, Rothstein JM: Muscle mutability. Part 1: general concepts and adaptation to altered patterns of use. Phys Ther 62:1773, 1982

11. Hennig R, Lomo T: Firing patterns of motor units in normal rats. Nature 314:164, 1985

12. Buller AJ, Eccles JC, Eccles RM: Differentiation of fast and slow muscles in the cat hind limb. J Physiol 150:399, 1960

13. Salmons S, Vrbova G: The influence of activity on some contractile characteristics of mammalian fast and slow muscles. J Physiol (Lond) 201:535, 1969

14. Dimengo JM: Surgical alternatives in the treatment of heart failure. AACN Clin Issues 9:192, 1998

15. Lucas CMHB, Debelaar ML, Vanderveen FH, et al: A new stimulation protocol for cardiac assist using the latissimus dorsi muscle. PACE 16:2012, 1993

16. Zajac Fe, Faden JS: Relationship among recruitment order, axonal conduction velocity, and muscle-unit properties of type-identified motor units in cat plantaris muscle. J Neurophysiol 53:1303, 1985

17. Fleshman JW, Munson JB, Sypert GW, et al: Rheobase, input resistance, and motor-unit type in medial gastrocnemius motoneurons in the cat. J Neurophys 46:1326, 1981

18. Kent-Braun JA, le Blanc R: Quantitation of central activation failure during maximal voluntary contractions in humans. Muscle Nerve 19:861–869, 1996

19. Stevens JE, Binder-Macleod SA, Snyder-Mackler L: Characterization of the human quadriceps muscle in active elders. Arch Phys Med Rehabil (in press).

20. Snyder-Mackler L, De Luca PF, Williams PR, et al: Reflex inhibition of the quadriceps femoris muscle after injury or reconstruction of the anterior cruciate ligament. J Bone Joint Surg 76-A(4):555–560, 1994

21. Binder-Macleod SA, Snyder-Mackler L: Muscle fatigue: Clinical implications for fatigue assessment and neuromuscular electrical stimulation. Phys Ther 73:902–910, 1993

22. Reed BV: Wound healing and the use of thermal agents. p. 3. In Michlovitz SL (ed): Thermal Agents in Rehabilitation. 3rd Ed. FA Davis, Philadelphia, 1996

23. Nicks DK, Beneke WM, Key RM, et al: Muscle fiber size and number following immobilization atrophy. J Anat 163: 1, 1989

24. Veldhuizen JW, Verstappen FTJ, Vroemen JPAM, et al: Functional and morphological adaptations following four weeks of knee immobilization. Int J Sports Med 14:283, 1993

25. Vandenborne K, Elliott MA, Walter GA, et al: Longitudinal study of skeletal muscle adaptations during immobilization and rehabilitation. Muscle Nerve 21:1006, 1998

26. Leivseth G, Clausen T, Everts ME: Effects of reduced joint mobility and training on Na,K-ATPase and Ca-ATPase in skeletal muscle. Muscle Nerve 15:843, 1992

27. Heslinga JW, te-Kronnie G, Huiging PA: Growth and immobilization effects on sarcomeres: a comparison between gastrocnemius and soleus muscles of the adult rat. Eur J Appl Physiol 70:49, 1995

28. Appell HJ: Skeletal muscle atrophy during immobilization. Int J Sports Med 7:1, 1986

29. Heslinga JW, Huijing PA: Effects of short length immobilization of medial gastrocnemius muscle of growing young adult rats. Eur J Morphol 30:257, 1992

30. Williams PE: Use of intermittent stretch in the prevention of serial sarcomere loss in immobilized muscle. Ann Rheum Dis 49:316, 1990

31. Kannus P, Jozoa L, Kvist M, et al: The effect of immobilization on myotendinous junction: an ultrastructural, histochemical and immunohistochemical study. Acta Physiol Scand 144: 387, 1992

32. Oki S, Desaki J, Matsuda J, et al: Capillaries with fenestrae in the rat soleus muscle after experimental limb immobilization. J Electron Microsc Tokyo 44:307, 1995

33. Kauhanen S, Leivo I, Michelsson JE: Early muscle changes after immobilization. An experimental study on muscle damage. Clin Orthop 297:44, 1993

34. Booth FW, Criswell DS: Molecular events underlying skeletal muscle atrophy and the development of effective countermeasures. Int J Sports Med, suppl, 18:S265, 1997

35. Nicholson WF, Watson PA, Booth FW: Glucose uptake and glycogen synthesis in muscles from immobilized limbs. J Appl Physiol 56:431, 1984

36. Haggmark T, Jansson E, Eriksson E: Fiber type area and metabolic potential of the thigh muscle in man after knee surgery and immobilization. Int J Sports Med 2:12, 1981

37. Kondo H, Miura M, Itokawa Y: Antioxidant enzyme systems in skeletal muscle atrophied by immobilization. Pflugers Arch 422:404, 1993

38. Kannus P, Jozsa L, Kvist M, et al: Expression of osteocalcin in the patella of experimentally immobilized and remobilized rats. J Bone Miner Res 11:79, 1996

39. Houde JP, Schulz LA, Morgan WJ, et al: Bone mineral density changes in the forearm after immobilization. Clin Orthop 317:199, 1995

40. Bikle DD, Harris J, Halloran BP, et al: Skeletal unloading induces resistance to insulin-like growth factor I. J Bone Miner Res 9:1789, 1994

41. AbiEzzi SS, Foulk RA, Harwood FL, et al: Decrease in fibronectin occurs coincident with the increased expression of its integrin receptor alpha5beta1 in stress-deprived ligaments. Iowa Orthop J 17:102, 1997

42. Harwood FL, Amiel D: Differential metabolic responses of periarticular ligaments and tendon to joint immobilization. J Appl Physiol 72:1687, 1992

43. Dowdy PA, Miniaci A, Arnoczky SP, et al: The effect of cast immobilization on meniscal healing: an experimental study in the dog. Am J Sports Med 23:721, 1995

44. Padgett LR, Dahners LE: Rigid immobilization alters matrix organization in the injured rat medial collateral ligament. J Orthop Res 10:895, 1992

45. Djurasovic M, Aldridge JW, Grumbles R, et al: Knee joint immobilization decreases aggrecan gene expression in the meniscus. Am J Sports Med 26:460, 1998

46. Palmoski MJ, Perrione E, Brandt KD: Development and reversal of proteoglycan aggregation defect in normal canine knee cartilage after immobilization. Arthritis Rheum 22:508, 1979

47. Jurvelin J, Diviranta I, Tammi M, et al: Softening of canine articular cartilage after immobilization of the knee joint. Clin Orthop 207:246, 1986

48. Schollmeier G, Uhthoff HK, Sarkar K, et al: Effects of immobilization on the capsule of the canine glenohumeral joint. A structural functional study. Clin Orthop 304:37, 1994

49. Holloszy JO, Coyle EF: Adaptations of skeletal muscle to endurance exercise and their metabolic consequences. J Appl Physiol 56:831, 1984

50. Holloszy JO: Biochemical adaptations in muscle. Effects of exercise on mitochondrial oxygen uptake and respiratory enzyme activity in skeletal muscle. J Biol Chem 242:2278, 1967

51. Morgan TE, Cobb LA, Short FA, et al: Effects of long-term exercise on human muscle mitochondria. p. 87. In Pernow B, Saltin B (eds): Muscle Metabolism during Exercise. Plenum, New York, 1971

52. Kraemer WJ, Patton JF, Gordon SE, et al: Compatibility of high-intensity strength and endurance training on hormonal and skeletal muscle adaptations. J Appl Physiol 78:976, 1995

53. Staron RS, Johnson P: Myosin polymorphism and differential expression in adult human skeletal muscle. Comp Biochem Physiol 106B:463, 1993

54. Goldberg A, Etlinger JD, Goldspink DF, et al: Mechanisms of work-induced hypertrophy of skeletal muscle. Med Sci Sports 7:248, 1975

55. Staron RS, Karapondo DL, Kraemer WJ, et al: Skeletal muscle adaptations during the early phase of heavy resistance training in men and women. J Appl Physiol 76:1247, 1994

56. Frontera WR, Meredith CN, O'Reilly KP, et al: Strength training and determinants of VO₂ max in older men. J Appl Physiol 68:329, 1990

57. Pyka G, Lindenberger E, Charette S, et al: Muscle strength and fiber adaptation to a year long resistance training program in elderly men and women. J Gerontol 49:M22, 1994

58. Sipila S, Elorinne M, Alen M, et al: Effects of strength and endurance training on muscle fiber characteristics in elderly women. Clin Physiol 17:459, 1997

59. Taaffe DR, Pruitt L, Phka G, et al: Comparative effects of high- and low-intensity resistance training on thigh muscle strength, fiber area, and tissue composition in elderly women. Clin Physiol 16:381, 1996

60. Hather BM, Tesch PA, Buchanan P, et al: Influence of eccentric actions on skeletal muscle adaptations to resistance training. Acta Physiol Scand 143:177, 1991

61. Adams GR, Hather BM, Baldwin KM, et al: Skeletal muscle myosin heavy chain composition and resistance training. J Appl Physiol 72:911, 1993

62. Hakkinen D, Newton RU, Gordon SC, et al: Changes in muscle morphology, electromyographic activity and force production characteristics during progressive strength training in young and older men. J Gerontol Biol Sci 53:8415, 1998

63. Narici MV, Hoppeler H, Kayser B, et al: Human quadriceps cross-sectional area, torque and neural activation during 6 months strength training. Acta Physiol Scand 157:175, 1996

64. Sipila S, Siromonen H: Effects of strength and endurance training on thigh and leg muscle mass and composition in elderly women. J Appl Physiol 78:334, 1995

65. MacDougall JD, Sale DG, Moroz JR, et al: Mitochondrial volume density in human skeletal muscle following heavy resistance training. Med Sci Sports 11:164, 1979

66. Tesch PA, Larsson L: Muscle hypertrophy in body builders. Eur J Appl Physiol 49:301, 1982

67. Tesch PA, Karlsson J: Muscle fiber type characteristics of m. deltoideus in wheelchair athletes. Comparison with other trained athletes. Am J Phys Med 62:239, 1983

68. Gonyea WJ: Muscle fiber splitting in trained and untrained animals. Exp Sports Sci 8:19, 1980

69. Gordon EE, Kowalski K, Fritts W: Changes in rat muscle fiber with forceful exercise. Arch Phys Med Rehabil 48:577, 1967

70. Ploutz LL, Tesch PA, Biro RL, et al: Effects of resistance training on muscle use during exercise. J Appl Physiol 76:1675, 1994

71. Tesch PA, Komi PV, Hakkinen K: Enzymatic adaptations consequent to long-term strength training. Int J Sports Med, suppl, 8:66, 1987

72. Tesch PA, Thorsson A, Colliander EB: Effects of eccentric and concentric resistance training on skeletal muscle substrates, enzyme activities and capillary supply. Acta Physiol Scand 140:575, 1990

73. Houston ME, Froese EA, Valeriote SP, et al: Muscle performance, morphology and metabolic capacity during strength training and detraining: a one leg model. Eur J Appl Physiol 51:25, 1983

74. Larsson LG, Grimby G, Karlsson J: Muscle strength and speed of movement in relation to age and muscle morphology. J Appl Physiol 46:451, 1979

75. Danneskoild-Damsoe B, Kofod V, Munter J, et al: Muscle strength and functional capacity in 77–81 year old men and women. Eur J Appl Physiol 52:123, 1984

76. Larsson L: Histochemical characteristics of human skeletal muscle during aging. Acta Physiol Scand 117:469, 1983

77. Aniansson A, Grimby G, Hedberg M, et al: Muscle morphology, enzyme activity and muscle strength in elderly men and women. Clin Physiol 1:87, 1981

78. Frontera WR, Meredith CN, O'Reilly KP, et al: Strength conditioning in older men: skeletal muscle hypertrophy and improved function. J Appl Physiol 64:1038, 1988

79. Fiatarone MA, O'Neill EF, Ryan ND, et al: Exercise training and nutritional supplementation for physical frailty in very elderly people. N Engl J Med 330:1769, 1994

80. Nelson ME, Fiatarone MA, Morganti CM, et al: Effects of high-intensity strength training on multiple risk factors for osteoporotic fractures. JAMA 272:1909, 1994

81. Ryan AS, Treuth MS, Hunter GR, et al: Resistive training maintains bone mineral density in postmenopausal women. Calcif Tissue Int 62:295, 1998

82. Jones DA: Strength of skeletal muscle and the effects of training. Br Med Bull 48:592, 1992

83. DeLorme TL: Restoration of muscle power by heavy-resistance exercises. J Bone Joint Surg 27:645, 1945

84. Costill DL, Coyle EF, Fink WF, et al: Adaptations in skeletal muscle following strength training. J Appl Physiol 46:96, 1979

85. Moritani T, deVries HA: Potential for gross muscle hypertrophy in older men. J Gerontol 35:672, 1980

86. Stone MH: Muscle conditioning and muscle injuries. Med Sci Sports Exerc 22(4):457–462, 1990

87. Kraemer WJ, Duncan ND, Volek JS: Resistance training and elite athletes adaptations and program considerations. J Orthop Sports Phys Ther 28:110, 1998

88. Manal TJ, Snyder-Mackler L: Practice guidelines for anterior cruciate ligament rehabilitation: a criterion-based rehabilitation progression. Oper Tech Orthop 6:190, 1996

89. Snyder-Macker L, Delitto A, Bailey S, et al: Quadriceps femoris muscle strength and functional recovery after anterior cruciate ligament reconstruction: a prospective randomized clinical trial of electrical stimulation. J Bone Joint Surg 77-A:1166–1173, 1995

90. Snyder-Mackler L, Ladin Z, Schepsis AA, et al: Electrical stimulation of thigh muscles after reconstruction of the anterior cruciate ligament. J Bone Joint Surg 73-A:1025–1036, 1991

91. Snyder-Macker L, Delitto A, Stralka SW, et al: Use of electrical stimulation to enhance recovery of quadriceps femoris muscle force production in patients following anterior cruciate ligament reconstruction. Phys Ther 74:901–907, 1994

92. Hakkinen D, Komi PV: Training-induced changes in neuromuscular performance under voluntary and reflex conditions. Eur J Appl Physiol 55:147, 1986

93. Moritani T, deVries HA: Neural factors vs. hypertrophy in time course of muscle strength gains. Am J Phys Med Rehabil 58:115, 1979

94. Milner-Brown HS, Stein RB, Lee RG: Synchronization of human motor units: possible roles of exercise and supraspinal reflexes. Electroencephalogr Clin Neurophysiol 38:245, 1975

95. Sale DG: Neural adaptation to resistance training. Med Sci Sports Exerc, suppl, 20:S135, 1988

96. Higbie EJ, Cureton KJ, Warren GL, et al: Effects of concentric and eccentric training on muscle strength, cross-sectional area, and neural activation. J Appl Physiol 81:2173, 1996

97. Fees M, Decker T, Snyder-Mackler L, et al: Upper extremity weight-training modifications for the injured athlete. Am J Sports Med 26:732–742, 1998

98. Axe MJ, Linsay K, Snyder-Mackler L: The relationship between knee hyperextension and articular pathology in the anterior cruciate ligament deficient knee. J Sports Rehabil 5:120–126, 1996

CHAPTER 4
Upper Quarter Evaluation: Structural Relationships and Interdependence

Bruce Greenfield

As physical therapists, we are concerned about the process of disablement, or the consequences of disease on the musculoskeletal system. The consequences of disease can lead to impairments and functional limitations. Impairments are the discrete losses or alterations in anatomy, structure, and action in body parts.[1] Examples of impairments include loss of range of motion and muscle strength, abnormal posture, muscle spasms, and pain. Impairments may lead to functional limitations or restriction of the ability to perform a physical action, activity, or task in an efficient or expected manner.

Impairments of the motor system often result in secondary joint and soft tissue changes. The main areas of dysfunction—the cervical spine, the shoulder complex, the thoracic outlet, and the craniomandibular complex—may be involved simultaneously, especially in chronic conditions. Muscle imbalances and postural abnormalities may predispose to or perpetuate a particular musculoskeletal lesion.

The myriad changes related to musculoskeletal impairments often confuse clinicians and hamper treatment. The discussion in this chapter of the interrelationships of structure and function in the upper quarter is designed to end this confusion. Elements of an upper quarter screening evaluation are reviewed as a systematic method of evaluating all structures that could contribute to or be the sole cause of the patient's chief complaint. Two case studies illustrates the use of the upper quarter screening evaluation in a patient who presents with shoulder pain and dysfunction.

Structural Interrelationships in the Upper Quarter

The upper quarter includes the occiput, the cervical and upper thoracic spine, the shoulder girdle, the upper ex-

tremities, associated soft tissues, and related nerves and blood vessels. The relationships among these structures are such that changes in the position and function of one structure may influence the position and function of another. A cursory review of functional anatomy will help clarify these relationships.

Functional Anatomy

The shoulder girdle, which consists of the clavicle, humerus, and scapula, is largely suspended by muscles to allow mobility. The only direct connection of the shoulder girdle to the axial skeleton is through the clavicle. The clavicle articulates at its medial and more movable end with the sternum, and at its lateral end, through a slightly movable sliding joint, with the scapula.[2]

The clavicle is important as a brace that keeps the shoulder joint positioned far enough laterally to allow movements of the humerus. The movements of the scapula and humerus are dependent on each other. Limited excursion of the free limb at the glenohumeral joint under normal circumstances is dependent on movements of the scapula. Forward, upward, and downward movements of the humerus are typically accompanied by a turning of the glenoid cavity in the corresponding direction. The mobility of the scapula, in turn, depends in part on the mobility of its one bony brace, the clavicle.[2]

The occiput, mandible, cervical spine, and shoulder girdle are joined by numerous soft tissue and muscular attachments. The superficial and deep fibers of the cervical fascia join the superior nuchal line of the occipital bone, the mastoid process, and the base of the mandible above to the acromion, clavicle, and manubrium sterni below. Muscles partly responsible for scapular movement, namely, the upper fibers of the trapezius and the levator scapulae, connect the occiput and cervical spine to the superior lateral and superior medial borders of the scapula, respectively. Anteriorly, the sternocleidomastoid muscle attaches from the mastoid process of the cranium to the sternum and clavicle.[3]

The deep muscles in the cervical and thoracic spine can be divided anatomically and functionally into a longer and a shorter group.[4] The muscles of the longer group, which includes the iliocostalis, longissimus, and spinalis muscles, originate and insert across several segments. These muscles function as prime movers for spinal extension, as well as counteract the forces of gravity in the spinal column during upright posture.

The shorter group, which includes the multifidus, rotatores, interspinales, and intertransversarii, arise from and insert more closely into the intervertebral joints. These muscles function during spinal movement by stabilizing and steadying the bony segments.[4,5] According to Basmajian,[5] during movement and standing, the shorter or intrinsic muscles in the back act as dynamic ligaments by adjusting small movements between individual vertebrae. Movements of the vertebral column are performed by the larger muscles with better leverage and mechanical advantage.[5]

The deep suboccipital muscles connecting the axis, atlas, and occipital bones are the rectus capitis posterior minor and major and the obliquus capitis superior and inferior.[4] These muscles have a high innervation ratio, with approximately three to five fibers innervated by one neuron. These muscles, therefore, rapidly alternate tension within milliseconds, allowing for subtle postural adjustments in the head and neck during standing.[4] Joint stiffness or degenerative joint disease that alters suboccipital joint mobility influences suboccipital muscle function. Muscle dysfunction commonly accompanies degenerative joint disease. Jowett and Fiddler[6] demonstrated, in the presence of degenerative spinal disease, histochemical changes in the multifidus muscle resulting in an increase in slow twitch muscle fibers. They concluded that the multifidus, in the presence of spinal segmental instabilities and joint disease, functions less as a dynamic spinal stabilizer than as a postural muscle.[6] One may speculate that degeneration in the craniovertebral joints may alter the phasic capabilities of the suboccipital muscles to a more postural mode. The result may be a loss of the quick muscle reaction necessary for normal upper quarter equilibrium and control.

An important area of soft tissue connections is that between the cranium, mandible, hyoid bone, cervical spine, and shoulder girdle. The cranium and the mandible are joined by the temporalis and masseter muscles. The mandible is joined to the hyoid bone by the suprahyoid muscles including the digastric, stylohyoid, mylohyoid, and geniohyoid. The infrahyoid muscles connect the hyoid bone to the shoulder girdle and indirectly, through soft tissue connections, to the cervical spine.[3] These muscles include the sternohyoid, sternothyroid, thyrohyoid, and omohyoid. Specifically, the hyoid bone is joined to the scapula by the omohyoid muscle and to the sternum and clavicle by the sternohyoid muscle.[3]

Using a model substituting pieces of elastic for muscles, Brodie demonstrated how tension in one group of muscles may result in tension in another group.[7] The mandible, during the normal standing posture, remains balanced with the cranium through tensile forces produced by normal function of the supra- and infrahyoid muscles.[8] The activity of these muscles is related to those of the neck and trunk, as well as to the direction of the gravitational forces acting on the system. Changes in head position in a relaxed subject will alter the position of the mandible at rest. When the head is inclined backward, the mandible moves away from the maxilla into a retruded position.[9] The influence of the cervical spine on the position and function of the mandible is well documented.[10–13] Further discussion of this relationship will be presented later in this chapter and in Chapter 4.

Specialized mechanoreceptors are numerous in the cervical facet joint capsules, as well as in the skin overlying these joints.[14] Afferent impulses for the static and dynamic regulation of body posture arise from the receptor systems in the connective tissue structures and muscles around these joints.[15] Muscle tone is regulated by these and other afferent impulses in upper quarter joint structures including capsules, the synovial membrane, ligaments, and tendons. Activation of these specialized receptors and pain receptors during musculoskeletal dysfunction may alter motor activity in the neck and limb musculature. Subsequent changes in muscle tone about the head, neck, and shoulder girdle result in distortions in posture, movement patterns, and joint mobility.

Summary

The upper quarter functions as a mechanical unit, interconnected by numerous soft tissue links. These links, or articulations, are functionally and reflexly interdependent on one another. The simple act of picking up a pencil involves movement at the head, neck, shoulder, elbow, hand, and fingers. Performance of a precision task requires adequate freedom of motion in the different joints (arthrokinematics), proper muscle control and length, and proper neurophysiologic responses. The relative alignment of body segments influences motor function. Alignment of body segments is a function of postural control. Normal posture is the state of muscular and skeletal balance that protects the supporting structures of the body against injury and deformity and occurs in the presence of normal joint and soft tissue mobility.[16] Maintaining good alignment in the upper quarter, therefore, is necessary for normal function. Good alignment allows for normal joint integrity and muscle balance and promotes normal arthrokinematic movements. Long-term changes in normal postural alignment resulting in muscle imbalances and compromising joint arthrokinematics may result in motor dysfunction and pathology.

■ Posture

When referring to posture, an important distinction should be made between dynamic and static posture. Although, one can argue that all posture to some degree is dynamic, for our purposes dynamic posture refers to positional changes that occur during function, while static posture is the position of a subject during relaxed, standing, sitting, or lying down.

Relaxed, standing posture is defined by Steindler[17] in terms of the relationship of the parts of the body to the line and center of gravity. For example, in the sagittal plane, the ideal erect posture is one in which the line of gravity corresponds with the following points: (1) midpoint of the mastoid process, (2) a point just in front of the shoulder joints, (3) the greater trochanter (or a point just behind it), (4) a point just in front of the center of the knee joint, and (5) a point just in front of the ankle joint (Fig. 4–1).

The maintenance of normal posture is influenced by the forces of weightbearing (e.g., leg length difference, uneven terrain) and several physiologic processes including respiration, deglutition, sight, vestibular balance, and hearing.[18-20] Solow and Tallgren[18] found, during cephalometric postural recording, that subjects looking straight into a mirror held their head and neck approximately 3 degrees higher than did subjects using their own feeling

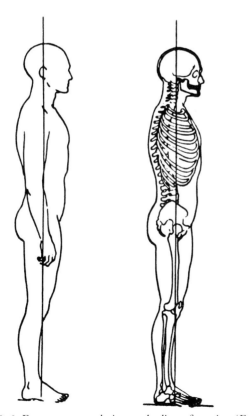

Figure 4–1. Erect posture relative to the line of gravity. (From Basmajian,[5] with permission.)

of natural head balance. Vig et al.[19] demonstrated that experimental nasal obstruction in humans resulted in progressive extension of the head and that removal of the obstruction resulted in a return to the normal baseline head position. Cleall et al.[20] demonstrated that a consistent pattern of head extension and flexion during normal swallowing is altered in subjects with a grade II malocclusion and tongue thrust.

Relaxed, standing posture, therefore, is dynamic, requiring constant neurophysiologic and accommodative adjustments. These normal adjustments maintain balance of equal weight in front of and behind the central gravity line. In more accurate, mechanical terms, the moment of the forces anterior to the central gravity line must equal the moment of forces posterior to that line.[21] Therefore, if more weight of a body part is displaced forward of the central gravity line, there must be an equal shift of another body part backward. Thus, if the pelvis shifts anteriorly, lumbar lordosis and thoracic kyphosis are increased. The cervical spine shifts forward, resulting in decreased midcervical lordosis. Backward bending occurs in the occipitoatlantal joint, so that one is in a position to look straight ahead.[21]

Similarly, body weight in the frontal plane must be equally divided between the two legs, and in the normal posture equal weight is supported by each foot. A considerable margin of lateral shift of the central gravity line is possible, however, because each leg can support all of the body's weight at any time. A lateral shift, in the presence of uneven terrain or a leg length difference, of parts of the body away from the central gravity line results in compensatory shifts somewhere else. For example, if one side of the pelvis drops, a lateral curve is created in the lumbar spine to the opposite side and a compensating convexity to the same side higher up in the spine.[21] These accommodative shifts maintain the upper quarter within the central gravity line, allowing for normal balance and function.

Neurophysiology and Normal Posture

Vestibular sensation results in part from the orientation of the semicircular canals in the head. The head is held so that the horizontal semicircular canals are actually in a horizontal plane. Proprioceptive impulses from nerve endings in ligaments, joint capsules, tendons, and muscles also form a very large part of the input pattern and are most closely related to postural tone.[14,15] Muscle spindles are the specialized receptors involved in tendon reflexes. Postural or antigravity muscles are richly supplied with muscle spindles. When muscles are lengthened—for example, the posterior cervical muscles when the central gravity line in the cervical spine shifts forward—the parallel muscle spindles also are lengthened. This lengthening stimulates the muscle spindles to send afferent impulses to the homonymous alpha motor neurons, which carry excitatory impulses to the related muscles. Afferent impulses may also send inhibitory impulses through inter-neurons to alpha motor neurons of antagonistic muscles, causing reflex inhibition of the anterior cervical or prever-tebral muscles.[15,21] Other afferent fibers from the muscle spindles carry impulse patterns of approximate mus-cle length to the central nervous system, where these patterns are integrated in higher centers with patterns of changing tension and position that have originated in other proprioceptors.[15]

Summary

Posture during weightbearing consists of subtle accom-modative movements to maintain the body segments along the central gravity line. Normal posture, therefore, depends on a variety of factors including normal joint arthrokinematics, muscle balance, and normal neurophys-iologic responses. Muscular contractions, required to maintain normal balance, are controlled and coordinated by the nervous system. Changes in joint range of motion (ROM) or muscle function may interfere with the normal accommodative responses necessary to maintain normal posture. Poor accommodative responses may result, in turn, in long-term postural deviations, pain, muscle im-balances, and pathologic conditions.

■ Interdependence of Function and Structure During Normal Posture

An excellent example of the interdependence of function and structure in the upper quarter is illustrated during shoulder elevation.

Shoulder elevation, or elevation of the humerus, is commonly described with reference to several different body planes: the coronal or frontal plane, the sagittal plane, and the plane of the scapula.[22] The plane of the scapula is approximately 30 to 45 degrees anterior to the frontal plane.[21] Movement of the humerus in this plane allows the muscles surrounding the glenohumeral joint to function in an optimal length–tension relationship.

Elevation of the humerus in the plane of the scapula depends on smooth, synchronous motion involving every component of the shoulder girdle complex. Normal scap-ulohumeral rhythm requires full ROM at each joint and well-coordinated muscle balance. The ratio of humeral to scapular motion is a matter of controversy, but many authors agree that the humerus and scapula move in rhythm so that, for every 15 degrees of elevation of the arm, 10 degrees is provided by elevation at the glenohu-meral joint and a corresponding 5 degrees by rotation of the scapula. Thus, full overhead elevation of the arm (180 degrees) requires 60 degrees of scapular rotation and 120 degrees of glenohumeral elevation.[23]

Movement of the scapula is accompanied by move-ment of the acromioclavicular (AC) and sternoclavicular (SC) joints. Movement of the SC joint is most evident from 0 to 90 degrees of elevation, and that of the AC joint primarily before 30 degrees and beyond 135 degrees. Half of the scapular rotation (30 degrees) is reached by clavicular elevation. The remaining 30 degrees occurs by rotation of the crank-shaped clavicle exerting pull on the coracoid process through the coracoclavicular liga-ments.[23,24]

Elevation of the humerus results from a series of muscular force couples acting at the glenohumeral and scapulothoracic joints. A force couple is formed when two parallel forces of equal magnitude but opposite direc-tion act on a structure, producing rotation.[25]

Rotation at the glenohumeral joint is produced by the upward pull of the deltoid and by the combined inward and downward pull of the rotator cuff muscles. Similarly, scapular rotation results from the upward pull of the upper fibers of the trapezius and the downward pull of the lower fibers of the trapezius. The serratus anterior also helps to rotate and glide the scapula along the thoracic wall.[23]

Elevation of the upper extremities results in motion in the cervical and upper thoracic spine, as well as in the atlantoaxial joint.[26,27] Unilateral elevation of an upper extremity in the plane of the scapula results in rotation of the midcervical spine to the ipsilateral side.[27] Pure rotation does not occur in the midcervical spine but is accompa-nied by side flexion to the ipsilateral side. Contralateral side flexion with ipsilateral rotation occurs at the occipi-toatlantal joint and upper thoracic spine to enable the head to remain in the sagittal plane. This counterrotation occurs only in the axially extended or neutral position. In the presence of a forward head posture, these compen-satory motions are lost and excessive forces are placed on the midcervical spine.[26]

Overhead work requiring bilateral elevation of the upper extremities results in extension of the head and thorax. This "habitual extension" induces flexion of the upper thoracic spine, extension of the midcervical spine, and extension of the atlanto-occipital joint, thus restoring the weight of the skull in the line of gravity.[26] Specifically, during midcervical extension, the superior articular facets slide posteriorly and inferiorly on the inferior facets, as well as tilting posteriorly, thus increasing the anterior interspace of the facet joint.[26] The posterior tilting of the related spinal segment is restrained by the intervertebral disk and its associated longitudinal ligaments and by the osseous impact of the posterior neural arches, as well as the capsule of the facet joints.[26,27]

The forces generated during limb, trunk, and neck movements are also responsible for the repeated piston-like movement of the nerve complex in the interverte-bral foramen of the cervical and upper thoracic spine. Overstretching of the nerve roots, according to Sunder-land,[28] is prevented by the nerves' elastic properties, as well as by their attachment by fibrous slips to gutters in the corresponding transverse processes. Overstretching or friction on the nerve roots often occurs in the presence of postural deviations, such as the forward head posture.

Postural Deviation and Tissue Changes

A musculoskeletal impairment, according to Janda,[29] produces a chain of reflexes that involve the whole motor system. The reflex changes and functional impairment not only may result in clinical manifestations of pain arising from impaired function but also may influence the results of the whole process of motor reeducation.

Changes in muscle function play an important role in the pathogenesis of many painful conditions of the motor system and are an integral part of postural defects. Certain muscles usually respond to dysfunction by tightening or shortening, whereas others react by inhibition, atrophy, and weakness. Muscles that have become tight tend to pull the body segments to which they attach, causing deviations in alignment. The antagonistic muscles may become weak and allow deviation of body parts due to their lack of support. These muscle responses follow typical patterns and have been described by Janda.[29]

The structures of connective tissue, bone, and muscle adapt to alterations in function. When stresses are applied to a bone, the trabeculae within that bone develop and align themselves to adapt to these lines of stress (Wolff's law).[30] Pressure within the physiologic limits of force exerted by the musculature stimulates or enhances osteogenesis.[31] Excessive pressure causes necrosis with delayed osteogenesis. Pressure exerted perpendicular to the axis of a long bone is more likely to cause resorption of bone, whereas pressure acting in the line of the bone axis is more likely to cause osteogenesis.[30] Therefore, postural deviations causing malalignment and asymmetric stresses on bone and cartilage can result in reabsorption and degeneration.

Continued asymmetric stresses on soft tissues can result in degeneration. Salter and Field[32] found in animal models that continuous compression of opposing joint surfaces causes pressure necrosis of articular cartilage. Tabary et al.[33] experimentally shortened soleus muscles in guinea pigs and demonstrated resultant hypoextensibility and a decreased number of sarcomeres. These authors suggested that reduction of the number of sarcomeres in a shortened muscle is an adaptation to faulty posture. The connective tissue response to immobility is well documented.[34,35] Changes in the joint capsule include loss of glycoaminoglycan and water, random deposition of newly synthesized collagen with abnormal cross-linking, and infiltration of joints by fibrofatty material. The results are increased joint stiffness and altered arthrokinematics. Similar changes may occur in joint capsules shortened as a result of long-term postural deviations.

Abnormal Posture and Shoulder Dysfunction

The Guide to Physical Therapy Practice published by the American Physical Therapy Association (APTA) describes preferred practice patterns containing generally accepted elements of patient management that physical therapists provide for patient diagnostic groups.[36] Diagnostic groups are classified by clustering primary impairments together with a patient's functional loss. The Guide to Physical Therapy Practice identifies 11 diagnostic groups for musculoskeletal rehabilitation. Included among these diagnostic groups is impaired posture. Impaired posture includes appendicular postural deficits, cumulative effects of poor habitual posture in addition to poor work-related posture, pregnancy-related postural changes, and scoliosis or other excessive spinal curvatures. Patients with functional limitations secondary to impaired posture present with associated muscle weakness or imbalance, associated pain, structural or functional deviation from normal posture, and suboptimal joint mobility.

The forward head posture typifies a postural impairment reflective of muscle imbalance that may result in pain and suboptimal mobility. For example, the relationship between forward head posture and pain was examined in 88 otherwise healthy subjects by Griegel-Morris et al.[37] Subjects with increased thoracic kyphoses and rounded shoulders had an increased incidence of interscapular pain, and those with a forward head posture had an increased incidence of cervical interscapular and headache pain. Forward head posture is characterized by protracted and medially rotated scapulae, internal rotation at the glenohumeral joints, increased kyphoses of the upper thoracic spine, increased cervical spine lordosis, and craniomandibular backward bending. A second variation of forward head posture is characterized by reversal of the cervical lordoses, or flattening out of the midcervical spine, without craniomandibular backward bending. This type of forward head posture occurs commonly after a cervical injury.[38]

The muscles and other soft tissues of the upper quarter change in response to changes in forward head posture. Excessive compression of the facet joints and posterior surfaces of the vertebral bodies occurs, as well as excessive lengthening, with associated weakness of the anterior vertebral neck flexors and tightness of the neck extensors. Additional changes include shortening of the suboccipital and suprahyoid musculature and lengthening of the infrahyoid muscles with elevation of the hyoid bone. Increased tension in the suprahyoid muscles pulls the mandible posteriorly and inferiorly, increasing the distance between the maxilla and the mandible. The temporalis, masseter, and medial pterygoid muscles must contract against the shortened antagonistic muscles to close the jaw. Excessive tension in the muscles of mastication can result in myofascial strain and painful trigger points.[39]

Stomatognathic problems are discussed further in Chapter 5.

Elevation of the hyoid increases tension on the omohyoid muscle and its attachment to the upper portion of the scapula. With the head moving anteriorly and the posterior aspect of the occiput moving posteriorly and inferiorly, there is shortening of the upper trapezius muscle and of the levator scapulae. Shortening of these muscles results in scapular elevation.[5]

The increased thoracic kyphosis tends to abduct or protract the scapulae and lengthen the rhomboid and lower trapezius muscles while shortening the serratus anterior, latissimus dorsi, subscapularis, and teres major muscles. Also, the increased scapular abduction shortens the pectoralis major and minor muscles, which, by their attachment to the coracoid process of the scapula, tend to pull the scapula over the head of the humerus. The humerus rotates internally, shortening the glenohumeral ligaments and the anterior shoulder capsule.[40]

Muscle tone changes in response to afferent impulses from the joint capsule, resulting in inhibition or facilitation of selected muscles. Several muscle imbalances result because a tight muscle inhibits its antagonist.[29] Weakness of the lower trapezius muscle may result from shortening of the upper trapezius and levator scapulae muscles, whereas inhibition of the rhomboid muscles may occur in response to shortening of the teres major muscle. Increased glenohumeral internal rotation shortens the glenohumeral medial rotators, with lengthening and inhibition of the lateral rotators. These changes in normal muscle length may result in alteration of the normal scapulohumeral rhythm.[29]

Weakness of the supraspinatus, infraspinatus, and teres minor alters the force couple at the glenohumeral joint during elevation of the humerus. The function of these muscles in maintaining the humeral head at the glenoid fossa and resisting the upward pull of the deltoid is lost. Repetitive upward pull of the deltoid during glenohumeral elevation results in abutment of the humeral head and associated soft tissues against an unyielding coracoacromial ligament. Impingement of the rotator cuff tendons may result in inflammation, with subsequent pain and loss of function.[41]

Diminished scapular rotation during elevation of the humerus results from muscle imbalances at the scapulohumeral articulation. Increased strain is placed on the rotator cuff muscles to elevate the arm overhead. The result may be inflammation of the rotator cuff tendons. Overactivity of the rotator cuff muscles to compensate for reduced scapular rotation results in painful trigger points.[42]

Abnormal Posture and the Cervical Spine

Forward head posture produces compensatory motions in the cervical and upper thoracic spine, as well as in the atlantoaxial joint. Unilateral elevation of an upper extremity, as mentioned previously, results in rotation with ipsilateral side bending in the midcervical spine.[26] Compensatory contralateral side flexion with ipsilateral rotation occurs in the upper thoracic spine and in the occipitoatlantal joint to maintain the head and neck in the central gravity line. However, these compensatory motions occur only in the axially extended or neutral position. The forward head posture results in increased flexion in the upper thoracic spine and extension in the upper cervical spine. Compensatory motions, therefore, are lost, and excessive forces are placed on the midcervical spine during unilateral elevation of the upper extremity. Traumatic changes in the intervertebral disk and neural arches may result in transverse intradiskal tears, most commonly seen at the C5-C6 and C6-C7 segments. Degeneration of the intervertebral disk leads to reabsorption and approximation of the related segments.[26,31] Osteophytic spurs may develop in the uncovertebral joints as well as the posterior facet joints. The result during repetitive extension and rotation of the degenerated midcervical spine is friction of the nerve roots by osseofibrous irregularities in the intervertebral foramen or traction on nerve roots fixed in the gutters of the related transverse processes.[26,28]

Pressure or traction on a nerve can result in mechanical irritation of that nerve, producing pain and dysfunction.[28] The initial response of a nerve to mechanical irritation, according to Sunderland,[28] is an increase in the intrafunicular pressure in the nerve, obstructing venous drainage and slowing capillary drainage. Capillary circulation slows and intrafunicular pressure rises. The incarcerated nerve fibers are compressed, and their nutrition is impaired by hypoxia to the point where they become hyperexcitable and begin to discharge spontaneously.[28] Spontaneous firing of selective large, myelinated fibers occurs, resulting in hyperesthesia in the related dermatome. A steady increase in intrafunicular pressure can result in spontaneous firing of γ-efferents, leading to hypertonicity of the segmentally related muscles.

Chronic anoxia damages the capillary endothelium, with leakage of protein through the capillary walls, fibroplasia, and intraneural scarring.[28] In patients with a long history of recurrent sciatica, Lindahl and Rexed[43] observed histologic changes at the L5 and S1 nerve roots, including hyperplasia of the perineurium with infiltration of lymphocytes and degeneration of nerve fibers. Resultant demyelination of selected nerve fibers may increase the sensitivity of segmentally related structures. According to Gunn,[44] deep muscle tenderness may be secondary to denervation sensitivity of nociceptors at the neurovascular hilus. Long-term denervation can result in decreased total collagen in the segmentally related soft tissues and muscles.[43] Muscle atrophy occurs, with progressive destruction of the fiber's contractile element, resulting in decreased fiber diameter and decreased speed of muscle contraction. Changes in collagen content and degenerated muscle fibers can increase the susceptibility of the related tissues to micro- or macrotears, resulting in inflammation and dysfunction. Lee[26] has suggested denervation of the C6 nerve root in the cervical spine as a possible extrinsic cause of lateral epicondylitis. Examination of a musculoskeletal lesion should therefore include the local contractile and noncontractile tissues, as well as the integrity of the related spinal and/or peripheral nerve.

Abnormal Posture and Entrapment Neuropathies

Thoracic Outlet

Compression of the nerves of the brachial plexus and of the great vessels in the region of the thoracic outlet may occur in a variety of ways, some caused in part by poor posture.

The clavicle holds the shoulder up, out, and back, thus producing a short, broad outlet canal. The angle between the anterior and middle scaleni muscles is broad enough to allow passage of the nerve roots of the brachial plexus. The loss of muscle tone and drooping shoulders seen in persons with forward head posture can result in depression of the anterior chest wall. The depression of the sternum pulls the anterior thoracic cage down. This, in turn, pulls the shoulder girdle down, forward, and closer to the chest wall. As a result, the angle between the scaleni muscles is decreased, and the outer end of the clavicle and the shoulder girdle are pulled closer to the lateral chest wall, as well as down and forward. These changes decrease the width and increase the length of the outlet canal, which makes the nerve trunks of the brachial plexus and the subclavian artery more vulnerable to compression or kinking as they pass through the scaleni triangle[45] (Fig. 4–2). Thoracic outlet problems are discussed further in Chapter 6.

Dorsal Scapular Nerve

The dorsal scapular nerve arises from the upper trunk of the brachial plexus and pierces the body of the scalene medius muscle. The scaleni muscles are prime movers of the cervical spine. When the myoligamentous system (i.e., the stabilization mechanism for vertebral function) is inadequate, the prime movers go into compensatory hyperactivity.

Myoligamentous laxity may result from increased tension in the anterior cervical spine with a forward head posture. Hyperactivity and hypertrophy of the scalene muscle may result in entrapment of the dorsal scapular nerve. When the dorsal scapular nerve is compressed at the entrapment point in the scalene medius muscle, the slack necessary to compensate for head and arm motion is prevented.[40] A tense nerve moving against taut muscles can set up the initial mechanical irritation in the nerve.[28] The resultant nerve ischemia, as outlined previously, can result in scapular pain, as well as diffuse pain that radiates down the lateral surface of the arm and forearm.[28,34,43] Soft tissue changes in response to denervation neuropathy may result along the segmental distribution of the nerve.[44]

Suprascapular Nerve

The suprascapular nerve is derived from the upper trunk of the brachial plexus, which is formed from the roots of C5 and C6. The nerve passes through the suprascapular notch at the upper border of the scapula. The notch is roofed over by the transverse scapular ligament. This nerve supplies the supraspinatus muscle, the glenohumeral and acromioclavicular joints, and the infraspinatus muscle.

The forward head posture, resulting in increased scapular abduction and medial rotation, may cause traction in the brachial plexus at the origin of the suprascapular nerve[40-42] (Fig. 4–3). The abducted position increases

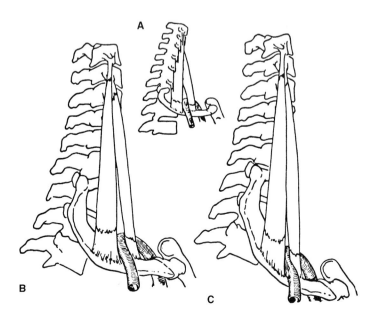

Figure 4–2. The descent of the sternum with maturation and aging. (A) Position at birth; (B) position in an adult man; (C) position in an adult woman. (From Overton,[45] with permission.)

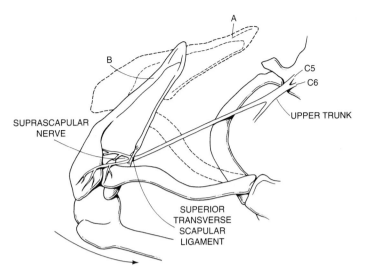

Figure 4–3. The effect of shoulder abduction on the course of the suprascapular nerve. (A) Position of the scapula when the arm is in the anatomic position; (B) position of the scapula when it is abducted across the thoracic wall. (From Thompson and Kopell,[55] with permission.)

the total distance from the origin of the nerve to the suprascapular notch, placing tension on the suprascapular nerve.

Changes in normal scapulohumeral rhythm in such conditions as frozen shoulder may result in suprascapular nerve neuropathy. Limitation of glenohumeral motion in frozen shoulder forces a greater range of scapular motion for a desired degree of shoulder motion. This abnormal excursion of the scapula may induce a neuropathy at the entrapment point of the suprascapular nerve. Pain may be felt in the lateral and posterior aspects of the shoulder, with secondary radiation down the radial nerve axis to the region of the common extensor group.[40]

Summary

Impairment of upper quarter function may result in, and from, postural deviations. The interdependence of the motor system suggests that a functional disturbance produces a chain of reflexes that may involve the whole upper quarter. Therefore, although upper quarter dysfunctions appear locally, the subsequent success of treatment may necessitate evaluation of the motor system as a whole.

■ Upper Quarter Evaluation

Elements of an upper quarter evaluation offer a systematic method of evaluating all structures that could contribute to or be the sole cause of the patient's chief complaint. History taking should precede the physical evaluation. Proper interpretation of each test designed to differentiate tissues and structures is based on our knowledge of anatomy, mechanics, and typical etiologic and pathologic processes, as well as our clinical processes.

History

History-taking procedures for individual joints and joint complexes have been described elsewhere.[45–48] Routine

questions are asked to determine the onset of the problem, the area and nature of the pain, the behavior of pain (what activities increase or decrease the intensity or alter the type of pain), previous treatment, functional losses, and associated health problems.

Common musculoskeletal disorders usually manifest with pain.[46] Because the different lesions that produce pain and impairment about the shoulder and upper extremities may have their origin in the cervical spine, the thoracic outlet, the craniomandibular area, or the arm itself, the clinician must have knowledge of the patterns of pain referral.

Embryology

Many structures are innervated by nerve fibers from more than one spinal segment. Limb buds in the developing embryo comprise a mass of undifferentiated mesenchymal cells. The anterior primary divisions of the spinal nerves invade the developing limb buds to innervate the muscle masses. Because of the intertwining of segmental nerves throughout the regional plexus, and because the muscle masses tend to divide or fuse with one another, a muscle typically receives innervation from more than one segment, and a segmental nerve tends to innervate more than one muscle.[3]

Overlapping of myotomes, dermatomes, and sclerotomes results from a change in the orientation of the developing limb buds from a position in the frontal plane at approximately 90 degrees of abduction, with the palms facing forward, to the fetal position.[3] The growth of the arm bud draws the lower cervical and uppermost thoracic segments out into itself. The scapula and surrounding muscles are derived from the middle and lower cervical segments, whereas the overlying skin and ribs are formed from the thoracic segments. Therefore, pain felt in the upper posterior part of the thorax into the shoulder and upper limb has a cervical or scapular origin, and pain felt in the upper posterior thorax radiating into the upper chest has an upper thoracic origin.[48]

Patterns of Pain Referral

Several authors have investigated the patterns of pain referral.[42,49–52] Robinson[49] found that similar patterns of referred pain in the upper extremity area were reproduced by stimulating different structures in the cervical spine. Robinson exposed the anterior portions of the cervical vertebrae and the adjacent muscles of patients under local anesthesia. The same referred pain was reproduced by plucking with a needle the anulus fibrosus of more than one intervertebral disk. Similarly, identical pain was reproduced by plucking the edge of the longus colli muscle. Feinstein et al.[50] studied patterns of deep somatic pain

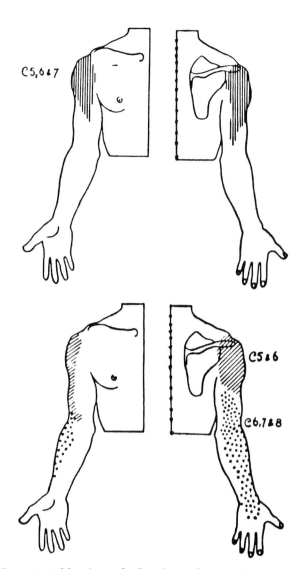

Figure 4–5. Mappings of referred pain from local irritation of the serratus anterior (oblique hatching) and the latissimus dorsi (stippling). (From Kellgren,[51] with permission.)

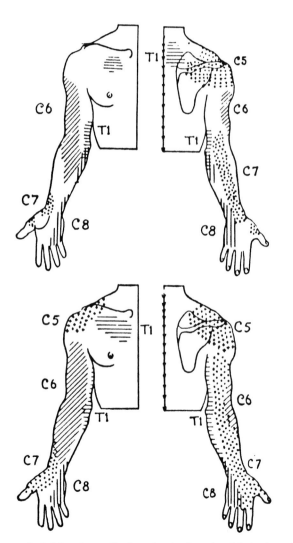

Figure 4–4. Mappings of referred pain from local irritation of the rhomboids (crosses), the flexor carpi radialis (oblique hatching), the abductor pollicis longus (stippling), the third dorsal interosseus (vertical hatching), and the first intercostal space (horizontal hatching). (From Kellgren,[51] with permission.)

referral after paravertebral injections of a 6 percent saline solution from the occiput to the sacrum. Pain distributions were found to approximate a segmental plan, although the pain patterns overlapped considerably and differed in location from the conventional dermatomes.

Studies by Kellgren[51] identified specific reproducible patterns of pain activated when selective connective tissues and muscle structures were irritated (Figs. 4–4 and 4–5). Inman and Saunders[52] demonstrated that pain resulting from the stimulation of joints and other structures deep to the skin had no superficial component. These authors used needles with or without hypertonic saline to produce pains that commonly arise from the deeper structures. Such a pain, Inman and Saunders concluded, unlike that of a cut in the skin, cannot be localized with any precision. The distance of radiation, they found, varied proportionately with the intensity of the stimulus. Activation of trigger points in muscles about the shoulder and neck was shown by Travell and Simons[42] to refer pain consistently to the hand, wrist, and elbow, as well as to produce pain at the site of the lesion.

To summarize, pain arising from the muscles, deep ligaments, and joints of the cervical spine and shoulder girdle area tends to be referred segmentally. Because of the similarity of the type and distribution of pain referred to the upper extremities from different structures, the clinician should consider every case with careful attention to all potential pain-producing structures and tissues.

Upper Quarter Screening Examination

The following screening examination was developed by Personius at the Medical College of Virginia (Fig. 4–6). The goal is to scan quickly the entire upper quarter to

---

Patient _____

Date _____

Observation and Inspection
1. Body build: endo _____ , ecto _____ , meso _____ ; ht _____ ; wt _____
   Unusual features _____
2. Assistive devices _____
3. Skin _____
4. Upper Quarter Functions
   Position _____
   Use _____
5. Posture
   Lateral _____
   Posterior _____
   Anterior _____

Function Tests

1. Cx ROM   active   OP
   FB   ___ M ___ : ___ P _____   ___ P _____
   BB   ___ M ___ : ___ P _____   ___ P _____
   LRot ___ M ___ : ___ P _____   ___ P _____
   RRot ___ M ___ : ___ P _____   ___ P _____
   LSB   ___ M ___ : ___ P _____   ___ P _____
   RSB   ___ M ___ : ___ P _____   ___ P _____
   Comp ___ M ___   ___ P _____
   Trac ___ M ___   ___ P _____

2. Neuro
   Motor
        C1   ___
        C2,3 ___
        C3,4 ___
        C5   R ___ = L ___
        C6   ___   ___
        C7   ___   ___
        C8   ___   ___
        T1   ___   ___

   Sensory
        Dizziness: yes   no
        Tinnitus: yes   no
        Light Touch & Pinprick   R   LT   L   R   PP   L
        C4   ___   -   ___   ___   -   ___
        C5   ___   -   ___   ___   -   ___
        C6   ___   -   ___   ___   -   ___
        C7   ___   -   ___   ___   -   ___
        C8   ___   -   ___   ___   -   ___
        T1   ___   -   ___   ___   -   ___

   Reflex   R   L
        C5,6   ___   ___
        C7   ___   ___

3. Vascular
   Radial Pulse
   Thoracic Outlet

4. Peripheral Joints
   Shoulder
        UE Elevation   ___ M ___ : ___ P _____   (OP) _____
        Locking Position ___ M ___ : ___ P _____
        Quadrant Position ___ M ___ : ___ P _____
   Elbow   (OP)
        Flex RL   ___ M ___ : ___ P _____   ___ P _____
        Ext   ___ M ___ : ___ P _____   ___ P _____
   Forearm
        Sup   ___ M ___ : ___ P _____   ___ P _____
        Pro   ___ M ___ : ___ P _____   ___ P _____
   Wrist
        Flex ___ M ___ : ___ P _____   ___ P _____
        Ext   ___ M ___ : ___ P _____   ___ P _____
        RD   ___ M ___ : ___ P _____   ___ P _____
        UD   ___ M ___ : ___ P _____   ___ P _____

Figure 4–6. Upper quarter screening examination. (Courtesy of Walter J. Personius, Department of Physical Therapy, Medical College of Virginia. From Moran and Saunders,[47] with permission.)

rule out problems and note areas that need more specific testing. The entire examination should require no more than 5 minutes.

The first three steps are self-explanatory. The fourth step requires a brief explanation on how the arm is held and used. For example, a patient with a painful, stiff shoulder tends to hold the arm adducted and internally rotated across the body. Elevation at the glenohumeral joint may be compensated for by increased elevation at the scapula.

Postural evaluation in step 5 requires observations for postural deviation such as a forward head posture. From behind, the therapist should observe the positions of the scapulae for protraction, retraction, elevation, or winging of the medial border, as well as the relative positions of the cervical spine on the thorax and the cranium on the cervical spine. Deviations from the midsagittal spine (scoliosis, rotation, or tilting of the head and neck) should be recorded.

Laterally, the alignment of the upper quarter segments should be compared with the hypothetical plumb mentioned previously. Increased cervical inclination or increased cervical lordosis with backward bending of the cranium on the cervical spine indicates postural deviations and potential dysfunction. Anteriorly, the position of the cervical spine and cranium relative to the midsagittal plane should again be noted. Positional changes at the shoulder (internal or external rotation, elevation, or depression) together or relative to each other are recorded.

In the next step, the function of the cervical spine is examined with respect to the mechanics (degree and quality of motion) and pain (location and severity). After each active motion, overpressure is applied while the pain is located and its severity is assessed. Janda[53] has suggested

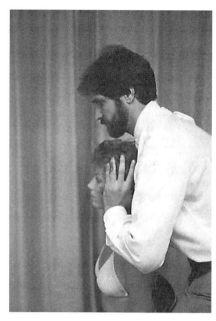

Figure 4–8. Axial distraction as part of the screening evaluation.

that rotation should be tested in ventro- and dorsiflexion, as well as in the vertical position. If the cervical spine is maximally flexed, the segments below C2 and C3 are blocked, and therefore the movement restriction is a sign of dysfunction of the upper cervical segments. Conversely, during maximum dorsiflexion the upper segments are blocked. The limitation of rotation is then a symptom of dysfunction of the segments distal to C2 and C3. Also, axial compression (Fig. 4–7) and axial distraction (Fig. 4–8) are applied manually by the clinician to provoke or change the patient's symptoms. The cervical spine tests are performed to identify or exclude pathology originating in the cervical region.

The neurologic, sensory, and vascular examinations have been described elsewhere.[45–48] The vascular examination includes tests (Adson's, costoclavicular, hyperabduction) to rule out vascular or neural entrapment in the areas of the thoracic inlet.[54]

Each peripheral joint is tested for mechanics and pain during overpressure. The locking position (Fig. 4–9) and the quadrant position (Fig. 4–10) are performed on the shoulder to test for impingement and anterior capsule inflammation and/or laxity, respectively. Reproduction of the patient's symptoms is recorded.

Palpation should be added to the screening evaluation to differentiate and recognize changes in skin, subcutaneous tissue, ligaments, and muscles.[53] Patterns of pain referral should be recorded. Special attention should be paid to the muscles. Spasm, tenderness, hyperirritability, tightness, or hypotonia should be noted. A characteristic and specific chain of muscle changes and imbalances should be assessed. A proposed sequence of palpation in the head and neck is as follows: trapezius and levator scapulae, followed by the scaleni, sternocleidomastoid,

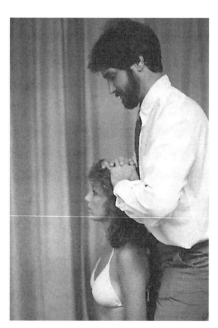

Figure 4–7. Axial compression as part of the screening evaluation.

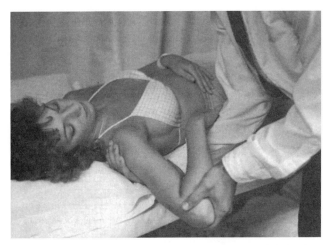

Figure 4–9. Locking maneuver: internal rotation and abduction of the shoulder.

and suprahyoid muscles, followed in turn by the lateral and medial pterygoid, masseter, and temporalis muscles.[53]

In conclusion, the screening examination affords the clinician a quick, precise scan of upper quarter structure and function. A specific test that provokes the patient's symptoms alerts the clinician to the potential site of the musculoskeletal lesion, to be followed by a thorough evaluation of that area.

CASE STUDIES

The following cases provide examples of the manner in which an upper quarter screening examination is integrated into an overall clinical evaluation. It is the author's belief that an upper quarter evaluation will often yield additional information on the impairment contributing to or perpetuating a patient's functional loss, to be included in the overall treatment program.

CASE STUDY 1

This first case illustrates the use of components of upper quarter screening in a patient with shoulder pain and dysfunction. An initial history is followed by a physical therapy evaluation. The upper quarter screening is incorporated in the physical therapy evaluation. An assessment outlines the physical therapy problem list, impairments or treatment goals, and plan. Actual treatments are beyond the purview of this chapter and are not reviewed. The reader is encouraged to review subsequent chapters in this text that examine specific treatment techniques.

History

The patient is a 36-year-old woman who developed gradual right shoulder pain and stiffness. She is right-hand dominant and works as a secretary in a law firm. She reports that her pain started approximately 6 months earlier, after she painted a room in her house. Since that time her shoulder has become progressively more painful and stiff. Her pain is located along the lateral and anterior aspects of her shoulder and radiates along the right cervical spine and right interscapular area. She describes her pain as a diffuse dull ache, which becomes sharp during elevation of her right extremity. Her pain and stiffness are worse in the morning and tend to decrease when she begins to move her arm. However, at the end of her work day, she reports that the pain, particularly along the cervical and interscapular areas, is worse. She has difficulty sleeping on that shoulder at night. She is taking anti-inflammatory medicine. Significant past and current medical histories were unremarkable. She enjoys tennis but is unable to play because of her shoulder problem.

Upper Quarter Screening

Posture: forward head posture with rounded shoulders (protracted and medially rotated scapulae). The right scapula was slightly elevated relative to the left.

Function tests: cervical right rotation slightly limited and painful, with overpressure at the end of the range. However, this test, as well as the cervical compression or distraction tests, did not reproduce the patient's pain.

Passive mobility testing: restricted segmental mobility in the mid- and upper thoracic spine and midcervical spine.

Neurologic, sensory, and reflex tests: negative.

Vascular tests (i.e., thoracic outlet tests): negative.

Shoulder tests: bypassed until later in the evaluation.

Peripheral joints: ROM and overpressure in related peripheral joints did not reproduce the patient's pain.

Palpation: elevated tone with muscle trigger points were palpated in the muscle bellies of the right upper trapezius, rhomboids, and subscapularis muscles. Palpation of the trigger point in the upper trapezius muscle

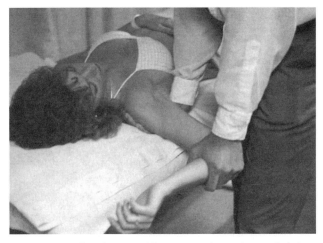

Figure 4–10. Quadrant position: external rotation and abduction of the shoulder.

reproduced the patient's right cervical pain. Palpation of the trigger point in the rhomboid muscles reproduced the interscapular pain. Palpation of the subscapularis trigger point reproduced most of the anterior and lateral shoulder pain.

Active/passive ROM in right shoulder: limited in capsular pattern, with external rotation most limited, followed by abduction in the plane of the scapula, followed by internal rotation. In this case, internal rotation was tested by having the patient reach behind her back and by assessing the spinal level she could touch with her thumb. All movements were painful and stiff concomitantly at the end of the range. Her passive external rotation was most limited with the extremity positioned at neutral abduction, with more external rotation available from 60 to 90 degrees of abduction.

Scapulohumeral rhythm: lateral rotation of the scapula initiated within the initial 30 degrees of humeral elevation.

Accessory testing: limited inferior and anterior glenohumeral joint glides.

Resisted tests: moderately weak but painless for shoulder abduction and external rotation.

Special tests: impingement test negative; quadrant test difficult to perform because of anterior glenohumeral joint tightness.

Palpation: tender anterior glenohumeral capsule.

Assessment

1. Medical diagnosis: adhesive capsulitis.
2. Stage of reactivity: moderate.
3. Physical therapy problem list
   a. Restricted passive/active ROM in right shoulder, both physiologic and accessory movements.
   b. Decreased strength in shoulder abduction and external rotation.
   c. Postural changes (i.e., forward head posture with rounder shoulders perpetuating muscle imbalances about the shoulder). Spinal segmental restrictions perpetuating forward head posture.
   d. Myofascial pain with active trigger points as secondary sources of shoulder pain. The trigger point in the subscapularis reflected chronic tightness and resulted in limited external rotation of the humerus in the neutral position. The elevated tone and trigger point in the right upper trapezius also reflected muscle tightness, and resulted in an elevated scapula and right cervical spine pain and limitation. The trigger point in the rhomboid muscles resulted from stretch weakness caused by the protracted scapula.

Goals of Treatment

1. Restore active/passive ROM to right shoulder.
   Treatments:
   • Stretch subscapularis.

• Mobilize glenohumeral anterior and inferior capsules.
   • Strengthen rotators and force the couple mechanism in both the glenohumeral joint and the scapulothoracic junction.
2. Decrease myofascial pain.
   Treatment: eliminate trigger points in upper trapezius rhomboid, and subscapularis muscles.
3. Improve upper quarter posture.
   Treatment: promote axial extension.
   • Mobilize segmental restrictions in mid- and upper thoracic spine and midcervical spine.
   • Correct muscle imbalances (i.e., stretch tight muscles and strengthen weak antagonists).

Summary

This case represents a typical shoulder dysfunction that is complicated by upper quarter changes. Failure to evaluate the structure and function of the upper quarter thoroughly and systematically in this patient would result in failure to resolve a large component of her pain and dysfunction and would perpetuate her shoulder problem. The upper quarter screening was incorporated into the total physical therapy evaluation, and certain steps in the upper quarter evaluation were omitted or implemented later in the overall evaluation.

CASE STUDY 2

John is a 34-year-old carpenter with a diagnosis of lateral epicondylitis in the right elbow. The problem began 2 weeks ago after the patient began working on a job renovating a house. The patient is right-hand dominant. His pain is described as a dull ache located along the lateral aspect of the elbow. The patient describes the pain as radiating along the lateral aspect, posterior surface of the forearm, and proximal to the middle one-third of the upper arm. The patient reports occasional tingling and numbness in the same area of the pain in his arm and forearm.

The symptoms are worsened with repetitive gripping and with reaching activities.

Upper Quarter Screening

Posture: lateral or sagittal plane alignment of the cervical spine and upper thoracic spine is unremarkable. In the frontal plane (anterior view), the cervical spine is in slight right-side bending and left rotation.

Function tests: cervical spine right rotation and side bending with overpressure reproduces paraesthesia in the right upper extremity. The cervical compression test reproduces paraesthesia in the right upper extremity. Cervical distraction eliminates right upper extremity paraesthesia.

Neurologic exam: manual muscle testing indicates the following:

	Right	Left
Lateral shoulder rotation	5/5	5/5
Abduction of shoulder	5/5	5/5
Elbow flexion	4/5	5/5
Elbow extension	4/5	5/5
Wrist extension	3+/5	5/5
Wrist flexion	4/5	4/5
Forearm supination	4/5	5/5
Forearm pronation	5/5	5/5
Finger abduction	4/5	5/5
Finger adduction	4/5	5/5

Manual muscle testing produces right lateral elbow pain for wrist extension and forearm supination on the right.

	Deep Tendon Reflexes	
	Right	*Left*
Biceps C5	normal	normal
Triceps C6	decreased	normal
Brachioradialis C7	decreased	normal

Sensation: decreased to light touch and pinprick along the posterior aspect of the right proximal arm and forearm to the wrist.

Thoracic outlet tests: positive for right upper extremity pain and paraesthesia with the Adson's and costoclavicular tests. However, no signs and symptoms of vascular compromise were present, including diminished radial pulse.

Palpation: elevated tone and muscle spasms in the right scalene and sternocleidomastoid muscles. Palpation along the cervical spine elicited tenderness along the lower cervical posterolateral facet joints at the C6-C7 and C7-T1 levels.

Peripheral joints: shoulder has full ROM and no pain; the elbow has full motion; passive wrist and finger flexion with forearm pronation reproduces right lateral elbow pain.

Accessory testing: side glide of C6 on C7 and C7 on T1 to the left is painful and limited.

Resisted tests: painful, with resisted wrist extension and forearm supination.

Palpation: tender along the right lateral epicondyle and proximal muscle–tendinous junction of the wrist and finger extensor muscles.

Assessment

1. Medical diagnosis: lateral epicondylitis of the right elbow. The screening evaluation indicates a second-ary problem characterized by a C7 nerve root radiculopathy. The findings that indicate this problem include positive spine provocation tests that reproduce paraesthesia along the C7 dermatome, tenderness at the C6-C7 interspace, and sensory motor and reflex changes consistent primarily with C7 spinal innervation.
2. Stage of reactivity: moderate for both the lateral epicondyle and cervical radiculopathy.
3. Physical therapy problem list
   a. Tender lateral epicondyle.
   b. Pain with passive wrist extension, forearm supination, and finger flexion.
   c. Pain and mild weakness with wrist extension and forearm supination.
   d. Limited and painful cervical spine side bending and rotation to the right.
   e. Tender lower cervical facet joints.
   f. Spasms scalenes and sternocleidomastoid muscles.

Goals of Treatment

1. Eliminate tenderness of the right lateral epicondyle.
   Treatments: anti-inflammatory modalities including iontophoresis, ice massage, pulses or low-intensity, continuous ultrasound, and rest from harmful activities including repetitive gripping activities.
2. Increase passive wrist flexion, forearm supination, and finger flexion.
   Treatment: gradual low load stretch into the ranges identified in (2).
3. Increase pain-free wrist extension and forearm supination strength.
   Treatments: Begin with submaximal isometrics to the forearm supinators and wrist extensors and progress to partial range concentrics and finally full range eccentrics.
4. Reduce signs and symptoms of C7 radiculopathy.
   Treatment: cervical traction.
5. Increase passive and active cervical side bending and rotation.
   Treatment: cervical mobilization using an initial grade of 1 and 2 for the left side glide at C6 through T1. As reactivity decreases, progress to grades 3 and 4.
6. Eliminate muscle spasms in right scalenes and sternocleidomastoid muscles.
   Treatments: heat; continuous ultrasound, soft tissue massage, and stretching.

Summary

This case illustrates a secondary problem that resulted in a considerable number of impairments in addition to those resulting from the lateral epicondylitis. Although a tentative medical diagnosis is given based on the physical therapy evaluation, this was done for continuity to present case findings, not to illustrate this author's general approach to patient care. If this were an actual situation, the author would contact the referring physician to discuss the additional clinical findings of the screening evaluation so that the physician can make the decision concerning an additional medical workup.

■ Summary

The information presented in this chapter underscores the importance of a screening evaluation as part of the overall physical therapy evaluation for musculoskeletal rehabilitation. The interdependent nature of the upper quarter indicates that impairments often occur in clusters, and several tissues and structures may be involved in producing pain and functional loss. The presenting signs and symptoms often are confusing, particularly to the novice practitioner. A systematic approach that briefly but concisely examines all relevant pain-producing tissues will help to clarify potential confusing presentations for effective treatment planning.

■ References

1. Dekker J, van Baar ME, Curfs EC, et al: Diagnosis and treatment in physical therapy: an investigation of their relationship. Phys Ther 73:568, 1993
2. Hollinshead WH: The Back and Limbs. Anatomy for Surgeons. Vol. 3. Harper & Row, New York, 1969
3. Warwick R, Williams P (eds): Gray's Anatomy. 35th British Ed. WB Saunders, Philadelphia, 1973
4. Grieve GP: Common Vertebral Joint Problems. Churchill Livingstone, New York, 1981
5. Basmajian JU: Muscles Alive. 4th Ed. Williams & Wilkins, Baltimore, 1979
6. Jowett RL, Fiddler MW: Histochemical changes in the multifidus in mechanical derangements of the spine. Orthop Clin North Am 6:145, 1975
7. Brodie AG: Anatomy and physiology of head and neck musculature. Am J Orthod 36:831, 1950
8. Rocabado M: Biomechanical relationship of the cranial, cervical and hyoid regions. J Craniomandib Pract 11:3, 1983
9. Mohl NO: Head posture and its role in occlusion. NY State Dent J 42:17, 1976
10. Ayub E, Glasheen-Wray M, Kraus S: Head posture: a study of the effects on the rest position of the mandible. J Orthop Sports Phys Ther 5:179, 1984
11. Gresham H, Smithells PA: Cervical and mandibular posture. Dent Rec 74:261, 1954
12. Darling PW, Kraus S, Glasheen-Wray MB: Relationship of head posture and the rest position of the mandible. J Prosthet Dent 16:848, 1966
13. Goldstein DF, Kraus SL, Williams WB, et al: Influence of the cervical posture on mandibular movement. J Prosthet Dent 52:3, 1984
14. Wyke B: Neurology of the cervical spinal joints. Physiotherapy 85:3, 1979
15. Guyton AC: Organ Physiology: Structure and Function of the Nervous System. 2nd Ed. WB Saunders, Philadelphia, 1976
16. Kendall HO, Kendall FP, Boynton D: Posture and Pain. Robert E. Krieger, Huntington, NY, 1977
17. Steindler A: Kinesiology of the Human Body: Under Normal and Pathological Conditions. 5th Ed. Charles C Thomas, Springfield, IL, 1955
18. Solow B, Tallgren A: Natural head position in standing subjects. Acta Odontol Scand 29:591, 1971
19. Vig PS, Showfety KJ, Phillips C: Experimental manipulation of head posture. Am J Orthod 77:3, 1980
20. Cleall JR, Alexander WJ, McIntyre HM: Head posture and its relationship to deglutition. Angle Orthod 36:335, 1966
21. Bailey HW: Theoretical significance of postural imbalance, especially the "short leg." J Am Osteopath Assoc 77:452, 1978
22. Johnston TB: Movements of the shoulder joint-plea for use of "plane of the scapula" as plane of reference for movements occurring at the humeroscapula joint. Br J Surg 25:252, 1937
23. Calliet R: Shoulder Pain. 2nd Ed. FA Davis, Philadelphia, 1981
24. Poppen N, Walker P: Normal and abnormal motion of the shoulder. J Bone Joint Surg 58(A):195, 1976
25. Frankel VH, Nordin M: Basic Biomechanics of the Skeletal System. Lea & Febiger, Philadelphia, 1980
26. Lee D: Tennis elbow. J Orthop Sports Phys Ther 8:3, 1986
27. Kapandji IA: The Physiology of Joints. 2nd Ed. Vol 3. Churchill Livingstone, London, 1974
28. Sunderland S: Traumatized nerves, roots and ganglia: musculoskeletal factors and neuropathologic consequences. p. 137. In Korr IM (ed): The Neurobiologic Mechanisms in Manipulative Therapy. Plenum, New York, 1978
29. Janda V: Muscles, central nervous motor regulation and back problems. p. 29. In Korr IM (ed): The Neurobiologic Mechanisms in Manipulative Therapy. Plenum, New York, 1978
30. Turek SL: Orthopaedic Principles and Their Application. 3rd Ed. JB Lippincott, Philadelphia, 1977
31. Eggers GWN, Shindler TO, Pomerat CM: Osteogenesis: influence of the contact-compression factor on osteogenesis in surgical fractures. J Bone Joint Surg 31:693, 1949
32. Salter RB, Field P: The effects of continuous compression on living articular cartilage: an experimental investigation. J Bone Joint Surg 42(A):31, 1960
33. Tabary JC, Tardieu C, Tardieu G, et al: Experimental rapid sarcomere loss with concomitant hypoextensibility. Muscle Nerve 4:198, 1981
34. Akeson WH, Amiel D, Mechanis GL, et al: Collagen cross-linking alterations in joint contractures: changes in the reducible cross-links in periarticular connective tissue collagen after nine weeks of immobilization. Connect Tissue Res 5:15, 1977
35. Woo S, Matthews JU, Akeson WH, et al: Connective tissue response to immobility: correlative study of biomechanical and biochemical measurements of normal and immobilized rabbit knees. Arthritis Rheum 18:3, 1975
36. Guide to Physical Therapy Practice. Part One: Description of patient/client management and Part Two: Preferred practice patterns. Phys Ther 77:1163, 1998.
37. Griegel-Morris P, Larson K, Mueller-Klaus K, et al: Incidence of common postural abnormalities in the cervical, shoulder, and thoracic regions and their association with pain in two age groups of healthy subjects. Phys Ther 72:6, 425–430, 1992
38. Manns A, Miralles R, Santander H: Influence of the vertical dimension in the treatment of myofascial pain dysfunction syndrome. J Prosthet Dent 50:700, 1983

39. Mannheimer JS, Anttansio R, Cinotti WR, et al: Cervical strain and mandibular whiplash: effects upon the craniomandibular apparatus. Clin Prev Dent 11:29–32, 1989

40. Kopell HP, Thompson WAL: Peripheral Entrapment Neuropathies. 2nd Ed. Robert E Krieger, New York, 1976

41. Penny JN, Welsh MB: Shoulder impingement syndromes in athletes and their surgical management. Am J Sports Med 9:11, 1981

42. Travell JG, Simons DG: Myofascial Pain and Dysfunction. The Trigger Point Manual. Williams & Wilkins, Baltimore, 1984

43. Lindahl O, Rexed B: Histologic changes in spinal nerve roots of operated cases of sciatica. Acta Orthop Scand 20:215, 1951

44. Gunn CC: Prespondylosis and some pain syndromes following denervation supersensitivity. Spine 5:2, 1980

45. Overton LM: The causes of pain in the upper extremities: a differential diagnosis study. Clin Orthop 51:27, 1967

46. Kessler RM, Hertling D: Management of Common Musculoskeletal Disorders. Harper & Row, Philadelphia, 1983

47. Moran CA, Saunders SA: Evaluation of the shoulder: a sequential approach. p. 17. In Donatelli R (ed): Physical Therapy of the Shoulder. Churchill Livingstone, New York, 1987

48. Cyriax J: Textbook of Orthopaedic Medicine. 7th Ed. Vol 1. Bailliere Tindall, London, 1979

49. Robinson RA: Brachalgia: a panel discussion. Proceedings of the International Congress on Orthopaedics and Trauma, Paris, France, 1966

50. Feinstein B, Langton JNK, Jameson RM, et al: Experiments of pain referred from deep somatic tissues. J Bone Joint Surg 36(A):5, 1954

51. Kellgren J: Observations of referred pain arising from muscle. Clin Sci 3:175, 1938

52. Inman VT, Saunders JB: Referred pain from skeletal structures. J Nerv Ment Dis 99:660, 1944

53. Janda V: Some aspects of extracranial causes of facial pain. J Prosthet Dent 56:4, 1986

54. Ridell DH: Thoracic outlet syndrome: thoracic and vascular aspects. Clin Orthop 51:53, 1967

55. Thompson WAL, Kopell HP: The effect of shoulder abduction on the course of suprascapular nerve. N Engl J Med 260:1261, 1959

CHAPTER 5
Influences of the Cervical Spine on the Stomatognathic System

Steven L. Kraus

Physical therapists see patients who present with a variety of upper quarter symptoms. Treatment for such symptoms may be helped by addressing the dysfunction of the cervical and upper thoracic spine, the shoulder girdle, and/or the upper extremity. During treatment of upper quarter dysfunction, the physical therapist will ask the patient if the treatments offered are affecting the symptoms. The patient's response will depend on the area and degree of dysfunction, the age and overall physical condition of the patient, and the skills of the therapist rendering the treatments.

During the initial evaluation and subsequent treatments, the physical therapist may question the reliability of a patient who complains of certain symptoms that may not be thought of as associated with upper quarter dysfunction. The patient may indicate that these symptoms are being relieved or aggravated as the upper quarter dysfunction is treated. Such seemingly unrelated symptoms cannot always be explained on the basis of referred pains or pathologic involvement. For the therapist trying to determine whether such unrelated symptoms are clinically possible, an understanding of how the cervical spine influences the stomatognathic system may provide some answers.

The suggestion that a specific dysfunction (e.g., of the cervical spine) can cause or contribute to a dysfunction in an adjacent area that results in a specific symptom(s) in the adjacent region (stomatognathic) must be made cautiously. The actual experience and expression of a symptom(s) by an individual involve a very complicated and detailed series of events that is yet to be fully understood. These events involve a variety of excitatory and inhibitory reflexes occurring at the spinal cord, brain stem, thalamus, and cortex of the central nervous system. With such a complex series of events occurring, the clinician seldom observes a specific dysfunction contributing to a specific symptom. A precise correlation between signs of dysfunction and symptoms is the exception rather than the rule. Dysfunction, in fact, can exist in the absence of any subjective complaints. It is not yet understood why some individuals with dysfunctions experience symptoms, whereas other individuals with the similar dysfunctions are asymptomatic.

The treatment goals that physical therapists establish for patients vary, depending on their clinical experience and expertise. A common treatment goal is to achieve normal function and positioning. It is a general belief that once normal function and position are achieved in the area being treated, a reduction or alleviation of symptoms will follow. But what are the normal values for the upper quarter region? For example: What is a normal head-neck-shoulder girdle posture? What is normal muscle tone? What is normal active-passive mobility of the cervical spine? What is normal passive range of motion of the cervical spine? The word normal implies conformity with the established norm or standard for its kind. If one were to apply this definition to an asymptomatic population, one would probably find that what is normal or average actually consists of varying degrees of dysfunction. By definition, then, when we attempt to restore normal function, we may actually be moving toward an ideal condition that does not commonly exist. Evaluating for what we as therapists consider normal in a patient would seemingly help us to identify those patients who are abnormal. However, this conclusion assumes that we have the tools and techniques to help us in this clinical decision-making process. Major obstacles to overcome are the establishment of reliability, validity, and predictive values of our examination procedures. What purpose does an examination technique or procedure have if it cannot separate a normal population from a symptomatic population with some degree of reliability and validity? Physical therapy currently has few tools/procedures that are reliable and valid for the cervical spine.

Goals established for patients should be what is functional for the individual, not what is normal or abnormal based on the examination. Improving individual function in conjunction with decreasing symptoms would be more appropriate goals. Clinically, it is not possible to resolve all dysfunctions. Achieving as much mobility as is consistent with stability and educating the patient on appropriate exercise (i.e., flexibility, endurance, strength) and means of prevention by patient education are reasonable goals for most patients. These goals will help patients to maintain an individual asymptomatic physiologic adaptive range.

The treatment techniques used and their sequence depend largely on the experience and level of expertise of the physical therapist. Caution should be exercised before asserting that one treatment approach is better than another for a particular dysfunction or symptom. The effectiveness of physical therapy treatments in a clinical environment has seldom been evaluated through rigorous experimentation. Clinically controlled studies also need to consider the measurement of pain, which remains elusive. The application of a particular technique or treatment approach is largely based on clinical opinions. Sichers[1] warned us many years ago that "clinical success does not prove anything but the acceptability of the method employed; any attempt to prove an anatomical concept by clinical success is merely a rationalization and certainly is not to be regarded as truly scientific evidence." The approach to treatment for functional involvement should be noninvasive unless the neurological assessment suggests otherwise. Treatment should not be given if the clinician is not willing to treat the complications that may result.

The objective of this chapter is to heighten the reader's awareness of the influence of the upper quarter, primarily the cervical spine, on the stomatognathic system. The clinical symptoms associated with dysfunction of the stomatognathic system are discussed. Cervical spine dysfunction indicates altered mobility, position, and tissue tension of the cervical spine. Altered head-neck positioning that often is seen with cervical spine dysfunction will be referred to as an acquired forward head posture (AFHP). An AFHP develops in response to but is not limited to trauma, sleeping postures, sitting postures, lack of exercise, and/or lack of postural awareness. An AFHP is one that can possibly be corrected to a more upright head posture. On the other hand, a forward head posture that is genetically/congenitally determined is therefore more than likely normal. Correction of a genetic/congenital forward head posture is not possible by physical therapy intervention.

I do not want to mislead the reader into believing that the following interrelationships have been documented. Documentation does confirm that a neurophysiologic and anatomic relationship exists between the cervical spine and portions of the stomatognathic system. References to normal functional relationships are provided when possible. Any conclusions drawn about dysfunctional relationships and associated symptoms, and any mention of treatments, are entirely a matter of clinical opinion.

■ Stomatognathic System

The word stomatognathic is one that is not often used by physical therapists. *Stoma* is the Greek word for "mouth," and *stomato* denotes relationship to the mouth.[2]

Gnathos[2] likewise means "jaw," and gnathology[3] is the study of relationships of the temporomandibular joint (TMJ), the occlusion (teeth), and the neuromusculature. The phrase stomatognathic system refers to the muscles of mastication (the mandibular and cervical musculature), the tongue, the TMJ, the occlusion, and all associated vessels, ligaments, and soft tissues.

The stomatognathic system functions continuously during breathing and in the maintenance of an upright postural position of the mandible and tongue. The daily activity of this system is intermittently increased during such activities as chewing, talking, yawning, coughing, and licking the lips.

The following areas of the stomatognathic system are suggested to be directly influenced by cervical spine dysfunction:

- The upright postural position of the mandible
- The upright postural position of the tongue
- Swallowing
- Centric position (Centric position is the initial contact made between the maxillary and mandibular teeth when the mandible closes from an upright postural position.[4] Ideally, this initial contact is the maximum intercuspation, otherwise known as centric occlusion.[4])

Upright Postural Position of the Mandible

The rest or upright postural position of the mandible (UPPM) is maintained nearly 23 hours a day. When the mandible is in this position, the teeth are held slightly apart. The vertical space (freeway space) between the tips of the mandibular anterior teeth and the maxillary anterior teeth is on average about 3 mm. In the anteroposterior/mediolateral relationship of the UPPM to the maxilla, the mandibular teeth are positioned just below the point of contact (maximum intercuspation) of the maxillary teeth (Fig. 5–1).

In the UPPM, the muscles and soft tissues attaching to the mandible are in a state of "equilibrium."[5] The least amount of muscle and soft tissue effort is then needed to elevate the mandible from the UPPM to maximum intercuspation. Once movement of the mandible has occurred toward achieving tooth-to-tooth contact or after any other functional movements of the mandible, the

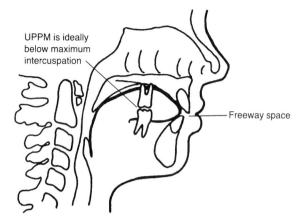

UPPM is ideally below maximum intercuspation

Freeway space

Figure 5–1. The upright postural position of the tongue and mandible. UPPM, upright postural position of the mandible. (From Kraus,[54] with permission.)

mandible will return to the UPPM. Essentially all movement begins and ends in the UPPM.[6] Individuals who talk or eat excessively, or who have acquired certain habits such as chewing gum or biting their fingernails, will spend less time with the mandible in the UPPM. Individuals who brux or clench their teeth will spend even less time with the mandible in this position. Less time spent in the UPPM means that more muscle and soft tissue activity is occurring. Such an increase in muscle activity over time is not therapeutic.

Cervical Spine Influences

Many short- and long-term factors have been suggested to influence the UPPM.[7] However, head posture appears to have the most significant and immediate effect on the UPPM.[8] Several studies have been cited as demonstrating that changes in the UPPM occur in response to short-term changes in the position of the head on the neck.[9–11] It is proposed that cervical spine dysfunction influences the UPPM.[11] Positioning or mobility changes associated with acute or chronic cervical spine dysfunction influencing the UPPM have not yet been documented.

The mandible can be visualized as being engulfed in the web of muscles and soft tissue attaching to it. The presence of cervical spine dysfunction together with the influence of gravity changes the mandibular position by altering the tone and tension of the muscle and soft tissue attaching to the mandible.[11] It has been suggested that this altered muscle and soft tissue tone acts to develop a force of elevation and retrusion on the mandible.[11] Whether cervical spine dysfunction actually contributes to the elevation and retrusion of the mandible is immaterial. The point of concern to the clinician is that the UPPM in the presence of cervical spine dysfunction may be different than it is with a cervical spine having good mobility and position. To what degree and for how long a change in vertical, anteroposterior/mediolateral posi-

tioning occurs with the UPPM will depend on the degree of cervical spine involvement.[11]

Symptoms

A common symptom relating to a change in the UPPM is the patient's complaint that "I don't know where or how to rest my jaw." This complaint may result from cervical spine dysfunction influencing the UPPM. Cervical spine dysfunction changing the UPPM may give the patient the perception of not knowing where to position the jaw.

This perception of not knowing how or where to rest the mandible may also be influenced by the occlusion. Studies have shown significant differences between individuals with respect to the occlusal receptors' sensory threshold.[4] Occlusal receptors provide a great deal of proprioceptive feedback to the mandibular muscles, which in turn influence the UPPM.[4] As previously stated, the vertical, anteroposterior/mediolateral position of the UPPM should be below maximum intercuspation. Patients whose UPPM is strongly influenced by muscle memory of occlusal contacts[4] will not allow for much variability in their UPPM. Cervical spine dysfunction changes the UPPM. The end result is that both the occlusion (whether normal occlusion or malocclusion) and the cervical spine have an influence on the UPPM. The occlusal and cervical spine influences on the mandible may decrease the patient's individual physiologic adaptive range, resulting in symptoms. Therefore, a patient's symptom may be alleviated by removing one or both influencing factors (i.e., the occlusion [intraocclusal appliance] or the cervical spine dysfunction [restore function]).

A consequence of not knowing where to rest the mandible may be that the patient tries to "brace" the mandible. The patient may brace the anterior mandibular teeth against the anterior maxillary teeth. Bracing the mandible gives the patient some point of reference for jaw positioning. Bracing does require isometric contraction of the mandibular muscles, but it should not be confused with bruxism. Some patients, however, place their teeth in maximum intercuspation (clenched) as another way of having some point of reference with the mandible. The symptoms expressed by such a patient are those associated with muscle hyperactivity (myalgia) of the mandibular muscles. The patient may also complain of a decrease or tightness in jaw movement.

Upright Postural Position of the Tongue

The tongue is composed of two muscle groups, extrinsic and intrinsic. The extrinsic muscles suspend the tongue from the skull (styloid process) to the anterior portion of the mandible. The mandible itself is also suspended from the skull. The intrinsic tongue muscles begin and end within the tongue and have no attachment to skeletal structures. The only intrinsic muscle of the tongue to be mentioned is the genioglossus because it is the only muscle that protrudes the tongue,[12] and most electromyographic (EMG) documentation has been performed on the genioglossus. Clinical observations to be covered will emphasize tongue protrusion.

The tongue is active during almost all oral and mandibular functions. When the stomatognathic system is in a state of equilibrium, the upright postural position of the tongue (UPPT) is up against the palate of the mouth.[13] In this position, the tip of the tongue will touch the back side of the upper incisors lightly, if at all (Fig. 5–1). The UPPT enhances the UPPM. As Fish has stated,[14] "the rest position of the mandible is related to the posture of the tongue."

Cervical Spine Influences

Cervical spine dysfunction has been proposed to influence the UPPT in several ways. The main supports of the extrinsic tongue muscles are the styloid process at one end and the front of the mandible at the other end (Fig. 5–2). The tongue can be visualized as being suspended like a sling between the styloid process and the mandible.[15] If an AFHP is present with cervical spine dysfunction, the cranium extends (rotates posteriorly) on the upper cervical spine.[16] The styloid process, being a part of the cranium, moves anteriorly as posterior rotation of the cranium occurs as a result of the AFHP (Fig. 5–2).

As previously stated, cervical spine dysfunction may create forces that elevate and retrude the mandible. Such a change in the UPPM with an AFHP causes the two points of attachment of the extrinsic muscles to come closer together (Fig. 5–2). This positional change of both the styloid process and the mandible causes the tongue to move from the top of the palate (the UPPT) to an abnormal position at the floor of the mouth. A change in the resting length of the extrinsic muscles of the tongue will more than likely change the resting length of the intrinsic muscles.

Besides a change in the length of the extrinsic muscles, a change in EMG activity of the genioglossus secondary to a change in head-neck positioning will occur. Studies have documented that a change in mandibular position will alter genioglossus (intrinsic muscle) activity mediated through the TMJ receptors.[17,18] Mandibular position is altered by a change in head position (AFHP). It is conceivable, then, that a change in head posture that alters the UPPM will in turn alter the TMJ receptors influencing genioglossus activity.

A second way in which head and neck position may alter genioglossus activity is through the tonic neck reflex. Extension of the head on the neck has been shown to produce an increase in genioglossus activity.[19] Backward bending (extension) of the head on the upper cervical spine occurs in the AFHP (Fig. 5–2). In a study using normal subjects, a change from a neutral head posture to a more anterior head posture (AFHP) resulted in a significant change in resting genioglossi EMG activity and maximal isometric genioglossi EMG activity.[20] These data suggest that changes in head-neck positioning (i.e., from neutral to an AFHP) may have an effect on genioglossi muscle activation thresholds. Therefore, the previous discussions suggest that the AFHP can cause an in-

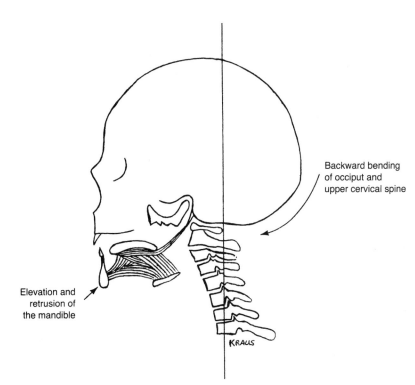

Backward bending of occiput and upper cervical spine

Elevation and retrusion of the mandible

KRAUS

Figure 5–2. Forward head posture (FHP) with a cutaway section of the mandible for easier viewing of the tongue and its muscles. The primary insertions of the extrinsic tongue muscles are to the styloid process and the anterior portion of the mandible. The arrows represent the proposed anatomic positional changes that occur secondary to FHP. The result is that the two points of insertion for extrinsic muscles come closer together, influencing the upright postural position of the tongue.

crease in genioglossus activity, either indirectly through the TMJ receptors or directly through the tonic neck reflex.

Cervical spine dysfunction will result in the tongue lying on the floor of the mouth, with the tip of the tongue pressing against the posterior side of the anterior mandibular teeth.

Symptoms

Patients often are not aware of where they position their tongues at rest until they are asked. When cervical spine dysfunction is present, the patient often states that the tongue is lying in the floor of the mouth, with the tip of the tongue pressing against the back side of the bottom teeth. Some patients, when asked to place the tongue up against the palate of the mouth (in the UPPT), may say that such a position feels awkward or difficult.

An altered tongue position contributes to symptoms of fullness or tightness in the floor of the mouth and/or the front of the neck. The pressing of the tongue against the teeth contributes to discomfort felt in the angle of the mandible. This discomfort is often mistaken for discomfort stemming from the TMJ. The reader can experience such discomfort by pressing the tip of the tongue against the front teeth for a period of time.

Maintaining the UPPT will keep the teeth out of the maximum intercuspated position. If the teeth were to come together, the patient could not maintain the UPPT. This natural phenomenon of the tongue up and teeth apart is enhanced in most patients by an overbite. An overbite occurs when the maxillary anterior central incisors overlap the mandibular anterior central incisors by approximately 1 to 1½ mm. If the patient maintains the correct UPPT, he or she must keep the teeth apart; otherwise, the patient will either bite the tip of the tongue or move the tongue away from its upright postural position. Therefore, an altered rest position of the tongue secondary to cervical spine dysfunction may facilitate the coming together of the teeth, resulting in hyperactivity of the elevator muscles of the mandible. Patients may then complain of myalgia of the mandibular muscles, especially the elevator muscles of the mandible.

Finally, in the supine position, the tonic activity of the genioglossus is markedly increased.[21] This increased activity plays an important role in maintaining an open air passage in the oropharyngeal region in the supine position.[21] Supine sleeping with proper support is best for the cervical spine. Cervical spine dysfunction with or without proper cervical support influences the UPPT. To maintain an adequate airway, the patient may lie on the stomach to keep the tongue out of the oropharyngeal area. The prone-lying position, which places a great deal of stress on the cervical spine tissues, may produce or increase cervical symptoms. One way to discourage the prone-lying position is to maintain the tongue in its upright postural position, thereby maintaining an open air-

way. Training the patient to maintain the UPPT will have to be performed first during waking hours. Achieving good mobility and positioning of the cervical spine, educating the patient on the normal UPPT, and providing good cervical support at night will encourage supine and/or side-lying sleeping postures. I have observed clinically that when the previously mentioned therapies are offered, nocturnal clenching/bruxism may decrease in patients.

Swallowing

Although it is generally acknowledged that swallowing involves nearly all the muscles of the tongue, the muscles that seem to be of particular importance are the geniohyoid, the genioglossus, the mylohyoid, and the anterior digastric.[22] Of these four muscles, emphasis will be placed on the activity of the genioglossus. Swallowing, or deglutition, is the process by which a fluid or solid is passed from the mouth to the stomach. There are three stages of swallowing: oral, pharyngeal, and esophageal.[23] The oral stage is voluntary and involves passage of the bolus to the fauces (passage from the mouth to the pharynx). The other two stages of swallowing are involuntary. During a 24-hour period, we swallow subconsciously many times. The amount of subconscious swallowing added to the number of times we swallow during eating and drinking adds up to a significant amount of muscle activity even when performed correctly.

The oral stage is the only stage of swallowing for which some documentation is available regarding the influence of positional changes of the head and neck. It is also the only stage over which we have conscious control to correct altered swallowing patterns. For these reasons, the oral stage will be the only stage covered.

During the normal oral stage of swallowing (Fig. 5–3), once the fluid or solid is in the mouth, the tip of the tongue moves forward and upward to contact the palatal mucosa behind the upper incisors.[24] With the tip of the tongue kept stationary, the rest of the tongue, like a wave in the ocean, reaches the junction of the hard and soft palates.[25] At this point, the oral stage of swallowing ends, with the tongue resting once again in its upright postural position.

Cervical Spine Influences

The UPPT has been described as the foundation of all swallowing movements.[25–27] Cervical spine influence on the UPPT has been discussed. Because swallowing begins and ends in the UPPT, the entire oral stage of swallowing will be altered in the presence of cervical spine dysfunction.

During an altered sequence of swallowing, the patient often will push the tip of the tongue off the back side of the upper or lower incisors. The tongue pressing anteriorly diminishes the effectiveness of the middle and posterior parts of the tongue in pressing up at the junction of

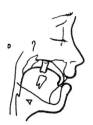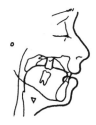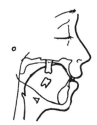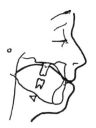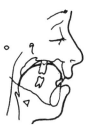

Figure 5–3. Normal sequence of swallowing depicted in five stages. (From Kraus,[54] with permission.)

the hard and soft palates. Continuation of an altered sequence of swallowing contributes to an increase in the duration of swallowing. The duration of normal swallowing ranges from 1.42 to 2.74 seconds.[28] It has been suggested that swallowing can occur with the teeth either together or apart.[29] It is my belief that in the presence of good mobility and positioning of the cervical spine, swallowing should occur without tooth contact. Cervical spine dysfunction, as previously discussed, influences the UPPM and UPPT and causes the oral stage of swallowing to be altered. Cervical spine dysfunction therefore may contribute to an increase in tooth contact time for each swallow. Prolonged tooth contact contributes to muscle hyperactivity of the tongue and mandibular muscles.

To appreciate the influence of head posture on swallowing, simply look up and then swallow. You will find it difficult to swallow. However, you may find it slightly easier to swallow if you press the tip of your tongue firmly against the back side of your upper or lower incisors. This tongue position encourages more dysfunction. Now bring your eyes level but exaggerate the AFHP. Again you will find it more difficult to swallow correctly with the middle to posterior third of the tongue pressing against the palate of the mouth.

Symptoms

Symptoms associated with an altered sequence of swallowing secondary to cervical spine dysfunction consist of difficulty in swallowing (food gets caught in the throat or there is a fullness in the throat) or tightness in the front of the neck. Secondary symptoms are related to myalgia of the tongue and masticatory muscles. Some patients will feel as though their tongue is swollen. Patients may complain of biting their tongue because of the lack of coordination between tongue positioning, swallowing, and chewing.

Centric Position

Occlusion refers to the way teeth meet, fit, come together, or touch. Much has been written about malocclusion of the teeth and the relationship between occlusion and myofascial pain and/or TMJ disorders.[30–32] The modification of occlusal relationships is regarded by some dentists as a specific and definitive treatment for muscle and TMJ involvement.[33,34] Some individuals consider occlusal modification to be specific treatment because it deals directly with the presumed etiologic factor and definitive because it eliminates or corrects the occlusal problem. On the basis of this concept, some clinicians treat patients with muscle and TMJ involvement by altering the occlusion in different ways. Occlusal relationships may be altered by any one technique or a combination of techniques including equilibration (selective grinding to modify the occlusion), orthodontics, or full-mouth reconstruction.

The rationale behind altering the occlusion is based on several biomechanical hypotheses. Some believe that malocclusion causes displacement of the mandible and that proper occlusal treatment allows repositioning of the mandible to its optimal position.[35,36] The other, more popular theory holds that malocclusion initiates neuromuscular reflexes of accommodative activity in the masticatory muscles. Such muscle activity in response to the malocclusion is suggested to lead to muscular fatigue and spasm.[37,38]

However, many individuals with obvious malocclusion have no dental, muscle, or joint complaints.[39,40] In fact, malocclusion is the rule rather than the exception. Because of this common observation, a theory of physiologic versus pathologic occlusion has been espoused.[40] By definition,[40] a "physiologically acceptable occlusion is one free of patient complaints and recognizable pathological conditions, by the dentist, at the time of examination."

When to treat or not to treat the occlusion in the absence or, for that matter, the presence of symptoms is largely a matter of clinical judgment. It has been shown that the same types of occlusal disharmonies are distributed equally among populations of patients with muscle and/or TMJ symptoms and among randomly selected normal individuals.[41] It has also been shown that four of five patients with muscle and/or TMJ symptoms are women; however, no consistent differences with respect to occlusion have been shown to exist between the sexes.[42]

When muscle and/or TMJ symptoms do appear, it becomes important for the dentist to use reversible treatments, for example, by using an interocclusal appliance.[43,44] Other forms of treatment such as equilibration and orthodontics are irreversible. Interocclusal appliances must be designed, applied, and modified for the individual patient; otherwise, orthodontic movement of the teeth can occur, which should be avoided in the symptomatic patient. It should be recognized that the patient's response to either occlusal adjustment or splint therapy is a complex interaction between the psychology of the patient, the type of treatment offered, and how the treatment may be influenced by other adjacent areas. Simply to suggest that a response by a patient to treatment of the occlusion, or for that matter to treatment of any dysfunctional problem, is a cause-and-effect phenomenon is not justified.[1,45]

With such differences in opinion as to the role of occlusion in producing symptoms, the dentist and the physical therapist should be alert to other adjacent areas that influence how the teeth approach maximum intercuspation (centric occlusion). An area often overlooked by the clinician that may decrease the patient's ability to adapt to a malocclusion is the cervical spine.[10,44] Treating patients with symptoms related to the muscle and/or the TMJ will require dealing with more than just the occlusion. To help the patient achieve a pain-free functional physiologic adaptive range, it is necessary to treat not only the occlusion by reversible procedures but also those areas that influence how the teeth come together. One such area believed to influence how the teeth come into maximum intercuspation is the cervical spine.

Cervical Spine Influences

How cervical spine dysfunction influences centric position (the initial contact made between the upper arch and lower arch of teeth) can be understood by appreciating the influence that the cervical spine has on the adaptive (habitual) arc of closure. The adaptive arc of closure is an arc directed by a conditioned reflex[40]: "The entire proprioceptive neuromuscular mechanism sets up the conditioned reflex and guides this arc of closure."

What is acknowledged by the dentist is that at one end of this arc is the occlusion. Ideally, the teeth should meet in maximum intercuspation as the mandibular teeth approach the maxillary teeth during closure. If any portion of a tooth or teeth makes contact before maximum intercuspation, this is considered a form of malocclusion. Such interference or premature contact stimulates the mechanoreceptors of the periodontium (the tissues investing and supporting the teeth).[4] This, in turn, causes abnormal recruitment of the muscles of mastication to reposition the mandible in a more favorable position as maximum intercuspation is approached.[4,44] The neuromuscular system, by positioning the mandible to avoid interference, changes the adaptive arc of closure. A change in the adaptive arc of closure occurs at the expense of additional muscle activity.[44] As previously suggested, when such interference cannot be accommodated by the neuromuscular system, muscular symptoms develop. Muscle hyperactivity contributes to symptoms arising

from the muscle and is also believed to be a cause of temporomandibular disorders.

However, what is often totally overlooked in this ordering of events is the other end of the adaptive arc of closure. The end of the arc from which jaw closure begins is the UPPM. Posselt stated, "The conclusion that the rest position can generally be considered a position on the path of closing movement is almost self-suggestive."[46] Cervical spine dysfunction changes the UPPM.[11] As Mohl stated regarding head and neck posture, "We must logically conclude that, if rest position is altered by a change in head position, the habitual path of closure of the mandible must also be altered."[47] Cervical spine dysfunction may alter the arc of closure so that the initial teeth contact occurs somewhere other than at the maximum intercuspation.[11] Such a change in the path of closure will cause premature contacts of the teeth before maximum intercuspation. If premature contacts secondary to a malocclusion eventually cause muscle and/or TMJ symptoms, premature contacts secondary to cervical spine dysfunction may also result in muscle and/or TMJ symptoms. The neuromuscular system will try to accommodate such interferences. When such accommodative responses are exhausted and muscle and/or TMJ symptoms develop, the cervical spine needs to be evaluated and treated.

Symptoms

Symptoms of cervical spine dysfunction are those that have been attributed to a malocclusion (interferences before achieving maximum intercuspation). A physiologic occlusion may be present, yet there is interference of the mandibular teeth approaching the maxillary teeth to maximum intercuspation. An interference secondary to cervical spine dysfunction is referred to as a pseudomalocclusion.[11] Clinically, a combination of malocclusion and pseudomalocclusion is very common, thus complicating the clinical picture even more.

Bruxism is considered by some investigators to be a symptom of malocclusion. Bruxism is the clenching or grinding of the teeth when the individual is not chewing or swallowing.[48] Bruxism has been implicated in producing a variety of symptoms such as headache, TMJ and myofascial pain, tooth mobility, and occlusal wear.[49] Bruxism has been associated with the presence of occlusal interferences.[4] Cervical spine dysfunction may contribute to one form of occlusal interference, the manner in which teeth come into contact. This form of occlusal interference may initiate bruxism or at least mandibular muscle hyperactivity. Other causes of bruxism (muscle hyperactivity) have been suggested to be related to daily stress and emotional tension.[50]

Patients may also complain of their "bite" (occlusion) being off. The dentist may not find any indication that this complaint is related to the occlusion. In this case, the patient's perception is of a pseudomalocclusion caused by cervical spine dysfunction. Some patients may feel that they cannot bring their posterior teeth together on one or both sides even after an occlusal adjustment or during splint therapy. Again, the cervical spine may be implicated.

If a patient is undergoing splint therapy with a dentist and is not responding, the following should be considered[11]:

1. The splint is not indicated, but therapy of the cervical spine is.
2. The splint is indicated, but because of the degree of cervical spine dysfunction present, adaptation to the splint is not possible unless cervical spine dysfunction is treated before and/or during the use of the splint.
3. The splint does not have those features that facilitate acceptance by the patient with cervical spine dysfunction.

■ Treatment

The physical therapist should always perform an evaluation of the cervical spine to determine if treatment is needed. The specifics of the evaluation are not within the scope of this chapter; the reader is referred to the references.[51] The treatment of the cervical spine used to reduce its influence on the stomatognathic system is the same treatment offered for involvement of the cervical spine alone. Even if the patient does not complain of any of the symptoms of dysfunction of the stomatognathic system, instructing the patient on the normal function of the stomatognathic system will enhance treatment of the cervical spine.

Awareness Exercises for the Stomatognathic System

The patient needs to be told what is normal jaw and tongue positioning at rest. First, instruct the patient on the normal rest position of the tongue. The tongue should be up against the mouth, with the tip lightly touching, if at all, the back side of the upper central incisors (Fig. 5–1). Patients tend to overcompensate, so inform the patient not to press the tongue hard against the roof of the mouth.

The UPPM (rest position) is with the teeth apart. As discussed earlier, if the patient's tongue is up and an overbite exists, the teeth will be apart. The patient should not be concerned with how far apart the teeth are. Inform the patient not to work hard at keeping the teeth apart ("Just let the jaw float"). Reassure the patient that the position with the tongue up and the teeth apart will become easier as the cervical spine dysfunction is treated.

Patients who have developed an altered sequence of swallowing secondary to cervical spine dysfunction will need to be instructed on the normal sequence of swallowing. Swallowing will be practiced with water. Inform the patient to practice swallowing with the teeth slightly apart.

In stage 1 (Fig. 5–3), the tongue drops from its normal rest position to allow water to enter the mouth.

In stage 2, the tip of the tongue is directed to its rest position. Emphasize to the patient that no pressure should be felt from the tip of the tongue pressing upward or forward against the teeth.

In stage 3, the main force of swallowing occurs with the middle third (middle to posterior) of the tongue. From stage 2 to stage 3, the patient should feel the tongue moving like a wave in the ocean.

Stage 4 is essentially the end of stage 3, as the water is pressed into the pharynx, where involuntary control takes over.

Stage 5 is the completion of the swallowing cycle. The tongue is in its rest position, and the teeth are apart.[52]

A pseudomalocclusion is treated by treating the cervical spine. The therapist should not dwell on the patient's perception of his or her occlusion too often after the initial evaluation. Occasionally asking the patient about how the bite feels is acceptable. Otherwise, repeated mention of the bite, especially if the patient has a keen sense of his or her occlusion, may result in too much awareness by the patient. This is important to realize, because even after occlusal therapy, malocclusion may still persist.

The awareness exercises should be practiced several times during the day. Awareness exercises must be practiced with good head and neck posture. If good head and neck posture cannot yet be achieved, the patient should practice with the existing head and neck posture at that time. Above all, do not have the patient force a good head and neck posture.

CASE STUDY

History

Ms. A is an active 43-year-old writer whose chief complaint was pain in the neck, jaw, and throat areas. Ms. A reported that her symptoms began insidiously 2 years previously. During the 3 months immediately preceding her complaint, her symptoms increased in intensity to the point where they interfered with her work. Ms. A reported that she exercised regularly, including walking and jogging, and other than her symptoms, she felt that she was in good health.

Ms. A consulted with her family physician 2 months prior to presentation to see if there were any treatments that would resolve her symptoms. The physician took a series of standard cervical spine radiographs. The physician reported that the radiographs showed a little arthritis, but overall they were normal. The physician diagnosed her problem as cervicalgia and prescribed physical therapy treatments.

The patient's responses to questions regarding the frequency, intensity, and duration of her symptoms were as follows:

Neck Pain

Frequency: Constant.

Intensity: Variable (i.e., worse in the morning, eased off by noon, and slowly increased as the day progressed); on an intensity scale of 0 to 10, low was 4 and high was 8.

Duration: Constant.

Jaw Pain

Frequency: The patient stated, "The jaw pain is always there, but I have gotten used to it. However, I seem to notice my jaw pain more when I experience an increase in my neck pains."

Intensity: 8.

Duration: Lasted for several hours, then subsided to the point where she no longer noticed it.

Throat Pain

Frequency: Several times a week.

Intensity: The patient stated that it was not an actual pain but more of a "nagging tightness" in her throat. It got to the point where she felt that it was hard to swallow.

Duration: Lasted for several hours.

The patient's responses to questions about what increased or decreased her symptoms will now be summarized.

Neck Pain

Increase: The patient stated, "Stress will increase my symptoms." With more direct questioning, the patient became aware of certain neck movements that bothered her, such as looking up and looking over her shoulder when backing her car out of the driveway. As a writer, she sat for 6 to 7 hours a day at a computer, which she believed was a factor in her afternoon pain.

Decrease: Patient reported that she could decrease her symptoms by taking two aspirins twice a day and a hot shower.

Jaw Pain

Increase: Patient stated that her jaw pain increased when her neck pains increased. Patient denied any clenching and bruxing but was aware of tightness in her jaw on awakening. When the patient became aware that tense jaw muscles are strongly correlated with parafunctional activity, and that the teeth-together position is not normal, she acknowledged that she must be doing some parafunctional activity at night and possibly during the day but was completely unaware of it.

Decrease: Her jaw pain seemed to decrease when her neck pains decreased.

Throat Pain

Increase: The patient could not identify anything that would increase her throat pains other than the stress of making deadlines for her writing assignments.

Decrease: The patient recognized that taking several deep breaths reduced her throat pains.

Questions pertaining to her sleeping patterns revealed that the patient woke up several times a night with neck pains. She reported that she slept on several pillows, with the top one rolled up in an attempt to support her neck. She reported experiencing significant neck pains and jaw tightness in the morning.

The patient was asked what she believed was necessary to relieve her symptoms. She responded, "My neck feels like it needs to be stretched several inches longer."

The patient was asked how she would recognize if physical therapy was helpful to her. She responded, "I would recognize improvement if I could get one full night's sleep without pain waking me up."

Physical Examination

The patient's neck pain, as well as 50 percent of her jaw pain, were reproduced during the examination of the cervical spine. Palpation of the upper trapezius and levator scapulae muscles bilaterally, palpation over the greater occipital nerve bilaterally, and performance of passive intervertebral overpressure techniques of sidebending and rotation at the C2-C3 and C3-C4 segments bilaterally reproduced the patient's neck and jaw pain. Active movements were within normal limits. Repeated movements of cervical extension and rotation to the left began to produce an irritating feeling in the patient's neck. A significant reduction in the neck and jaw pain occurred while manual traction to the cervical spine was performed in the standing position. The remaining 50 percent of the jaw pain was reproduced during palpation over the masseter muscle bilaterally. The throat pain was reproduced by having the patient exaggerate her AFHP, and in this posture the patient was asked to take 10 to 15 sips of water from a cup. Examination of the TMJs revealed no capsular or intercapsular involvement.

Summary of the History and Physical Examination

The patient was screened by her family physician for any major medical problems that could be a source of her symptoms. From the history and physical examination, it appeared that the patient's symptoms were caused by a nondiseased/nonspecific condition of the cervical spine. The physical therapy diagnosis for such a condition is cervical spine dysfunction. The physical therapist should be alert to the fact that the neck, jaw, and throat symptoms may require intervention by an orthopaedist (i.e., muscle and/or facet joint injections or medication), a dentist (a nonrepositioning intraoral appliance), and an otolaryngologist, respectively, if improvement was not made with physical therapy treatments within a reasonable period of time.

Treatment and Prognosis

Treatment consisted of educating the patient regarding her condition. The patient was informed that her condition was dysfunction (tight muscles and joints) and that her symptoms could be managed if she was willing to modify her work and sleeping environments. Awareness exercises of proper tongue and mandibular rest positions were covered in detail. Instructions on the proper swallowing patterns as an exercise were given. Instructions on sleeping positions using a cervical pillow support and detailed instructions on sitting postures were reviewed. Based on the patient's response to the history and physical examination, as well as her activity level, the patient was judged not to have significant tissue inflammation. Modalities were not used. Instead, manual therapy consisting of rotational, diagonal, and spiral movement patterns with and without stretch was initiated and continued throughout the period of physical therapy treatments. Joint manipulation at the C2-C3 and C3-C4 segments was performed at the end of the third week.

The patient responded well to the first 4 weeks (twice per week) of treatments. At the end of the fourth week, the patient was reporting sleeping 4 out of 5 nights a week. The patient was also taking aspirin only 2 days a week. After an additional 2 weeks of therapy, the patient was reporting overall 85 percent improvement in neck pains and 100 percent improvement in throat pains. The subjective improvement was verified by reassessing the objective findings of the physical examination. However, after 6 weeks of therapy, the patient was reporting only 50 percent improvement in her jaw pain. By this time, the patient had become more aware that she was doing parafunctional activities through the awareness exercises of tongue and mandibular rest positions. After the referring physician was consulted, the patient was referred to an experienced dentist, who constructed an intraoral appliance with the proper features that would control and minimize the adverse effect of parafunctional activities. The appliance was used only at night. With the use of the appliance and continued therapy once a week for 6 more weeks, her remaining jaw pains improved.

After a total of 12 weeks, the patient's symptoms were controlled by her exercise program plus a home program of stretching and strengthening exercises to the cervical spine. Most important, the patient recognized warning signs that her symptoms may be recurring and knew what she needed to do to help herself. The patient was discharged but was informed that if she had any problems, she was to give her physical therapist and/or physician a call.

■ Summary

This chapter expresses clinical opinions about the influence of the cervical spine on key portions of the stomatognathic system, which is often not recognized by the clinician. By understanding how the cervical spine influences the stomatognathic system, certain symptoms may be better understood.

The indirect influence of the cervical spine on the TMJ has been covered. The cervical spine influences mandibular positioning and mobility and thus, indirectly, the TMJ. The cervical spine plays a key role in the treatment of a symptomatic TMJ. Regardless of the capsular and/or intercapsular involvement, treatment of the cervical spine will decrease muscle hyperactivity/imbalances of the stomatognathic area. Most treatment for a symptomatic TMJ involves reduction of muscle hyperactivity. If inflammation of the TMJ cannot be reduced and/or an internal derangement of the TMJ appears to be a factor perpetuating joint inflammation, an intraoral appliance from a dentist may need to be considered.[53]

Muscles of the stomatognathic system have been discussed only as needed, not to deemphasize the importance of the muscles, because muscles are, in fact, the key to interrelating the cervical spine with the stomatognathic system. The topic of cervical spine influence on masticatory muscle activity has been covered in detail elsewhere.[11]

The symptoms discussed in this chapter are those symptoms originating from the stomatognathic system in response to cervical spine dysfunction. The reader should be alert to referred symptoms from the cervical spine to the stomatognathic system.[11]

Treatment of stomatognathic dysfunction involves patient education and instruction on awareness exercises. Treatment of cervical spine dysfunction must also be offered. Involvement of the masticatory muscles and the TMJ beyond that responsive to physical therapy treatment requires consultation with a dentist.

■ References

1. Sichers H: Positions and movements of the mandible. J Am Dent Assoc 48:620, 1954
2. Dorland's Medical Dictionary. 26th Ed. WB Saunders, Philadelphia, 1981
3. Nasedkin J: Occlusal dysfunction: screening procedures and initial treatment planning. Gen Dent 26:52, 1978

4. Ramfjord SP, Ash M Jr: Occlusion. 2nd Ed. WB Saunders, Philadelphia, 1971

5. Yemm R: The mandibular rest position: the roles of tissue elasticity and muscle activity. J Dent Assoc South Africa 30:203, 1975

6. Kazis H, Kazis A: Complete Mouth Rehabilitation. Henry Kimpton, London, 1956

7. Atwood DA: A critique of the rest position of the mandible. J Prosthet Dent 16:848, 1966

8. Mohl N: Head posture and its role in occlusion. Int J Orthod 15:6, 1977

9. Mohamed SE, Christensen LV: Mandibular reference positions. J Oral Rehabil 12:355, 1985

10. Funakoshi M, Fujita N, Takehana S: Relations between occlusal interference and jaw muscle activities in response to change in head position. J Dent Res 55:684, 1976

11. Kraus S: Cervical spine influences on the craniomandibular region. p. 367. In Kraus S (ed): TMJ Disorders: Management of the Craniomandibular Complex. Churchill Livingstone, New York, 1988; and p. 325. In Kraus S (ed): TMJ Disorders: Management of the Craniomandibular Complex. 2nd Ed. Churchill Livingstone, New York, 1994

12. Sauerland EK, Mitchell SP: Electromyographic activity of intrinsic and extrinsic muscles of the human tongue. Tex Rep Biol Med 33:258, 1975

13. Proffit W: Equilibrium theory revisited: factors influencing position of the teeth. Angle Orthod 48:172, 1978

14. Fish F: The functional anatomy of the rest position of the mandible. Dent Practitioner 11:178, 1961

15. Grant JCB: A Method of Anatomy. 6th Ed. Williams & Wilkins, Baltimore, 1958

16. Kendall H, Kendall F, Boynton D: Posture and Pain. Robert E Krieger, Malabar, FL, 1967

17. Lowe A: Mandibular joint control of genioglossus muscle activity in the cat and monkey. Arch Oral Biol 23:787, 1978

18. Lowe A, Johnston W: Tongue and jaw muscle activity in response to mandibular rotations in a sample of normal and anterior open bite subjects. Am J Orthod 76:565, 1979

19. Bratzlavsky M, Vander Eecken H: Postural reflexes in cranial muscles in man. Acta Neurol Belg 77:5, 1977

20. Milidonis M, Kraus S, Segal R, et al: Genioglossi muscle activity in response to changes in anterior/neutral head posture. Am J Orthod Dentofacial Ortho 103:1, 1993

21. Sauerland E, Harper R: The human tongue during sleep: electromyographic activity of the genioglossus muscle. Exp Neurol 51:160, 1976

22. Hrycyshyn A, Basmajian J: Electromyography of the oral stage of swallowing in man. Am J Anat 133:333, 1972

23. Guyton AC: Textbook of Medical Physiology. 3rd Ed. WB Saunders, Philadelphia, 1967

24. Cleall J, Alexander W, McIntyre H: Head posture and its relationship to deglutition. Angle Orthod 36:335, 1966

25. Cleall J: Deglutition: a study of form and function. Am J Orthod 51:566, 1965

26. Barrett H, Mason R: Oral myofunctional disorders. CV Mosby, St. Louis, 1978

27. Logemann J: Evaluation and Treatment of Swallowing Disorders. College-Hill Press, San Diego, CA, 1983

28. Cunningham D, Basmajian J: Electromyography of genioglossus and geniohyoid muscles during deglutition. Anat Rec 165:401, 1969

29. Bole C: Electromyographic kinesiology of the genioglossus muscles in man. Thesis, Ohio State University, 1969

30. Shore NA: Occlusal Equilibration and Temporomandibular Joint Dysfunction. JB Lippincott, Philadelphia, 1959

31. Mann A, Pankey LD: Concepts of occlusion. The PM philosophy of occlusal rehabilitation. Dent Clin North Am 621, 1963

32. Dawson PE: Evaluation, Diagnosis and Treatment of Occlusal Problems. CV Mosby, St. Louis, 1974

33. Krogh-Poulsoen WG, Olsson A: Occlusal disharmonies and dysfunction of the stomatognathic system. Dent Clin North Am 10:627, 1966

34. Posselt UOA: Physiology of Occlusion and Rehabilitation. 2nd Ed. FA Davis, Philadelphia, 1968

35. Granger ER: Occlusion in temporomandibular joint pain. J Am Dent Assoc 56:659, 1958

36. Dyer EH: Importance of a stable maxillomandibular relation. J Prosthet Dent 30:241, 1973

37. Ramfjord SP: Bruxism: a clinical and electromyographic study. J Am Dent Assoc 62:21, 1961

38. Zarb GA, Thompson GW: Assessment of clinical treatment of patients with temporomandibular joint dysfunction. J Prosthet Dent 24:542, 1970

39. Barghi N: Clinical evaluation of occlusion. Tex Dent J 96:12, 1978

40. Huffman R, Regenos J, Taylor R: Principles of Occlusion: Laboratory and Clinical Teaching Manual. 3rd Ed. H&R Press, Columbus, OH, 1969

41. Posselt U: The temporomandibular joint syndrome and occlusion. J Prosthet Dent 25:432, 1971

42. Carraro JJ, Caffesse RG, Albano EA: Temporomandibular joint syndrome. A clinical evaluation. Oral Surg 28:54, 1969

43. Greene C, Laskin D: Splint therapy for the myofascial pain-dysfunction syndrome: a comparative study. J Am Dent Assoc 81:624, 1972

44. Razook S: Nonsurgical management of TMJ and masticatory muscle problems. p. 113. In Kraus S (ed): TMJ Disorders: Management of the Craniomandibular Complex. Churchill Livingstone, New York, 1988; and Razook S, Laurence E. Nonsurgical management of mandibular disorders. p. 125. In Kraus S (ed): TMJ Disorders: Management of the Craniomandibular Complex. 2nd Ed. Churchill Livingstone, New York, 1994.

45. Goodman P, Greene C, Laskin D: Response of patients with myofascial pain-dysfunction syndrome to mock equilibration. J Am Dent Assoc 92:755, 1976

46. Posselt U: Studies on the mobility of the human mandible. Acta Odont Scand 10:1, 1952

47. Mohl N: Head posture and its role in occlusion. NY State Dent J 42:17, 1976

48. Ramjford SP, Kerr DA, Ash MM: World Workshop in Periodontics. p. 233. University of Michigan Press, Ann Arbor, MI, 1966

49. Solberg W, Clark G, Rugh J: Nocturnal electromyographic evaluation of bruxism patients undergoing short term splint therapy. J Oral Rehabil 2:215, 1975

50. Rugh JD, Solberg W: Psychological implications in temporomandibular pain and dysfunction. Oral Sci Rev 7:3, 1976

51. Kaput M, Mannheimer J: Physical therapy concepts in the evaluation and treatment of the upper quarter. p. 339. In Kraus S (ed): TMJ Disorders: Management of the Craniomandibular Complex. Churchill Livingstone, New York, 1988

52. Kraus S: Physical therapy management of TMJ dysfunction. p. 139. In Kraus S (ed): TMJ Disorders: Management of the Craniomandibular Complex. Churchill Livingstone, New York, 1988

53. Kraus S: Evaluation and management of temporomandibular disorders. In Saunders HD (ed): Evaluation, Treatment and Prevention of Musculoskeletal Disorders. 2nd Ed. Viking Press, Minneapolis, 1993

54. Kraus S: Tongue-Teeth-Breathing-Swallowing: Exercise Pad. Stretching Charts, Inc., Tacoma, WA, 1987

CHAPTER 6

Dysfunction, Evaluation, and Treatment of the Cervical Spine and Thoracic Inlet

Steven A. Stratton and Jean M. Bryan

Many patients present to physical therapy with complaints of pain caused by cervical dysfunction. The cervicothoracic region is complex and requires a thorough evaluation to treat the disorder appropriately. The clinician must understand the applied anatomy and biomechanics of this region to recognize pathology. This chapter covers the pertinent anatomy and kinesiology of the cervical and upper thoracic spine, the evaluation procedure, and the correlation of findings to initiate treatment.

■ Functional Anatomy

Upper Cervical Spine

The joints of the upper cervical spine region, also known as the craniovertebral joints, include the occipitoatlantal (OA) joint, the atlantoaxial (AA) joint, and the articulations between the second and third cervical vertebrae (C2-C3) including the facet joints, intervertebral disk, and joints of von Luschka. Clinically, the upper cervical spine is considered a functional region because of the interdependency of these joints associated with movement.

The Atlas

The first and second cervical vertebrae have characteristics that make them different from the more typical cervical vertebrae, C3 to C7. The atlas (C1) is best thought of as a "washer" between the occiput and the axis (C2).[1] The two distinguishing features of the atlas are its long transverse processes and its lack of a spinous process. The superior articulating surfaces, which articulate with the

paired, convex occipital condyles, are concave both anteroposteriorly and mediolaterally. The articulating surfaces are oval[2] (Fig. 6–1).

The Axis

Besides being the largest cervical vertebra of the upper cervical region, the axis (C2) has several other distinguishing features (Fig. 6–1). Its most striking landmark is the odontoid process (the dens), which passes up through the middle of the atlas, articulates with the anterior arch, and acts as a pivot for the OA joint. The axis also has a large vertebral body. The superior articular facets are oriented superiorly and laterally, are convex anteroposteriorly, and are flat transversely. The spinous process of the axis is bifid, like that of other cervical vertebrae, but is larger in mass. The inferior articular processes of C2 are attached below the pedicle, face inferiorly and anteriorly, and correspond to the superior articular processes of C3. Both the C1 and C2 transverse processes have a vertical foramen for the vertebral artery.[2]

Occipitoatlantal and Atlantoaxial Ligaments

Alar Ligaments

The alar ligaments are irregular, quadrilateral, pyramid-like trunks that attach from the medial occipital condyle to the lateral surface of the dens (Fig. 6–2). The function of the alar ligament is to assist in controlling movements of extension and rotation.[1,3] During extension of the head, the alar ligament is stretched; during flexion, it is relaxed. During rotation of the OA joint, the ligament of the opposite side is stretched and drawn against the dens of the axis. For example, with rotation to the right, the left alar ligament is stretched and the right alar ligament is

The opinions expressed herein are solely those of the authors and are not to be construed as reflecting official doctrine of the U.S. Army Medical Department.

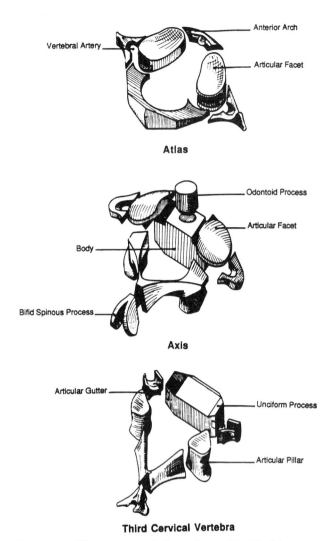

Atlas

Vertebral Artery
Anterior Arch
Articular Facet

Odontoid Process
Articular Facet
Body
Bifid Spinous Process

Axis

Articular Gutter
Uniform Process
Articular Pillar

Third Cervical Vertebra

Figure 6–1. The upper cervical vertebrae. (Modified from Kapandji,[2] with permission.)

relaxed. During sidebending, the alar ligament on the same side relaxes and the opposite alar ligament causes a forced rotation of the axis to the sidebending side. The forced rotation is due to the attachment of the alar ligament to the dens[1,2] (Fig. 6–3).

Cruciform Ligament

The cruciform ligament consists of a horizontal transverse ligament of the atlas and the vertical attachments to the occiput and axis, respectively called the transverso-occipital and transversoaxial ligaments. The transverse ligament arises from the medial surfaces of the lateral mass of the atlas and guarantees physiologic rotation of C1-C2 while protecting the spinal cord from the dens.[2] The other ligaments of the craniovertebral complex—the tectorial membrane, anterior longitudinal ligament, OA ligament, facet capsules, and ligamentum nuchae—all help to provide support; however, only certain ligaments restrict flexion and extension[1] (Fig. 6–2, Table 6–1).

Occipitoatlantal Motion

The upper surface of the occipital condyles is concave; thus, arthrokinematically, movement of the occiput on the atlas requires opposite joint glide in relation to physiologic movement.[4] The articulations are divergent at approximately 30 degrees, so that the joint surfaces are not in the true sagittal plane. The sagittal axial angle of the joints is 50 to 60 degrees in the adult. The sagittal angle of the joint axes from the occipital condyles, as described by Ingelmark,[5] reveals a 28 degree divergence of the articular surfaces anteriorly (Fig. 6–4). Werne[3] described the OA joint as condyloid, with free flexion and extension (nodding) and limited sidebending. Flexion and extension take place around a transverse axis and sidebending around a sagittal axis. Flexion and extension range from 16 to 20 degrees and are limited by bony structures. Sidebending measures approximately 4 to 5 degrees. Maximum sidebending is possible with the head in a slightly flexed position; when the head is extended, sidebending is prohibited by the alar ligaments.[6]

Different findings have been reported in the literature regarding the possibility of rotation at the OA joint. Fielding et al.,[6,7] Werne,[3] White and Panjabi,[8] and Penning[9] found no rotation. Recent investigations reveal one-side axial rotation between C0 and C1 in the range of 3 to 8

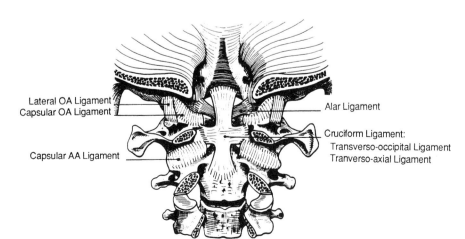

Lateral OA Ligament
Capsular OA Ligament

Capsular AA Ligament

Alar Ligament

Cruciform Ligament:
Transverso-occipital Ligament
Tranverso-axial Ligament

Figure 6–2. Ligaments of the upper cervical spine complex. OA, occipitoatlantal; AA, atlantoaxial. (Modified from Kapandji,[2] with permission.)

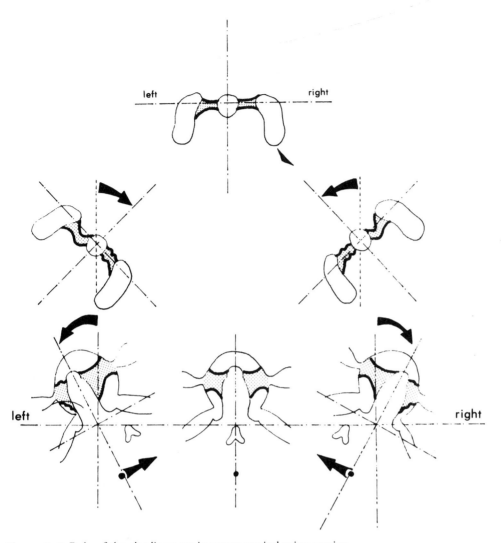

Figure 6–3. Role of the alar ligament in upper cervical spine motion.

□□□□ □ □ □ □

Table 6–1. Structures That Restrict Occipitoatlantal and Atlantoaxial Joint Range of Motion About the Transverse Axis

Flexion	Extension
Bony limitation	Bony limitation
Posterior muscles of the neck	Anterior muscles of the neck
Longitudinal fibers of the cruciform ligament	Sternocleidomastoid and scalene muscles
Tectorial membrane	Tectorial membrane
Nuchal ligament	Alar ligaments
Posterior longitudinal ligament	Anterior longitudinal ligament

degrees. Clark and colleagues[10] have found an average of 4.8 degrees. Dvorak and colleagues,[11] using computed axial tomography in vivo, noted an averaged one-side axial rotation of 4.3 degrees. Panjabi and associates[12] found 8 degrees using three-dimensional analysis. Dupreux and Mestdagh[13] contend that up to 5 degrees of rotation exists, with an average of 3.2 degrees. Attempts to explain this rotation often describe the atlas as a washer, interposed between the occiput and atlas like a meniscus, which would imply a gliding or linear movement[1] (Table 6–2).

Atlantoaxial Motion

The AA joint has four articulations for movement: the bursa atlantodentalis together with the middle and two lateral articulations. The bursa atlantodentalis is a space between the transverse ligament of the atlas and the dens of the axis. The middle AA articulation is located between the dens of the axis and the posterior surface of the anterior arch of the atlas. Most movement at the AA joint occurs at the lateral AA articulations, which are the supe-

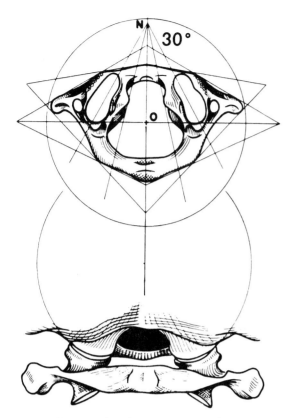

Figure 6–4. Occipitoatlantal joint sagittal axis from the occipital condyles. (Modified from Kapandji,[2] with permission.)

rior articular surfaces between the atlas and axis.[2] The articular surfaces of the atlas are convex, and those of the axis are relatively flat.[1] The range of motion to each side is 40 to 50 degrees, which constitutes half of the total rotation of the cervical spine.[6] Werne[3] reported 47 degrees of rotation to one side, whereas Panjabi and colleagues[12] measured 38.9 degrees. As in the OA joint, rotation is limited primarily by the alar ligaments. Only minimal (10 to 15 degrees) flexion-extension occurs because of the bony geometry and the securing ligamentous structures.

Sidebending between C1 and C2 is possible only with simultaneous rotation about the axis.[1] Lewit[14] and Jirout[15] described this movement as forced rotation that is mainly a result of the physiologic function of the alar ligaments. When forced rotation is produced, there is lateral displacement of the articular margin of the lateral joint of the atlas as compared with the lateral margin of the axis.[2] Sixty percent of axial rotation of the entire cervical spine and occiput is found in the upper cervical spine (C0-C2).[16]

Third Cervical Vertebra

The third cervical vertebra is typical of the remaining cervical vertebrae, C3 to C7 (Fig. 6–1). The vertebral body is wider than it is high, and its superior surface is raised laterally to form the uncinate processes (uncovertebral joints or joints of von Luschka). The inferior vertebral surface resembles the superior surface of the inferior vertebra, and the anterior border shows a beak-like projection facing downward. These articular processes, which are part of the posterior arch, have both superior and inferior articulating facets. The superior facet is oriented superiorly and posteriorly and corresponds to the inferior facet of the overlying vertebra; the inferior facet faces inferiorly and anteriorly and corresponds to the superior facet of the underlying vertebra. These articular processes are attached to the vertebral body by the pedicles so that the spaces between the processes form the articular pillar. The transverse processes form a gutter and contain a transverse foramen for passage of the vertebral artery (Fig. 6–1). The two lamina, which are oblique inferiorly and laterally, meet in the midline to form the bifid spinous process.[2] In the upper cervical spine complex, the articular surfaces for the OA and AA joints are in a horizontal plane, but C2-C3 articular processes or facets have an abrupt frontal oblique slope.[17]

Motion of the C2-C3 Segment

Motion of the C2-C3 segment is representative of the typical cervical vertebral segment, with an intervertebral

Table 6–2. Active Range of Motion of the Upper Cervical Spine

	Active Range of Motion (degrees)			
Vertebral Unit	Flexion	Extension	Sidebending[a]	Axial Rotation[a]
C0-C1 (occipitoatlantal joint)	0–15	0–20	5–0–5	8–0–8
C1-C2 (atlantoaxial joint)	0–10	0–10	3–0–3	40–0–40

[a]Range available on either side of neutral.

disk and eight plane articulations, including the four articular (apophyseal) facets and four uncovertebral joints (joints of von Luschka). The axis of motion is through the nucleus pulposus and allows freedom of movement in all three planes. Because of the orientation of the articular facets, sidebending and rotation occur concomitantly in the same direction.[2] Because of this concomitant motion, pure rotation or pure sidebending is impossible. The sliding of the joint surface depends on the rotation perpendicular to the axis. The relative amount of rotation or sidebending that occurs depends on the obliquity of the articular surfaces in the frontal plane. The more horizontal the joint surface, the more rotation will occur; the more vertical the joint surface, the more sidebending will occur. At the second cervical vertebra, there are 2 degrees of coupled axial rotation for every 3 degrees of sidebending.[18] The most abrupt change in joint obliquity occurs at the C2-C3 facet. Grieve[17] noted that all cervical facet joints are oriented so that the cervical facet joint surfaces converge in the region of the eyes.

Motion of the C3-C7 Segments

The midcervical spine allows the greatest ranges of motion in the neck (Table 6–3). The inclination of the facet surfaces of these vertebrae is 45 degrees to the horizontal plane. The lower segments are steeper than the upper segments. As in the C2-C3 segment, sidebending and rotation occur concomitantly in the same direction because of the oblique plane of the articular surfaces. However, at each motion segment there is opposite gliding of the articular surfaces. For example, with right rotation or

right sidebending, the left superior articular facet glides superiorly and anteriorly, while the right superior articular facet glides posteriorly and inferiorly on their adjoining inferior articular surfaces.[1] The total amount of sidebending in this region is 35 to 37 degrees, and total rotation is 45 degrees. With pure flexion and extension, both superior facets at each motion segment glide in the same direction. With flexion, both facets move superiorly; with extension, both move inferiorly. Total range of flexion and extension in the lower cervical column is 100 to 110 degrees.[2] At the seventh cervical vertebra, there is 1 degree of coupled axial rotation for every 7.5 degrees of sidebending.[18]

Upper Thoracic Spine

The upper thoracic spine must be included in any discussion of the cervical spine because the movement of the lower cervical spine occurs in conjunction with that of the upper thoracic spine. Gross cervical spine movements include upper thoracic spine motion as a result of the distal attachment of the cervical muscles to as low as T6 in the case of the splenius, longissimus, and semispinalis cervicis and semispinalis capitis muscles.[19] To accommodate the more frontal orientation of the thoracic articular facets, the seventh cervical vertebra makes a transition in its plane of facet motion. Besides having all the characteristics of a typical vertebra, a thoracic vertebra has specific characteristics that distinguish it from a cervical vertebra. Thoracic vertebrae have no uncovertebral joints, bifid spinous processes, or intertransverse foramina. The attachments of the ribs to the thoracic vertebral bodies

□□□□□ □ □ □ □

Table 6–3. Limits and Representative Values of Ranges of Rotation of the Middle and Lower Cervical Spine

Interspace	Combined Flexion-Extension ($\pm x$-axis rotation)		One-Side Lateral Bending (z-axis rotation)		One-Side Axial Rotation (y-axis rotation)	
	Limits of Ranges (degrees)	Representative Angle (degrees)	Limits of Ranges (degrees)	Representative Angle (degrees)	Limits of Ranges (degrees)	Representative Angle (degrees)
Middle						
C2-C3	5–16	10	11–20	10	0–10	3
C3-C4	7–26	15	9–15	11	3–10	7
C4-C5	13–29	20	0–16	11	1–12	7
Lower						
C5-C6	13–29	20	0–16	8	2–12	7
C6-C7	6–26	17	0–17	7	2–10	6
C7-T1	4–7	9	0–17	4	0–7	2

(Data from White and Panjabi.[16])

allow stability at the expense of mobility, with motion of the facet articulations occurring more in the frontal plane. The spinous processes incline inferiorly.[2]

Ribs

The first two ribs are atypical in that they have only one facet. The first rib is the most curved and is usually the shortest rib. This rib slopes obliquely downward and forward from the vertebra toward the sternum. Because of the costovertebral orientation primarily in the transverse plane, movements occur in a superior-inferior direction, with a resultant "pump-handle" effect, with secondary movement in the medial-lateral direction described as "bucket-handle" movement. The second rib is about twice the length of the first but has a similar curvature. The first rib is the site of insertion for the anterior and middle scalene muscles and the site of origin for the subclavius and the first digit of the serratus anterior. The second rib is the site of origin for the serratus anterior and the site of insertion for the posterior scalene and serratus posterior superior muscles.[19]

A typical rib has two articulations with the corresponding vertebra; the costovertebral joint articulates with demifacets on the vertebral bodies, and the costotransverse joint articulates between the rib tubercle and the transverse process of the underlying vertebra. The costovertebral joint is a synovial joint with condyloid movement because the head of the rib is convex and moves on the concave costal facets of the vertebra. The costotransverse joint is a simple synovial joint, which allows a gliding movement. Both of these joints are reinforced by strong ligaments.[19,20]

During breathing, the axis of the costovertebral joints of the upper ribs lies close to the frontal plane, allowing an increase in the anteroposterior diameter of the thorax. Because of the fiber orientation of the scalene muscles superior to the first two ribs, these muscles can elevate these ribs and influence rib motion.[20]

Vertebral Artery

The vertebral artery enters the costotransverse foramen of C6 (sometimes that of C5) and traverses to the axis through the costovertebral foramina of the individual vertebrae. After entering the costotransverse foramen of the atlas, the artery exits and penetrates the atlanto-occipital membrane and dura mater in the region of the foramen magnum at the occiput.[19] Functionally, the vertebral artery is important because the decreased blood supply in the basilar region of the brain stem reduces one of the main blood supplies to the brain. Selecki[21] observed that after 30 degrees of rotation, there is kinking of the contralateral vertebral artery, occurring first as the vertebral artery exits from the transverse foramina. It becomes more marked as the angle of rotation is increased. At 45 degrees of neck rotation, the ipsilateral artery also begins to kink.[21]

Typical neurologic symptoms of vertebrobasilar artery insufficiency include dizziness, tinnitus, visual disturbances, and nausea.[22,23] Occlusion of the vertebral artery may occur either at the suboccipital region or at the C6 level.[24]

Thoracic Inlet

Clinicians usually refer to the thoracic inlet as the thoracic outlet; however, from a strictly anatomic point of view, the thoracic outlet is the opening at the inferior portion of the rib cage and the diaphragm.[19] The thoracic inlet is the superior opening of the rib cage, bounded posteriorly by the first thoracic vertebra, anteriorly by the superior border of the manubrium, and laterally by the first ribs. The structures that pass through the inlet include, centrally, the sternohyoid muscle, sternothyroid muscles, thymus, trachea, esophagus, and thoracic ducts. Behind these ducts and just in front of the vertebral column are the longus colli muscles and the anterior longitudinal ligament. Laterally, the inlet contains the upper lung and neurovascular structures, which join the lowest trunk of the brachial plexus. Within the thoracic inlet, the vagus nerve deserves special attention because this nerve provides parasympathetic innervation to the pharynx and visceral organs.[19] The complex anatomy of the thoracic inlet and the intimate relationship of the bony, soft tissue, and neurovascular structures within the inlet provide multiple opportunities for compression. The term *thoracic inlet* (outlet) *syndrome* refers to the compression of neurovascular structures to include arteries, veins, and/or the upper or lower trunk of the brachial plexus.[25]

■ Musculoskeletal Dysfunction and Trauma

Postural Abnormality

The most common postural deviation affecting the cervical spine is the forward head posture. This posture involves increased kyphosis of the thoracic spine, with resultant increased lordosis of the cervical spine and increased backward bending in the upper cervical complex.[26] Over time, persons with forward head posture adjust their head position and decrease the midcervical lordosis.[27] The increased backward bend of the upper cervical complex results from the body's attempt to keep the eyes horizontal.[17] In doing so, the head is anterior to the vertical plumbline (the ideal postural alignment). This postural deviation puts abnormal stress on the soft tissues and changes the weightbearing surfaces of the vertebrae, especially in the suboccipital and cervicothoracic areas. Forward head posture causes muscle length adaptation, which results in altered biomechanics such that normal motions produce abnormal strain.[28] The muscles most often affected are the levator scapulae, upper trapezius, sternocleidomastoid, scalene, and suboccipital muscles.

Factors contributing to a forward head posture include poor postural habits and pain. We acquire these poor postural habits at a young age when we learn that slumping the upper back requires no energy expenditure. Adolescent girls who are taller and more developed than their peers also develop this posture. In older patients, this posture may be related to working at an incorrect height or in poor lighting. The second factor contributing to this posture is pain. Many patients with chronic cervical pain compensate by thrusting their head forward in an attempt to move away from their pain. Along with a forward head posture, patients present with associated postural changes in the head, neck, trunk, and shoulder region, such as a retruded mandible, rounded shoulders, and protracted scapulae with tight anterior muscles and stretched posterior muscles. Because of this direct relationship between pain and posture, postural correction is an appropriate treatment goal for most patients with chronic cervical pain[28] (Fig. 6–5).

Somatic Dysfunction

By far the most common cervical pathology seen by manual therapists is vertebral motion restriction or somatic dysfunction. The term *somatic dysfunction* is used by the osteopathic profession to refer to altered function of the components of the musculoskeletal system. Many terms such as *loss of joint play*,[29] *chiropractic vertebral subluxa-tion*,[30] *joint dysfunction*,[29] *joint blockage*,[31] and *acute facet lock*[32] describe restrictions of vertebral motion. The osteopathic profession has adopted somatic dysfunction terminology to represent a specific joint restriction in three dimensions. Specifically describing the loss of joint movement by its location in relationship to position or by its lack of movement allows administration of treatment specific to the restriction.[33,34]

Many theories attempt to explain vertebral motion restriction. These theories range from entrapment of the synovial material[35] or a meniscoid,[36] to hypertonic contracted or contractured musculature,[37] to changes in nervous reflex activity such as sympathicotonia[38] or gamma bias,[39] to abnormal stresses on an unguarded spine.[40] To date, no clear scientific evidence exists to explain what causes somatic dysfunction. However, one conceptual model, the biomechanical model, does help explain the clinically observable relationship between two vertebral segments or within a group of vertebral segments. This model conceptually defines the inability of the facet joints to open or close, either individually or bilaterally. This methodology allows consistency for a single examiner between patients and between multiple examiners with the same patient. Probably the most important reason for using this model is that it is an excellent method for distinguishing structural and functional asymmetries.[33] Jull et al.[41] have demonstrated the accuracy of manual diagnosis for determining symptomatic cervical zygapophyseal joint pain syndromes.

According to this manual medicine model, if some pathology interferes with the ability of both the right and the left facet of a given segment to open, that segment will have restriction of forward bending movement. Conversely, if some pathology prevents both facets from closing, there will be backward bending restriction of that segment. If only one facet is unable to open, forward bending movement will be restricted because the facet cannot open, but sidebending movement to the contralateral side will also be limited. In determining segmental vertebral motion, if both facets are functioning symmetrically, the excursion of the paired transverse processes should be symmetric through forward and backward bending.[42]

Cervical Spondylosis

Cervical spondylosis is the result of wear and tear on the weightbearing structures of the cervical spine. This degenerative process is generally considered to occur first in the articular cartilage but is not limited to the cartilage. Bland[43] uses cervical osteoarthritis to describe all joint involvement, including all secondary manifestations in vertebrae, tendons, ligaments, capsules, muscles, and hyaline cartilage, without the overall assumption that the primary disorder begins in the cartilage. This wear-and-tear phenomenon is attributed to repetitive microtraumas to cartilage from sustained impact loading on the

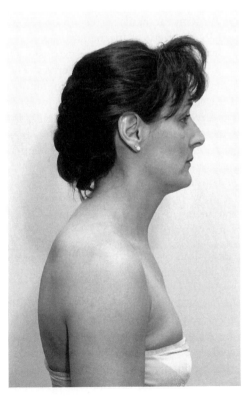

Figure 6–5. The forward head posture.

bone.[43–46] Changes first occur in the deepest, calcified layer of cartilage, where subchondral bone hyperplasia begins as an irregular advance of ossification into the cartilage. This change becomes evident radiographically as increased bone density and sclerosis. At the vascular borders where cartilage, bone, synovium, and periosteum meet, a proliferation of bone formation begins, concentrated at the edges of the articular cartilage. These intra-articular osteophytes grow outward and tend to increase the lateral dimensions of the bone ends, increasing the joint cavity and stretching the capsule. These bony rims may trespass on pain-sensitive structures. These peripheral osteophytes are covered by a layer of fibrocartilage and are larger than they appear on radiographs because of this radiotranslucent covering. Typically, degeneration occurs at the uncovertebral joints (joints of von Luschka), facets, intervertebral disks, vertebral bodies, and hyaline cartilage plates.[17,47]

Rib Dysfunction

Dysfunction of the upper costovertebral joints may cause pain in the cervical spine in the posterior triangle region. Greenman[20] stated that the first and second ribs, being atypical, can contribute to pain in the cervicothoracic region. Costovertebral motion allows both pump-handle and a bucket-handle movement, as described earlier. If the first and second ribs cannot complete a normal range of motion, several patterns of restriction are possible. The most common dysfunctions are inhalation and exhalation restrictions. If the first rib is not able to complete its anteroposterior range of motion, the motion of all the underlying ribs will be restricted. Most often a rib becomes dysfunctional as a result of the position assumed when a thoracic vertebra is asymmetrically restricted. The result is a slight rotation of a rib, with rotation of the corresponding thoracic vertebra secondary to its inability to follow the rib in a straight plane. With rotation of the thoracic vertebra, the rib also rotates because of the attachment of the ligaments and intercostal muscles above and below the rib. If the vertebra remains rotated, soft tissue around the rib will compensate and adapt to this abnormal position so that the rib becomes hypomobile. If motion is restored to the vertebra, the rib may not return to its normal position because of this soft tissue adaptation. This situation is called torsional rib dysfunction.[34]

The first rib can also subluxate superiorly because there are no structures above it to limit its superior excursion. This dysfunction can contribute to myriad symptoms including cervicothoracic pain, difficulty with deep breathing, restricted cervical rotation and sidebending, and possibly the numbness, tingling, and vascular complaints seen with thoracic inlet syndrome. Often the fibromyositis described in the upper trapezius muscle is accompanied by dysfunction of the first and second ribs.

Thoracic Inlet Syndrome

As mentioned earlier, thoracic outlet syndrome should be termed thoracic inlet syndrome to be anatomically correct in describing the superior opening of the thoracic cavity. This syndrome includes a multitude of symptoms involving the neck and upper extremities that are believed to be caused by proximal compression of the subclavian artery and vein and the brachial plexus. Probable etiologies for compression of the neurovascular structures include a cervical rib, a subluxated first thoracic rib, a shortened anterior scalene muscle, and anomalous fibromuscular bands. Other structures that can be involved in compression are any bony or soft tissue abnormality including malunion of a fractured clavicle, Pancoast's tumor of the apex of the lung, altered posture, tight pectoralis minor muscles, and anomalous thoracic vertebral transverse processes. Secondary causes associated with thoracic inlet syndrome include trauma, occupational stress, obesity, and pendulous breasts.[25]

Vertebrobasilar Insufficiency

The vertebrobasilar arterial system supplies the spinal cord, meninges and nerve roots, plexuses, muscles, and joints of the cervical spine. Intracranially, the basilar portion supplies the medulla, cerebellum, and vestibular nuclei.[19] This arterial system can be compromised at several points during its course: as it passes through the transverse foramina of the upper six cervical vertebrae; as it winds around the articular pillar of the atlas; as it pierces the posterior OA membrane; or as it enters the foramen magnum to unite with the basilar artery. Blood flow can be diminished by a variety of mechanical disorders, which can be classified as either intrinsic or extrinsic. The most common intrinsic disorder is atherosclerosis. The basilar artery is the most commonly affected component, followed by the cervical portion of the vertebral artery. Usually seen as a complication of atherosclerosis, thrombosis of the vertebrobasilar arteries can result from an embolus that usually lodges in the distal branches of the system, particularly the posterior cerebral artery.[17]

An extrinsic disorder compromises a blood vessel, restricting flow by compressing its external wall and thereby narrowing its lumen. This compression can result from the following:

1. An anomalous origin of the vertebral artery from the subclavian, causing the vertebral artery to be kinked and occluded during rotation of the neck.
2. Constriction of the vertebral artery by bands of the deep cervical fascia during rotation of the neck.
3. An anomalous divagation of the vertebral artery from its course through muscle and transverse foramina of the vertebrae, or compression or angulation caused by projecting osteophytes. The most com-

mon site of compression is at the C5-C6 level, with a lower incidence at the C6-C7 level.

When this system is compromised, patients present with nystagmus, vertigo, blurred vision, giddiness, nausea, pallor, dysphagia, pupil dilation, and cervical pain.[17,22,23] Because compromise of the vertebral artery can occur both in the craniovertebral region and in the area where the artery passes through the transverse foramen, all patients presenting with cervical pain should be screened for vertebrobasilar artery insufficiency. Manual therapists emphasize the need to test this system in patients with upper cervical complaints; however, serious compromise can also occur with damage to the middle and lower cervical regions.[17,24,48] A vertebral artery test for assessing vertebrobasilar insufficiency, described under the objective portion of the examination, must always be performed before any manual therapy of the cervical spine is attempted.

Cervical Disk

Cervical disk disease may cause symptoms similar to those of facet involvement and/or neurologic signs caused by root or cord compression. The typical history involves insidious onset after performing a relatively minor physical activity or maintaining a prolonged position—for example, taking a long car trip, sleeping in an uncomfortable hotel bed, holding the phone with one's shoulder, or working overhead. The pain is usually unilateral and may be felt anywhere in the cervical or scapular area.[45,46,49]

Cloward[50] described the typical referred pain pattern of cervical disk involvement. The pain usually starts in the cervical area and then diminishes and quickly extends to the scapula, shoulder, upper arm, and then possibly the forearm and hand.[50] The symptoms of a cervical disk lesion are provoked in a manner similar to those in a restricted facet joint, in that certain cervical movements are painful and others are pain-free; however, the pattern of painful and pain-free movements does not follow the pattern for a restricted joint.[51]

Painful or restricted neck movements may be intermittent over several months. Initially, the patient may experience only a paresthesia, but when the nerve root becomes involved, the pain is more defined and can be reproduced with extreme neck movement. Sustained holding of these neck positions will exacerbate arm paresthesia and pain.[43,45] Clinical presentation of root involvement has been described as acute radiculopathy from a posterolateral bulging disk, an acute disk extrusion, or an exacerbation or preexisting trespass in patients with radiographic evidence of spondylosis. Besides nerve root symptoms, the tendon reflex may be depressed or absent, or muscle weakness within the myotome may exist. If the disk material is extruded and occupies enough of the spinal canal to put pressure on the cord, the patient may show myelopathic signs such as spasticity, a positive plantar response, clonus, and spastic quadriparesis or paraparesis.[46]

Trauma

All patients presenting with a history of trauma to the cervical region should have radiographs performed to rule out any fractures. Aside from fractures, discussion of which is beyond the scope of this chapter, a common clinical presentation of patients with cervical trauma is the *whiplash syndrome*. This term was introduced to describe the total involvement of the patient with whiplash injury and its effects.[32,52,53] The typical mechanism of injury involves flexion-extension injuries of the cervical spine that result from sudden acceleration and deceleration collision forces on a vehicle in which the patient is riding. The magnitude of this collision force is determined by the mass of the vehicle and its rate of change of velocity. The shorter the impact time, the greater the rate of change of velocity or acceleration. As the acceleration becomes greater, the force of the impact likewise increases. The faster a vehicle is moving at the time of impact, the greater the impact forces.[54]

A head-on collision causes deceleration injuries, with the head and neck moving first into hyperflexion and terminating when the chin touches the chest. Following Newton's third law, after hyperflexion the head and cervical spine rebound into extension. These reciprocal flexion-extension movements continue until the forces are finally dissipated.

Side-on collisions cause lateral flexion of the cervical spine, with movement ceasing as the ear hits the shoulder. In rear-end collisions the car accelerates forward, causing the front seat to be pushed into the trunk of the occupant. This force causes the trunk to be thrust forward. The unrestrained head stays at rest, moving into relative backward bending as the trunk moves forward. This backward bending of the head and cervical spine continues until the occiput strikes the headrest or the thoracic spine. Many patients describe the impact as being so great that their car seat was broken, or their glasses or dentures were thrown into the back seat, or the movement into hyperextension was so great that they came to rest facing the rear of the vehicle. Rebound into flexion occurs after the car stops accelerating and is complemented by contraction of the flexor muscles.[54]

The amount of actual damage to anatomic structures depends on the position of the head in space at the time of impact, the forces generated, and the histologic makeup of the tissues. In experimental studies simulating rear-end automobile accidents, the following lesions occurred:

1. Tearing of the sternocleidomastoid and longissimus colli muscles
2. Pharyngeal edema and retropharyngeal hematoma

3. Hemorrhage of the muscular layers of the esophagus
4. Damage to the cervical sympathetic plexus
5. Tearing of the anterior longitudinal ligament
6. Separation of the cartilaginous endplate of the intervertebral disk
7. Tears of the facet joint capsules
8. Hemorrhage about the cervical nerve roots and spinal cord, with possible cerebral injury

The extent of damage seen in hyperflexion (head-on collision) injuries is similar. Damage can include tears of the posterior cervical musculature, sprains of the ligamentum nuchae and posterior longitudinal ligament, facet joint disruption, and posterior intervertebral disk injury with nerve root hemorrhage.[17,54]

Depending on the magnitude and direction of forces at the time of impact, patients may present with any combination of these hyperflexion and hyperextension injuries, as well as damage to the thoracic, lumbar, and temporomandibular joint (TMJ) regions. Whiplash symptoms usually begin within 24 hours after the accident. The patient may describe headache, posterior neck pain, and referred scapular pain. Pain may radiate down the arm, mimicking thoracic inlet syndrome. Other complaints include upper thoracic and pectoral pain, weakness, dysphagia, dyspnea, TMJ dysfunction, and cerebral complaints such as insomnia, fatigue, nervousness, tenseness, decreased concentration span and memory, and hyperirritability. Many patients describe dizziness, which may be associated with a high-frequency hearing loss. They may also have tinnitus and visual disturbances.[17] Because of the complexity of this syndrome, if these patients are not evaluated thoroughly and treated appropriately, they may develop postural adaptations, psychogenic overlay, and chronic manifestation of any of the above symptoms.

Myofascial Pain Syndrome

Myofascial pain disorders are not well understood because of the use of a variety of terms to describe similar clinical findings. The different terms used may have the same, similar, or totally different meanings. *Myofascial pain syndrome*, also referred to as *myofascial syndrome* and *myofascitis*, involves pain and/or autonomic responses referred from active myofascial trigger points with associated dysfunction. Other terms such as *myositis, fibrositis, myalgia*, and *fibromyositis* have multiple meanings.[55] Some authors use these terms to identify myofascial trigger points; others use them to label clinical manifestations.[56] To avoid further confusion, the definition of myofascial pain syndrome used here refers to the trigger point, as described by Travell and Simons.[56] A myofascial trigger point is a hyperirritable spot, usually within a taut band of skeletal muscle or in the muscle's fascia, that is painful on compression and that can give rise to characteristic referred pain, tenderness, and autonomic phenomena. Normal muscle does not have these trigger points.[56]

A clinical manifestation of myofascial trigger points is a typical referred pain pattern from the trigger point. On examination, findings include a local spot tenderness (the trigger point) and a palpably tense band of muscle fibers within a shortened and weak muscle. The trigger point may also respond to rapid changes in pressure; this has been described as the pathognomonic local twitch response. Direct pressure over a trigger point will reproduce the referred pain patterns. Travell and Simons[56] contend that a myofascial trigger point begins with muscular strain and later becomes a site of sensitized nerves, increased local metabolism, and reduced circulation. A myofascial trigger point is to be distinguished from a trigger point in other tissues such as skin, ligament, and periosteum. Myofascial trigger points are classified as either active or latent. An active trigger point causes pain, whereas a latent trigger point causes restriction of movement and weakness of the affected muscle and may persist for years after apparent recovery from an injury. However, a latent trigger point is predisposed to acute attacks of pain because minor overstretching, overuse, or chilling of the muscle may cause a latent trigger point to become active. This symptomatology is not found in normal muscle.[56]

Referred Pain

Pain that is perceived in a location other than its origin is termed *referred pain*.[57] Nearly all pain is referred pain. It is referred segmentally, as in a dermatomal distribution, or is specific to the tissue involved, as in left upper extremity pain with myocardial infarction. Recognition of the embryologic derivation of tissues from the same somite is important in identifying many of the segmentally referred pain patterns. For example, as the upper limb bud grows, it draws the lower cervical and upper thoracic segments out into itself. Thus, the scapula and its muscles are derived from the middle and lower cervical segments, whereas the skin overlying the scapula and ribs is formed from the thoracic segments; therefore, pain perceived in the upper posterior thoracic region may have a cervical origin. Also, tissues other than visceral organs may have a specific reference pattern of pain that cannot be ascribed to a segmental distribution.[51] Most practitioners are familiar with patients who complain of suboccipital headache and describe a reference pattern to the frontal region of the cranium.

Although clinical expectation is based on the assumption that a somatic nerve goes to a specific anatomic region, pain in that peripheral distribution can only be due to abnormalities of the spinal segment associated with that nerve. This assumption may be true; however, other pain patterns have been identified. Miller[58] suggested that pain does not really occur in the hands, feet, or head, but rather in the patient's conscious image of his or her hands, feet, or head. This theory suggests that pain and referred pain are central phenomena. A classic example is the phantom pain experienced by some amputees. Supporting this idea of referred pain as a central phenomenon, Harman[59] found that anginal pain referred to the left arm was not abolished by a complete brachial plexus block with local anesthesia. Referred pain has been evoked experimentally in areas previously anesthetized by regional nerve block.[60] Bourdillon[61] suggests that the central mechanism involves both the spinal cord and higher centers.

According to Cyriax,[51] if pain is segmentally referred, a lesion at a cervical level will produce pain in all or part of that cervical dermatome. For example, a C5 nerve root compression may produce pain in the neck, midneck, shoulder, and/or lateral upper arm. All these areas are supplied by the C5 dermatome. Although this relationship appears clear-cut, some research and clinical experience show that the pain reference appears to be segmental in nature yet does not always correspond to dermatome or myotome distributions.[17,62–64] Because some referred pain patterns are not easily ascribed to particular segments, the clinician must perform a detailed, specific examination to determine the source of the pain. Experienced therapists are familiar with specific reference patterns that have several separate possible sources. An example is the clinical presentation of unilateral pain along the trapezial ridge (yoke area), which may be produced by dysfunction of the OA joint, the C4-C5 segment, or the joints of the first rib. Treatment of these dysfunctions may relieve the symptoms; however, any two or all three sites may have to be treated before the signs and symptoms are eliminated.[61] Dwyer et al.[65] produced pain patterns from the cervical zygapophyseal joints in normal volunteers, which further substantiates the view that the cervical joints are sources of referred pain. Feinstein et al.[60] described patients with frontal headache referred from the OA joint.

Some general characteristics of segmentally referred pain are that the pain is usually referred distally from the cervical spine; the pain never crosses the midline; and the extent of the pain is controlled by the size of the dermatome and the location of the tissue involved. A tissue that does not follow segmental reference is the dura mater. Again considering the C5 dermatome, a lesion at the nerve root level can result in a larger dermatomal reference pattern than a lesion of a C5-derived tissue at the shoulder level.[51] A lesion at the cervical level may cause pain anywhere from the head to the midthorax, and the pain often pervades several dermatomal levels. Symptoms are usually central or unilateral[51,57] (Fig. 6–6).

Other Pathologies

This discussion of cervical pathologies is by no means all-inclusive; other pathologies of nonmusculoskeletal origin can also elicit cervical pain. Some of these disorders, if not recognized, can have serious consequences. The clinical picture seen in these disorders differs significantly from symptoms of musculoskeletal origin. These differences

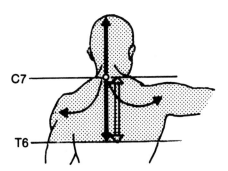

Figure 6–6. Extrasegmental reference of the dura mater.

include the presence of night pain, as seen with metastatic disease; cord signs such as Lhermitte's sign, the positive plantar response, and ankle clonus, as seen in myelopathies; nuchal rigidity, as seen in spinal meningitis or subarachnoid hemorrhage; and brachial plexus tension signs, as seen in brachial plexus neuritis or stretch injuries. Unrelenting, pulsating pain may be seen in a patient with an aortic aneurysm. Patients with advanced rheumatoid arthritis may present with the neck in the characteristic "cocked robin" position because of unilateral subluxation of the AA joint. Systemic infections may enlarge the lymph nodes and cause neck pain, as seen in sinusitis, pharyngitis, otitis media, mediastinitis, and dental abscess. Other symptoms not usually seen with pain of musculoskeletal origin include unrelenting pain, severe symptoms after a trivial insult, and neurologic symptoms including blurred vision, visual field deficit, and loss of motor control.[66,67]

■ History and Physical Examination

Patient History

The importance of careful and precise history taking cannot be overemphasized. The clinician will ultimately base a treatment plan on the patient's presenting signs and symptoms. The history should always precede the evaluation because areas of emphasis during the examination will be determined by the history. Hoppenfeld[68] stated that this selective examination, based on a good history, produces the highest yield of information about clinical disease in the shortest time.

Asking concise, clinically relevant questions is a far more complex skill than the actual techniques of physical examination. Learning how to ask those questions by reading textbooks or listening to lectures is difficult. Good history taking is both an art and a science. A closed-end question asks for a yes or no answer. Many practitioners, in an attempt to hurry the interview, will guide the patient in answering by the way they ask the questions. A yes or no response may reflect only a portion of what the patient may really want to say. The questioning process should use open-ended rather than closed-ended questions to allow the patient to answer in his or her own words. Instead of asking, "Do you have pain?" the question could be phrased as "Where do you have discomfort?" The second question requires the patient to formulate his or her own answer and will probably yield more useful information than the first question. This approach helps keep the examiner from jumping to conclusions and forces the examiner to attend to the patient as a person rather than as a disease entity.

While taking the history and performing the evaluation, the clinician should record the findings in a format that is easy to interpret and familiar to other health professions. The "subjective, objective, assessment, and plan" (SOAP) note format meets these criteria. It can be used for initial evaluations, progress notes, and discharge summaries. Although notes are important for communicating with other professionals, this record is also invaluable to the clinician as a quick reference on each patient.

The patient's chief complaint or complaints should be documented carefully. Initially, the patient should be allowed to tell his or her own story for several minutes without interruption; otherwise, important details may be pushed aside in his or her mind. The clinician may then need to guide the patient's comments with a question such as "How did your neck problem begin?" to get a chronologic picture of the symptoms. The clinician needs to ask open-ended questions to find out important details about the symptoms such as the time of day they occur, the location of the pain, and the relation of symptoms to other events. In evaluating the cervical and upper thoracic spine, the clinician should follow the general rule of evaluating the joints above and below the joint being examined and should ask the patient questions concerning the cranium, TMJ, and shoulder. The actual analysis of the patient's symptoms follows a logical sequence for any musculoskeletal evaluation.

Identifying the Patient's Complaints

Identifying the patient's cervical complaint is a logical introduction to establishing rapport between the therapist and the patient. Documenting the chief complaint includes noting the location of the symptoms and how the patient describes the symptoms.[69] The total area in which the patient has pain needs to be documented. Therefore, the area and depth of symptoms should be mapped out on a body chart for future reference. The patient should also be questioned about the nature of the pain. Typically, superficial electric shock-like pain is from a dermatomal reference; deep, aching, diffuse pain may be from either a myotomal or a sclerotomal reference.[51] Upper extremity numbness or tingling may help pinpoint the involvement of a specific nerve root.

Present History

The patient's current history needs to be established before the past history. The examiner should consider the precipitating factors related to the onset of current symptoms. Again, the patient should have the opportunity to say what he or she thinks may have caused the problem before the clinician begins systematic questioning. If a specific injury occurred, the clinician should try to determine the exact mechanism of injury. The clinician should also ask about the onset (whether immediate or delayed) and the degree of pain. This information will assist in implicating specific tissues. For example, injured muscle or vascular tissue will cause immediate pain, whereas injury to noncontractile structures may cause delayed onset of symptoms.[70] This information will allow the clinician to focus on what special tests should be performed during the examination.

Behavior of Symptoms

Asking the patient to describe his or her symptoms over a 24-hour period is valuable in establishing what activities aggravate or relieve the symptoms and how long the symptoms last. It also provides a baseline for future comparison. The clinician needs to know about the frequency and duration of the patient's symptoms (i.e., whether they are constant or intermittent). If dysfunction is present, specific movements should exacerbate or relieve the symptoms and rest should decrease them. Answers to the clinician's questions will reveal what positions, movements, and activities exacerbate or relieve symptoms and provide additional information about the nature of the problem, the tissue source of irritation, and the severity of the condition. If rest does not relieve the symptoms and the patient describes them as constant and unrelenting, the cause of the problem may not be musculoskeletal.

Past History

If the patient has experienced similar symptoms in the past, that information is vital to the examiner. Clear information about the frequency and onset of symptoms, the recovery period, and the treatment of previous episodes will help establish the correct diagnosis and treatment plan. Other details of the patient's past medical history such as cardiac problems, trauma, and surgeries, and bony pathologies such as arthritis and osteoporosis, may also be pertinent and affect treatment plans. The patient's social history is also an important consideration (Fig. 6–7).

Review of Systems

The patient's current symptoms can be easily influenced by visceral or neurologic involvement; therefore, the clini-

Symptom	Yes	No	Comments
1. Fever/chills/sweats	——	——	
2. Unexplained weight loss	——	——	
3. Fatigue/malaise	——	——	
4. Change in physical features	——	——	
5. Bruising/bleeding	——	——	
6. Vertigo/dizziness	——	——	
7. Dyspnea	——	——	
8. Nausea/vomiting	——	——	
9. Change in bowel habits	——	——	
10. Dysuria	——	——	
11. Urinary frequency changes	——	——	
12. Numbness/tingling	——	——	
13. Night pain	——	——	
14. Syncope	——	——	
15. Weakness	——	——	
16. Sexual dysfunction	——	——	
17. History of smoking	——	——	
18. History of substance abuse	——	——	
19. History of illness	——	——	
20. History of surgery	——	——	
21. Medications	——	——	
22. Family medical history	——	——	
23. Change in lifestyle	——	——	

Figure 6–7. Review of systems.

cian needs to ask questions concerning gastrointestinal function, including recent weight loss, abdominal pain, change in bowel habits, or blood in the stool. Questions dealing with the genitourinary system include asking about polyuria, dysuria, blood in the urine, or problems with sexual function or menses. Questions pertaining to the cardiopulmonary systems include asking about ease of breathing, coughing, palpitations, hemoptysis, and chest pain. To rule out central nervous system disorders, the clinician should ask about lack of coordination, seizures, dizziness, tremors, and headaches (Fig. 6–7).

All the above information will give the practitioner a general idea about the patient's cervical problems. However, some specific questions will not only give information about the problem but also help rule out more serious pathologies.

1. Is the patient experiencing any headaches? Several disorders can cause headache. However, headaches from cervical spine problems usually present with specific referral patterns. Problems at the first cervical level usually cause headaches in a characteristic pattern at the base and top of the head. The second cervical level tends to refer ipsilateral pain retro-orbitally in the temporal region. Lower cervical problems will frequently refer to the base of the occiput.[70]

2. Is the patient experiencing dizziness, especially on rotation or extension of the spine? These symptoms may be due to vertebral artery occlusion or inner ear

disorders.[71] Disorders of the cervical spine can also cause vertigo.[72]

3. Is the patient experiencing bilateral numbness or tingling of the hands or feet? Bilateral symptoms should lead the therapist to suspect either a large space-occupying lesion pressing on the spinal cord or a systemic disorder causing neuropathies, such as diabetes or alcohol abuse.[66]

4. Does the patient experience difficulty in swallowing? Anterior space-occupying lesions can cause retropharyngeal compromise. With a history of trauma, swelling may be the space-occupying lesion.[66,67]

5. Does the patient experience any electric shock-like pain? If the head is flexed and the patient experiences such pain down the spine, the therapist should consider the possibility of inflammation or irritation of the meninges (Lhermitte's sign).[49,66]

6. What kind of pillow does the patient sleep on? Cervical symptoms are often increased when a foam or very firm pillow is used, as a result of loss of cervical lordosis or abnormal pressure placed against the neck caused by lack of support.[17]

■ Objective Testing

Besides the upper quarter screening examination (Table 6–4), the clinician needs specific objective information about the cervical spine. This information allows the prac-

□□□□□ □ □ □

Table 6–4. Upper Quarter Screening Examination

Standing
  Posture
  Gait
  Reverse hands overhead
  Hands behind back
Sitting
  Vital signs (temperature, pulse, blood pressure)
  Observation of lips, nails, hair, lesions
  Head
    Eyes—observation, acuity, visual fields, pupillary reaction,
      near reaction
    Ears—observation, palpation, acuity
    Nose—observation, breathing, sinuses, smell
    Mouth—gums, teeth, tongue, gag reflex
  Neck
    Observation
    Soft tissue and lymph node palpation
    Salivary glands
    Carotid pulses
    Trachea/thyroid gland
  Upper extremity
    Skin
    Pulses
    Lymph node—epitrochlear
    Muscle tone/definition
  Thorax
    Breathing/respiration
    Axillary lymph nodes
    Auscultation/palpation/percussion
  Temporomandibular joint
    Open/close/lateral movement
    Jaw reflex

Cervical spine
  Active range of motion
    Rotation
    Sidebending
    Flexion
    Backward bending
    Quadrant
  Compression/distraction
  Resisted motions (all three planes)
Scapula
  Active elevation/protraction/retraction/depression
  Resisted elevation
Shoulder/elbow/wrist/hand
  Active range of motion
  Overpressure
Neurologic
  Resisted myotomes
    Shoulder abduction C5-C6 (axillary nerve)
    Elbow flexion C5-C6 (musculocutaneous nerve)
    Elbow extension C7 (radial nerve)
    Wrist extension C6 (radial/ulnar nerves)
    Thumb extension C8 (radial nerve)
    Finger abduction/adduction T1 (radial/median
      nerves)
  Reflexes
    Muscle stretch reflexes
      Biceps C5-C6
      Brachioradialis C6
      Triceps C7
    Pathologic (Hoffmann's)
  Cutaneous sensation
Supine
  Palpation
  Passive mobility testing C-spine
  Inhalation/exhalation rib cage testing

titioner to confirm the subjective findings and identify the area causing the patient's symptoms. Further, more specialized objective testing will help isolate the structure or structures at fault. As mentioned in the section on patient history, according to the upper quarter screen format, the TMJ, shoulder, and thoracic spine joints should be cleared during the cervical spine examination. The neurologic examination should include muscle stretch reflexes; sensation testing incorporating light touch, pinprick, and two-point discrimination; and specific muscle testing if weakness was found in the screening examination. The following special tests should be performed only if warranted by the patient's history or findings during the upper quarter screen (Table 6–5).

Range-of-Motion Assessment

Observation of active cervical range of motion will give the clinician a general impression of movement dysfunc-

tion. For example, active sidebending that is restricted in the first few degrees from neutral position suggests a restriction in the upper cervical complex. In contrast, restriction at the end range of sidebending suggests a restriction in the mid- to lower cervical region.[73] If active movements are full and pain-free, introduce overpressure to stress the structures further to clear that specific range of motion.

When there is restriction in range of motion, establishing an objective and reliable baseline assessment of the limitation of motion is important. Objective measurement of active range of motion of the neck can be obtained through a variety of techniques including electrogoniometers, bubble and gravity goniometers, protractors, radiographs, and computed tomography.[74] Some of these techniques are more readily available and easier to use than others and have high reliability. One technique that meets all three of these criteria is the CROM (Cervical

□□□□□ □ □   □

Table 6–5. Schematic for Objective Examination of the Cervical and Upper Thoracic Spine

Range-of-Motion Tests	Special Tests	Thoracic Inlet Syndrome Tests
Active ROM of cervical and upper thoracic spine	Cervical distraction	Adson's
Functional occipitoatlantal range of motion	Cervical compression	Costoclavicular
Functional atlantoaxial range of motion	Vertebral artery	Hyperabduction

Foraminal closure
    Upper cervical
    Mid- and lower cervical
	Layer palpation
	    Transverse process
	    Spatial orientation, upper
	        thoracic spine
	    Trigger points
		3-Minute elevated arm exercise

Passive mobility
    Translation occipitoatlantal, atlantoaxial, midcervical
    Transverse process positioning through flexion/
        extension in upper thoracic spine
    Spring testing or ribs
	Neurologic examination
	    Motor testing
	    Sensation testing
	    Muscle stretch reflexes	

Active respiratory motion	Radiographs	

Range of Motion Device) (see Fig. 6–8). The CROM is a plastic device which is fixed to the patient's head and aligned according to the three planes of movement. Sagittal and frontal plane motions are measured using gravity goniometers. The transverse plane measurement involves a compass goniometer and a shoulder-mounted magnetic yoke.[74] Several studies have addressed the reliability of the CROM and found it to be satisfactory.[75,76] The CROM has also been used to establish normal cervical range-of-motion values (see Table 6–6).

Functional Active Testing

Several combined active movements can alert the practitioner to regions of the cervical spine that may be restricted. For example, in assessing the movement of the upper cervical spine, the OA joint can be tested grossly by fully rotating the cervical spine and asking the patient to nod his or her head while the clinician looks for asymmetric movement between the two sides (Fig. 6–9 A,B). A gross test of the AA joint consists of asking the patient to sidebend as far as possible and, while sidebent, to rotate the head in the opposite direction; the clinician looks for restricted movement (R. Erhard, personal communication) (Fig. 6–10). To test motion in the midcervical spine, ask the patient to sidebend the head and, while maintaining that range, to introduce flexion and extension. These tests only tell the practitioner whether further mobility testing is required.

Foraminal Closure Tests

Combined cervical rotation and sidebending to the same side together with extension narrows the intervertebral

foramen and puts the mid- and lower cervical facet joints in the closed-packed position.[4,40,73] If this maneuver reproduces the patient's symptoms (i.e., neck, interscapular, or upper arm pain), the cervical spine is implicated (Fig. 6–11). With respect to referred pain, the more distally the pain is referred from the cervical spine, the neck is held in normal lordosis while the patient actively bends the upper cervical complex backward and maintains that position[73] (Fig. 6–12). If the patient's symptoms are reproduced, the test is positive.

Cervical Compression/ Distraction Tests

The cervical compression test is performed by placing the head in slight flexion and sidebending and exerting a downward compressive force through the head[68] (Fig. 6–13). To further test the integrity of bony and soft tissue relationships, place the neck into a combined movement pattern of sidebending, extension, and rotation in the same direction and exert a compression force. This variation is done if the first procedure has not produced any symptoms. If no symptoms are produced by placing the neck in a closed-packed position and then exerting a compression force, the clinician can be satisfied that no major musculoskeletal pathology exists. By approximating the articular surfaces, the compression test assesses foraminal patency and joint relationships. If a motion segment loses its normal anatomic spatial relationships, pain-sensitive tissue may be compromised. Therefore, the compression test is positive if this maneuver elicits articular or neural signs. Conversely, a distraction force, which separates the joint surfaces and stretches the adjacent soft tissues,

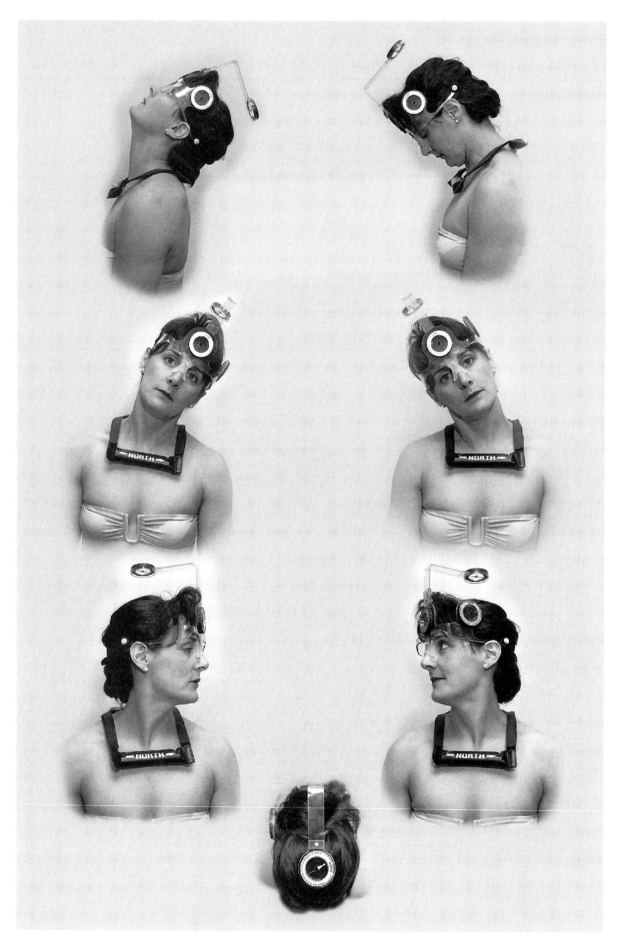

Figure 6–8. Active cervical range of motion using the CROM device.

□□□□□□ □ □

Table 6-6. Normal Values of Cervical Range of Motion Using the CROM

Age	Flexion	Extension	Lateral Flexion	Rotation
10	67	86	49	76
20	64	81	46	72
30	61	76	43	68
40	58	71	40	65
50	55	66	36	62
60	52	62	33	58
70	49	58	30	55
80	46	54	27	52
90	43	49	24	49

should decrease symptoms from a tissue that was being compromised by compression. A cervical distraction test is performed by having the seated patient lean against the clinician, who stands behind the patient. The clinician slightly grasps the patient's head over the mastoid processes and, while maintaining the head and neck in a neutral position, lifts the patient's head so that the patient's body weight provides the distraction. This distraction test is positive when the patient's symptoms are decreased[70] (Fig. 6–14).

Vertebral Artery Test

Provocative testing of vertebrobasilar sufficiency is necessary if the head is going to be moved through extremes of motion. The vertebral artery should be tested in both a weightbearing and a nonweightbearing position.[24] The weightbearing position is done with the patient seated; place the patient's head in a neutral position and have the patient actively rotate the head to both sides (Fig. 6–15). If no symptoms are produced, place the head and neck in extension and have the patient go through active rotation. If active movement does not produce symptoms, the examiner slowly moves the head passively, asking the patient to report any symptoms experienced during the test. The nonweightbearing test is performed with the patient supine and the head supported by the examiner off the edge of the table. From this position, the head is passively extended and rotated to either side (Fig. 6–16). This position of extension and rotation is maintained for 10 to 15 seconds while the examiner observes the patient's eye movements (nystagmus) and looks for asymmetric pupil changes. Patient reports of any unusual sensations such as dizziness, giddiness, lightheadedness, or visual changes are also positive test findings.[1,24] A variation of

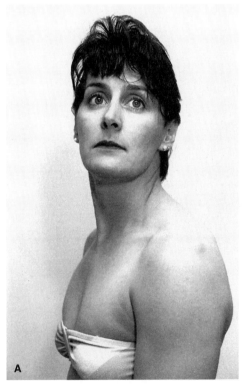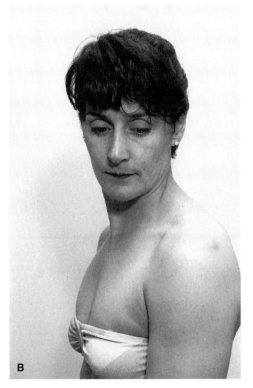

Figure 6-9. Functional active testing of the occipitoatlantal joint. A, extension; B, flexion.

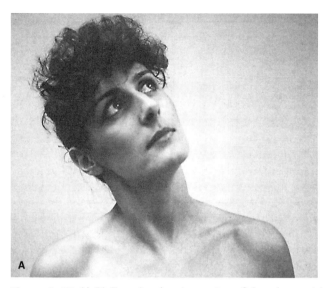

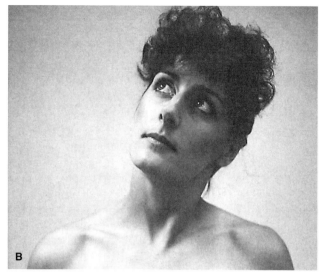

Figure 6–10. (A,B) Functional active testing of the atlantoaxial joint.

this test is to have the patient count backward out loud. If the patient has diminished blood flow, he or she will usually stop talking before other symptoms are manifested.

Upper Limb Tension Test

Elvey[77] demonstrated on cadavers during autopsy that movement of and tension on cervical nerve roots, their investing sheaths, and the dura occur with movement of the arm in certain planes. The maximum tension on the brachial plexus and on C5, C6, and C7 nerve root complexes occurs with glenohumeral joint horizontal abduc-

tion and external rotation, elbow and wrist extension, forearm supination, shoulder girdle depression, and side-bending of the cervical spine to the opposite side. Butler[78] advocated the use of four upper limb tension tests (ULTTs):

1. ULTT1—median nerve dominant tension test using shoulder abduction

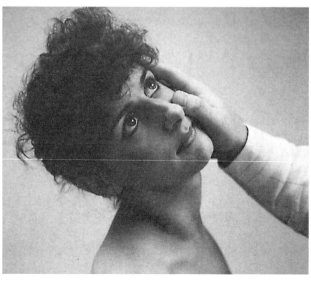

Figure 6–11. Mid- and lower cervical foraminal closure test.

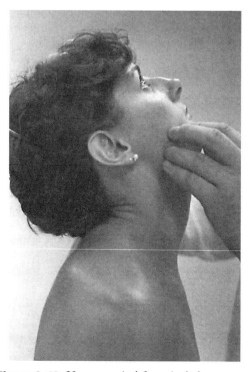

Figure 6–12. Upper cervical foraminal closure test.

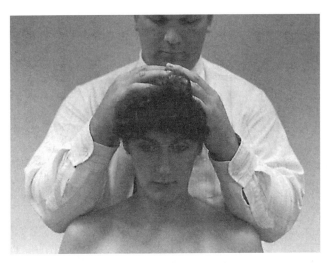

Figure 6–13. Cervical compression test.

2. ULTT2a—median nerve dominant tension test using shoulder girdle depression and external rotation of the shoulder
3. ULTT2b—radial nerve dominant tension test using shoulder girdle depression and internal rotation of the shoulder
4. ULTT3—ulnar nerve dominant tension test using shoulder abduction and elbow flexion

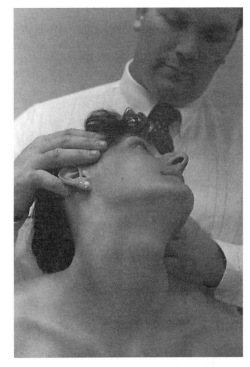

Figure 6–15. Weightbearing vertebral artery test.

The tension tests are powerful nervous system tensioning maneuvers that bias to a particular nerve trunk. The ULTT1 positions the patient supine, with the shoulder girdle held in neutral position, the arm abducted to 110 degrees, the forearm supinated, and the wrist and fingers extended. The shoulder is externally rotated, and then the elbow is extended. With this position maintained, cervical sidebending first away from and then toward the limb being tested are added (Fig. 6–17). Margarey[79] reported that in performing this test, when sidebending of the neck was toward the side of the arm

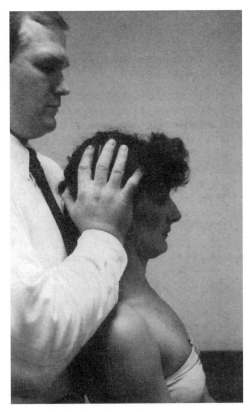

Figure 6–14. Cervical distraction test.

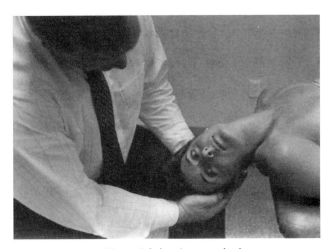

Figure 6–16. Nonweightbearing vertebral artery test.

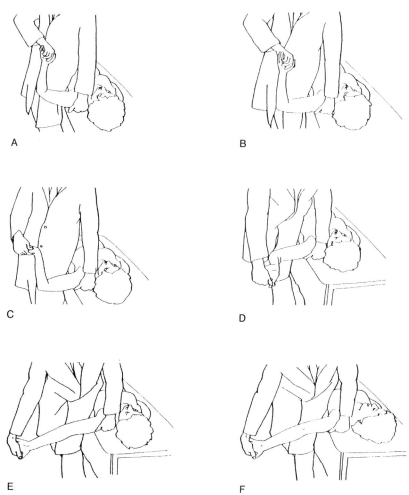

A

B

C

D

E

F

Figure 6–17. (A–F) Upper limb tension test (ULTT1). (From Butler,[78] with permission.)

being tested, the patient's symptoms decreased 70 percent of the time. This test assists the clinician in identifying the source of vague or recalcitrant shoulder or upper arm pain. If this maneuver reproduces the patient's arm pain, the test can be broken down into its parts to see which component actually insults the brachial plexus.[78,80]

ULTT2a is a predominantly median nerve bias tension test. The patient lies supine, with the scapula free of the table. The examiner's thigh rests against the patient's elbow. The patient's shoulder girdle is depressed, the shoulder is abducted 10 degrees, the elbow is extended, and then the arm is externally rotated. The position is maintained, and the patient's wrist/fingers/thumb are extended. The most common sensitizing addition is shoulder abduction (Fig. 6–18).

The ULTT2b radial nerve bias test has the same starting position as the ULTT2a test; the difference consists of adding internal rotation of the entire arm (also involving forearm pronation). At this point, the position is held while the patient's wrist is flexed, followed by thumb flexion and ulnar deviation (Fig. 6–19).

The ULTT3 is an ulnar nerve biased tension test. ULTT3 differs from ULTT1 and 2 in that it introduces

elbow flexion followed by wrist/finger extension[78] (Fig. 6–20).

Passive Mobility Testing

Besides the physical examination of the cervical spine, the clinician needs to assess passive motion from a manual medicine viewpoint. To understand the passive movement of the cervical spine, a review of spinal mechanics is appropriate.

Vertebral motion is described by facet function; however, the intervertebral disk and soft tissues also participate in motion. The available motion was described by Fryette[81] in terms of three basic laws of motion. The first law states that when the anteroposterior curve is in a neutral position (where facets are not engaged), bending to one side is accompanied by rotation to the opposite side. This law is in effect in typical thoracic and lumbar spines. The second law states that when the anteroposterior curve is flexed or extended, sidebending and rotation occur in the same direction. This law is seen in the typical cervical spinal segment and is in effect in the typical thoracic and lumbar spine. Fryette's third law states that

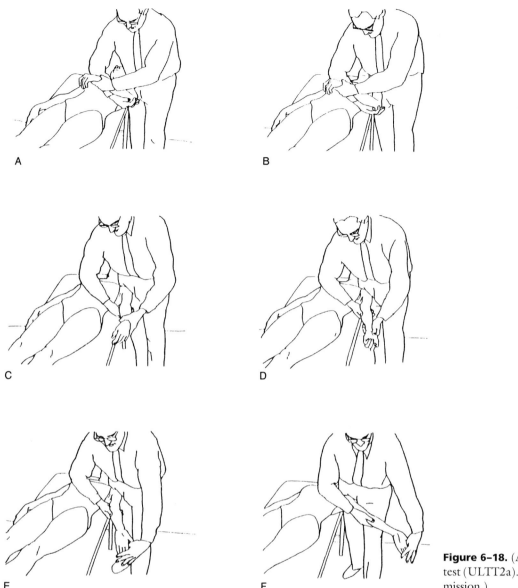

A

B

C

D

E

F

Figure 6–18. (A–F) Upper limb tension test (ULTT2a). (From Butler,[78] with permission.)

when motion is introduced in one direction, motion in all other directions is restricted. This law is evident when rotation in a forward head posture is compared with rotation with the head aligned over the trunk. Even though rotation occurs in the horizontal plane, rotation will be restricted with a forward head posture because of the accentuation of flexion of the lower cervical spine and extension of the upper cervical spine.[33,34]

Motion can be described in terms of the superior vertebra moving on the inferior vertebra during a motion segment. In the cervical spine, passive movement can be evaluated by using translation in the frontal plane. By side gliding a cervical vertebra, the clinician imparts a sidebending force. For example, with a left side glide of C4 on C5, a right sidebending movement occurs. Because sidebending and rotation occur concomitantly, the clini-

cian is also assessing rotation to the right. This translation maneuver allows the operator to assess the quantity of movement as well as end-feel resistance. Because rotation and sidebending occur in the same direction in the mid-cervical spine, according to Fryette's second law, the ability to sidebend and rotate must be determined both in flexion and in extension. By comparing translation to the right and to the left, the clinician can assess the total movement available at that segment.[82,83]

Restricted motion can be described either by the location of the superior segment in space or by the motion that is restricted. The location or position of the superior segment is described using the past participle (e.g., ex-tend*ed*, flex*ed*, rotat*ed*, and side*bent*). The suffixes used for physiologic motion restriction are exten*sion*, flex*ion*, rotat*ion*, and sidebend*ing*. For example, in C4 vertebral

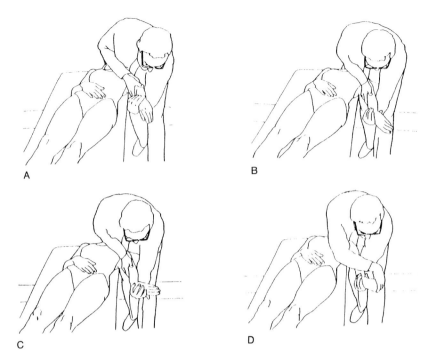

Figure 6–19. (A–D) Upper limb tension test (ULTT2b). (From Butler,[78] with permission.)

motion on C5 for right sidebending, the right inferior articular process of C4 biomechanically glides inferiorly and posteriorly on the superior articular process of C5. At the same time, the left inferior articular process of C4 glides anteriorly and superiorly on the superior articular process of C5 (Fig. 6–21). If right sidebending is restricted, the superior segment (C4) is left sidebent or in a relative position of left sidebending. The positional diagnosis is described in terms of the restriction in three planes. If right sidebending is restricted, right rotation at that segment will also be restricted, since rotation and sidebending are concomitant movements in the midcervical spine. The motion in the sagittal plane that causes the superior segment to glide down and back is extension.

At this point, the clinician assessing a patient with a right sidebending restriction at C4-C5 would not be able to ascertain whether the restriction is at the right or the left facet. However, by testing active movements, the clinician may be able to determine which facet is restricted. For example, a patient who has restricted and painful right sidebending will probably also have restricted and painful right rotation. Evaluating extension and flexion will help determine right or left involvement. If the right facet is unable to go through its full active range of motion, extension movement will also be restricted; however, if the left facet is unable to glide up and forward, flexion will be restricted and painful. In theory, this presentation is plausible; however, patients do not always present in this classic mode because accommodation for loss of active movement can be accomplished at adjacent segments.[42]

When discerning the loss of passive mobility, assessing the end-feel resistance will assist the examiner in determining what tissue or structure may be limiting the range of motion. Describing the end-feel as a barrier that is restricting motion may be helpful. This restriction may be due to one or more factors: skin, fascia, muscle, ligament, joint capsule, joint surface, or loose bodies. The examiner must be able to differentiate normal from abnormal barriers. A normal barrier at the limit of active motion will have resilience to passive movement that is caused by stretching of muscle and fascia. If the examiner imparts a passive stretch to the anatomic limits of the tissue, a harder end-feel will be noted. Passive stretch beyond the anatomic limits will result in violation of the tissue—a ligamentous tear, a fracture, or a dislocation. By learning to recognize normal restriction of passive movement, the examiner can identify resistance within the normal limits of cervical range of motion. With practice, the examiner can assess and quantify this resistance objectively.[83,84] (For more information on end-feels, see Chapter 7.)

For the purpose of passive motion testing, the cervical spine can be divided into atypical cervical joints (i.e., the OA and AA joints) and the typical cervical joints from the inferior surface of C2 to C7. In testing the OA joint, the examiner holds the patient's head between his or her palms and thenar muscles while using the index fingers to palpate for movement of the atlas. This position will assure the operator that movement is localized between the occiput and the atlas. By introducing translatory movement, sidebending can now be assessed. If the OA joint is localized in

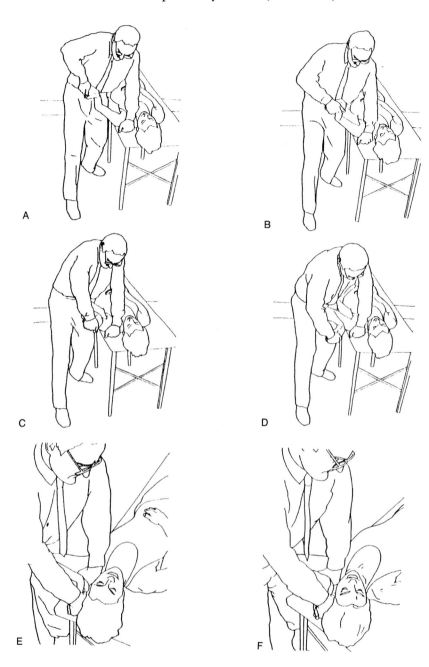

Figure 6–20. (A–F) Upper limb tension test (ULTT3). (From Butler,[78] with permission.)

flexion by acutely tipping the head forward, translation can be performed both to the right and to the left. Flexion of the neck and right translatory movement of the head test for restriction of flexion, left sidebending, and right rotation. The motion restriction is felt when resistance is encountered during the translatory movement. To test for backward bending restriction, the OA joint is localized by acutely tipping the head upward, making sure that extension has not occurred below the level of the atlas. From this position, translatory movement is introduced to both sides (Fig. 6–22). The examiner is testing the ability of the OA joint to produce extension together with sidebending-rotation movement to opposite sides. Backward bending and

translation to the left tests for extension, right sidebending, and left rotation movement of the occiput at the atlas. These four maneuvers, translating the head to the right and left in both the flexed and extended positions, test for all the motion restrictions found within the OA joint.[82,83]

Because rotation is the primary motion available at the AA joint, passive mobility evaluation of this joint will be confined to testing rotation.[6] To test rotation at C1-C2, the head is flexed in an attempt to block as much rotational movement as possible in the typical cervical spine, and rotation is then introduced to the right and to the left until resistance is encountered. If resistance is encountered before the expected end range, a presump-

NECK EXTENDED TO LEVEL

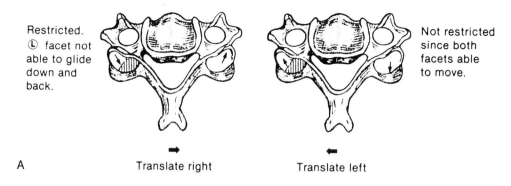

Restricted. Ⓛ facet not able to glide down and back.

Not restricted since both facets able to move.

A

Translate right

Translate left

NECK FLEXED

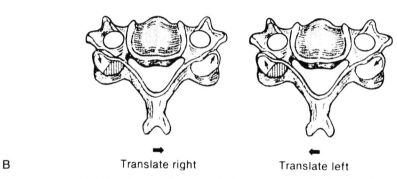

B

Translate right

Translate left

Figure 6–21. (A,B) Translation of C4 on C5 illustrating a motion barrier. Arrows indicate the direction of the superior facet moving on the inferior facet. Diagonal lines indicate areas of joint restriction (loss of range). The facets in the open position are able to glide freely in both directions.

tive diagnosis of limited rotation of the atlas on the axis can be made.[82,83]

To test for movement of the typical cervical segments (C2-C7), translation is performed in the flexed and extended positions. For testing purposes, the examiner palpates the articular pillars of the segment to be tested. Then the cervical spine is either flexed or extended to the level being tested, followed by translation to the right or the left. With the examiner's palpating fingers on the articular pillows of C2, the head is carried into extension, and right translation is introduced until C3 begins to move under the examiner's finger. This tests the ability of the left C2-C3 facet joint to close (extension, left sidebending, and left rotation). The segment is also evaluated in flexion with right and left translation (Fig. 6–23). These translatory movements can be repeated at all remaining cervical segments.[82]

The upper thoracic spine can be assessed for motion restriction by locating the transverse processes of a vertebral segment and determining their position in space through full flexion and extension. Using the second thoracic vertebra, the examiner's thumbs are placed on each transverse process, and during forward and backward bending, the excursion of the paired transverse processes is assessed. If, during forward bending, the examiner notes that the right transverse becomes more prominent and, with backward bending, the two transverse processes become more equal, the right facet is closed and cannot open. When the right facet is restricted in the closed position and is unable to open, that segment has restriction of forward bending, left sidebending, and left rotation.[34,83]

The upper ribs can also be assessed for their ability to move symmetrically. If the thoracic spine has been assessed and determined to be moving normally, any asymmetric motion of the ribs would be considered rib dysfunction. Two methods used to assess restricted rib motion are springing of the rib cage and evaluation of rib motion during full inspiration and expiration. Springing the thoracic cage is a gross measure of mobility; resistance to spring alerts the examiner to dysfunction within that area of the rib cage. The second method is determining the key rib limiting the ability of the rib cage to produce an anteroposterior (pump handle) and a mediolateral (bucket handle) excursion. In performing this test, the examiner places both open hands over the anterior

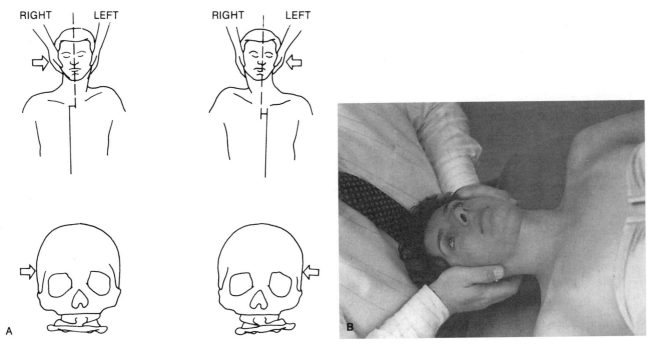

Figure 6–22. (A) Occipitoatlantal joint translation; (B) translation of the occipitoatlantal joint in extension.

chest wall, with the index fingers touching the clavicles. The patient is instructed to take a deep breath, and the examiner assesses the ability of the rib cage to move symmetrically throughout the pump-handle motion (Fig. 6–24). If one side of the rib cage stops moving before the other, that restricted side is the dysfunctional side. To assess the bucket-handle motion, the examiner places both cupped hands inferior to the clavicle but superior to the nipple line. Again, asymmetric motion is assessed

during inspiration, and the side that stops first is considered the restricted side (Fig. 6–25). Although pump-handle movement is the main motion in the upper rib cage, restrictions of bucket-handle movement will be greater and easier to detect than the pump-handle movement.[34,83] Then the examiner's fingers are placed on the first rib to determine if that is the segment that is restricting inhalation. Each segment is assessed until the level of asymmetry is found. That level is considered the key rib limiting motion (Fig. 6–26). Exhalation is assessed in the same manner; the side that stops moving first is considered restricted, and the key rib is then identified, starting inferiorly and moving superiorly.[34,83]

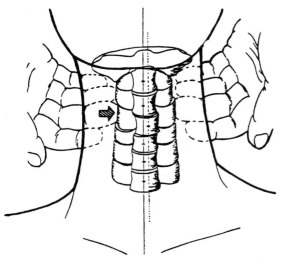

Figure 6–23. Hand positioning for translation of the midcervical spine (C3 and C4).

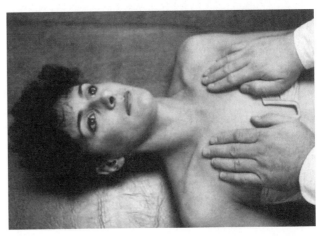

Figure 6–24. Assessing upper rib cage pump-handle motion.

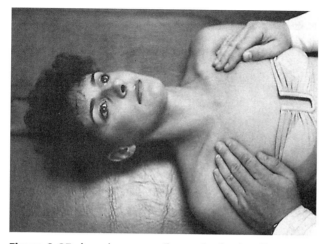

Figure 6–25. Assessing upper rib cage bucket-handle motion.

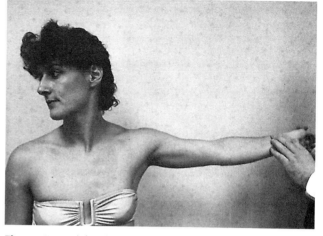

Figure 6–27. Adson's test for thoracic inlet syndrome.

Thoracic Inlet Tests

Many tests have been described to assess compromise of the thoracic inlet. The following provocative tests—Adson's test and the costoclavicular, hyperabduction, and 3-minute elevated arm exercise tests—have been identified as the most sensitive in locating the site of the compromise. Adson's test evaluates the anterior scalene muscle's role in compression of the subclavian artery. This test is performed by holding the arm parallel to the floor, turning the head first away and then toward the arm while holding a deep breath. Meanwhile, the examiner monitors the radial pulse; a positive test is indicated by an obliteration or decrease in the pulse rate, as well as reproduction of the patient's symptoms[85] (Fig. 6–27). A variation of Adson's test is sitting erect with the chin tucked in, with the arm being tested in extension and grasping the edge of the table. The head is sidebent and rotated away. The radial pulse is monitored while the patient holds a deep breath (C. Steele, personal communication) (Fig. 6–28).

The costoclavicular test, or exaggerated military position, has been described as compressing the subclavian

vessels and/or the brachial plexus in the narrow space between the first rib and the clavicle. To perform this test, the patient is seated with the arms held comfortably at the sides; the shoulder girdle is then retracted and depressed. Simultaneously, the examiner monitors for a change in the radial pulse. A positive test is indicated by an obliteration of or decrease in pulse rate and/or onset of symptoms[86] (Fig. 6–29).

The hyperabduction maneuver involves passive circumduction of the upper extremity overhead while the examiner monitors the radial pulse. Like Adson's test, this test is considered positive if the pulse rate changes and/or symptoms are elicited[87] (Fig. 6–30). The

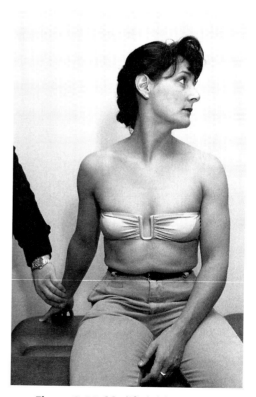

Figure 6–28. Modified Adson's test.

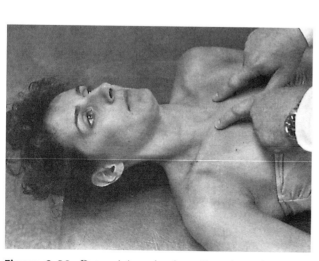

Figure 6–26. Determining the key rib resistor in pump-handle movement.

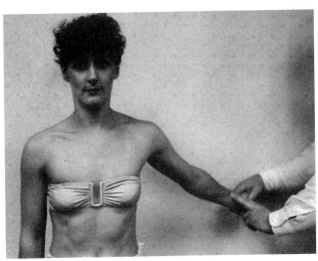

Figure 6–29. Costoclavicular test for thoracic inlet syndrome.

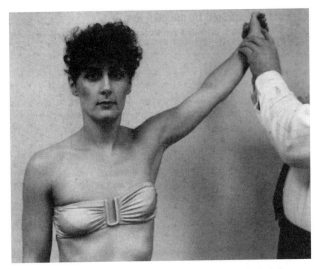

Figure 6–30. Hyperabduction maneuver for thoracic inlet syndrome.

3-minute elevated arm exercise test is performed with the patient seated, arms abducted and elbows flexed 90 degrees, and the shoulder girdle slightly retracted. The patient is then asked to open and close the fists slowly and steadily for a full 3 minutes. The examiner watches for dropping of the elevated arms or a decreased exercise rate before the patient's symptoms begin. Roos[88] stated that this test evaluates involvement of all the neurovascular structures, and a positive test is indicated by the patient's inability to complete the full 3 minutes as well as the onset of symptoms (Fig. 6–31).

Palpation

Cyriax[51] has advocated doing palpation as the last part of an examination to preclude premature conclusions and incomplete examinations. However, in testing passive cervical mobility, the examiner is also gathering information on tissue tensions and specific structures. A thorough knowledge of cervical anatomy is necessary to perform a complete palpation examination. The examiner must view the anatomy in three dimensions before palpating any anatomic structure. Structures should be palpated from their origin to their insertion. Many structures cannot be differentiated when tissues are healthy; however, pathologically altered tissue can usually be distinguished. The ability to palpate anatomic structures, especially in the cervical spine, takes hours of practice and concentration. The examiner should always palpate by layers, identifying every structure in one layer before attempting to palpate deeper structures. If the examiner has a good mental picture of all the muscles, ligaments, and soft tissues in the cervical area, he or she can identify individual structures.[1]

Palpation gives the examiner information about the size, consistency, temperature, and location of a structure and about swelling, bony changes, or soft tissue changes such as nodules or scar tissue. Crepitus of bony surfaces can be easily detected, and temperature changes can be appreciated. All these clinical findings are important ob-

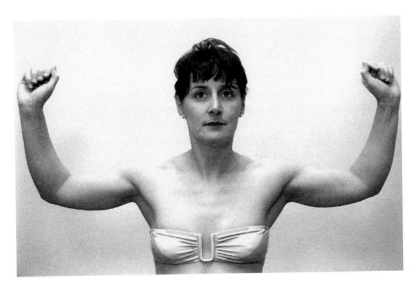

Figure 6–31. Three-minute elevated arm exercise test for thoracic inlet syndrome.

jective information. Palpation and point tenderness are viewed in terms of the patient's sensation, but more importantly, the objective sensation of the examiner (what the examiner "feels") should be guided by sound anatomic knowledge and adequate application of pressure with regard to area, force, and direction. The clinician must remember, however, that point tenderness of a structure may also provide misinformation. Palpation should be done only after the tissue at fault has been identified by testing its function. Treating point tenderness without identifying and treating the cause of the symptom is not an acceptable treatment approach.[51]

Correlation of Findings

After completing the objective examination, the clinician should be able to make assumptions about possible pathology or movement dysfunction that are corroborated by both the subjective and objective findings. The evaluation process depends on the clinician's ability to make inferences based on his or her knowledge and experience, as well as the information obtained from the patient history and the examination. The clinician's inferences are the basis for appropriate clinical decision making. With the information received from the patient and the objective examination, the clinician is now able to establish meaningful short- and long-term goals and to plan treatment to meet these goals.

■ Treatment

A complete, detailed description of treatment procedures for all cervical spine problems is beyond the scope of this chapter. Instead, the intent is to alert the clinician to the different treatment procedures available. Although specific treatment procedures are addressed, treatment should always include patient education on posture, neck hygiene, and recreational and workplace ergonomics. This patient education and patient responsibility for self-care are an integral part of any successful intervention.

Modalities

The decision to use physical agents must be based on appropriate treatment goals; however, the use of physical agents alone will rarely alleviate the cause of the patient's complaints. Mennell[29] stated that the only problems "cured" by physical therapy are rickets treated with ultraviolet therapy and joint dysfunction treated with joint mobilization.[68] As with the rest of the spine, heat is still the treatment of choice for acute cervical problems when, in fact, cryotherapy is more effective in acute situations to decrease pain, swelling, and muscle spasm.[89] Aside from these acute situations, any modality including both superficial and deep heat, electricity, and cold laser can be used as adjunctive therapy to decrease pain, promote relax-

ation, or prepare the tissues before other therapeutic procedures are used.

Traction

Mechanical or manual traction of the cervical spine separates the vertebrae of the cervical spine, affecting both articular and periarticular structures. Mechanical traction allows the clinician to give a specific poundage of traction over a given time, whereas manual traction allows the therapist to better localize the traction to the vertebral segments affected and requires less time for treatment. In setting up cervical traction, the therapist must be aware of several factors: the weight of the head, the angle of pull, the position of the patient, and the poundage of the traction pull. Accurate knowledge of these components is necessary to control the stress that is being applied in a particular direction to the cervical spine and soft tissues.[90,91] As a precaution, traction is usually initiated at a relatively low poundage and is directed to the vertebral segments involved; therefore, a standard position for the cervical spine for traction is not appropriate. Because most movement is achieved when a joint is positioned in its midrange, actual distraction will vary, depending on the segment being treated. The OA and AA joints should be treated in a neutral or a slightly extended head and neck position.[92] By introducing more flexion, lower cervical spine segments can be isolated.[90]

Research reveals that traction forces greater than 20 lb separates the vertebrae by 1 to 1.5 cm per space, with the greatest separation occurring posteriorly as flexion is increased. The normal cervical lordosis is eradicated with traction forces of 20 to 25 lb. At a constant angle, a traction force of 50 lb produces greater separation than 30 lb, but the amount of separation is not significantly different at 7, 30, or 60 seconds.[91] Intermittent traction produces twice as much separation as sustained traction. If separation of vertebral bodies is desired, high traction forces for short periods of time will achieve that goal. When traction forces are removed, restoration of normal dimensions is four to five times quicker in posterior structures than in anterior structures. As would be expected, less separation occurs in 50-year-olds than in normal 20-year-olds.[93-95]

The behavior of the patient's symptoms during traction is important, especially if the symptoms decrease. Even if traction reduces the symptoms, there is no guarantee that the symptoms will remain relieved after treatment. However, relief of symptoms during treatment is a sign that traction will benefit that patient.

Soft Tissue Mobilization

Regardless of the cervical spine pathology, the clinician must always consider the soft tissue component of the problem. If body parts have maintained an abnormal relationship for some time, following Wolff's law,[96] soft tissue will adapt accordingly (see Chapter 1). All soft tissues must be recognized: skin, fascia, capsule, and muscle. Several soft tissue mobilization procedures are available, including stretching, myofascial release, fluorimethane spraying and stretching, rolfing, deep massage, strain-counterstrain,[97] and craniosacral therapy.[98]

Joint Mobilization

Indications for joint mobilization include loss of active and passive range of motion, joint asymmetry, and tissue texture abnormality. Passive mobility testing during the evaluation will identify the joints to be treated. Chapter 7 discusses specific techniques such as oscillations, articulations, and muscle energy techniques. Indirect techniques such as strain-counterstrain, functional technique, and craniosacral therapy are also available.

Therapeutic Exercise

Active rehabilitation is of vital importance for restoration of function; however, patients cannot typically "work out" neck pain. An appropriate treatment plan should include restoration of normal, painless joint range of motion followed by correction of muscle weakness or imbalance, resumption of normal activities, and then prevention of recurrent problems. Too often treatment ends after normal, pain-free motion is restored. Exercise restores adequate control of movement, and increased muscle strength provides increased dynamic support to the spine.

The choice of specific exercises is just as important as the decision to initiate cervical exercises. The spinal musculature, which is composed mainly of slow-twitch oxidative muscle fibers, has a role in maintaining body relationships. After restoration of normal muscle length, appropriate strengthening exercise should include isometric and endurance activities.

Supports

Cervical collars and supports do have their place in treatment program planning; however, they are appropriate only in acute conditions and in segmental instability. The amount of external support needed should be dictated by the objective examination.

CASE STUDIES

CASE STUDY 1

Rarely does the clinical presentation of cervical pain have a single underlying cause. The following case study describing an actual patient is a typical example of this point.

Subjective Examination

A 32-year-old woman presented to physical therapy with complaints of cervicothoracic pain referring into the left upper extremity. She had been working as a word processing secretary; her symptoms started 6 months previously. She reported no specific incident that might have brought on her symptoms, except for sitting at a computer terminal 5 hours a day.

The patient's chief complaints were stiffness and pain in the posterior neck that traveled along the trapezial ridge into the left superior and lateral shoulder. She described numbness along the lateral upper arm, the forearm, and the ulnar side of the left hand. The symptoms in her left upper extremity were aggravated when she attempted to lift a heavy object or use her arms overhead. Her upper back pain was aggravated when she sneezed. She related difficulty sleeping at night, with inability to find a comfortable position; she was using a down feather pillow.

During a 24-hour period, the patient noticed stiffness on awakening in the morning. As the day progressed, she experienced discomfort only if she was very active or sat too long (35 minutes or more) at the computer terminal without getting up.

Her history revealed a similar episode of pain in 1978, which lasted for more than 1½ years after the patient began working at a word processing machine. When she was promoted and no longer worked at a word processor, her symptoms disappeared. She had experienced no neck symptoms since that initial episode until this episode occurred. She related a history of trauma to the cervicothoracic region 11 years previously, when she fell off a motorcycle, landing directly on her buttocks. Ten months previously, she had fallen down one flight of stairs, with minimal musculoskeletal complaints. She denied having any history of bowel or bladder dysfunction, headaches, dizziness, difficulty swallowing, weight loss, or pregnancy.

The patient was not currently being treated for any other medical condition, although she had had an epigastric hernia repair 6 years prior to presentation. She reported that stress played an important role in determining how she felt; she noticed a direct relationship between increased stress and exacerbation of her symptoms. In her current job, she noticed less cervical pain after her boss bought her a Pos Chair (Congleton Workplace Systems, Inc., College Station, TX), which improved her head and neck alignment.

Objective Examination

The patient presented in no acute distress but with guarded upper quarter movement. She had a forward head posture, with rounding of the shoulder girdle complex. Active range of motion of both upper extremities was within normal limits; however, extreme elevation of the arms increased discomfort in the cervicothoracic region. Active range of motion of the cervical spine was restricted in left rotation (30 percent) and left sidebending (25 percent). Right rotation was full but produced pain along the left upper trapezius ridge. Backward bending was within normal limits but produced discomfort in the posterior neck region. Forward bending was restricted, with two fingerbreadths of distance between the chin and the anterior chest wall at maximum flexion. Right sidebending was full and pain-free.

Neurologic testing revealed 2+ muscle stretch reflexes in both upper extremities. Sensation to light touch, pinprick, and two-point discrimination was intact in the upper quarter. Gross muscle testing revealed weakness in the following muscles: left biceps brachii, good minus (4/5), and left triceps brachii, good (4/5). The triceps muscle contraction appeared to give way secondary to the pain felt by the patient in the cervicothoracic region.

Several special tests revealed positive findings. The foraminal closure test (quadrant) was positive for the lower cervical spine on the left and produced pain along the upper trapezius, and on the left side the pain was reproduced in the right neck region. The left upper limb tension test was slightly positive, with reproduction of neck and shawl pain. The cervical compression test was negative. The cervical distraction test decreased the patient's neck and shoulder pain. A vertebral artery test was negative. Clearing tests for the TMJ shoulder, elbow, wrist, and hand were unequivocal.

Radiographs taken at the time of the examination revealed flattening of lordosis at the midcervical spine and posterior spurring of the vertebral body at the C4-C5 level, with foraminal encroachment at C4-C5 greater on the right than on the left (Fig. 6–32).

Passive mobility testing demonstrated restrictions at the left OA joint with translation to the left in flexion (extended, rotated right, sidebent left). The right AA joint was restricted with passive rotation to the right with the neck bent fully forward (rotated left). Translation of the cervical spine from C2 to C7 revealed restriction at the C2-C3, C4-C5, C5-C6, and C6-C7 levels. Translation of the C2-C3 level to the left in extension (flexed, rotated left, sidebent left) was diminished. The C4-C5, C5-C6, and C6-C7 levels were restricted in translation to the right in extension (flexed, rotated right, sidebent right). Asymmetry of the upper thoracic region was revealed by palpation of the transverse processes at the T1-T2 and T2-T3 levels. The transverse process at T1 was more posterior on the left in flexion of the head and upper trunk (extended, rotated left, sidebent left) than when the neck and trunk were placed in extension. The T2 transverse process was more prominent on the right in flexion (extended, rotated right, sidebent right). Inhala-

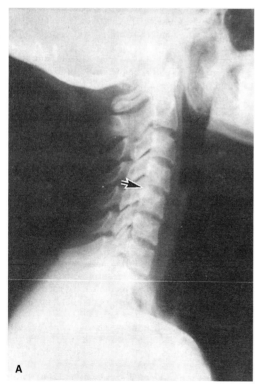 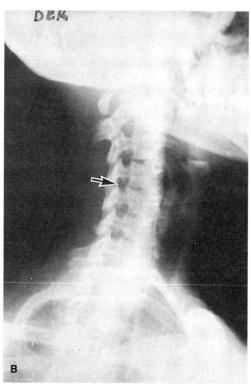

Figure 6–32. Cervical radiographs. (A) Lateral view. Arrow shows C4-C5 spurring. (B) Oblique view. Arrow shows bony encroachment at the C4-C5 intervertebral foramen.

tion/exhalation testing of the anterior rib cage showed less movement on inhalation on the left, with the left first and second ribs revealing the most restriction.

Palpation revealed tightness in the posterior cervical musculature, suboccipital muscles, scalene muscles, trapezius, and levator scapulae muscles. Flexibility testing revealed tightness of the levator scapulae, pectoralis major, and scalene muscles. A trigger point was identified in the midsubstance of the upper trapezius muscle.

Assessment

The findings were consistent with cervical spondylosis with left C5 radiculopathy, upper cervical dysfunction, forward head posture, and upper rib and thoracic dysfunction.

Treatment Plan

Treatment goals included decreasing the patient's symptoms, improving her posture, and increasing range of motion in the cervical and thoracic spine and upper ribs. Other important treatment goals were patient education about work simplification, awareness of the need for lifetime postural correction, and avoidance of potentially harmful activities.

To accomplish these goals, the following treatment plan was administered:

1. Intermittent supine cervical traction using a Saunders[28] harness at 16 lb, 30-second pull, followed by 12 lb, 10-second pull, for a total treatment time of 20 minutes (static traction with intermittent increases)
2. High-voltage electrical stimulation massage of the upper trapezius, upper thoracic, and posterior cervical regions for 10 minutes
3. Postural instruction in correct head and neck alignment during all activities
4. Basic instruction in proper sleeping postures; encouragement of continued use of a down feather pillow
5. Soft tissue mobilization of the paracervical, suboccipital, levator scapulae, scalene, and upper trapezius muscles
6. Joint mobilization of the upper thoracic spine with the patient supine and the head supported; muscle energy technique to decrease upper cervical spine joint restrictions

Treatment Progression

The patient was seen every other day, three times a week, for a total of six treatments. The initial treatment included traction and high-voltage massage and posture education. Subsequent treatments focused on the soft tissue and joint dysfunctions. After this treatment regimen, the patient was asymptomatic and resumed her normal activities.

Because this was the patient's first episode of radicular referred symptoms, home cervical traction would not be recommended unless the symptoms recurred.

CASE STUDY 2

This chapter has discussed the importance of performing a thorough examination, not only to determine if a patient is a candidate for physical therapy, but also to provide appropriate treatment according to the signs and symptoms found during the evaluation. This case study stresses the importance of taking a thorough history before starting treatment.

With the advent of direct access, a physical therapist or any other health practitioner should no longer rely on another person's interpretation of subjective and objective findings on a patient. Obtaining a complete, correct clinical picture allows the clinician to design an appropriate treatment plan.

Subjective Examination

This case study describes a 53-year-old businessman who presented to our clinic with complaints of left shoulder pain and left upper extremity burning and numbness. He had been referred to our clinic by a general practitioner with a diagnosis of left cervical radiculopathy. The prescription for physical therapy treatment read "evaluate and treat."

The patient reported a gradual onset of intermittent superior left shoulder pain for the past 4 months. His symptoms began as a diffuse ache in the left shoulder, which increased progressively in intensity. The patient recalled no specific incident or unusual activity that could have contributed to his current symptoms. He started to notice the pain traveling along the inside of his left upper extremity to his fourth and fifth digits, with numbness in the same distribution. He began to feel achiness along the medial aspect of the left scapula. Occasionally, he felt discomfort along the left trapezial ridge. He denied having any neck pain. While eating, he often noticed the feeling that something was stuck in his throat. He reported having difficulty sleeping for the past 2 months; for the past 2 weeks, he reported having to get out of bed to find relief for his left upper extremity numbness and pain.

The patient reported that his physician ordered cervical spine radiographs, which revealed moderate degenerative disk and joint disease at the C5-C6, C6-C7, and C7-T1 levels bilaterally, with minimal intervertebral foramina osteophytosis encroachment at the C5-C6 level on the left and the C6-C7 level on the right. The patient was given a nonsteroidal anti-inflammatory medication, which did not relieve his pain. Holding the left upper extremity in an awkward position usually aggravated his symptoms, mainly the numbness in the medial hand. He had difficulty grasping heavy objects with his nondominant left hand, especially his briefcase. The patient had been smoking one pack of cigarettes per day since the age of 15. He drank wine at every dinner and several six-packs of beer on the weekends. His typical work week had traditionally been 55 hours long, but for the past month he was working only 35 hours weekly because of increased pain. His medical history revealed no major sickness, an appendectomy at age 15, and a negative family history.

Objective Examination

Objective examination found an older man who appeared to be in distress. He was holding his left arm against his rib cage and was trying not to move the left upper extremity. He had increased thoracic kyphosis, rounded shoulders, protracted scapulae, and a forward head posture. His blood pressure taken while sitting was 162/84 mmHg; pulse was 82; respiration was 20; and oral temperature was 98.8°F. Active range of motion of the cervical spine showed restriction of movement in all three cardinal planes. Cervical range of motion measured with CROM inclinometer revealed 28 degrees right sidebending with pain referred along the left medial brachium and forearm to the medial hand. Left sidebending was 34 degrees. Cervical rotation was 44 degrees right and 42 degrees left. Cervical forward bending was 40 degrees; cervical forward bending was 40 degrees; cervical backward bending was painful and diminished 48 degrees. Active range of motion of left shoulder flexion was 155 degrees, and shoulder abduction was 152 degrees. Neck palpation re-

vealed swelling in the left posterior triangle, with tenderness on pressure. Palpation of other soft tissues demonstrated tightness and tenderness of the following muscles: sternocleidomastoid, anterior and middle scalenes, upper trapezius, levator scapulae, left splenius capitis and cervicis, and suboccipital muscles. The left cervical foraminal encroachment test increased his left lateral trapezial pain. Compression and distraction tests of the cervical spine were unremarkable. Manual muscle testing revealed weakness in the following muscles: left interossei dorsales (3+/5), left interossei palmares (3+/5), lumbricales I and II (4/5) and III and IV (3+/5), flexor digiti minimi (3+/5), opponens digiti minimi (3+/5), abductor digiti minimi (3+/5), left pronator teres (4/5), left flexor digitorum superficialis I and II (4/5) and III and IV (3+/5), flexor pollicis longus (4/5), abductor pollicis brevis (4+/5), flexor pollicis brevis (4/5), adductor brevis (3+/5), opponens pollicis (4/5), shoulder external rotation right (4/5) and left (4/5), and grip strength using a hand-held dynamometer (right, 95 lb; left, 35 lb). Symmetric hyporeflexive muscle stretch reflexes were in the upper quarter. The patient's sensation to pinprick was significantly reduced along the ulnar distribution of the left hand. Hoffman's sign was negative bilaterally. The left upper limb tension test was positive with sidebending of the head to the right without placing the left arm in a stretched position.

With the significant clinical features of a history of smoking, difficulty swallowing, lower trunk brachial plexopathy, sleep disturbance, and severe pain in the shoulder and scapula, it was suggested that the patient return for

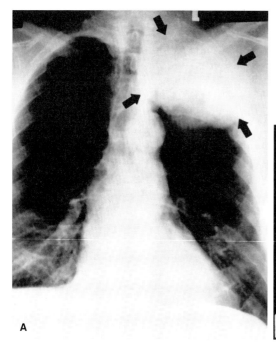
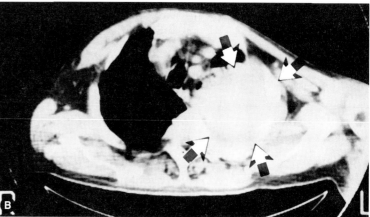

Figure 6–33. (A) Chest radiograph showing Pancoast's tumor (arrows). (B) Computed tomography scan demonstrating tumor (arrows) in the superior pulmonary sulcus.

further evaluation by the referring physician. The physician was telephoned with the findings. It was obvious from this discussion that a short, scanty evaluation had been performed by the physician. A chest radiograph and possibly a computed tomography scan was suggested.

The patient was sent for a chest radiograph (Fig. 6–33A), which revealed a large tumor in the superior pulmonary sulcus. It was diagnosed by computed tomography scan as a Pancoast's tumor (Fig. 6–33B).

Summary of Case Study

This case study illustrates the importance of performing a thorough examination on every patient. Given the findings of the examination, this patient was not a proper candidate for physical therapy. He should have been sent to a specialist immediately instead of to a physical therapist. A proper initial examination would have directed the patient to proper medical attention. The literature[99] has reported Pancoast's tumors presenting as cervical radiculopathy. However, the clinical features of this patient's history and physical examination warranted further study.

■ Summary

A complete evaluation of the cervical spine must begin with a thorough understanding of its functional anatomy and biomechanics. With this background, the examiner will have a clear mental picture of the structures and the interdependency of the structures being examined. However, this mental image is sharpened and honed only with study, practice, and experience. The clinician must address all potential sources of the patient's complaints, which may go beyond the physical sources. Physiologic and psychosocial factors can play an important role in the patient's symptoms. A detailed discussion of all cervical and upper thoracic spine pathology is beyond the scope of this chapter; however, the clinician must always remember that not all cervical symptoms are musculoskeletal in origin. Those patients whose pain is not musculoskeletal in origin should be referred to the appropriate physician for further evaluation.

The cervical and upper thoracic spine is indeed complex, and no two patients are alike. Each patient presenting with cervical and upper thoracic pain must be evaluated according to his or her own signs and symptoms.

■ References

1. Dvorak J, Dvorak V: Manual Medicine Diagnostics. Thieme-Stratton, New York, 1984
2. Kapandji I: Physiology of the Joints. 2nd Ed. Vol. III. The Trunk and Vertebral Column. Churchill Livingstone, Edinburgh, 1974
3. Werne S: Studies in spontaneous atlas dislocation. Acta Orthop Scand, suppl 23:1, 1957
4. Kaltenborn FM: Mobilization of the Extremity Joints. Examination and Basic Treatment Techniques. 3rd Ed. Olaf Norlis Bokhandel, Oslo, 1980
5. Ingelmark BE: Ueber den craniocervicalen Uebergang bei Menschen. Acta Anat, suppl 23:1, 1957
6. Fielding JW: Cineroentgenography of the normal cervical spine. J Bone Joint Surg 39(A):1280, 1957
7. Field JW, Hawkins RJ, Hensinger RN, et al: Deformities. Orthop Clin North Am 9:955, 1978
8. White A, Panjabi MM: The basic kinematics of the human spine. Spine 3:13, 1978
9. Penning L: Functional Pathology of the Cervical Spine. Excerpta Medica Foundation, Amsterdam, 1968
10. Clark CR, Goel VK, Galles K, et al: Kinematics of the occipito-atlanto-axial complex. Trans Cervical Spine Res Soc 10:210, 1986
11. Dvorak J, Panjabi MM, Gerber DG, et al: Functional diagnostics of the rotatory instability of the upper cervical spine: an experimental study in cadavers. Spine 12:197, 1987
12. Panjabi M, Dvorak J, Duranceau J, et al: Three dimensional movements of the upper cervical spine. Spine 13:726, 1988
13. Dupreux R, Mestdagh H: Anatomic functionelle de l'articulation sousoccipitale. Lille Med 19:122, 1974
14. Lewit K: Blockierung von Atlas-Axis und Atlas-Occiput im Robild und Klink. Z Orthop 108:43, 1970
15. Jirout J: Changes in the atlas–axis relations on lateral flexion of the head and neck. Neuroradiology 6:215, 1973
16. White A, Panjabi MM: Clinical Biomechanics of the Spine. 2nd Ed. JB Lippincott, Philadelphia, 1990
17. Grieve GP: Common Vertebral Joint Problems. Churchill Livingstone, Edinburgh, 1979
18. Lysell E: Motion in the cervical spine. Acta Orthop Scand, suppl 123:69, 1969
19. Warwick R, Williams PL (eds): Gray's Anatomy. 35th British Ed. WB Saunders, Philadelphia, 1973
20. Greenman PE: Manipulative therapy for the thoracic cage. Osteop Ann 140:63, 1977
21. Selecki BR: The effects of rotation of the atlas on the axis: experimental work. Med J Aust 1:1012, 1969
22. Tatlow TWF, Bammer HG: Vertebral artery compression syndrome. Neurology 7:331, 1957
23. Coman WB: Dizziness related to ENT conditions. p. 303. In Grieve GP (ed): Modern Manual Therapy of the Vertebral Column. Churchill Livingstone, Edinburgh, 1986
24. Grant ER: Clinical testing before cervical manipulation—can we recognize the patient at risk? Paper presented at the World Confederation of Physical Therapy, Sydney, Australia, 1987
25. Howell JW: Evaluation and management of the thoracic outlet syndrome. p. 133. In Donatelli R (ed): Physical Therapy of the Shoulder. Churchill Livingstone, New York, 1987
26. Kendall FP, Kendall-McCreary E: Muscles: Testing and Function. 3rd Ed. Williams & Wilkins, Baltimore, 1983
27. Rocabado M: Diagnosis and Treatment of Abnormal Craniocervical and Craniomandibular Mechanics. Rocabado Institute, Knoxville, TN, 1981
28. Saunders HD: Evaluation, Treatment and Prevention of Musculoskeletal Disorders. 2nd Ed. Viking Press, Minneapolis, 1985
29. Mennell JM: Joint Pain. Little, Brown, Boston, 1964
30. Schafer RC: Chiropractic Management of Sports and Recreational Injuries. Williams & Wilkins, Baltimore, 1982
31. Lewit K: Manipulative Therapy in Rehabilitation of the Motor System. Butterworths, Boston, 1985

32. Seimon LP: Low Back Pain: Clinical Diagnosis and Management. Appleton-Century-Crofts, East Norwalk, CT, 1983
33. Greenman PE: Vertebral motion. Mich Osteopath J 6:31, 1983
34. Mitchell FL, Moran PS, Pruzzo NA: An Evaluation and Treatment Manual of Osteopathic Muscle Energy Procedures. Institute for Continuing Education in Osteopathic Principles, Valley Park, MD, 1979
35. Bogduk N, Engel R: The menisci of the lumbar zygapophyseal joints: a review of their anatomy and clinical significance. Spine 9:454, 1984
36. Kos J, Wolf J: Die "Menisci" der Zwischenwirbelgelenke und ihre mogliche Role bei Wirbelblockierung. Manuelle Med 10:105, 1972
37. Janda V: Muscles, central nervous regulation and back problems. p. 27. In Korr IM (ed): Neurobiologic Mechanisms in Manipulative Therapy. Plenum Press, New York, 1978
38. Korr IM: Sustained sympathicotonia as a factor in disease. p. 229. In Korr IM (ed): Neurobiologic Mechanisms in Manipulative Therapy. Plenum Press, New York, 1978
39. Korr IM: Proprioceptors and somatic dysfunction. J Am Osteopath Assoc 74:638, 1975
40. Calliet R: Neck and Arm Pain. FA Davis, Philadelphia, 1981
41. Jull G, Bogduk N, Marsland A: The accuracy of manual diagnosis for cervical zygapophyseal joint pain syndromes. Med J Aust 148:233, 1988
42. Greenman PE: Restricted vertebral motion. Mich Osteopath J 7:31, 1983
43. Bland JH: Disorders of the Cervical Spine: Diagnosis and Medical Management. WB Saunders, Philadelphia, 1987
44. Hirsh LF: Cervical degenerative arthritis. Possible cause of neck and arm pain. Postgrad Med 74:123, 1983
45. Bateman JE: The Shoulder and Neck. 2nd Ed. WB Saunders, Philadelphia, 1978
46. Brain WR, Northfield D, Wilkinson M: The neurological manifestations of cervical spondylosis. Brain 75:187, 1952
47. Cyriax JH: Cervical spondylosis. Butterworths, London, 1971
48. Grieve GP: Manipulation therapy for neck pain. Physiotherapy 65:136, 1979
49. Cloward RB: Cervical discography: a contribution to the etiology and mechanism of neck, shoulder and arm pain. Ann Surg 150:1052, 1959
50. Cloward RB: The clinical significance of the sinuvertebral nerve. J Neurol Neurosurg Psychiatr 23:321, 1960
51. Cyriax JH: Textbook of Orthopaedic Medicine. 8th Ed. Vol. I. Diagnosis of Soft Tissue Lesions. Bailliere Tindall, London, 1983
52. McNab I: The whiplash syndrome. Orthop Clin North Am 2:389, 1971
53. Hohl M: Soft tissue injuries of the neck in automobile accidents. J Bone Joint Surg 56(A):1675, 1974
54. Bower KD: The patho-physiology and symptomatology of the whiplash syndrome. p. 342. In Grieve GP (ed): Modern Manual Therapy of the Vertebral Column. Churchill Livingstone, Edinburgh, 1986
55. Yunus M, Masi AT, Calabro JJ, et al: Primary fibromyalgia (fibrositis): clinical study of 50 patients with matched normal controls. Semin Arthritis Rheum 11:151, 1981
56. Travell JH, Simons DG: Myofascial Pain and Dysfunction: Trigger Point Manual. Williams & Wilkins, Baltimore, 1983
57. Cyriax JH, Cyriax PJ: Illustrated Manual of Orthopaedic Medicine. Butterworths, Boston, 1983
58. Miller J: How do you feel? Listener 100:665, 1978
59. Harman JB: Angina in the analgesic limb. Br Med J 2:521, 1951
60. Feinstein B, Langton JNK, Jameson RM, et al: Experiments on pain referred from deep somatic tissues. J Bone Joint Surg 36(A):981, 1954
61. Bourdillon JR: Spinal Manipulation. 3rd Ed. Butterworth-Heinemann, London, 1982
62. Inman VT, Saunders JB: Referred pain from skeletal structures. J Nerv Ment Dis 90:660, 1944
63. Campbell DG, Parsons CM: Referred head pain and its concomitants. J Nerve Ment Dis 99:544, 1944
64. Wall PD: The mechanisms of pain associated with cervical vertebral disease. p. 201. In Hirsch C, Zotterman Y (eds): Cervical Pain. Pergamon Press, Oxford, 1971
65. Dwyer A, Aprill C, Bogduk N: Cervical zygapophyseal joint pain patterns I: a study in normal volunteers. Spine 15:453, 1990
66. Collins RD: Dynamic Differential Diagnosis. JB Lippincott, Philadelphia, 1981
67. D'Ambrosia RD: Musculoskeletal Disorders, Regional Examination and Differential Diagnosis. 2nd Ed. JB Lippincott, Philadelphia, 1986
68. Hoppenfeld S: Physical Examination of the Spine and Extremities. Appleton-Century-Crofts, New York, 1976
69. Boissonnault WG: Examination in Physical Therapy Practice: Screening for Medical Disease. Churchill Livingstone, New York, 1991
70. Gould JA, Davies GJ (eds): Orthopaedic and Sports Physical Therapy. CV Mosby, St. Louis, 1985
71. Bogduk N: Cervical causes of headache. p. 289. In Grieve GP (ed): Modern Manual Therapy of the Vertebral Column. Churchill Livingstone, Edinburgh, 1986
72. Ryan GM, Cope S: Cervical vertigo. Lancet 2:1355, 1955
73. Maitland GD: Vertebral Manipulation. 4th Ed. Butterworths, London, 1977
74. Youdas JW, Garrett TR, Suman VJ, et al: Normal range of motion of the cervical spine: an initial goniometric study. Phys Ther 72:770, 1992
75. Rheault W, Albright B, Byers C, et al: Intertester reliability of the cervical range of motion device. J Orthop Sports Phys Ther 15:147, 1992
76. Youdas JW, Carey JR, Carrett TR: Reliability of measurements of cervical spine range of motion: comparison of three methods. Phys Ther 71:98, 1991
77. Elvey RL: The investigation of arm pain. p. 530. In Grieve GP (ed): Modern Manual Therapy of the Vertebral Column. Churchill Livingstone, Edinburgh, 1986
78. Butler DS: Mobilisation of the Nervous System. Churchill Livingstone, Melbourne, 1991
79. Margarey ME: Examination of the cervical spine. p. 503. In Grieve GP (ed): Modern Manual Therapy of the Vertebral Column. Churchill Livingstone, Edinburgh, 1986
80. Kenneally M: The upper limb tension test: an investigation of responses amongst normal asymptomatic subjects. Unpublished thesis, School of Physiotherapy, South Australia Institute of Technology, 1983
81. Fryette HH: Principles of Osteopathic Technique. Academy of Applied Osteopathy, Carmel, CA, 1954
82. Greenman PE: Motion testing the cervical spine. Mich Osteopath J 8:32, 1983
83. Greenman PE: Principles of Manual Medicine. Williams & Wilkins, Baltimore, 1989
84. Greenman PE: Barrier concepts and structural diagnosis. Mich Osteopath J 3:28, 1982
85. Hirsch LF, Thanki A: The thoracic outlet syndrome. Meeting the diagnostic challenge. Postgrad Med 77:197, 1985

86. Falconer MA, Weddell G: Costoclavicular compression of the subclavian artery and veins. Lancet 2:539, 1943

87. Wright IS: The neurovascular syndrome produced by hyperabduction of the arms. Am Heart J 29:1, 1945

88. Roos DB: Congenital anomalies associated with thoracic outlet syndrome. Am J Surg 132:171, 1976

89. Knight KL: Cryotherapy: Theory, Technique, and Physiology. Chattanooga Corp., Chattanooga, TN, 1985

90. Colachis SC, Strohm BR: A study of tractive forces and angle of pull on vertebral interspaces in the cervical spine. Arch Phys Med Rehabil 46:820, 1965

91. Colachis SC, Strohm BR: Cervical traction: relationship of traction time to varied tractive force with constant angle of pull. Arch Phys Med Rehabil 46:815, 1965

92. Daugherty RJ, Erhard RE: Segmentalized cervical traction. p. 189. In Kent BE (ed): International Federation of Orthopaedic Manipulative Therapists Proceedings, Vail, CO, 1977

93. Valtonen EJ, Moller K, Wiljasalo M: Comparative radiographic study of the effect of intermittent and continuous traction on elongation of the cervical spine. Ann Med Int Fenn 57:143, 1968

94. Colachis SC, Strohm BR: Effect of duration of intermittent cervical traction on vertebral separation. Arch Phys Med Rehabil 47:353, 1966

95. Valtonen EJ, Kiurn E: Cervical traction as a therapeutic tool: a clinical analysis based on 212 patients. Scand J Rehabil Med 2:29, 1970

96. Glimcher MJ: On the form and function of bone: from molecules to organs. Wolff's law revisited. p. 617. In Veis A (ed): The Chemistry and Biology of Mineralized Connective Tissues. Elsevier/North Holland, New York, 1981

97. Jones LH: Strain and Counterstrain. American Academy of Osteopathy, Colorado Springs, CO, 1981

98. Upledger JE, Vredevoogd JD: Craniosacral Therapy. Eastland Press, Seattle, 1983

99. Vargo MM, Flood KM: Pancoast tumor presenting as cervical radiculopathy. Arch Phys Med Rehabil 71:606, 1990

CHAPTER 7
Differential Assessment and Mobilization of the Cervical and Upper Thoracic Spine

Robert B. Sprague

The purposes of this chapter are (1) to present a description of a differential assessment between the cervical spine and the thoracic spine and (2) to present methods for mobilization of the cervical and upper thoracic spine.

Types of Assessment and Clinical Reasoning

To learn a new technique and then apply it to a patient without accurate assessment is completely the wrong idea. If the patient gets better, the improvement is simply the result of random, dumb luck. Assessment, or evaluation, is the cornerstone of effective clinical practice. There are three types of assessment: (1) daily clinical assessment, (2) analytical assessment, and (3) differential assessment.

Daily clinical assessment is an unremitting process that occurs in every quality clinic. Patients are assessed; techniques are assessed; therapists are assessed; facilities are assessed; equipment is assessed; and programs are assessed. For the subjective examination (SE), an effective format to facilitate the flow of the clinical assessment is (1) the nature and kind of the disorder, (2) the area or areas of the symptoms, (3) the behavior of the symptoms, (4) the present and past history, and (5) the special questions. For the physical examination (PE), an effective format is (1) special tests, (2) active physiological movement tests, (3) passive physiological movement tests, and (4) passive accessory movement tests.

Clinical hypothesis categories, as described by Jones,[1-3] provide a guideline for all types of assessment. These categories are (1) the source of the patient's symptoms, (2) factors contributing to the disorder, (3) precautions and contraindications, (4) management, (5) prognosis, and (6) mechanisms of the symptoms. They are tested consistently during the SE, during the PE, and during treatment. Details about the categories are found elsewhere.[1-7]

Analytical assessment is the cognitive foundation of the clinical reasoning processes. It is a continuous process that enhances *all* effective clinical functions; it is in a sense the thinking about our thinking, the reason why we do what we do. It is a series of accumulating thoughts that result in overt acts by therapists. The acts are heard as questions in the SE and PE, seen as objective tests in the PE, and finally seen as treatment. It is a process of thinking, planning, and executing to prove or disprove a hypothesis. It is a way to an answer. Analytical assessment is the key to self-improvement. Without it nothing happens; theories and dogma are accepted without question, and progress is nil.

Differential assessment is largely hypotheses testing, which takes place before, during, and after all phases of the patient's visit. There are at least four ways to complete a differential assessment: (1) charts and tables, (2) traditional diagnostic tests, (3) physical differentiation, and (4) questioning and examining during the SE, PE, and treatment. What is the source of the patient's disorder? Where must the treatment be directed to be effective?

Charts and tables that list, compare, or discuss signs and symptoms of various disorders are readily available in textbooks and journals. Traditional diagnostic tests, such as X-rays and CAT scans, may be available for study. Results of these tests may be helpful in determining the source of the patient's disorder. The results may also be misleading.

Jones defines physical differentiation as that which "involves altering the pain provoking position, or movement in such a way, that one structure is implicated as source, while another is eliminated from contention."[6] The purpose of physical differentiation is to so stress one area that the symptoms are produced from that area alone; thus, the other area(s) are ruled out as a source of the disorder. A key to differential assessment is to differentiate the source of the symptoms manually rather than labeling the disorder as a syndrome based on a collection of symptoms. The T-4 syndrome is an example of labeling a disorder.[8]

Careful questioning and examination of the patient during the SE, PE, and treatment is the most common way to accomplish a differential assessment. If the source of the disorder is not clarified this way, other ways are explored.

Clinical reasoning is the process of making clinical decisions. Both vertical and lateral thinking are usually involved. Vertical thinking is characterized by logical, sequential, predictable, and what might be called conventional thinking. Lateral thinking is not necessarily sequential, and it is unpredictable. Lateral thinking involves restructuring, the escape from old patterns and the creation of new ones; it is concerned with the generation of new ideas and with looking at things in a different way. While vertical thinking stays within a problem space, lateral thinking tends to restructure the problem space. Vertical thinking is hindered by the necessity to be right at each stage of the thought process and the attempt to rigidly define everything. Lateral thinking is based on the notion that premature formation and expression of an idea may inhibit its natural development.

■ The Need to Differentiate

The need to differentiate is generated by the requirement to direct treatment, whatever the mode, at the source of the patient's disorder. To treat the wrong area is simply unproductive. The tempest of managed care and the results of outcome studies have made this need more obvious. Differentiation is usually required when (1) the physician has rendered a nonspecific diagnosis, (2) the diagnosis appears to be in question, and/or (3) the therapist decides that the patient's disorder may be multistructural and/or multisegmental.

In uncomplicated presentations, the source of the disorder is clarified during the SE and an initial hypothesis is formed. This hypothesis is confirmed, rejected, or modified during the PE, and/or during treatment. In complicated presentations, clarification of the source of the disorder is often delayed until treatment; the hypothesis is then tested at subsequent visits. The questioning techniques in the SE, the examination techniques in the PE, and the techniques used for treatment may all influence the outcomes of the differential assessment.

Two terms, which may require clarification, are *comparable sign* and *asterisks*. The comparable sign "refers to a combination of pain, stiffness and spasm which the examiner finds on examination and considers to be comparable with the patient's symptoms."[9] The comparable sign may be thought of as both a comparable sign and comparable symptom. The sign is visible to or palpable

by the therapist, and the symptom is felt by the patient. Asterisks (*) "are not mandatory for treatment by passive movement to be quickly successful. Their only purpose is to highlight the important aspects that can be used to guide the assessment of the effectiveness of the treatment—it speeds up the whole process."[9]

The cervical spine and the thoracic spine are intimately related anatomically and functionally. When patterns of patient presentations are complicated, it may be necessary to examine each area individually. For presentation of cervical-thoracic differentiation, the sections to follow are labeled "Cervical (Doubtful Thoracic)" and "Thoracic (Doubtful Cervical)." *Her* is used to refer to the therapist and *he* is used for the patient for convenience. No gender bias is intended.

■ Cervical (Doubtful Thoracic)

Nature and Kind of the Disorder

Is the *nature* of his disorder an annoyance, an impairment, or disabling? What *kind* of disorder is it: pain, stiffness, weakness, instability, or incoordination? An input questionnaire,[10] completed by the patient, provides information to estimate the nature and kind of the disorder. If he knows the source of his symptoms, he will implicate the cervical spine. In general, chronic symptoms are more difficult for him to describe accurately than acute symptoms. If cervical instability is present, words like *unsafe*, *give way*, and/or *slipping out* are used. The history, if there was significant trauma, may suggest instability. Extensive work on cervical instability is presented by Aspinwall.[11] Words like *tired* and *fatigue* suggest weakness. Difficulty walking suggests spinal intermittent claudication, recently investigated by Kikuchi et al.[12] The painful neck is a common complaint; however, it isn't always a pain disorder, but rather a stiff neck that has pain. Pain may not be the dominant factor; when stiffness lessens, the pain often lessens. When movement is restored, pain subsides.[13]

Area(s) of Symptoms

Cervical symptoms are often ipsilateral, referring into the medial scapular area, the supraspinatous fossa, and/or the posterior arm, forearm, and/or hand. Symptoms referred from the upper, middle, and lower cervical spine will differ, but dermatome and myotome charts are often of little help in localizing the lesion. Cervicogenic headaches are a common complaint. Many of these headaches have their origin at C3 or above,[14] but headaches may also originate from C6 through T4.[8] Variations in the sites of headaches may be due to referral from the dura and/or from the muscles.[15]

Generally speaking, symptoms from a deformed cervical disc are felt deeply, and symptoms from an apophyseal joint(s) are felt relatively superficially. The patient can often point to the site of apophyseal pain with accuracy, but not to the site of discogenic pain. Acute cervical pain is often, but not always, worse distally. Paresthesia is common but is not always recognized as significant by the patient. Ocular dysfunctions such as visual accommodation, visual convergence, and disorders of pupil function may be present in patients with cervical disorders.[16]

Behavior of Symptoms

Symptoms are usually increased by neck movements, especially sustained or quick movements. Symptoms are sometimes relieved by reaching overhead or by lifting up the ipsilateral elbow. At times, neck postures alter upper extremity symptoms. Upper limb tension tests often reproduce cervical symptoms.[8] Patients with cervical disorders usually prefer to sleep on the affected side.

History of Symptoms

The area of onset is the cervical spine, and if symptoms spread, the spread is toward the ipsilateral shoulder. Often stiffness is noticed prior to the onset of pain. Both gradual and sudden onset is common. Patients, if questioned thoroughly, often recall a previous neck stiffness. Prior treatment to the thoracic spine has failed to produce any relief. Patients with a discogenic neck disorder often wake *with* their neck pain, as opposed to those with a cervical "lock," who are often awoken *by* their neck pain.[17,18] There is no history of trauma in cervical lock, compared to a neck sprain.[19] The history of many cervical disorders reveals repetitive microtrauma to the cervical spine from chronic poor posture or patterns of postural activities.[20, 21]

Physical Examination

The plan is to reproduce the symptoms from the cervical spine and to clear the thoracic spine. Active physiologic, passive physiologic, and passive accessory test movements are used to examine both the cervical and thoracic spines. Later, one of the test movements will probably be used as a treatment technique; the treatment logically evolves from the examination.

Reproduction of the comparable sign is desirable but not mandatory, especially in the irritable patient. Irritable patients have intense symptoms, symptoms which are produced or made worse by mild activities, constant symptoms, or long-lasting, intermittent symptoms which settle slowly. In the nonirritable patient, it may be necessary to add vigor to the examination to reproduce the comparable sign—for example, upper and lower cervical quadrants, axial compression, and/or axial distraction. Compression may implicate weightbearing structures (intervertebral disc or the apophyseal joints); axial distraction may implicate ligaments and/or muscles believed to be under stretch.[22]

Agreement between the objective findings of the therapist and the subjective responses of the patient is important to verify the source of the disorder. If the features of the examination do not fit, that is, if there is no subjective and objective agreement, then the examination may be faulty. After the PE of the cervical spine, signs should be reassessed to determine the effects of the examination; the cervical signs should change.

The thoracic spine is cleared with appropriate overpressures in flexion, extension, bilateral sidebending, and bilateral rotations. Reassessment of the thoracic spine after the PE shows no change unless thoracic signs are cervical in origin.

Hypothesis Testing and Treatment

If the cervical hypothesis is true, signs in the cervical spine are comparable and reproducible. Thoracic signs are minimal and are not comparable. Initially, treat the most comparable cervical sign; then reassess both areas. To confirm the cervical hypothesis, both the cervical spine and the thoracic spine should improve if thoracic signs are cervical in origin. If the cervical spine improves and clears and the thoracic spine does not, then reject the cervical (doubtful thoracic) hypothesis and treat the thoracic spine; both areas are at fault.

The lower cervical spine and the upper thoracic spine should move simultaneously. In treating the lower cervical spine, it is often beneficial to treat the upper thoracic spine as well. Restoring movement to upper thoracic spine generally allows the lower cervical spine to move more effectively.

■ The Thoracic Spine

The cervical and thoracic regions are so closely related anatomically and functionally that they may require examination as a single unit.[3] Theoretically, there are coupled movements between the two regions; cervical and thoracic rotation and sidebending occur in a pattern. Assessment of coupled movements provides an opportunity to correlate theoretical knowledge and clinical findings. It also provides an opportunity to determine how treatment of one area may affect another, untreated area.

■ Thoracic (Doubtful Cervical)

Kind and Nature of the Disorder

Within the spine, the thoracic spine is least understood by most therapists and least investigated by researchers, but the findings of palpation are often easy to find and interpret.[23] Disorders range from trivial complaints to serious, disabling disorders. Pain, stiffness, and weakness are among the most common complaints. The patient's own words reveal extremely useful information regarding the kind and nature of the patient's problem.

Area(s) of Symptoms

In addition to soft, neural, and muscle tissues, there are seven joints at each level of the thoracic spine—more articulations than occur at any other spinal region.[24] Sometimes symptoms are visceralogenic (heart, lungs, diaphragm) and/or vertebralogenic.[25] The thoracic spine houses the sympathetic nervous system except lumbar levels 1 and 2; the costovertebral joints and other tissues are adjacent to the sympathetic trunks; thus, mechanically induced sympathetic symptoms are possible.[26,27] Hyperhydrosis, hypotrophic changes, and other symptoms are present in chronic cases.[16]

Thoracic symptoms occur in (1) the anterior and posterior chest wall; (2) the groin and posterior thigh (T10-T12); (3) following the ribs; and (4) the anterior and posterior arm (T1). Midthoracic symptoms are often neurogenic, most likely from the dura, nerve root, and/or nerve root sleeves. The cervical and thoracic spines both refer into the interscapular area. Levels T2 to T7 may produce a vertex headache.

Complete charts of typical thoracic symptoms are available.[25] Deep central back pain radiating through the chest, producing central anterior chest pain, appears to arise from the intervertebral disc if the pain is neuromuscular in origin. Unilateral thoracic pain, radiating horizontally around the chest wall, is probably due to unilateral joint structures: the zygapophyseal, costovertebral, and/or costotransverse joints. Unilateral thoracic pain radiating along the line of the rib usually originates from the nerve root, and, if acute, is likely to be worse either laterally on the chest wall or anteriorly in the distal part of the affected dermatome.[28]

Behavior of the Symptoms

Patients often complain of difficulty breathing, especially inspiration. Activities involving thoracic rotation and extension frequently produce symptoms. To a lesser extent, activities requiring stabilization of the thoracic spine are informative.

History

Insidious onset is common. It is often attributed to intrinsic forces of chronic poor posture, including disuse, misuse, and overuse. Obvious causal factors are (1) motor vehicle accidents, (2) postsurgical condition, and (3) excessive physical activity. Visual disturbances, probably from mechanical deformation or chemical irritation of the sympathetic chain, may be present. Adverse neural tension signs are common, especially in chronic cases.

Physical Examination

The vigor of the PE is determined by the outcome of the SE. Active physiologic, combined physiologic, passive physiologic, passive accessory, and neurotension tests are informative. The slump test produces pain in 90 percent of normal subjects at the T8 and T9 levels.[25] The long-sitting position usually isolates the thoracic spine better than sitting on the edge of the treatment table. The sympathetic slump test assesses disorders of the autonomic nervous system.[29,30]

For a physiologic differentiation test, rotate the cervical spine without rotating the thoracic spine; then add to the cervical rotation only thoracic rotation. Assess the symptoms at each interval of change and then reverse the order of the tests to confirm or reject the results. For an accessory test, the intent is to try to move one segment locally.[25] For a thoracic segment to be significantly rotated, the transverse processes *and* the spinous process of the segment should show asymmetry; deviation of the spinous process alone may be normal asymmetry. Deep-set and high-set spinous processes should be considered suspicious.[25] Reproduction of the comparable sign, coupled with significant palpation abnormalities, strengthens the hypothesis of local thoracic injury.

Evidence of thoracic cord myelopathy calls for reflex tests, clonus tests, and tests of lower limb coordination. To reproduce an evasive comparable sign, try the slump test in the long-sitting position, with thoracic sidebending away from the disorder coupled with a deep inspiration.[29] For indirect neural tension tests of the thoracic spine, use the straight-leg raise, passive neck flexion, and prone knee bend. See Butler et al.[8,29,31] and Pecina et al.[32] for details of nerve tension tests and tunnel syndromes.

Hypothesis Testing and Treatment

If the thoracic hypothesis is true, signs in the thoracic spine are comparable and reproducible. Cervical signs are minimal and not comparable. Initially, treat the most comparable thoracic sign; then reassess both areas. To confirm the thoracic hypothesis, both the thoracic spine and the cervical spine should improve if cervical signs are thoracic in origin. If the thoracic spine improves and clears and the cervical spine does not, then reject the thoracic (doubtful cervical) hypothesis and treat the cervical spine; both areas are at fault. Assessment of outcomes at the next visit (day 2 assessment) is useful in chronic thoracic cases, especially if the transverse accessory test provokes symptoms.[25]

■ Mobilization of the Cervical and Upper Thoracic Spine

Mobilization of the cervical and upper thoracic spine, with the intent of relieving pain or increasing range of motion, or both, may be performed actively or passively using a variety of procedures and techniques. There is little evidence that passive techniques alone provide lasting relief of pain and a permanent increase in range of motion. Studies[33–37] of the effectiveness of spinal manipulation demonstrate the limitations of this form of treatment. Therefore, it seems logical, from both a clinical and an economic point of view, to provide the patient with a treatment protocol that will have a lasting effect. Physical therapists, in cooperation with their medical colleagues, have made significant progress toward providing such treatment.

This section presents an integrated approach to the assessment and treatment of the upper spine. The emphasis is on clinical assessment by the therapist and on treatment that fosters patient participation, self-treatment, and the prevention of recurrent pain. The greater part of this section relies heavily on the approaches presented by Robin McKenzie,[38,39] Geoffrey Maitland,[25] and James Cyriax.[40] However, other methods of treatment borrowed from a variety of sources are also introduced.

McKenzie[38,39] proposes that therapists first use active movements performed by the patient, supplementing these with passive movements when required. However, therapists may elect to use passive movements first, supplemented by active movements as required.[39] It is quite possible that joints that are very stiff or very painful will require passive movement prior to active movement. When active movements produce a desirable treatment effect, the patient is on his way toward improved function and independence.

The use of mobilization dates back to the days of Hippocrates.[41] The birth of orthopaedic medicine, according to Cyriax,[40] was in 1929. Orthopaedic manual therapy, as described by Cookson and Kent,[42] first became popular in Europe and Australia in the middle of the 20th century, largely as a result of the work of Freddy Kaltenborn, John Mennell, and Geoffrey Maitland. Robin McKenzie[43] first published his theories in 1972. Stanley Paris is thought by many physical therapists to be largely responsible for introducing mobilization concepts in the United States during the 1960s.

It is recognized that not all lesions of the upper spine are related to the articulations alone. Thus, an effective program of treatment will often include other techniques for the soft tissues. It is also acknowledged that not all lesions of the upper spine are mechanical. Thus, an effective program of treatment will frequently include physical agents or rest and analgesics for the treatment of the chemical or inflammatory component of the patient's pain. A discussion of physical agents, connective tissue massage, cranial sacral therapy, or other approaches is beyond the scope of this chapter.

Generally speaking, a physical therapist may elect one of two approaches to assess a patient. One approach is to conduct an SE and a series of objective tests with the intent of reaching a tentative diagnosis, which may lead

to the identification of a suspected structure at fault. The treatment is then aimed at this suspected structure. The therapist feels very comfortable and secure in addressing the problem in such a definite manner. In this approach, usually called the diagnostic approach, the techniques used in treatment help to confirm or deny the diagnosis.

The second approach is to respect the medical diagnosis rendered by the referring physician, with appropriate precautions, and then to conduct an SE and a series of objective tests with the intent of recording the changes in the patient's signs and symptoms. No specific structure is designated as being at fault, and the treatment rendered is adjusted according to the patient's individual response. It is quite permissible to hypothesize what is at fault, but the nature and progression of the treatment depend on the clinical behavior of the patient's problem. This approach is usually called the signs-and-symptoms approach or the nonpathologic approach.

It is suggested that, from a historical perspective, diagnosis is subject to whims of the times. During the 1950s, for example, the diagnosis of fibrositis was very popular; now there is some doubt about whether that condition even exists. Then there is the chronic debate among practicing therapists concerning the relative involvement of the apophyseal joint and the intervertebral junction. It may well be that, in the next decade, the neurocentral joints of Von Luschka will be the focus of our attention on the cervical spine. The current pathology appears to be subject to an eternal succession of changes.

From an academic and clinical point of view, physical therapists must understand diagnoses and pathologies. The stages of repair, referenced more thoroughly later in this chapter, are clearly related to proper management. It is proposed that individual therapists may use either or both methods—the diagnostic approach or the signs-and-symptoms approach—depending on their preference. In this chapter, the emphasis will be on the latter, with some reference to the former approach when appropriate.

■ The McKenzie and Maitland Approaches

Some areas of agreement and difference between the approaches of McKenzie and Maitland are apparent. Both approaches are rooted in James Cyriax's principles. In 1950 Cyriax[44] advocated the use of heavy lumbar traction coupled with strict maintenance of lumbar lordosis. In both approaches, there appears to be a bias in the direction of spinal extension. McKenzie's extension principle,[38,43,45] may be comparable to Maitland's[25] central vertebral pressures or posteroanterior central vertebral movements.

It is acknowledged clearly that the two approaches are different. Spinal traction is advocated more by Maitland than by McKenzie. The Maitland approach relies heavily on the use of passive movement performed by the therapist, whereas the McKenzie approach relies heavily on the use of active movement performed by the patient.

Both approaches are largely nonpathologic, with heavy reliance on treatment of the clinical signs and symptoms, compared with treatment by diagnosis or using the theories of biomechanics. Consequently, for each approach the therapist must be highly skilled in both types of assessment, objective and subjective. For example, subjective assessment of the changes in the patient's symptoms during treatment, based on information supplied by the patient, is essential in assessing the effects of the test movements. One clear exception to the nonpathologic nature of McKenzie's approach is the theory that the derangement syndrome is caused by deformation of the intervertebral disk. The theory that the disk is responsible for the derangement is in agreement with Cyriax's teachings. In fact, Cyriax[41] stated that the intervertebral disk is responsible for 90 percent of all low back pain.

McKenzie and Maitland seldom designate a specific structure responsible for spinal stiffness. They apparently see no need to join the endless debate regarding which specific structure is at fault. If the movement used in treatment is correct, the symptoms and/or the signs will be influenced positively. For example, when treating the pain of derangement, if repeated passive or active sidebending to the painful side of the cervical spine reduces, centralizes, and eliminates the patient's pain, this movement is the preferred one and should be used as an initial treatment until it is no longer effective. When treating stiffness, if the repeated sidebending away from the painful side, performed either passively or actively, produces the patient's pain, and subsequently increases his range and does not worsen his symptoms, then the movement is the preferred one and should be used as a major part of treatment until it is no longer effective.

■ Definitions

Most physical therapists use standard medical terminology. However, the advent of specialization within the profession has generated a body of knowledge and, concurrently, a particular language peculiar to each specialization. For example, for some therapists the term *dysfunction* has more specific meaning than simply *loss of function*. To oversimplify, dysfunction in the McKenzie approach means a lack of movement caused by adaptive shortening of tissues. Provided that this definition is accurate as a clinical assessment, the treatment rendered follows a particular pattern with certain expectations. Thus, it is imperative that therapists speak the same language to communicate their thoughts, theories, and treatment rationales.

In the sections on assessment and treatment that follow, certain terminology is consistently used. Therefore, in the interests of clarity, this terminology is defined and illustrated.

Mechanical and Chemical Pain

Pain is not a primary sensation, like vision, hearing, and smell, but rather an abnormal affective state accurately described as an unpleasant emotional state. This emotional state is aroused by unusual patterns of activity within the nociceptive receptor system and is subject to different degrees of facilitation and inhibition.[46] The nociceptive receptor system is sensitive to mechanical and chemical tissue activity. Thus, if this largely inactive receptor system is stimulated by the application of sufficient mechanical forces to stress, deform, or damage it, mechanical pain is produced. However, if the system is irritated by sufficient concentrations of chemical substances such as lactic acid or potassium ions, chemical pain is produced. Thus, in a clinical situation, it is quite possible to have either chemical, mechanical pain, or both concurrently.

Generally, mechanical pain is constant and variable or intermittent and often is affected by movement or position. Movements, either passive or active, that reduce the mechanical deformation also reduce the patient's symptoms. Patients whose problem is mechanical usually will report that there is some time during the day or night when they are symptom-free, or when their symptoms are significantly reduced or increased. Careful questioning by the therapist will frequently reveal that pain reported by the patient to be constant is, in fact, intermittent.

Chemical or inflammatory pain is more constant and is less affected by movement or position. Seldom is chemical pain reduced by either passive or active movements, because the movements have little positive effect on the chemical irritants. Chemical pain is often increased by movement and reduced by rest. Chemical pain is also obviously more responsive to medications that reduce the inflammatory process. For example, if a patient has active cervical arthritis and the main complaint is a constant burning ache together with reduced range of motion, even gentle attempts to increase this range by movement may increase the ache and either have no effect on the range or reduce it.

However, a second patient may present with the same medical diagnosis, correctly rendered, but with the main complaint of intermittent pain coupled with reduced range. Attempts to increase this patient's range of movement in the proper direction will decrease the pain and often increase the range concurrently. The latter patient often complains of increased symptoms, including occipital headache on arising in the morning. Symptoms often are limited to the first hour on awakening in the morning. Further, the patient will report that the symptoms are either decreased or eliminated with movement, and frequently he or she experiences pain only after periods of inactivity.

Many patients present with pain that has both a chemical and a mechanical component. These patients complain of both pain and stiffness. It is suggested that the two components of their pain, chemical and inflammatory, are closely related and interdependent (i.e., the chemical component may be the cause of the mechanical component). With the presence of both mechanical and chemical components, the therapist must make a therapeutic decision to treat either one component or both. It is quite possible that reduction of one component will have a positive effect on the other. For example, gentle low-grade movements applied to an apophyseal joint that is mechanically deformed may reduce the deformation and consequently the mechanical pain. The movements have no obvious effects on the chemical irritation, but at least the chemical irritation is not increased. Because the mechanical component of pain has been reduced, the range is increased and the patient regains function without an exacerbation of the pain.

In this example, the therapist has chosen to treat the stiffness caused by the mechanical deformation and, concurrently, to respect (by not increasing) the patient's inflammatory pain. Provided that the patient retains some of the increased function, it is reasonable to assume that the same treatment should be repeated until the patient's progress plateaus. It is suggested that, in certain circumstances in which the components of mechanical and chemical pain are present, treatment of one component may have a positive effect on the other. Further, it is suggested that to treat only one component may result in an incomplete recovery. For example, treating only the chemical component of the patient's pain with physical agents may have no effect, or an incomplete effect, on the mechanical component. Thus, the stage is set for recurrent bouts of the same problem because of a likely regression of the patient's condition.

In summary, active, acute inflammatory pain in the cervical spine, as elsewhere, often requires rest, immobilization, and physical agents. As the healing process progresses and scar tissue forms, the area requires appropriate active or passive movement in proper doses. As the chemical pain abates and the patient presents with dominant mechanical pain, the area requires more vigorous movement. Excellent and detailed discussions of the relation-ships among the healing processes and treatment modes may be found in writings by Cummings et al.[47] and Evans.[48] A summary of the relationships among the stages of healing, joint reactivity to movement, and treatment modes is presented in Table 7–1.

Elimination of the mechanical pain by proper treatment logically leads to the need to restore full function. Adequate muscle strength and flexibility to provide quality movement and reconditioning of the entire body for life's activities are essential. The use of appropriate treatment methods at the proper time to eliminate the chemical and mechanical pain, with progression through the reconditioning program, requires the skills of a talented therapist. This complete progression, managed well, is *effective* physical therapy.

Three Syndromes: Pain, Stiffness, and the Centralization Phenomenon

In the nonpathologic approaches, in which changes in clinical signs and symptoms, with due respect for the medical diagnosis and contraindications, are used to select techniques and determine the progression of treatment, obvious principles and theories underlie the clinical assessments and treatments. The terms *posture, dysfunction, derangement*, and the *centralization phenomenon*, as described by McKenzie,[39] deserve explanation. Maitland[25] uses the terms *pain* and *stiffness*, which may vaguely be compared to derangement and dysfunction, respectively. The proposed relationships among these terms may provide some limited, but clinically useful, guidelines for assessment and treatment.

The terms *posture, dysfunction*, and *derangement* have very specific meanings in the McKenzie approach. Although not all patients fit neatly into a particular category, the use of the three terms provides a framework from which are generated essential clinical principles. For example, in treating dysfunction, defined in simplified terms as adaptive shortening of structures that hinders function, the purpose of the treatment is to lengthen the adaptively shortened structures to restore function. The patient's

□□□□□□ □ □

Table 7–1. Treatment Modes Related to Reactivity and Stages of Scar Tissue Formation

Stages	Reactivity	Treatment
Inflammation	Pain, then resistance	Rest Immobilization Grade I and II movements
Granulation Fibroplastic (healing)	Pain and resistance simultaneous	Active range-of-motion exercises Grade I and II movements
Maturation	Resistance, then pain	Passive range-of-motion exercises Grade III, IV, and V movements

(Adapted from Paris,[88] with permission.)

symptoms should be produced and the limitations of function established. In the treatment of derangement, defined simply as a disturbance of the normal anatomic relationship within the intervertebral disk, the purpose of treatment is to reduce, centralize, and eliminate the patient's pain. Maintenance of reduction, restoration of function, and prevention of recurrences follow logically.

In the treatment of the posture syndrome, defined briefly as end-range strain on normal tissues, the purpose of treatment is to remove the end-range strain by correcting the patient's poor posture. The patient must become keenly aware and convinced of the cause of the symptoms.

In the Maitland approach, the therapist is obligated to decide, among other possibilities, whether she is treating the patient's pain or the patient's stiffness, respecting the pain. This decision is based on many subjective and objective assessment variables including joint irritability, the patient's perception of the nature of the problem, the relationship between range and pain, and the effects of passive movement during treatment. If pain is the dominant factor of concern to the patient, and if pain rather than resistance or stiffness prevents full range of motion, the therapist elects to treat the patient's pain. Thus, the success or failure of the treatment is based on its ability to reduce, centralize (where applicable), and eliminate the pain. This is not meant to imply that the treatment of pain in the cervical spine is limited to cases in which the pain is produced by deformation of the intervertebral disk. There are structures other than the disk that are commonly capable of producing sufficient pain to warrant the treatment of the pain alone. The analogy between the two approaches in the treatment of derangement (McKenzie) and in the treatment of pain (Maitland) is definitely limited.

A very weak analogy between the two approaches in the treatment of dysfunction (McKenzie) and in the treatment of stiffness (Maitland) may be postulated. In a case in which lack of movement, for example, is theoretically caused by decreased gliding of an apophyseal joint and the patient complains mainly of stiffness or perhaps mild discomfort, treatment may be directed at the dysfunction or stiffness while respecting the discomfort. In this case, lack of movement concerns the patient most. Thus, the therapist has the latitude to reproduce the patient's discomfort during treatment with the intent of increasing the patient's range and reducing stiffness. A positive treatment effect is possible using either approach, provided that the end-range pain or discomfort produced during treatment, by either active or passive exercises, does not linger unreasonably. A certain amount of post-treatment soreness is acceptable and expected. If there is no increase in range as a result of the stretching of adaptively shortened tissues after a reasonable number of treatments, the treatment has been unsuccessful.

It is acknowledged that most patients present with both pain and stiffness, and the decision as to which is the dominant complaint is often difficult. If in doubt, treat the pain; only time (not the patient) is lost if the decision is incorrect. Subsequent assessments will reveal no gain from the treatment, and in most cases the role of the pain was exaggerated by the patient, by the therapist, or both. With the new knowledge that the treatment of the pain was ineffective, therapist and patient may well decide to change the treatment and begin to treat the stiffness while respecting the pain. If this decision is made, it is most advisable that the patient agree with the therapist. Patient compliance and understanding are both increased, not to mention happiness. An unhappy patient rapidly becomes a no-show and/or conveys an unfavorable message to the referring physician.

The three syndromes, as described by McKenzie,[38,39] are also described in handouts by the faculty of the McKenzie Institute at appropriate courses. Therapists are encouraged to refer to them. However, reading material is no substitute for course participation or supervised clinical practice.

McKenzie[38] described the centralization phenomenon as a movement of pain from the periphery toward the midline of the spine. This mechanical pain, originating from the spine and referred distally, centralizes as a result of certain repeated movements or the assumption of certain positions. The movements that cause this phenomenon then may be used to eliminate radiating and referred symptoms. Centralization occurs only in the derangement syndrome during reduction of the mechanical deformation. This centralization of pain in patients whose symptoms are of recent origin may occur within a few minutes. When centralization takes place, there is often a significant increase in central spinal pain. For example, decreased arm pain is traded for a temporary increase in neck pain.

In a study of approximately 100 patients with low back pain, Donelson et al.[49] reported that occurrence of the centralization phenomenon had been documented. Centralization was found to be reliable in evaluating the nature of the disorder, selecting the appropriate mechanical treatment, and predicting eventual outcomes. Those patients whose pain centralized at the initial examination had an excellent prognosis for recovery. Those patients whose pain did not centralize or, worse yet, peripheralized usually had a poor prognosis for recovery.

Although Donelson et al.[49] reported the centralization phenomenon in regard to the lumbar spine, I have repeatedly observed, along with other authors, the same behavior in the cervical spine. Repeated movements, either active or passive, performed in one direction will often produce an increase in peripheral pain. Other movements, usually performed in the opposite direction, will reduce the peripheral pain and centralize the symptoms. Cervical traction may be effective in some cases in producing the centralization phenomenon; however, the lasting effects of traction without other procedures in retaining centralization are open to question. However, patient procedures (active exercises), when successful in producing centralization, are preferred to cervical traction because of the ease with which self-treatment can be accomplished outside the therapist's office. There are circumstances in which centralization is not possible with either active or passive exercises, and under these circumstances, cervical traction may serve as a bridge to exercises. In other words, traction may be the treatment of choice until the exercises can produce a desirable effect. However, patients do not get better with traction alone.[50]

Active Procedures and Therapist's Techniques

Active procedures are those movements performed by the patient. They are similar to active exercises, but not identical, because some active procedures may be largely passive. In the cervical spine, retraction and extension performed in the supine position, coupled with small rotations at the limit, are assisted by gravity and may require little or no active muscle action. If the patient applies overpressure, an active component is introduced into the procedure. In the lumbar spine, the press-up movement is mainly a passive procedure, without active involvement of the erector spinae or gluteal muscles. With active muscle contractions, full available range may not be obtained and the assessment becomes distorted. Side-bending or lateral flexion of the head performed in the sitting position is also assisted by gravity, and relaxation of the muscles within the cervical spine often enhances a positive treatment effect.

Therapists must instruct the patient carefully in the proper method of performing active procedures. It is often necessary to demonstrate the exact movement desired. Instruct the patient to report any changes in symptom behavior that take place during and immediately after the procedure. The precise status of the symptoms before the procedure is required for proper assessment. The consistency of test-retest (assessment) is affected by the patient's pretest posture.

Extension of the cervical spine is usually performed starting in a retracted position. If consistency of the starting position (i.e., proper retraction) is not maintained, the assessment may be inaccurate. A potentially successful procedure thought to be ineffective because of inaccurate instruction by the therapist is wrongly abandoned or, worse yet, the approach is faulted.

Therapists' techniques are those movements performed on the patient by the therapist. They are passive and, in most respects, are mobilizations using either passive physiologic techniques or passive accessory techniques. In the McKenzie approach, therapists' techniques are used as an adjunct to active procedures when needed to produce a desired treatment effect. The application of therapists' techniques may promote dependence on the therapist, and their use may reduce the effectiveness of self-treatment. Therapists' techniques, in contrast to active procedures, provide an extrinsic force, whereas active procedures provide an intrinsic force generated by the

patient. Because the patient may, in part, be responsible for his own problem, either by chronic poor posture or other self-inflicted abuse, it is the patient's responsibility to treat his own problem using active procedures. It is also believed that a well-educated patient who understands the problem, including the mechanical model, will most likely able be to prevent or reduce future bouts of spinal pain. Thus, the patient stands a reasonable chance of ending or reducing recurrent cycle of repeated bouts of spinal pain.

Therapists' techniques are usually performed as oscillating or repeated movements in a preferred direction. Movements may be sustained when a sustained position produces desirable effects. Sustained movements may also be used as provocative tests in an attempt to reproduce the patient's comparable sign. There are endless variations in the speed, direction, and/or rhythm of a technique. The degree of clinical skill required to apply and assess most of the techniques described by McKenzie may not be as high as that required to apply and assess the techniques described by Maitland. This is not meant to imply that one approach is superior; it is merely an observed difference between the two approaches. There is an appropriate place within the healing arts for both approaches. History will be the judge of any differences in effectiveness and efficiency. There is no room for exclusion based on the myth of elitism.

Direction of a Procedure or Technique

There are few, if any, absolutes or correct techniques or procedures based on theories. General guidelines and contraindications provide the clinician with reasonably logical methods of selecting techniques or procedures. General guidelines and contraindications may be used in determining the desirable direction of the forces. These guidelines are based on the correct mechanical diagnosis (rendered by the physical therapist) using the McKenzie approach. In general, the guidelines are based on current knowledge of pathology, the known mechanical disorders of the vertebral column, the medical diagnosis, and the changes in symptoms and signs. For the cervical and thoracic spine, Maitland[25] provides guidelines for the sequence of techniques and primary uses for mobilizing techniques. He recommends the use of cervical traction for an acute cervical condition in which there is severe arm pain with markedly limited neck movements to the painful side. Once the pain is under control with the use of traction, the therapist may elect to change techniques to address the residual stiffness, respecting the pain. This is not meant to imply that techniques are used only to treat stiffness, because the low-grade techniques (grades I and II) are used frequently and effectively to treat pain. The treatment of pain using passive movement is thoroughly described by Maitland.[25]

Some clinicians believe that one of the advantages of the Maitland approach is its efficacy in treating pain. For example, passive accessory movements are frequently used in the part of the range that is totally free of pain or discomfort. As the patient's pain decreases and signs of movement improve, the technique can be taken further through the range and the amplitude of the technique increased. Some clinicians are surprised when gentle rotation movements of the cervical spine, often performed away from the painful side in the painless part of the range, produce a significant improvement in the pain behavior and range on the painful side. The patient will often report only a feeling of mild strain on the painful side during application of the technique. As this strain is reduced, the active movement toward the painful side increases when it is assessed after treatment or between episodes of therapy. The stretching of the painful side in a carefully controlled manner by rotation away from the painful side is also described elsewhere.[18,51]

Guidelines for determining the preferred direction of a technique are provided by the McKenzie[38] approach. These guidelines are reasonable, practical, and clinically effective, provided that the mechanical diagnosis is accurate. The physical therapist classifies the patient as having a postural, dysfunction, or derangement syndrome. This classification is based in part on the physician's diagnosis appropriately weighed together with the information provided from the therapist's subjective and objective assessments. Both assessments are discussed later in this chapter.

Besides providing guidelines for the preferred direction of a technique, the teachings of McKenzie provide a reasonable and logical rationale for the progression of a technique. The direction of a gentle therapeutic movement in advance of more vigorous techniques has been determined to be proper. For example, in treating a recent derangement, if movement in the direction of flexion of the lower cervical spine increases the patient's peripheral symptoms, this is most likely the wrong direction. Theoretically, the flexion movement has made the patient worse by increasing the mechanical deformation. However, if movement in the direction of extension of the lower cervical spine decreases and centralizes the patient's symptoms, this is most likely the preferred direction. Theoretically, the extension movement has made the patient better by reducing the mechanical deformation of the structure(s) causing the patient's pain. This illustration assumes, for the sake of clarity, that the lateral compartment's contribution to the pain is irrelevant (i. e., it is unnecessary to effect movement in the frontal plane to gain centralization). Provocation and reduction of symptoms generate useful information. If movement is provided in the preferred direction, the patient will get better regardless of the underlying theories.

How are the direction, vigor, and frequency of a technique determined? Part of the answer lies in the correctness of the mechanical diagnosis and in the clinical assessment. The three syndromes—posture, dysfunction, and derangement—are all treated differently, and the intent of the procedure or technique is peculiar to each syndrome.

The posture syndrome has no pathology. In other words, the pain is produced by abnormal stress on normal tissue. Normal tissue, when stretched to the limit, produces pain. When the deformation or stretch is removed, the pain goes away. Hyperextension overpressure of a metacarpophalangeal joint is used to illustrate pain of postural origin, provided that the joint is normal. Remove the overpressure and the pain stops; the postural strain has been removed.

Because there is no structural anomaly and no loss of joint motion, there is no need to worry about the direction or progression of a technique. Such therapy is contraindicated because there is nothing to stretch (no dysfunction) and nothing to reduce (no derangement). There is something to balance by removing the deforming stress of end-range strain. For example, assume that the average head weighs 9 lb and the average neck cephalad to C7 weighs 3 lb. The total potential deforming force at C6-C7 is then equal to the total weight of 12 lb times the lever arm distance from the center of gravity of the combined masses. Thus, if the head and neck mass is 2 in. forward of the fulcrum at C6-C7, then the moment of the force at C6-C7 is 2 ft-lb.

If this deforming force is present 16 hours a day (during waking hours only), the stage is set for mechanical deformation, either elastic or plastic, depending on the time elapsed. Removal of this sustained end-range stretch of normal tissues will eliminate the patient's pain. Thus, correction of the patient's poor posture is all that is required to treat the posture syndrome effectively. No phonophoresis, manual techniques, or electrical currents are needed. The patient simply must learn how to remove the deforming force. Compliance, which is enhanced by a clear demonstration explaining the cause of the pain, is the key. The intent of the posture instruction is to remove the deforming force by teaching the patient how to sit, stand, and lie correctly, with a balanced posture. Balanced posture must be devoid of end-range strain.

In the derangement syndrome, the intent of the technique or procedure is to reduce, centralize, and eliminate the patient's pain. The direction, mode (sustained or oscillating), and amplitude of techniques, procedures, and postures are dictated by selecting movements and positions that reduce the derangement. Reliance on the centralization phenomenon is essential. A temporary increase in central spinal pain, accompanied by a simultaneous decrease in peripheral pain, is acceptable.

In the dysfunction syndrome, the intent of the technique or procedure is to reproduce the pain of dysfunction and to increase the range of motion as a result of appropriate repeated stretching. The direction of the procedure or technique is dictated by selecting movements that reproduce the pain of dysfunction most effectively. The adaptively shortened structures are stretched over a period of time, and function slowly improves. Treatment or exercise soreness is normal, but this soreness should not linger or interfere with subsequent exercise or treatment sessions. The pain of dysfunction or stiffness is slow to resolve, as is the pain of a frozen shoulder.

Suggested Mechanisms for Relief of Pain and Increase in Range of Movement

Nyberg[52] presented three possible mechanisms by which spinal manipulation may work: the mechanical effects, the neurophysiologic effects, and the psychological effects. The term *manipulation* has a multitude of meanings, and there is little agreement in the literature that could lead to universal acceptance. In this chapter, manipulation is defined in its broadest sense, which includes the use of refined motion performed either by the therapist (technique) or by the patient (procedure). Within the boundaries of this definition, we explore the mechanical and neurophysiologic effects. The psychological effects, although important, are beyond the scope of this chapter.

Mechanical Effects

It is established that new scar tissue can be influenced by movement applied at the appropriate time in the proper direction. Both Evans[48] and Cummings et al.[47] have described the beneficial effect of remodeling new collagen. It is also quite possible that hypomobile joints that have been underexercised for an extended time can be influenced positively by movement. One possible mechanism is the stretching or rupture of abnormal cross-links that were formed between fibers.

Another mechanical effect, proposed by McKenzie,[38] consists of influencing annular or nuclear material by removing the forces causing the mechanical deformation and applying an appropriate reductive force. The mechanical deformation is reduced or eliminated by the use of repeated movements, usually performed in the direction opposite to the one that caused the mechanical deformation. For example, if the deforming force was flexion, the reductive force would be extension, or vice versa. It is further hypothesized that, when the intervertebral disk is at fault, the pain is centralized, reduced, and eliminated in response to the appropriate repeated movements. Studies by Donelson et al.[49] addressing this centralization phenomenon lend credibility to this theory. One advantage of the McKenzie approach is that, in most cases, the patient is able to perform these repeated movements independent of the therapist.

One clinical problem frequently encountered in practice, which is largely mechanical in nature, is the common kyphus deformity in the lower cervical and upper thoracic spine. Older patients present with a markedly forward head and significant loss of movement. Younger patients present with the same deformity but only moderate loss of movement. One theory that may explain some of the differences between the two age groups involves the concept of plastic and elastic mechanical deformation.

Deformation in a material is defined as displacement of atoms from their equilibrium position as a result of a load.[53] The deformation is elastic if the displaced atoms return to their equilibrium position when the load is removed and plastic if they do not.[54] Thus, elastic deformation is nonpermanent and totally recovered on release of the applied load, whereas plastic deformation is permanent and nonrecoverable after release of the applied load.[55]

It is suggested that, in the older patient with a flexed lower cervical spine and an extended upper cervical spine, recovery of full function is impossible, in part because of plastic deformation. The opposite results can be expected in most younger patients. It is also essential, in treating both age groups, to attain and retain proper posture with a desirable cervical lordosis. The proper posture will either correct the elastic deformation or reduce the progression of the plastic deformation. The elimination of chronic postural loads that most likely produce deformation of tissues is an essential part of a comprehensive treatment program.

Neurophysiologic Effects

Another theory dating back to the work of Peterson[56] suggests that appropriate movements may have a positive effect on the neurophysiologic activity of the tissues. For example, in the cervical spine, according to Wyke,[57] there are three types of mechanoreceptors. Type I receptors, in the superficial layers of the fibrous capsule of the joints, are stimulated by end-range movements of the joints; type II receptors, in the deeper layers of the fibrous capsule of the joints, are stimulated by midrange movements of the joints; and type IV, the nociceptive afferents, are responsible for producing the unpleasant emotional experience commonly called pain.

The stimulation of either type I or type II mechanoreceptors, through an involved network of neural connections, is believed to be capable of modulating the experience of pain. Repeated movements, either active or passive, when performed either at the end of the range or in the midrange, are capable of reducing pain and allowing for increased movement.

Subjective Examination

Skillful assessment separates the successful clinician from the technician. Without assessment, treatment is the blind application of techniques without guidelines; success is a matter of luck rather than skill. Planning and progression are haphazard, without direction, and the therapist and the patient are often confused about the purpose or the expected outcome of the treatment. The practitioner, the patient, and the profession suffer needlessly. Some of our medical colleagues who rely only on the use of medications to treat mechanical problems of the spine may benefit from a lesson on assessment.

The SE involves more than a classical history. Although the information is collected by talking with the patient, as opposed to measuring objective changes, the quality of the information needed far exceeds the recording of simple facts. For example, the accurate completion of a pain drawing or a body chart on a patient with an assortment of neck, head, upper extremity, and upper thoracic symptoms may consume 10 minutes of skilled questioning and clarification. The relationships, if any, among the different symptoms must also be sorted out. The present and past histories of the disorder have yet to be addressed.

In general, the six major parts of the SE (often abbreviated C/O, C, or S) are (1) the nature and kind of the disorder, (2) the area of symptoms, (3) behavior of the symptoms, (4) the past history, (5) the present history, and (6) special questions. Accurate definition of the area of symptoms includes the precise location on the body chart of all the patient's abnormal sensations, including their depth, their surface location, and the extent of their spread peripherally. It is often helpful, when the therapist has completed the body chart, to clarify where the symptoms stop—for example, by asking, "You mean that, below your elbow, your right forearm feels the same as your left forearm—there are no abnormal sensations in either forearm?" Clarification of the distal extent of the symptoms will then allow the therapist to refer to the elbow symptoms as the barometer for determining centralization in a derangement syndrome.

Symptom behavior, both diurnal and nocturnal, provides the therapist with an understanding of the nature of the problem. Are the symptoms constant or intermittent? If constant, do they vary in intensity? If symptoms caused by mechanical deformation are completely abolished during certain periods of the day, the mechanical deformation has been removed. Once the symptoms appear to be mechanical, the effects of movement and posture on the symptoms can be established. For example, are the symptoms better or worse when the patient is sitting, moving, lying, or standing? Ask the patient to compare symptoms in the morning with symptoms in the evening. Is sleep disturbed? If so, to what extent? For example, "Are you unable to fall asleep or is your sleep disturbed?" If so, "How frequently are you awoken?" Pain at night may reflect inflammatory problems, other medical problems, or poor sleeping posture in need of correction. Coughing and sneezing increase intrathoracic pressure, and the behavior of symptoms during those maneuvers is essential information. If the patient's responses to questions about the behavior of symptoms are not clear, possibly because of the chronic nature of the complaints or the minor nature of the problem, the relative worsening of symptoms may be ascertained. It may

be necessary to rephrase or repeat questions to get a clear picture.

The past or previous history, as compared with the recent history of current neck pain, is established. For recurrent problems, it is important to clarify the severity and frequency of past bouts to determine if the problem is progressive. Repeated progressive bouts with exacerbations in the absence of trauma strongly suggest a derangement syndrome. It is also helpful for the therapist to know the condition of the cervical spine before the most recent bout. If there have been repeated insults, from either intrinsic or extrinsic trauma, it is quite possible that the neck may never move normally in response to the current treatment because of chronically hypershortened tissue or some other irreversible residual deformity.

Prior treatment for the same or previous conditions, and the efficacy of the prior treatment, may provide a clue as to what will be successful this time. It is also helpful to know what, if anything, has been done for the present problem and the effects, if any. Patients will frequently report that they get limited benefit from a particular exercise, and on further investigation, it is found that fine tuning of the exercise produces a more positive treatment effect. For example, the direction of the self-treatment, discovered by the patient, may have been correct, but the depth of movement or the frequency of exercises was insufficient. All that was needed was to go further into the range more often.

Questions regarding special diagnostic tests such as radiography, computed tomography (CT), and magnetic resonance imaging (MRI) should be unbiased; simply ask, for example, "Have you had recent x-rays?" The therapist would like to know the results and where the radiographs may be located to know if problems for which certain treatments are unsuitable have been ruled out. Cyriax[58] feels that radiographic findings can be misleading, as they often show an irrelevant abnormality unrelated to the present problem or fail to show any soft tissue deformation. The patient is led to believe that there is absolutely nothing wrong. There is no positive correlation between the findings on radiography and the clinical state of the patient.[59]

The patient's general health is explored to discover serious pathology that may have been undetected by the referring physician and to determine the relevance of known health problems. Does the patient look unwell, and has there been a recent unplanned weight loss? Is there a history of rheumatoid arthritis, which may suggest laxity of the transverse ligament? Are there any systemic diseases, including recent surgery and cardiorespiratory diseases, which will restrict the patient's ability to do active exercises? Are there symptoms of vertebral artery disease?

Questions regarding medications, including steroids, are asked to determine the effects of the medications on the patient's pain and to estimate any systemic effects of the drugs. The occasional use of mild analgesics that eliminate the pain suggests a moderately painful condition, whereas regular use of strong analgesics that only reduce the pain suggests a more painful condition. Long-term use of steroids may weaken the connective tissue. Patients who report suspected osteoporosis deserve gentle treatment, especially in the thoracic spine.

On completion of the SE, the therapist has gleaned extensive and relevant information in an efficient manner to the extent that she is able to establish, in many cases, a tentative conclusion. When the questions and answers flow in a fluid and logical manner, a particular structure is often implicated. The assessment has been successful to this point. A summary of the SE is presented in Table 7–2.

The PE will confirm, deny, or modify the therapist's tentative hypotheses. For example, headaches are well known to be associated with lower cervical spondylosis and upper cervical joint arthrosis. Empirical evidence favors the upper joints as being at fault.[60] Many patients will complain of a stiff neck and a morning headache at the base of the occiput or late-day headaches behind the ipsilateral eye or on the vertex of the head. Granted, there are many variations to these headache patterns, but let us assume that the occipital headache comes from the lower cervical spine, the headache behind the ipsilateral eye comes from C2, and the headache on the vertex of the head comes from C1. During the SE, the patient has indicated the areas of the neck where he feels pain and the areas of the headaches. There are no upper extremity or interscapular symptoms. The clear areas are marked by a check or a tic on the body chart. A popular diagnosis is either lower cervical spondylosis or upper cervical arthrosis. Subsequent movement tests and palpations are aimed at reproducing the pain of the stiff neck and a very

small portion of the headache symptoms. It is most likely that the stiff neck and the headache are related, but it is also possible that they are two separate entities. If the relationship was not clarified during the SE, it will most likely be clarified during the PE.

In a review of cervical radiculopathy, Dillin et al.[61] reported that cervical disk herniation is most common at the C5-C6 level, followed by C6-C7, C4-C5, C3-C4, and C7-T1. Earlier, Cyriax[40] reported that protrusions were rare at C2-C3, uncommon at C4, C5, and C7, and very common at C6. Thus, it is likely that either the C6 or the C7 nerve root is involved.

There are many hypotheses regarding the proximate cause of these lower cervical lesions. Ligamentous lengthening with periosteal lifting, chronic lower cervical spine flexion deformation with weakening of the posterior annular wall, osteophyte formation, and alteration of the length and tone of the cervical musculature are the explanations most frequently suggested.

It has been the author's experience that, regardless of the treatment approach favored by the therapist, most treatment is ineffective unless the patient assumes a balanced posture 24 hours a day. Thus, sitting, standing, and lying postural awareness is essential. Few patients, except in the acute state of a disorder, are unable to benefit from reduction of the chronic forward head posture. It is indeed frustrating for both the patient and the therapist to see no consistent significant reduction of symptoms when the treatment is appropriate but the chronic stress of poor posture remains a dominant factor. In fact, many patients will get significant relief from their symptoms by postural correction alone.

□□□□□ □ □ □ □

Table 7–2. Summary of Subjective Assessment[a]

Type of disorder (pain, stiffness, weakness, etc)

Location of the patient's symptoms, including the extent of peripheralization (recorded on the body or pain chart)

Nature of the symptoms, including frequency, original location, and degree of disability

Cause of the problem, if known (trauma, systemic disease, insidious)

Behavior of the symptoms over a 24-hour period, including the effects of different postures

Effects of changes in intrathoracic pressures

Present or recent history

Past history including treatment, if any

Patient's general health, results of any medical tests, and medications and their effect

Other relevant information peculiar to the patient

[a]It is assumed that the patient has already completed a brief medical history and that this information has been reviewed by the therapist.

■ Objective Assessment or Physical Examination

Definition

The objective assessment or PE is sometimes abbreviated O (in the SOAP notation), O/A (objective assessment), or O/E (on examination). This part of the total assessment follows the SE in which the therapist has gathered a complete description of the patient's presenting symptoms. The PE is a series of appropriate active and passive movement tests aimed at collecting additional data that will confirm or deny the therapist's tentative hypotheses reached during the SE. A typical PE consists of active physiologic movements, passive physiologic movements, passive accessory movements, and special tests, as needed.

Purpose

The general purpose of the PE is to assess movement and symptom behavior, that is, limitations, deviations, aberrations, and the effects, if any, of the movements on the patient's symptoms. Any deviation from normal movement and all symptom changes are noted. Future changes in the patient's condition can then be measured against the benchmarks of objective signs and subjective symptoms. Movement loss may be graded as major, moderate, minor, or none. The loss may also be expressed as a percentage of normal or expressed in degrees.

Besides assessing movement, a second purpose of the PE, especially when treating stiffness, is to reproduce the patient's comparable sign. For example, if the patient's chief complaint is a moderate midcervical pain and this same pain is reproduced by overpressure into the quadrant position, the quadrant position may be used later to assess the effects of the treatment.

A third purpose of the PE is to determine the preferred direction of treatment movements. Repeated movements that reduce, centralize, and eliminate the patient's symptoms are the movements to use in treating derangements. Repeated movements that temporarily produce, but do not worsen, the patient's symptoms are the movements to use in treating dysfunction. If no movements, either passive or active, can be found that produce the desirable effect on the patient's symptoms, either the patient may not be a good candidate for this treatment or the examination is faulty.

Instructions to Patients

The relative vigor and extent of the PE depend on the irritability of the patient's symptoms. If the cervical or thoracic spine is judged to be irritable, the examination must be gentle and limited to a few necessary movements. The patient with an acute nerve root irritation, with symptoms extending below the elbow, deserves a gentle examination. However, a nonirritable and moderately painful condition will require a more vigorous and extensive examination. Few patients require all the test movements to satisfy the purpose of the examination.

The therapist must know the status of the patient's symptoms immediately before starting the examination and at the conclusion of each test movement. Thus, the patient is asked to describe pretest symptoms and to report clearly any change in symptoms during and immediately after each test movement. It is also important for the patient to understand that, in most circumstances, some test movements may make the symptoms worse and others may make them better. The more accurately the patient is able to convey any changes to the therapist, the more informative will be the examination and, quite likely, the more effective will be the treatment.

Special Tests Before the Physical Examination

If the symptoms extend below the elbow, a neurologic examination must be completed before the PE is conducted. If the patient complains of dizziness or other associated symptoms, an essential part of the examination

consists of tests that estimate the integrity of the vertebrobasilar system. When these tests are performed before the PE, the effects, if any, of the examination itself may be assessed at the conclusion of the examination. Without a pretest, there is no benchmark from which to measure.

Corrigan and Maitland[23] described two clinical tests of the vertebral arteries. The first is to sustain the three positions of rotation to each side and extension. Symptoms may occur while in the sustained positions or on release. The second test is to have the patient rotate the trunk beneath the motionless head. For example, the therapist stabilizes the patient's head while the patient twists the trunk in the standing position fully from side to side, without moving the feet, or the movement is performed with the patient sitting on a swivel chair. The second test may eliminate the effect of inner ear movement. Other tests for vertebral artery insufficiency, published by the German Association of Manual Medicine,[62] are the extension tests, Hautant's test, De Klejn's test, and Underberger's tests.

Dizziness and reflex disorders of posture and movement can also be caused by degenerative, inflammatory, or traumatic disorders of the joints and muscles of the cervical spine. These structures are richly supplied with proprioceptive nerve endings.[60, 63, 64] Thus, dizziness is not always vertebrobasilar in origin.

Proper radiographic evaluation of suspected atlantoaxial instability is imperative before any vigorous objective assessment is attempted. Afflictions of this joint do occur, especially in Down syndrome, rheumatoid arthritis, ankylosing spondylitis, psoriatic arthritis, and posttraumatic conditions. Vigorous examinations or treatment, where instability exists, have had disastrous complications dating back to early reports by Blaine.[65]

According to Dvorak et al.,[66] it is not difficult to diagnose instability of the upper cervical spine caused by lesions of the transverse ligament. Functional radiographic studies, including CT scanning in maximal flexion of the cervical spine, provide indirect information about the integrity of the transverse ligament. In a cadaver study using 12 specimens, the same investigators reported that, after a one-sided lesion of the alar ligament developed, there was a 30 percent increase in original rotation to the opposite side. The increased movement was divided equally between C0-C1 and C1-C2. It was concluded that irreversible overstretching or rupture of the alar ligaments can result in rotatory hypermobility of the upper cervical spine. The alar and transverse ligaments could be differentiated on CT images in axial, sagittal, and coronal views.

Observation of the Cervical Spine

The patient usually sits on the narrow end of the treatment table to enable the therapist to observe from either side and from the front. Note the general sitting posture, static deformity, asymmetry, and skin condition. Also note the patient's willingness to move and any tenderness or swelling.

Test Movements

Before any test movements are assessed, the present symptoms in the sitting position must be recorded. For each test movement, estimate movement loss and the relationship between the patient's symptoms and his range. It is helpful, for the sake of consistency in recording data, for the therapist to establish a routine sequence. A routine in the order of testing movements also helps avoid omissions.

The normal method of testing active physiologic movements, in the McKenzie approach, is to test a movement once and then to repeat the same test movement several times. The joints must be moved sufficiently far into the range to produce a valid response to the test. A sequence of testing is as follows: protraction, flexion, retraction, retraction and extension, bilateral sidebend, and bilateral rotation.

Active movements may be sustained or oscillated to produce the desired effect. For the sake of patient education, it is often necessary to ask the patient to repeat a movement that makes him worse and then to repeat a movement that makes him better. The practical lesson learned by the patient creates a lasting impression, which will foster compliance.

One method of testing active physiologic movements, in the Maitland approach, is to have the patient move to the pain (when treating pain) or to move to the limit (when treating stiffness). It is important to clarify and accurately record the relationship between range and pain. A sequence of testing in balanced posture is flexion, extension, lateral flexion and bilateral rotation. Movements may also be tested in different parts of the flexion/extension range.

Movements may be sustained and overpressured as needed. The quadrants (a combination of extension with sidebending and rotation to the same side) for the upper and lower cervical spines may be tested if previous tests have been negative. Compression and distraction are used when necessary. Passive physiologic movements may also be tested in the supine position. Tests of the pain-sensitive structures in the intervertebral canal and static tests for muscle pain are performed as applicable.

The patient is then placed in a prone position for palpation tests including temperature and sweating, soft tissue palpation, position of vertebrae, and passive accessory intervertebral movement tests. The passive accessory intervertebral movements are described later in the section on Treatment Procedures and Techniques. The therapist marks important findings on the chart with an asterisk. The effects of the examination are then assessed both subjectively and objectively by retesting one or two movements. The patient's chart is also reviewed for reports of relevant medical tests.

For treating pain, the technique that reduces (and in some cases centralizes and eliminates) the pain is used as the treatment technique. For treating stiffness, the technique that produced the comparable sign but did not make it worse is used as the treatment technique. A concurrent increase in range is also a desirable treatment outcome when treating stiffness. After treatment, the patient is reassessed.

The patient is then warned of possible exacerbations, requested to report details of the behavior of symptoms between now and the next visit, and given instructions in neck care.

For both approaches, the complete objective assessment involves testing other joints, including the glenohumeral joints, which may be responsible for the production of the patient's symptoms. These tests involve active quick tests and passive accessory tests as needed.

Not all active physiologic test movements are illustrated in this chapter. However, many of the procedures and techniques illustrated later in the chapter are used as part of the objective assessment.

The Thoracic Spine

Active physiologic and passive accessory movements are tested using the same principles of assessment as those presented for the cervical spine. Techniques and procedures for the thoracic spine are presented later in this chapter.

A summary of the physical examination is presented in Table 7–3.

■ Treatment Procedures and Techniques

Principles

Treatment procedures or techniques are usually selected during the PE. Confirmation or denial of the original selection takes place at the second visit. It may be necessary to fine tune the procedure by, for example, correcting

□□□□□ □ □ □

Table 7–3. Summary of the Objective Assessment[a]

Neurologic and vertebral artery tests
Active physiologic movements
Passive accessory movements
Passive physiologic movements
Special tests (i.e., quadrants and tension tests)

[a]Not all these tests are performed on every patient. The therapist determines the extent of the examination on the basis of the information gleaned during the subjective assessment.

faults in the patient's performance of the procedure. If the patient has made significant progress, both objectively and subjectively, at the second visit there is no need to modify the procedure. However, if the patient is the same or worse at the second visit, the therapist is obligated to reevaluate the tentative conclusion reached at the initial visit and revise the treatment as needed. The patient with derangement should be seen daily until his pain is controlled by active procedures.

The following general principles will help guide the therapist in the selection of techniques or procedures, in the progression of treatment, and in the estimation of expected progress.

1. Use procedures to reduce the symptoms of derangement or to produce the symptoms of dysfunction with the knowledge that the patient understands the purpose of the procedures. The symptoms of derangement are expected to be reduced quickly, and the symptoms of dysfunction are expected to be reduced slowly. In derangement, once the symptoms are reduced, the next three phases of treatment are maintenance of the reduction, restoration of function, and prevention of recurrences.

2. In most cases, if not all, the learning of a new posture is essential to the success of a treatment program. For the patient to continue to use poor posture habits, which perpetuate chronic mechanical deformation, will only delay recovery or produce treatment failures.

3. The use of a therapist's technique may promote dependence on the therapist. Techniques are needed when the application of procedures has been exhausted or when the patient's progress has plateaued. A therapist's technique is useful in the treatment of derangement when the application of extrinsic forces is needed to gain or maintain a reduction.

4. Regardless of the approach selected, active exercises performed by the patient on a regular and continuing basis are one of the keys to preventing recurrent spinal pain and/or aborting future attacks of spinal pain. It is reasonable to expect that most patients are able and willing to do about four different exercises on a regular basis if they can see the benefits of the exercises.

5. One of the most difficult tasks faced by the practicing therapist is to create an effective and efficient home exercise program that will be followed meticulously by a happy patient. This taks is particularly challenging to both the therapist and the patient when it involves the conversion of a therapist's technique into an effective active exercise.

6. In very general terms, it is reasonable to expect that most patients will retain, from one treatment session to another, about 50 percent of the gain that was achieved at a treatment session. Optimally, this gain will be both a subjective and an objective improvement. The actual rate of improvement achieved by individual patients will vary, but the average gain for each patient is useful in determining the prognosis. Patients are more secure and satisfied with their treatment program when they are aware of the expected outcome.

7. Not all patients are suitable candidates for physical therapy. All approaches have their limitations, and it is the therapist's responsibility to identify unsuitable candidates and to offer a reasonable explanation and recommend viable alternatives. To do otherwise is irresponsible.

8. The true success of an approach is not measured by the date of return to work or by symptom-free behavior. Spinal pain is self-limiting in most of the population. The true success of an approach is measured, in part, by the effectiveness of the approach in preventing or reducing the severity of recurrent bouts of spinal pain.

9. Physical therapists have been guilty of seeing patients too often but not long enough. Once the patient has gained control of the symptoms, the frequency of visits may be significantly reduced. However, to be confident that an effective program of prevention is actually working, it is necessary to see the patient for rechecks over a reasonable period of time. In other words, the simple relief of pain is not sufficient evidence for discharging a patient.

10. Physical therapists should remain within the framework of organized medicine. Although independent practice without referral is an attractive concept, it does not appear to be the ultimate answer for the profession or for the patient. Physical therapy has much to gain in terms of quality of care and professional respectability by retaining a cooperative relationship with physicians. We are on the brink of a new era of effective treatment. Our professional research and clinical skills are reaching new heights. To separate from organized medicine, with all its faults, would in some respects put us into the role of "lay manipulators," as described by Cyriax.[40]

Techniques and Procedures

There are thousands of procedures and techniques. Maitland and McKenzie have described most of the ones that follow. They have contributed enromously to the delivery of effective and efficient assessment and treatment.

The following techniques and procedures for the cervical and upper thoracic spine are those I use most frequently. This presentation is not intended to be comprehensive or exclusive. Although the proper application of procedures or techniques contributes to the success of the treatment, the relative importance of proper assessment far exceeds the importance of proper technique. There are no limits to the nature and variations of procedures and techniques, and what may work for one therapist may be ineffective for another.

Books and journal articles are poor methods for learning procedures or techniques because the communication between teacher and learner is one-way. Techniques and procedures are learned most effectively either in well-supervised workshops or in supervised clinical practice, where instant feedback is provided. Practicing techniques on an experienced therapist, who understands the intent of the technique, is an excellent teaching and learning situation. Treating patients under supervision is also invaluable.

Procedures for the Cervical Spine

The procedures illustrated in Figures 7–1 to 7–4 and 7–7 to 7-14 are described by McKenzie.[39,67]

Typical Slumped Posture

In the typical slumped posture (Fig. 7–1), the patient sits in an unbalanced posture with a loss of lumbar lordosis, increased thoracic kyphosis, and a forward head posture. Such posture is believed to cause deformation of the spine. Correction of this poor posture, including the restoration of normal lumbar lordosis, normal cervical lordosis, and normal thoracic kyphosis, is an essential part of the treatment program for all but a very few patients.

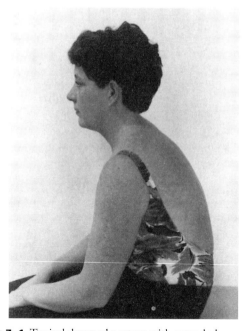

Figure 7–1. Typical slumped posture with extended upper cervical and flexed lower cervical spine. Note also the absence of lumbar lordosis, the markedly forward head, and the protracted shoulders.

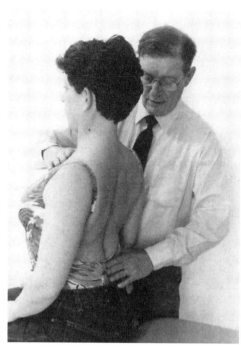

Figure 7–2. Teaching the patient the proper lumbar lordosis, which for most people is about 10 percent off the end-range of extension.

Teaching Proper Sitting Posture (Lumbar Lordosis)

The therapist assists the patient, either from in front or from the side, to attain normal lumbar lordosis (Figs. 7–2 and 7–3). This balanced lumbar posture provides a foundation on which to establish proper cervical and thoracic postures. Use of the slump overcorrection exercise, as described by McKenzie,[38] helps the patient become aware of his posture deficit. Removing the forces that cause mechanical deformation is key to successful treatment of mechanical spine pain. Restore the hollow and help the patient sit with a normal lordosis.

Cervical Retraction

Cervical retraction, dorsal glide, or posterior glide (Fig. 7–4) is performed to help reduce the forward head posture. It is normal for the patient to have difficulty learning this procedure, probably because of poor muscle control; therefore, the therapist must often demonstrate the proper method of doing the procedure and reinforce the proper execution of the exercise at subsequent visits. The patient may add overpressure to the movement by pushing on the maxilla or the mandible in a posterior direction. Cervical retraction is often combined with extension of the lower cervical spine and flexion of the upper cervical spine as a procedure for treating stiffness or reducing pain. Cyriax[68] described retraction as anteroposterior glide.

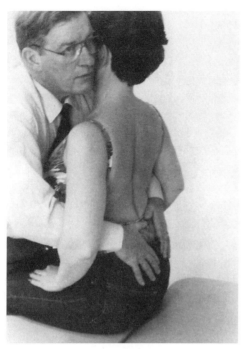

Figure 7–3. Teaching the patient the proper lumbar lordosis by enhancing an anterior pelvic tilt. An awareness of this tilt is important in learning proper posture.

Flexion of the Upper Cervical Spine

Flexion of the upper cervical spine (Fig. 7–5) is usually performed with the head in the retracted position. The purpose of this procedure is to stretch the upper cervical spine. The patient is able to provide overpressure by push-

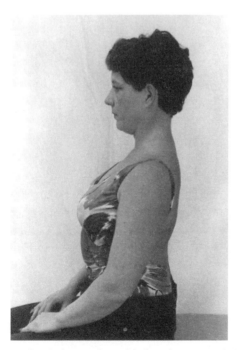

Figure 7–4. Cervical retraction added to the proper sitting posture of normal lumbar lordosis.

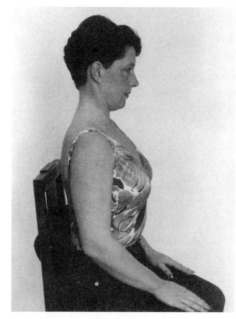

Figure 7–5. Flexion of the upper cervical spine added to the retraction movement. The patient nods the head to stretch the upper cervical spine.

ing on the maxilla or mandible in the direction of flexion. This procedure is often used to treat flexion dysfunction of the upper cervical spine. This procedure, like many other procedures, may also be performed lying prone, with or without support (cervical roll) of the lower cervical spine.

Flexion of the Lower Cervical Spine

Flexion of the lower cervical spine (Fig. 7–6), in combination with flexion of the upper cervical spine, is performed by having the patient move his chin toward the sternum. This procedure is used to treat flexion dysfunction of the lower cervical and upper thoracic spine. Theoretically, it is also used to reduce the pain in an anterior derangement and to restore flexion movement after the reduction of a posterior derangement. When treating the lack of flexion movement, when a posterior derangement is stable, flexion of the lower cervical spine must be followed by retraction and extension movements to prevent a recurrence of the posterior derangement. When instituting flexion procedures, the expected strain-pain of dysfunction should not remain worse as a result of the procedure.

Sidebending or Lateral Flexion in Sitting

The patient performs generalized sidebending (Fig. 7–7), usually in the retracted position, as a physiologic movement. The movement may be used as a treatment procedure for sidebending dysfunction or to reduce and centralize the pain of derangement. Often, but not always, the symptoms of lower cervical spine derangement can

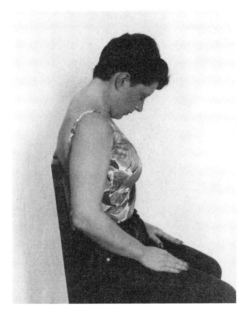

Figure 7-6. Flexion of the lower cervical and upper thoracic spine performed in sitting. The patient brings the chin toward the sternum, with the mouth closed, whereas in flexion of the upper cervical spine, the chin is moved in the direction of the neck (nodding).

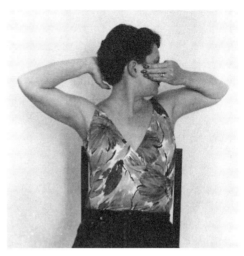

Figure 7-8. Rotation overpressure to the left. The patient applies the end-range movement using both hands. The patient's left hand is placed on the maxilla in an attempt to reduce the stress on the temporomandibular joint. It is also important for the patient to keep the elbows in the position shown to facilitate feedback regarding the vigor of the overpressure. Movement of the upper cervical spine can often be enhanced by having the patient place the hands on the upper portion of the trapezius muscle to stabilize the middle and lower cervical spine (not illustrated).

be reduced by sidebending to the painful side. Likewise, the symptoms of dysfunction can be produced by side-bending away from the painful side. However, the direction of a procedure is always dictated by careful assessment of the changes in the signs and symptoms. Sidebending may also be performed while lying supine.

Rotation with Overpressure

The patient applies overpressure in the direction of rotation, usually with the head retracted[39,67] (Fig. 7–8). This general physiologic movement is often restricted in the

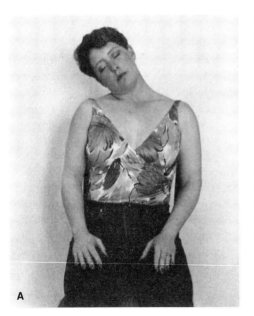

Figure 7-7. (A,B) Sidebending or lateral flexion of the cervical spine. The patient is instructed to bend sideways and bring the ear toward the shoulder, as opposed to rotation movements, where the patient turns the nose toward the shoulder.[36] The curve of the neck, on the side away from the movement, is of superior quality in left (B) compared to right (A) sidebending. Assessment of sidebending and rotation often yields similar results; therefore, it is not always necessary to assess both movements.

upper cervical spine by arthrosis and in the lower cervical spine by spondylosis. Generally, rotation is most effective in producing movement in the upper cervical spine, and sidebending is most effective in producing movement in the lower cervical spine.

Lower Cervical Spine Extension Performed in Retraction

The patient first retracts the head and then moves into extension (Fig. 7–9). One or both of these movements are frequently blocked in derangement. Retraction performed in different positions of flexion, as needed, may be a required variation before extension is possible. This procedure is used to reduce posterior derangement. For extension dysfunction, it is used to help restore lost movement into extension. Testing of the vertebral arteries is often required before using this procedure. The procedure may also be performed supine. The patient should be encouraged to reach the full limit of the range and to perform small rotations at the limit of extension.[67]

Lower Cervical Spine Extension Performed in Lying

In the lying position, the effects of gravity are reduced compared with the effects in the sitting position (Fig. 7–10). The method of performing the procedure and the uses for the procedures are similar to those for extension performed in retraction in the sitting position (Fig. 7–9).

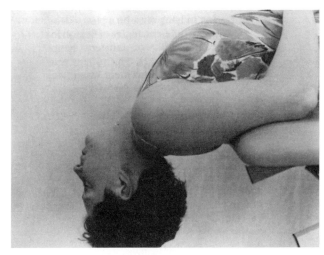

Figure 7–10. Lower cervical spine extension performed in a lying position. This procedure usually follows retraction in a lying position and usually includes rotations performed at the limit of extension.[39,67] It is important for the edge of the table to be at the level of T4 to allow for movement in the upper thoracic spine. When returning from extension to neutral position, the patient should lift the head with the hand and not perform the return movement actively. The patient should also rest in the neutral position on the table for about 30 seconds before sitting up. In sitting up, the patient should turn onto one side and sit up sideways to avoid neck flexion instead of sitting straight forward.

Retraction in Lying

Retraction in lying (Fig. 7–11) is used mainly for the treatment of neck pain. This procedure, as well as others, may be performed with a sustained position and/or oscillations with appropriate precautions.

Sidebending or Lateral Flexion in Lying

Sidebending in lying must be a pure sidebend, but it may be performed at different angles of flexion for reduction

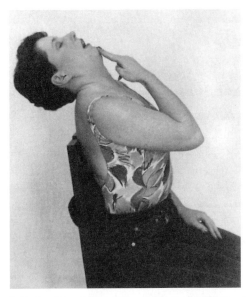

Figure 7–9. Lower cervical spine extension performed in the retracted position. The patient is holding a finger on the chin as a reminder to retain the retraction while moving into extension. A high-backed chair, which stabilizes the middle thoracic spine, helps the patient to do this procedure correctly.

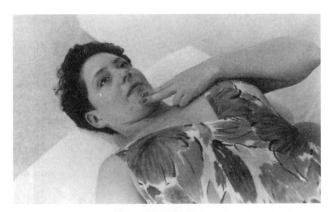

Figure 7–11. Retraction in lying. The patient is lying flat on the table. Upper cervical spine flexion may also be performed in this position. Some patients who are unable to gain any positive treatment effects from doing this procedure while sitting will benefit from doing this procedure in a lying position.

and centralization of unilateral symptoms in derangement (Fig. 7–12). The patient usually has better control of this movement when lying rather than sitting. When treating dysfunction, movement is usually away from the painful side. There are times when this procedure will result in an increase of active flexion or extension movement.

Extension in Lying with Cervical Retraction

Cervical retraction and extension may produce movement down to T4, and repeated extension in lying may produce movement up to T4 (Fig. 7–13). Combining these procedures into one exercise is most useful in treating extension dysfunction of the spine.

Patient Procedures for the Thoracic Spine

Thoracic Rotations in Sitting

To perform thoracic rotations in sitting (Fig. 7–14), the patient sits straddling the end of the table, facing the table. The intent of the procedure is to produce rotation in the thoracic spine, not to rotate the cervical or lumbar spine. This procedure is used for unilateral pain and stiffness. Often the patient rotates toward the painful side when treating pain and away from the painful side when treating stiffness. Thoracic spine disorder as a cause of angina-like pain has been described by Lindahl and Hamberg.[69]

Thoracic Extension in Lying or Standing

The intent of thoracic extension in lying or standing (Fig. 7–15) is to enhance extension of the thoracic spine using the weight of the body against a bolster.

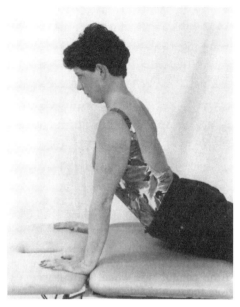

Figure 7–13. Extension in the lying position with cervical retraction. This combined procedure is best taught in parts. The patient first perfects the lumbar procedure and then adds the cervical and thoracic procedures. Many patients extend their upper cervical spine when doing this exercise, sometimes with reckless abandon. Substitution of cervical retraction for upper cervical extension is helpful in preventing treatment soreness.

Klapp's Crawling Position (Prayer Position)

The crawling or prayer position (Fig. 7–16), when performed properly, is a passive extension of the thoracic spine performed in the prone position. The force is provided by the weight of the body. This procedure is used as an alternative or supplement to those previously described (Fig. 7–15).

Therapist's Techniques for the Cervical Spine

Palpation in Supine

The upper cervical spine is palpated with the patient lying supine, if possible. (Fig. 7–17). In the neutral posture, with the patient supine, the therapist can feel abnormalities of tissue tension and joint restriction. The cervical spine may also be palpated in the prone-lying position.

Manual Cervical Traction

Cervical traction, or longitudinal movement cephalad, may be applied manually or mechanically (Fig. 7–18). Manual traction is frequently used when very gentle movement is required and/or to help determine the force, position, and mode (sustained or intermittent) of mechanical traction. There is evidence that traction can be both beneficial and harmful.[70]

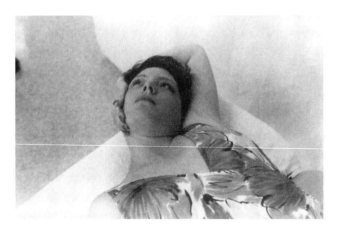

Figure 7–12. Left sidebending in lying. The head is usually moved toward the desired side without allowing any rotation. The left arm is used, as illustrated, to provide overpressure when needed.

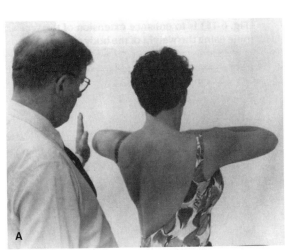
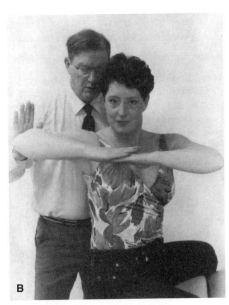

Figure 7–14. Thoracic rotations in sitting. (A) Rotation to the left; (B) rotation to the right. The patient in (B) straddles the end of the treatment table, facing the table. To reduce cervical rotations, the patient's head moves with the thoracic spine instead of facing forward. The patient must keep the chin in line with the hands, as shown in (B). End-range is accomplished by asking the patient to hit the therapist's hand with the elbow.

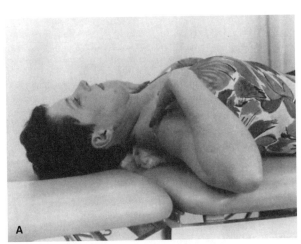
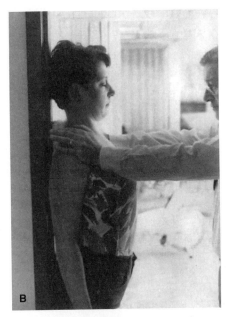

Figure 7–15. Thoracic extension performed (A) while lying and (B) while standing. In (A) the patient is lying supine on a firm surface with a bolster under the affected area. A bench press table (not illustrated) is most efficient because it is narrow and allows the patient to move into the posture correction position of shoulder horizontal extension. The patient should inhale when moving into horizontal extension. The same exercise may be performed by standing at the edge of a doorway (B). A bolster between the scapulae helps to localize the force. Overpressure may be added by the therapist or by a spouse by pushing on the patient's shoulders bilaterally.

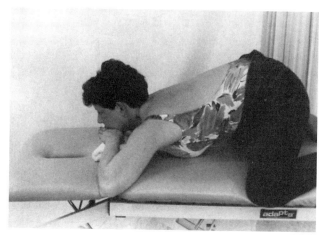

Figure 7–16. Klapp's crawling position (modified). The patient's hands are placed under the chin instead of reaching out forward. The modified position places more force on the cervical spine than does the unmodified, or prayer, position. The thighs should be kept vertical, and an extension strain should be felt in the middle thoracic spine.

Retraction and Extension in Lying

Retraction and extension in lying (McKenzie) are used in treating posterior derangements (Fig. 7–19). If tolerated, it is desirable to start the extension movement from the retracted position and/or to precede the retraction movement often with static traction. End-range extension is required, and overpressure is applied in small rotary movements.

Sidebending in Sitting

The therapist stands behind the patient, who is sitting erect on a firm chair. The intent of the technique is to

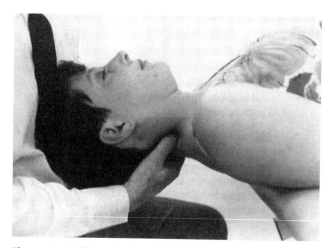

Figure 7–17. Palpation in the supine position. The patient's head is comfortably supported by the therapist over the edge of the treatment table. Palpation for abnormal joint and muscle signs may be performed in either the supine or the prone position (Figs. 7–23 to 7–28). Passive physiologic intervertebral movements may also be performed in this position.

localize the sidebending at a particular level of the cervical spine. Figure 7–20 illustrates sidebending left of C7 on T1. A variation of the technique, designed to improve stabilization, is for the patient to sit on a treatment table with the therapist standing behind him. The therapist

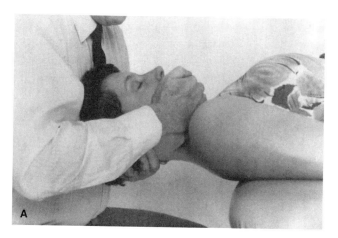

A

B

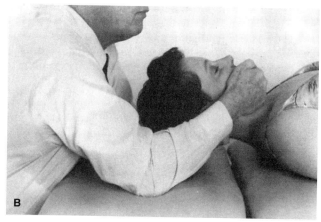

C

Figure 7–18. Manual cervical traction performed in the horizontal position using three different methods: (A) with the patient's head over the edge of the table; (B) with the patient lying on the table; (C) using pivotal traction. In (A) the therapist provides the force by leaning backward. In (B) the force comes from flexion of the therapist's elbows. In (C) force comes from the patient's head pushing against the therapist's fingers.

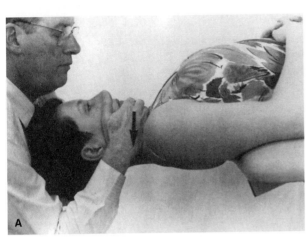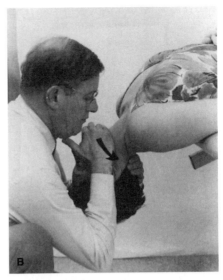

Figure 7–19. Retraction and extension in the lying position. The patient is unsupported to about T4. (A) A traction force is applied and held, and then the neck is retracted. (B) While in the retracted position, the neck is slowly extended. Small rotary movements are frequently applied in overpressure. Continuous assessment of the changes in symptoms is essential.

then places her foot on the treatment table adjacent to the patient's hip on the side of the intended movement. The patient then rests his arm on the therapist's thigh (not illustrated).

This technique is useful when full-range sidebending is needed in the treatment of dysfunction. Because the spinous process of C7 moves left in normal right rotation, the technique is also useful in treating rotation dysfunc-

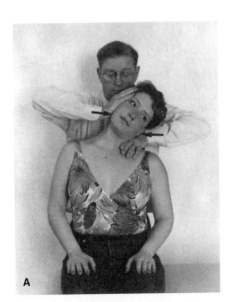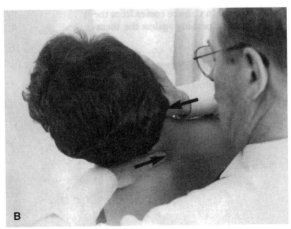

Figure 7–20. Sidebending in the sitting position. The patient's neck is near or at the end of retraction. In left sidebending (A), the patient's head is sidebent to the limit of the available range, and the force is applied by the therapist's right hand. (B) The spinous process of T1 is stabilized by the therapist's left thumb. It is important for the therapist to hold her shoulders abducted, with the elbows out to the side (A), to obtain optimum tactile feedback from the patient.

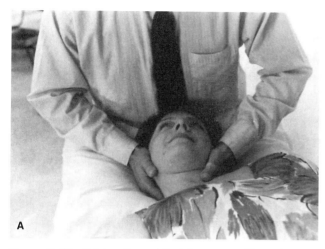
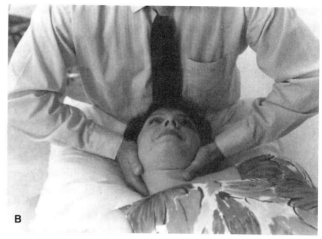

Figure 7–21. Sidebending while lying on a pillow. (A) Left sidebending; (B) further left sidebending. The patient is lying supine on a pillow, and the therapist stands at the head of the treatment table. The patient's neck is supported from both sides. The therapist's left hand may act as a fulcrum for the sidebending. The force for the movement comes from the therapist's right hand. The left side is closed down, and the right side is opened or stretched.

tion of the lower cervical spine. For example, to help restore right rotation, the spinous process of C7 is at first stabilized on the right, and the neck is sidebent to the right while the spinous process of C7 is moved left.

Sidebending in Lying on a Pillow

The patient lies supine, with his head on a pillow (Fig. 7–21). The therapist stands at the head of the table and supports the patient's neck from both sides. Positioning the head on a pillow allows the therapist to perform very gentle movements into sidebending while allowing the pillow to slide on the table. This technique is useful in treating pain when other positions are not tolerated.

Grade II and IV Rotations

The patient's head is properly cradled, and the therapist stands at the head of the treatment table (Fig. 7–22). Maitland[55] states that rotation is one of the most useful

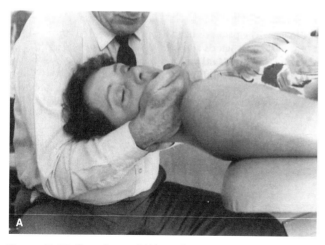
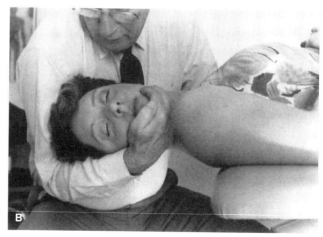

Figure 7–22. Rotations of (A) grade II and (B) grade IV. The therapist cradles the patient's head at the occiput and at the chin. Grade II is a midrange rotation, and grade IV an end-range rotation. The therapist should be able to do this technique with one hand at a time if the position is correct. Note that the patient's head is in contact with the therapist's chest and the anterior surface of the shoulder. Gentle oscillations are given at the proper position of the range. The angle of flexion or extension may also be varied to produce an optimum treatment effect.

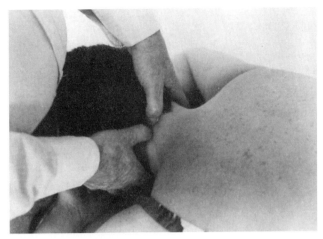

Figure 7–23. Posteroanterior unilateral vertebral pressure to C0-C1. (↓). Force is applied in the direction of the patient's ipsilateral eye. Therefore, the therapist must lean over the patient's head. The therapist's thumbs are placed on, above, or below the joint. Medial and lateral inclinations are other variations.

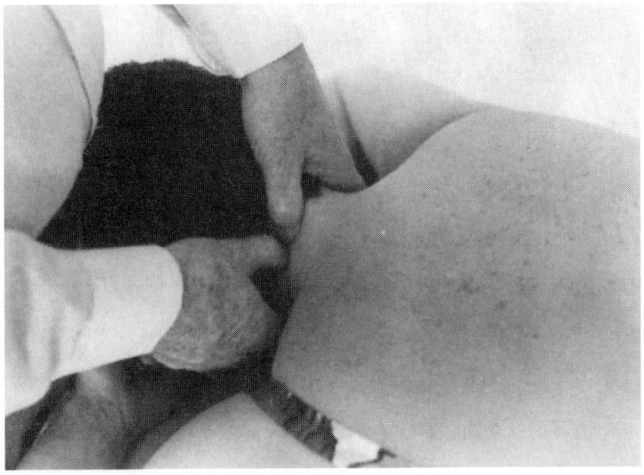

Figure 7–24. Posteroanterior unilateral vertebral pressure to C2-C3. (↓). Force is applied on the left articular pillar of C2 to move C2-C3. The patient's head is in neutral rotation. The therapist's arms are directed about 30 degrees medially to prevent the thumbs from slipping off the articular pillar. (From Maitland,[25] with permission.)

techniques for the cervical spine. It is most useful in treating unilateral stiffness, with the movement usually in the direction away from the painful side. It is quite possible that the restrictions causing the stiffness are being stretched when the painful side is being opened by rotation away from the pain. Grade II movements are useful in the reduction of treatment soreness, and grade IV movements are useful in the treatment of stiffness, respecting the patient's pain. Grade I and grade III movements are also useful methods of treatment. (That grades I and III are not illustrated is not meant to imply lack of use of the techniques.)

Selected passive accessory intervertebral movements, as described by Maitland,[25] are presented in Figures 7–23 to 7–29.* Further information about these and other techniques is also presented by Maitland in his many writings.[71–81] Selected techniques are presented that provide a brief introduction to the approach. Examples are offered of how the techniques are used in concert with patient procedures. The skillful transfer between the use of the therapist's techniques and the use of the patient's procedures is always challenging.

For the techniques presented in Figures 7–23 to 7–29, the patient lies prone, with the forehead resting on the overlapped and supinated hands. The therapist uses either the tips or the pads of the thumbs to provide an oscillating movement in the desired direction. The movement force is generated by movement of the therapist's shoulders and/or trunk, and this force is transmitted through the arms to the thumbs, which act as eccentric springs. No intrinsic muscle action should take place in

the therapist's thumbs or hands because accurate feedback from the patient is destroyed by such action.

The Nelson Technique

The Nelson technique for traction and improved extension of the cervical-thoracic junction and upper thoracic spine (Fig. 7–30) is taught in the McKenzie approach. The Nelson technique is used only after confirmed premanipulative testing for providing extrinsic reductive or stretching forces in the lower cervical and upper thoracic

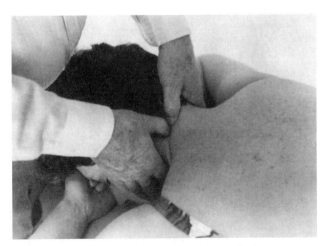

Figure 7–25. Posteroanterior unilateral vertebral pressure to C1-C2 (↓ in 30 degrees of rotation left). Force is applied as in Figure 7–24, except that the patient's head is turned 30 degrees to the left. Rotation at C1-C2 is enhanced in this rotated position. (From Maitland,[25] with permission.)

---

* Arrows indicate the direction of the technique; the arrow pointing down indicates the posteroanterior direction.

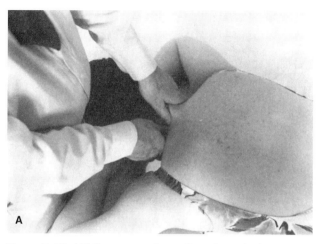
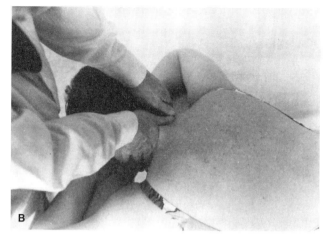

Figure 7–26. (A) Posteroanterior unilateral vertebral pressure to C5-C6. These techniques may also be directed medially, laterally, (B) cephalad, or caudad as variations.

spine. Other procedures or techniques, if required, are used before this technique to obtain and/or retain centralization of symptoms. This procedure cannot be performed on patients with significant shoulder pathology because of the discomfort produced in moving the shoulders into end-range horizontal extension and external rotation. Well-muscled persons are very difficult to position properly. This technique is described by Laslett.[82]

Extension Mobilizations

The intent of the extension mobilization technique (Fig. 7–31), also taught in the McKenzie approach, is to provide central posteroanterior movement of the involved segment and gentle distraction. It is used on C2 through T4 to effect an extension movement. Asymmetric variations are often used to treat unilateral or asymmetric pain or stiffness. This technique is also described by Laslett.[82]

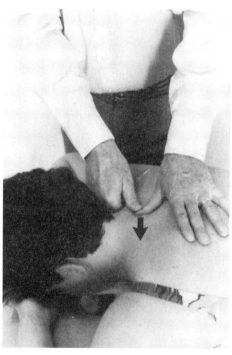

Figure 7–27. Transverse vertebral pressures to C7 (←). Force is applied on the lateral surface of the spinous process of C7. Here the force is applied through the therapist's right thumb to the nonactive left thumbnail. The pad, not the tip, of the nonactive thumb is used for the patient's comfort. The therapist's right forearm should be held near parallel to the surface of the treatment table to provide movement in the desired direction. Often in treatment of stiffness, the patient rotates the neck to the limit of the available range. The technique is then performed at the pathologic limit (not illustrated).

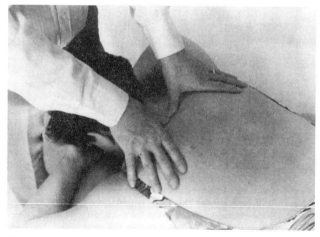

Figure 7–28. Posteroanterior central vertebral pressures directed on C7 (↓). The therapist's two thumbs, often in contact with each other, cradle the spinous process; for gentle techniques, the tips of the thumbs may be used to localize the movement. To apply the technique in the pain-free range, the neck may have to be placed in slight flexion. Prominent spinous processes are often the source of the patient's complaint.

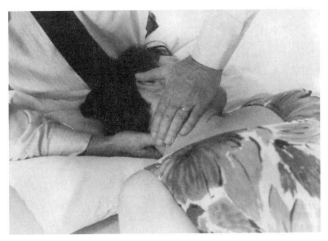

Figure 7–29. A combined technique using left rotation and unilateral posteroanterior pressures on the right side of C2. Shown is an example of a physiologic and an accessory movement performed simultaneously. It is frequently necessary to combine movements to reproduce the comparable sign. The same movements are then used as a treatment technique to reduce pain and/or increase the range. In general, the technique performed at the lowest grade that produces the desired treatment effect is preferred. The lowest grade provides for smooth, controlled rather than rough, random movement.

Thoracic Spine Techniques

Transverse Vertebral Pressures on T4

The technique for applying transverse vertebral pressure to T4 ($\leftarrow$) is similar to the technique shown for transverse vertebral pressures on C7 (Fig. 7–32). The technique is usually directed toward the side of pain.[26] When dysfunction is being treated, the patient's comparable sign is reproduced, and the range of physiologic movements is often increased. Although the accessory movement is in a frontal plane, physiologic movements in the sagittal plane (i.e., flexion or extension) are often improved.

Posteroanterior Central Vertebral Pressures to T4

The technique for applying posteroanterior central vertebral pressure to T4 ($\downarrow$) is similar to that shown for posteroanterior central vertebral pressures on C7, except that in this case the force is usually not directed laterally (Fig. 7–33). This technique is used commonly for central or symmetric symptoms and may be used for vague or generalized unilateral symptoms.[25] It is one of the most useful techniques for the thoracic spine and is often followed by a more vigorous technique, illustrated later.

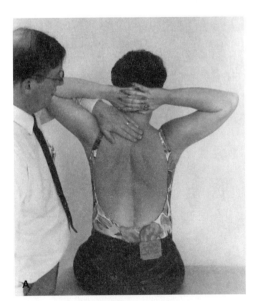
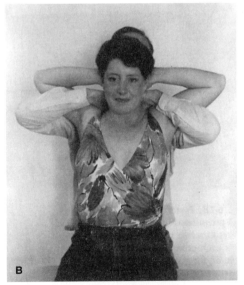

Figure 7–30. The Nelson technique for traction and improved extension of the cervical-thoracic junction and the upper thoracic spine. (A) The index and middle fingers of the therapist's left hand are placed over the spinous process of C7. The same two fingers of the therapist's right hand are then placed on top of these fingers. A posteroanterior force is directed cephalad by the therapist's arms and hands through the index and middle fingers of both hands. This force is generated by pushing on C7 and pulling the patient's shoulders into horizontal extension. The traction force is applied by attempting to lift the patient off the table. At the peak of the traction force, the therapist applies the extension force. (B) Note that the shoulders of the therapist and the shoulders of the patient are at the same level.

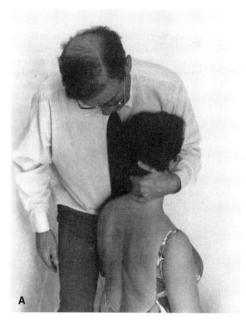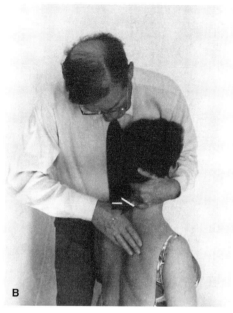

Figure 7–31. Extension mobilization. The patient should be sitting in a high-backed chair (not illustrated). (A) The patient's head is cradled by the therapist's left hand and forearm against the therapist's chest. The therapist's little finger is placed on the spinous process of the appropriate vertebra. (B) The therapist's right thumb, or right pisiform-hamate groove, is then placed securely on her left little finger. The movement desired is gentle traction, provided by the therapist's left arm, combined with posteroanterior central vertebral pressures, provided by the thumb or hand. The patient's head should remain stable.

Intervertebral Rotatory Posteroanterior Movements of T1-T4

The technique of intervertebral rotatory posteroanterior movements of T1-T4 provides a method for producing desirable movement without direct contact on the spinous processes (Fig. 7–34). It is suggested that localized movement, depending on the placement of the hands, may be produced in the costotransverse joints, the costovertebral joints, the intervertebral (apophyseal) joints, and the intervertebral junction. It is common for even gentle techniques to produce local sounds of release and for the patient to gain rapid relief from symptoms using this technique.

Figure 7–32. Transverse vertebral pressures to T4 (←). Force is applied on the lateral surface of the spinous process of T4. The force is applied through the therapist's right thumb to the nonative left thumbnail. The pad, not the tip, of the nonactive thumb is used for the patient's comfort. Note that the patient's arms are at the sides to enhance relaxation of the thoracic spine.

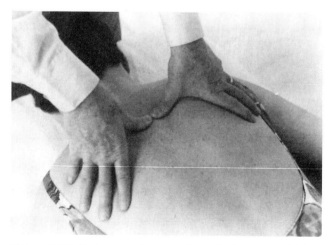

Figure 7–33. Posteroanterior central vertebral pressures (↓) to T4. The therapist's two thumbs, often in contact with each other, cradle the spinous process. For gentle techniques, the tips of the thumbs may be used to localize the movement.

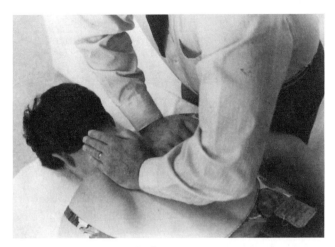

Figure 7–34. Intervertebral rotatory posteroanterior movements of T1-T4. Force is applied bilaterally through the therapist's hypothenar eminences to the spaces between the spinous processes and the medial borders of the scapulae. A combination of clockwise and counterclockwise movements is applied in a posteroanterior direction. The force may also be directed cephalad, caudad, and laterally.

Thoracic Rotations

Thoracic rotations may be tested with the patient standing (mostly lower movement), sitting (Fig. 7–35), and lying. For stretching stiff structures, rotation is often performed in the direction away from the symptomatic side. Assess-ment of the individual patient and his response to movement tests dictate the proper direction.

Longitudinal Movement and Extension in Sitting

The generalized technique of longitudinal movement and extension may be performed with the patient sitting (Fig. 7–36) or standing. Because of the nonspecific nature of the technique, it is most useful in treating generalized stiffness of the middle thoracic spine. Greater specificity may be achieved with the technique described next.

Posteroanterior Manipulation of T4

The technique of posteroanterior manipulation of T4 ($\downarrow$), which must be learned and practiced under the supervision of an experienced therapist, is one of the most useful techniques for the upper and middle thoracic spine (Fig. 7–37). When successful, the patient experiences dramatic relief. It is suggested not only that stiff joints are loosened but that thoracic spine derangements may be reduced by selected use of this technique. Reduction, if achieved, must be retained by the consistent use of the patient's procedures.

Thoracic spine disorders as a cause of angina-like pain have been described by Lindahl and Hamberg.[83] This technique has been useful in treating this type of disorder. This technique is described in detail by Maitland,[25] Mc-Guckin,[84] and Flynn.[85]

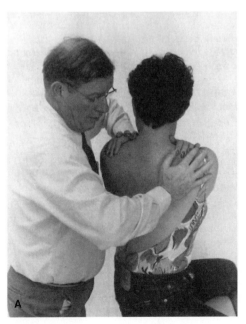
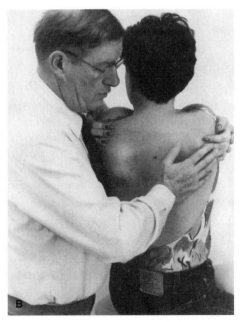

Figure 7–35. Thoracic rotation to the left. (A) Generalized thoracic rotation. The patient sits straddling the end of the treatment table, with the arms folded in front of the chest. (B) More localized overpressure in the middle thoracic spine.

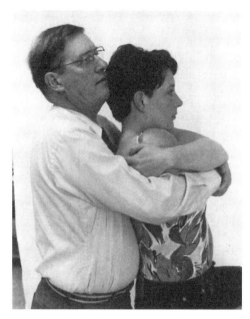

Figure 7–36. Longitudinal movement and extension in sitting. The patient sits straddling the end of the treatment table. The longitudinal movement is provided by partially lifting the patient off the table. The extension movement is provided by the therapist leaning backward and applying overpressure (when desired) through her chest.

CASE STUDIES

CASE STUDY 1

The use of passive movement techniques coupled with active exercises is the main emphasis of this case study.

Initial Assessment

Subjective Examination

The patient was a 33-year-old female factory worker who spent most of her time operating a forklift. She had a headache in the occipital region and neck pain extending from C1 to T4, which spread bilaterally and equally to the area of the glenohumeral joints. She had no upper extremity symptoms. Initially, her symptoms were constant but variable. They were worsened by sitting, driving a forklift, and doing housework. They were reduced by lying in the fetal position and by taking a hot bath. The patient's sleep was disturbed because she had increased pain when turning her head from side to side. Both coughing and sneezing increased her symptoms temporarily.

Her symptoms commenced as a result of shoveling cullet (broken glass). She was first seen for this examination 18 months after the initial injury but had never been symptom-free for more than a few hours since the original injury. Radiographs were negative. She had received chi-ropractic treatments and physical therapy elsewhere. She was fully employed at the time of these treatments.

Physical Examination

The patient's general cervical flexion was limited to 50 percent of normal. Lower cervical extension was blocked by pain at 15 degrees. Left cervical rotation was 55 degrees, and right cervical rotation was 65 degrees. Extension reproduced the patient's comparable sign in the C7 area centrally.

The patient's posture was poor, with a marked forward head on a long neck with a definite cervical-thoracic kyphus. Her upper thoracic spine was held in excessive flexion, and she had forward shoulders bilaterally.

Repeated test movements into protraction of the head made her C7 pain worse. Repeated retractions of her head increased her headache and increased her C7 pain, both temporarily. She was very stiff in both of these movements (i.e., she had great difficulty performing the test movements except in the early part of the ranges).

Passive accessory movements and passive physiologic movements revealed the following: (1) The C7 spinous process was rotated to the patient's left. Attempted correction by pushing the spinous process to the patient's right (in a transverse grade II+ passive movement) reproduced her C7-area symptoms. (2) Her headache was reproduced by passive posteroanterior pressures in the suboccipital muscles bilaterally. (3) The upper thoracic spine was very stiff and painful locally at each level, especially in extension-type articulations. (4) Overpressure in left cervical rotation also reproduced the C7-area pain. (5) Extension of the lower cervical spine was blocked at the C7 level.

Interpretation

This patient presented with marked hypomobility secondary to known trauma. Her poor posture, coupled with excessive stiffness, suggested that she may have had a posture problem before the trauma. Her main complaints were reproduced with passive accessory movements and/or passive physiologic movements. It was suggested that she had marked hypomobility caused by shortening of joint structures and soft tissue secondary to the trauma.

Treatment

The primary goals of treatment were to eliminate the patient's headache, restore normal movement to her cervical and upper thoracic spine, and restore other functional components such as strength and endurance. Treatment consisted of posture correction, passive mobilization, and active exercises, including an explanation of the rationale to the patient. She remained fully employed.

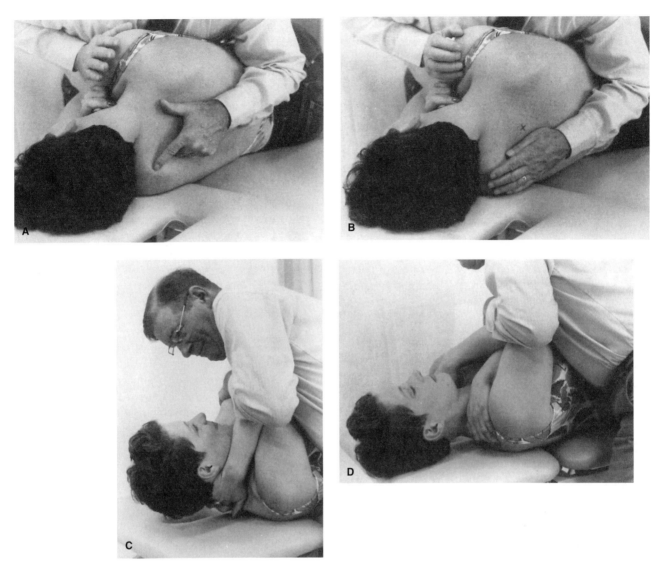

Figure 7–37. Posteroanterior manipulation (↓) of T4. (A) The therapist's hand placement for the central technique; (B) the therapist's hand placement for the unilateral technique; (C) positioning of the patient in neutral flexion and extension for the level to be treated; (D) application of force through the patient's elbows. At this point, the patient exhales. The hand of the therapist under the patient provides the localization of the technique. In (C) and (D), the therapist's right hand is under the patient.

WEEK 1

The patient was seen twice the first week. C7 was passively mobilized transversely to the right on both days to increase left rotation and possibly extension, The patient was taught upper cervical spine flexion to reduce her suboccipital headache. She was also taught the slump/overcorrection to correct her posture.

RESULTS. Left rotation increased from 55 to 70 degrees. The patient's posture started to improve, especially her body awareness. She tolerated the active exercises and was able to reduce but not eliminate her headache.

WEEK 2

The patient was also seen twice this week. The upper thoracic spine was mobilized vigorously, and the C7 transverse pressures were continued. Retraction, extension, and rotation of the cervical spine performed actively in lying were initiated.

RESULTS. The patient's headache disappeared. Cervical rotations were near normal limits, and active lower cervical spine extension increased from the initial 15 degrees to about 60 degrees. The patient was very encouraged and highly motivated. Her pain of hypomobility decreased.

WEEK 3

The patient was seen once this week. All active exercises were continued, and T4 was vigorously mobilized centrally but not manipulated.

RESULTS. The patient was progressing well in all areas, except that T4 was painful locally and very stiff. She probably needed to be manipulated unless active exercises reduced the dysfunction at T4.

WEEK 4

The patient was seen twice, and T4 was manipulated at the first visit. All active exercises were rechecked and progressed as tolerated.

RESULTS. Cervical-thoracic extension improved to near-normal limits, but right rotation of the upper thoracic spine was limited by 10 degrees. Active right rotation exercises for the thoracic spine were added.

WEEK 5

The patient was seen once. Thoracic rotations were near normal limits. Cervical-thoracic extension was clear. A manual muscle test of the neck and shoulder girdle revealed a fair plus lower trapezius on the right. Strengthening exercises were initiated. Upper limb tension tests and the slump test were normal.

RESULTS. Range of movement for the cervical and upper thoracic spine was normal. Posture was good. Isolated lower trapezius weakness was the only known deficit.

WEEK 6

Recheck of the weak trapezius showed a good plus. All exercises were rechecked. The patient was to be seen only as needed. She remained symptom-free and was discharged.

CASE STUDY 2

The use of passive movement techniques and active exercises used to eliminate a cervical headache is the focus of this case study. Edeling's work is an excellent reference on assessment and treatment of headaches.[89]

Initial Assessment

Subjective Examination

The patient was a 53-year-old domestic laundry worker. Her main complaint was an intermittent, severe upper cervical headache with spread to the right temporal region, coupled with a feeling of lightheadedness and dizziness. The symptoms, when present, usually lasted for about 2 hours. The patient's headache commenced 2½ years earlier for no apparent reason, and at times her pain, when at its worst, involved her whole head.

Her headache was worsened by cold air, bending her head forward as when ironing, and, most significantly in her mind, 2 to 5 minutes after she entered a store. Her headache was reduced or eliminated by wearing a soft cervical collar. Her sleep was not disturbed, and coughing and sneezing signs were negative. Previous treatment consisted of the neck collar, isometric exercises, and anti-inflammatory medications. The medications did not help. The isometric exercises, at times, reduced the patient's headache.

A CT scan showed that the patient had degenerative disk disease of C6-C7. She reportedly had high blood pressure under control with medication. She also claimed to have a nervous disorder and prior heart disease, with no symptoms at this time. She was referred for evaluation and treatment.

Physical Examination

Cervical range of movement was within normal limits, and there was no reproduction of symptoms with these test movements. The patient did have a moderate forward head, with extension of the upper cervical spine and flexion of the lower cervical spine. Palpation of her neck using passive accessory movements reproduced her headache by right unilateral vertebral pressures on the articular pillar of C2, moving C2 on C1.

Treatment

WEEK 1

The patient was seen twice the first week and was taught active postural excercises to reduce her forward head. Upper cervical flexion with partial retraction was chosen because the patient reported, at her first visit, that this exercise reduced her headache. She was instructed to do the exercise frequently and to stop or reduce the exercise if any of her symptoms were aggravated. At the second visit, her neck was palpated in detail, and C1-C2 on the right was mobilized using grade II for three bouts. The joint resistance diminished, and local pain was eliminated.

RESULTS. At her second visit, the patient stated that her exercises were helpful, but she believed that the headache was unchanged because she had to use the collar as usual. She responded well to the passive accessory movement on C1-C2.

WEEK 2

At her third visit, the patient reported that she had not worn the collar for 1 week and that her headache was well controlled by her exercises. She had created a modification of her exercise that she believed stretched her headache area. Essentially, she had combined upper cervical flexion (her original exercise) with left sidebending to produce a desirable stretch at C1-C2 on the right.

WEEK 3

At her fourth visit, the patient reported that her headache was no problem because the symptoms were less frequent, less severe, and did not spread beyond the local area of C1-C2. Her neck was palpated and appeared to be normal for her age, with no reproduction of symptoms beyond normal local pressure/strain. She was discharged with instructions to continue her exercise program and was advised to report if her exercises did not eliminate her headache.

■ Summary

Two major topics were covered in this chapter: (1) a differential assessment between the cervical spine and the thoracic spine and (2) methods for mobilization of the cervical and upper thoracic spine. The methods for mobilization relied heavily on the teachings of McKenzie,[38,39] Maitland,[25] and Cyriax.[40] The three syndromes of posture, dysfunction, and derangement, as described by McKenzie,[38,39] may be loosely related to the treatment of pain and stiffness, as described by Maitland.[25]

The individual therapist may elect to use active procedures followed by passive procedures or passive procedures followed by active procedures to relieve pain and restore function. Suggested mechanisms to relieve pain and to increase range were described.

The SE, PE, and methods of treatment were described and illustrated. Guidelines and principles for the direction of a technique or procedure were presented. Further information regarding the details of these approaches may be found in the writings of McKenzie,[38,39,43,45,67,86] Maitland,[25,71–81] and Cyriax.[40,44,68,87]

■ References

1. Jones M: Clinical reasoning in physical therapy. Phys Ther 72:875–884, 1992
2. Jones M: Clinical reasoning process in manipulative therapy. pp. 471–490. In Boyling J (ed): Grieve's Modern Manual Therapy. Churchill Livingstone, New York, 1994
3. Jones M, Christensen N, Carr J: Clinical reasoning in orthopedic manual therapy. p. 89. In Grant R (ed): Physical Therapy of the Cervical and Thoracic Spine. Churchill Livingstone, New York, 1994
4. Anderson M, Stevens Practice B, Richards J, et al: Cervical spine. pp. 727–788. In Myers R (ed): Saunders Manual of Physical Therapy Practice. WB Saunders, Philadelphia, 1995
5. Higgs J, Jones M (eds): Clinical Reasoning in the Health Professions. pp. 35–104. Butterworth-Heinemann, Boston, 1995
6. Jones M, Jones H: Cervical-shoulder differentiation (course handout). Cayuga Professional Education Association, Trumansburg, NY, 1993
7. Tichenor C, Davidson J, Jensen G: Cases as shared inquiry: model for clinical reasoning. J Phys Ther Ed 9(2):57–62, 1995
8. Butler D: Mobilization of the Nervous System. Churchill Livingstone, New York, 1991
9. Maitland G: Peripheral Manipulation. Butterworths, Oxford, 1991
10. Vernon H, Mior S: The neck disability index: a study of reliability and validity. J Manip Physiother 14:409–415, 1991
11. Aspinall W: Clinical testing for the craniovertebral hypermobility syndrome. J Orthop Sports Phys Ther 12(2):47–54, 1990
12. Kikuchi S, Watanabe E, Hasue M: Spinal intermittent claudication due to cervical and thoracic degenerative disease. Spine 21(3):313–318, 1996
13. Isaacs E: Should physical therapists diagnose?: a neurologist's viewpoint. J Phys Ther Ed 9(2):63–64, 1995
14. Schoensee S, Jensen G, Nicholson G, et al: The effect of mobilization on cervical headaches. J Orthop Sports Phys Ther 21(4):184–196, 1995
15. Hack G, Koritzer R, Robinson W, et al: Anatomic relation between the rectus capitis posterior minor muscle and the dura mater. Spine 20(23):2484–2486, 1995
16. Brown S: Ocular dysfunction associated with whiplash injury. Aust Physiother 41(1):59, 1995
17. Maitland G: Acute locking of the cervical spine. Aust J Physiother 24:103–109, 1978
18. Sprague R: The acute cervical joint lock. Phys Ther 63(9):1439–1444, 1983
19. Saunders D: Evaluation, Treatment and Prevention of Musculoskeletal Disorders. Educational Opportunities, Eden Prairie, MN, 1985
20. Demetra J: Pathologies of the cervical spine. Orthopedic physical therapy home study course 96-1, pp. 1–17. Orthopedic section, American Physical Therapy Association, Washington, DC, 1996
21. Grant R, Forrester C, Hides J: Screen based keyboard operation: the adverse effects on the nervous system. Aust Phys Ther 41(2):99–107, 1995
22. Reif R: Evaluation and differential diagnosis of the cervical spine. Orthopedic physical therapy home study course 96-1, pp. 1–26. Orthopedic and sports section, American Physical Therapy Association, Washington, DC, 1996
23. Corrigan B, Maitland G: Practical Orthopedic Medicine. Butterworths, Oxford, 1983
24. Blair J: Examination of the thoracic spine. p. 536. In Grieve G (ed): Modern Manual Therapy: The Vertebral Column. Churchill Livingstone, New York, 1986
25. Maitland G: Vertebral Manipulation. Butterworths, Oxford, 1986
26. Grieve G: The autonomic nervous system in vertebral pain patterns. pp. 293–308. In Boyling J (ed): Grieve's Modern Manual Therapy. Churchill Livingstone, New York, 1994
27. Slater H, Butler D, Shacklock M: The dynamic central nervous system: examination and assessment using tension tests. pp. 587–606. In Boyling J (ed): Grieve's Modern Manual Therapy. Churchill Livingstone, New York, 1994
28. Magarey M: Examination of the cervical and thoracic spine. p. 109. In Grant R (ed): Physical Therapy of the Cervical and Thoracic Spine. Churchill Livingstone, New York, 1994
29. Butler D, Slater H: Neural injury in the thoracic spine: a conceptual basis for manual therapy. p. 313. In Grant R (ed): Physical Therapy of the Cervical and Thoracic Spine. Churchill Livingstone, New York, 1994
30. Slater H, Vicenzino B, Wright A: "Sympathetic slump": the effects of a novel manual therapy technique on peripheral sympathetic nervous system function. J Man Manip Ther 2(4):156–162, 1994

31. Butler D, Shacklock O, Slater H: Treatment of altered nervous system mechanics. pp. 693–704. In Boyling J (ed): Grieve's Modern Manual Therapy: The Vertebral Column. Churchill Livingstone, New York, 1994

32. Pecina M, Nemanie J, Markiewitz A: Tunnel Syndromes, Peripheral Nerve Compression Syndromes. 2nd Ed. CRC Press, Boca Raton, FL, 1996

33. Laslett M: Use of manipulative therapy for mechanical pain of spinal origin. Orthop Rev 16:8, 1987

34. Haldeman S: Spinal manipulative therapy: a status report. Clin Orthop 179:62, 1983

35. Ottenbacher K, DiFabio R: Efficacy of spinal manipulation/mobilization therapy. Spine, suppl 9, 10:833, 1985

36. Cherkin D, et al: A comparison of physical therapy, chiropractic manipulation, and provision of an educational booklet for the treatment of patients with low back pain. N Engl J Med 339:1021, 1998

37. Bove G, Nillson N: Spinal manipulation in the treatment of episodic tension-type headache. JAMA 280:1576, 1998

38. McKenzie R: The Lumbar Spine. Spinal Publications, Waikanae, New Zealand, 1981

39. McKenzie R: The Cervical and Thoracic Spine. Spinal Publications, Waikanae, New Zealand, 1990

40. Cyriax J: Textbook of Orthopedic Medicine. 6th Ed. Williams & Wilkins, Baltimore, 1975

41. Basmajian J (ed): Manipulation. Traction and Massage. 3rd Ed. Williams & Wilkins, Baltimore, 1985

42. Cookson JC, Kent B: Orthopedic manual therapy—an overview. II. The spine. Phys Ther 59:259, 1979

43. McKenzie R: Manual correction of sciatic scoliosis. NZ Med J 76:484, 1972

44. Cyriax J: Treatment of lumbar disk lesions. Br Med J 2:1434, 1950

45. McKenzie R: Prophylaxis in recurrent low back pain. NZ Med J 89:22, 1979

46. Wyke B: The neurology of low back pain. p. 56. In Jayson M (ed): The Lumbar Spine and Back Pain. 3rd Ed. Churchill Livingstone, New York, 1987

47. Cummings G, Crutchfield C, Barnes M: Orthopedic Physical Therapy Series—Soft Tissue Changes in Contractures. Vol. 1. Stokesville Publishing, Atlanta, GA, 1983

48. Evans P: The healing process at the cellular level: a review. Physiotherapy 66:256, 1980

49. Donelson R, Silva G, Murphy K: Centralization phenomenon: its usefulness in evaluating and treating referred pain. Spine 15:211, 1990

50. Saunders H: Evaluation, Treatment and Prevention of Musculoskeletal Disorders. Anderberg-Lund, Minneapolis, 1986

51. McNair J: Acute locking of the cervical spine. p. 357. In Grieve G (ed): Modern Manual Therapy of the Vertebral Column. Churchill Livingstone, Edinburgh, 1986

52. Nyberg R: Role of physical therapists in spinal manipulation. p. 36. In Basmajian J (ed): Manipulation, Traction and Massage. 3rd Ed. Williams & Wilkins, Baltimore, 1985

53. Thornton P, Calangelo V: Fundamentals of Engineering Materials. Prentice-Hall, Englewood Cliffs, NJ, 1985

54. Callister W: Materials Science and Engineering. John Wiley & Sons, New York, 1985

55. Smith C: The Science of Engineering Materials. 3rd Ed. Prentice-Hall, Englewood Cliffs, NJ, 1986

56. Peterson B (ed): The Collection of Papers of Irivin M. Korr. American Academy of Osteopathy, Colorado Springs, CO, 1979

57. Wyke B: Neurology of the cervical spine. Physiotherapy, suppl. 10, 65:72, 1979

58. Cyriax J: Illustrated Manual of Orthopedic Medicine. Butterworths, London, 1983

59. Gore D, Sepic S, Gardner G, et al: Neck pain: a long term follow-up of 205 patients. Spine, suppl 1, 12:1, 1987

60. Bogduk N: Cervical causes of headache and dizziness. p. 289. In Grieve G (ed): Modern Manual Therapy of the Vertebral Column. Churchill Livingstone, Edinburgh, 1986

61. Dillin W, Booth R, Cuckler J, et al: Cervical radiculopathy: a review. Spine, suppl 10, 11:988, 1986

62. German Association of Manual Medicine: Memorandum on the prevention of accidents arising from manipulative therapy of the cervical spine. April 1979

63. Grieve G: Common Vertebral Joint Problems. Churchill Livingstone, Edinburgh, 1981

64. Wyke B: Articular neurology: a review. Physiotherapy 58:94, 1972

65. Blaine E: Manipulative (chiropractic) dislocation of the axis. JAMA 1356, 1925

66. Dvorak J, Panjabi M, Gerber M, et al: CT-functional diagnostics of the rotary instability of the upper cervical spine. Spine, suppl 3, 12:197, 1987

67. McKenzie R: Treat Your Own Neck. Spinal Publications, Lower Hut, New Zealand, 1983

68. Cyriax J: Textbook of Orthopaedic Medicine. Vol. 2. Williams & Wilkins, Baltimore, 1971

69. Lindahl O, Hamberg J: Thoracic spine disorders as a cause of angina-like pain. Pract Cardiol, suppl 2, 10:62, 1984

70. DeLacerda F: Cervical traction. p. 683. In Grieve G (ed): Modern Manual Therapy of the Vertebral Column. Churchill Livingstone, Edinburgh, 1986

71. Maitland G: Application of manipulation. Physiotherapy 56:1, 1970

72. Hickling J, Maitland G: Abnormalities in passive movement: diagrammatic representation. Physiotherapy 3:105, 1983

73. Maitland G: The hypothesis of adding compression when examining and treating synovial joints. J Orthop Sports Phys Ther 2:7, 1980

74. Maitland G: Negative disc exploration. Aust J Physiother, suppl 3, 25:129, 1979

75. Maitland G: Manipulation: individual responsibility. Physiotherapy 1:2, 1972

76. Maitland G: The treatment of joints by passive movement. Aust J Physiother, suppl 2, 19:65, 1973

77. Maitland G: Relating passive movement treatment to some diagnoses. Aust J Physiother, suppl 3, 20:129, 1974

78. Maitland G: Palpation examination of the posterior cervical spine: the ideal, average and normal. Aust J Physiother, suppl 3, 28:3, 1982

79. Maitland G: Examination of the cervical spine. Aust J Physiother, suppl 2, 25:49, 1979

80. Maitland G: Manipulation-mobilization. Physiotherapy 52:382, 1966

81. Maitland G: Musculoskeletal Recording Guide. Virgo Press, Adelaide, South Australia, 1978

82. Laslett M: The rationale for manipulative therapy in the treatment of spinal pain of mechanical origin. Unpublished workshop manual. Mark Laslett. 211–213 White Swan Rd., Mt. Rosekill, Auckland 3, New Zealand, 1986

83. Lindahl O, Hamberg J: Thoracic spine disorders as a cause of angina-like pain. Pract Cardiol, suppl 2, 10:62, 1984

84. McGuckin N: The T4 syndrome. p. 370. In Grieve G (ed): Modern Manual Therapy of the Vertebral Column. Churchill Livingstone, Edinburgh, 1986

85. Flynn T: The thoracic spine and rib cage. Butterworth-Heinemann, Boston, 1996

86. Stevens B, McKenzie R: Mechanical diagnosis and self treatment of the cervical spine. p. 271. In Grant R (ed): Physical Therapy of the Cervical and Thoracic Spine. Churchill Livingstone, New York, 1988

87. Cyriax J: Illustrated Manual of Orthopaedic Medicine. Butterworths, Boston, 1983

88. Paris SV: Extremity Dysfunction and Mobilization. Institute Press, Atlanta, GA, 1980

89. Edeling J: Manual therapy for chronic headache. 2nd Ed. Butterworth Heinemann, Boston, 1994

CHAPTER 8

Dysfunction, Evaluation, and Treatment of the Shoulder

Steven C. Janos and William G. Boissonnault

It is well recognized that pain in the shoulder and shoulder girdle is very common in the general population, with a reported prevalence of 15 to 25 percent in patients 40 to 50 years of age.[1,2] With the contemporary explosion of physical fitness activities, these numbers will very likely increase.

This chapter presents a brief overview of the functional anatomy of the shoulder region, an examination scheme for the area, and an in-depth look at three common shoulder pathologies: frozen shoulder, rotator cuff injuries, and anterior glenohumeral joint instability. The description of the pathologies will include pathohistologic changes, common clinical signs and symptoms, and treatment considerations. For further information related to assessing and treating shoulder dysfunction, see Chapter 4.

■ Functional Anatomy

The anatomic and biomechanical complexity of the shoulder region can make assessment and treatment of shoulder dysfunction difficult, but also very interesting and challenging to the clinician. By better understanding the mechanics of the individual structures about the shoulder, we are able to identify those that may be the primary source of symptoms and dysfunction, as compared to similar structures in the surrounding area. Inman et al.[3] demonstrated the interdependence of glenohumeral joint and shoulder girdle motions for elevation of the upper extremity to 180 degrees. Using straps to prevent scapulothoracic motion and clavicular elevation, they showed that shoulder abduction was restricted to 90 and 120 degrees, active and passive, respectively. Inman et al. also manually prevented clavicular rotation, which limited active shoulder flexion and abduction to approximately 110 degrees. The fact that the glenohumeral, sternoclavicular, acromioclavicular, and scapulothoracic joints all contribute to shoulder movement makes a detailed clinical assessment of each of these joints and associated soft tissue structures a necessity. A working knowledge of the anatomy and mechanics of each of these regions is the basis for many of the examination techniques and for the understanding of many of the shoulder disorders seen clinically.

Humerus

The price for the tremendous mobility of the shoulder complex is poor stability. This is particularly true at the glenohumeral joint. In contrast to the hip joint, little support is supplied by the osseous elements, the humeral head and glenoid fossa. Sarrafian[4] stated that because the concave glenoid fossa is relatively flat and only one-quarter the size of the convex humeral head, no element of stability is provided by the bony articulation.

The humeral head makes up essentially one-third of a sphere and is oriented medially, cephalically, and posteriorly. It has been noted to have an "angle of inclination" of 135 degrees to the humeral shaft in the frontal plane. It also has a 30 degree "angle of torsion" facing posterior to the frontal plane. This is also sometimes referred to as *retrotorsion* or *retroversion*. The humeral head is separated from the shaft by the anatomic neck. The hyaline cartilage of the humeral head is thickest centrally and thinnest peripherally. Other bony areas of note that are clinically palpable and associated with tissues that are commonly seen as clinical problems are the greater and lesser tuberosities (rotator cuff and adductor insertions) and the intertubercular sulcus (bicipital groove—a floor for the long head of the biceps and an attachment region for the pectoralis major, latissimus dorsi, and teres major). The deltoid tuberosity is also palpable and is the site of the insertion of the deltoid muscle. It is important to note this landmark, for although it is a common pain referral site for subacromial joint problems, it is rarely a problem locally.

Scapula

The glenoid fossa is pear-shaped, shallow, and relatively flat and is oriented 10 degrees cephalically in the frontal plane. This position appears to help offset the bony instability of the glenohumeral joint, primarily in the caudal direction.

The orientation of the glenoid fossa in relation to the remainder of the scapula may also be a factor in glenohumeral joint stability, however. Saha[5] related the retrotilted position of the glenoid fossa to a reduced inherent risk of anterior dislocation of the humeral head. The orientation of the scapula on the thorax may also influence glenohumeral joint stability regarding inferior dislocation of the humeral head.[6] With the upper extremity in a dependent position, the glenoid fossa faces laterally, anteriorly, and superiorly. Because of this superior inclination, for the humeral head to subluxate inferiorly it must also displace laterally.[7] The glenoid labrum is attached to the periphery of the glenoid fossa and serves to deepen the functional fossa by about 2.5 mm. It is also an attachment site for the joint capsule. It is fibrocartilage superiorly, anteriorly, and posteriorly and more of a capsular thickening inferiorly. The hyaline cartilage of the fossa is thinnest centrally and thickest peripherally. This structural arrangement is the opposite of that of the humeral head and, once again, shows the synergism of joint structures. Other points of note are the supraglenoid and infraglenoid tubercles, which serve as the origin points for the long head of the biceps and long head of the triceps, respectively.

Joint Capsule

The glenohumeral joint capsule is relatively thin, allowing approximately 2 to 3 cm of joint distraction in a dissected specimen.[8] It is weakest anteriorly and inferiorly. The joint capsule is reinforced superiorly and anteriorly by the coracohumeral and glenohumeral ligaments, respectively. The middle portion of the glenohumeral ligament appears to be situated to prevent anterior dislocation of the humeral head with the glenohumeral joint at rest and in some abduction, with the inferior glenohumeral ligament best able to resist anterior humeral head translation with the shoulder positioned in greater abduction and external rotation.[9] Therefore, by preventing lateral displacement, structures oriented in the horizontal plane, such as the superior joint capsule, superior glenohumeral ligament, and coracohumeral ligament, could prevent inferior subluxation of the humeral head in the anatomic position. Because of the horizontal orientation of the supraspinatus and the posterior deltoid, these muscles may also contribute to this mechanism.

There are several "openings" in the capsule, the two most notable being anterior. The first is anterior/superior over the intertubercular groove for the exit of the long head of the biceps. The second is more caudal and opens to become the subscapular bursa. The third communicates posteriorly with the infraspinatus bursa. As with other synovial joint capsules, a "negative pressure" is noted inside the joint, giving the glenohumeral joint some additional stability.

Rotator Cuff

The rotator cuff muscles also reinforce the joint capsule.[5,10] They are intimately blended with the capsule for added strength and support and are approximately 2.5 cm in length. The subscapularis adds support anteriorly, especially when the arm is positioned near the body.[9] The teres minor and the infraspinatus help stabilize the posterior aspect of the glenohumeral joint[5]; the supraspinatus stabilizes the superior aspect. The inferior aspect of the joint is not reinforced by muscles or capsular ligaments, making it the weakest area (Fig. 8–1). The rotator cuff muscles provide dynamic stability by muscle contraction with attachment to the capsule, and they adjust capsular tension. Additionally, they help to stabilize the joint via compression of the glenohumeral joint, and they work in synergy with the deltoid as part of a force couple to allow full range of motion of shoulder girdle elevation.

The supraspinatus is active in the resting position and is believed to assist dynamically in resisting downward displacement of the humeral head. The rotator cuff interval is the space between the supraspinatus and subscapularis portions of the cuff. It is a cleft between the coracohumeral/superior glenohumeral ligament and the middle

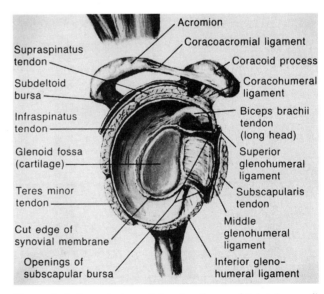

Figure 8–1. Lateral view of the glenohumeral joint (opened) illustrating the anatomic relationship between the rotator cuff, capsular ligaments, and glenoid labrum. (From Netter,[75] with permission.)

glenohumeral ligament. It is commonly used as a port of entry during arthroscopic glenohumeral joint surgery. The long head of the biceps also appears to be involved in the dynamics of the glenohumeral joint. It is not involved in resisting primary downward displacement of the humeral head at rest, but it assists in abduction of the shoulder as external rotation is imparted through the range of motion of elevation, and it assists in depression of the humeral head later in the movement of abduction.

Limiting superior displacement of the humeral head is the coracoacromial arch. This arch forms the superior border of the subacromial joint, a physiologic joint described by Kessel and Watson.[8] The acromion process and the coracoacromial ligament form the superior portion of this arch. The rotator cuff tendons and the greater tuberosity of the humerus form the inferior border of this joint, and the subacromial (subdeltoid) bursa acts as the joint cavity. Soft tissue structures, such as the supraspinatus and infraspinatus tendons, lying between the two unyielding joint borders are at risk for impingement or compressive injuries in the presence of abnormal glenohumeral joint mechanics or trauma (Fig. 8–2).

The anatomic joints of the shoulder girdle include the acromioclavicular (ACJ) and sternoclavicular joints (SCJ). Being the sole bony connection between the upper extremity and the trunk, the SCJ is designed to withstand significant forces. In fact, because of the strength of the supporting periarticular structures, excessive forces transmitted through the upper extremity are more likely to cause a fracture of the clavicle rather than a dislocation of the SCJ.[11,12]

The fibrocartilaginous disk and the costoclavicular ligament are the principal stabilizers of the SCJ, firmly anchoring the medial end of the clavicle to the manubrium and the first rib and its costal cartilage.[13,14] Little stability is afforded by the articulation itself, as the articular surfaces lack congruity. The upper portion of the medial end of the clavicle can extend well above the sternal portion of the articulation. The disk and the costoclavicular ligament prevent medial and superior migration of the clavicle as forces are transmitted toward the SCJ.[14] The SCJ capsule is reinforced superiorly, posteriorly, and anteriorly by ligaments, with the anterior aspect of the joint being the least supported. Therefore, although uncommon, SCJ dislocation is more likely to occur in the anterior direction than in the posterior or superior direction.[14] Generally, during clavicular movements, the capsular ligaments become lax on the side of the joint corresponding to the direction in which the clavicle is moving and taut on the opposite side. For example, during retraction the posterior aspect of the capsule and the supporting ligament become lax, while the anterior structures become taut.

Like the SCJ, the ACJ relies heavily on an accessory ligament, the coracoclavicular ligament, for stability. The conoid and trapezoid portions of the coracoclavicular ligament firmly attach the lateral end of the clavicle to the coracoid process of the scapula. This strong ligament prevents superior migration of the clavicle in relation to the acromion in response to forces being transmitted through the upper extremity or directly through the acromion (e.g., during a fall).[4,5,12,14] The relatively weak ACJ capsule is also supported superiorly by a capsular ligament.

Shoulder Motion: Elevation

The most often studied shoulder movement has been elevation in the frontal plane or in the plane of the scapula. The plane of the scapula is described as being approximately 30 to 45 degrees anterior to the frontal plane.[15] Shoulder abduction is generally considered to consist of 90 to 120 degrees of glenohumeral joint motion and approximately 60 degrees of upward scapular rotation.[4,16,17] There is agreement that the initial 25 to 30 degrees of abduction occur primarily at the glenohumeral joint, while the scapula seeks a stable position.[4,17] Afterward, both the shoulder girdle and the glenohumeral joint contribute to the movement in what has been described as scapulohumeral rhythm.

Poppen and Walker[11] studied the position of the humeral head in relation to the glenoid fossa during elevation of the arm in the plane of the scapula. The humeral head translated in a superior direction an average of 3 mm during the initial 30 to 60 degrees of the motion. Afterward, the position of the humeral head on the glenoid was relatively constant, translating 1 to 2 mm in

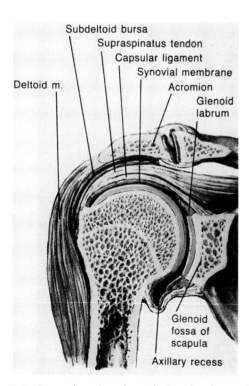

Figure 8–2. Coronal section through the glenohumeral joint illustrating the anatomic relationship between the supraspinatous muscle and the overhanging acromion. (From Netter,[75] with permission.)

either a superior or an inferior direction. This was thought to be caused by the medially and inferiorly directed pull of the teres minor, infraspinatus, and subscapularis muscles. These muscles form a functional group, which depresses the head of the humerus to counteract the superior and lateral pull of the deltoid.[4,10] The teres minor, the infraspinatus, and the subscapularis are active throughout the abduction range, as is the deltoid.[4] The deltoid and the supraspinatus are considered the prime movers for glenohumeral joint abduction. Each muscle is capable of elevating the arm independently, but with a resultant loss of power.[18] Glenohumeral joint external rotation is necessary for normal shoulder abduction. The rotation allows the greater tuberosity and accompanying rotator cuff tendons to clear the acromion, the coracoacromial ligament,[10,17] and/or the superior ridge of the glenoid fossa.[19] Components of the rotator cuff—the teres minor and the infraspinatus—are thought to account for the external rotation, as their activity increases throughout the abduction range, whereas the subscapularis activity tends to peak at about 90 degrees of the motion.[13] Extensibility of the inferior and anterior periarticular structures of the glenohumeral joint is necessary for angular displacement of the humerus away from the inferior aspect of the glenoid, with corresponding inferior glide of the humeral head, and for the external rotation that must occur.[20]

Shoulder girdle contributions to shoulder elevation are important for many reasons. Besides adding to the abduction range, the 60 degrees of upward scapular rotation on the thorax helps maintain an optimal length-tension relationship between muscles acting across the glenohumeral joint[4,10,16] and allows the glenoid fossa to remain in a stable position in relation to the humeral head.[16,17] The amount of upward scapular rotation is equal to the amount of movement occurring at the clavicular joints.[14] Saha described the initial 20 degrees of scapular rotation as occurring at the ACJ as the scapula moves on the clavicle. This produces tension within the coracoclavicular ligaments, resulting in clavicular rotation at the SCJ. This clavicular rotation, which allows for another 40 degrees of upward scapular rotation, is therefore passive in nature, relying on normal ACJ mechanics.[14]

Clavicular elevation occurring at the SCJ during the initial 90 degrees of abduction is also important for the general position of the scapula on the thorax.[4] For clavicular elevation to occur, inferior displacement of the sternal end of the clavicle is necessary. This movement occurs primarily between the clavicle and the fibrocartilaginous disk.[14] The trapezius, the rhomboids, the serratus anterior, and the levator scapulae muscles form the axioscapular muscle group, which is responsible for scapular stability and motion.[4] The serratus anterior, the lower and middle trapezius, and the rhomboids stabilize the medial border of the scapula, preventing winging from occurring during abduction.[4,10] The serratus anterior also works in concert with portions of the trapezius to rotate the scapula upward on the thorax.[4,10]

The other shoulder motions have not been studied as extensively as abduction; therefore, only a brief comparison between flexion and abduction is presented. Although flexion is somewhat like abduction in that similar contributions at the glenohumeral joint and shoulder girdle are necessary for full range of motion, differences between the two movements exist. Inman et al.[3] stated that approximately 60 degrees of flexion occurs before significant scapular motion begins, as opposed to 30 degrees of abduction. Inman et al.[3] demonstrated that there was less middle trapezius activity with flexion than with abduction, which would allow the scapula to migrate further laterally on the thorax during flexion. Blakely and Palmer[15] found internal rotation of the humerus to be an important concurrent motion for full flexion to occur, whereas external rotation is important for full abduction to occur. Basmajian and Bazmant[9] stated that the anterior deltoid and the clavicular portion of the pectoralis major are the prime movers for flexion. Both of these muscles are also internal rotators. Finally, Saha[5] described an anterior and superior movement of the humeral head on the glenoid during flexion, which again differs from the humeral head displacement noted during abduction.

Description of the other shoulder motions is beyond the scope of this chapter. These other motions, however, are specifically related to shoulder dysfunction, which is discussed later in the chapter.

■ Examination and Evaluation of the Shoulder

Evaluation of the shoulder follows the same principles used in examination of any joint in the body. It is assumed that a subjective examination and an upper quarter screening examination have been completed and that the findings have led to the decision to look at the shoulder in more detail. The cervical spine is an important region to be screened because local cervical dysfunction may cause referred pain to the shoulder. Kellgren[16] demonstrated the referral of pain to the glenohumeral joint area from the midline cervical and thoracic spine ligaments. Glenohumeral joint pain has been noted primarily with irritation of the interspinous ligament associated with the motion of C4-C5 segments but also with irritation of ligaments of the C7-T1 and T1-T2 segments. In a similar study, Campbell and Parsons[17] demonstrated referral of pain to the shoulder area, with irritation of ligaments and joints of the upper and midcervical regions. See Chapter 4 for a description of an upper quarter screening examination that indicates tests for the cervical spine. Table 8–1 presents a proposed examination scheme for the shoulder region.

Observation and Inspection

The initial observation and inspection of the shoulder are often referred to as the postural portion of the examina-

□□□□□ □ □ □

Table 8–1. Examination of the Shoulder Girdle

Observation/inspection
  Standing
  Sitting

Palpation
  Standing
  Sitting
  Supine
  Prone

Active and passive range (physiologic)
  Shoulder girdle
    Elevation
    Depression
    Protraction
    Retraction
  Glenohumeral joint
    Forward flexion
    Abduction
    Internal rotation
    External rotation
    Extension
    Horizontal flexion
    Horizontal extension
    Hand behind back
    Hand behind head

Accessory movements
  Glenohumeral joint
    Distraction
    Compression
    Anterior glide
    Posterior glide
    Inferior glide
  Subacromial joint
    Distraction
    Compression

Accessory movements (*cont.*)
  Acromioclavicular joint
    Anterior glide/distraction
    Posterior glide/compression
    Cephalic glide
    Caudal glide
  Sternoclavicular joint
    Distraction
    Compression
    Anterior glide
    Posterior glide
    Cephalic glide
    Caudal glide
  Scapulothoracic joint
    Distraction
    Cephalocaudal glide
    Mediolateral glide
    Mediolateral rotation

Resisted tests (isometric)
  Cardinal planes (shoulder/elbow)
  Specific manual muscle testing

Special tests
  Locking position
  Quadrant test
  Biceps tendon testing (Yergason's and Speed's tests)
  Apprehension test
  Drop arm test
  Empty can test
  Andrew's Anterior Instability Test
  Sulcus sign
  Relocation test
  Load and shift test

tion. It is important to remember not to diagnose a problem solely on the basis of a patient's posture in a given area. The real importance of posture lies in its relationship to function, which is studied later in the examination. For the shoulder, it is important to look at the trunk and neck positions with both sitting and standing. The position of the scapula relative to the trunk should be inspected. Excessive protraction is probably most commonly seen, followed by excessive elevation. Next, the position of the humerus relative to both the scapula and the trunk should be noted. Often the humerus sits anteriorly relative to the scapula. Hypertrophy and atrophy of the musculature of the shoulder region should be noted, as should other soft tissue changes. In more chronic shoulder dysfunction, one will often note atrophy of the deltoid, along with hypertrophy of the upper trapezius in an attempt to compensate for this weakness.[21,22] In observing soft tissue and bony landmarks, it is important that the patient be relaxed and that the arms be free to

hang at the side if possible. If the arm stays supported, one could miss a possible elevated clavicle indicative of an acromioclavicular separation.

Palpation

Palpation should start superficially and proceed to deeper structures. One should look for changes in soft tissue and bony contours, skin temperature and moisture, and swelling and thickening of soft tissue. Pain and tenderness are important findings but can be misleading. A systematic approach should be taken when palpating major bony and muscle landmarks around the shoulder.[23] Alterations in muscle tone should be noted, as well as any hypertrophy of bony landmarks such as the greater and lesser tuberosities, the acromion, and the bicipital groove region when involved in a chronic impingement syndrome. The joint lines of the ACJ, SCJ, and glenohumeral joint should be found and palpated for abnormalities.[23] The examiner should also assess soft tissue mobility of the muscles and tendons around the shoulder. This is analogous to accessory motion testing of joints. Normal mobility may be lost secondary to spasm, swelling, or fibrosis.

Active Range of Motion

Always start with the big picture. Look at what happens to the patient's entire body on active range of motion of the shoulder girdle. As in assessing active motion at any joint complex, one should look for provocation of symptoms and note the quantity and quality of movement. Ideally, one should observe shoulder motion from the anterior, posterior, and lateral positions to note changes in both quality and quantity. Poor quality may manifest as any of the following: a hitch during range; an arc of pain with impingement of the rotator cuff and subacromial bursa between 70 and 120 degrees of abduction; trunk over- or undercompensation; or improper rhythm of movement between the scapula and the humerus. As an example, excessive protraction and upward rotation of the scapula on elevation are common. The examiner must then determine if the problem is scapular muscle weakness, or if the scapula is merely compensating for a glenohumeral problem, or both. While the patient performs these movements, one should also palpate each of the joints of the shoulder girdle for quality of movement, crepitation, popping, clicking, or snapping.

Passive Range of Motion

Again, the examiner should assess the quantity and quality of movement, as well as the end-feel imparted to the examiner's hands by the structures limiting the movement. Normal end-feels at the glenohumeral joint are classified as capsular.

For both passive physiologic and accessory movements, the examiner must be aware of the starting position

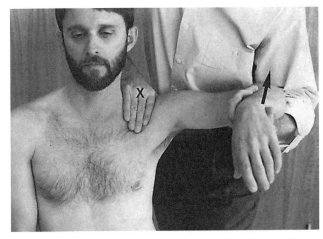

Figure 8-4. Abduction overpressure at the glenohumeral joint.

for testing, as well as stabilization on production of movement. As an example, in producing passive physiologic abduction, the therapist needs to align the humerus in the plane of the scapula before abducting the humerus (Fig. 8-3). If the arm is brought straight up in the body's frontal plane, in most cases the movement produced will be one of abduction as well as horizontal extension.

Proper stabilization is also important. When one looks at glenohumeral motion, the scapula must be well stabilized (Figs. 8-4 to 8-9). It is not, the range of movement will be greater, the end-feel not as specific, and provocation of symptoms not as reliable. Ideally, the examiner should move the shoulder through its range, both with scapular stabilization for the glenohumeral joint and without stabilization for the ACJ, SCJ, and scapulothoracic joint. For both active and passive range of motion, one should be noted whether, with restricted motion, a pattern exists. At the shoulder, the capsular pattern of restriction in order of limitation is external rotation, abduction, and internal rotation.

In testing passive accessory movements at the shoulder, information similar to that elicited during passive

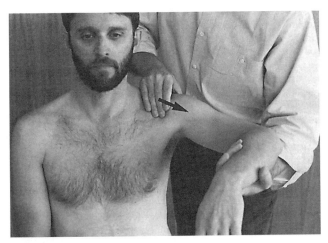

Figure 8-3. Passive abduction. The humerus is in the same plane as the scapula (approximately 30 degrees of flexion). This is closer to pure abduction.

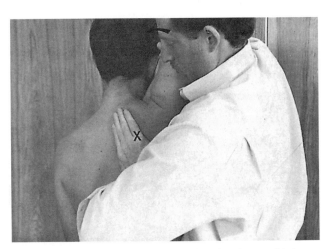

Figure 8-5. Flexion overpressure at the glenohumeral joint.

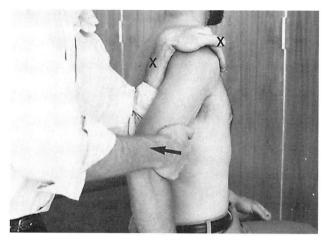

Figure 8–6. Extension overpressure at the glenohumeral joint.

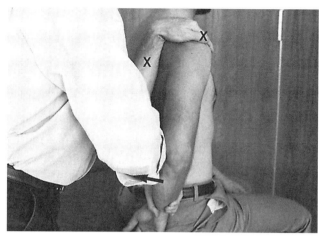

Figure 8–9. Overpressure for the functional movement of placing the hand behind the back (extension, adduction, internal rotation).

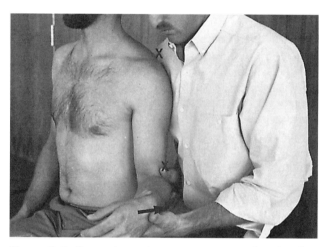

Figure 8–7. External rotation overpressure at the glenohumeral joint.

physiologic testing should be gained (Figs. 8–10 and 8–11).

Resisted Testing

The two goals of resisted testing are provocation of symptoms and assessment of the strength of the muscle-tendon unit. To be sure that pain is reproduced from the contractile unit involved, the examiner should avoid joint movement during testing. This can be especially difficult at the shoulder because of its great mobility. For resisted testing there, the humerus is placed at the patient's side in a neutral position. Resistance should be provided slowly while observing and palpating for possible movement. If pain is not an issue, standard manual muscle testing can be used to better assess the strength of specific muscles.

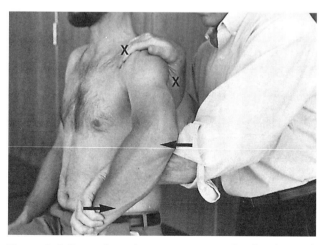

Figure 8–8. Internal rotation overpressure at the glenohumeral joint. The arm is slightly abducted so that the hand will clear the patient's body.

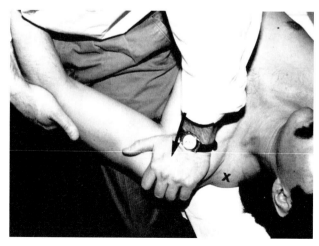

Figure 8–10. Example of passive accessory movement testing of the glenohumeral joint: posterior glide of the humerus, scapula stabilized.

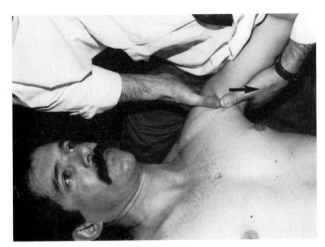

Figure 8–11. Caudal glide of the humerus with no scapular stabilization.

Special Tests

An assortment of special tests are used in the examination of the shoulder.

Empty Can Test

This test is used to isolate the supraspinatus muscletendon unit. The arm is abducted in the plane of the scapula to 90 degrees, with the humerus in internal rotation. Resisted testing to abduction may demonstrate pain and/or weakness implicating the supraspinatus tendon, but it also will compress all other subacromial structures as well. Therefore, as with many other special tests, the results must be considered in relation to all other examination findings.

Locking and Quadrant Tests

Locking and quadrant tests have been described by Maitland.[18] In the locking position (Fig. 8–12), the greater

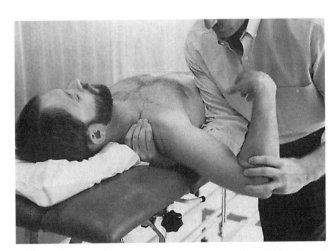

Figure 8–12. Locking position. The scapula is stabilized, and the humerus is slightly rotated internally and placed in slight extension, then abducted until a firm stop is reached.

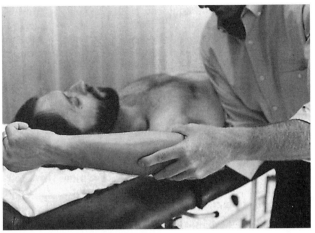

Figure 8–13. Quadrant position. From the locking position, the humerus is allowed to externally rotate slightly and flex while the arm is slowly abducted. A small hill or arc of movement is felt at approximately 30 degrees from the fully abducted position. Both the locking and quadrant positions place stress on the subacromial structures (rotator cuff, bursa, coracoacromial arch), as well as on the glenoid labium. Both tests are used to provoke symptoms and to determine the feel of the joint at the point of resistance.

tuberosity and its rotator cuff attachments are caught within the subacromial space so that any further movement into lateral rotation, abduction, or flexion is impossible. The quadrant position (Fig. 8–13) is a continuation of the locking position, allowing some flexion and external rotation as the arm is abducted. A small hill or arc of movement can be felt at approximately 30 degrees from the fully abducted position.

Biceps Tendon Tests

Tedinitis of the long head of the biceps tendon should be revealed by standard testing at the shoulder, but occasionally the information is confusing. *Speed's Test* consists of resisted testing of shoulder flexion/abduction with the elbow extended and supinated. Weakness and pain in the anterior aspect of the shoulder suggest involvement of the biceps tendon and/or the superior labrum. In *Yergason's Test,* the patient resists elbow flexion and supination while externally rotating the shoulder against resistance. If the biceps tendon is unstable in the bicipital groove it may subluxate, and the patient will experience pain.

■ Instability Testing

Apprehension Test

To test for chronic anterior glenohumeral dislocation, slowly abduct and externally rotate the patient's arm to a position where it may easily dislocate. If the shoulder is ready to dislocate, the patient will begin to hesitate and guard against the movement. The patient should also be asked if this movement reproduces the sensation that occurs when the shoulder pops out.

Sulcus Sign Test

The status of the superior, inert structures of the glenohumeral joint is assessed with this examination procedure. With the arm at the side and with the patient typically sitting, the examiner palpates the subacromial region and proceeds to pull the humerus in a downward or caudal direction. Excessive movement (greater than 1–2 cm, depending on the individual) and/or symptom reproduction implicates one or more of the following: the superior glenohumeral ligament, coracohumeral ligament, superior joint capsule, and superior labrum.

Load and Shift Test

With the patient sitting and the examiner standing behind the patient and to the side, the humeral head is first compressed into the glenoid in a medial direction; then, with the heel of the hand, an anterior glide is imparted. This test grossly looks at potential anterior instability and may implicate one or more of the following structures: the anterior joint capsule, anterior labrum, and middle glenohumeral ligament, and to a lesser extent, the superior and inferior glenohumeral ligaments. This test can also be modified to assess the posterior stability of the joint.

Other Anterior Instability Tests

There are many other special tests that can be used to assess the stability of the glenohumeral joint. The *Andrews Anterior Instability Test* places the shoulder in approximately 130 degrees of abduction and lateral rotation toward end-range. In this position the examiner stabilizes the distal part of the humerus with one hand and, with the other hand, grasps the superior/lateral humeral head and lifts it in an anterior direction. Excessive range of movement (of which there should little to none) and/or symptom reproduction implicates one or both of the following structures: the inferior glenohumeral ligament and the anterior labrum. The *Relocation Test* is similar to the Andrews Anterior Instability Test and incorporates a good problem-solving strategy that can be used in many other testing procedures throughout the body. The shoulder is taken to the end-range of lateral rotation in a position of 90 degrees of abduction, and symptoms are elicited. Then the test is repeated with a posteriorly directed glide of the humeral head imparted to the shoulder. If the symptoms are relieved, anterior instability is implicated as the source of the problem.

Additionally, local gliding procedures of the joints of the shoulder in various directions are invaluable in determining instability and symptom reproduction.

These procedures can be modified to be as simple or complex as the examiner deems necessary.

Drop Arm Test

The drop arm test is used to diagnose complete tears of the supraspinatus tendon. It is positive if the patient is unable to lower the arm slowly from a position of 90 degrees of abduction.

It is not just performing all of these tests that makes for a good shoulder examination, but performing them well. A wealth of information can be gained from each part of the examination if one is sensitive in using both the eyes and the hands.

■ Frozen Shoulder

The diagnosis of frozen shoulder provides the therapist with little information except that the patient usually has a stiff, painful shoulder. The condition, whose onset is often insidious and idiopathic,[24] is usually progressive. There is general agreement that the glenohumeral joint capsule is the site of the lesion, although some authors hypothesize that bicipital tenosynovitis[25,26] and rotator cuff injuries[25,27,28] precede the capsular involvement.

Pathologic changes in the glenohumeral joint capsule are often believed to result in shoulder stiffness.[29] Adhesive capsulitis has been described as a condition that includes a thickened, fibrotic glenohumeral joint capsule adherent to the humeral head and obliteration of the capsular axillary pouch. Loss of the axillary pouch in the early stages of frozen shoulder has also been described. Arthrography supports the contention that glenohumeral joint capsule extensibility is lost in these patients. Normal shoulder joint volume capacity is 20 to 30 ml, whereas a capacity of 5 to 10 ml is present in patients with frozen shoulder.[24,30] Arthrography has also demonstrated loss of the axillary pouch, the subscapular bursa, and the long head of the biceps sheath.[29,30] Histologic events that could result in the loss of capsular extensibility may include abnormal cross-bridging between newly synthesized collagen fibers and preexisting fibers and loss of critical fiber distance caused by a significant decrease in hyaluronic acid and water content.[26,27] Some authors have also described a postimmobilization fatty fibrous connective tissue scar, creating intra-articular adhesions within synovial joints, which could also result in decreased mobility.[26,28]

A capsular pattern of restricted passive motion and abnormal glenohumeral joint accessory movements are among the physical examination signs that suggest glenohumeral joint capsule involvement. Cyriax defined joint capsule dysfunction as arthritis, which at the shoulder is represented by external rotation as the most limited motion followed by abduction and internal rotation.[24] The arthrographic evidence of loss or reduction of the axillary pouch and anterior joint capsule extensibility[25] corresponds to the finding that external rotation and abduction are the most restricted movements, because normal extensibility of these portions of the joint capsule is necessary for the two motions to occur.[31] The arthrographic findings also correspond to the commonly found restriction of glenohumeral joint accessory movements, namely, inferior and anterior glides. This does not preclude other accessory movements from being restricted, including lateral distraction, which stresses the entire capsule.

The therapist must consider factors other than the glenohumeral joint capsule when assessing shoulder stiffness. ACS, SCS, and scapulothoracic joint dysfunction may contribute to decreased or painful shoulder motion. Fibrotic changes and adhesions affecting the rotator cuff, the long head of the biceps, and the subacromial bursa have also been associated with loss of shoulder motion.[25-27,30] Adaptive muscle shortening caused by the pattern of restricted motion and the commonly observed patient posture, which includes the shoulder held in an adducted and internally rotated position, may contribute to the stiffness associated with frozen shoulder. Physical examination findings often include tightness of the internal rotator and adductor muscle groups of the shoulder, with particular involvement of the pectoralis major, the latissimus dorsi, and the teres major. Stretch weakness of the scapular muscles such as the middle and lower trapezius and the rhomboids is also often found. The protracted shoulder girdle posture and the increased scapulothoracic joint motion often observed in these patients may account for the stretch weakness. These muscle imbalances may contribute to the altered glenohumeral joint mechanics, providing additional abnormal stresses to the capsule and associated structures such as the rotator cuff muscles and subacromial bursa.

Physical therapy treatment must address these imbalances to maximize shoulder function during the rehabilitation process. Differentiation between muscle and capsular tightness is important because the two tissues respond to different types of manual stretching. The end-feel detected during assessment of passive physiologic and accessory movements at the glenohumeral joint will help the therapist determine the nature of the restriction. A patient with frozen shoulder will usually require both joint and soft tissue mobilization and stretching techniques for improving shoulder range of motion. The brachial plexus is another important structure to be screened in patients presenting with shoulder pain and stiffness. Elvey[32] described methods for placing different components of the brachial plexus and associated peripheral nerves under a tensile load. Adhesions or obstructions restricting the nerve tissue's mobility during cervical or upper extremity movements may result in pain and stiffness in the shoulder area.

Besides assessing the nature of the shoulder dysfunction, the therapist must determine if the shoulder symptoms are local or referred. Many local structures could be the source of the patient's pain, including bone, joint capsule, ligaments, myofascial units, or bursa. An examination scheme based on Cyriax's theory of diagnosis by selective tension,[24] plus the accessory movement techniques and special tests already described, should help the therapist determine which structure(s) is involved.

Assessment of patients with frozen shoulder requires examination of many anatomic regions. If these different areas are not at least screened, the source of the patient's symptoms and the dysfunction directly related to the symptoms could be missed completely, making treatment success unlikely.

Management

Decreasing pain and shoulder stiffness is the ultimate treatment goal for this patient population. The treatment modalities used depend on which stage of the frozen shoulder cycle the patient is in: early (acute) or late (chronic). In the early stage, decreasing the inflammation and the associated pain and muscle guarding is the primary goal. Many modalities are suggested for relief of acute pain and muscle guarding, including transcutaneous electrical nerve stimulation (TENS), cryotherapy, phonophoresis, and iontophoresis.[33,34] Active-assisted, active, and passive exercises also play an important role in the early rehabilitation of these patients. Increasing local blood flow by exercising the shoulder to the patient's tolerance may decrease local edema and congestion.[35] These procedures may assist removal of metabolic waste products, which may be responsible for the stimulation of local nociceptors. A decrease in nociceptor activity may lessen pain perception and muscle guarding. These forms of exercise may also result in neuromodulation of the nociceptive input due to stimulation of type I or II mechanoreceptors.[36,37] Pendulum exercises can be very effective active-assisted home exercises for muscle relaxation. These exercises are also safe, as the patient has complete control over how vigorously the upper extremity is exercised. Besides the immediate glenohumeral joint area, muscle guarding is often detected in the cervical and shoulder girdle regions.[38] Therefore, an exercise that incorporates gentle movement throughout these regions can be very effective for muscle relaxation.

Feldenkrais[39] described several such exercises for the entire body. An example of an exercise that may benefit the patient with frozen shoulder is as follows: The patient lies on the uninvolved side, with the involved upper extremity supported by the patient's body. Visualizing a clock dial painted on the lateral surface of the involved shoulder, the patient gently oscillates the shoulder toward the ear (12 o'clock) and then toward the hip (6 o'clock) within the pain-free range of motion. Movement between any pair of numbers on the clock can be attempted. At the clinic, this exercise can be active-assisted or passive, with the therapist guiding the limb and shoulder girdle through the range. Passive shoulder movements, either physiologic or accessory, as described previously for the examination, should be of grade I or II range, as described by Maitland.[18] These techniques can be very effective in decreasing pain and muscle guarding. Constant reassessment of the patient's symptoms and objective findings is essential to prevent overtreatment or inappropriate treatment. Reassessment of muscle tone, tissue temperature, and selected active and passive movements, paying particular attention to the passive end-feel, can alert the therapist to an adverse reaction to the treatment being performed.[40] Any increase in the cardinal signs of inflammation, spasm end-feel, or pain occurring early in the passive range of motion is a warning that the treatment was or is too vigorous.

Patient education is also an important part of early-phase rehabilitation. The patient must understand the warning signs of too vigorous home exercises to prevent a flare-up of symptoms. The patient also needs to understand the importance of proper posture to help reduce stress on the entire involved upper quarter. In the early stages, improved head-neck, shoulder girdle, and truck positions may decrease activity in the cervical and scapular muscles, which are trying to support these regions. This decreased muscle activity may help relieve local symptoms while also allowing for more normal shoulder motion. In the later, chronic stage of frozen shoulder, the patient should be aware of how the commonly seen forward head posture, with the upper extremity internally rotated and adducted, can propagate muscle tightness and weakness, resulting in abnormal glenohumeral joint mechanics. Postural reeducation and rehabilitation may include use of a lumber pillow and thoracolumbar mobility treatment techniques to facilitate the assumption of a less physically stressful posture. All the above treatments are designed to enhance the wound-healing process and decrease the physical stress on all the tissues in the shoulder region. If they are successful, the pain and muscle guarding will be decreased to a level at which the specific dysfunction can begin to be treated.

The primary goal during the late stage of frozen shoulder is to normalize shoulder movement. Improving soft tissue mobility throughout the glenohumeral joint and shoulder girdle region; joint mobility at the glenohumeral joint, the ACJ, and the SCJ; and muscle strength and coordination throughout the glenohumeral joint and shoulder girdle regions are all important treatment considerations. The objective examination findings will reveal the specific treatment needs of each patient. See Chapter 13 for joint mobilization techniques that may be useful with the frozen shoulder patient. Movement grades III and IV, as described by Maitland[18] for accessory and physiologic movements, should be used to stress the involved tissue. High-velocity thrust techniques can also be a useful tool, in the hands of a skilled clinician, to restore glenohumeral joint motion (Fig. 8–14). Because of the adaptive shortening of other soft tissue structures, muscle stretching and soft tissue mobilization techniques are essential for restoration of motion. Soft tissue restrictions are com-

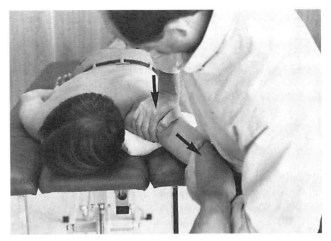

Figure 8–14. Example of a grade V technique for increasing end-range elevation.

monly found in the anterior glenohumeral joint and shoulder girdle regions, the inferior glenohumeral joint, and the ipsilateral cervical spine areas as a result of the poor posture commonly seen. As previously stated, rotator cuff adhesions are common, and stretching of these muscles may be important for restoration of motion. An excellent reference for muscle-stretching techniques is that by Evjenth and Hamberg.[41] Modalities such as ultrasound to facilitate tissue stretch and heat to promote relaxation are useful adjuncts to manual stretching techniques.[34] Muscle-strengthening and coordination exercises are also necessary for normalizing shoulder motion. Stretch weakness and disuse atrophy are often found throughout the glenohumeral joint and scapular regions.

Feldenkrais and proprioceptive neuromuscular facilitation (PNF) exercises are extremely useful for restoring coordination and motor control to the involved areas, a necessary adjunct to strengthening exercises. The therapist should consider Janda's[37] theory that attempting to strengthen weak muscles without stretching tight antagonistic muscle groups could result in enhancement of the imbalance.

There are few controlled studies in the literature on treatment for frozen shoulder, and often no mention is made of whether the patients were in the early or late stage. Hamer and Kirk[34] compared the results of cryotherapy and ultrasound, with both patient groups also receiving active and passive exercises. Both groups demonstrated improved shoulder range of motion and decreased pain, but there was no significant difference between the groups. Bulgen et al.[38] investigated four groups of patients, all of whom used pendulum exercises. Each group also received either no additional treatment, ice packs and proprioception neuromuscular facilitation (PNF) techniques, joint mobilization, or intra-articular steroids. All four groups noted decreased pain, and after 6 months of treatment, there was no significant difference between the groups. Other studies demonstrate similar findings in which various modalities or combinations of therapeutic interventions relieve pain and improve shoulder mobility.[29,30,35] Treating patients with frozen shoulder can be a long, complicated process because of the nature of the pathology and the intricate relationships among the shoulder and other upper quarter structures. Therapists should base their choice of treatment on the specific examination findings and on the techniques that they have found to be most useful in addressing the individual patient's needs.

■ Rotator Cuff Injuries

The rotator cuff performs many functions. Passively, the muscles of the rotator cuff stabilize the glenohumeral articulation; actively, they are dynamic stabilizers, firmly seating the humeral head within the glenoid fossa so that more superficial muscles, such as the deltoid, can move the glenohumeral joint optimally.[7,10] Along with this function, studies have suggested that the rotator cuff contributes between one-third and one-half of the power of the shoulder in abduction and at least 80 percent of the power in external rotation.[4,11]

As we have seen, the glenohumeral joint is an extremely mobile articulation. Unfortunately, it has long been recognized that to have great mobility, one must sacrifice stability, and contributions to both functions are demanded of the rotator cuff. This fact alone makes it more prone to injury. Injury to the musculotendinous cuff is common and occurs with one or more of the following: (1) trauma, (2) overuse, and (3) attrition or aging.[42–44] It is important to be aware of which of these conditions may be involved because this information will impact on later treatment and prognosis.

Trauma can be differentiated according to the type of force involved: tension or compression. A forceful and usually sudden contraction of the rotator cuff is an example of a tensile stress. The main component of tendon is the fibrous protein collagen. In mature tendon, completely acellular areas are common. To achieve the high tensile strength necessary to transmit muscular force efficiently, the collagen is arranged into parallel arrays of fiber bundles oriented along its lines of stress.[45,46] Tendon of any kind has the most tensile stress applied to it when its associated muscle contracts, especially when the contraction is of the lengthening or eccentric type.[47] When tendon is extended beyond its point of elasticity, which is at approximately 8 percent extension of total length, overstretching and rupture of some collagen fibers occur. This type of injury to the rotator cuff is not unusual given its important function as a stabilizer of the glenohumeral articulation.

Compressive trauma is most commonly seen as a fall on an outstretched arm, driving the humerus and cuff up into the coracoacromial arch. The resultant bruising and inflammatory response will compromise the function of the involved muscle-tendon unit. In general, rotator cuff injuries are seen arthroscopically as incomplete tears on the undersurface of the muscle-tendon unit. There is minimal to no well-defined demarcation between the supraspinatus, infraspinatus, and teres minor muscles to allow easy indentification.[22,42]

Throwing has been shown to be one of the movements that most consistently produces rotator cuff tears, with and without other associated pathologic conditions. In a study of the throwing motion in athletes, of 178 baseball players reviewed, 122 (68 percent) had rotator cuff tears. Of that number, 100 (82 percent) had supraspinatus muscle involvement; 75 (61 percent) of these injuries were limited to the supraspinatus muscle, and 25 (20 percent) were combined supraspinatus and infraspinatus muscle injuries.[13,43,44] The deceleration phase of the throwing motion seems to be the causative factor when the rotator cuff is attempting to stabilize the glenohumeral joint.

■ Impingement Syndrome

A second and quite common type of rotator cuff pathology is the overuse or impingement syndrome. This involves impingement of the rotator cuff and overlying subacromial bursa against the anterior edge of the acromion and its associated coracoacromial arch. This is one of the most common problems that afflict the shoulder. The term *impingement syndrome* is descriptive but not very helpful in actually diagnosing and treating the patient. It is defined as a symptom complex involving structures that make up the subacromial physiologic joint space; it may consist of primary or secondary compressive or tensile disease. Basically, it implicates one or more of the following structures: the acromion process, coracoacromial ligament, subacromial bursa, rotator cuff, and the long head of the biceps/labrum.[3]

Primary compressive disease is most common and results from one or more of the following etiologies:

1. Acromial morphology
2. Thickened coracoacromial ligament
3. Rotator cuff imbalance/weakness or imcompetence
4. Degenerative spurs/fibrosis of the subacromial space
5. Hypertrophy/inflammation of the rotator cuff[48]

Additionally, secondary compressive disease is seen quite often with glenohumeral instablity.[49,50]

Clinical findings usually involve reproduction of symptoms with activities that place the arm overhead and cause the shoulder to reach across the body. An arc of pain between 70 degrees and 120 degrees indicates that the subacromial space is being compressed at its closed-packed position of 90 degrees of abduction. Often frank weakness is noted, as well as an alteration in the scapulohumeral rhythm. Excessive scapular motion attempts to compensate for glenohumeral incompetence and pain.

Secondary glenohumeral instability is also commonly associated with impingement.

Neer[49,50] described three progressive stages of impingement. Stage I usually occurs in individuals younger than 25 years of age but may occur at any age in those who are engaged in excessive overhead use of the arm. The pathologic changes seen are edema and hemorrhaging of the subacromial bursa. If impingement continues the condition becomes chronic, producing thickening and fibrosis of the bursa and tendinitis of the cuff. Stage II disease is commonly seen in patients 25 to 40 years of age. Stage III disease results from further impingement, producing degeneration or complete or incomplete tears of the rotator cuff. Often this impingement of the cuff is a result of poor shoulder girdle mechanics. It may be due to hypomobility (shortening of soft tissues), hypermobility (lengthening of soft tissues, damage to glenoid labrum), or a strength imbalance of one or more muscles about the shoulder girdle.

The supraspinatus tendon is the most susceptible because of its location and because there is an area of relative avascularity close to its insertion. Microangiographic studies have revealed a profuse blood supply to the rotator cuff tendons except for a portion of the supraspinatus. This tendon has a so-called critical zone: an area of hypovascularity near its humeral insertion not unlike that of many tendons with a circular cross section elsewhere in the body. It has been hypothesized that the relative ischemia in this zone can produce changes mimicking tendon degeneration.[49,50]

Aging causes progressive degeneration of all elements of the rotator cuff. The attachment to bone and the tendon fibers exhibit disorganization with fragmentation, and in addition to decreased vascularity, there is a loss of tendon cellularity.[22,42] This limits the ability of the tendon to adapt to stresses and decreases its ability to heal after injury. Tensile strength is decreased with age, and calcification at the bony insertion is common.

Variations in the anatomy of the subacromial region may render some individuals even more prone to degenerative cuff disease. Soon after injury, a vicious cycle begins. Damage to the cuff leads to impairment of its normal function; it can no longer provide the normal glenohumeral fulcrum and abnormal upward displacement of the humeral head occurs, which results in further impingement, with capillary compression and additional tendon damage.[42,51] It has also been postulated that ACJ disease plays a role in initiating the impingement process and that disease in this joint in conjunction with rotator cuff tears may have an incidence of well over 50 percent. A gradually enlarging osteophyte from a posttraumatic or degenerative ACJ or an extracapsular mechanical erosion of the inferior joint capsule may also lead to subacromial impingement and rotator cuff pathology.[52,53]

Examination

Clinical findings at the shoulder in a patient with a rotator cuff problem can vary greatly. There is no list of positive findings that one will always see when the rotator cuff is involved. Some conditions are common among many patients with rotator cuff problems. We will discuss these findings and their treatment, but we will also mention other possible findings.

We mentioned earlier that the infraspinatus and supraspinatus are most commonly involved. Active elevation can be painful near end-range secondary to lack of motion and pinching or secondary to hypermobility, or there can be an arc of pain between 70 and 120 degrees secondary to midrange compression under the coracoacromial arch.

Poor-quality movement between the scapula and the humerus is also common, especially during the lowering or eccentric phase of elevation, when increased stress is placed on the tendon. The scapula tries to compensate for this with increased movement to remove the force from the rotator cuff. This may take place because of pain and/or weakness.

More often than not, the patient complains of a single, fairly consistent location of pain. The pain is usually localized to a relatively small area of the lateral (slightly anterior or posterior), proximal humerus and is reported to be either a sharp pain or a burning sensation. There is also usually a larger referral area of pain (a generalized dull ache) laterally, down to the region of the deltoid insertion. Many times the pain moves from a lateral site anteriorly or posteriorly. This change in location may suggest a combination of a cuff problem with instability of the glenohumeral articulation, most commonly anteriorly.[54,55]

Classically, passive movements that stretch or compress the involved tendon also provoke the symptoms. Compression injuries as well as overuse (impingement) syndromes weaken the tendon and usually lead to thickening and increased scarring of the cuff secondary to a chronic inflammatory reaction.

Many times tension forces alone do not provoke a patient's symptoms, but compression of the tendon will give rise to pain. Tension forces include passive stretch of a tendon or isometric contraction of the associated muscle. Compression forces include weightbearing on the extremity or movements that compress the involved tendons.

Isometric muscle testing of abduction and/or external rotation often reproduces pain and more often shows weakness. It is important to note the position of the shoulder at the moment of resisted muscle testing. If the humerus is placed in a position of 90 degrees of abduction and the cuff is made to contract and hold there, the cuff receives both compressive and tensile forces under the coracoacromial arch.

Passive accessory movement testing of the glenohumeral joint may reproduce pain as well as demonstrate hypo- or hypermobility. Movements such as cephalic glide of the humerus compress the rotator cuff; inferior glide and lateral distraction stretch the supraspinatus; posterior glide stretches the infraspinatus and teres minor portions of the cuff. One may attempt to differentiate between a partial cuff tear and tendinitis based on clinical findings. Tendinitis more often is aggravated by compressive and compressive/shear-type examination procedures. If one session of appropriate manual intervention dramatically reduces or eliminates all signs and symptoms (even pain and weakness on resisted testing), one may assume that a cuff tear was not the problem. Minor cuff tears may show good improvement in one session, but signs and symptoms are not eliminated.

The more chronic the problem, the more likely one is to find dysfunction at the ACJ and SCJ as well (Table 8–1). Magnetic resonance imaging (MRI) is proving to be an effective means of evaluating the shoulder. The tendinous rotator cuff is well displayed, the cuff muscles can be evaluated for atrophy, and the location of the musculotendinous junction can be visualized to determine the extent of muscular retraction in cases of massive rotator cuff tears. Tears of the glenoid labrum are also easily identified and are commonly associated with instability. T_1-weighted images are most useful for display of anatomic details and the evaluation of bone marrow. T_2-weighted images identify fluid (e.g., within the glenohumeral joint or rotator cuff tendons). Often, imaging with both T_1 and T_2 weighting is required to characterize different tissues by their changes in signal characteristics. This modality not only can assist in decision making for conservative versus surgical repair of these lesions but can also provide guidance in determining if arthroscopic or open repair is indicated.[56]

Treatment

Treatment of rotator cuff injuries depends upon the type and severity of the clinical signs. Treatment can be divided into conservative and surgical care.

Conservative treatment is indicated for cuff tendinitis as well as for partial-thickness tears. Depending on the severity of signs and symptoms, rest in some form is indicated. This consists of immediate avoidance of all aggravating positions and movements. It may include the use of a sling to immobilize the shoulder for a few days if any use of the arm produces symptoms. At this stage the use of ice, nonsteroidal anti-inflammatory drugs, and/or local steroid injection may also be indicated.[49,51,52]

It is important to determine early on if the shoulder has an acute or a chronic inflammatory reaction. Acute inflammation is marked by primarily fluid changes (i.e., edema or bleeding) and a stimulus of brief duration. A chronic inflammatory response is marked by fibrous changes with little fluid and a stimulus that persists.[45] For the rotator cuff, this stimulus is usually some abnormality of shoulder movement or an irritating activity. The prognosis for a quick, full recovery with conservative care is not as good for a large tear, a chronic condition, or an older individual. After cuff injury, rupture of some collagen fibers occurs, accompanied by cell damage. Healing is initiated by the invasion of the area by cells that remove debris and synthesize a new connective tissue matrix. Tendon is a dense, regular connective tissue and is therefore mechanically well suited to transmit tensile loads, but it has a low cell count and a poor vascular supply and therefore is not a quick healer. Increased tensile strength during healing is enhanced by controlled passive motion; the strength (ultimate load) increases to 35 percent of the value for intact tendons after 84 days, whereas complete immobilization results in an increase to only 21 percent. The greatest amount of tensile force put on tendon is derived from contraction of its associated muscle. Therefore, active and resisted movements should be withheld until the tendon is strong enough.

Besides rest and medication, there are many physical therapy modalities (e.g., ice, heat, ultrasound, high-voltage galvanic stimulation, transcutaneous electrical nerve stimulation) that can control inflammation and decrease swelling, edema, and pain. These are definitely indicated during the course of rehabilitation of the shoulder, with the eventual goal of restoring normal strength, movement, and function.

Management

Short-term treatment of impingement syndrome is quite rewarding, with marked improvement in symptoms and motion accomplished within several sessions. Local treatment with ice/heat, ultrasound/iontophoresis, and massage affect the subacromial region quickly and effectively. Additionally, gentle passive movement (in particular anterior-posterior gliding) in the loose-packed position can restore normal motion immediately.[57] The difficulty lies in attempting to sort out the reason(s) for the impingement and restoring as normal function as possible to prevent recurrance. This typically involves more long-term stretching, resistance exercises, and modification of activities.

Hypomobility, or a lack of normal motion at the glenohumeral joint, is a common problem. If the joint is not free to move passively, the rotator cuff cannot be expected to perform its normal dynamic function. It is important to determine whether the restrictions are secondary to muscle or inert tissues about the joint (capsule, ligaments, labrum, etc.). This information should be obtained from palpation and by looking at the pattern of restricted movement, as well as from the end-feel on passive testing. The rotator cuff may be stretched locally at the joint with accessory movement treatment techniques, or the muscle-tendon unit may be lengthened with soft tissue stretching techniques. These may include different forms of massage, as well as physiologic muscle-stretching techniques (Fig. 8–15). In either case, active-resisted exercise using the muscles that maintain the newly gained range should follow immediately, and a home program should be designed to do the same. This should be true both for single movements (i.e., flexion-extension) and more functional motions such as reaching behind the back. This motion commonly tends to be limited, especially when the supraspinatus is involved. Reaching behind the back both elongates the muscle-tendon unit and compresses it as it is pulled under the coracoacromial arch with internal rotation. Pain and limitation on horizontal flexion are also common when the infraspinatus is involved for similar reasons.

Probably more common than stiffness is hypermobility at the glenohumeral joint with involvement of the rotator cuff. With this problem, treatment becomes more difficult and progresses more slowly. Treatment is now aimed at muscle reeducation and strengthening of the entire shoulder girdle. For the rotator cuff, this type of treatment should be based on the following:

1. Type of tissue (tendon)
2. Function (stabilization and movement of the humerus)
3. Type of dysfunction (instability versus hypomobility)
4. Severity of the lesion (extent of the tear, whether acute or chronic)

Once active movement is pain-free, resistive concentric exercise is indicated. Isometric "holds" should be incorporated at different points of the range as progress warrants. Movement should be slow so that the cuff can control the motion. This is followed by slow, eccentric exercise,[47] incorporating rotation into the movements whenever possible (e.g., PNF diagonals). As the patient progresses, faster speeds are incorporated into the exercise

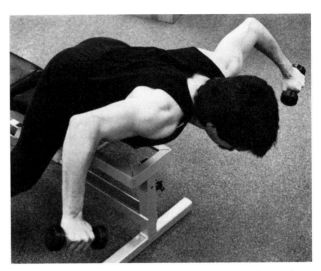

Figure 8–16. Prone shoulder horizontal extension (prone laterals). Isolated resisted exercise training for both the posterior and lateral rotator cuffs, as well as the scapular retractors.

program. It is important that constant tension be kept on the muscle and tendon during each set of exercises and that the axis for the particular movement be located at the individual's own joint. Examples of this kind of exercise include manual resistance, dumbbells, cables, and Theraband (Figs. 8–16 and 8–17). This automatically limits the use of machines with fixed axes of motion (e.g., Cybex, Universal, Nautilus). All human joints have a changing axis during motion, and the glenohumeral joint is no exception. Again, the problem here is unstable motion, and movement *must* take place about the normal physiologic axis. A later progression should also include weightbearing exercise (push-ups, modified dips, etc.).

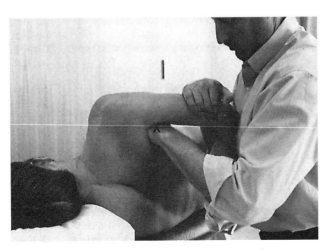

Figure 8–15. Stretching of the supraspinatus muscle.

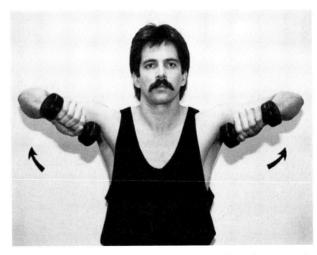

Figure 8–17. Lateral raises. This is an excellent basic exercise for strengthening the entire rotator cuff, as well as for improving the coordination of appropriate scapulohumeral position and rhythm.

Surgery

When conservative care fails to produce the desired result, surgical intervention may be indicated. This is usually the case with complete cuff tears or chronic, persistent problems in an active individual.[50,51]

The most minor and least involved procedure is arthroscopy and shaving of any small defects in the cuff. Anterior acromioplasty (removal of a portion of the anterior and inferior acromium) with limited detachment of the deltoid presently appears to be the most direct, least potentially harmful, and perhaps most effective procedure for persistent rotator cuff tendinitis. This decompressive procedure offers the possibility of satisfactory pain relief and return to normal daily function. Neer[50] reported satisfactory results in 15 of 16 patients treated by anterior acromioplasty. Results do not seem to be as good for competitive athletes. Tibone et al.[52] reported that 76 percent of the patients studied could not return to their preinjury throwing status or overhead sport after surgery.

A variety of procedures have been advocated to close large defects in the rotator cuff and restore function. Grafting methods include the use of a free biceps tendon, the coracoacromial ligament, freeze-dried cadaver rotator cuff, bovine tendon or ligament tissue, and a variety of synthetic materials.[58] Any of these procedures requires more extensive surgery and usually offers a less optimistic prognosis than the procedures mentioned previously. Any surgical procedure should be followed by extensive rehabilitation.

Rotator cuff disease is a common and important source of shoulder symptoms. The cuff mechanism functions not only to stabilize the shoulder but also to provide power for movement. The pathogenesis of rotator cuff disease is associated with trauma, overuse, and attrition or aging. The supraspinatus and the infraspinatus are most commonly involved. Treatment consists usually of graded rest as well as, eventually, a comprehensive exercise program to restore strength and stability to the area.

■ SLAP Lesions

Superior labral anterior-posterior (SLAP) lesions of the glenoid labrum have become increasingly common sources of shoulder pain and dysfunction. The SLAP lesion is a detachment lesion of the glenoid labrum. It can be associated with impingement-like syndromes, as well as with glenohumeral instabilities. SLAP lesions are most commonly due to a fall or a blow to the shoulder. They also occur in throwing athletes and are associated with the follow-through portion of the activity secondary to high tensile stresses on the shoulder. Occupations requiring heavy lifting also have been reported to involve a higher incidence of SLAP lesions.[59,60] Slight detachment of the superior/posterior labrum may be normal in older adults. Associated conditions that are often seen are rotator cuff pathology (40 percent) and anterior glenohumeral instability.[59]

SLAP lesions may be classified into one of four categories:

Type I Fraying and degeneration of the superior labrum, with a normal long head of the biceps structure.

Type II Detachment of the superior labrum and biceps insertion from the supraglenoid tubercle. This is the most common type of SLAP lesion, but it may resemble a normal variant.

Type III A bucket-handle tear, with the biceps anchor intact.

Type IV A vertical tear of the superior labrum which extends into the biceps.

The typical clinical finding is pain with overhead activity. In general, the signs and symptoms may mimic those of impingement syndrome.[60] Glenohumeral instability, especially anterior, is often associated with SLAP lesions. Complaints of clicking, popping, and/or locking of the shoulder are not uncommon.

It is important to note that treatment of SLAP lesions[62] is no different from treatment of any other mechanical problem noted at the shoulder. Treatment of signs and symptoms takes first priority. Commonly, excessive translation is observed at the glenohumeral joint.[61,63] Therefore, treatment may be aimed at stabilizing the joint, with mobilization of surrounding hypomobile joints, while improving strength and control dynamically with exercise. But given the nature of the disorder, if conservative treatment does not provide relief of symptoms and improvement in function, surgical intervention may be indicated. Debridement and repair of the defect is usually done arthroscopically, often in conjunction with other procedures.[64,65]

■ Anterior Glenohumeral Instability

Instability at the shoulder is a common clinical problem, with anterior instability seen most often. The relatively small size and shallowness of the glenoid cavity, the position of the glenoid fossa (facing laterally and forward), and the advantage of the external rotators over the subscapularis combine to make the shoulder susceptible to dislocations in the forward, medial, and inferior directions.[4,66] Anterior instability can be subdivided into two groups: acute traumatic anterior dislocation and recurrent anterior dislocation or subluxation.

Acute traumatic anterior dislocation is an injury predominantly of young adults, particularly athletes. It is usually caused by forced external rotation and extension of the shoulder; the humeral head is driven forward and frequently avulses the cartilaginous glenoid labrum and capsule from the anterior aspect of the glenoid cavity.[66-68] The association between acute traumatic anterior shoulder dislocations and lesions of the rotator cuff has long been recognized. The exact incidence of cuff ruptures is unknown, but McLaughlin and MacLellan[54] suggested that the incidence may be as high as 70 percent in patients older than 40 years of age. A single episode of anterior dislocation is relatively more common in the older patient population. This group is more likely to suffer injury secondary to a fall on an outstretched arm, with the dominant arm involved twice as often as the nondominant arm. The older population also has a higher risk of nerve and vascular injury.[69]

Recurrent anterior dislocation or subluxation is much more common in the younger population for several possible reasons. The underlying mechanism seems to be either an anterior one, consisting of stretching of the anterior capsule or avulsion of the glenoid labrum (usually occurring in younger patients), or a posterior one (occurring in older patients), consisting of tendon rupture of the rotator cuff.[70] Because rotator cuff tears associated with anterior dislocation are more common in older patients, they tend to give way first, possibly sparing the anterior structures (capsule, labrum, glenohumeral ligaments). In younger patients, an anterior intracapsular pouch is formed, and healing is generally poor. This is also true for the labrum. It may be supposed as well that older patients are less prone to encounter situations that provoke anterior dislocation than are younger patients and therefore have a lower incidence of dislocation.[67-69]

Clinical Examination

In the acute traumatic situation, the patient will have a history of a specific activity or event that caused the dislocation, usually involving a fall on an outstretched arm or forced movements of abduction, extension, and external rotation. The patient will be unable to use the arm and often will support it with the opposite extremity. With recurrent dislocation or subluxation, the patient will report sudden attacks of shoulder pain that occur with certain movements. The patient may state that he or she feels a clicking sensation, that the shoulder "pops out," and that lately these episodes have occurred more frequently. The objective examination will usually show some general atrophy around the involved shoulder girdle. Passive physiologic and accessory movement testing most often reveals hypermobility or instability about the glenohumeral joint, especially with external rotation and anterior glide testing. In assessing accessory movements in these patients, it is important to start with the humeral head in a neutral position, for often it will rest somewhat anterior to the glenoid fossa. This may give false information and confuse the diagnosis. The apprehension test at the shoulder often reveals a painful, hypermobile shoulder and may reproduce the patient's symptoms. It is important to remember the incidence of rotator cuff injury in the patient with anterior shoulder instability, especially in the older population. Resisted testing at the shoulder may show signs of a rotator cuff tear. It is not uncommon for a stretch injury of the axillary nerve to occur after an acute episode of anterior dislocation. Deltoid weakness as well as altered sensation in a small area of skin over the lateral shoulder is to be expected. Clinically, we find this also to be true for patients with recurrent anterior dislocation, although the findings are more subtle.

Radiographic evaluation will help to provide additional objective information on anterior shoulder instability. The Hill-Sachs lesion is a posterolateral notch defect (compression fracture) in the humeral head that is created by impingement of the articular surface of the humeral head against the anteroinferior rim of the glenoid fossa. It is the most common radiographic finding in the patient with recurrent anterior dislocation.[55,71]

The Bankart lesion is a cartilaginous or osseous defect in the anterior margin of the glenoid rim or an ectopic bone formation at this site produced by an anterior or inferior translation of the humeral head against the glenoid rim.[71]

Treatment

Conservative treatment should be the first choice in most cases of anterior shoulder instability. This may be subdivided into four basic areas:

1. Address signs of inflammation.
2. Normalize the quality of motion at the glenohumeral joint.
3. Normalize the quantity of motion at surrounding joints.
4. Strengthen the shoulder girdle and related musculature.

Once the acute signs of irritation (heat, swelling, spasm, pain) have decreased, intervention to help restore the quality of movement at the glenohumeral joint should begin. Passive movements through a normal range of motion without pushing the end-range are incorporated first. Also at this time, assessment and normalization of the quantity of movement at the surrounding joints (the ACJ, the SCJ, the scapulothoracic joint, and the cervical and thoracic spine) are begun to help decrease abnormal stresses applied to the glenohumeral joint. Shortened musculature also needs to be lengthened. Often the patient with chronic involvement will demonstrate tight anterior chest musculature secondary to a forward shoulder posture.

A good strengthening program should start with slow, controlled movements and isometrics, progressing to more eccentric contractions and finally to higher-speed activities if needed, depending on the individual patient (Fig. 8–18). Ideally, we strive for strong, and well-balanced musculature throughout the upper quarter. However, some areas often require special attention.

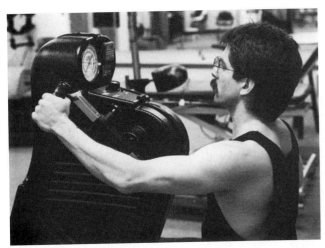

Figure 8–18. Upper Body Ergometer (UBE, Lumex Inc., Cybex Division, Ronkonkoma, NY) used for general upper body conditioning, as well as for improving dynamic stabilization at the shoulder.

It is important that the posterior scapular musculature be strong and well coordinated with the rest of the shoulder girdle. To maintain good joint congruency, the scapula must be able to elevate and rotate with the humerus and must not be allowed to protract excessively, especially with abduction, extension, and external rotation.

A second important muscle group to strengthen is the rotator cuff. We have already mentioned the high incidence of cuff injury involved with anterior shoulder instability. The external rotation component of the cuff (supraspinatus, infraspinatus, teres minor) helps to keep the humerus posterior in the glenoid on contraction. It also helps to maintain joint congruence by compressing the humerus into the glenoid.

The third muscle involved is the subscapularis. It may control anterior instability at the shoulder by passively acting as an anterior barrier to the humeral head, as well as a dynamic stabilizer to control external rotation.

When conservative care has failed to give the desired outcome or if tissue damage is severe, several surgical procedures may be used for anterior instability at the shoulder. Arthroscopic repair/reconstruction and open repair are both used to restore more normal biomechanical function. In the Putti-Platt procedure, the capsule and the subscapularis muscle are divided and then overlapped. The Bankart procedure repairs and shortens the anterior capsule at the glenoid. Both procedures are designed to leave the patient with some limitation of external rotation, thereby maintaining anterior stability.[71–73]

In the Bristow procedure, a block of bone taken from the tip of the coracoid process, with its attached tendons, reinforces the anterior part of the joint. The bone block is placed near the front of the glenoid at the anterior neck of the scapula with screw fixation. It provides an anterior block and produces a dynamic musculotendinous sling, holding the humeral head posteriorly with the arm in abduction and external rotation. This procedure allows a quicker return of range of motion and has a low redislocation rate.[74]

For any of the preceding procedures to be successful, a comprehensive rehabilitation program must follow. For the most part, the program should include the same treatment guidelines outlined for conservative care.

Anterior instability at the shoulder, whether a primary acute dislocation or recurrent episodes of anterior dislocation of the humerus, is a common clinical problem. It usually involves both the rotator cuff (primarily in the older patient) and the anterior joint structures (primarily in the younger patient). Conservative treatment involves passive motion and eventual strengthening of the posterior scapular muscles and the rotator cuff. Surgical intervention primarily involves tightening of anterior joint structures.

CASE STUDIES

CASE STUDY 1

An 18-year-old male college baseball pitcher was seen with complaints of lateral-superior right shoulder pain. Symptoms were brought on by throwing the baseball hard for variable periods of time. Physical examination of the shoulder showed generalized hypermobility but nonpainful active range of movement. Passive testing revealed reproduction of symptoms with internal rotation overpressure as well as with quadrant position testing. On resisted testing, the patient was found to have four-fifths strength into abduction and external rotation, but without pain. He also had a positive upper limb tension test on the right for limitation of movement and a different type of posterior shoulder pain.

Treatment consisted of passive movements to normalize internal rotation, quadrant testing, and a resistive training program to address the weakness. Over the course of 3 weeks, the patient's pain decreased but the weakness did not change. He was referred for examination to an orthopaedic physician, and a MRI scan was ordered. The scan revealed mild subacromial bursitis, normal rotator cuff structures, and, most interesting, a ganglionic swelling of the suprascapular nerve (Figs. 8–19 and 8–20). This last finding explains the abduction and external rotation weakness that could have caused the bursitis during the vigorous throwing movements. Continued conservative care produced good results, including decreased complaints of pain, increased strength, and no provocation of symptoms on objective tests.

CASE STUDY 2

A 62-year-old woman was seen for continued shoulder exercises after surgical repair of a torn left rotator cuff.

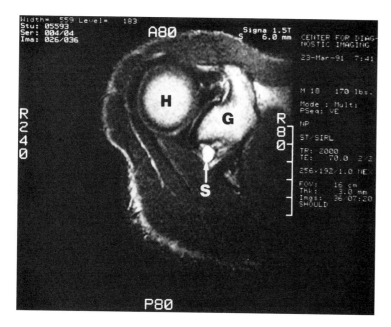

Figure 8–19. An 18-year-old baseball pitcher. T_2-weighted MRI scan. Axial view of the right shoulder visualizing the humeral head (H), the glenoid portion of the scapula (G), and the swelling of the suprascapular nerve (S).

When seen initially, she was 12 weeks postoperative and had been seeing another therapist regularly for exercise and stretching.

On examination, marked atrophy of the left glenohumeral joint musculature was noted, and the left humeral head appeared to be subluxed caudally. Active elevation of the shoulder was limited to 80 degrees and was nonpainful, but the patient showed marked scapular compensation. Also, when the humeral head was palpated during this motion, the head appeared to be moving excessively, both anteriorly and cephalically.

Passive accessory movements of the glenohumeral joint showed excessive anterior and inferior glide and moderate limitation into posterior glide. When the humeral head was held posteriorly by the therapist, active elevation was increased to 120 degrees and passive elevation to 140 degrees. Finally, resisted testing showed two-fifths abduction strength and trace external rotation strength at the left shoulder. The patient also had a positive drop arm test.

The patient was asked to return to her surgeon, and the therapist's findings were communicated to the refer-

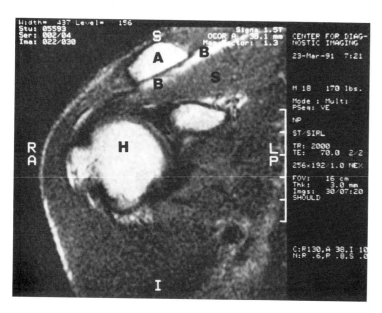

Figure 8–20. An 18-year-old baseball pitcher. T_2-weighted MRI scan. Coronal view of the right shoulder visualizing the humeral head (H), the acromion (A), the supraspinatus tendon (S), and the mild swelling of the subacromial bursa (B).

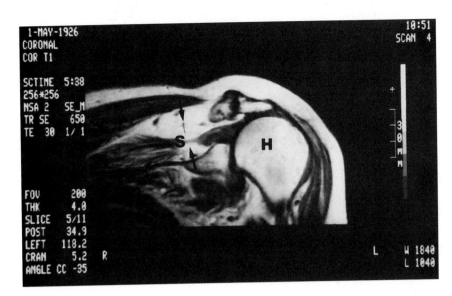

Figure 8–21. A 62-year-old patient who had had prior rotator cuff repair in the left shoulder. T_1-weighted MRI scan. Coronal view visualizing the humeral head (H) and complete rerupture of the supraspinatus (S).

ring physician. Subsequent MRI testing of the left shoulder revealed rerupture of the rotator cuff (Fig. 8–21).

■ Summary

Physical therapists see many patients who present with shoulder pain and dysfunction. To evaluate and treat these patients adequately, the clinician must not isolate the shoulder from the rest of the upper quarter. Therefore, an upper quarter screening examination before a detailed assessment of the shoulder region may be beneficial to the clinician. Three common shoulder pathologies seen by physical therapists—frozen shoulder, rotator cuff pathology, and anterior dislocations—were presented in this chapter. This information is important for the therapist because the nature of the pathology may influence treatment planning and goals. Ultimately, however, the signs and symptoms obtained during the evaluation will dictate the specific treatment techniques chosen for each patient. If the examination scheme presented in this chapter is carried out carefully, the clinician should have all the information needed to initiate a proper treatment program.

■ References

1. Westerling C, Jousson BG: Pain from neck-shoulder region and sick leave. Scand J Soc Med 8:131, 1980
2. Maeda K: Occupational cervicobrachial disorder and its causative factors. J Hum Ergol 6:193, 1977
3. Inman V, Saunders M, Abbott L: Observations of the function of the shoulder joint. J Bone Joint Surg 26(A):1, 1944
4. Sarrafian S: Gross and functional anatomy of the shoulder. Clin Orthop 173:11, 1983
5. Saha AK: Dynamic stability of the glenohumeral joints. Acta Orthop Scand 42:491, 1971
6. Turkel S, Panio M, Marshall J, et al: Stabilization mechanisms preventing anterior dislocation of the glenohumeral joint. J Bone Joint Surg 63(A):1208, 1981
7. Kent B: Functional anatomy of the shoulder complex: a review. Phys Ther 51:867, 1971
8. Kessel L, Watson M: The painful arc syndrome. J Bone Joint Surg 59(B):166, 1977
9. Basmajian J, Bazmant F: Factors preventing downward dislocation of the adducted shoulder joint. J Bone Joint Surg 41(A):1182, 1959
10. Last RJ (ed): Anatomy: Regional and Applied. 6th Ed. Churchill Livingstone, New York, 1977
11. Poppen NK, Walker PS: Normal and abnormal motion of the shoulder. J Bone Joint Surg 58(A):195, 1976
12. Lucas DB: Biomechanics of the shoulder joint. Arch Surg 107:425, 1973
13. Bechtol C: Biomechanics of the shoulder. Clin Orthop 146:37, 1980
14. Saha AK: Theory of Shoulder Mechanism: Descriptive and Applied. Charles C Thomas, Springfield, IL, 1961
15. Blakely RL, Palmer ML: Analysis of rotation accompanying shoulder flexion. Phys Ther 64:1214, 1984
16. Kellgren J: On the distribution of pain arising from deep somatic structures with charts of segmental pain areas. Clin Sci 4:35, 1939
17. Campbell D, Parsons C: Referred head pain and its concomitants. J Nerv Ment Dis 99:544, 1944
18. Maitland GD: Peripheral Manipulation. 3rd Ed. Butterworths, Boston, 1991
19. Loyd JA, Loyd HM: Adhesive capsulitis of the shoulder. Arthrographic diagnosis and treatment. South Med J 76:879, 1983
20. Turek S: Orthopaedics, Principles and Their Application. JB Lippincott, Philadelphia, 1977
21. Lippmann RK: Frozen shoulder; periarthritis, bicipital tenosynovitis. Arch Surg 47:283, 1943
22. Macnab I: Rotator cuff tendinitis. Ann R Coll Surg Engl 53:271, 1973

23. Janos SC, Bacro TR: Surface Anatomy. CD-ROM. Medical University of South Carolina, Greenfield, South Carolina, 1999

24. Cyriax J: Textbook of Orthopaedic Medicine, 7th Ed. Vol 1. Bailliere Tindall, London, 1978

25. Reeves B: Arthrographic changes in frozen shoulder and post-traumatic stiff shoulders, Proc R Soc Med 59:827, 1966

26. Akeson WH, Amiel D, Woo S: Immobility effects of synovial joints: the pathomechanics of joint contracture, Biorheology 17:95, 1980

27. LaVigne A, Watkins R: Preliminary results on immobilization: induced stiffness of monkey knee joints and posterior capsule. Perspectives in Biomedical Engineering. Proceedings of a Symposium of the Biological Engineering Society. University of Strathclyde, Glasgow, June 1972. University Park Press, Baltimore, 1973

28. Soren A, Fetto JF: Contracture of the shoulder joint. Arch Orthop Trauma Surg 115:270–272, 1996

29. Bunker TD: Frozen shoulder:unravelling the enigma. Ann R Coll Surg Engl 79:210–213, 1997

30. Leppala J, Kannus P, Sievanen H, et al: Adhesive capsulitis of the shoulder (frozen shoulder) produces bone loss in the affected humerus, but long-term bony recovery is good. Bone 22:691–694, 1998

31. Kapandji IA: The Physiology of the Joints. Vol. 1. Upper Limb. Churchill Livingstone, Edinburgh, 1982

32. Elvey R: Treatment of conditions accompanied by signs of abnormal brachial plexus tension. Paper presented at the Neck and Shoulder Symposium: Manipulative Therapy, Australia, 1983

33. Mannheimer J, Lampe G: Clinical Transcutaneous Electrical Nerve Stimulation. FA Davis, Philadelphia, 1984

34. Hamer J, Kirk JA: Physiotherapy and the frozen shoulder: a comparative trial of ice and ultrasonic therapy. NZ Med J 83:191, 1976

35. Melzer C, Wallny T, Wirth CJ, et al: Frozen shoulder—treatment and results. Arch Orthop Trauma Surg 114:87–91, 1995.

36. Wyke BH. Articular neurology—a review. Physiotherapy 58:94, 1972

37. Janda V: Central nervous motor regulation and back problems. p. 27. In Korr IM (ed): The Neurobiologic Mechanisms in Manipulative Therapy. Plenum Press, New York, 1978

38. Bulgen DY, Binder AL, Hazleman BL, et al: Frozen shoulder: prospective clinical study with an evaluation of three treatment regimens. Ann Rheum Dis 43:353, 1984

39. Feldenkrais M: Awareness Through Movement. Harper & Row, New York, 1972

40. Nicholson GG: The effects of passive joint mobilization on pain and hypomobility associated with adhesive capsulitis of the shoulder. J Orthop Sports Phys Ther 6:238, 1985

41. Evjenth O, Hamberg J: Muscle Stretching in Manual Therapy. Vols. I and II. Scand Book AB Alfta, Sweden, 1984

42. Gross TP: Rotator cuff injuries. Orthop Rev 15:33, 1986

43. Poppen NK. Walker TS: Forces at the glenohumeral joint in abduction, Clin Orthop 135:165, 1978

44. Cofield. RH: Rotator cuff disease of the shoulder. J Bone Joint Surg 67(A):974, 1985

45. Robbins SL, Angell M: Basic Pathology. WB Saunders. Philadelphia, 1976

46. Frank C, Woo SLY, Amiel D, et al: Medial collateral ligament healing: multidisciplinary assessment in rabbits. Am J Sports Med 11:379, 1983

47. Standish W, Rabinovich R, Curwin L: Eccentric exercise in chronic tendinitis, Clin Orthop 208:65, 1986

48. Brewer B: Aging of the rotator cuff. Am J Sports Med 7:102, 1979

49. Neer CS II: Impingement lesions, Clin Orthop 173:70, 1983

50. Neer CS II: Anterior acromioplasty for the chronic impingement syndrome in the shoulder, J Bone Joint Surg 54(A):41, 1972

51. Post M, Cohen J: Impingement syndrome. Clin Orthop 207:126, 1986

52. Tibone J, Jobe F, Kerland R, et al: Shoulder impingement syndrome in athletes treated by an anterior acromioplasty. Clin Orthop 198:134, 1985

53. Hyvonen P, Lohi S, Jalovaara P: Open acromioplasty does not prevent the progression of an impingement syndrome to a tear. Br Editorial Soc Bone Joint Surg 80-B:813–816, 1998

54. McLaughlin HL, MacLellan DI: Recurrent anterior dislocation of the shoulder. II. A comparative study. J Trauma 7:191, 1967

55. Pavlov H, Warren R, Weiss C, et al: The roentgenographic evaluation of anterior shoulder instability. Clin Orthop 194:153, 1985

56. Seeger LL: Magnetic resonance imaging of the shoulder. Clin Orthop 244:48, 1989

57. Conroy DE, Hayes KW: The effect of joint mobilization as a component of comprehensive treatment for primary shoulder impingement syndrome. JOSPT 28:3–14, 1998

58. Ozaki J, Fujimoto S, Masuhara K, et al: Reconstruction of chronic massive rotator cuff tears with synthetic materials. Clin Orthop 202:173, 1986

59. Payne LZ, Deng X, Craig EV, Torzilli PA, et al: The combined dynamic and static contributions to subacromial impingement. Am J Sports Med 25:801–817, 1997

60. Snyder SJ, Karzel RP, Del Pizzo W, et al: SLAP lesions of the shoulder. Arthroscopy: J Arthrosc Related Surg 6:274–279, 1990

61. Pagnani MJ, Deng X, Warren RF, et al: Effect of lesions of the superior portion of the glenoid labrum on glenohumeral translation. J Bone Joint Surg 77-A:1003–1010, 1995

62. Smith DK, Chopp TM, Aufdemorte TB, et al: Sublabral recess of the superior glenoid labrum: study of cadavers with conventional nonenhanced MR imaging, MR arthrography, anatomic dissection, and limited histologic examination. Radiology 201:251–256, 1996

63. Berg EE, Ciullo JV: A clinical test for superior glenoid labral or "SLAP" lesions. Clin J Sports Med 8:121–123, 1998

64. Berg EE, Ciullo JV: The SLAP lesion: a cause of failure after distal clavicle resection. Arthroscopy: J Arthrosc Related Surg 13:85–89, 1997

65. Segmuller HE, Hayes MG, Saies AD: Arthroscopic repair of glenolabral injuries with an absorbable fixation device. J Shoulder Elbow Surg 6:383–392, 1997

66. Wuelker N, Korell M, Thren K: Dynamic glenohumeral joint instability. J Shoulder Elbow Surg 7:43–52, 1998

67. Steinbeck J, Liljenqvist U, Jerosch J: The anatomy of the glenohumeral ligamentous complex and its contribution to anterior shoulder instability. J Shoulder Elbow Surg 7:122–126, 1998

68. Paletta GA, Warner Jon JP, Warren RF, et al: Shoulder kinematics with two-plane x-ray evaluation in patients with anterior instability or rotator cuff tearing. J Shoulder Elbow Surg 6:516–527, 1997

69. Hawkins RJ, Bell RH, Hawkins RH, et al: Anterior dislocation of the shoulder in the older patient. Clin Orthop 206:192, 1986

70. Craig EV: The posterior mechanism of acute anterior shoulder dislocations. Clin Orthop 190:212, 1984

71. Warner Jon JP, Beim Gloria M: Combined Bankhart and HAGL lesion associated with anterior shoulder instability. Arthroscopy: J Arthrosc Related Surg 13:749–752, 1997

72. McIntyre LF, Caspari RB, Savoie FH: The arthroscopic treatment of multidirectional shoulder instability: two-year results of a multiple suture technique. Arthroscopy: J Arthrosc Related Surg 13:418–425, 1997

73. Torchia ME, Caspari RB, Asselmeier MA, et al: Arthroscopic transglenoid multiple suture repair: 2 to 8 year results in 150 shoulders. Arthroscopy: J Arthrosc Related Surg 13:609–619, 1997

74. Salter RB: Textbook of Disorders and Injuries of the Musculoskeletal System, 3rd Ed. pp. 589–593. Williams & Wilkins, Baltimore, 1999

75. Netter FH: Anatomy, physiology, and metabolic disorders, p. 34. In CIBA Collection of Medical Illustration. Vol. 8. Musculoskeletal System. CIBA-GIGY Corp., Summit, NJ, 1987

CHAPTER 9

Arthroscopic Surgery of the Shoulder

Rick K. St. Pierre

Shoulder arthroscopy is the direct viewing of the glenohumeral joint with a videoscope.[1] Johnson[2] stated that the advent of shoulder arthroscopy has increased diagnostic accuracy by allowing direct visualization of pathologic lesions, applying to the shoulder joint the surgical techniques developed for the knee. Caspari et al.[3] noted that, during the past 15 years, developments in arthroscopic techniques in the shoulder have paralleled those in the knee, providing excellent visualization of the joint with minimal morbidity. Andrews et al.[4] found that although the usual diagnostic modalities of radiography, arthrography, radioactive scanning, and magnetic resonance imaging increased their knowledge of the shoulder, these techniques did not compare with the understanding of the intra-articular anatomy and pathology that they acquired with the use of the arthroscope. Shoulder arthroscopy facilitates the diagnosis and treatment of pathologic intra-articular conditions.

The indications for shoulder arthroscopy have been expanding in the past few years with the evolution of new techniques. Andrews et al.,[4] Snyder and Pattee,[5] and Johnson[2] described the following indications: rotator cuff lesions, glenoid labrum tears, biceps tendon tears, synovitis, loose bodies, shoulder instability, and chronic shoulder pain refractory to conservative treatment. More recently, the indications for arthroscopic surgery have been expanded to include complete rotator cuff tears, soft tissue and bony impingement, and both anterior and posterior shoulder instability.[6–14] Currently, Rahhal et al.[15] have determined that shoulder arthroscopy-detected glenohumeral pathology would have been missed without arthroscopic evaluation. They were concerned that the prognosis and alternative operative treatment regimens would have been significantly affected without arthroscopic evaluation. In addition, Baker and Liv[13] found that the assisted mini-open technique for the treatment of complete rotator cuff tears preserves the deltoid attachment, improves cosmesis, and reduces pain better than open surgical rotator cuff repairs. In early clinical trials, Thadbit[14] reported good to excellent results with arthroscopic laser surgery used to treat anterior instability.

Indications for arthroscopic surgery of the shoulder have significantly increased within the last 2 to 3 years, with new surgical techniques to treat glenoid labrum tears, shoulder instability, impingement, and complete rotator cuff tears.[6–21] This chapter describes the operative technique, arthroscopic anatomy, and surgical treatment of pathologic lesions of the shoulder.

■ Surgical Technique

Glenohumeral Joint

This procedure is performed on an outpatient basis under sterile conditions in the operating room. General anesthesia is used with endotracheal intubation. The patient is placed in a lateral decubitus position with the chest and pelvis stabilized with a bean bag. The involved arm is suspended in an abducted and forward-flexed position using a traction glove with 10 to 15 lb of traction weight. The arm is abducted 70 degrees and forward-flexed 20 degrees. The shoulder is then prepared and draped in a sterile manner (Fig. 9–1).

The bony landmarks are used to localize the posterior arthroscopic portal, located 3 cm inferior and 1 cm medial to the posterior tip of the acromion in the soft spot between the infraspinatus and teres minor. An 18-gauge needle is used to distend the shoulder joint with saline. The spinal needle is then removed, and a 1 cm skin puncture is made at the insertion point. With a blunt trochar, the arthroscopic cannula is inserted into the shoulder joint (Fig. 9–2). The arthroscope is then inserted through the posterior portal into the shoulder joint, with the inflow connected to the arthroscope sheath to maintain distention of the shoulder joint. An arthroscopic inflow pump system is used for continuous distention of the shoulder joint, minimizing the number of accessory portals and instrumentation of the joint.

Accessory portals are made anteriorly for the introduction of operative instruments. The anterior portal is established under direct visualization after localization with an 18-gauge spinal needle directed into the interval soft spot between the coracoid process and the acromion. Placement of the portal is verified by direct intra-articular visualization with the arthroscope in the posterior portal (Fig. 9–3). Operative instruments are then inserted through the anterior portal into the shoulder joint. If necessary, a second anterior portal may be placed adjacent to the first for the insertion of additional operative instruments. The anterior portal is the working instrumentation portal for debridement and stabilization procedures (Fig. 9–4). At the end of the procedure, the glenohumeral joint is drained and the arthroscope is removed. Sterile dressings are applied, and the extremity is placed in a sling for 1 to 2 days.

Subacromial Bursoscopy

Under sterile conditions, the arm position is changed to 30 degrees of abduction and 5 degrees of forward flexion. The arthroscopic cannula with a blunt trochar is then inserted through the posterior portal, directed at a 10 to 15 degree caudal angle, and advanced into the subacromial bursa. The pump inflow system is then attached to the arthroscope cannula. The bursa is visualized and, if there is difficulty with visualization, a lateral portal is established with an 18-gauge spinal needle 3 cm laterally and 1 cm posterior to the anterolateral corner of the acromion. An arthroscopic shaver system is then inserted through the lateral portal for resection of inflammatory tissue, scar tissue, and redundant bursa tissue, allowing visualization of the subacromial bursa and permitting arthroscopic bursoscopy. If there is soft tissue or bony impingement, a decompression acromioplasty is then performed, switching back and forth between the posterior and lateral portals, with the inflow from the infusion pump attached to the arthroscope cannula. At the end of the procedure, both the shoulder joint and the subacromial bursa are copiously irrigated and then injected with a local anesthetic. Sterile dressings are applied, and the extremity is placed in a sling for 1 to 2 days for comfort.

■ Arthroscopic Anatomy

Glenohumeral Joint

Arthroscopic anatomy of the shoulder has been described by many authors.[2,4,22–24] They agree that it is essential to have a thorough knowledge and understanding of the gross anatomy of the shoulder prior to performing arthroscopic surgery (Fig. 9–5). After the surgeon has a thorough knowledge and understanding of the gross anatomy of the shoulder, he or she can correlate this knowledge with knowledge of the arthroscopic anatomy. For successful arthroscopic surgery, it is essential that the shoulder joint be thoroughly and systematically examined. The biceps tendon is the orienting structure that must be traced from its origin on the superior aspect of the glenoid to its exit at the bicipital groove[23] (Fig. 9–6). The articular surface of the humeral head and the glenoid fossa are then inspected for areas of chondromalacia. Attention is then focused on the glenoid labrum, a cartilaginous structure forming the border of the glenoid fossa.[22] The glenohumeral ligaments are visualized next. They are thickenings of the anterior capsule and provide stability to the anterior inferior capsule.[24] The subscapularis tendon and bursae are then visualized between the superior and middle glenohumeral ligaments. Next is the evaluation of the rotator cuff. The supraspinatus component of the rotator cuff is seen superior to the biceps tendon (Fig. 9–7). The infraspinatus and teres minor components of the rotator cuff can be seen by directing the arthroscope posteriorly and superiorly.[4]

In portal placement, it is essential to know the anatomy. Any variance in portal placement can lead to significant neurologic or vascular injury. Incorrect posterior portal placement may lead to injury to the axillary and/or suprascapular nerves. Incorrect anterior portal placement may lead to injury to the musculocutaneous nerve, the brachial plexus, and/or the thoracoacromial vessels. Incorrect placement of the lateral portal used for arthroscopic acromioplasties may lead to injury to the axillary nerve, cephalic vein, and/or thoracoacromial artery.[18,19]

Subacromial Bursa

Recently, arthroscopic anatomy of the subacromial bursa has been well defined.[6–10,18,19] With the arthroscope inserted through the posterior portal, the subacromial bursa is thoroughly visualized (Fig. 9–8). If there is difficulty with visualization, a lateral portal is established and an arthroscopic bursectomy is performed to allow visualization of the subacromial bursa (Fig. 9–9). For orientation, the anterior inferior surface of the acromion and the attachment of the coracoacromial ligament are initially visualized.[6–10,18,19] Further inspection of the subacromial bursa through the posterior portal reveals the rotator cuff tuber-

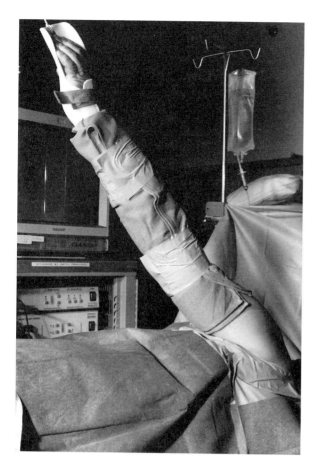

Figure 9–1. The standard arthroscopy position with the patient in the lateral decubitus position, with the arm in 70 degrees of abduction and 10 degrees of forward flexion.

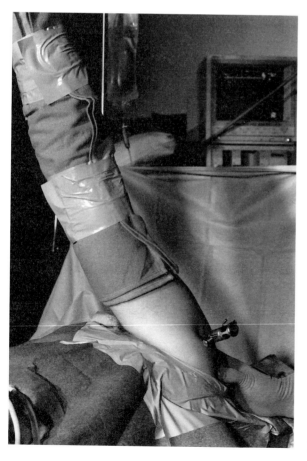

Figure 9–2. The arthroscopic cannula inserted through the posterior portal into the shoulder joint.

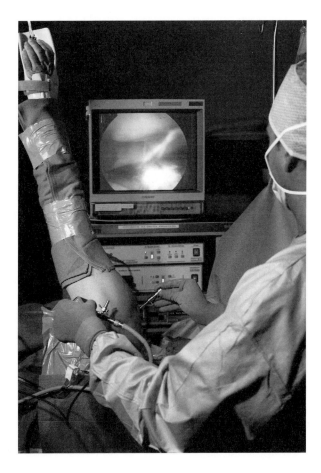

Figure 9–3. The location of the anterior portal is established under direct visualization with the arthroscope.

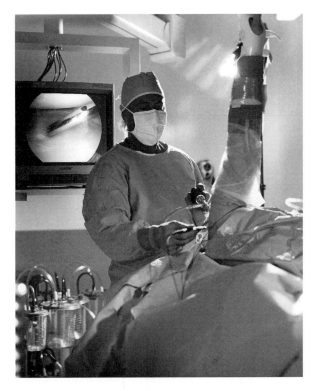

Figure 9–4. Operative arthroscopy is performed with the arthroscope in the posterior portal and the Holmium laser in the anterior portal. The surgical procedure is performed with the surgeon viewing one of the two video monitors.

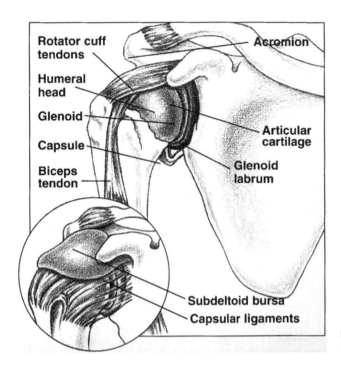

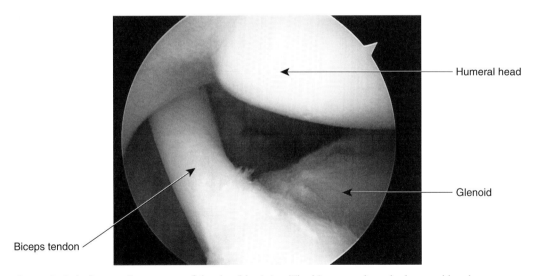

Figure 9–5. Linear drawing of the anatomic structures that can be treated with arthroscopic surgery.

Figure 9–6. Arthroscopic anatomy of the shoulder joint. The biceps tendon, the humeral head, and the glenoid can be seen.

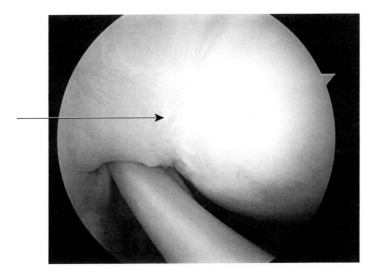

Figure 9–7. The articular surface of the supraspinatus tendon is evaluated with its insertion into the humeral head.

osity insertion, the supraspinatus tendon of the musculocutaneous junction, and the fat pad at the acromioclavicular joint.[6–10,18,19] The arthroscope is then inserted through a lateral portal for further visualization of the bursa. Through the lateral portal the shape of the acromion is determined, including the posterior surface of the supraspinatus and infraspinatus tendons. An assessment can then be made of a partial rotator cuff tear at the bursal surface, soft tissue impingement, bony impingement, or inflammatory bursitis.[6–10,18,19]

■ Surgical Treatment of Pathologic Lesions

Resection of glenoid labrum tears, debridement of rotator cuff tears and biceps tendon tears, removal of loose bodies, chondroplasties of the humeral head and glenoid fossa, and synovectomies can all be performed using the two-portal technique with the arthroscopic inflow attached to the arthroscope cannula using the inflow pump system.

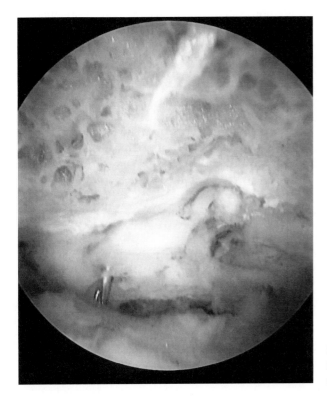

Figure 9–8. Impingement findings during bursoscopy reveal inflammation and degeneration around the coracoacromial ligament and the undersurface of the acromion.

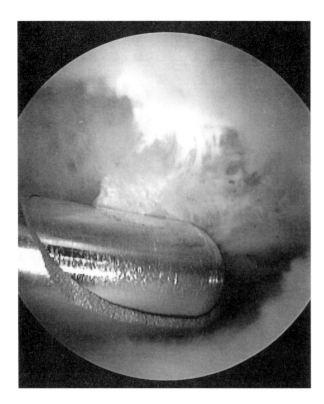

Figure 9–9. A motorized shaver is inserted from the lateral portal to allow visualization of the subacromial bursa.

The most common pathologic lesion is a torn glenoid labrum. The labrum may be injured by impingement between the humeral head and the glenoid.[17,19,23] Andrews and Carson[25] noted that all 73 throwing athletes who underwent arthroscopic examination of the shoulder showed tears of the glenoid labrum. Glenoid labrum tears may be resected with intra-articular knives, punches, motorized shavers, and the Holmium laser. The labrum is visualized with the arthroscope in the posterior portal, and the tear is excised through an anterior portal (Fig. 9–10A). The mobile fragment is resected and a contoured rim established (Fig. 9–10B).[3,17,19,23]

The next most common pathologic lesion is a partial-thickness rotator cuff tear. The arthroscope is used to inspect the undersurface of the tear (Fig. 9–11A). The loose fragments of rotator cuff are debrided with a motorized resector down to healthy, bleeding tissue (Fig. 9–11B). Caspari et al.[3] noted that arthroscopic debridement may result in dramatic relief of pain. Andrews et al.[26] demonstrated that 85 percent of the patients in their series returned to their preoperative athletic activities after arthroscopic debridement of an incomplete rotator cuff tear.

Removal of loose bodies from the shoulder is performed using the same techniques as in the knee. The arthroscope is inserted posteriorly, with the loose bodies removed anteriorly with a grasping clamp. Smaller loose bodies may be removed with the motorized shaver. Partial and complete synovectomies may also be performed with

the motorized shaver system. Similarly, degenerative and rheumatoid arthritis can be treated with arthroscopic debridement using the motorized synovial resector. Chondroplasties of the humeral head and glenoid fossa reduce pain, catching, and swelling in the shoulder joint. Caspari et al.[3] demonstrated that the technique is more effective in the shoulder than in the knee because the shoulder is a nonweightbearing joint.

■ New Techniques

Recent advances in arthroscopic shoulder surgery have occurred in the treatment of anterior instability, impingement syndrome, complete rotator cuff tears, and the use of the arthroscopic Holmium laser.

Arthroscopic Laser Surgery

A laser (light amplification by stimulated emission of radiation) produces a beam of protons that is monochromatic, coherent, and columnated. The laser energy is absorbed by cellular water and converted into heat. This vaporizes the tissue, with little or no thermal damage. The Holmium laser is currently being used for resection of glenoid labrum tears, for debridement of humeral head and glenoid chondromalacia, and for tissue tightening and collagen shrinkage.[14,20,21] Advantages of the laser include no

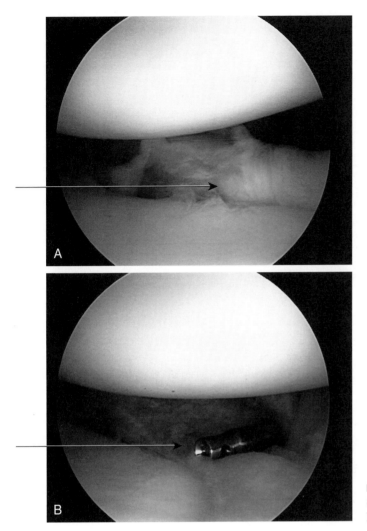

Figure 9–10. (A) Tear of the anterior glenoid labrum; (B) surgical resection of the glenoid labrum tear with the Holmium laser.

mechanical trauma to cartilage and other tissues; greater access to limited, restricted areas of the joint; and the ability to resect, ablate, smoothe, and coagulate tissue with one surgical instrument. Synovectomy, bursectomy, and acromioplasty of the shoulder are more easily performed with laser instrumentation[8] (Fig. 9–12). Postoperative pain and swelling are minimized, the inflammatory response is diminished, and patient recovery proceeds quickly with laser-assisted shoulder and subacromial arthroscopic surgery.

Lasers are extremely beneficial when used properly. Complications associated with laser use are most frequently caused by an inappropriate pairing of the laser system with the target tissue or poor surgical technique.[20]

Laser-Assisted Capsular Shift

The newest advance in arthroscopic laser surgery is the treatment of shoulder instability.[14,21] The Holmium YAG laser is used to stabilize the shoulder by shrinking the capsular tissue. The laser is used to paint a cross-

redundant collaginous material in the capsule to reduce its volume and redefine its shape. The precision of the laser beam allows preservation of normal healthy tissue while ablating only diseased or injured tissue. Currently, the laser-assisted capsular shift (LACS) procedure for capsular redundancy related to shoulder instability is an outpatient surgery that takes less than 45 minutes to perform. Laser settings of 1 joule and 10 Hz are used to achieve the desired visual shortening of the glenohumeral ligaments and capsule as the laser is brought into near-tissue contact. The patient's arm is placed in a sling for 1 week to allow the inflammation to subside. One week postoperatively, the patient is placed on an intensive neuromuscular rehabilitation regimen for strengthening of the rotator cuff and parascapular muscles.

Arthroscopic Acromioplasty

Recently, arthroscopic techniques have been used successfully in anterior acromioplasty, which is a subacromial decompression procedure.[6–10,19] In an anterior acromio-

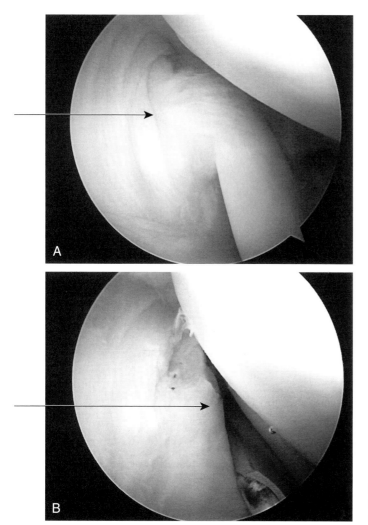

Figure 9–11. (A) Partial-thickness rotator cuff tear; (B) postsurgical resection of the partial-thickness rotator cuff tear debrided to healthy tissue.

plasty, the anterior third of the acromion is debrided of tissue, and the coracoacromial ligament and bony spur on the undersurface of the acromion are resected to decompress the rotator cuff from impingement wear (Fig. 9–13). Arthroscopic acromioplasty is an effective alternative to open surgery, since disturbance of soft tissues, particularly of the deltoid muscle, is minimal.[6–10,19]

Following arthroscopic acromioplasty, the patient is placed on a supervised shoulder rehabilitation program. The goals of therapy are to relieve pain and restore shoulder motion and strength equal to those of the uninvolved side. On the first postoperative day, the sling is removed and passive-assisted motion is started. Dependent pendulum exercises are instituted as comfort allows, and progressive strengthening exercises are begun about 2 weeks after surgery. Depending on the patient's response, normal activities, including sports, may be resumed 6 weeks after decompression. Currently, shoulder arthroscopy with subacromial decompression has shown consistent results equal to or better than those of open acromioplasty, with the additional benefit of accelerated rehabilitation.[6–10,19]

Arthroscopically Assisted Rotator Cuff Repairs

A major advantage of arthroscopically assisted rotator cuff repairs is the preservation of the deltoid attachment, with surgery limited to the rotator cuff units. This surgical specialization improves cosmesis and pain relief and allows earlier return to full activity. Recent results of arthroscopically assisted mini-open rotator cuff repairs are promising.[11–13,15] The surgical technique for these repairs has been described by Levy et al.[11] The rotator cuff is repaired under a tension-free condition, with the arm at the patient's side.

Postoperative immobilization involves a shoulder immobilizer. Rehabilitation is started on the first postoperative day, with passive range-of-motion exercises emphasized for the first 3 weeks. Active-assisted range-of-motion exercises begin 3 weeks postoperatively. At 6 to 8 weeks resistance exercises are instituted, with progression to restricted activities at 3 to 4 months on average. Preliminary reports on arthroscopically assisted rotator cuff repairs have shown results comparable to those of

Text continued on page 179

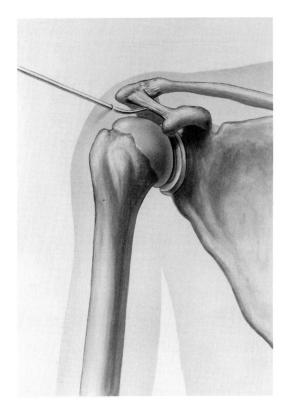

Figure 9–12. Diagram demonstrating the use of the Holmium laser for resection of the coracoacromial ligament.

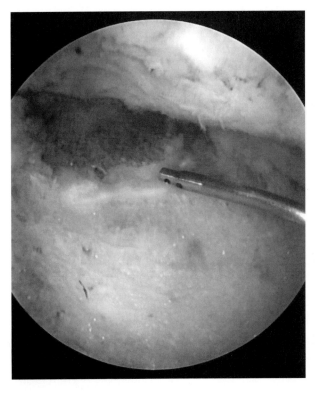

Figure 9–13. The anterior acromion is visualized following sub-acromial decompression with the Holmium laser.

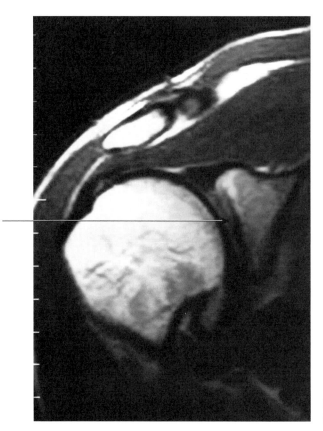

Figure 9–14. MRI scan of an anterior superior glenoid labrum tear.

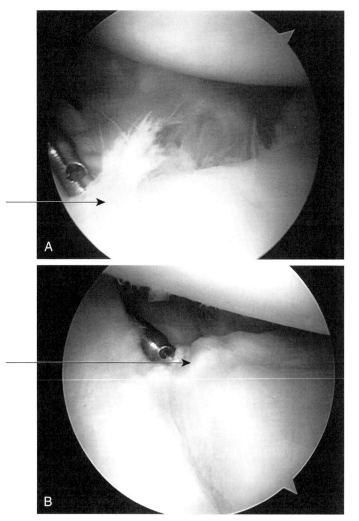

Figure 9–15. (A) Anterior glenoid labrum tear; (B) postoperative resection of the anterior glenoid labrum tear with the Holmium laser.

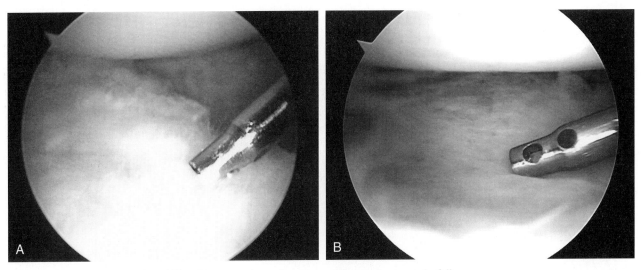

Figure 9–16. (A) Anterior instability from capsular redundancy; (B) anterior capsule following LACS.

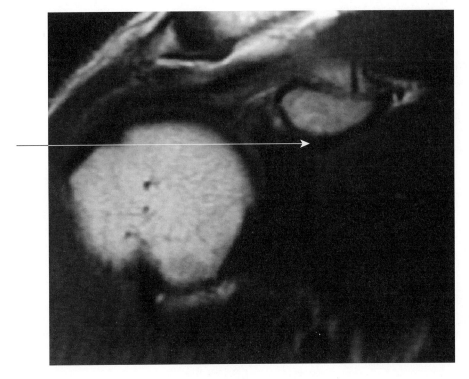

Figure 9–17. MRI scan with subacromial impingement on the rotator cuff.

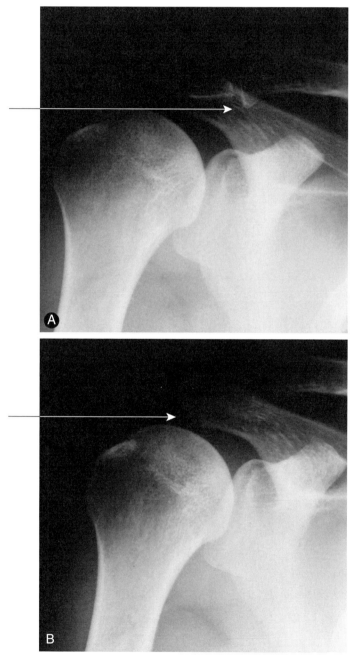

Figure 9–18. (A) Preoperative anteroposterior x-ray of the shoulder with subacromial impingement; (B) postoperative anteroposterior x-ray of the shoulder after arthroscopic subacromial decompression and distal clavicle resection.

the open repair in terms of pain relief and functional improvement.[11–13,15]

In comparison with open rotator cuff repairs, arthroscopically assisted repairs offer many advantages. These advantages include inspection and treatment of any glenohumeral joint abnormalities, subacromial decompression with concomitant treatment of the acromioclavicular joint lesions, preservation of the deltoid attachment during rotator cuff repair, shorter hospitalization time, and earlier return to function.[13]

CASE STUDIES

CASE STUDY 1

Glenoid Labrum Tear

A 23-year-old catcher for the Cincinnati Reds developed severe right shoulder pain, catching, popping, and weakness when throwing over a 3 month period. He was initially treated with anti-inflammatory medication, injections, ultrasound, and iontophoresis. He was referred for surgery since he had no improvement in his shoulder condition after 3 months of a conservative treatment regimen. Physical examination revealed that he had both audible and palpable popping and clicking, consistent with a glenoid labrum tear. He had a negative supraspinatus stress test for a rotator cuff tear, as well as a negative apprehension test and a negative relocation test for shoulder instability. His magnetic resonance imaging (MRI) scan revealed an anterior superior glenoid labrum tear (Fig. 9–14). Arthroscopic outpatient laser surgery was performed. Arthroscopic findings revealed a tear of the anterior superior glenoid labrum, with a normal rotator cuff and a normal anterior capsule (Fig. 9–15A). There

was no scarring, inflammation, or impingement in the subacromial bursa. Arthroscopic laser resection of the anterior superior glenoid labrum tear was performed (Fig. 9–15B). Following surgery, a comprehensive shoulder rehabilitation program and subsequent throwing program were prescribed. Three months postoperatively, the patient was clocked throwing 90 miles per hour with no pain, popping, clicking, fatigue, or weakness. He was called up from the Double A leagues to the Triple A leagues and told that he was a strong candidate for major league play.

CASE STUDY 2

Anterior Instability

A 21-year-old college baseball pitcher sustained an anterior dislocation of his right shoulder when sliding into second base. He was initially treated with immobilization for 4 weeks, followed by a comprehensive rehabilitation program for 3 months. Following his rehabilitation program, he experienced three more anterior dislocations of his right shoulder. He was referred for operative treatment to stabilize his anterior right shoulder instability. An arthroscopic LACS was performed to treat the recurrent anterior instability (Fig. 9–16A,B). Postoperatively, the patient was immobilized for 1 week, followed by a 2 month supervised shoulder rehabilitation program. Three months postoperatively, the patient was playing full-time, throwing with normal velocity and no pain. His 3 month postoperative visit revealed that he had full range of motion with normal strength and a negative apprehension test, as well as a negative relocation test. Six months postoperatively he was drafted by a professional baseball team.

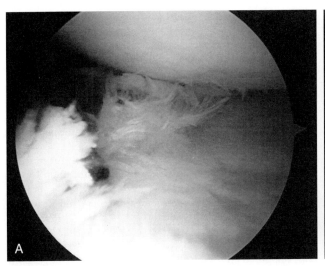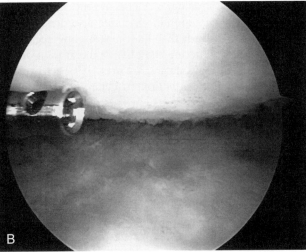

Figure 9–19. (A) Preoperative fragmented glenoid labrum tear with glenohumeral chondromalacia; (B) postoperative laser chondroplasty and resection of the glenoid labrum tear.

CASE STUDY 3

Impingement

A 35-year-old man complained of left shoulder pain, weakness, and catching of 3 years' duration. He stated that he was unable to play golf or tennis or to perform any overhead motions without severe pain. His physical examination revealed that he had a positive impingement test with subacromial spurring. An MRI scan of the shoulder confirmed the subacromial impingement (Fig. 9–17). An arthroscopic laser acromioplasty was performed to treat the impingement syndrome (Fig. 9–18A,B). Postoperatively, the patient was placed on a supervised shoulder rehabilitation program for 6 weeks. Two months later, he was aggressively playing tennis and golf, with normal motion and no pain.

CASE STUDY 4

Glenohumeral Chondromalacia Impingement

A 51-year-old man complained of moderate to severe right shoulder pain of 2 years' duration that was unresponsive to injections, medications, and physical therapy. He was unable to lift weights or exercise for 16 months due to severe right shoulder pain. An MRI scan of his shoulder demonstrated significant impingement, as well as degenerative changes of the glenohumeral joint. He was treated with an arthroscopic laser chondroplasty of his glenohumeral joint and an arthroscopic laser acromioplasty (Fig. 9–19A,B). Postoperatively, following a 6 week shoulder rehabilitation program, he was able to lift weights and exercise with only minor discomfort.

■ Summary

Arthroscopy of the shoulder is an effective means of diagnosing and treating common shoulder disorders. It is technically more difficult than knee arthroscopy because of the difficulty of entering the glenohumeral joint and avoiding nearby neurovascular structures.[4,19,24] With experience and meticulous attention to detail, arthroscopic techniques can be used to diagnose and treat multiple shoulder conditions, including partial-thickness and complete rotator cuff tears, glenoid labrum tears, biceps tendon tears, loose bodies, rheumatoid and degenerative arthritis, anterior instability, and impingement syndrome. However, it is essential to know the neurovascular anatomy of the shoulder. Any variance in portal placement can lead to significant neurologic or vascular injury.[18,19] In the short term, the results are comparable to those obtained with extensive open procedures.[2,6–17,25,26] Even though the technique is rapidly advancing and expanding, there is still a need for further research and refinement.

With the development of new, sophisticated arthroscopic equipment and techniques, including the Holmium laser, arthroscopic surgery of the shoulder is now as universal as arthroscopic surgery of the knee.

■ References

1. Zarins B: Arthroscopy of the shoulder: technique. p. 76. In Zarins B, Andrews JR, Carson WG (eds): Injuries to the Throwing Arm. WB Saunders, Philadelphia, 1985
2. Johnson L: The shoulder joint: an arthroscopist's perspective of anatomy and pathology. Clin Orthop 223:113, 1987
3. Caspari RB, Whipple TL, Meyers JF: Shoulder arthroscopy. p. 87. In Grana WA (ed): Update in Arthroscopic Techniques. Aspen Publishers, Rockville, MD, 1984
4. Andrews JR, Carson WG, Ortega K: Arthroscopy of the shoulder: technique and normal anatomy. Am J Sports Med 12:1, 1984
5. Snyder SJ, Pattee GA: Shoulder arthroscopy in the evaluation and treatment of rotator cuff lesions. p. 47. In Paulos LE (ed): Techniques in Orthopaedics. Aspen Publishers, Rockville, MD, 1988
6. Paulos LE, Franklin JL: Arthroscopic shoulder decompression: development and application. A five-year experience. Am J Sports Med 18:235, 1990
7. Sampson T: Precision acromioplasty in arthroscopic subacromial decompression of the shoulder. Arthroscopy 7:301, 1991
8. Imhoff A, Ledermann T: Arthroscopic subacromial decompression with and without the Holmium YAG-laser: a prospective comparative study. J Arthrosc Related Surg 11(5):549, 1995
9. Altchek DL, Wassen RF, Wickjewjcz TL, et al: Arthroscopic acromioplasty. J Bone Joint Surg 72A:1198, 1990
10. Ellmon H: Arthroscopic subacromial decompression: Analysis of one-to-three year results. Arthroscopy 3:173, 1987
11. Levy HJ, Uribe JW, Deleney LG: Arthroscopically-assisted rotator cuff repair: Preliminary results. Arthroscopy 6:55, 1990
12. Liv SH: Arthroscopically-assisted rotator cuff repair. J Bone Joint Surg 76B:592, 1994
13. Baker CL, Liv SH: Comparison of open and arthroscopically-assisted rotator cuff repairs. Am J Sports Med 23(1):99, 1995
14. Thadbit G III: Treatment of unidirectional and multidirectional glenohumeral instability by laser-assisted capsular shift. Paper presented at the meeting of the California Orthopedic Association. Squaw Creek, NV, May 1994
15. Rahhal SE, Snyder SJ, Stetson WB: The benefits of arthroscopy in the evaluation and treatment of full-thickness rotator cuff tears. Submitted for publication
16. Glousman RE: Shoulder arthroscopy in the throwing athlete. Operative Tech Orthop 1:155, 1991
17. Altcek DW, Wassen RF, Wickiewicz TL, et al: Arthroscopic labral debridement: a three-year follow-up study. Am J Sports Med 20:702, 1992
18. Snyder SJ: A complete system for arthroscopy and bursoscopy of the shoulder. Surg Rounds Orthop (7):57, 1989
19. Snyder SJ: Shoulder Arthroscopy. McGraw-Hill, New York, 1994
20. Vongsness CT, Smith CF: Arthroscopic shoulder surgery with three different laser systems: an evaluation of laser applications. Arthroscopy 6:696, 1995

21. Hayashi K, Markel MD, Thadbit G III, et al: The effect of thermal heating on the length and histological properties at the glenohumeral joint capsule. Am J Sports Med 24(5): 640, 1996

22. Carson WG: Arthroscopy of the shoulder: normal anatomy. p. 83. In Zarins B, Andrews JR, Carson WB (eds): Injuries to the Throwing Arm. WB Saunders, Philadelphia, 1985

23. Neviaser TJ: Arthroscopy of the shoulder. Orthop Clin North Am 18:361, 1987

24. Pettrone FA: Shoulder Arthroscopy. p. 300. In Pettrone FA (ed): AAOS Symposium on Upper Extremity Injuries in Athletes. CV Mosby, St. Louis, 1986

25. Andrews JR, Carson WG: Operative arthroscopy in the throwing athlete. p. 89. In Zarins B, Andrews JR, Carson WB (eds): Injuries to the Throwing Arm. WB Saunders, Philadelphia, 1985

26. Andrews JR, Broussard TS, Carson WG: Arthroscopy of the shoulder in the management of partial tears of the rotator cuff: a preliminary report. Arthroscopy 1:117, 1985

CHAPTER 10
The Elbow Region

David C. Reid and Shirley Kushner

Anatomy

The elbow joint is a unique multifaceted articulation between the capitellum and trochlea of the distal end of the humerus and the radial head and olecranon of the proximal radius and ulna. Nevertheless, it is classically described as a uniaxial hinge joint. This belies the complexity of the anatomy, which is, additionally, closely related to the superior radioulnar joint. Both articulations share the same joint capsule, and the joint spaces are continuous.[1] If one appreciates this unusual arrangement of three articulations within one joint space, it is easier to understand why the response of the elbow joint to trauma, exercise, heat, and massage is sometimes surprising, often unusual, and, unfortunately, not always good.[1-3]

Capsule and Ligaments

The capsule is a thin structure, reinforced and thickened by the lateral (radial) and medial (ulnar) collateral ligaments, which resist and prevent excessive abduction and adduction stresses and movements (Fig. 10–1). These ligaments do not, however, impede pronation and supination, and some abduction of the ulna always accompanies pronation.

Valgus stability is provided equally by the medial collateral ligament, by the anterior capsule, and by the bony configuration in extension, whereas at 90 degrees of flexion the contribution of the anterior capsule is assumed mainly by the medial collateral ligament.[4] Varus stress is resisted primarily by the anterior capsule and bony articulation, with only a minor contribution from the radial collateral ligament; this arrangement changes very little throughout the range.[4]

Distraction stresses, which are most significant in high-velocity throwing maneuvers, are resisted primarily by the anterior capsule in extension and the ulnar collateral ligament in flexion[4] (Table 10–1). This information, obtained by necessity from cadaver studies, underscores the considerable contribution to stability made by muscle in the living state.[5] Furthermore, careful dissection reveals that many of the fibers of the so-called collateral ligaments of the elbow are continuous with the collagenous septa of the muscles crossing the joint. Indeed, relatively few ligamentous fibers go directly from bone to bone. The collagen of the radial collateral ligament, for example, belongs to the septa within and around the muscles of the anterolateral muscle group, and the annular ligament to the sheath around the muscle fasciculi of the supinator muscle.[5] A comparable relationship is seen between the muscle fasciculi and the collagenous connective tissue of the ulnar collateral ligament and the common flexor origin. It is the intimate association of the connective tissue of ligament and overlying muscle at the elbow that makes pathology at the site of the muscle insertion sometimes difficult to isolate from the noncontractile portion of the joint. This important concept of muscle fasciculi connected in series with collagenous fibrous strands, blending into the ligament, gives a basis for considering a single musculoligamentous unit as contributing to the dynamic stability of many joints.[5,6]

Arthrology

Classification

The elbow joint is a compound paracondylar joint in that one bone, the humerus, articulates with two others that lie side by side by way of two distinct facets. The humeroulnar component is a modified sellar articulation (convex in one direction and concave at right angles to this first plane). The humeroradial component is an unmodified ovoid (convex or concave in all planes). The proximal radioulnar articulation, by contrast, is a modified ovoid.[7]

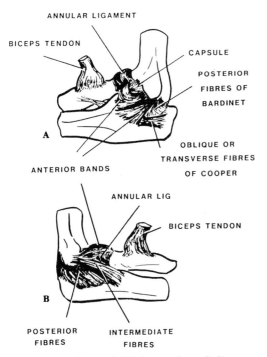

Figure 10–1. (A) The medial (ulnar collateral) ligament. The very strong anterior fibers are in two bundles, reinforcing the annular ligament. (B) Similarly, the lateral (radial collateral) ligament reinforces the annular ligament. Although shown as discrete fibers, in reality the collagenous connections with the overlying intermuscular septa form a musculotendinous unit. (Modified from Kapandji,[6] with permission.)

Resting and Closed-Packed Positions

The resting position of a joint is defined as that position in which the joint capsule is most relaxed and the greatest amount of joint play is possible. The resting position is central to the concept of joint mobilization procedures. In pathologic states, it actually represents the position of maximum intra-articular volume and, hence, the position adapted to minimize capsular tension with effusion and thus reduce pain.

In the humeroulnar joint, the resting position is with the elbow flexed to 70 degrees and the forearm supinated 10 degrees; this position is most frequently adopted with capsulitis of the elbow. The resting position of the humeroradial joint is in elbow extension and forearm supination. In the superior radioulnar joint, the resting position is 35 degrees of supination and 70 degrees of elbow flexion. The position for mobilization of joint play movements is therefore specific for the individual articulation within the elbow joint, although pathology seldom isolates the joint so specifically.

The closed-packed position is the position of the joint in which the capsule and ligaments are tight or maximally tensed; there is maximal contact between articular surfaces, and the surfaces cannot be separated by distractive forces. Testing and mobilization cannot be performed in this position.[8,9]

In the humeroulnar joint, the closed-packed position is with the elbow extended and the forearm supinated. In the humeroradial joint, the closed-packed position is at 90 degrees of flexion and 5 degrees of supination. In the superior radioulnar joint, this position is 5 degrees of supination, where the interosseous membrane is tightest.[8]

The capsular pattern is a proportional pattern of limitation of movement at a joint. Initially triggered by pain, effusion, and synovial irritation and subsequently reinforced and established by capsular shortening and contractures, it is usually accepted as an indication of capsular or intra-articular disease. In the elbow, flexion is usually more restricted than extension, but with time they may become equal. Once marked limitation of flexion and extension is present, pronation and supination may become equally restricted. There are many extrinsic factors, which make a very significant degree of individual variation common at the elbow.

Movement and Joint Play

Joint play or accessory movements are essential for normal function and full range of motion. There is a small amount of side-to-side movement of the ulna on the trochlea of the humerus in flexion and extension. Abduction of the forearm occurs as a conjunct motion with extension and pronation; conversely, adduction occurs together with flexion and supination. There is as well a forward and

Table 10–1. Percentage Resistance to Applied Stress

Structure	Valgus Stress		Varus Stress		Distraction	
	Extension	*90° Flexion*	*Extension*	*90° Flexion*	*Extension*	*90° Flexion*
Medial collateral ligament	31	54			6	78
Lateral collateral ligament			14	9	5	10
Capsule	38	10	32	13	85	8
Osseous	31	33	55	75		

(Data from Morrey and Kai-Nan.[4])

backward movement of the head of the radius on the capitellum.

Supination and pronation occur at both the radiohumeral joint and the proximal radioulnar joint. A backward and forward accessory movement occurs as the radial head moves on the radial notch of the ulna, and the ulna moves forward and backward on the radius.[7,9]

Range of Motion

The lower end of the humerus is offset in two planes. The angulation in the coronal plane, the carrying angle, alters the axis of flexion and extension so that the forearm sweeps through an arc, facilitating hand-to-mouth movement (Fig. 10–2). The humeral trochlea groove is spiral and is the main factor that dictates the arthrokinematics.[6] Anteriorly, the groove is vertical and parallel to the longitudinal humeral axis. Posteriorly the groove runs obliquely, forming the carrying angle of between 5 and 20 degrees.[9]

Flexion and extension is an impure swing. Flexion is associated with conjunct humeroulnar adduction, whereas extension is of necessity associated with conjunct humeroulnar abduction.

The capitelloradial articulation is an unmodified ovoid, but the degrees of freedom are limited by the ligamentous attachment of the radius to the ulna; hence the radiohumeral articular pathway follows the axis dictated by the anatomy of the humeroulnar joint. Restoration of these angles after fracture allows resumption of normal range of motion. Fortunately, fractures in this area occur most frequently in children; although present-

ing the potential problem of injury to the growth plates, these fractures usually resolve by restoration of the delicate anatomy by remodeling, provided that adequate initial reduction is achieved.

The normal range of flexion–extension is approximately 150 to 160 degrees, with about 10 degrees of hyperextension commonly present, particularly in women. Active flexion is usually limited by opposition of the soft parts but occasionally by bone on bone. Passive flexion is limited by tension of the posterior capsule and passive tension of the triceps. Extension is limited by contact of the tip of the olecranon in its contiguous fossa in the posterior lower humerus. At about the time of apposition, the anterior capsule tightens and tension develops in the elbow flexors so that bony impact is attenuated. If extension continues, ligament rupture must occur, or the olecranon may fracture, leading to a posterior dislocation.[6]

When elbow pathology is treated with splinting, flexion is usually chosen as the resting position; therefore, loss of extension is a common feature after immobilization. The anterior band of the ulnar collateral ligament has been implicated as one of the prime limiting factors in humeroulnar motion.[10,11] More recently, plication of the anterior band of the ulnar ligament in cadaver studies has failed to support this concept, and it is more likely, particularly in pathologic states, that adhesions and adaptive shortening of the adjacent anterior capsule are more important.[12] Although joint mobilization techniques to the hypomobile humeroulnar articulation may help restore normal arthrokinematics, it is probably through the influence on the joint capsule as well as the collateral ligament.[9,12,13] Where normal range is possible, the position of active extension is some 5 to 10 degrees short of that obtainable by forced extension. This reflects the contribution of the muscle, as demonstrated by experiments using myoneural blocking agents.[14] The unwillingness of living subjects to allow terminal extension reflects MacConaill's statement that, in living subjects, positions just short of the closed-packed state are used rather than the full closed-packed position.[9]

The superior radioulnar joint again highlights the subtle differences in anatomy that make the elbow joint difficult to treat. In this case, 80 percent of the articular surface consists of the annular ligament as opposed to articular cartilage. This ligament is tough and cone-shaped and will usually prevent dislocation in the adult. The imperfectly formed radial head of the very young child, in contrast, may be easily dislocated by excessive traction with rotation.

The axis for pronation and supination passes from the center of the radial head to the pit adjacent to the styloid process of the ulna distally. This compound movement, involving the three articulations at the elbow as well as the distal radioulnar joint and the radiocarpal articulation, can obviously be compromised by pathology

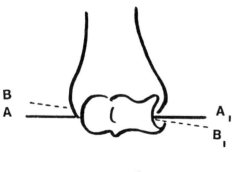

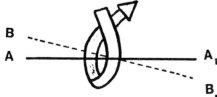

Figure 10–2. Because of the configuration of the trochlea, the axis of movement changes progressively from horizontal (A–A₁) in flexion to oblique (B–B₁) in extension. This results in midline movement in flexion and the carrying angle in extension in most individuals. (Modified from Kapandji,[6] with permission.)

at any of these joints. Normal range encompasses 90 degree of both pronation and supination.

The elbow is a highly congruous joint, which nevertheless depends significantly on its soft tissue restraints during its complex motions. Indeed, the ligaments of the elbow have to resist considerable valgus and, to a lesser degree, varus stresses that accompany rapid flexion and extension. In many throwing activities, for instance, elbow motion exceeds 300 degrees per second, and it is of little wonder that chronic overuse syndromes occur at this joint.[15]

Muscle Action

During flexion, there is considerable interplay between the biceps, brachialis, and brachioradialis muscles, with all three working to various degrees at different ranges and speeds and between individuals. Hence, it is not surprising that many studies on their actions appear, at first glance, contradictory.[1,2] The following main points emerge:

1. The biceps and the brachialis are both muscles of considerable bulk, which add power and are the prime movers of flexion.[15,16]
2. The body tends toward economy; therefore slow movements, without added resistance, may be performed by one or the other of these muscles or by a diminished amount of work by both.
3. The biceps may actively supinate the arm while flexion is taking place, unless this is counteracted.[16,17]
4. In rapid movements, the brachioradialis may act in two ways, initially as a shunt muscle, overcoming centrifugal forces acting at the elbow and then by adding power to increase the speed of flexion. It does this most efficiently in the midprone position.[2,16]
5. The common flexor mass from the medial epicondyle may weakly assist the prime movers or become hypertrophied to assist in flexion in cases of paralysis of the proximal muscles.[1]

Of the three heads of the triceps, the medial head seems to be the most consistent in its action over the extensor mechanism of the elbow.[2,16] The long and lateral heads provide extra strength for this motion but may be relatively silent electrically for slow, low-power movements.[2,16] The triceps is most powerful when the elbow and shoulder are simultaneously extended. Deep extensions from the triceps insert into the capsule of the posterior recess of the joint and help pull the redundant synovium away during extension, thus avoiding impingement.[1] This is similar to the articularis genu mechanism over the suprapatellar pouch at the knee.

The pronator quadratus needs the power offered by the pronator teres for most everyday and all resisted pronation activities.[1] Similarly, the biceps, in most actions,

supplements the power of the supinator.[16,17] This is particularly true of high-speed motion.[2]

■ Assessment

An adequate history and examination to rule out cervical spine and shoulder pathology is mandatory (Fig. 10–3). Specific factors in the history such as age, occupation, pastime, pattern of pain, and functional difficulties should be used to focus the examination on the probable diagnoses. Examples include the complaint of intermittent locking with loose bodies and dislocation of the radial head in children younger than 6 years of age. After the history has been obtained, examination of the elbow is performed.

Observation

The patient's elbow is observed for swelling, contours, color, and carrying angle. The carrying angle is normally 5 to 10 degrees in men and 10 to 15 degrees in women. Also, have the patient place the arms at 90 degrees of forward flexion at the shoulder and observe the elbow–wrist relationships in pronation and supination. These relationships may be altered after abduction and adduction lesions develop.

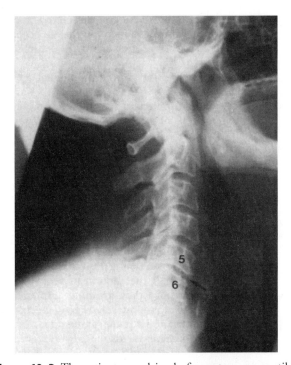

Figure 10–3. The patient complained of symptoms compatible with lateral epicondylitis. Further interrogation and examination unmasked cervical pathology. The radiograph confirmed C5-C6 degenerative changes (arrow). Although local injection ended the elbow problem, recurrence is likely unless the neck dysfunction is also attended to.

Range of Motion

Active Motion

Flexion is tested in supination and is normally 150 degrees. Extension is normally to 0 degrees in men and up to 5 degrees in women, but 15 degrees of hyperextension in women or children is not uncommon. Supination and pronation are tested with the shoulder adducted and the elbow held against the trunk to rule out shoulder rotation. These movements range from 0 degrees at the neutral position to 80 or 90 degrees.

Passive Motion

The movements are tested with particular attention to the end-feel. The flexion end-feel is one of soft tissue

approximation, whereas that of extension is bone to bone; the end-feel of pronation and supination is one of soft tissue stretch. The forearm should be held proximal to the wrist to rule out movement in this joint.

Muscle Tests

Resisted movements are tested isometrically in a neutral position. The test is repeated for five contractions to uncover subtle weaknesses in neurologic conditions, such as nerve root palsies. Minimal to maximal resistance is applied. Minimal resistance causing pain is indicative of a contractile lesion, whereas if pain is elicited only with maximal resistance, one must also consider inert structures due to increased articular pressure.

Primary selective tissue tension tests will determine which muscle group is involved. Secondary tests will assist

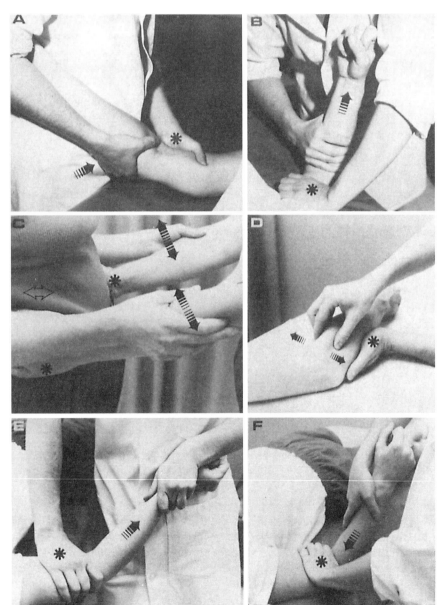

Figure 10–4. Tests for accessory movements. Asterisks indicate the fixed point and the arrow indicates direction of movement. (A) Lateral and medial ulnar glide; (B) ulnar distraction; (C) flexion and extension of the radial head; while the patient's hands are fixed on the therapist's hips, forward and backward motion helps produce flexion and extension at the patient's elbows; (D) dorsal and ventral glide of the radial head; (E) distraction of the radial head; (F) compression of the radial head.

in pointing to the specific muscle involved. For example, if resisted elbow flexion is painful, the biceps, brachioradialis, or brachialis muscle may be involved. Now, if pain is elicited on pronation to neutral from full supination, the brachioradialis is likely at fault. If resisted supination from neutral increases the pain, it is likely that the biceps is involved.

Wrist flexion and extension strength tests must be included, along with all elbow motions, because of the proximal insertions of the forearm musculature on the epicondyles and supracondylar ridges.

Ligamentous Tests

The collateral ligaments should be tested 15 to 30 degrees short of full extension and may also be tested in midflexion, because with moderate pathology there may only be signs in selected positions where tension is maximal.

Accessory Movement Tests

The suspect elbow is compared with the normal one, with attention to end-feel. The following tests are performed:[8,13]

1. Lateral and medial glide of the ulna on the humerus is tested just short of full extension (Fig. 10–4A).
2. Distraction of the ulna on the humerus is carried out with 70 degrees of flexion and 35 degrees of supination (Fig. 10–4B).
3. Flexion and extension of the radial head on the humerus are performed while passively flexing and extending the elbow by the movement of the therapist's body (Fig. 10–4C).
4. Dorsal and ventral glide of the radial head on the ulna is performed in 70 degrees of elbow flexion and 35 degrees of supination (Fig. 10–4D).
5. Distraction of the radial head on the humerus is performed in 70 degrees of flexion and 35 degrees of supination (Fig. 10–4E).
6. Compression of the radial head on the humerus is performed in 70 degrees of flexion and 35 degrees of supination (Fig. 10–4F).
7. The extension adduction quadrant is 10 degrees from full extension (Fig. 10–5A).
8. The extension abduction quadrant is 10 degrees from full extension (Fig. 10–5B).
9. The flexion abduction quadrant is 10 degrees from full flexion and supination (Fig. 10–5C).

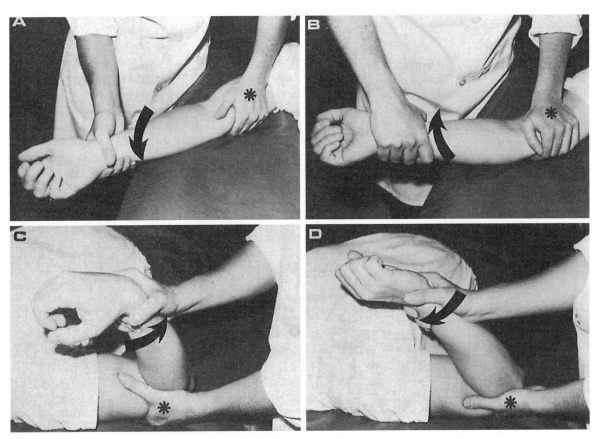

Figure 10–5. Accessory movement tests. Asterisks indicate the fixed point. (A) Extension adduction quadrant; (B) extension abduction quadrant; (C) flexion abduction quadrant; (D) flexion adduction quadrant.

10. The flexion adduction quadrant is 10 degrees from full flexion and pronation (Fig. 10–5D).

Palpation

Palpation should be systematic and should include all bony points, tendons, and ligaments, with attention to crepitus, pain, boggy edematous changes, and abnormal contours.

Other Tests

Reflexes will have been tested during the cervical scan and include the biceps (C5), brachioradialis (C6), and triceps (C7). These reflexes are compared with those on the opposite side and noted as either hyperreflexic, normal, hyporeflexic, or absent. Dermatomes are also tested with the cervical scan. Generally, the lateral elbow is C5, the anterior elbow is C6, the posterior elbow is C7, and the medial elbow is T1 and T2. The dermatomes at the elbow, however, are nonspecific, and there is considerable individual variation and overlap.

Special tests for specific pathologic entities conclude the examination and are discussed below in the context of the appropriate conditions.

■ Conditions

Tennis Elbow Syndrome

Definition

By definition, tennis elbow (lateral epicondylitis, lateral elbow stress syndrome) is a lesion affecting the origin of the tendons of the muscles that extend the wrist. Like many medical terms, its usage is often ill-defined, and the term tends to mean different things to different people (Table 10–2). The term *tennis elbow* has been loosely used to encompass posterior and medial symptoms, which have been referred to as posterior and medial tennis elbow, respectively, adding confusion to an already complicated topic.[18-21] Tennis elbow will here refer only to lateral epicondylitis and associated common extensor origin tendinitis.

Pathology and Symptoms

The exact nature of the pathology at the common extensor origin is open to question, and it is likely that several basic etiologic entities giving rise to slightly different pathologic changes in the tissue may present a fairly similar clinical picture[22-24] (Table 10–2). The three main sites of pathology are the common extensor origin, the radiocapitellar joint, and the radioulnar joint, with fibrillation and chondromalacic changes. Furthermore, neurogenic causes such as C6 radiculopathy and, more locally, radial tunnel entrapment of the posterior interosseous nerve

□ □ □ □ □ □ □   □

Table 10–2. Pathology of Lateral Tennis Elbow[a]

Region	Possible Pathology
Proximal	Periostitis
	Common extensor origin
	Tendinitis
	Microtearing with painful granulation
	Degenerative changes in tendon
Joint	Lateral ligament strain
	Radiohumeral bursitis
	Inflammation of annular ligament
	Hypertrophic synovial fringe
	Degenerative changes in radial head cartilage
	Extension/abduction ulnohumeral lesions
Neural	Cervical radiculopathy
	Posterior interosseous nerve entrapment

[a] These causes of elbow pain have all been implicated in the tennis elbow syndrome.

must be considered. With C6 root involvement secondary to dysfunction at the C5-C6 segment, weakness results at the radial wrist extensors, leaving them prone to injury. The patient's clinical picture resembles that of a true tennis elbow that is resistant to treatment. While the elbow is treated, simultaneous attention must be given to the cervical spine (Fig. 10–3). Only then will the patient respond.[24] The problem as well as the patient must be treated. In view of the high success rate of local limited release of the common extensor origin and the recovery at surgery of granulation tissue and scar tissue from this area, this site of pathology probably accounts for most cases.

Whatever the etiology, there is generally an element of overuse or overstress; 45 percent of tennis players who practice or play daily experience problems.[25] Tennis elbow syndrome is also an occupational hazard in individuals who frequently perform forceful pronation and supination motions, heavy lifting, or repetitive hammering activities.

There is a local tenderness on the outside of the elbow at the common extensor origin, with aching and pain in the back of the forearm; the condition is aggravated by continual use. Special tests include resisted wrist extension, which precipitates pain at the extensor origin (Fig. 10–6). Performing the test in full elbow extension will decrease the number of false-negative results. Painful resisted extension of the middle and ring fingers implicates the extensor digitorum communis, and painful resistance of wrist extension and radial deviation points to the extensor carpi radialis longus and brevis. A further test for tennis elbow is to stretch the insertion by holding the elbow in extension and performing passive wrist flexion and pronation. A positive test is one that elicits pain at the common origin.

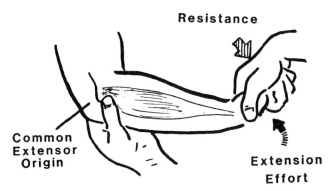

Resistance

Common Extensor Origin

Extension Effort

Figure 10–6. Palpation over the common extensor origin while resisting extension elicits the patient's symptoms in lateral epicondylitis. The test may be even more sensitive when performed in full extension.

The treatment will be outlined in detail for the tennis player, but many of the principles may be extrapolated to other situations. Both sexes are affected equally, and the condition rarely occurs before the age of 20 years. Less experienced players who have poor stroke technique but who play frequently are the group at risk. The average age of players who develop tennis elbow is 40 years. This reflects, first, the typical microcirculatory changes in the blood supply at the myotendinous junction of the extensor muscles at the elbow and, second, an increasing number of joint symptoms occurring with age rather than true tennis elbow.

Etiology and Treatment

The etiology and treatment of tennis elbow can be considered under three headings: playing style, anatomic factors, and equipment. An understanding of these etiologic features suggests a logical approach to therapy.

Playing style

A poorly executed backhand is mainly implicated. The forearm is used as the power source rather than the kinetics of the body and weight transfer from the body to the shoulder.

A typical faulty backhand has no forward weight transfer, and the front shoulder is usually elevated. The trunk leans away from the net at the time of impact, and the racket head is down. The elbow and wrist extend before impact, and the power source is forearm extension in the pronated position. The stroke is usually a nonrhythmic, jerky movement, with sharp pronation in the follow-through. When the ball is hit incorrectly, the forces are transmitted as an acute strain up and along the muscle mass to the extensor origin at the elbow.[21] Repetitive stresses may eventually cause the small tears and inflammation that are reflected in the pain associated with tennis elbow.

Anatomic studies confirm that the extensor carpi radialis brevis (ECRB) is under maximum tension when con-

tracting while the forearm is pronated, the wrist flexed, and the ulna deviated.[25] The head of the radius rotates anteriorly against the ECRB during pronation, where a bursa is frequently located, and this may explain why some individuals experience pain at the head of the radius, perhaps secondarily to inflammation of the bursa.[25]

In the serve, there is usually slightly less stress on the lateral side of the elbow than with the backhand. First, the use of a backhand grip forces the arm into a hyperpronated position, thereby stressing the extensor origin. Second, some tennis players who have played seriously for many years have increased the bulk of their extensor muscles considerably but may have lost full flexibility. Therefore, they experience increased stresses at the completion of the stroke.[23]

A frequent error is an exaggerated effort to hit the ball hard. Maximum speed is imparted to the ball by good style, keeping the eye on the ball and hitting it on the "sweet spot" in the center of the racket. Very little is to be gained by sacrificing style for power. Usually the result of overpowering the stroke is failure to transfer the body weight, thus relying on the forearm as the main source of strength, often aggravating a preexisting condition further.

As far as technique is concerned, then, the stroke most implicated in tennis elbow is firmly established as the backhand. Investment in a few tennis lessons to improve one's technique should be considered. The development of a two-handed backhand may also alleviate the problem for some players with chronic repetitive symptoms.

Many more experienced players run into trouble with their forehand and top spin. The common error is to roll the racket head over the ball in an attempt to produce top spin. This motion produces excessive strain because the impact is sustained in the hyperpronated position. Supination follows, with the ball in contact with the strings for only 0.004 second. This is not long enough to impart adequate top spin. The more correct long stroking maneuver, starting low and ending high, with a good follow-through, is more effective and produces less stress.

During the serve, the racket head travels at 300 to 350 mph before ball impact, at which time it abruptly slows to about 150 mph. With poor use of the trunk and legs, the forearm once again absorbs too much stress.[25]

When recovering from tennis elbow, the patient should commence with the easiest strokes, try not to be too competitive, and play only with people who are willing to have an easy game.

Anatomy

Many individuals play tennis with less than optimal grip strength. Indeed, the average woman has a forearm girth of 9 in. and a grip strength of about 50 lb, whereas the average man has a forearm girth of 11 in. and a grip strength of approximately 80 lb. By contrast, the professional tennis player usually has a forearm girth of about

12 in. and a grip strength of 105 lb.[21] The strength of the normal wrist extensors should be about 50 percent of the flexor strength.[22] The wrist flexors have been found to be the strongest, followed by the radial deviators, the ulnar deviators, and then the extensors. The supinators are normally stronger than the pronators.[9] In regular tennis players, the extensor muscles should be strengthened, so that they are at least 50 percent and probably closer to 75 percent of flexor strength. An even grip, taking care not to allow the thumb to be placed along the axis of the shaft, will assist in even distribution of forces.

Equipment

In individuals with incipient or established symptoms, the racket should be strung to only 52 to 55 lb.[25] This will allow the impact to be spread over slightly more time and decrease the forces transmitted to the forearm muscles.[26] Sixteen-gauge catgut is more resilient than nylon and has the ability to lessen the shock of the impact of the ball. However, gut is expensive and loses resilience quickly; 16-gauge nylon is probably the best compromise.

A racket handle that is too large or too small may produce an uneven force distribution across the hand and hence to the muscles. This problem may be particularly applicable to women, whose average hand size is about 4⅛ in. A measurement taken from the proximal hand crease to the tip of the ring finger along its radial border gives an indication of grip size.[21]

Heavy-duty or rubber-centered balls impart more concentrated moments of force and may aggravate the symptoms. Regular-duty balls are recommended. Playing with balls soaked from landing in puddles may also trigger problems.[25]

It is hard to give advice in regard to the racket itself. Both wooden and metal rackets have their merits and disadvantages. The very heavy wooden rackets should be avoided by all but the most experienced players. Nirschl[21] advises a midsize graphite racket weighing only 12 to 12.5 oz. Graphite absorbs the shock of ball impact better than wood, and the midsize racket has a larger "benevolent" or "sweet" zone, the area on the strings where minimal torque is produced on impact.[25] The lighter racket allows players to position more quickly and lessens the chance of hitting late.[27] However, balanced weight, hand size, and stringing are all more significant factors. Most of all, good style, hitting the ball in the sweet spot in the center of the racket, can do more to reduce stresses on the forearm than any change of racket can.

General Treatment

Treatment is aimed at relief of inflammation, promotion of healing, reducing the overload forces, and increasing upper extremity strength, endurance, and flexibility.[21,25] The following are some important points in preventing and treating tennis elbow.

Before practicing, warm up slowly and perform adequate stretching exercises to the forearm and hand. Some-times rubbing ice onto the common extensor origin before playing may help.

Wearing a tennis arm band (epicondylar splint) of nonelastic fabric, lined with foam rubber to prevent slipping, may reduce the stresses on the common extensor origin. When muscle expansion is limited the contraction force is reduced, decreasing irritation of the muscle. This band must be wide enough (3 to 3.5 in.); the narrower widths are usually not as effective.[28] The band should be applied lightly while tensing the muscles of the arm. If the elbow band is applied while the muscles are relaxed, it may cut off the circulation. The band should be comfortable with the forearm relaxed. The band should not be applied too far proximally, but rather over the major muscle belly about two fingers' breadth distal to the elbow flexor crease. The efficacy of these bands in decreasing pain during many activities has been well documented.[29,30]

Occasionally, a wrist resting splint can be made and adapted for whatever the occupation or sport of the individual entails. This moderate defunctioning of some of the wrist extensor contraction may allow a resistant clinical problem to resolve slowly, with considerable comfort, during the activities of daily living.

Physiotherapy treatment initially consists of assessment, modification of activity, ice, and electrical stimulation.[24]

To assess objectively the severity of a clinical complaint, keep in mind that grip strength correlates very well with a visual pain scale and functional incapacity. Even measuring grip strength with the aid of a simple sphygmomanometer cuff, preinflated to 20 mm Hg, can give a reasonable assessment of the pain threshold and progress of treatment.[31–33] Electrotherapeutic modalities such as laser, ultrasound phonophoresis with 10 percent hydrocortisone, interferential therapy, high-voltage galvanic stimulation, and transcutaneous electrical nerve stimulation (TENS) have all been advocated to relieve pain and inflammation. Cure rates ranging from 55 to 90 percent have been reported.[31] Topical application of dimethyl sulfoxide has also been suggested.[32,33] Manual therapy techniques such as transverse frictions, joint mobilization and manipulation, myofascial release, and strain and counterstrain techniques may be used[34,35] (Table 10–3). Mobilization techniques are covered in Chapter 13.

Whatever the treatment used, as resolution occurs and the patient returns to his or her sport or occupation, exercise will form a mainstay of treatment, as complete rest is seldom indicated. Reduced physical activity leads to reduction in strength, so that on resuming the activity, a recurrence of the injury could be precipitated by stresses of lesser magnitude than those that caused the initial insult.[36]

Isometric exercises for the wrist extensors, with the elbow in flexion, moving closer to extension as pain permits, can be used in the acute phase.[35] As pain permits, concentric and then eccentric strengthening using free weights or surgical tubing will be performed. Isokinetic

Table 10-3. Comparison of Manipulation Techniques

	Author					
	Mills	*Cyriax I*	*Cyriax II (Mills)*	*Kaltenborn*	*Mennell*	*Stoddard*
Lesion	Frayed or detached orbicular ligament in acute cases. Adhesions in chronic cases	Partial tear at tenoperiosteal junction of extensor carpi radialis brevis	Inadequate healing. Scar in extensor carpi radialis brevis at tenoperiosteal junction	Lateral epicondylitis	Painful scar in common extensor tendon	Adhesions binding origin of extensor digitorum communis to radial collateral ligament
Position	Lying. General anesthetic	Sitting. No anesthetic. After 5–10 minutes of deep friction	Sitting. Following 10–15 minutes of deep friction	Sitting or supine. No anesthetic	Standing. Prior injection of local anesthetic	Supine
Manipulation	Forced extension of elbow. Wrist and fingers fixed. Forearm pronated	Elbow fully extended. Forearm supinated. Fixation at medial elbow. Varus thrust at lateral wrist	Should be abducted and medially rotated. Forearm pronated, wrist flexed. Fixated at wrist. Extensor thrust at elbow	Fixation at wrist. Varus thrust at extended elbow	Fully flexed and pronated wrist and elbow. Elbow extension with forced overpressure	Shoulder abducted 90°. Pronate and supinate to identify maximum tension in extensor digitorum communis. Varus thrust at elbow by forearm adduction
Indication	Minimal loss of range of motion of elbow extension. Tested with full wrist and finger flexion in pronation. Local epicondylar or radiohumeral joint tenderness	Pain over the lateral epicondyle or common extensor tendon origin	Tenoperiosteal variety. Pain on resisted wrist extension and radial deviation	Lateral epicondylitis. Restricted movement of the radial head	Painful area at common extensor origin on palpation	Chronic cases. No response to hydrocortisone injection. Pain on gripping
Contraindication	Gross limitation of extension. Full range of motion		Loss of full elbow extension. Osteoarthrosis. Loose bodies, traumatic arthritis	Inability to extend fully		Acute condition. Rest pain. Restriction of elbow extension
Frequency	Usually one manipulation	Three times per week. Average of four treatments. Range: 1–9 treatments	2–3 times per week until cure. Range: 4–12 sessions			

(From Kushner and Reid,[35] with permission.)

191

strengthening eccentrically and concentrically may also be used. Not only are the flexors and extensors strengthened, but also the radial and ulnar deviators, pronators, and supinators.

Curwin and Stanish[36] have developed a program to combine stretching and eccentric strengthening of the wrist extensors. Exercising the muscle eccentrically allows it to withstand greater resistance and prevent injury, which occurs by eccentrically loading an inflexible muscle. The patient warms up with local heat or general exercise. The wrist extensors are stretched passively three times for 30 seconds. Three sets of 10 eccentric contractions are performed with a weight of 1 to 5 lb; surgical tubing may also be used as an effective way of applying resistance. The stretches are repeated and ice is then applied. This 20-minute session is repeated daily for about 3 weeks.

Before returning to the sport or occupation, the patient mimics the backhand, forehand, and serve, or the specific tasks of the occupation, using surgical tubing or pulleys for resistance. Throughout the physiotherapy treatment, shoulder and trunk strength and range of motion are maintained, as is the patient's cardiovascular fitness, if applicable.

Injection of a steroid preparation can be very effective, provided that the lesion is well localized.[31] This treatment is best supplemented with oral anti-inflammatory medication and may be repeated at 1-month intervals for up to 3 months or until the patient is asymptomatic. Considerable care is needed with the injection technique to avoid skin atrophy. It must be stressed that simply injecting the patient with steroids does not constitute complete treatment. Assessment and modification of precipitating factors, as well as exercise therapy, are usually necessary.

When nonoperative management fails, release of the fascia and part of the common extensor origin may be considered. Variations of the procedure involve increasingly radical releases, to include part of the annular ligament of the superior radioulnar joint, and the ECRB or the fascial band at the proximal edge of the supinator.[37] These variations in the extent of the procedure reflect confusion as to the exact site of the pathology.[38]

Postoperative rehabilitation involves a short period of gentle active motion and, at 3 weeks, increasing range of motion, strengthening, and stretching exercises.

Medial Epicondylitis

Etiology

Medial epicondylitis (epitrochleitis, golfer's elbow, medial tennis elbow) is probably a tendinopathy of the common flexor origin including the pronator teres. Pain is located over the medial epicondyle and is exacerbated by resisted wrist flexion and pronation. Pain is also elicited on passive wrist extension and supination. It is an overuse syndrome related to throwing sports, golf, and occupa-

tions such as carpentry that involve repetitive hammering or screwing. Chronic symptoms may eventually lead to contractures, with inability to fully extend or supinate.[39]

Treatment

Restoration of lost range of motion are an important part of the treatment. In the acute phase, ice, ultrasound, and other physical modalities may be used in conjunction with anti-inflammatory medication. Any course of treatment must culminate in a strengthening program. The stretching and strengthening routine described for tennis elbow is used, but the direction of motion is reversed.[36] Injection of a steroid preparation into the area is performed with care because of the propensity for skin atrophy in this area as well as the proximity of the ulnar nerve. In recalcitrant cases, a release of the common origin is possible, with surprisingly little measurable loss of functional strength.

Injuries to the Throwing Arm (Medial Tension Overload Syndrome)

Throwing Action

The throwing mechanisms used in different sports have more biomechanical similarities than differences, and baseball pitching is frequently used to demonstrate these principles and their effect on the supporting anatomy. Three stages are defined, namely, the cocking phase or windup, the acceleration phase (better considered as divided into early and late), and the follow-through[40,41] (Fig. 10–7).

Cocking phase
The shoulder is abducted to about 90 degrees and simultaneously taken into extreme external rotation with extension. The elbow is flexed to approximately 45 degrees and the wrist extended.

Early acceleration
The trunk and shoulder are brought rapidly forward, leaving the forearm and hand behind, prestressing all the structures at the elbow and, in particular, the ulnar collateral ligament.

Late acceleration
As vigorous contraction of the shoulder flexors and internal rotators, with early co-contraction of the elbow extensors and wrist flexors, takes place, the forearm and wrist are accelerated to add speed to the throw. The maneuver results in a whipping action, throwing significant additional stress onto the medial elbow (Fig. 10–7).

Follow-through
Follow-through begins with the missile release and varies somewhat with the type of throw, but it is characterized by stress on the structures around the olecranon.

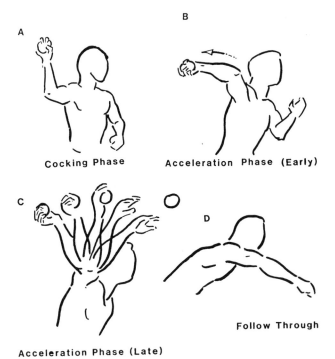

Figure 10–7. (A–D) The throwing mechanism is common to many sports. Stress is initially put on the shoulder and elbow, with a final distraction force largely damped by muscle and ligamentous structures at the elbow.

□□□□□ □ □ □

Table 10–4. Throwing Injuries of the Elbow

Type of Injury	Possible Pathology

Medial tension overload	Muscular
	  Overuse
	  Fascial compression syndrome
	Ligamentous and capsular
	  Ulnar traction spur
	  Loose bodies
	  Medial epicondylitis
	  Joint degeneration

Lateral compression injuries	Osteochondritis dissecans Capitellar fractures Loose bodies Lateral epicondylitis Joint degeneration

Extensor overload	Acute
	  Triceps strain
	  Olecranon fracture
	Chronic
	  Bony hypertrophy
	  Stress fracture
	  Olecranon fossa loose bodies
	  Joint degeneration

(Modified from Slocum,[41] with permission.)

Injuries

The sequence of events described, when repeated many times, may result in a series of pathologic changes, best considerd under the headings of acute and chronic (Table 10–4). The lateral joint line experiences compressive forces during throwing, while shear forces are generated posteriorly in the olecranon fossa, and tensile forces develop along the medial joint line.[15]

Acute Injuries

Muscular Strains. Minor muscular strains are common, presenting with point tenderness to palpation and pain with resisted contraction. These injuries, usually to the common flexor group, are frequently self-limiting, requiring only modified rest, ice, and treatment by electrical modalities and gentle stretching. With healing, progressive strengthening is added to ensure adequate ability to return to function without reinjury. Flexion contractures, which predispose to muscle strains, are present in more than half of all adult professional pitchers.[15]

Major tears or ruptures, usually of the forearm flexors, must be recognized because surgery may be required (Fig. 10–8). Usually deformity and a palpable defect, as well as considerable ecchymosis, will alert the clinician to the correct diagnosis. In the muscular individual, a transverse sulcus may be present at the anterior border of the lacertus fibrosus (bicipital aponeurosis), and this normal groove should not be confused with a rupture of the pronator teres or common flexor muscle belly. Very rarely, the biceps tendon may rupture distally; this is compatible with acceptable function in the noncompetitive individual. However, surgical repair gives the best results in the heavy manual laborer and the athlete.

Medial Collateral Ligament Sprains. Repetitive valgus stress in pitchers and javelin throwers may produce acute inflammation of the medial collateral ligament. Point tenderness over the medial joint line and an absence of instability help to make this diagnosis. Treatment is the same as for muscular strains.

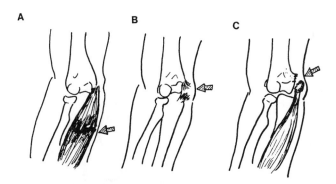

Figure 10–8. Acute stress to the medial elbow may result in (A) a muscle belly tear, (B) a ligament sprain, or (C) an avulsion fracture, which, in the skeletally immature, may be an epiphyseal injury.

Avulsion of the Medial Epicondyle. Before epiphyseal closure, rapid strong contraction of the forearm flexors is capable of avulsing the medial epicondyle (Fig. 10–8). Tenderness in the region of the medial condyle in an adolescent should arouse suspicion of this injury. Failure to detect it may lead to increasing varus deformity. When there is extreme tenderness, prophylactic splinting of the elbow for 2 weeks is a safe precaution. A repeat radiograph at this time may show callus. A widely displaced fragment may require surgical reattachment.

Chronic injuries

The effects of repeated valgus stress of the elbow are most pronounced in the professional pitcher, particularly if the individual began his career at an early age. Clinically, elbow flexion contractures occur in up to 50 percent of professional pitchers, and an increased carrying angle is seen in about 3 percent.[40–42] Repeated stresses result in attenuation of the medial collateral ligament with laxity (Fig. 10–9). Pain and swelling, catching, and locking are often manifestations of additional bony and joint surface changes. X-ray examination may reveal loose bodies, particularly in the olecranon fossa; hyperostotic changes and osteophytes around the posteromedial olecranon process; and traction spurs at the attachment of the medial collateral ligament to the ulna. Oblique views and tomograms may be necessary to elucidate all these changes. Occasionally, the joint symptoms are accompanied by ulnar nerve neuritis or neuropathy secondary to repeated minor traction stresses or chronic scarring. Surgical excision of osteophytes and removal of loose fragments may be necessary to restore range of motion and a fully functional elbow.

Little leaguer's elbow

The young pitcher is exposed to the risks already outlined, as well as the additional risk of epiphyseal injury. Originally, the term *little leaguer's elbow* referred to an epiphysitis of the medial epicondylar epiphysis related to the repeated trauma of pitching. This stress is greatly increased by throwing curve balls and other breaking pitches, which require more forceful pronation of the wrist. The clinical features of little leaguer's elbow include pain and tenderness with loss of full extension. Characteristic changes are accelerated growth of the medial side as well as fragmentation of the medial epicondylar epiphysis.[42,43] The term *little leaguer's elbow* has since come to encompass all stress changes involved in pitching in the skeletally immature individual. These changes include compression of the lateral joint, which may trigger changes of osteochondritis dissecans of both the capitellum and the radial head. It is important to recognize this condition early because adequate rest from repeated stresses may allow resolution of the problems. Failure to protect the joint may result in the formation of loose fragments, pain, deformity, and possibly arthrosis.

The incidence of this problem is unknown and varies widely in reported series.[44] In 1972, before major rule changes were adopted to protect the youngsters, accelerated growth and separation of the medial epicondylar epiphysis were present in up to 90 percent of little league pitchers between the ages of 9 and 14 years in Southern California. These same changes were seen in fewer than 10 percent of children of the same age who did not play baseball.[44]

Osteochondritis dissecans, particularly of the capitellum, is reported in other sports, notably gymnastics, where the arms frequently function as weightbearing extremities under stress.[44,45]

Treatment

Treatment is initially aimed at decreasing inflammation with ice and rest, as dictated by the signs and symptoms. Electrical modalities to decrease pain and inflammation are used. These may include TENS, high-voltage galvanic stimulation, ultrasound, interferential, current, and laser.

If the patient is partially immobilized, active range-of-motion therapy commences in the whirlpool. Gentle resisted isometric exercises to pain are started. Once immobilization is discontinued, strengthening with surgical tubing or free weights is begun, progressing to isokinetic strengthening, push-ups, and pull-ups. Shoulder range-of-motion and isometric exercises are performed throughout the rehabilitation period.

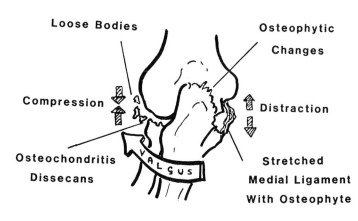

Loose Bodies

Osteophytic Changes

Compression

Distraction

Osteochondritis Dissecans

VALGUS

Stretched Medial Ligament With Osteophyte

Figure 10–9. Repetitive valgus stresses associated with throwing produce stretching and instability on the medial side, with shearing forces on the olecranon. The result is growth defects in the young and degenerative changes in the adult.

Injuries in throwing sports are decreased and prevented by attention to flexibility, decreasing muscle imbalances, and correcting the throwing technique. Proper use of body mechanics will alter the stress on the elbow. Overhead rather than sidearm and curveball throws should be taught. Whipping and snapping of the elbow should be discouraged. The frequency and length of time each player is allowed to pitch should be decreased. Javelin throwers may have to change their technique or hold to reduce the stresses on the medial joint.[46] Prophylactic taping to prevent hyperextension and decrease valgus stresses may be appropriate when the individual returns to practice.

Care of the throwing arm includes[46]:

1. Gently stretching and massaging the elbow and shoulder before throwing
2. Performing throwing actions without the ball
3. Commencing with gentle throwing while wearing a warm-up jacket
4. Gradually increasing the velocity of the throw
5. After throwing, replacing the warm-up jacket, performing gentle stretching, and allowing a period of time to cool down
6. Applying ice after each throwing session

Osteochondrosis of the Capitellum

Etiology

Osteochondrosis of the capitellum (Panner's disease, osteochondrosis deformans, osteochondritis) may be directly related to trauma or to changes in the circulation; this is the so-called Panner's disease of aseptic or avascular necrosis.[47,48] There has been much debate as to the etiology of this condition; cartilage rests, bacterial infection, vascular insufficiency, primary fracture with separation, and hereditary factors have all been espoused.[45–49] However, the evidence always seems to lead back to some form of disordered endochondral ossification in association with trauma or vascular impairment. Certain common features prevail. More than 90 percent of the lesions occur in males, fewer than 5 percent are bilateral, and the dominant arm is virtually always involved in unilateral cases. In children younger than the age of 8 years, the lesions are similar to those described by Panner, with changes in density and fragmentation of the capitellum, whereas in older children and adolescents, loose bodies are more frequent.

Osteochondritis is rarely seen before the age of 5 years, when the chondroepiphysis of the capitellum has an abundant nutrient vascular supply.[48] The lesion usually becomes manifest clinically when the capitellar nucleus is supplied only by one or two discrete vessels with no obvious anastomosis.[44] The path of these vessels from the posterior surface of the chondroepiphysis is through unossified epiphyseal cartilage to the capitellum, and they are therefore situated, at least part of the way, in compressible cartilage.

The circulation is vulnerable until fusion of the ossific nucleus occurs in the late teens. Repeated minor trauma may damage the tenuous vasculature and may account for the prevalence of this condition in young baseball pitchers, gymnasts, and javelin throwers. Whatever the underlying etiology, the ultimate outcome may be healing, nonhealing, or loose body formation.

The main presenting symptoms are usually pain, swelling, limitation of range of motion in a noncapsular pattern, and sometimes clicking and locking. Interestingly, the patient may display a soft end-feel when extension is blocked by the displaced fragment and a hard end-feel when flexion is limited.[34] The diagnosis can usually be made from plain radiographs.

Treatment

Nonoperative treatment requires rest from stress and, very rarely, a short period of immobilization with a splint. Treatment is the same as outlined for throwing injuries. The indications for surgery include a locked elbow, loose fragments, or failure of conservative therapy to relieve symptoms. Surgical treatment may include removal of loose fragments, excision of the capitellar lesions, and curettage to bleeding bone.[50] Usually, joint motion is restored or improved with manual therapy, a graduated strengthening and stretching program, and adequate therapy. A return to organized competitive sport is possible, provided that there have not been excessive joint changes.[50]

Ligament Ruptures and Dislocations

Acute Ligament Tears

Acute ligament tears without dislocation are relatively rare but occasionally result from valgus or varus stresses in sport or recreation. The medial collateral ligament appears to be more vulnerable, and this injury is surprisingly easy to overlook in the acute stage unless there is an index of suspicion and careful valgus and varus stressing is carried out with the elbow flexed at 15 degrees[51] (Fig. 10–10). Often, acute medial collateral ruptures are associated with some ulnar nerve paresthesias. Disability and restriction of range of motion can be prevented and adhesions minimized by early protected range-of-motion exercises in minor cases; surgical repair may be considered in more significant tears. For some individuals, a functional brace eliminating valgus or varus stress allows resumption of quite strenuous activities moderately early.

Lee[24] has described Fryette's abduction ulnohumeral lesion secondary to a fall on an outstretched hand, in which the ulna is forced into extension and abduction, increasing the carrying angle. Subsequently, the radius glides distally at the radioulnar joints, increasing tension

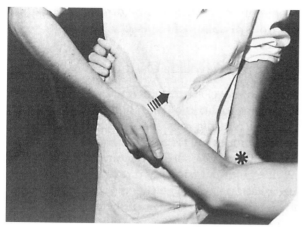

Figure 10–10. Elbow abduction or valgus stress performed at 15 to 20 degrees of flexion to test the integrity of the ulnar collateral ligament. The asterisk indicates the fixed point.

on the radioulnar ligaments and the interosseous membrane. The radius carries the hand distally with it, increasing tension on the ulnar collateral ligament at the wrist. The wrist is held in an ulnarly deviated position (Fig. 10–11). The radial wrist extensors attempt to pull the hand into functional alignment, and the overuse of these muscles results in tennis elbow-like symptoms. Although these symptoms may be a direct result of the trauma to the elbow, in the above circumstances they represent a dysfunction from a concomitantly sustained lesion to the wrist. The wrist lesion may be related to the well-

described carpal shift and carpal collapse subsequent to ligament damage from a fall on the outstretched hand. This lesion must also be distinguished from the well-recognized congenital ulnar negative variance, which may lead to wrist and sometimes elbow pain. The appropriate examination for this condition is observation of the elbow–wrist relationship in pronation. The third digit and metacarpal are held at an angle of 5 to 15 degrees to the axis of rotation of the forearm. Tests for accessory movements at the wrist and elbow will confirm the findings. Radial deviation is restricted at the radiocarpal joint, as is adduction at the ulnohumeral joint.

The articular dysfunction should be treated first with manual therapy, restoring ulnohumeral adduction; the ulnar collateral ligaments and radial wrist extensors should be addressed as well.

Dislocations

Radius and ulna

A fall on the outstretched hand may result in elbow dislocation, frequently associated with fracture of the olecranon or the coronoid process. After reduction, careful examination of the ulnar nerve is necessary, followed by immobilization in a sling for about 3 weeks. At this time, gentle range-of-motion exercises can be begun.

Radial head in adults

In the adult, dislocation of the radial head has a significant tendency to recur. Careful scrutiny of the lateral and anteroposterior films after reduction is mandatory. Immobilization for 3 to 6 weeks in flexion is usually necessary. Any evidence of imperfect reduction is an indication for operative intervention.

Radial head in children

The imperfectly formed radial head may allow subluxation or dislocation in association with damage and unfolding of the immature annular ligament (pulled elbow, nursemaid's elbow; Fig. 10–12). Distraction with rotation of

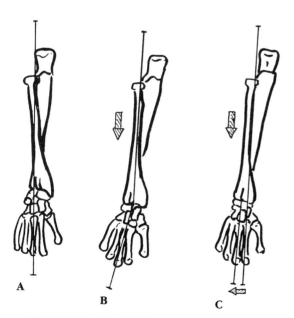

Figure 10–11. Abduction ulnohumeral lesion. (A) The normal functional axis of rotation is disrupted; (B) initial adaptation to an abduction ulnar lesion, by distal movement of the radius, forces the carpus into 5 to 15 degrees of ulnar deviation; (C) secondary compensation results in a carpal shift, producing chronic elbow and possible wrist symptoms. This is best demonstrated by examining the outstretched pronated hand.

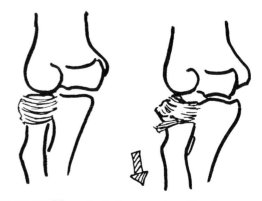

Figure 10–12. The pulled elbow produced by distraction-rotation forces damages the annular ligament, allowing all or part of it to be carried into the joint.

the radius caused by swinging the child by the arms gives rise to one of the names for this condition. Reduction is usually easily accomplished by elbow flexion and rotation of the forearm or may even occur spontaneously. The main features of successful treatment are demonstration of reduction by a normal radiograph and restoration of range of motion and prompt resolution of pain. An inadequately reduced radial head will go on to significant overgrowth and deformity, culminating in serious disability of the elbow joint.

Myositis Ossificans

The proximity of attachment of the fleshy brachialis and triceps to the joint, and the complex nature of the three articulations in one capsule, give the elbow a propensity for stiffness and myositis ossificans after trauma. Usually a fracture or dislocation is involved, but occasionally direct contusion is the precipitating factor. The therapist must constantly be aware of the syndrome of increasingly pain and decreasing range during rehabilitation of elbow trauma. The therapist may frequently be the first to recognize the evolution of this condition by detecting a subtle difference in the feel of the motion or an increasingly firm mass in the muscle. At the first sign of this problem, soft tissue radiographs should be taken as a baseline and repeated at 2-week intervals if the elbow fails to improve. Heat should be discontinued, anti-inflammatory medication begun, and rest with the exception of gentle active range-of-motion exercises instituted. No resisted exercises should be performed. With stabilization of the condition, as evidenced by decreasing inflammation, bone mass, and pain, gentle therapy is reinstituted and plays an important role in safely pacing the return to full activity. More often, with fractures around the elbow, the myositic ectopic bone is present on removal of the cast after 3 to 6 weeks of immobilization. With maturity of the ectopic bone, as evidenced by a bone scan, surgical excision may be the best treatment to restore a significant loss of range of motion.

Nerve Entrapment, Neuritis, and Neuropathies

Ulnar Nerve

The ulnar nerve is well protected by the bulk of the medial head of the triceps above the elbow and is rarely involved in humeral shaft fractures. However, it is more susceptible to damage in connection with supracondylar and epicondylar fractures (Table 10–5). In passing from the anterior to the posterior compartment of the arm, the ulnar nerve may be involved in fibrous compression or adhesion to the medial intermuscular septum. This septum slopes from a wide base at the medial epicondyle, where it is thick and unyielding, to a weak, thin edge, at varying distances more proximally on the humeral shaft. If the nerve is

□ □ □ □ □ □   □

Table 10–5. Factors Contributing to Ulnar Nerve Decompression

Etiology	Pathophysiology
Neuritis	Tension through repetitive elbow flexion Subluxating nerve
Neural pressure	Perineural adhesions Congenital variations (e.g., bifid nerve) Exostosis and osteophytes Medial intermuscular septum Flexor carpi ulnaris, superficial and deep aponeurosis
Trauma	Fractures Dislocations Callus Progressive valgus deformity Prolonged bed rest Leaning on elbow (repetitive minor trauma) Saturday night palsy (traction or pressure)
Predisposing conditions	Peripheral neuritis Anatomy Rheumatoid arthritis Osteoarthritis

rerouted by surgery to the anterior aspect of the elbow, it may be drawn across or compressed on the firm edge of the septum unless mobilized sufficiently proximally. This may explain some surgical failures with anterior transposition of the ulnar nerve.[52]

Behind the epicondyle, the ulnar nerve is superficial and is particularly vulnerable to direct injury. Dislocations, contusions, traction injuries, fractures of the epicondyle, callus, osteophytes from the radiocapitellar articulation and olecranon, and subluxation of the nerve with flexion and extension may all contribute to neuritis or neuropathy.[53] Simple ganglia and benign tumors such as lipomas have also been implicated in neural compression.

The cubital tunnel, as traditionally described by Feindel and Stratford,[54] is an osseoaponeuritic canal behind the medial epicondyle. It is formed by the epicondyle, the olecranon, the medial collateral ligament, and an aponeuritic arch giving origin to, and formed by, the two heads of the flexor carpi ulnaris. This tunnel may be considered to extend distally to varying degrees between the two heads of the flexor carpi ulnaris and may have a superficial and a deep component to the arch, both of which must be released to ensure adequate surgical decompression in resistant cases of tardy ulnar palsy.[1,53,55] This osseoaponeuritic canal has a varying lumen, being wide in extension and narrow during flexion of the elbow. Prolonged flexion, with the associated mild traction on the nerve, may cause sufficient pressure to result in transient paresis in the absence of external pressure, as can repeated rapid movements of the elbow, as seen in pitching or serving in volleyball. Contraction of the flexor carpi ulnaris may narrow the tunnel by pulling on the aponeuritic portion and narrowing the interval between the two heads.[1,53]

In sport, the most common malady involving the nerve at the elbow is a frictional neuritis with mainly sensory symptoms of pain and numbness in the classic ulnar distribution of the little finger and the contiguous side of the ring finger. The nerve may be hypersensitive to tapping behind the elbow, exacerbating the distal symptoms. Untreated, the symptoms may progress, and there may be signs of wasting of the intrinsic muscles of the hand, often most noticeable as atrophy of the first dorsal interosseous muscle, reducing the bulk of the web space. Soon, weakness of grip starts to accompany the increasing clumsiness in fine prehension, which was initially due to poor stereognosis. Sensation is decreased at the palmar and dorsal surfaces of the little finger and the ulnar half of the ring finger. Two-point discrimination can be measured and recorded and will deteriorate with increasing pathology. In the normal hand, compass points set 3 to 4 mm apart are clearly distinguished as separate stimuli (Fig. 10–13). Testing of the adductor pollicis reveals weakness, as a positive Froment's sign. Weakness of the interossei results in inability to squeeze the little finger to the rest of the hand, a positive Wartenburg's sign (Fig. 10–13).

Treatment will depend on the frequency, duration, intensity, magnitude, and etiology of the symptoms. If the neuritis is secondary to repeated blows, as in wrestling, or to pressure, as with a student studying and writing, a well-constructed pad may help. If the neuritis is frictional, it may be sufficient to block terminal extension for a period of time by initially taping the elbow. Persistent symptoms should not be allowed to continue or progress.

Complete rest from the offending activity supplemented by anti-inflammatory medication will usually help the acute case. In more chronic situations, the diagnosis and exact location are confirmed by radiography, and nerve conduction studies and surgical treatment are considered.

Decompression and transposition of the ulnar nerve are the main alternatives, and exact knowledge of the anatomy is needed if success is to be achieved.[56] With tumors or stenosis of the cubital tunnel, decompression is usually adequate; however, sufficient distal release is mandatory to ensure division of both the superficial and deep aponeuroses.[55] If there are large osteophytes, callus, a subluxating nerve, significant nerve changes and severe clinical signs, or a situation of repeated local trauma, transposition may be a better alternative to ensure minimal continued tension on the nerve. Adequate proximal release is necessary to avoid tension across the medial intermuscular septum.[55] If transposition is desirable but would entail devascularization of too great a section of nerve, medial epicondylectomy with nerve decompression may be the most suitable alternative.[54] This is a particularly useful technique in athletes with large arm girths and in whom over 20 cm of nerve would have to be mobilized for adequate transportation.[53,57] Removal of the condyle does not alter grip strength or elbow flexor power after adequate rehabilitation.[53,54]

Median Nerve

Median nerve entrapment about the elbow is a rare phenomenon, although cases have been reported after posterior dislocation. When it does occur, it is usually in children, and recognition of the problem is usually delayed.[58] Progressive involvement of the nerve in developing callus after distal humeral fractures has also been recorded.[58]

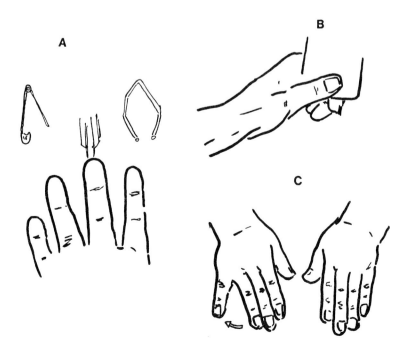

Figure 10–13. Tests for frictional neuritis. (A) Sensory function may be tested for pain and light touch using a safety pin and two-point discrimination (normal is 3 to 4 mm at the fingertip) with calipers or a paper clip; (B) weakness of the adductor pollicis is detected by Froment's sign and is compensated for by flexing the thumbtip as the paper is pulled away; (C) a positive Wartenburg's sign with inability to obtain close adduction of all fingers.

Rarely, the nerve may become compressed above the elbow as it passes under the anomalous ligament of Struthers, which attaches to a spur in the lower third of the humerus. Because of its anterior location, the median nerve may be subjected to direct blows, particularly in some sports. However, the result is generally neuropraxia and infrequently axonotmesis, and patients usually recover without surgical intervention.

There may be decreased sensation to the lateral three digits and the palm or decreased motor and sensory conduction. Awareness of the potentially more serious injury, with careful initial neurologic assessment and meticulous assessment of pinch and grip strength and two-point discrimination during the early rehabilitation phase, will allow diagnosis of a persistent defect or progressive median nerve function deterioration and point to the need for electromyographic evaluation and potential nerve exploration. In severe nerve injury, a functional splint may be required until recovery is achieved. Active range of motion must be maintained.

Anterior Interosseous Nerve

Entrapment or damage of the anterior interosseous branch of the median nerve is more frequent than injury to the main nerve. It may be involved in scar formation after trauma or fracture, usually as the nerve passes between the two heads of the pronatur teres. Fractures and dislocation of the radius and ulna may also precipitate injury. Infrequently, ganglia or soft tissue tumors such as lipomas may compress the nerve. The deficit is purely motor, involving the flexor pollicis longus and the flexor digitorum profundus to the index and middle fingers and the pronator quadratus. The inability to carry out a tip-to-tip pinch is the diagnostic sign. Attempts to pinch a sheet of paper or a card between the thumb and index finger result in pulp-to-pulp apposition. The patient may also have some difficulty pronating with a flexed elbow. Recovery after release or spontaneously after trauma is to

be anticipated. Rehabilitation is directed at strengthening the grip.[59]

Radial and Posterior Interosseous Nerves

The radial nerve is most vulnerable in the spiral groove of the humerus. Midshaft humeral fractures always jeopardize the nerve during both the initial trauma and subsequent callus production. Less frequently, the nerve is damaged by direct blows to the lateral aspect of the distal arm just as it dives into the bulk of the brachioradialis and the extensor carpi radialis longus. The most common site of pathology in the forearm is at the point at which the main motor branches of the radial nerve continue as the posterior interosseous nerve (Fig. 10–14). Just before entering the plane between the deep and superficial heads of the supinator muscle, the nerve may be involved in the so-called arcade of Frohse.[60] This is probably a fairly rare syndrome. During extension and pronation, the ECRB and the fibrous edge of the superficial part of the supinator are seen to tighten around the nerve. The resulting entrapment has been referred to as the radial tunnel syndrome and is believed to be important in the differential diagnosis of a tennis elbow that is resistant to treatment (Fig. 10–14).

In a series reported by Roles and Maudsley,[60] clinical findings were fairly uniform. At the onset, the patient usually complained of the classic signs and symptoms of lateral epicondylitis, namely, tenderness over the common extensor origin, pain on passive stretching of the extensor muscles, and pain on resisted extension of the wrist and fingers. After all the usual therapies, these patients are often left with pain radiating up and down the arm, weakness of grip, tenderness over the radial nerve, and pain on resisted extension of the middle finger, which tightens the facial origin of the ECRB[60,61] (Fig. 10–14). It has also been suggested that resisted supination is generally much more painful than resisted wrist extension because of the contraction of the supinator muscle.[24] Nerve con-

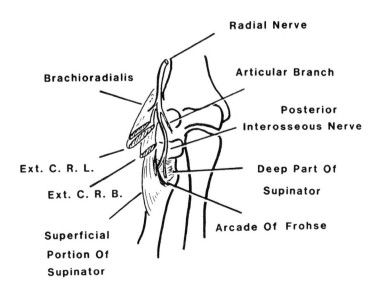

Figure 10–14. Possible site of entrapment of the posterior interosseous nerve at the level of the arcade of Frohse. Ext. C.R.B., extensor carpi radialis brevis; Ext. C.R.L., extensor carpi radialis longus.

duction studies should show significant delay in motor latencies measured from the spiral groove to the medial portion of the extensor digitorum communis. Recognition of the few but significant resistant cases of tennis elbow allows prompt, effective treatment by surgical release of the entrapment.

Olecranon Pathology

Olecranon Bursitis

The olecranon bursa, lying as it does superficial to the insertion of the triceps tendon, can be irritated either by a single episode of trauma, such as a fall on the point of the elbow, or by repetitive grazing and weightbearing, as is often seen in students or in wrestling. The acute bursitis may present as a swelling over the olecranon process, varying in size from a slight distention to a swelling that could be the size of a small chicken's egg. Depending on the acuteness of the inflammatory reaction, there is a variable amount of heat and redness associated with this swelling.

The important diagnostic differential here is between a simple posttraumatic bursitis and an infected olecranon bursa. The former may be treated with ice and elastic wrap and different forms of well-fitting protective pads and will usually, with time, disappear by itself. The infected bursa, however, must be brought to prompt medical attention so that appropriate antibiotic therapy can be started and drainage instituted if necessary. Failure to do this may lead to a spreading cellulitis and an infection involving a large part of the forearm or the upper arm. The proximity of the bursa to the elbow joint itself actually makes treatment all the more urgent. Repeated posttraumatic bursitis may lead of fibrin deposits in the bursa. These may eventually metaplase into a cartilage-like material and form tiny seeds within the bursa itself. These then form a source of aggravation even with minor friction, and a perpetual painful bursitis may be set up. In these instances, conservative treatment is no longer warranted, and surgical excision of the bursa should be considered.

Stress Fractures of the Olecranon

The valgus and varus overload during forceful throwing action has been dealt with in the section on ''Injuries to the Throwing Arm.'' However, stress fractures of the olecranon, while uncommon, must be borne in mind as part of the differential diagnosis.[62] Individuals usually experience pain in the elbow of the throwing arm for some weeks or months before the lesion is obvious on radiography. The etiology is linked to the explosive forces applied to the olecranon during the final phases of delivery and perhaps the impingement of the olecranon process against the base and medial wall of the olecranon fossa.[63] These injuries are disastrous for competitive athletes because, if ignored, they may complete themselves during a throw, and if the fracture line is sufficiently distal, dislocation may occur. Complete cessation of throwing is usually necessary. If the lesion is treated very early, throwing may be resumed in 8 to 12 weeks. However, significant stress fractures or complete fractures may take up to 4 months to heal sufficiently for resumption of throwing if internal fixation is used. Splinting or casting is usually not required. Excision of a very proximal stress fracture of the tip of the olecranon, the most frequent site, allows resumption of throwing at 8 weeks. Fractures treated conservatively may take up to 18 months before throwing is resumed successfully if the lesion is well established.[58]

A similar lesion is a fracture separation of the olecranon epiphysis in children, and an even more rare situation is fracture separation of an incompletely fused olecranon physis in adults.[64] The proximal ulnar ossification center appears at age 8 years in girls and 10 years in boys and usually unites with the ulnar shaft at ages 14 and 16 years, respectively. The size of the olecranon ossification center varies from a small flake to up to 25 percent of the olecranon.[65] The secondary ossification center may also be bipartite. Usually, the physis closes from deep to superficial, with rarely a deep posterior cleft persisting. It is this cleft that may form the start of a stress fracture or a weakened area, which may occur secondary to a direct blow. The etiology is usually a direct blow from a fall, frequently in a football player. These are difficult injuries to treat, frequently requiring bone grafting as well as open reduction and internal fixation, because there is a propensity to fibrous union.[64]

Tendon Avulsions and Ruptures

Triceps

Injuries involving avulsion or rupture of the triceps tendon are among the least frequent tendon injuries, and major ruptures of the belly of triceps are even more uncommon.[66,67] The mechanism is essentially the same for both sites, namely, a decelerating stress superimposed on the contracting triceps muscle either through a fall on the outstretched hand or due to sudden contact during an extension maneuver such as a karate chop. Significant tears of the tendon must be recognized immediately because a successful functional outcome depends on early surgical repair. Delayed repair is possible but technically more difficult and has less chance of an excellent result. Recognition is through loss of active extension, a palpable gap, pain, and a large hematoma going on to diffuse swelling and ecchymosis.[68] In tendon avulsion, a small fleck of olecranon is often seen on the plain radiograph, and where there is doubt as to the diagnosis, computed tomography accurately visualizes the pathology. Muscle belly tears usually involve only the medial head, and usually nonoperative treatment produces a satisfactory outcome.[66]

It is well to recall that a normal tendon must sustain considerable force before it will rupture; hence, avulsion of the insertion is an expected event when the trauma is sufficient. For this reason, rupture of the substance of the tendon should lead to a search for associated pathology. Conditions such as rheumatoid arthritis, systemic lupus erythematosus, hyperparathyroidism, xanthomatous degeneration, and hemangioepithelioma as well as sytemic steroids and local steroid injections may all predispose the tendon to rupture.

Biceps

Biceps ruptures at the elbow are extremely rare, and while they are compatible with normal function in a relatively sedentary individual, surgical repair is probably best carried out early in young or very active patients. The diagnosis is based on the inability to palpate the tendon and by altered muscle delineation. Hemorrhage is often considerable and may obscure the diagnosis unless an adequate index of suspicion is maintained. This injury is sometimes associated with a radial head dislocation, and both injuries need therapy.

Brachialis

Most tears of the brachialis are partial, but isolated complete tears may infrequently occur. Dislocation of the elbow is the most common associated injury. The major significance of brachialis rupture is the propensity to myositis ossificans or delayed instability of an associated unrecognized elbow dislocation.

Extensor or Flexor Muscle Mass

Rapid violent contraction in association with a blow to the forearm may lead to rupture of the flexor or extensor muscle mass. Usually this injury is comparable with return to excellent function when treated nonoperatively. Treatment includes splinting and gentle range-of-motion, muscle-strengthening, and functional exercises. Avulsion of the muscles from their tendons at the musculotendinous junction should be repaired operatively, and these injuries are usually associated with an excellent surgical outcome. Early mobilization and therapy are the keys to success.

Compartment Syndromes

Volkmann's Ischemic Contracture

Classic Volkmann's ischemic contracture is associated with supracondylar fractures in children, and this entity is discussed in Chapter 11. It is useful to recall, however, that it may also occur with severe bleeding from trauma to the forearm, with crushing injuries, or from a tight cast or bandage for any reason. Awareness of the impending disastrous situation and prompt attention to complaints of numbness, swelling, and discoloration of the fingers with increasing pain will avert a very unhappy outcome.

Other Compartment Syndromes

Traditionally, compartment syndromes of the forearm have been synonymous with the more dramatic Volkmann's ischemic contracture secondary to dislocation of the elbow or supracondylar fractures. However, in 1959 Bennett described a fascial compartment compression syndrome secondary to overuse.[66] Repetitive pitching, for example, can lead to a syndrome of medial elbow and forearm pain secondary to swelling and edema within the tight forearm fasical compartments. Recognition of the problem, with adequate rest, sufficient warm-up, and carefully spaced intervals between activity, is usually successful, but in recalcitrant cases fasciotomy may be required.[39]

Systemic Conditions

A selection of systemic conditions are mentioned to emphasize the need for constant awareness of the broad differential diagnosis of elbow pain; treatment for these conditions will not be outlined.

Mainly Monoarticular Conditions

Osteoarthrosis
Osteoarthrosis of the elbow may be the result of repeated minor trauma in such occupations as mining and working with compressed air hammers, and through recreation and sport with repetitive throwing. Mild osteoarthrosis may be relatively painless, although it may be accompanied by loss of extension and occasionally ulnar nerve symptoms.

Chrondromatosis
The elbow, along with the knee and shoulder, is the most frequent site of chondromatosis. The presentation may be pain, limitation of motion, or, more usually, catching and locking. Synovectomy may be necessary to restore function to the joint.

Pigmented villinodular synovitis
Although this uncommon disease of the synovium occurs primarily at the knee, the elbows and ankles are the next most frequent joints involved. Repeated hemarthrosis may be the presenting sign. Treatment may involve synovectomy with very persistent therapy postoperatively if joint range is to be maintained.

Diseases of the blood and arthropathies
With the exception of the knee, the elbow is probably the joint most frequently involved in hemophiliacs.[69] Repeated joint bleeds destroy the synovium and joint sur-

face. Normal growth is disturbed, with marginal overgrowth of the radial head; early loss of joint range, deformity, and sometimes ankylosis are all possible sequelae of the disease.[68] Similarly, although less commonly, the elbow may be involved in hemoglobinopathies such as sickle cell anemia and thalassemia. In contrast to most elbow pathology, contractures caused by severe, advanced hemophilia may respond to prolonged stretching techniques using slings and pulleys or spring-loaded splints. For these specialized techniques, the reader is referred to the classic articles by Duthie et al.[69] and Dickson.[70]

Mainly Polyarticular Conditions

Rheumatoid arthritis

In only about 3 percent of cases does rheumatoid arthritis present for the first time with elbow symptoms. However, after 3 years of disease, almost 50 percent of patients have elbow involvement, and this proportion increases with time. These prevalence figures also probably hold for juvenile chronic arthritis. About 20 percent of rheumatoid patients have rheumatoid nodules, which classically develop on the extensor surface of the olecranon and the proximal ulna. Nodules in association with seropositive disease often indicate a bad clinical course.[68] Whereas the adult disease is characterized by severe painful synovitis and ultimately much joint destruction, bony ankylosis is more common in children with juvenile chronic arthritis.

Seronegative arthropathies

The seronegative arthropathies include ankylosing spondylitis, Reiter's syndrome, and the reactive arthropathies. In this seronegative group are the arthropathy complicating Crohn's disease and ulcerative colitis, Behçet's syndrome, and Whipple's disease. Generally, the elbow is involved only in patients in whom the disease is widespread and chronic, and usually only one side is affected. The exception is the very destructive psoriatic arthropathy, in which the elbow is frequently involved.[68]

Gout

It is rare for gout to present initially with elbow involvement, but in severe gout almost one-third of patients have involvement of the joint and of the extensor surface of the forearm, and the olecranon is the most common site of gouty tophi.

Chondrocalcinosis

Chondrocalcinosis is an x-ray diagnosis based on visualization of calcification in the joint capsule or cartilage. Chondrocalcinosis of the elbow joint is frequently indicative of hyperparathyroidism but may occur in ochronosis, hemochromatosis, gout, and Wilson's disease. Elbow involvement is seen in approximately one-third of patients with calcium pyrophosphate deposition disease, or pseudogout, where the deposit is mainly in the capsule.

Tumors and Infections

Neoplasms around the elbow, whether primary or metastatic, are rare. Nevertheless, they are an important part of the differential diagnosis in situations in which the pain and swelling do not resolve in response to normal treatment regimens or when the radiologic appearance is abnormal. Similarly, although infection is rare, local extension of infection from intravenous therapy may involve the elbow.

■ Summary

A superficial discussion of the elbow joint necessarily understates the complexity of the anatomy. Arising out of the subtle biomechanics, the proximity of muscle belly attachments, and the multiple articulations is the propensity for loss of range and myositis ossificans. Loss of function at this joint seriously impairs the versatility of the hand and compromises the useful range of the whole upper limb segment, because, unlike in the shoulder, wrist, and fingers, very little compensatory adjustment is possible. For this reason, early diagnosis and very careful, well-planned, and meticulous therapy are essential to successful treatment. Failure to pick up subtleties of diagnosis or of the changing pathologic state and the institution of mistimed or inappropriate therapy have the potential to result in permanent significant disability. The exclusion of pathology in C5, C6, and C7 must always be kept in mind with elbow pain syndromes. This chapter has attempted to explain the more commonly seen conditions, with a guide to treatment approaches.

■ Acknowledgments

We thank Jim Meadows for his advise and assistance.

■ References

1. Reid DC: Functional Anatomy and Joint Mobilization. 2nd Ed. University of Alberta Press, Edmonton, 1975
2. Basmajian JV: Muscles Alive: Their Function Revealed by Electromyography. 2nd Ed. Williams & Wilkins, Baltimore, 1967
3. Thompson HC, Garcia A: Myositis ossificans: aftermath of elbow injuries. Clin Orthop 50:129, 1967
4. Morrey BF, Kai-Nan A: Articular and ligamentous contributions to the stability of the elbow joint. Am J Sports Med 11:315, 1983
5. VanMameren H, Drukker J: A functional anatomical basis of injuries to the ligamentum and other soft tissues around the elbow joint. Transmission of tensile and compressive loads. Int J Sports Med, suppl., 5:88, 1984
6. Kapandji IA: The Physiology of the Joints. 5th Ed. Vol. 1. Churchill Livingstone, Edinburgh, 1982
7. MacConaill MA: A structurofunctional classification of articular units. Ir J Med Sci 142:19, 1973

8. Kaltenborn F: Mobilization of the Extremity Joints. 3rd Ed. Olaf Norlis Bokhandel, Oslo, 1980

9. MacConaill MA: Arthrology. p. 429. In Warwick R, Williams PL (eds): Gray's Anatomy. 35th Ed. WB Saunders, Philadelphia, 1975

10. Schwab G, Bennett J, Woods G, et al: Biomechanics of elbow instability; the role of the medial collateral ligament. Clin Orthop 146:42, 1980

11. Gutieriez L: A contribution to the study of limiting factors of elbow extension. Acta Anat 56:145, 1964

12. Schuit D, McPoil TG, Knecht HG: Effect of tightened anterior band of the ulnar collateral ligament on arthrokinematics at the humeroulnar joint. J Orthop Sports Phys Ther 8:123, 1986

13. Maitland G: Peripheral Manipulation. 2nd Ed. Butterworth, Boston, 1977

14. Cummings GS: Comparison of muscle to other soft tissue in limiting elbow extension. J Orthop Sports Phys Ther 5:170, 1984

15. Jobe FW, Nuber G: Throwing injuries of the elbow. Clin Sports Med 5:621, 1986

16. Pauly JE, Rushing JL, Schering LE: An electromyographic study of some muscles crossing the elbow joint. Anat Rec 1:42, 1967

17. Rasch PI: Effect of position of the forearm on strength of elbow flexion. Res Q Am Assoc Health Phys Educ 27:333, 1956

18. Runge F: Zur Genese und Behandlung des Schreibekrampfes. Berl Lin Wochenschr 10:245, 1973

19. Morris HL: The rider's sprain. Lancet 133:29, 1882

20. Innes CA: Letter to the editor. Lancet 210:5, 1882

21. Nirschl RP: Muscle and tendon trauma: tennis elbow. p. 42. In Morrey BF (ed): The Elbow and Its Disorders. WB Saunders, Philadelphia, 1985

22. Van Swearingen JM: Measuring wrist muscle strength. J Orthop Sports Phys Ther 4:217, 1983

23. Briggs CA, Elliott BG: Lateral epicondylitis. A review of structures associated with tennis elbow. Anat Clin 7:149, 1985

24. Lee DG: Tennis elbow: a manual therapist's perspective. J Orthop Sports Phys Ther 8:134, 1986

25. Legwold G: Tennis elbow: joint resolution by conservative treatment and improved technique. Phys Sports Med 12:168, 1984

26. Liu YK: Mechanical analysis of racquet and ball during impact. Med Sci Sports Exerc 15:388, 1983

27. Elliot BC: Tennis: the influence of grip tightness on reaction impulse and rebound velocity. Med Sci Sports Exerc 14:348, 1982

28. Froimson AI: Treatment of tennis elbow with forearm support band. J Bone Joint Surg 53(A):183, 1971

29. Burton AK: Grip strength and forearm straps in tennis elbow. Br J Sports Med 19:37, 1985

30. Burton AK, Edwards VA: Electromyography and tennis elbow straps. Br Osteopath J 14:83, 1982

31. Halle JS, Franklin RJ, Karalfa BL: Comparison of four treatment approaches for lateral epicondylitis of the elbow. J Orthop Sports Phys Ther 8:62, 1986

32. Percy EC, Carson JD: The use of DMSO in tennis elbow and rotator cuff tendinitis: a double blind study. Med Sci Sports Exerc 13:215, 1981

33. Burton K: Grip strength as an objective clinical assessment in tennis elbow. Br Osteopath J 16:6, 1984

34. Cyriax J: Textbook of Orthopaedic Medicine. 5th Ed. Vol. 1. Diagnosis of Soft Tissue Lesions. Williams & Wilkins, Baltimore, 1970

35. Kushner S, Reid DC: Manipulation in the treatment of tennis elbow. J Orthop Sports Phys Ther 7:264, 1986

36. Curwin S, Stanish WD: Tendinitis: Its Etiology and Treatment. Collamore Press, Lexington, MA 1984

37. Ingham B: Transverse friction massage for relief of tennis elbow. Physician Sportsweek 9:116, 1981

38. Boyd HB, McLeod AC: Tennis elbow. J Bone Joint Surg 55(A):1183, 1973

39. Cabrera JM, McCue FC: Non-osseous athletic injuries of the elbow, forearm and hand. Clin Sports Med 5:681, 1986

40. Woods GW, Tullos HS, King JW: The throwing arm: elbow injuries. J Sports Med 1:43, 1973

41. Slocum DB: Classification of the elbow injuries from baseball pitching. Tex Med 64:48, 1968

42. Wilson FD, Andrews JR, Blackburn TA, et al: Valgus extension overload in the pitching elbow. Am J Sports Med 11:83, 1983

43. Adams JE: Injuries to the throwing arm—a study of traumatic changes in the elbow joints of boy baseball pitchers. Calif Med 102:127, 1965

44. DeHaven KE, Evarts CM: Throwing injuries of the elbow in athletes. Orthop Clin North Am 4:801, 1973

45. Singer KM, Roy SP: Osteochondrosis of the humeral capitellum. Am J Sports Med 12:351, 1984

46. Roy S, Irvin R: Sports Medicine Prevention Evaluation, Management and Rehabilitation. Prentice-Hall, Englewood Cliffs, NJ, 1983

47. Panner HJ: A peculiar affection of the capitellum humeri resembling Calve-Perthes' disease of the hip. Acta Radiol 10:234, 1929

48. Haraldsson S: On osteochondrosis deformans juvenilis capituli including investigation of intraosseous vasculature in distal humerus. Acta Orthop Scand, suppl. 38, 1959

49. Lindholm TS, Osterman K, Vankka E: Osteochondritis dissecans of the elbow, ankle and hip: a comparative survey. Clin Orthop 148:245, 1980

50. McManama GB, Micheli LT, Berry MV, et al: The surgical treatment of osteochondritis of the capitellum. Am J Sports Med 13:11, 1985

51. Norwood LA, Shook JA, Andrews JR: Acute medial elbow ruptures. Am J Sports Med 9:16, 1981

52. Carpendale MT: The localization of ulnar nerve compression in the hand and arm—an improved method of electromyography. Arch Phys Med Rehabil 47:325, 1966

53. Dangles CJ, Bibs JZ: Ulnar nerve neuritis in a world champion weightlifter. Am J Sports Med 8:443, 1980

54. Feindel W, Stratford J: The role of the cubital tunnel in tardy ulnar palsy. Can J Surg 1:287, 1958

55. Wojtys EM, Smith PA, Hankin FM: A cause of neuropathy in a baseball pitcher. Am J Sports Med 14:422, 1986

56. Broudy A, Leffert R, Smith R: Technical problems with ulnar nerve transposition at the elbow: findings and results of re-operation. J Hand Surg 3:85, 1978

57. Neblett C, Elini G: Medial epicondylectomy for ulnar nerve palsy. J Neurosurg 32:55, 1970

58. Rappaport NH, Clark GL, Bara WF: Median nerve entrapment about the elbow. Adv Orthop Surg 8:270, 1985

59. Van Der Wuff P, Hagmeyer RH, Rijnders W: Case study: isolated anterior interosseous nerve paralysis: the Kiloh-Nevin syndrome. J Orthop Sports Phys Ther 6:178, 1984

60. Roles NC, Maudsley RH: Radial tunnel syndrome. J Bone Joint Surg 54(B):499, 1972

61. Spinner M: The arcade of Frohse and its relationship to posterior interosseous nerve paralysis. J Bone Joint Surg 50(B):809, 1968

62. Hulkko A, Orava S, Nikula P: Stress fractures of the olecranon in javelin throwers. Int J Sports Med 7:210, 1968

63. London JT: Kinematics of the elbow. J Bone Joint Surg 63(A):529, 1981

64. Kovac J, Baker BE, Mosher JF: Fracture separation of the olecranon ossification centre in adults. Am J Sports Med 13:105, 1985

65. Kohler A: Roentgenology: The Borderlands of the Normal and Early Pathology in the Skeleton. William Wood, New York, 1928

66. Kunichi A, Torisu T: Muscle belly tear of the triceps. Am J Sports Med 12:485, 1984

67. Sherman O, Snyder ST, Fox JM: Triceps tendon avulsion in a professional body builder. Am J Sports Med 12:328, 1984

68. Bach BR, Warren RF, Wickiewicz TL: Triceps rupture—a case report and literature review. Am J Sports Med 15:285, 1987

69. Duthie RB, Matthews JM, Rizza CR, et al: The Management of Musculoskeletal Problems in Haemophiliacs. Blackwell Scientific, Oxford, 1972

70. Dickson RA: Reversed dynamic slings—a new concept in the treatment of post-traumatic elbow flexion contractures. Injury 8:35, 1976

CHAPTER 11
Dysfunction, Evaluation, and Treatment of the Wrist and Hand

Blanca Zita Gonzalez-King, Dorie B. Syen, and Brenda Lipscomb Burgess

Many of us never stop to wonder what it would be like if we were to lose the use of our hands, either partially or totally. We often take for granted that we are able to perform the fine motor skills needed to close the buttons on our shirts, drive ourselves to work, or caress the face of someone we care about. For the person who injures his or her hand, these things may not be possible. However, it is up to us as therapists to provide the most effective treatment program directed toward optimizing function. To do so, we must consider the osseous structures, musculotendinous units, nerve supply, vascular supply, and fascia. The first part of this chapter examines the anatomy and kinesiology of the wrist and hand, and the second part reviews the evaluation. Finally, case studies are presented that demonstrate the integration of the information in the clinical setting.

■ Osseous Structures

Wrist

Distal Radioulnar Joint

The palmar surface of the distal radius is flat and smooth. Lister's tubercle is located on the dorsal aspect. The radial surface ends as the radial styloid, and the medial facet has a concavity, the sigmoid notch, which is covered with hyaline cartilage, for articulation with the ulna. The distal surface of the radius is basically triangular, with a long articulating surface secondary to the distal position of the radial styloid. It is concave in both the anteroposterior and lateral planes. It has two facets on its distal surface for articulation with the scaphoid and lunate[1] (Fig. 11–1).

The ulna is covered with hyaline cartilage on its dorsal, lateral, and volar surfaces. The ulnar styloid projects from the posterior aspect of the ulna. It does not participate in the wrist joint and is separated from the triquetrum by the triangular fibrocartilage and ulnocarpal meniscus. The distal radioulnar joint capsule is lax, allowing pronation and supination. The two bones are held together by the triangular fibrocartilage complex and the interosseous membrane.[2]

Carpal Bones

Historically, the carpus has been viewed schematically as having two rows made up of eight carpal bones. The distal row is composed of the trapezium, trapezoid, capitate, and hamate, and the proximal row is composed of the scaphoid, lunate, triquetrum, and pisiform. Each bone, except the pisiform, has six surfaces, the posterior and anterior of which are usually roughened and irregular for ligamentous attachment (Fig. 11–2).

Scaphoid
The scaphoid is the most radial carpal bone and acts as a connecting link between the proximal and distal carpal rows. Most of its surface is covered with hyaline cartilage for different articulations. The proximal facet for the radius is the largest. The medial surface has two facets, one for articulation with the capitate and one for articulation with the lunate. The distal pole is divided by a ridge into two articulating surfaces for the trapezium and trapezoid. The nonarticular surface is narrow and is often referred to as the *waist* of the scaphoid. It is a site of different ligamentous attachments. The dorsal radiocarpal ligament and the radial collateral ligament attach to the dorsal surface, and the flexor retinaculum attaches to the volar surface.

Lunate
The lunate has a deep, concave surface on its distal aspect for articulation with the capitate. Its proximal surface is convex for articulation with the radius. It articulates

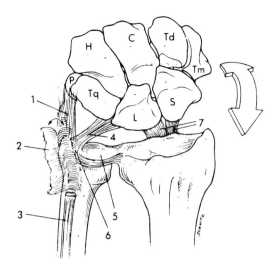

Figure 11–1. Dorsal view of the flexed wrist, including the triangular fibrocartilage. 1, Ulnar collateral ligament; 2, retinacular sheath; 3, tendon of extensor carpi ulnaris; 4, ulnolunate ligament; 5, triangular fibrocartilage; 6, ulnocarpal meniscus homologue; 7, palmar radioscapholunate ligament. P, pisiform; H, hamate; C, capitate; Td, trapezoid; Tm, trapezium; Tq, triquetrum; L, lunate; S, scaphoid. (From Strickland,[1] with permission.)

medially with the triquetrum and laterally with the scaphoid.

Triquetrum

The triquetrum is shaped like a pyramid. Its distal surface is concave for articulation with the hamate, and its proximal surface is convex for articulation with the triangular fibrocartilage. There is a roughened area on its distal surface that serves as the site of attachment for the ulnar collateral ligament. Its lateral surface is covered with hyaline cartilage where it articulates with the lunate. Its palmar surface has an oval facet for articulation with the pisiform.

Pisiform

The pisiform is the only carpal bone to receive a tendon insertion from a forearm muscle (flexor carpi ulnaris [FCU]). It is small and rounded on most of its surfaces. Part of the transverse carpal ligament attaches to it, as does the abductor digiti minimi (AbDM). It has one articulating surface for the triquetrum.

Trapezium

The distal surface of the trapezium, which articulates with the first metacarpal, is referred to as a *saddle joint*. Its medial surface has two facets for articulation with the second metacarpal and trapezoid. Proximally, it articulates with the scaphoid. The trapezium has a tuberosity for attachment of the flexor retinaculum and a deep groove on its palmar surface that acts as a tunnel for the flexor carpi radialis (FCR) tendon.

Trapezoid

The trapezoid is the smallest carpal in the distal row. It articulates with the scaphoid, trapezium, second metacarpal, and capitate.

Capitate

The capitate is located at the center of the carpus and is the largest of all the carpal bones. It is the center of wrist motion in all planes. The proximal head is convex for articulation with the scaphoid and lunate. Its medial surface articulates with the hamate. The distal surface is divided by two ridges that form three facets for articulation with the second, third, and fourth metacarpals. The volar and dorsal surfaces are roughened for ligament attachments.

Hamate

The hamate's most distinguishable feature is the hook that projects from the palmar surface for attachment of the flexor retinaculum. The hook also constitutes the medial wall of the carpal tunnel and the distal and lateral wall of Guyon's canal. The flexor digiti minimi (FDM) and opponens digiti minimi (OppDM) muscles originate from the hook of the hamate. Proximally, it articulates with the lunate and distally with the fourth and fifth metacarpals. It articulates with the triquetrum on its ulnar aspect and the capitate on its radial aspect.[2–4]

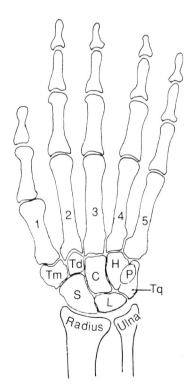

Figure 11–2. Volar view of the right wrist. The proximal row contains the scaphoid (S), lunate (L), triquetrum (Tq), and pisiform (P). The distal row contains the trapezium (Tm), trapezoid (Td), capirate (C), and hamate (H). (From Cailliet,[21] with permission.)

Wrist Ligaments

The wrist ligaments provide much support to the carpal bones as the latter transmit forces and allow motion at the radiocarpal and intercarpal joints. The volar ligaments are thick and strong, and the dorsal ones are thinner and less numerous.

Taleisnik[3] classified the ligaments as either extrinsic (those originating or inserting outside the carpus) or intrinsic (the entire ligament is situated within the carpus) (Table 11–1). The extrinsic group is further divided into proximal and distal. The proximal extrinsic ligaments include the radial collateral, volar radiocarpal, ulnocarpal complex, and dorsal radiocarpal ligaments (Fig. 11–3). The radial collateral ligament originates from the volar margin of the radial styloid. It crosses the wrist volar to the axis of rotation and attaches to the scaphoid tuberosity and into the walls of the tunnel for the FCR tendon. Although it is not a true collateral ligament, just as the wrist is not a hinge joint, it is partly responsible for the stability of the distal pole of the scaphoid. The volar radiocarpal ligaments consist of the superficial and deep ligaments. The superficial ligament assumes a V shape, with its apex at the capitate and lunate. The two arms diverge proximally to insert on the radius and ulna. There are three deep volar radiocarpal ligaments, which are named according to their origin and insertion. These include the radiocapitate, which is the most lateral and may send some fibers to the scaphoid; the radiolunate, which originates at the base of the radial styloid and inserts onto the lunate; and the radioscapholunate, which inserts primarily onto the lunate and more weakly onto the scaphoid. The space between the superficial and deep

volar radiocarpal ligaments is referred to as the *space of Poirier* and is an area of weakness on the volar aspect of the wrist secondary to a lack of a volar lunocapitate ligament. This is a common site of lunate dislocation. The ulnocarpal complex is composed of the triangular fibrocartilage, the ulnocarpal meniscus, the ulnolunate ligament, the ulnar collateral ligament, and the extensor carpi ulnaris (ECU) sheath. The ulnocarpal meniscus acts as a spacer between the ulnar styloid and wrist. It originates on the dorsal corner of the radius and inserts onto the triquetrum. The triangular fibrocartilage shares its origin with the ulnocarpal meniscus. It inserts onto the base of the ulnar styloid. The ulnolunate ligament originates at the anterior border of the triangular fibrocartilage complex and inserts onto the lunate. The fourth component of the ulnocarpal complex is the ulnar collateral ligament, which originates at the base of the ulnar styloid and inserts onto the triquetrum. The dorsal radiocarpal ligament originates at the dorsal edge of the radius. It is usually composed of two fascicles that insert onto the lunate and triquetrum. The distal extrinsic ligaments form a strong ligamentous structure that connects the third metacarpal to the capitate.[2,5]

The intrinsic ligaments originate and insert onto the carpal bones and are characterized as short, intermediate, or long. The short intrinsic ligaments are solid and bind the carpal bones of the distal row into one single unit. The intermediate intrinsic ligaments connect the scaphoid and the trapezium, the lunate and the triquetrum, and the scaphoid and the lunate. These ligaments span the joints where most intercarpal motion occurs. The long intrinsic ligaments are either volar or dorsal. The dorsal

□□□□□ □ □ □

Table 11–1. Classification of Wrist Ligaments

Extrinsic ligaments	Proximal (radiocarpal)	Radial collateral		
		Volar radiocarpal	Superficial	Radioscaphoid-capitate
			Deep	Radiolunate
				Radioscaphoid-lunate
		Ulnocarpal ligamentous complex		Meniscus (radio-triquetral)
				Triangular fibrocartilage
				Ulno lunate ligament
				Medial collateral ligament
	Distal (carpo-metacarpal)	Radiocarpal dorsal		
Intrinsic ligaments	Short	Volar		
		Dorsal		
		Interosseous		
	Intermediate	Lunate-triquetral		
		Scaphoid-lunate		
		Scaphoid-trapezial		
	Long	Volar intercarpal (deltoid, V, radiate, or arcuate)		
		Dorsal intercarpal		

(From Taleisnik,[5] with permission.)

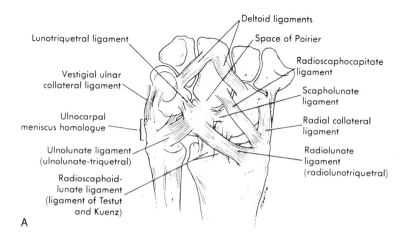

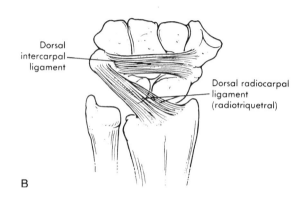

Figure 11–3. (A) Palmar wrist ligaments; (B) dorsal wrist ligaments. (From Strickland,[1] with permission.)

ligaments originate at the triquetrum and insert onto the trapezium and trapezoid. The volar one has been referred to as the *deltoid* or V *ligament*. It attaches to the neck of the capitate and fans out proximally to insert onto the scaphoid laterally and the triquetrum medially. Some fibers may or may not be present between the capitate and the lunate.[2,5]

Arthrokinematics

In 1919, Navarro proposed the concept of a *columnar* or vertical wrist to explain its function and the relationship between the carpals. The vertical column was composed of the lunate, capitate, and hamate. The scaphoid, trapezium, and trapezoid belonged to the lateral column, and the triquetrum and pisiform made up the medial column. In 1988, Taleisnik[5] also addressed the importance of considering the wrist in this manner but modified Navarro's theory somewhat by including the entire distal row and the lunate in the central column, while the scaphoid and the triquetrum were the lateral and medial columns, respectively. Sennwald[6] disputes Taleisnik's theory, for he argues that, based on the work of other authors and on cadaver studies, there is no connection between the lunate and the capitate. All authors do agree, however, that the distal row acts as a single unit, for the bones in that row are all held together by intercarpal ligaments.[5,6]

Wrist flexion and extension occur at both the radiocarpal and intercarpal rows. Most flexion occurs at the midcarpal row, and most extension takes place at the radiocarpal joint. During extension, the radiocapitate ligament tightens and causes the scaphoid and capitate to dorsiflex. The lunate dorsiflexes as well, although the arc of motion of the scaphoid is greater than the arc of motion of the lunate. During flexion, the lunate rotates 30 degrees and the scaphoid rotates 60 degrees. In terms of radial and ulnar deviation, Flatt et al.[7] used cadavers and live subjects to determine that radial deviation occurs primarily at the intercarpal joint and that ulna deviation occurs at both the radiocarpal and intercarpal joints. During radial deviation, the scaphoid palmar flexes to avoid the radial styloid tuberosity. The lunate is brought dorsally and also becomes slightly palmar flexed. During ulnar deviation, the scaphoid appears elongated, for its proximal pole glides in a palmar direction. The lunate also rotates dorsally and radially. The triquetrum glides distally onto the slope of the hamate.[4,6–8]

Hand

The bones of the hand form three arches. Two are transversely oriented and one is longitudinally oriented. The center of the transverse proximal arch is the capitate, and the distal transverse arch passes through the metacarpal heads and is the more mobile of the two. The transverse arches are connected by the rigid portion of the longitudinal arch, which includes the second and third fingers, the second and third metacarpals, and the central carpus.

Metacarpophalangeal Joints

The metacarpophalangeal (MP) joints are diarthroidal, with three planes of motion: flexion and extension, abduction and adduction, and circumduction. The heads of the metacarpals are asymmetric, with a greater slope on the radial aspect than on the ulnar aspect. The collateral ligaments (Fig. 11–4) arise from the dorsolateral aspect of the metacarpal heads and insert onto the palmar lateral aspect of the proximal phalanx. These ligaments are not true collateral ligaments, as they do not cross directly over the joint axis. The ligaments are composed of two bundles. The more central (cord) portion inserts directly into the proximal phalanx. The more palmar (accessory) portion inserts into the volar plate. The collateral ligaments are lax when the MP joint is in extension and tighten in flexion as they are stretched over the heads of the metacarpals. As a result, the MP joints have little joint play in flexion but can abduct and adduct when the MP joints are in extension. The volar plate is loosely attached

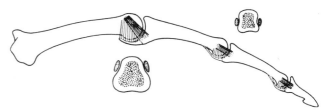

Figure 11–5. The collateral ligaments at the MP joints are lateral, oblique ligaments. In contrast, the lateral ligaments of the IP joints are true collateral ligaments and are under almost equal tension during both flexion and extension. (From Beasley,[12] with permission.)

to the metacarpal and slides proximally during flexion. It is strongly attached to the proximal phalanx. This arrangement, along with the position of the collateral ligaments, allows increased extension and circumduction at the MP joints. The volar plates of fingers two through five are connected by the transverse metacarpal ligament.[1,9]

Interphalangeal Joints

The interphalangeal (IP) joints are hinge joints with 1 degree of freedom for flexion and extension. The heads of the proximal and middle phalanges are convex, and the bases of the middle and distal phalanges are concave. The collateral ligaments at the IP joints are true collateral ligaments (Fig. 11–5). They pass directly through the axis of rotation as they cross the joint and maintain their tension during both flexion and extension. This contributes to increased lateral stability at the IP joints. The collateral ligaments at the proximal interphalangeal (PIP) joint and distal interphalangeal (DIP) joint also have a cord and an accessory portion that insert into the volar plate and phalanx. However, at the DIP joint, these bundles can overlap as much as one-third, which results in increased stability at the DIP joint compared with the PIP joint. The volar plate attachment at the PIP joint is a bony one. It is securely attached at its proximal end by the check-rein ligaments, which minimize PIP joint hyperextension. At the DIP joint, the volar plate insertion is a membranous one that allows for some hyperextension. The transverse retinacular ligament links the lateral bands from either side of the finger and the volar plate to prevent dorsal dislocation.[1,9]

Thumb

The carpometacarpal (CMC) joint of the thumb is a saddle joint with three planes of motion. The base of the first metacarpal is concave in the anteroposterior plane and convex in the lateral plane. There are four ligaments that provide stability at the joint. Three are capsular ligaments and are oblique in orientation. These include the anterior oblique, dorsoradial, and posterior oblique ligaments. The anterior oblique is the strongest and connects the first metacarpal and trapezium. It is lax during flexion

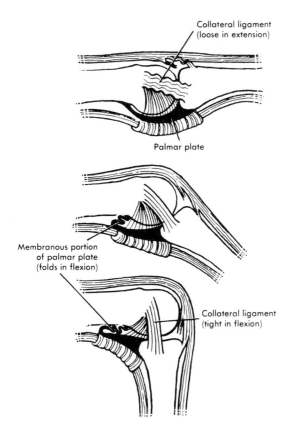

Figure 11–4. At the MP joint level, the collateral ligaments are loose in extension but become tightened in flexion. The proximal membranous portion of the palmar plate moves proximally to accommodate for flexion. (From Strickland,[1] with permission.)

and taut during extension. The posterior oblique is weaker, which results in decreased stability on the dorsal aspect of the joint. The extracapsular or Y ligament arises from the volar aspect of the trapezium, bifurcates, and attaches to the bases of the first and second metacarpals. It helps maintain the first metacarpal on the trapezium. It is also referred to as the *intermetacarpal ligament*.[1,10]

■ Muscles and Tendons

Muscles acting on the wrist and hand are classified as either extrinsic (the muscle belly is in the forearm) or intrinsic (the muscle belly is within the hand).

Extrinsic Flexors

The extrinsic flexors form a prominent mass of three layers on the medial side of the upper part of the forearm. The superficial layer is composed of the pronator teres (PT), FCR, FCU, and palmaris longus (PL). The FCR is the main wrist flexor and inserts onto the base of the third metacarpal. It is innervated by the median nerve. The FCU inserts onto the pisiform and fifth metacarpal. It assists with wrist flexion but is primarily an ulnar deviator of the wrist. It is innervated by the ulnar nerve. The PL is innervated by the median nerve and inserts into the palmar fascia. It is absent in 10 to 15 percent of the population. The middle layer in the forearm is composed of the individual muscle bellies of the flexor digitorum sublimis (FDS). This unique arrangement allows for individual PIP joint flexion for which it is responsible. The FDS is also innervated by the median nerve. The muscle belly of the flexor digitorum profundus (FDP) lies deep to the FDS in the forearm and flexes the DIP joints. The FDP tendons of the third, fourth, and fifth fingers are interconnected tendons with one muscle belly, which prohibits independent DIP joint flexion in those fingers. Independent DIP joint flexion of the index finger, however, is possible. At the level of the distal palmar crease, the tendons of the FDS and FDP to each finger enter a fibrous digital sheath, which extends from the palmar ligament of the MP joint to the insertion of the FDP into the base of the distal phalanx. The tendon sheaths protect the tendons and provide a smooth gliding surface by virtue of their synovial lining, nourish them through synovial diffusion, and maintain the tendons close to the bones and joint for increased efficiency. In the distal palm, the tendon of the FDS bifurcates, and the FDP passes through it to become superficial. The FDS then inserts onto the margins of the middle phalanx. The ulnar two tendons of the FDP are innervated by the ulnar nerve, whereas the radial two tendons are innervated by the median nerve. There is a pulley system consisting of five sturdy annular pulleys (A1–A5) that hold the flexor sheaths close to the bone and three cruciate pulleys, which are thin and pliable to permit flexibility of the tendon sheath (Fig.

11–6). The flexor pollicis longus (FPL) also lies in the deep layer on the forearm. It inserts onto the distal phalanx of the thumb and flexes the IP joint (and, to some extent, the MP joint) of the thumb. It is innervated by the median nerve.[9–11]

Extrinsic Extensors

The extrinsic extensors originate from the lateral epicondyle and dorsum of the forearm and include the extensor carpi radialis brevis (ECRB), extensor carpi radialis longus (ECRL), extensor carpi ulnaris (ECU), extensor digitorum communis (EDC), and extensor digiti minimi (EDM). In the forearm and dorsum of the hand, the muscles and their tendons lie in loose tissue. At the wrist, the extensors are held in place by the extensor retinaculum, which forms six compartments through which the extensor tendons travel (Fig. 11–7). The first compartment lies along the radial styloid process and contains the abductor pollicis longus (APL) and extensor pollicis brevis (EPB). The APL originates from the proximal part of the ulna, the interosseous membrane, and the middle one-third of the radius and inserts onto the first metacarpal. It radially abducts the first metacarpal and assists with radial deviation. The EPB originates from the interosseous membrane and the dorsum of the radius and inserts into the proximal phalanx. It extends the MP joint. This is the compartment involved in de Quervain syndrome. The second compartment contains the tendon of the ECRL and ECRB. The ECRB inserts centrally at the base of the third metacarpal and is the primary wrist extensor. The ECRL inserts onto the second metacarpal and contributes minimally to wrist extension and more to radial deviation. The third compartment houses the extensor pollicis longus (EPL) tendon, which takes a 45 degree turn at Lister's tubercle and inserts onto the distal phalanx of the thumb. It is responsible for thumb IP joint exten-

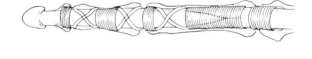

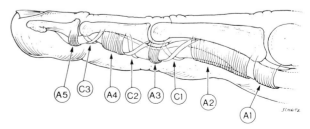

Figure 11–6. There are five annular (A) and three cruciate (C) pulleys. A2 and A4 are the largest and most important. (From Cannon et al.,[92] with permission.)

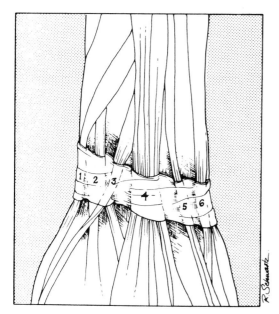

Figure 11-7. The extensor retinaculum at the wrist forms a roof over the six extensor compartments. (From Jupiter,[91] with permission.)

and continues distally as the central slip to insert into the base of the middle phalanx. Thus, it is a primary extensor of the MP joint. It gives off fibers to the intrinsic tendons before its insertion on the middle phalanx to form the lateral bands that extend distally and insert onto the base of the distal phalanx. The lateral bands are responsible for IP joint extension. The EI lies on the ulnar aspect of the EDC and is responsible for independent extension of the index finger. The EDM is usually composed of two or three separate tendon slips and is housed in the fifth dorsal compartment. It inserts into the dorsal hood of the fifth finger. It is a primary extensor of the fifth finger (responsible for independent extension of the fifth finger) and assists with abduction. The tendon of the ECU passes through the sixth dorsal compartment and inserts onto the fifth metacarpal.[9-11]

Intrinsics

The intrinsic muscle group consists of muscles that are associated with highly coordinated and refined movements. The group consists of the thenar, hypothenar, and interossei-lumbrical muscles.

Thenar Muscles

There are four thenar muscles, which are divided into two groups, lateral and medial, depending on their position relative to the FPL tendon (Fig. 11-8). The three muscles to the lateral side are all innervated by the median nerve and include the opponens pollicis (Opp), flexor pollicis brevis (FPB), and abductor pollicis brevis (APB). These muscles are involved in fine positioning of the thumb and

sion but does exert some influence at the MP joint as well. The fourth compartment holds the tendons of the EDC and extensor indicis (EI). The EDC arises from the lateral epicondyle, and the EI arises from the dorsum of the ulna. The EDC consists of a series of tendons with a common muscle belly. The tendons are interconnected on the back of the hand, and as a result, no one MP joint can extend independently of the others. The tendon inserts into the extensor aponeurosis over the MP joint

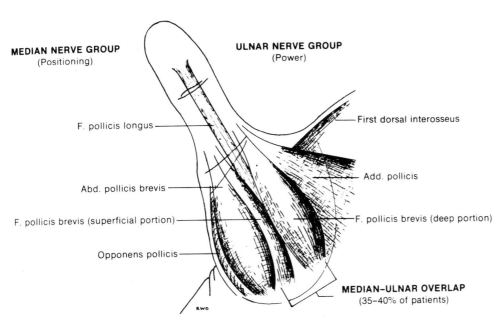

Figure 11-8. There are three muscle groups in the thumb that lie lateral to the FPL tendon and two groups that lie medial to it. (From Beasley,[12] with permission.)

coordinated movement. The APB is the most superficial. It arises from the scaphoid, trapezium, and transverse carpal ligament and inserts into the radial aspect of the proximal phalanx. It is responsible for palmar abduction and slight MP joint flexion and assists with IP joint extension, as some of its fibers insert into the extensor mechanism. The FPB has a superficial head located lateral to the FPL tendon and a deep head located medial to it. The lateral head originates from the transverse carpal ligament and trapezium and inserts into the proximal phalanx. It is primarily an MP joint flexor. The Opp originates from the transverse carpal ligament and trapezium and inserts along the radial side of the first metacarpal. It rotates the thumb, allowing the thumb pad to come in contact with the pad of the index. The two muscles to the ulnar side of the FPL tendon give the thumb its strength and are innervated by the ulnar nerve. The deep head of the FPB originates from the floor/wall of the carpal tunnel and one or more of the carpal bones of the distal row and inserts into the base of the proximal phalanx. It flexes the and assists with abduction and opposition. The adductor pollicis (Add) has a dual origin. One head (transverse) arises from the palmar border of the third metacarpal, and the other head (oblique) arises from the capitate, trapezoid, trapezium, and the bases of the first, second, and third metacarpals. Both heads insert into the proximal phalanx and are responsible for thumb adduction.[11,12]

Hypothenar Muscles

The three hypothenar muscles are innervated by the ulnar nerve and provide independent movement to the fifth finger. The AbDM arises from the pisiform and pisohamate ligament and inserts into the base of the proximal phalanx. Like its counterpart in the thumb (APB), it also sends some fibers to the extensor mechanism. As a result, it assists with extension in addition to abducting and flexing the fifth finger. The FDM arises from the hamate and transverse carpal ligament and inserts into the proximal phalanx. It flexes the MP joint. The OppDM originates from the hamate, traverses the carpal ligament, and inserts along the ulnar border of the fifth metacarpal. It allows one to bring the pad of the fifth finger into opposition.[11,12]

Interossei-Lumbrical Muscles

Three volar and four dorsal interossei are primarily responsible for adduction and abduction, respectively. Both groups have similar origins from adjacent metacarpals, pass volar to the axis of rotation at the MP joint (thus assisting with MP joint flexion), and insert into the lateral aspect of the proximal phalanx. They then continue distally, cross the PIP joint dorsal to the axis of rotation, join the fibers from the other side of the finger to form

the lateral bands, and insert into the base of the distal phalanx (Fig. 11–9). All the interossei are innervated by the ulnar nerve and are responsible for IP joint extension.[9–11]

The lumbricals originate from the tendons of the FDP. They pass radially and volarly to the MP joint and insert into the extensor mechanism. Like the interossei, they are responsible for MP joint flexion and IP joint extension. The lumbricals to the index and long fingers are innervated by the median nerve, and those to the ring and small fingers are innervated by the ulnar nerve.[10,11]

Thus, digital extension is a combination of extrinsic and intrinsic function (Fig. 11–10). At the MP joint, extension is purely an extrinsic function (EDC). At the PIP joint, it is a combination; when the MP joints are in flexion, the EDC is the primary extensor, but the intrinsics assist. If the MP joints are held in extension, the EDC is exerting all its force at the MP joint, and as a result, IP joint extension is purely a function of the interossei and lumbricals. DIP joint extension is purely an intrinsic function. A third contributor to IP joint extension is Landsmeer's ligament, which arises on the surface of the flexor sheath along the proximal phalanx, passes volar to the axis of rotation at the PIP, and inserts into the extensor mechanism distally.[9–11]

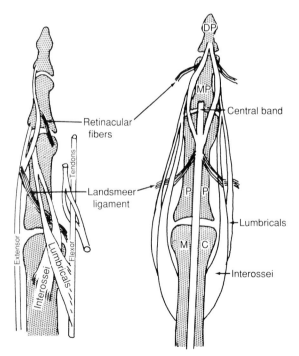

Figure 11–9. Extensor apparatus of the fingers. The EDG tendon inserts into the middle phalanx as the central band. Before that, it sends fibers into the lateral bands on each side of the finger that converge over the middle phalanx and insert onto the dorsal aspect of the distal phalanx. (From Cailliet,[21] with permission.)

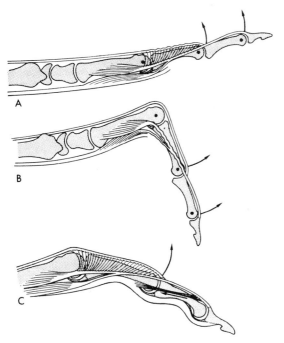

Figure 11–10. The IP joints have a dual extensor mechanism. (A) MP extension makes the extrinsic extensor mechanism redundant and less effective for IP extension while it reciprocally tightens and increases efficiency of the intrinsic system for IP extension. (B) MP flexion renders the intrinsic system inefficient for IP extension but tightens the extrinsic system to improve its efficiency. (C) A third IP extensor system is through the oblique retinacular ligament, which passes volar to the axis of rotation of the proximal phalangeal joint and thus is tightened by extension of this joint. Because it inserts into the extensor mechanism distally, tightening the ligament will assist with distal phalangeal extension. (From Beasley,[12] with permission.)

■ Nerves

The motor and sensory function of the wrist and hand is supplied by the median, ulnar, and radial nerves (Fig. 11–11).

Median Nerve

The median nerve is known as the *precision nerve.* It enters the forearm and innervates the pronator teres (PT) as it passes between its two heads. It gives off a branch, the anterior interosseous, which travels distally along the interosseous membrane and innervates the FPL, the first and second profundus, and the pronator quadratus. The nerve becomes superficial in the distal forearm after innervating the FDS and FCR and then enters the palm through the carpal tunnel. After passing through the carpal tunnel, the nerve typically splits into a sensory and a motor branch. The motor branch, however, can originate at different points along the median nerve, including in the forearm, in the carpal tunnel, or distal to the carpal tunnel. It continues distally to innervate the thenar muscles and the first and second lumbricals. The sensory branch provides sensation to the palmar surface of the palm and the lateral three and one-half fingers.[4,9–11]

Ulnar Nerve

The ulnar nerve is known as the *power nerve.* After passing through the cubital tunnel, it innervates the FCU and the third and fourth FDPs. It becomes superficial at the wrist and enters the hand through Guyon's canal. At that point, it divides into a sensory and a motor branch. The sensory branch is superficial and supplies sensation to the small finger and medial aspect of the ring finger. The motor branch innervates the hypothenar muscles and then continues deep and distal to innervate the interossei, the third and fourth lumbricals, the deep head of the FPB, and the Add.[4,9–11]

Often, innervation to the deep and superficial heads of the FPB varies from one person to the next. The deep head of the FPB may be innervated by the median nerve, and the superficial head may be innervated by the ulnar nerve.

Radial Nerve

The radial nerve is considered a preparatory nerve, for it controls wrist extension for positioning and stabilizing the hand. The digital extensors open the thumb and fingers in preparation for grasping or manipulating an object. The nerve enters the forearm and penetrates the two heads of the supinator at the arcade of Frohse after supplying a motor branch to the brachioradialis, ECRL, and ECRB. At this point, the nerve branches into a sensory branch, which travels down the radial aspect of the forearm and

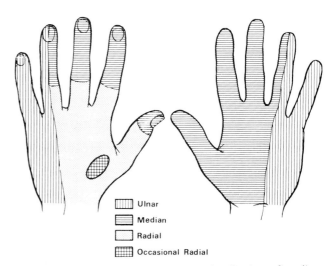

Figure 11–11. The normal cutaneous distribution of median, ulnar, and radial nerves. (From Salter,[15] with permission.)

supplies sensation to the radial aspect of the dorsum of the hand. The motor branch continues as the posterior interosseous to innervate the supinator, EDC, ECU, EI, EDM, EPL, EPB, and APL.[4,9-11]

Vascular Supply

Arterial System

The vascular supply to the wrist and hand is provided by the radial, ulnar, and common interosseous arteries. The last artery originates in the proximal forearm at the ulnar artery. It branches into an anterior portion, which in turn divides into a volar and a dorsal portion and a posterior portion. The volar branch of the anterior branch travels distally and joins with a small branch of the radial artery to form the transverse palmar carpal arch. The dorsal portion of the anterior interosseous artery supplies the dorsum of the wrist. It joins the posterior branch of the interosseous artery to supply the back of the hand through the dorsal carpal plexus, which also accepts a small branch from the radial artery. The ulnar artery arrives at the wrist along with the ulnar nerve. It divides into a large branch that forms the superficial palmar branch with a small branch from the radial artery. This lies directly deep to the palmar aponeurosis. This is the largest of the arterial arches. The superficial palmar arch gives off common palmar digital branches to the medial one and one-half fingers that bifurcate and continue along the sides of the fingers as radial and ulnar digital arteries. The radial artery enters the wrist and sends a small branch to join with the larger branch of the ulnar artery to form the superficial palmar branch, while the main portion of the radial artery joins with a smaller portion of the ulnar artery to form the deep palmar arch. The deep palmar arch supplies the lateral one and one-half fingers. Opposite each IP joint, each digital artery gives off a branch that passes under the strong attachment of the proximal end of the volar plate, joins its counterpart from the opposite side of the finger within the flexor sheath, and forms the vincula artery. This artery principally feeds the dorsal portions of the flexor tendons, with only a few branches reaching the anterior half of the tendon.[5,11,12]

Venous System

The hand is drained by two sets of veins. The superficial portion carries the greatest volume of blood and is best developed on the dorsum of the hand. This plexus drains into the cephalic and basilica veins. The small, deeper veins empty into the median antebrachial vein.[9]

Skin/Subcutaneous Fascia

Flexor Retinaculum

The flexor retinaculum (transverse carpal ligament) forms the roof of the carpal tunnel. Radially, it attaches to the trapezium and scaphoid, and medially, it attaches to the pisiform and hook of the hamate. Its function is to maintain the mechanical advantage of the finger flexors by preventing bowstringing.[2,11]

Extensor Retinaculum

The extensor retinaculum is a continuation of the deep fascia of the forearm. Over the dorsum of the hand, it has six septa, which form the six compartments through which the extensor tendons pass.[11]

Palmar Aponeurosis

The palmar aponeurosis is the continuation of the PL tendon. If the PL is absent, the fascia will not extend into the forearm. At the proximal palm, the fibers extend into the fingers and attach to the flexor sheath. The aponeurosis protects the underlying neurovascular and tendon structures. It fuses with the deep fascia at its medial and ulnar borders.[1,9,11]

Skin

The skin on the palmar aspect of the hand is highly specialized and thick. Papillary ridges are present but are best developed at the fingertips to increase friction for stable grasp. The skin on the palmar aspect of the hand is inelastic, as it is firmly attached to the underlying skeleton by many anchoring fibers. Its many sensory nerve fibers allow increased function of the hand based on a high level of sensory feedback. The skin on the back of the hand has few connecting fibers linking it to the underlying structure and is therefore more mobile. This is why swelling is so often more obvious on the back of the hand.[1,9]

Evaluation of the Wrist and Hand

The ultimate goal of rehabilitation is to restore optimal function in the minimal amount of time. A successful rehabilitation program is dependent on a selective treatment plan based on information obtained from the initial evaluation and periodic reassessments to evaluate changes. A sound knowledge of hand and wrist anatomy, as described, is a prerequisite to performing an informative and practical evaluation. The components of an evaluation (Table 11–2) consist of subjective and objective data.

History

The initial part of an evaluation is the history. It contains the patient's age, sex, handedness, occupation, and avocation and the time, description, and mechanism of injury.

□□□□□□ □ □

Table 11-2. Summary of Evaluation of the Hand and Wrist

History	
Patient profile	Age, sex, race, hand dominance, occupation, avocation, current work status, medical history
Problem profile	Date of onset, location, mechanism of injury
Medical treatment	Medications, diagnostic tests, physical therapy, surgeries, splinting
Pain profile	Type, location, frequency, duration, progression, what alleviates, what aggravates, analog scale
General observation	
Spontaneity of movement	Ease of use, substitutions
Asymmetry	Comparisons with noninvolved side
Gross deformity	Congenital, acquired
Abnormal posture	Protective, acquired
Muscle atrophy	Location
Upper extremity screening	
Cervical	Pain, mobility
Shoulder	Pain, mobility
Elbow	Pain, mobility
Inspection of the hand and wrist	
Skin	Color, moisture, nodules, lumps, creases, hair pattern
Wounds	Location, appearance, size, drainage
Nails	Appearance, alignment
Edema	Location
Scars	Location, appearance, size
Atrophy	Finger pulps, muscle
Digits	Absence, increased, amputation
Deformity	Congenital, acquired
Palpation	
Skin	Temperature, nodules, moisture mobility, contractures
Osseous structures	Tenderness of bone or ligaments, bumps
Muscle and tendons	Tenderness, nodules
Range of motion	
Active	Functional, goniometric, comparison with other side
Passive	Hypermobility, hypomobility, pain, end-feel
Accessory	Limitation, pain
Strength	
Functional	Grip, pinch
Muscle testing	Weakness, substitution
Isokinetic	Power, comparison with other side
Vascular	
Edema	Volumetric, circumferential measurement
Capillary refill	Quality
Arterial patency	Allen's test (wrist, digital)
Sensibility	
Localizing area	Tinel sign, mapping
Qualifying tests	Threshold, functional, objective
Standardized and functional tests	
Computerized evaluation	Grip, pinch, range of motion, recording sensibility, topographic data, computes impairment ratings, exercise functions
Work simulation	BTE, Lido work set
Dexterity and coordination	Different tests available, comparative norms
Special tests	

Abbreviation: BTE, Baltimore Therapeutic Equipment Company.

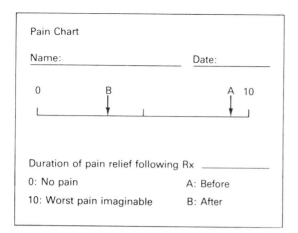

Pain Chart

Name: _____   Date: _____

```
0              B                        A    10
L_____|_____L
               ↓                        ↓
```

Duration of pain relief following Rx _____

0: No pain   A: Before
10: Worst pain imaginable   B: After

Figure 11–12. Pain chart. The degree of pain is measured by the patient on a visual analog 0–10 scale; 10 is the worst imaginable pain. (From Salter,[15] with permission.)

The history contains medical information from the referring physician including surgical procedures and their respective dates and any course of treatment, such as physical therapy and medications. This information is fairly straightforward if the problem is the result of macrotrauma such as a crush injury, laceration, or amputation; however, in cases of cumulative or repetitive trauma disorders, the subjective report becomes the main source of information before the examination. It is imperative that the evaluator listen to the patient and direct the patient through a series of nonsuggestive questions to prevent bias and ensure patient confidence and trust.

When and where did the problem begin? Was it sudden or did it have a gradual onset? What is the main problem? If the chief complaint is pain, questions are directed to define it; the patient is asked to localize the pain, describe when it occurs, and define its duration and intensity. What alleviates it? What aggravates the pain?

Has it changed since the initial onset? How does it affect the patient's work, activities of daily living (ADL), or recreational activities? Various visual, numerical, and descriptive methods of pain assessment such as the McGill pain questionnaire[13–15] are excellent means of attempting to objectify pain (Fig. 11–12). The clinician's choice may be influenced by the amount of time available to administer the test.

General Observation

While taking the history, the therapist should be observing the patient for any abnormalities of movement of the upper extremity. It is also important to observe for asymmetry, atrophy, and deformity. Inspect for abnormal posturing. Abnormal posturing could be secondary to pain and apprehension or could be related to bony or soft tissue injury (Fig. 11–13).

Upper Extremity Screening

Before the definitive hand and wrist evaluation is performed, the therapist needs to ensure that the more proximal structures are not the primary source of the problem or have not been secondarily involved. Many conditions that originate in the cervical area, shoulder, or elbow can manifest themselves in more distal structures. Cervical radiculopathy, brachial plexus injuries, myofacial pain, and systemic arthritic conditions are some examples.[16,17] An abbreviated examination of the cervical region, shoulder, and elbow[17] is performed to assess for limited range of motion, weakness, and/or localized or radicular pain. Based on findings from the history and the general observation, the screening may be limited to the patient's denying any problems in these areas when questioned. However, some patients may not be cognizant of involvement of the more proximal structures. A frozen shoulder is too

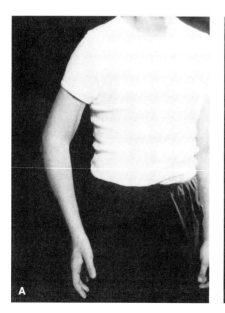

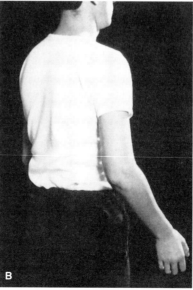

Figure 11–13. Abnormal posture of the hand. Note the increased supination and wrist extension and the decreased finger and thumb flexion as a result of a high median and ulnar nerve lesion. (From Salter,[15] with permission.)

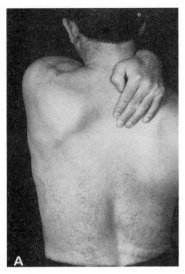
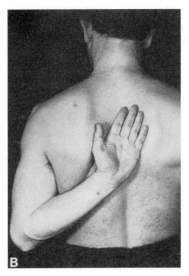
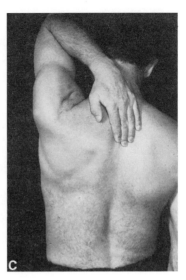

Figure 11–14. The motion of the shoulder can be quickly checked by asking the patient to touch the shoulder between the shoulder blades (A) over the contralateral shoulder, which is performed by flexion and adduction; (B) under the ipsilateral axilla, which demonstrates extension and internal rotation; and (C) over the ipsilateral shoulder, which demonstrates abduction and external rotation. (From Lister,[18] with permission.)

often a secondary complication of a wrist or hand fracture because the patient may have protectively held the hand close to the body during the immobilization period. With the patient performing functional movements of the cervical area, the shoulder,[18,19] (Fig. 11–14), and then the elbow, any pain, weakness, and limited range of motion will surface. Any positive findings warrant a complete, thorough assessment of the respective areas (refer to Chapters 5–10 for descriptions).

Inspection

The next important part of the evaluation is a more definitive inspection of the hand and wrist areas. The normal topography of the hand and wrist (Figs. 11–15 and 11–16) consists of anatomically related wrinkles, creases, mountains, and valleys. The hand has a resting "attitude" (Fig. 11–17) that reflects the balance of osseous support and muscle tone.[18–20] Edema, soft tissue or nerve injury, scarring, or pain can cause changes in normal posturing and ultimately affect hand function, whether temporary

Figure 11–15. Surface anatomy of the hand. (From American Society for Surgery of the Hand,[17] with permission.)

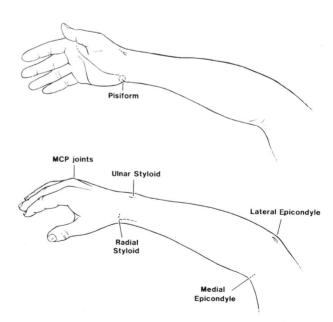

Figure 11–16. Bony prominences of the hand and forearm. (From Cannon et al.,[93] with permission.)

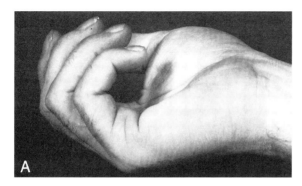

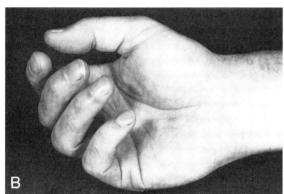

Figure 11–17. (A) A completely relaxed hand in the fully supinated position lies with the wrist in approximately 30 degrees of dorsal flexion and with a "cascade" of flexion in the fingers increasing from the index finger to a maximum at the joints of the small finger. (B) The thumb lies gently flexed so that its pulp lies in close approximation to that of the index finger. (From Lister,[18] with permission.)

or permanent. For example, a patient with a history of severe ulnar nerve compression at the wrist presents with hypothenar atrophy, "clawing" of the ulnar digits, and loss of the longitudinal arch (Fig. 11–18). Laceration of the flexor tendons of a finger clinically presents in an abnormal extension "stance" posture (Fig. 11–19). A droopy DIP joint (extensor lag) resulting from trauma could indicate a mallet finger[17-21] caused by rupture of the terminal extensor tendon (Fig. 11–20). Wrist drop (Fig. 11–21) is suspicious of radial nerve palsy.[14] The

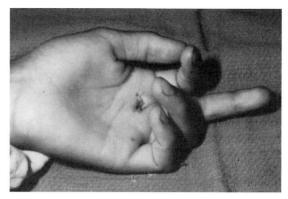

Figure 11–19. The posture of the middle finger in this anesthetized hand reveals division of both flexor tendons to that digit. (From Lister,[18] with permission.)

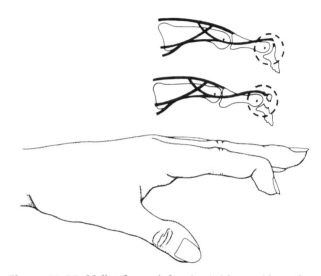

Figure 11–20. Mallet finger deformity (with or without fracture). (From American Society for Surgery of the Hand,[17] with permission.)

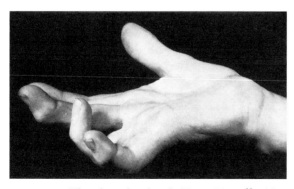

Figure 11–18. The ulnar claw hand. (From Lister,[18] with permission.)

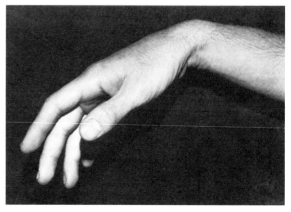

Figure 11–21. Wrist drop. The patient is unable to actively extend the wrist and finger MP joints. (From Lister,[18] with permission.)

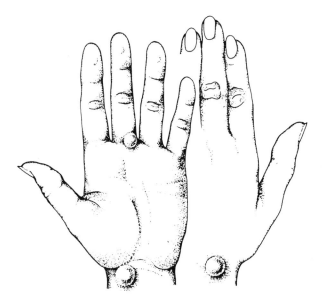

Figure 11–22. Ganglion cyst of the hand. (From American Society for Surgery of the Hand,[17] with permission.)

importance of good observation skills cannot be overemphasized.

As stated earlier, the dorsal skin surface of the hand is mobile and thin compared with the palmar surface, which is thick, glabrous, and irregular.[20] Inspect both surfaces for changes in skin texture, color, sweat patterns, callus formation, lumps, nodules, and masses. Record abnormal findings. Ganglion cysts are the most common soft tissue masses of the hand[17] (Fig. 11–22) and are commonly found on the dorsal or volar surfaces of the wrist and hand.

Also inspect the hand for loss of wrinkles or abnormal hair growth. Document the presence of any scars, their location and appearance, location of edema, or any open wounds. Edema with erythema and increased temperature are signs of inflammation or infection.[21] Paronychia, felon, and flexor tendon sheath infections are some common examples[17-21] (Fig. 11–23). A drawing of the hand to record abnormal findings is a valuable tool during initial and future reevaluations.

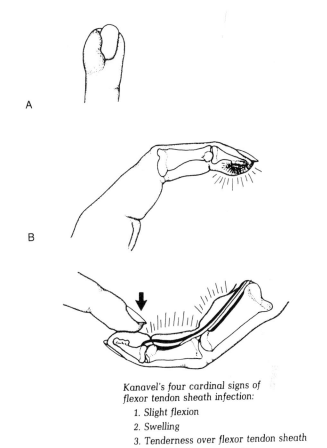

Kanavel's four cardinal signs of flexor tendon sheath infection:
1. *Slight flexion*
2. *Swelling*
3. *Tenderness over flexor tendon sheath*
4. *Pain on passive extension*

Figure 11–23. (A) Paronychia, (B) felon, (C) flexor tendon sheath infection. (From American Society for Surgery of the Hand,[17] with permission.)

Check the nails for abnormalities in appearance. Nail changes[22] can reflect systemic problems. Check for muscle atrophy and absent or extra digits. A thorough history and detailed inspection can often give clues to the problem even before other aspects of the evaluation are completed. A hypersensitive, painful, shiny, discolored, edematous hand 3 months after a Colles' fracture held in a protective posture may indicate the presence of reflex sympathetic dystrophy (Fig. 11–24).

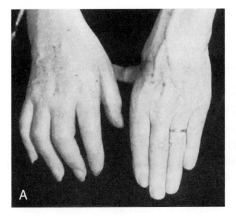
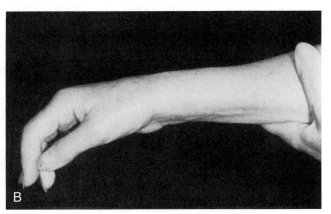

Figure 11–24. Reflex sympathetic dystrophy. (From Salter,[15] with permission.)

Palpation

Palpation often localizes the problem and usually supports the clinician's suspicions already created by the history and inspection. In the sequence of the examination, the problem site should be the last area addressed.[23,24]

The skin of the wrist and hand should be palpated for nodules, tenderness, and changes in temperature, moisture, or mobility. Palpate scars for sensitivity and mobility. Again, it is important to compare the noninvolved extremity. An old keloid scar located on the contralateral extremity should alert the clinician to the importance of early scar management and close monitoring of the scars on the involved extremity.

Palpate the forearm musculature for tenderness and trigger points. These muscles may refer pain to the wrist or hand[25] (Fig. 11–25).

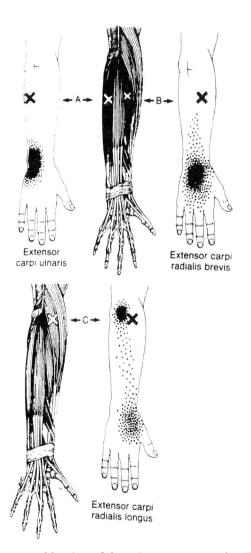

Figure 11–25. Mapping of the wrist extensor muscles (From Travell and Simons,[93] with permission.)

Most of the subcutaneous structures are palpable in the wrist and hand. The wrist is considered to be the "low back" of the upper extremity and warrants careful examination, especially when the patient presents with a general diagnosis of wrist pain. Hoppenfeld,[16] Beckenbaugh,[23] and Brown and Lichtman[24] suggested a methodic approach for examining the wrist, starting at the radial aspect, progressing dorsoulnarly, and ending at the volar radial side (Table 11–3).

Palpate the radial styloid and distal radius. A recent fracture or contusion will be tender. Next, palpate the anatomic snuffbox (Fig. 11–26). Tenderness in this area could indicate a navicular fracture[23,24] or a scapholunate ligamentous injury.

The first dorsal extensor compartment (EPB and APL) is palpable, as it forms the radial border of the snuffbox. Tenderness along the sheath is common with inflammatory disorders. Pain with active thumb flexion, tenderness at the radial styloid, and resistive thumb extension are usually indicative of stenosing tenosynovitis (de Quervain's tenosynovitis). A positive Finkelstein test may confirm this suspicion (Fig. 11–27). The test is performed by having the patient turn the thumb into the palm and then ulnarly deviate the wrist. Pain is elicited in the area of the radial styloid. In some very acute cases, thumb positioning alone can produce a positive test.[17,24,26]

The examination then moves distal to the snuffbox. Pressure is applied to the trapezium as the thumb is passively flexed. Pain in this area could signify ligamentous injury or, rarely, a fracture. Tenderness, capsular thickening, and painful axial compression of the first metacarpal bone indicate CMC arthrosis[17,24] (Fig. 11–28).

Next, palpate in the area of Lister's tubercle. At the radial aspect, the extensor carpi radialis and ECRB (second dorsal extensor compartment) are palpated for tenderness or swelling. They become prominent when the patient makes a tight fist. The EPL is palpable along the ulnar side of the radial tubercle as it courses distally and forms the ulna border of the anatomic snuffbox. Rupture of this tendon may occur secondary to a Colles' fracture, fatigue, or rheumatoid arthritis because of frictional forces at the tubercle during movements of the wrist and thumb. Manual muscle testing will confirm a rupture; however, with incorrect test positioning, the rupture may be missed because of substitution. The Add and the APB extend the IP joint of the thumb when the thumb is palmarly adducted.[24]

Palpable tenderness at the base of the second and third metacarpal bones may indicate ligamentous or bony injury. The Linsheid test can confirm instability: The metacarpal shafts are supported while force is applied in a palmar and dorsal direction at the metacarpal heads. A positive test produces pain in the CMC area.

Palpation of a fixed prominence at the second or third CMC joint may suggest a carpal boss (excess bone).

□□□□□ □ □ □

Table 11–3. Summary of Wrist Palpation

Wrist Area	Osseous Structures	Soft Tissues
Radial dorsal	Radial styloid Scaphoid Scaphotrapezial joint Trapezium First CMC joint	First dorsal extensor compartment (EPB and APL) Third dorsal extensor compartment (EPL)
Central dorsal	Lister's tubercle Scapholunate joint Lunate Capitate Base of 2nd and 3rd metacarpals CMC joints of index and long fingers	Second dorsal extensor compartment (ECRB and ECRL) Fourth dorsal extensor compartment (EDC) Fifth dorsal extensor compartment (EDM)
Ulnar dorsal	Ulnar styloid Distal radioulnar joint Triquetrum Hamate Base of 4th and 5th metacarpals	Triangular fibrocartilage complex Sixth dorsal extensor compartment (ECU)
Ulnar volar	Pisiform Hook of the hamate Triquetrum	FCU Ulnar nerve and artery (Guyon's canal)
Radial volar		Palmaris longus Carpal tunnel
	Tubercle of the trapezium Radial styloid	FCU Radial artery

Abbreviations: APL, abductor pollicis longus; CMC, carpometacarpal; ECRB, extensor carpi radialis brevis; ECRL, extensor carpi radialis longus; ECU, extensor carpi ulnaris; EDC, extensor digitorum communis; EDM, extensor digiti minimi; EPB, extensor pollicis brevis; EPL, extensor pollicis longus; FCU, flexor carpi ulnaris.
(Data from Hoppenfeld,[16] Beckenbaugh,[23] and Brown and Lichtman.[24])

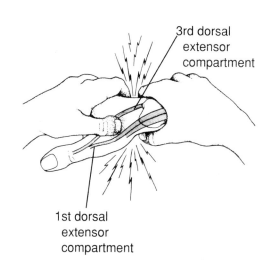

Figure 11–26. Fracture of the scaphoid with tenderness on deep palpation of the snuffbox area. (From American Society for Surgery of the Hand,[17] with permission.)

Associated ganglion cysts are common with carpal bosses.[26]

Next, the finger extensors (fourth dorsal extensor compartment) can be palpated on the dorsum of the wrist and along the dorsum of the metacarpals to their insertions distally.

The EI and the EDM tendons can be isolated and palpated by asking the patient to form the "hex" sign: With the long and ring fingers actively flexed, the index and little fingers are actively extended. Inflammatory conditions such as rheumatoid arthritis and peritendinitis make these structures tender to palpation and produce a boggy swelling. Next, palpate proximal to the third metacarpal within the sulcus of the capitate. Tenderness may indicate a fracture. Pain is referred to this area with scapholunate and triquetrolunate instability problems. Proximal to the sulcus is the lunate. With the wrist in flexion, the dorsal pole of the lunate becomes prominent. Tenderness in this area may be indicative of scapholnate ligamentous injury, fracture, ganglion cyst, or Kienbock's disease (avascular necrosis of the lunate).[24,26]

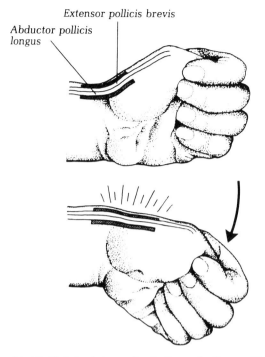

Extensor pollicis brevis

Abductor pollicis longus

Figure 11–27. Finkelstein's test for de Quervain disease. (From American Society for Surgery of the Hand,[17] with permission.)

these two bones, Guyon's tunnel, may be tender if pathology is present. Paresthesia produced with percussion in this area is indicative of ulnar nerve injury. Palpation of a pulsatile mass may indicate the presence of an aneurysm of the ulnar artery.[15,24] The ulnar artery is normally palpable just proximal to the pisiform.

The PL is palpable at the volar midwrist area. Check for tenderness. The carpal tunnel, which is located dorsal to the PL, may be tender. The most common pathology in that area is carpal tunnel syndrome. Percussion produces a positive median nerve Tinel's sign[23,24] (i.e., tingling in the area percussed, with radiation distally to the median innervated digits) (Fig. 11–29). Another test used to evaluate for carpal tunnel syndrome is Phalen's sign. Prolonged flexion of the wrist produces paresthesias in the median nerve distribution.

Moving radially, the tuberosity of the trapezium is palpable at the wrist crease and proximal to it, the tendon of the FCR longus. Tenderness of the tendon may be indicative of stenosing tenosynovitis. Just distal to the trapezial tuberosity, palpable tenderness may be the result of CMC ligamentous injury.[23,24,26] Lastly, the radial artery is palpated between the FCU and the radial styloid. Vascular tests are addressed later.

Just ulnar to the lunate, the triquetrum is palpable. As with the other carpal bones, tenderness may denote fracture or ligamentous injury.

Moving proximally, the distal radioulnar joint is palpable. Sensitivity at this joint may indicate fracture or ligamentous injury and pain, and clicking may be elicited with forearm movements.

Continuing ulnarly, the ulnar styloid is palpated. Often there is a fracture here in association with a Colles' fracture.[16] The ECU may be tender because of distal radioulnar arthritis. It can be the first and only clinical sign of rheumatoid arthritis.[24–27] Trauma or disease may produce a tear or rupture of the ECU; pain and clicking or snapping are common.[16,23]

Tenderness at the base of the fourth and fifth CMC joints may indicate fracture or ligamentous injury of the hamate. A similar Luscheid-type test is administered to confirm the suspicion of pathology at the CMC joints described.

Tenderness in the sulcus distal to the ulna between the ECU and FCU could denote triquetral injury and injury to the triangular fibrocartilage complex.[24]

Moving ulnarly and volarly, the pisiform is prominent at the wrist crease, and point tenderness could indicate fracture of the pisiform or triquetrum.

The FCU tendon is localized just proximal to the pisiform. Like other soft tissues, it can be tender in inflammatory conditions such as calcific tendinitis.[16]

The hook of the hamate is located just ulnar to the thenar crease and radial to the pisiform. Tenderness of the hamate may indicate a fracture. The area between

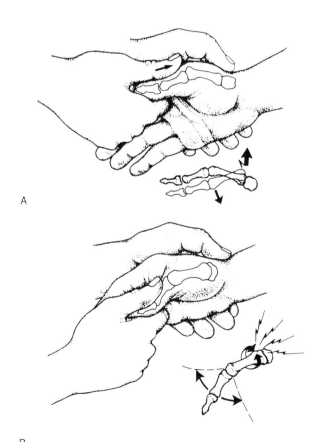

A

B

Figure 11–28. (A) Axial compression-adduction test; (B) axial compression and rotation test. (From American Society for Surgery of the Hand,[17] with permission.)

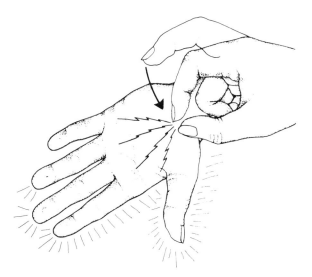

Figure 11–29. Tinel's test. (From American Society for Surgery of the Hand,[17] with permission.)

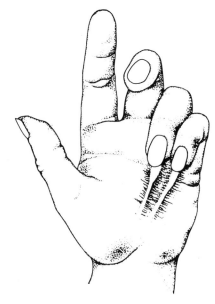

Figure 11–31. Dupuytren's contracture. (From American Society for Surgery of the Hand,[17] with permission.)

The examination then progresses from the wrist to the hand. The thenar and hypothenar eminences are palpated for discomfort or trigger points. Also, the palmar fascia is palpated for tenderness or masses. A tender nodule in the area of the palmar crease (or MP joint flexion crease of the thumb), along with patient complaints of the digit "catching" with movement, may suggest flexor tenosynovitis or what is commonly referred to as *trigger finger* or *trigger thumb*, respectively (Fig. 11–30). A contracture of the palmar aponeurosis with insidious onset and no history of injury is suggestive of Dupuytren's contracture (Fig. 11–31). There is usually an associated flexion contracture of adjacent digits distal to the lesion.[17,18,24]

Each of the MP and IP joints of the digits should be palpated dorsally, volarly, radially, and ulnarly. Tender-

ness at these joints may raise the suspicion to capsular or ligamentous injury. An acute injury will usually have some associated swelling or instability, and the patient may be apprehensive about moving the affected joint (Fig. 11–32).

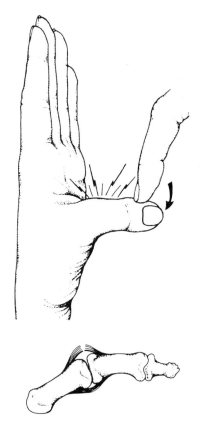

Figure 11–32. Rupture of the ulnar collateral ligament of the MP joint of the thumb. (From American Society for Surgery of the Hand,[17] with permission.)

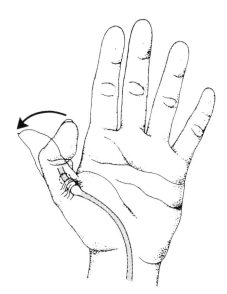

Figure 11–30. Trigger thumb. (From American Society for Surgery of the Hand,[17] with permission.)

Heberden's nodes (bony nodules), which appear on the dorsal and lateral areas of the DIP joints, are a common manifestation of osteoarthritis.[16,22] Bouchard's nodes (fusiform enlargement) at the level of the PIP joints dorsally are associated with rheumatoid arthritis and gastrectasis.[22]

Edema/Vascular Function

Edema is a common problem in hand injuries and can result in complications such as pain, stiffness, and disability. There are two popular methods for objectively measuring changes in hand size.[19,28,29] Circumferential measurements are performed at designated sites and recorded. The sites may vary, depending on the area of edema. It is important that tape placement be as consistent as possible from one session to another. Using anatomic creases is helpful. The other method is volumetric measurement (Fig. 11–33). A commercially available volumeter is filled with water to capacity and allowed to flow over until the spout stops dripping. The hand is immersed. The amount of water dispersed is collected in a receptacle, measured with a graduated cylinder, and recorded on a flow chart; the other hand is measured for comparison. It is suggested that both methods be used because each has its limitations.

The assessment of vascular function starts with inspection and palpation of the wrist and hand. Physical changes have already been observed and recorded. Besides these techniques, Allen's test (Fig. 11–34) is used to assess the patency of the radial and ulnar arteries at the wrist. Pressure is applied over the radial and ulnar arteries at the wrist volarly. The patient is asked to open and close the hand and then hold. The color of the palm changes. The pressure is released from the radial side, and the color of the palm should return to normal. This test is repeated for the ulnar artery. A similar test is used for the digital vessels. Capillary refill is assessed by pinching the finger

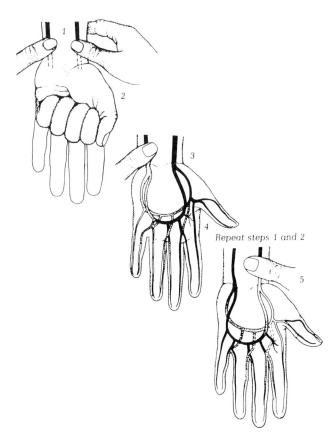

Repeat steps 1 and 2

Figure 11–34. Allen's test. (From American Society for Hand Surgery,[17] with permission.)

pulp or applying pressure over the nail, causing a blanching response. On release, the clinician monitors the quality of capillary refill, using a normal digit for comparison.

Cold intolerance testing can also be used to assess vascular function in patients with conditions such as Raynaud syndrome and reflex sympathetic dystrophy.

Range of Motion

The quantity and quality of movement can be assessed by measurement both actively and passively. Goniometric measurement is a reliable and reproducible method for recording joint motion.[20,21] Initial measurements should be recorded on a serial chart, along with follow-up recordings that show the patient's progress and status. This becomes a positive feedback system for the patient who often does not realize subtle improvement. Before beginning the goniometric recordings, screen the patient by having him or her perform bilateral functional movements. This allows the patient to exhibit movement capability and allows the clinician to screen for areas that may need detailed goniometric measurement. These active movements include (1) wrist flexion and extension and radial and ulnar deviation; (2) composite finger flexion followed by composite finger extension; (3) finger abduction and adduction; (4) thumb opposition to the finger tips; and (5) thumb flexion composite toward the MCP

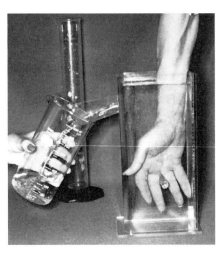

Figure 11–33. Volumetric measurement for edema. (From Lister,[18] with permission.)

of the little finger to the distal palmar crease, proximal to the small finger, followed by active extension of the thumb into the plane of the palm. If this screening is normal when compared with the noninvolved hand, this portion of the examination is complete. Abnormal findings indicate a need for more specific measurement. Depending on the time available and the status of the patient, gross measurements or total excursion measurements can be performed first (i.e., finger flexion to the palm and/or distal palmar crease; composite finger extension to a flat surface; thumb opposition to individual digits). A commercially available digi-o-meter (Smith & Nephew Rolyand Manufacturing, Inc., Menomonee Falls, WI, and North Coast Medical, Inc., Campbell, CA) or ruler (in centimeters) is used to assess these movements (Fig. 11–35). Old injuries that may affect joint mobility to either extremity should have been noted in the history and inspection.[17]

Individualized measurements of the digits require that the wrist and forearm be positioned in neutral to eliminate the influence of extrinsic musculature when the wrist changes position. The wrist is measured dorsally or laterally. The main factor in measurement is that placement is consistent and any deviation from the standard is documented with explanation. After abnormal active range of motion is recorded, passive range of motion is assessed for quantity and response. Pain and end-feels are noted.

Full passive range of motion but limited active range of motion alerts the clinician to muscle dysfunction, whether from trauma to the musculotendinous unit (e.g., rupture of the index FDP) or motor weakness from nerve injury. For example, postoperative extensor tendon repair at 8 weeks may have full passive range of motion but lacks 50 percent active range of motion secondary to limited tendon excursion because of scarring.

Accessory motion (see Chapter 13) is assessed for pain, and the type of restriction is also noted.

Strength

A functional assessment is made using standardized calibrated instrumentation.[30] The Jamar dynamometer (Therapeutic Baltimore Equipment Corporation, Baltimore, MD) (Fig. 11–36) is a tool that measures static grip. The pinch meter is used to measure pinch: lateral or key-three-jaw chuck, and pulp to pulp (Fig. 11–37). A testing procedure was developed by the Clinical Assessment Committee of the American Society for Surgery of the Hand to ensure test reliability and producibility.[28–30] With the arm positioned at the side, the elbow flexed to 90 degrees, and the forearm in midposition, the patient squeezes the dynamometer with one hand and then with the other; this procedure is repeated until three trials are completed. The trials are totaled, averaged, and recorded in inch-pounds or kilograms. There is usually a 15 to 20 percent difference between the dominant and nondomi-

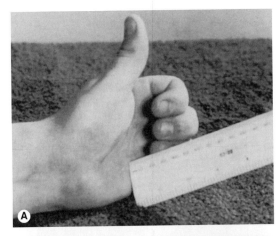

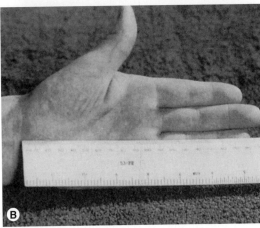

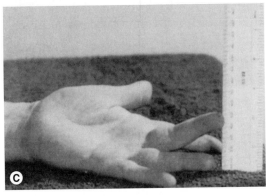

Figure 11–35. (A) Distance of the finger tips toward the palm. (B) Distance of the finger tips away from the scar or the wrist. (C) Distance of the finger tips from the table. This is finger extension deficit, usually caused by joint stiffness or adhesions. (From Salter,[15] with permission.)

nant extremities. Normative values have been established, but as with the other areas of any evaluation, the noninvolved extremity is the best source for comparison of the patient's norm.

In many situations, functional strength testing is sufficient to provide information on combined intrinsic and extrinsic muscle strength. With some hand problems, however, definitive muscle testing is needed. Results of muscle tests may vary, depending on the experience and

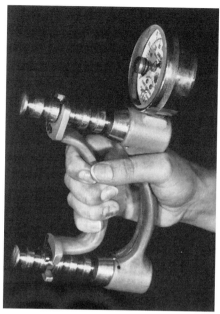

Figure 11–36. The Jamar grip dynamometer is used to record the strength of grasp. (From Lister,[18] with permission.)

interpretation of the clinician. For specific muscle testing procedures, please refer to Aulicino and DuPuy[19] and Evans.[20]

Isokinetic testing can be an adjunct to assessing muscle function and power of the wrist and hand. Commercially available equipment can be used to perform isokinetic testing. These devices may not be available in some clinics because of their cost or limited clinic space.

Sensibility

A desensitized hand is a vulnerable hand and one that must compensate functionally for sensory impairment. Severe nerve injuries warrant definitive evaluation to establish a baseline and monitor changes in nerve recovery.[31-36] Current academic and functional sensibility tests are constantly being researched to improve reliability and provide more functional information.[31] Most of these tests require a subjective response to a given stimulus, which can affect reliability. It is important to control as many variables as possible, such as minimizing environmental distractions, using consistency in method of application, using consistency in test selection, and limiting the number of examiners.[31-33] It has been reported that reliability improves if the same examiner performs all sensory tests.

Sensibility evaluation has been grouped into three test categories: threshold, functional, and objective. Of these, objective tests do not require a subjective response to the stimulus. Refer to Table 11–4 for a summary of some of these tests. The tests selected depend on the patient's problem, the experience of the evaluator, and the time available to administer the tests. A complete sensibility evaluation is not always needed, but the tests selected should reveal (1) the area of dysfunction, (2) the

quality of the protective sensation, and (3) the quality of the discriminative function. Based on knowledge of the hand and wrist anatomy and findings from the previous sections on evaluation of the hand, the clinician should already suspect specific nerve dysfunction.

The Tinel[34] test is a method of localizing the level of nerve injury. The suspected nerve is percussed from a distal to proximal direction. The patient reports a tingling sensation locally or radiating distally. In the case of a repaired nerve, Tinel's test is used to monitor nerve regeneration. As the nerve regenerates, the positive Tinel sign also moves distally. In compression neuropathies such as carpal tunnel syndrome, there is a positive Tinel's sign at the area of the volar carpal ligament with radiation to the index finger, the middle finger, and the radial half of the ring finger.

After the Tinel sign is documented, a "mapping" of the affected area is completed: With the patient's vision occluded, a blunt object is moved from an area of normal sensibility to the suspected area of abnormal sensibility; the patient is asked to inform the examiner when the stimulus starts to feel different. This area is outlined on the patient's hand and recorded on a hand diagram. As sensory dysfunction improves, the size of the affected area will decrease.

Once the affected area is mapped, protective sensation is assessed. The pinprick test is administered. A grid[30,35] diagram is used to document the patient's response. The sharp or dull end of the pin is randomly applied. The patient responds when he or she feels the stimulus and states whether it is sharp or dull. The exact response is recorded. The Weber two-point threshold discrimination test[16,21,30-33] is considered one of the more functional tests because it has been shown to correlate with hand use and ability. A Disk-Criminator (Disk-Discriminator, Baltimore, MD) is commercially available for two-point testing. It contains a series of blunt testing ends with different two-point spacing 2 to 15 mm apart. Starting with 2 mm, one or two points are randomly administered to the tip of the digit longitudinally and at right angles to the skin, avoiding skin blanching. The purpose of the test is to find the minimal distance perceived. Norms or ratings have been established.

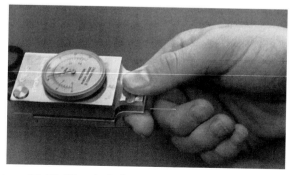

Figure 11–37. The pinch dynamometer is used to record pinch strength. (From Lister,[18] with permission.)

□□□□□ □ □ □

Table 11-4. Summary of Sensibility Tests

Stimulus	Sensation	Method	Response
Threshold tests			
Pinprick	Pain Protective	Apply randomly, sharp and dull	Correct Incorrect Absent
Temperature	Pain Protective	Apply test tubes with hot and cold liquids	Correct Incorrect Absent
Light touch	Pressure	Graded monofilaments	Touch thresholds associated with predetermined grams of pressure
Tuning fork	Vibration	256 cps applied 30 cps applied (compare with other side)	Absent Increased Decreased Same
Vibrometer	Vibration	Voltage meter, increase stimulus until perceived	Threshold recorded in volts
Functional tests			
Static two-point	Discriminative touch	Two points or one point randomly applied longitudinally	Normal 6–10 mm (fair) 11–15 mm (poor) One point (protective) Anesthetic
Moving two-point	Discriminative touch	8 mm applied from proximal to distal Decrease until 2 mm	Minimal perceived
Localization	Touch	Light touch	Map out response
Dellon modified pickup	Motor Discriminative	Prehension and placement of objects	Record time and quality
Objective tests			
Ninhydrin sweat	Sudomotor (sweating)	Ninhydrin prints made of the hands for comparison	0 = absent 3 = normal
Wrinkle	Sudomotor (wrinkling)	Hands soaked in warm water for 30 minutes	0 = absent 3 = normal

(Data from Callahan,[32] Dellon,[33] and Moran and Callahan.[36])

Another discriminative test, Dellon's[33] moving two-point discrimination test, is an indicator of functional recovery and clinically measures the quickly adapting fiber/receptor system. A two-point stimulus starting at a 8 mm distance is moved from a proximal to a distal direction along the finger tip. One point and two points are randomly administered; the two-point distance is gradually decreased to determine the minimal threshold perceived. The normal value is 2 mm, and the test is terminated at this point. Usually 7 to 10 trials are performed.[31–33]

The Semmes-Weinstein (North Coast Medical, Campbell, CA) monofilament instrument is used to assess light touch. It consists of 20 nylon monofilaments with different diameters having the same length. They are numbered from 1.65 to 6.65, which represents a logarithmic function of forces from 0.0045 to 448 g needed to bend the filament. Starting with the 2.83 filament, the instrument is applied perpendicular to the skin until it bends. One to three trials are administered until a minimal threshold is felt by the patient. It is time-consuming to perform the complete test, so a minikit has been developed that represents the cutoff point for functional levels. Results are recorded and color-coded.

The wrinkle (shrivel) test and the Ninhydrin sweat test are used to assess sudomotor function; however, they have limitations in predicting functional return of sensibility and are considered more academic. The Dellon modified Moberg pickup test is useful to assess motor and sensory functional integration. The patient is asked to pick up objects and place them in a container, first with the eyes open and then with the eyes closed, while being timed. The test is performed on the noninvolved hand and compared with the affected hand.

Standardized Testing/Computerization

Many standardized test systems are available to evaluate different aspects of hand function: prehension, dexterity, manipulation, speed, and fine motor coordination. The purpose of these tests is to observe and rate predetermined activities that can be compared with normative data. Some examples are the Bennett Hand Tool Dexterity Test, Purdue Pegboard Test, Minnesota Rate of Manipulation Test, Crawford Small Parts Dexterity Test, and the Jebson Standardized Test of Hand Function.[28-30] Test selection is based on the clinic's patient population and needs. Each of these tests has standardized norms to compare and rate the patient's performance.

There are two popular work simulator systems that can be used to evaluate a patient's ability to perform his or her job and ADL. The BTE Work Simulator (Therapeutic Baltimore Equipment Corporation, Baltimore, MD) and the Lido WorkSET (Loredan, Davis, CA) have evaluative and therapeutic applications. These systems are not appropriate for every clinic. Factors include patient population, clinic goals and financial limitations, and space availability. Simulators are frequently used in work capacity evaluation centers.

The computer age has influenced the area of hand rehabilitation. Computer software systems are now available that evaluate many aspects of hand function. Goniometers, dynamometers, and pinch gauges are interfaced with the software systems. Topographic changes including amputations and the location of scars and open wounds are part of the record system. Hand impairment ratings are calculated by the computer software based on the information recorded. Photography can also be incorporated into the evaluation to visually compare initial, subsequent, and final changes in topography.

A variety of commercial computer software programs are available to ease the administrative and record-keeping responsibilities of physical and hand therapy offices. These programs include documentation forms, internal peer review, patient education forms, professional scheduling, and clinical and financial outcome information. The need for these systems has been generated by changes in health care reform—specifically, managed care and the need to retrieve this type of information quickly and efficiently. Patient-centered outcome surveys are becoming the norm in many therapy clinics. FOTO, Inc. (Knoxville, TN 37939; 800-482-3686) and Mediserve Information Systems, Inc. (Tempe, AZ 85282; 800-279-8456) are examples of national and internal database systems, respectively. The data collected can be used as a research tool to analyze a clinic's effectiveness in all aspects of patient management.

Special Tests and Signs

Bunnel-Littler Test

The Bunnel-Littler test is used to determine intrinsic muscle tightness. With the MP joint in extension, the PIP joint is flexed. The MP joint is flexed, and the PIP joint flexed again. If the PIP joint is restricted with MP extension only, the intrinsic muscles are tight. Resistance to PIP joint flexion in both positions is indicative of capsular tightness.

Froment's Sign

Froment's sign is used to assess for ulnar nerve injury. The patient is asked to hold a piece of paper forcibly between the index proximal phalanx and the thumb while the paper is pulled away from the digits. A positive sign results in thumb IP joint flexion secondary to weakness of the adductor pollicis muscle and substitution of the FPL.

Retinacular Test

The retinacular test is used to determine retinacular ligmentous versus capsular tightness. The DIP joint is flexed with the PIP joint first in flexion and then in neutral. DIP joint tightness in both positions of the PIP joint is indicative of capsular restriction, whereas limited DIP joint tightness in neutral is positive for retinacular tightness.

Wartenberg's Sign

This is an indication of ulnar nerve paralysis or inflammation, with a resultant imbalance of weak palmar interossei and strong long extensor tendons. The little finger rests in abduction, and the patient is unable to adduct the digit actively after passive abduction.

Length-Tension Tests

Inability to perform complete active finger extension with full wrist extension is indicative of flexor extrinsic tightness. Conversely, inability to perform complete active finger flexion with full wrist flexion is indicative of extrinsic extensor tightness. Always check the noninvolved extremity for comparison.

■ Common Hand and Wrist Lesions

Distal Radial Fractures

Distal radius fractures are one of the most common fractures of the human skeleton and comprise about 33 percent of all fractures in emergency departments.[37-39] These injuries are predominant in two specific age groups: 6 to 10 years old and 60 to 70 years old. There is a higher incidence of females in the latter age group. Numerous classification systems have been developed to assist in determining the proper treatment. Some of those most commonly used may be categorized based on articular

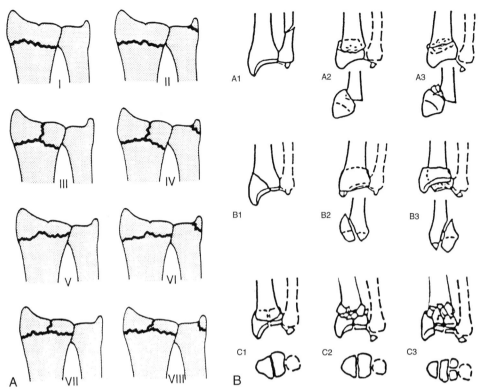

Figure 11–38. (A) Frykman's classification of distal radius fracture. Types I, II, V, and VII do not have an associated fracture of the distal ulna. Fractures III through VIII are intra-articular fractures. Higher-classification fractures have worse prognoses. (From Green,[95] with permission.) (B) The AO classification of distal radius fractures includes three main types, A, B, and C. Each type has three subtypes—1, 2, and 3—and each subtype has three further subtypes. Therefore, 27 total fracture patterns are described. The main type and principal subtype are shown here, comprising nine fracture patterns. The AO system is a useful classification both for treatment and prognosis. (From Leibovic,[43] with permission.)

joint involvement (Frykman,[40-44] Mayo,[42-44] Melone[43,44]), extent of communication (Older et al.[43,44]), radiographic appearance or degree of displacement (Universal, AO/ASIF[42-44]), or mechanism of injury (Fernandez[44]). The Frykman (Fig. 11–38A), Melone, Mayo, and AO (Fig. 11–38B) classifications are used most often. However, "because of the relative subjectivity involved in classifying distal radius fractures and the lack of inter- and intraobserver reliability, many surgeons classify distal radius fractures as displaced vs. nondisplaced, extra- vs. intra-articular, stable vs, unstable, and open vs. closed."[45]

Distal radius fractures are usually caused by a fall on the outstretched hand, producing a variety of fracture patterns. These include (1) *Colles'*: an extra-articular fracture of the radial shaft with dorsal or posterior displacement, giving the appearance of an upside-down dinner fork [38] (Fig. 11–39); (2) *Barton*'s: an intra-articular fracture with dorsal displacement of the dorsal lip of the radius[42]; (3) *Smith*'s: reversed Colles' fracture with volar displacement of the distal radius, giving it a "garden spade" deformity (Fig. 11–40); *Chauffeur*'s: fracture of the radial styloid, which may have various associated ligamentous and/or carpat fractures; and (5) pediatric epi-

physeal injuries.[42-45] In a Colles' fracture, the wrist usually lands in dorsiflexion and the forearm in pronation. The lunate acts as wedge to shear the radius off in a dorsal direction. The momentum of the body weight causes the distal fragment to displace radially and rotate in a supinatory direction with respect to the proximal bone end. The momentum often causes sprain of the ulnar collateral ligament and an avulsion fracture of the ulnar styloid process. Because of the mechanism of compressive forces in the radiocarpal joint, comminution and impaction of the distal fragment often occur.[38,41,43,44] In Smith's

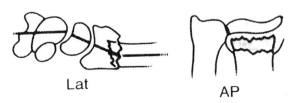

Figure 11–39. Diagramatic representation of the type of deformity seen in a Colles' fracture, showing dorsal comminution and displacement with shortening of the radius relative to the ulna. (From Green,[94] with permission.)

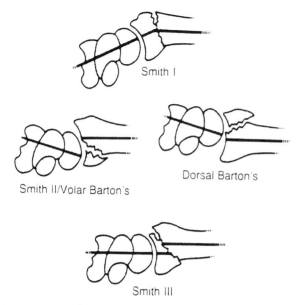

Figure 11–40. Thomas' classification of Smith's fractures. Type I Smith's fracture: an extra-articular fracture with palmar angulation and displacement of the distal fragment. Type II Smith's fracture: an intra-articular fracture with volar and proximal displacement of the distal fragment along with the carpus. Type III Smith's fracture: an extra-articular fracture with volar displacement of the distal fragment and carpus. (In type III, the fracture line is more oblique than in type I.) Smith's type II fracture is essentially a volar Barton's fracture. A dorsal Barton's fracture is illustrated for comparison, showing the dorsal and proximal displacement of the carpus and distal fragment on the radial shaft. (From Green,[94] with permission.)

fracture, the injury is classically believed to be caused by a fall on the back of the hand.[38,41,42]

Treatment goals for distal radius fractures are (1) restoration of articular congruity, (2) prevention of radial collapse, and (3) restoration and maintenance of articular tilt.[38] Accordingly, functional treatment goals[44] are to maximize joint mobility, maximize strength and dexterity, and minimize pain. Treatment options are closed reduction, percutaneous pinning, external fixation, and open reduction/internal fixation. Once the fracture is immobilized, attention should immediately shift to any current or potential secondary problems associated with this type of trauma. Consequently, according to Frykman,[41] "full finger motion must be permitted, significant edema or neurologic symptoms must be avoided, and frequent clinical follow-up is mandatory."

Medical Management

Medical management of the Colles' fracture is considerably more controversial than its diagnosis. Depending on the type of fracture, a closed manipulative reduction is usually carried out, restoring the radial length and dorsal angulation. The wrist is immobilized in slight palmar flexion and approximately 15 to 20 degrees of ulnar deviation.[40] There is controversy about whether the forearm

should be immobilized in pronation[44] or supination.[45] Frykman and Nelson[40] prefer the more pronated position. They believe that if forearm rotation is lost permanently, it is more functional for the forearm to be in pronation. The cast is sometimes placed above the elbow for 2 weeks, and then it is replaced with a short cast for another 3 to 4 weeks. In other cases, the elbow is left free. Special care should be taken when the elbow is left free; splinting in excessive pronation may result in a force that tends to pull the distal fragment into radial displacement and supination from tension on the brachioradialis when the elbow is extended.[36] Different noninvasive immobilization techniques including sugar-tong splints, short-arm casts, long-arm casts, and functional bracing are commonly used. No method has been shown to be statistically superior.[40] Regardless of which type of immobilization is used, full finger motion must be permitted, and close monitoring for edema and neurologic status is mandatory. The time of immobilization usually ranges from 6 to 8 weeks, and according to Beasley,[46] protective splinting should be maintained for another 6 to 8 weeks. The reduction of severely comminuted, unstable, or intra-articular distal radial fractures is extremely difficult to obtain with simple plaster immobilization. The most common methods used include percutaneous pins and external fixation. The external fixation methods are just as effective as percutaneous pins in maintaining reduction but also have the advantages of being lighter in weight and less restrictive, allowing finger and elbow mobility. The usual period of immobilization is 8 weeks.[40] Dynamic external fixators are now available to allow early wrist flexion and extension while maintaining radial length. A study done by Clyburn[47] in 1987 showed improved wrist motion with the use of this device.

Colles' fractures usually heal with some residual malalignment.[36,40] It is common to see a shortened radius or a distal radial displacement, with angulation or disruption of the relationship of the distal radioulnar joint articular surfaces. These malalignments result in a permanent loss of full wrist mobility. Other common resulting complications of the Colles' fracture are carpal tunnel syndrome, reflex sympathetic dystrophy, late rupture of the EPL tendon (Smith's fracture), and intrinsic contractures.[41] Each of these complications should be addressed early to avoid a more disabling result.

Physical Therapy Management

Therapy of Colles' fracture follows general healing fracture stages and rehabilitation principles. A detailed musculoskeletal evaluation is mandatory before initiating treatment (refer to the section on Evaluation of the Wrist and Hand earlier in this chapter). Reduction of edema is a priority after this type of fracture. The functional disuse of the hand and the required immobilization affect the pumping action of the muscles, resulting in venous stasis. The patient should be instructed about elevation of the upper extremity above the shoulder[48] and active range of motion of the uninjured joints. During the period of immobilization, special attention should be directed to maintaining the first web space and shoulder range of motion to avoid the development of adhesive capsulitis. The patient should also be instructed to report symptoms of severe pain, numbness, or "deadness" of the fingers, as well as persistent edema and shiny skin. These early signs of reflex sympathetic dystrophy need to be addressed as soon as possible to avoid the most disabling complication of wrist fractures. Once the immobilization is discontinued and if edema continues to be a problem, edema control should be continued. Several modalities are commonly used. A pulse galvanic muscle stimulator is used to activate the muscles around the affected edematous part. The physiologic rationale for this modality is that muscle pumping action could assist in the absorption process.[49] As recommended by Sorenson,[50] when using the pulse galvanic muscle stimulator, the negative pole is placed over the edematous area and the positive pole is placed proximally, usually over the median or ulnar nerve distribution on the upper arm, so that good muscle pumping action can be stimulated.

Another modality commonly used is the Jobst intermittent pressure glove (Jobst, Inc., Toledo, OH). The pressure should be at a point that the patient can tolerate well, not exceeding 60 to 66 mmHg. This glove is usually worn for 45 minutes to 1 hour. Retrograde milking massage, string wrapping techniques, and active range of motion are techniques recommended for use in edema control.[49] A combination of pulsated electric stimulation with the Jobst intermittent pressure glove can be effective in controlling edema. To maintain the fluid reduction gained in the treatment, the hand needs some gentle compressive dressing. Tubigrip (Seton Healthcare Group, Oldham, England) and Coban (3M Corp., St. Paul, MN) tape are the wraps most widely used. The patient should be taught how to use these wraps and cautioned not to wrap themselves too tightly, thereby compromising their circulation.

In most traumatic wrist injuries, it is desirable to start active mobilization of the joint before the bone and soft tissue are completely healed. Active wrist range of motion should be started as soon as the cast is removed, but splints are required to protect and support the wrist in its final stage of healing. The patient needs to receive specific written instructions and demonstration of the exercises prescribed as a home program. It is advisable to provide few exercises and a limited number of repetitions to ensure performance of the exercises. It is also recommended that the exercises be performed at least every 2 hours, with each session lasting for only 2 to 3 minutes. The patient should be observed for swelling or pain after the exercise program. The possible reasons for these adverse reactions could be too forceful range of motion, too long a period of exercise resulting in overstraining,

or not exercising often enough during the day, thus overworking when doing the exercises.[49]

Once the fracture is well healed, joint mobilization techniques can be initiated to restore the joint play and stretch the articular joint capsule. It is the joint play that allows normal physiologic performance of movement.[51] *Note of caution*: The therapist should not only be familiar with joint mobilization techniques, but should also have the skill to determine the forms of mobilization necessary to increase a specific range of motion, to evaluate the source of the pain, and to have a clear understanding of the wound-healing stages. For better understanding of mobilization techniques, refer to Chapter 13.

In this stage, the use of electrical muscle stimulation can increase muscle contraction and serve as an active assistive exerciser.[49] If pain is a complicating factor, the use of a transcutaneous electric nerve stimulator and interferential current may be helpful during performance of range-of-motion exercises. Many other modalities may need to be used to decrease pain, increase circulation, and alter the elasticity of tissues. The most widely used heat modalities are hot packs, placing the arm in an elevated position, paraffin, Fluidotherapy (Fluido Therapy Corp., Houston, TX), and warm water soaks. Whirlpool use with warm water is discouraged because the dependent position of the wrist and the heat increase swelling; however, it can be used at 95°F combined with active range-of-motion exercises performed in the water.[52] Ice is very helpful in extremely painful joints before range-of-motion exercises and after the treatment to decrease any joint reactivity.[53]

The treatment program should progress to resistive exercises when the fracture is well healed, the edema is controlled, and mobility is being improved. A progressive resistive exercise program for the elbow, wrist, and hand musculature needs to be used at this stage, and ADL should be incorporated as soon as joint mobility and strength allow.

The rehabilitation process needs to progress to coordination and endurance programs. Isokinetic/exercise equipment is useful to restore strength and endurance and to determine the strength of the affected wrist in comparison with the noninvolved wrist. Isokinetic exercise can be initiated at the 8th week after injury if the fracture is healed. To prepare the patient for the return to work, a job simulation program must be incorporated throughout the rehabilitation phase, and if necessary, a job analysis may need to be performed.

CASE STUDY

History

A 74-year-old right-hand-dominant housewife who fell as she was walking with her husband; she stubbed her toe on the curb and fell on her outstretched left hand. Pain developed immediately, with subsequent swelling of the left wrist. She was diagnosed with a left displaced, comminuted intra-articular distal radius fracture. She underwent closed reduction, and the extremity was placed in a sugar tong for 2 weeks. It was then removed, and a long arm cast was applied for an additional 4 weeks. A prefabricated wrist splint was applied after the cast was removed. The patient was also taking prescription pain medication as needed. Her main complaints were inability to bend the wrist, inability to make a full fist, wrist and hand pain with activity, and hypersensitivity of the finger tips. She rated the pain as 5 on a 0–10 verbal analog scale. The patient had moderate edema of the hand and also of the forearm and elbow. Volumetric measurement of the left hand was 90 ml more than the right. Circumferential measures revealed an increase of 2.5, 3.5, and 2.0 cm at the wrist crease, the elbow crease, and 2 inches below the elbow crease, respectively. She had limited active range of motion of all joints of the upper left extremity except for shoulder, elbow flexion, and forearm pronation compared to the right:

	Left	**Right**
Elbow extension	−35 degrees	−15 degrees
Forearm supination	−30 degrees	−90 degrees
Wrist flexion	−55 degrees	−85 degrees
Wrist extension	−20 degrees	−64 degrees
Ulnar deviation	−10 degrees	−30 degrees
Radial deviation	−10 degrees	−20 degrees

She had limited digital active and (passive range of motion) as follows:

Thumb CMC Extension 45 (60) Degrees, Abduction 40 (50) Degrees

	MCP	**IP/PIP**	**DIP**
Thumb	+15/30 (+20/30)	+20/25 (+25/55)	
Index	0/45 (0/60)	0/50 (0/70)	0/10 (0/45)
Middle	0/45 (0/55)	0/45 (0/75)	0/10 (0/50)
Ring	0/30 (0/60)	0/55 (0/90)	0/15 (0/55)
Little	0/30 (0/65)	0/55 (0/85)	0/20 (0/65)

Gross grip, lateral pinch and index pulp to pulp pinch averaged) 0, 1, and 0.5 lb, respectively, compared to 35,

10, and 7 lb for the right. The patient was unable to assume the three-jaw chuck testing position. She had marked tenderness throughout the wrist dorsally and volarly and tenderness of the IP joints of the fingers and the CMC of the thumb. Sensation was intact; she denied having any numbness or tingling but reported increased sensitivity of the volar finger tips. Functionally, she had limited use of the left hand and needed her husband to assist with ADLs.

Treatment

Initial treatment consisted of elevation, with cold packs to the hand, wrist, forearm, and elbow followed by retrograde massage and initiation of digital, wrist, forearm, and elbow active and gentle passive range-of-motion exercises. The patient was also started on digital tendon gliding exercises. A compressive glove was fitted for edema management to be worn during waking hours; the splint was adjusted for more wrist extension as tolerated, and the patient was given a written home program for cyotherapy one or two times daily, edema management, and range-of-motion exercises to be done every 3–4 hours. The patient was seen three times weekly for 2 weeks. By the end of the first week, her therapy program progressed to the use of moist heat as the pain and edema decreased, as well as hand putty and progressive resistive exercises for the wrist, forearm, and elbow using free weights. Functional activities such as clothes pin transfer, velcro board activity, putty pinches, and so on were added as tolerated. Joint mobilization was limited initially to techniques for pain reduction then advanced as pain and edema decreased. The patient had to go out of town for 1 month after completing 2 weeks of therapy. At that time, her therapy program was targeted at improving strength and range of motion. Her last therapy visit, 6 weeks after the initial visit and 3 months after the injury, demonstrated marked improvement in all areas. She had full elbow, forearm, and digital active range-of-motion. Wrist flexion was 60 degrees and extension was 45 degrees. Ulnar deviation was 15 degrees, and radial deviation was 25 degrees. The patient had regained 50 percent of grip and 75 percent of pinch strength of the right hand; the difference in volumetric measurement was only 20 ml, and circumferential measurements of the left hand were comparable to those of the right hand except for the wrist crease, which was now only 1.4 cm larger. The patient was independent with ADL but still had some wrist pain on lifting objects weighing over 7–10 lb. We were pleased with her progress and felt she would continue to improve with time and continued use of the left hand. The patient was discharged to a home program.

Carpal Tunnel Syndrome

The incidence of carpal tunnel syndrome (CTS) in the workplace has reached epidemic proportions, comprising

40.8 percent of all upper extremity repetitive motion disorders reported by the Bureau of Labor Statistics in 1994.[54,55] The association of CTS with work-related risk factors is a recurring theme of causation among workers, ergonomists, lawyers, and physicians. The majority of the literature that tries to establish this as a causal association fails to meet the appropriate standards of epidemiologic validity.[54,56,57]

CTS is a compression neuropathy of the median nerve at the level of the carpal tunnel, commonly associated with pain, numbness, and/or tingling that frequently disturb sleep.[58] (see Figure 11–41). This may result from an alteration in the osseous margin of the carpus secondary to fractures, dislocations, arthritis, or thickening of the transverse carpal ligament or from an increased volume of the carpal canal often believed to be the result of edema and tenosynovitis of the flexor tendons.[58,59] Studies by Schuind et al.[60] demonstrated no evidence of an inflammatory lesion in the synovium. The histologic lesions in idiopathic CTS found in their study were typical of connective tissue undergoing degeneration under repeated mechanical stresses.

Other cases of CTS result from trauma and from metabolic and anatomic abnormalities.[61] The most frequent traumatic cause of this condition is in association with a Colles' fracture. Median nerve neuropathy can occur at the time of injury from trauma to the nerve or during a period of immobilization if the maintained position causes pressure against the nerve. In an acute traumatic condition, immediate surgery is necessary to relieve and prevent nerve damage. Sunderland has postulated three stages of degeneration in cases of chronic progressive nerve compression.[35] In stage 1, progressive

obstruction of venous return occurs. The hypoxic nerve fibers become hyperexcitable and discharge spontaneously. Pain and paresthesias result from the imbalance of fiber activity or fiber dissociation. Nocturnal paresthesia is often present in this stage. The use of a night splint with the wrist in neutral (0 degree of extension) position is advocated in the management of CTS at this stage. Studies have confirmed that the position of wrist in flexion or extension increases pressure within the carpal canal.[62] It is hypothesized that decreasing neural pressure and tension by restricting joint position will reverse the neural process.[55]

In stage 2, capillary circulation slows so severely that anoxia damages the endoneurium. Edema occurs, promoting proliferation of fibroblasts and formation of constrictive endoneurial connective tissue. Segmental demyelination and axon thinning and destruction are found in individual nerve fibers. As the severity of the lesion increases, damage to the sensory and motor fibers occurs unless decompression takes place.

In stage 3, nerve fibers can undergo Wallerian degeneration, and the compressed nerve undergoes fibrosis, resulting in a reduction of the number of axons available for regeneration.

Clinical Presentation

The CTS patient often presents initially with symptoms of nocturnal pain and numbness, weakness or clumsiness in holding small objects, and diminished sensation in the thumb, index, and long fingers and in the radial aspect of the ring finger.[63] Although the symptoms often are intermittent, especially in the early stages, excessive use of the affected hand in highly repetitive activities, sustained wrist flexion or extension, and continued gripping or pinching activities may increase the severity of the symptoms. Silverstein et al., in what is regarded as a classic study, show the prevalence of CTS in work when high repetition and high force were present.[64] In the early stages, the patient is asymptomatic at rest and symptoms may be provoked by maneuvers that compress or place tension on the nerve, causing temporary ischemia to the nerve. At this stage the provocative maneuvers are the only positive findings in the clinical examination.[55] The changes caused by chronic compression occur slowly in the nerve, and the progression of changes occurs with the duration of compression. In a more advanced stage of neuropathy, two-point discrimination will be abnormal, and thenar muscles atrophy can be present.[54]

CTS is a combination of signs and symptoms, but there is no absolute clinical standard or definitive test to confirm its diagnosis.[54–65] The validity and reliability of many of the diagnostic tests used for CTS are not fully established. Electrophysiologic studies measuring median nerve function are the only objective way to show the nerve deficit. When properly used, these tests have sensi-

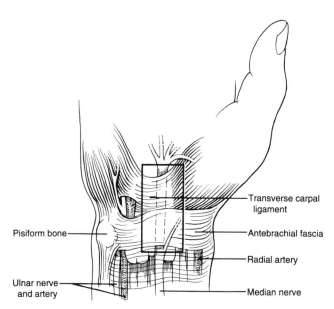

Figure 11–41. The median nerve passes through the carpal tunnel, along with nine flexor tendons. The transverse carpal ligament supports the median nerve and flexor tendons volarly. (Modified from Hunter et al.,[75] with permission.)

tivity and specificity of nearly 90 percent,[54,66–69] which is considered the gold standard.[66] Unfortunately, the majority of epidemiologic studies of CTS have not used these studies in the diagnosis.[54] Electrodiagnostic testing, although a valuable aid in the diagnosis of studies in the diagnosis of CTS, does not replace a carefully executed clinical assessment.[55] Patients with CTS frequently note unreliability of grip. Both muscle weakness and sensory deficits can contribute to this symptom. Thus, patients often complain of dropping objects or of difficulty grasping even before the occurrence of demonstrable weakness and long before the appearance of thenar atrophy. As median nerve damage progresses, thenar weakness may become more pronounced, and thenar atrophy may appear.[65] The muscles that receive median innervation distal to the carpal tunnel are the APB, Opp, flexor pollicis brevis (FPB), and lumbricals to the index and middle fingers. The APB is the muscle of choice in the motor examination because it is superficial, innervated solely by the median nerve, and the earliest muscle affected.[70] Early sensory changes may be detected by examination with the Semmens-Weinstein monofilament test (SWMF), which has relatively high specificity and sensitivity and provides a useful quantitative assessment of nerve function. Provocative testing can be useful in CTS. Phalen's test and Tinel's sign are the most common office-based clinical tests. However, a recent review of the literature[67] shows wide variation in their reported sensitivity and specificity. Estimates of the sensitivity of Phalen's test range from 10 to 88 percent, and those of Tinel's sign range from 26 to 79 percent. Estimates of the specificity of Phalen's test range from 47 to 100 percent and those of Tinel's sign range from 45 to 100 percent. A careful history and well-chosen elements of the clinical examination should lead to an accurate diagnosis.

The physical therapy evaluation should include a careful history and a visual inspection for pseudomotor changes and thenar muscle atrophy. Phalen's and Tinel's tests are the most commonly used provocative tests. Quantitative Phalen's assessment can also be done by performing a SWMT initially to obtain a sensory baseline. The SWMT is repeated with the wrist in gravity-assisted palmar flexion for 1 minute prior to the beginning of testing. Any change in the sensibility of the median nerve distribution is considered a positive quantitative Phalen's test.[71] Vibration may be the first sensory perception affected by median nerve compression.[65] Two-point discrimination is useful in the late stages of CTS. Thenar weakness usually does not occur until sensory loss is marked.[65] Motor examination in the patient with suspected CTS should exclude motor manifestations of more widespread neurologic dysfunction such as ulnar neuropathy, proximal median neuropathy, brachial plexopathy, or radiculopathy. Pinch strength (Ib) is measured with a pinch gauge (B&L Engineering, Santa Fe Springs, CA) as recommended by the American Society of Hand Therapists.[72]

Physical Therapy

Conservative Management

The purpose of conservative management is to reduce compressive forces on the median nerve, to decrease demands on the hand and wrist, and to reduce the inflammatory process. The goal of treatment is to decrease pain and paresthesia, increase or maintain muscle strength, maintain hand function, and educate the patient in the syndrome process, correct wrist and hand posture, and avoidance of provocative activities. A wrist splint in neutral position[62] is constructed for night wear. Commonly, a day-wear splint is worn during the first 3 to 4 weeks of treatment, but it is advisable to wean the patient off it as soon as inflammation and pain are reduced. Caution is needed since a study by Rempel et al. in 1994 reported that carpal tunnel pressures were higher with splint use at rest and during repetitive hand activities, perhaps suggesting some external compression.[73] A baseline sensory evaluation is performed initially, and a sensory progress evaluation every 6 weeks is recommended. Since heat has been shown to increase localized blood flow and to facilitate connective tissue extensibility, this modality is frequently used in CTS treatment to facilitate flexor tendon gliding. Cold, another modality that is widely used, produces analgesia and reduces inflammation and edema.[74] Other modalities such as electrical stimulation or ultrasound are commonly used to decrease the initial inflammation. The patient is encouraged to maintain his or her job with modifications as needed.

An exercise program should include elbow and shoulder range of motion, active and passive wrist range-of-motion, and flexor tendon and nerve gliding exercises. Tendon gliding exercises facilitate isolated excursion of each of the two tendons to each finger that passes through the carpal tunnel. The exercise is initiated from a position of full finger and wrist extension, followed by a "hook" fist position and continued by a straight fist position, maintaining the DIP joints in extension to obtain maximum flexor digitorum superficialis excursion. The exercise is completed by placing the hand in full fist position, providing maximum profundus tendon excursion. The nerve gliding exercise places the hand in six different positions, as described by Hunter and Belkin[75] (Fig. 11–42).

A recent study by Rozmaryn et al.[74] suggested that a program of nerve and tendon gliding exercises coupled with a traditional nonsurgical approach reduces CTS symptoms significantly. Once the inflammation and symptoms of nerve compression subside, progressive strengthening exercises for the wrist, elbow, and hand are initiated. Proper body mechanics and ergonomic evaluation of the job station are important aspects of CTS conservative management. Frequent resting periods during job performance are advised. Use of the night-wear splint should be continued for 4 to 6 more weeks after the initial symptoms are resolved.

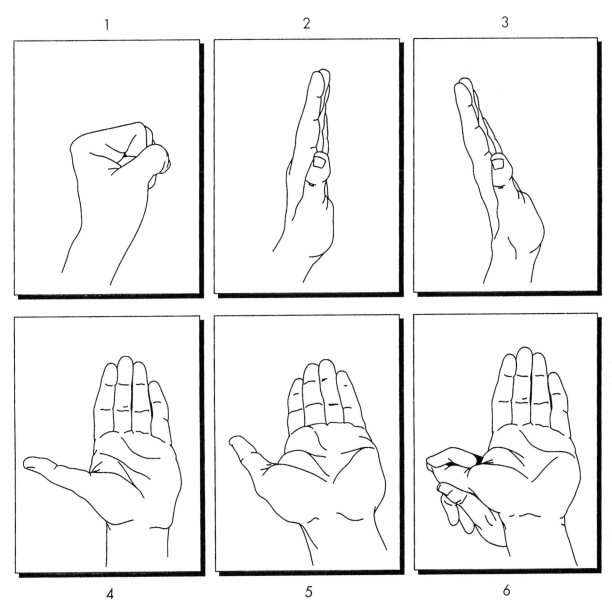

Figure 11–42. Nerve gliding exercises are initiated to facilitate mobilization of the median nerve. James Hunter, M.D., developed the exercises, and Julie Belkin, O.T.R., designed the home program. (Redrawn with permission from Totten PA and Hunter JM: Therapeutic techniques to enhance nerve gliding in the thoracic outlet and carpal tunnel syndromes. Hand Clin 7(3):505, 1991.)

Postoperative management

Therapeutic management of the patient after surgical decompression should be initiated as soon as the compressive dressing is removed, usually during the first 7 to 14 days postoperatively. Therapy goals in this stage should include edema control, maintenance of range of motion, and restriction of adhesion formation during the early fibroplasia phase. Edema control is initiated with a light compressive stockinette such as the Tubigrip stockinette, elevation of the involved hand, and retrograde massage if necessary. Active and passive wrist range-of-motion and differential tendon and nerve gliding exercises are initiated.[74] Exercises should be performed 10 repetitions each,

three to six times per day. A volar wrist splint positioning the wrist in 0 degrees of extension[62] is constructed for night wear or during strenuous activities. Scar mobilization is initiated as soon as the surgical scar is healed. Elastomer or silicone gelsheet[76] (Smith & Nephew Roly-and Manufacturing, Inc., Menomonee Falls, WI) is helpful in scar management. If nerve sensory disturbances result in prolonged paresthesia or hypersensitivity, desensitization exercises and fluidotherapy are recommended. A sensory baseline evaluation is performed, and a sensory progress reevaluation every 6 weeks is recommended. Light strengthening exercises with Theraputty or a hand exerciser can be initiated at 3 to 4 weeks postoperatively, but close monitoring of the patient's reactivity is necessary. Too early and too much exercise could result in tenosynovitis. The patient is encouraged to use his or her hand in light functional tasks as soon as this can be tolerated, using pain as a guideline.

A strengthening program including isotonic and isometric exercise is gradually progressed, and work simulation is initiated. The patient's physical capacity to perform his or her regular job should be assessed before the patient returns to work. It is necessary to educate the patient in proper body mechanics and in measurements to prevent recurrence of CTS. Many of these patients may need further therapy for pain control. Some respond well to a transcutaneous electric nerve stimulator (TENS), which can be rented for home use. Other modalities such as electric stimulation (i.e., high galvanic electric stimulation/interferential), contrast baths, ultrasound, and continuation of scar management have been helpful to patients with persisting pain. Often these patients need to learn to cope with chronic pain through pain management; others may require placement in a modified job.

CASE STUDY

History

A 32-year-old, female, right-hand-dominant insurance clerk underwent right carpal tunnel release after she failed to respond to 1 year of conservative management that included splinting, nonsteroidal anti-inflammatory medications, steroid injections, and workstation modification. She was immobilized for 10 days and referred to physical therapy for 4 weeks of treatment two times per week. The patient's main complaints were stiffness, numbness, and pain throughout the wrist and hand. She graded her pain as 6 on a visual analog scale of 0–10.

Evaluation

Observation demonstrated a well-healed surgical scar, but with diffuse edema throughout the hand. The patient was wearing a commercial cockup splint provided by her physician after suture removal.

Objective evaluation demonstrated a 25 ml difference between the affected and unaffected hands by volumetric measurements. The scar was markedly tender to palpation, dense, and with poor pliability. Tinel's sign was positive at the distal palmar crease. An SWMT revealed diminished protective sensation (4.31) of the thumb and decreased light touch of the index and long fingertips (3.61). A two-point discrimination test (Disk-Criminator) revealed 7 mm on the thumb and 5 mm on the index, long, ring, and little fingers.

The active range-of-motion measurements of the wrist were as follows:

	Right	Left
Flexion	40 degrees	70 degrees
Extension	18 degrees	60 degrees
Radial deviation	4 degrees	26 degrees
Ulnar deviation	10 degrees	34 degrees
Supination	45 degrees	80 degrees
Pronation	70 degrees	85 degrees

Composite flexion of the hand demonstrated 2 cm from the proximal palmar crease; however, passive range of motion (PROM) was full with moderate discomfort. Hand grip on the left hand measured 53.3 lb, but no torque was elicited with the right hand. Key pinch on the left hand was 20.6 lb. The patient stated that she has not attempted to use the right hand in any ADL or functional activities secondary to pain.

Treatment

Treatment was established with active and passive range-of-motion exercises for the wrist and hand, differential tendon and nerve gliding exercises, desensitization techniques, scar massage, fluidotherapy, and pulse ultrasound to the surgical area. Instructions in home exercises and in a contrast bath were provided.[74]

The patient was fitted with a compressive stockinette (Tubigrip), and an elastomer pad for scar remodeling was provided. A volar wrist splint in 0 degrees of extension was constructed for night wear. Treatment goals were to resolve edema, increase scar mobility, restore hand and wrist mobility, and promote sensory reeducation.

At the third week of treatment (5 weeks postoperatively), light strengthening exercises for the wrist and hand were initiated and the home program was upgraded. Reevaluation at this time demonstrated full composite fisting, the wrist active range of motion had improved 75 percent from the initial measurements, and the surgical scar was now supple and less tender to palpation. The patient now was able to develop a torque of 10 lb. with the right hand grip and 4.6 lb. of key pinch. The patient reported to be using her hand for ADL and light functional activities without discomfort.

At the sixth postoperative week, a new sensory test demonstrated normal sensibility of the index and long fingers, with remaining decreased light touch of the thumb (3.61). The hand grip improved from 10 lb. to 20 lb. At this time the patient returned to work on a 4 hour per day schedule, with typing limited to 15 minutes at a time. Specific recommendations and instructions for an ergonomically correct workstation were given.

The patient continued receiving therapy on a weekly basis for 4 more weeks, with progressive strengthening and endurance exercises to the entire right upper extremity. Therapy goals in this stage were to maximize right upper extremity strength and endurance and to facilitate the transition to full-time work. During this period, the patient gradually increased her working hours as well as her typing time. In the last week of therapy she was able to work 8 hours per day, with frequent rest periods and performance of stretching exercises as needed.

The patient was encouraged to continue the strengthening and stretching exercise program upon discharge. Reevaluation at this time demonstrated right wrist mobility equal to that on the left except for 10 degrees of limitation in extension. The right hand grip improved to 48.6 lb. and key pinch to 21.3 lb. The SWMT demonstrated full return of the median nerve, and two-point discrimination was 5 mm throughout the digits. The patient still experienced some discomfort over the surgical area, and her endurance for continuous work was limited to 45 minutes to 1 hour. However, she was satisfied with the result of the surgery and her improvement with therapy.

Boutonniere Deformity

The boutonniere deformity is the result of an injury of the extensor mechanism at the PIP joint, zone 111, when normal balance of forces of the extensor tendons and retinacular system is lost.[77]

The boutonniere deformity refers to a finger posture with the PIP joint flexed and the DIP joint hyperextended.[78] The deformity occurs when the common extensor tendon that inserts in the base of the middle phalanx is damaged and a volar sliding or subluxation of the lateral extensor bands occurs. (Fig. 11–43) These lateral extensor bands sublux volarly to the axis of the PIP joint when the spiral fibers and transverse fibers are ruptured. The head of the proximal phalanx herniates through the defect and assumes a flexed position as a result of an unopposed force of the flexor digitorum superficialis.[79] With progression of the deformity, proximal retraction of the extensor apparatus occurs; the extrinsic extensor tendon, released from the middle phalanx, transfers forces from the sagittal bands that enhance extension of the MP joint. Both extrinsic and intrinsic muscles transmit exaggerated forces through the conjoined lateral bands, resulting in hyperextension of the DIP joint.

Burton[80] describes three stages of the boutonniere deformity:

Stage 1. Dynamic imbalance, passively supple, in which the lateral bands are subluxated but not adherent anteriorly.

Stage 2. Established extensor tendon contracture in which the deformity cannot be passively corrected; the lateral bands are shortened and thickened, but the joint itself is not involved.

Stage 3. Secondary joint changes such as volar plate scarring and contracture, collateral ligament scarring, and intra-articular fibrosis.

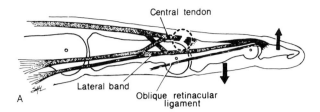

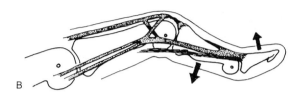

Figure 11–43. Pathomechanics of the boutonniere deformity. (A) As the central tendon either ruptures or attenuates, extensor tone is decreased at the dorsal base of the middle phalanx, allowing the PIP joint to drop into flexion. (B) As the joint flexes, the lateral bands move volar to the axis of motion. They will adhere in that position, and the central tendon heals in the attenuated position. The pathomechanics of the established boutonniere involve not only the attenuation of the central tendon, but the displaced, adherent, and foreshortened lateral bands resting volar to the axis of motion at the PIP joint. Excess extensor pull thus secondarily bypasses the PIP joint and is imposed dorsally at the DIP joint, causing a recurvature at this distal joint. (From Green,[94] printed with permission and adapted from Burton,[80] with permission.)

During the early stage of the deformity, the transverse retinacular ligament, oblique retinacular ligament, and check ligaments are loose. The oblique retinacular test is negative, and the prognosis for reversal of the deformity is more favorable with proper management.

The boutonniere deformity can result from a closed trauma when an involuntary forceful flexion of an actively extended finger occurs, commonly observed in sports activities such as: basketball,[81] or from injuries caused by division, rupture, avulsion, and laceration of the central extensor tendon. Other causes include full-thickness dorsal burns, rheumatoid arthritis, and Dupuytren's contracture.[82] In closed injuries, the characteristic boutonniere deformity may not be present at the time of the injury and usually develops during the 10- to 21-day period following injury. A painful, tender, and swollen PIP joint that has been recently injured should arouse suspicion.[77-80]

Treatment

There are conflicting opinions in the literature concerning direct repair and immobilization with K-wire versus conservative management of the open zone III injury. However, most authors recommend conservative treatment of the acute closed injury at this level, with uninterrupted immobilization of the PIP joint at 0 degrees of extension for 6 weeks.[77-83] Open and repaired injuries are mobilized as early as 3 to 4 weeks by some authors, with protective splinting between exercise sessions, and graded increments in range of motion are allowed between 3 and 6 weeks,[85,86] but most authors recommend continuous splinting for 6 weeks before motion is initiated. There are many surgical procedures for the management of the boutonniere deformity, depending on the stage and severity of the deformity. Passive extension of the PIP joint should be maximized before surgery. The most common procedures are the Eaton-Littler procedure, the Matev procedure, and the Littler-Eaton procedure.

Postoperative Management

Traditional management of acute open injuries can be divided in three stages:[82,84–87]

Zero to 6 weeks

The PIP joint is held with a K wire in 0 degrees of extension for initial immobilization in a cast for 3–4 weeks. The K wire and sutures are removed, and the PIP joint is splinted in extension. The MP and DIP joints now free from immobilization and are initiated in active exercises, but it is critical that the PIP joint be at absolute 0 degrees; otherwise, there will be some tension in the repair site, possibly creating some gapping, which may result in tendon healing in an elongated position. Wound care and digital edema control should be part of the initial treatment. Coban wrapping is commonly used to control edema. As soon as the wound closes, scar mobilization should be included in the treatment. Massage, elastomere molds, or silicone gelsheet (SGS) are commonly used. SGS has been found to reduce hypertrophic scars.[76]

If the lateral bands require no surgical repair, the distal joint is left free to prevent distal joint tightness, loss of extensibility of the oblique retinacular ligaments, and lateral band adherence.[88] Distal joint motion should be encouraged. As described by Burton, active blocked flexion of the DIP joint while the PIP joint is held at 0 degrees will gradually stretch the lateral band and oblique retinacular ligaments to their physiologic lengths.[80]

If the lateral bands are repaired, investigators have recommended that the DIP joint also be immobilized for 4 to 6 weeks; however, this can result in significant loss of distal joint motion. Evans[84] recommends initiation of lateral band gliding exercises by the third week by incorporating gentle intermittent traction to the DIP joint or by active DIP joint flexion combined with static splinting.

Six to 8 weeks

MP and DIP active exercises continue, followed by active gentle flexion and extension of the PIP joint. PIP joint flexion exercises should be initiated with caution because the immobilized extensor tendon will have little tensile strength and most likely will be adherent over the proximal phalanx, limiting gliding and elevating tension at the level of repair. The first week of PIP joint mobilization (regardless of whether motion is started at week 3, 4, 5, or 6) should emphasize active PIP joint extension. It is recommended that the MP joint be positioned in 0 degrees of extension while the PIP joint is actively ranged from full extension to no more than 30 degrees of flexion. If no extension lag develops, motion can progress to 40 to 50 degrees by the second week of motion, thereafter adding 20 to 30 degrees per week. Forceful flexion exercises are not appropriate, and development of lag should be addressed with increased extension splinting and decreased increments of flexion. A PIP extension splint is worn between exercise sessions. If there is no extensor lag, flexor forces can be directed to the stiff PIP joint by the use of a forearm-based dynamic splint that blocks the MP joint in extension and applies a light traction (less than 250 g) to the midphalanx level or by a hand-based static splint that blocks the MP joint in extension and encourages PIP joint flexion in the hook fist position. Or by applying a static extension splint to the DIP to negate the flexor digitorum profundus (FDP) force and manually blocking the MP joint, the patient is encouraged to actively flex the PIP joint.

Eight to 12 weeks

Active flexion and extension exercises continue for the MP, PIP, and DIP joints. Gentle resisted exercises are initiated at this time, with monitoring of the PIP joint for any extension lag development. If an extension lag occurs, the program should be regressed. Gradual weaning of the daytime extension splint occurs after 8 to 10 weeks, with buddy taping initially to allow the PIP joint to extend fully during the day. Night-time splinting for the PIP joint can continue for a couple of months more to prevent recurrence of the deformity.[80,84–87]

Conservative Management

Acute close injury

The PIP joint is placed in 0 degree of extension splint, leaving the DIP and MP joints free. The splint is worn 24 hours a day for 4 to 6 weeks. Care is taken to maintain the PIP joint in extension when the splint is removed for adjustments or during exercises. Different commercial splints have been suggested for the management of this deformity; they are the Bunnel Safety Pin splint, Capener splint, and LMB, Aluminum, and cylindrical casts.[77,80–87] Exercises, as described by Burton,[80] are initiated immediately. The exercise involves two sequential maneuvers. The first is active assisted PIP joint extension. This will stretch the tight volar structures, will cause the lateral bands to ride dorsal to the PIP joint axis, and will put longitudinal tension on the lateral bands and oblique retinacular ligaments. The second maneuver is maximal active forced flexion of the DIP joint while the PIP joint is held at 0 degrees or as close to that position as the PIP joint will allow. This will gradually stretch the lateral bands and oblique retinacular ligaments to their physiologic length.

By the end of the sixth week, gentle active range-of-motion exercises can begin for flexion and extension of the PIP joint. The progression of exercises and splinting is the same as that described for postsurgical management, with monitoring of any developing PIP joint extension lag.

Chronic Deformity

All efforts to decrease edema and pain and increase active and passive range of motion are attempted to avoid surgery. A splinting program recommended for treatment of the established boutonniere should be tailored to fit the tissue requirements. The goal is to obtain PIP joint extension while monitoring and upgrading DIP joint flexion range. Once the PIP joint restores the extension range, progression of the treatment follows the same steps as already described for postoperative management. The requirement for continued support of the PIP joint reflects postural stability of the finger. Splinting is recommended at night, until PIP joint extension can be sustained and there has been no deterioration during subsequent visits. The time required for rehabilitation of the boutonniere deformity by splinting and exercises can be prolonged. Resistant cases may require attention and supervision for 6 to 9 months.[87]

CASE STUDY

History

S.G., a 25-year-old, male, right-handed college student sustained a left little finger PIP joint subluxation while playing basketball. S.G. sought medical attention immediately following the injury. Radiologic studies indicated good joint alignment, and the finger was immobilized in full extension in an aluminum splint that he used continuously for 3½ weeks. At that time he was reevaluated by a physician, who recommended continuation of splint wear for another 2 weeks; however, S.G. decided to wear it occasionally. At the 6th week S.G. returned to see his physician since he was unable to fully extend the little finger. It was noticed that a pseudo-boutonniere deformity had developed. He was then referred to a physical therapy clinic for management of the dysfunction. He was treated for 3 weeks, which resulted in further increase of the deformity. At that time (9 ½ weeks post-injury) he was referred to our clinic for continuation of the treatment.

Physical Therapy Evaluation

S.G.'s complaints were inability to straighten the left little finger, inability to grip, constant pain, mostly over the radial aspect of the PIP joint, and persistent swelling of the finger; however, the major complaint was inability to play basketball, which he had played as a hobby two or three times a week.

Observation: The PIP joint was red and enlarged, and the finger was in flexion posture.

Objective evaluation: Circumferential measurement of the left PIP joint demonstrated an 0.5 mm difference when compared with the right.

Palpation: Point tenderness along the radial collateral ligament (RCL) and thickness of the PIP volar structures were present.

Active range of motion: S.G. was unable to actively extend the PIP joint. Goniometric measurement of the PIP joint demonstrated −28/66 degrees of extension/flexion. The DIP joint demonstrated 0/45 degrees compared to 0/90 degrees at the right PIP joint and 0/84 degrees at the DIP joint.

Passive range of motion: PIP extension limited in 6 degrees, DIP flexion was 60 degrees, and a mild joint capsule tightness was already present.

Special test: Positive oblique retinacular ligament (ORL) tightness. The PIP joint stress test was not significant. This test was performed because there was point tenderness along the RCL.

Treatment Goals

The goals of treatment were as follows:

Reduce pain and swelling

Prevent PIP joint flexion contracture

Prevent subluxation of lateral bands

Prevent ORL contracture

Allow soft tissue healing

Maintain range of motion of uninvolved digits

Return to previous level of function and sports participation.

Treatment

The finger was treated with deep tissue massage and pulse ultrasound to the RCL and volar joint area to reduce inflammation and promote healing.[89] A PIP 0 degree extension splint was constructed of Polyform, leaving free the DIP joint, and coban wrapping for edema control was applied. Instructions in active DIP joint flexion exercises to be performed every 2–3 hours, 15 repetitions each, and education about the deformity, importance of the role of continuous splinting, and self-assessment of finger vascularity were provided.

Reevaluation on the 3rd day demonstrated 3 mm difference in circumferential measurements, decreased tenderness over the RCL, and passive extension of 0. Instructions and initiation of exercises, as described by Burton[80] (already outlined), were done. S.G. was advised to remove the splint only during exercise sessions.

S.G. was seen on a weekly basis during the next 4 weeks for the outlined treatment, with monitoring of active range of motion and splint fit.

At the fifth week, S.G. reported resolution of pain. The central tendon strength was tested by asking him to flex the PIP joint to 20 to 30 degrees, followed by active extension; at this time, light resistance was applied to the middle phalanx. The extension motion was slow and hesitant, but he was able to maintain the PIP joint in extension. Due to the unsureness of the motion, he was advised to continue with the same program for another week. Ultrasound was discontinued at this point.

At the 6th week of continuous splint wear, active flexion exercises were initiated and progressed, as described in the postsurgical management. S.G. continued to wear the splint at all times except for exercises. The active PIP extension/flexion range was 0/32 degrees. The DIP flexion was 55 degrees.

By the 8th week of continuous splint wear, active range of motion was 0/50 degrees at the PIP joint and 0/70 degrees at the DIP joint, and the extensor tendon demonstrated good strength. S.G. was instructed to discontinue use of the splint during the day but continue wearing it at night. At this time he was allowed to return to play basketball with the splint on, but with the understanding that he was to start wearing it continuously if he noticed any loss of PIP joint extension range.

S.G. returned to the clinic 5 days later since he had lost the splint 3 days into the change of program. By then he demonstrated a 6 degree extension lag. A new splint was provided, and S.G. returned to continued wear of the splint for an additional 2 weeks. Full extension was restored within 3 days of splint wear.

By the 11th week, S.G. was weaned off day splinting, while night splint wear continued. Blocking exercises to all three joints were initiated. At the 12th week, light strengthening exercises to the hand were initiated. In addition, low-load prolonged stretching techniques by taping the finger in a comfortable passive flexion stretch while applying a paraffin bath,[90] and grade IV joint mobilization techniques were added to the program. The goals were to stretch the joint capsule and regain joint mobility.

At the 14th week of splint/exercise treatment, and 21½ weeks post injury, his therapy was discontinued, with a clear understanding that the splint would continue to be used at night for an additional 2 to 3 months and progressive hand strengthening exercises.

Discharge Summary

The MP joint's active range of motion measured +12/80 degrees of extension/flexion; that of the PIP joint was −2/74 degrees, and that of the DIP joint was 0/80 degrees. The left hand grip was 76.3 compared to 96.3 for the right hand grip. Palpation was pain-free through the joint, although he continued to demonstrate soft tissue density on its volar aspect.

In summary, the management of boutonniere deformity, either open or closed, is not difficult, but it requires an understanding of the anatomy of the extensor tendons and the pathomechanics of the deformity from the treating therapist. It also requires the patient's clear understanding of the importance of splint wear and a limited exercise program in the initial treatment. Educating the patient in the importance of 24 hour splint wear is probably the greatest challenge facing the therapist who treats this injury. The time required for rehabilitation of the boutonniere deformity by splinting can be prolonged. As stated by Burton,[80] for "those fingers that respond conservatively, the results equal or exceed that possible from surgery."

■ Summary

The complex anatomy and biomechanics of the wrist and hand can make rehabilitation either a challenge or drudgery. Successful rehabilitation avoids the complications associated with soft tissue damage or immobilization that results in functional impairment. The information presented in this chapter includes the anatomy and biomechanics of the wrist and hand, a comprehensive clarifying evaluation, and management of common injuries. It is designed to assist clinicians in developing and implementing effective and safe treatment within the constraints and relative time frame of soft tissue and fracture healing.

■ References

1. Strickland JW: Anatomy and kinesiology of the hand. p. 3. In Fess EE, Philips CA (eds): Hand Splinting: Principles and Methods. CV Mosby, St. Louis, 1987
2. Bogumill G: Anatomy of the wrist. p. 14. In Lichtman DM (ed): The Wrist and Its Disorders. WB Saunders, Philadelphia, 1988
3. Taleisnik J: The Wrist. Churchill Livingstone, New York, 1985
4. Sandzen SC: Atlas of Wrist and Hand Fractures. PSG Publishing, Littleton, MA, 1986
5. Taleisnik J: Ligaments of the carpus. p. 17. In Razemon JP, Fisk GR (eds): The Wrist. Churchill Livingstone, Edinburgh, 1988
6. Sennwald G: The Wrist. Anatomical and Pathophysiological Approach to Diagnosis and Treatment. Springer-Verlag, Berlin, 1887
7. Flatt AE, Youm Y, Berger RA: Kinematics of the human wrist. p. 45. In Razemon JP, Fisk GR (eds): The Wrist. Churchill Livingstone, Edinburgh, 1985
8. Weber ER: Wrist mechanics and its association with ligamentous instability. p. 41. In Lichtman DM (ed): The Wrist and Its Disorders. WB Saunders, Philadelphia, 1988
9. Tubiana R, Thomine J, Mackin E: Examination of the Hand and Wrist. CV Mosby, St. Louis, 1996
10. Jenkins DB: Hollinshead's Functional Anatomy of the Limbs and Back. WB Saunders, Philadelphia, 1998
11. Chase R: Anatomy and kinesiology of the hand. p. 13. In Hunter JM, Schneider LH, Mackin EJ, et al (eds): Rehabilita-

tion of the Hand. Surgery and Therapy. 3rd Ed. CV Mosby, St. Louis, 1990

12. Beasley RW: Hand Injuries. WB Saunders, Philadelphia, 1985

13. Melzack R: The McGill pain questionnaire. p. 41. In Melzack R (ed): Pain Measurements and Assessment. Raven Press, New York, 1983

14. Scott J, Huskeson E: Graphic representation of pain. Pain: 2:175, 1976

15. Salter MI: Hand Injuries: A Therapeutic Approach. Churchill Livingstone, Edinburgh, 1987

16. Hoppenfeld S: Physical Examination of the Spine and Extremities. Appleton-Century-Crofts, New York, 1976

17. American Society for Surgery of the Hand: The Hand, Examination and Diagnosis. 3rd Ed. Churchill Livingstone, New York, 1990

18. Lister G: The Hand: Diagnosis and Indication. 2nd Ed. Churchill Livingstone, Edinburgh, 1984

19. Aulicino P: Clinical examination of the hand. p. 53. In Hunter JM, Schneider LH, Mackin EJ, et al (eds): Rehabilitation of the Hand. Surgery and Therapy. 4th Ed. CV Mosby, St. Louis, 1995

20. Evans RB: Clinical examination of the hand. In Kasch MC, Taylor-Mullins PA, Fullenwider L (eds): Hand Therapy Review Course Study Guide. Hand Therapy Certification Commission, Garner, NC, 1990

21. Calliet R: Hand Pain and Impairment. 3rd Ed. FA Davis, Philadelphia, 1982

22. Magee D: Orthopedic Physical Assessment. WB Saunders, Philadelphia, 1987

23. Beckenbaugh RD: Accurate evaluation and management of the painful wrist following injury. p. 289. In Lichtman D (ed): The Wrist. The Orthopedic Clinics of North America, Vol. 15. WB Saunders, Philadelphia, 1984

24. Brown DE, Lichtman DM: Physical examination of the wrist. p. 74. In Lichtman DM (ed): The Wrist and Its Disorders. WB Saunders, Philadelphia, 1988

25. Moran CA, Saunders SR, Tribuzi SM: Myofascial pain in the upper extremity. p. 731. In Hunter JM, Schneider LH, Mackin EJ, et al (eds): Rehabilitation of the Hand. Surgery and Therapy. 3rd Ed. CV Mosby, St. Louis, 1990

26. Razemon JP, Fisk GR: The Wrist. Churchill Livingstone, Edinburgh, 1988

27. Brown DE, Lichtman DM: The evaluation of chronic wrist pain. p. 183. In Lichtman DM (ed): Symposium on the Wrist. The Orthopedic Clinics of North America, Vol. 15. WB Saunders, Philadelphia, 1984

28. Baxter-Petralia PL, Bruening LA, Blackmore SM, et al: Physical capacity evaluation. p. 93. In Hunter JM, Schneider LH, Mackin EJ, et al (eds): Rehabilitation of the Hand. Surgery and Therapy. 3rd Ed. CV Mosby, St. Louis, 1990

29. Cambridge-Keeling CA: Range-of-motion measurements of the hand. p. 93. In Hunter JM, Schneider LH, Mackin EJ, et al (eds): Rehabilitation of the Hand. Surgery and Therapy. 4th Ed. CV Mosby, St. Louis, 1995

30. Fess E: Documentation: essential elements of an upper extremity assessment battery. p. 185. In Hunter JM, Schneider LH, Mackin EJ, et al (eds): Rehabilitation of the Hand. Surgery and Therapy. 4th Ed. CV Mosby, St. Louis, 1995

31. Bell-Krotoski JA: Sensibility testing: state of the art. p. 575. In Hunter JM, Schneider LH, Mackin EJ, et al (eds): Rehabilitation of the Hand. Surgery and Therapy. 3rd Ed. CV Mosby, St. Louis, 1990

32. Callahan AD: Sensibility testing: clinical methods. p. 594. In Hunter JM, Schneider LH, Mackin EJ, et al (eds): Rehabilita-

tion of the Hand. Surgery and Therapy. 3rd Ed. CV Mosby, St. Louis, 1990

33. Dellon AL: Evaluation of Sensibility and Re-education of Sensation in the Hand. Williams & Wilkins, Baltimore, 1981

34. Tinel J: The "tingling" sign in peripheral nerve lesions (translated by EB Kaplan). In Spinner M (ed): Injuries to the Major Branches of Peripheral Nerves of the Forearm. 2nd Ed. WB Saunders, Philadelphia, 1978

35. Sunderland S: Nerves and Nerve Injuries. 2nd Ed. Churchill Livingstone, New York, 1978

36. Moran CA, Callahan AD: Sensibility measurement and management. p. 45. In Moran CA (ed): Hand Rehabilitation. Clinics in Physical Therapy. Churchill Livingstone, New York, 1986

37. Eglseder WA: Distal radius fractures. J Sout Ortho Assoc 6(4):289, 1997

38. Colles A: On the fractures of the carpal extremity of the radius. Edinb Med Surg J 10:182, 1914

39. Salter RB: Textbook of Disorders and Injuries of the Musculoskeletal System. Williams & Wilkins, Baltimore, 1970

40. Frykman G, Nelson E: Fractures and traumatic conditions of the wrist. p. 267. In Hunter JM, Schneider LH, Mackin EJ, et al (eds): Rehabilitation of the Hand. Surgery and Therapy. 3rd Ed. CV Mosby, St. Louis, 1990

41. Frykman G: Fracture of the distal radius including sequelae—shoulder-hand-finger syndrome, disturbance in the distal radioulnar joint, and impairment of nerve function: a clinical and experimental study. Acta Orthop Scand, suppl. 108:1, 1970

42. Andersen DJ, Steyers CM, El-Khouri GY: Classification of distal radius fractures: an analysis of interobserver reliability and intraobserver reproducibility. J Hand Surg 21(A):575, 1996

43. Leibovic SJ: Fixation for distal radius fractures. Hand Clin 13(4):665, 1997

44. Care SB, Graham TJ: Distal radius injuries. p. 69. In Jebson PJL, Kasdan ML (eds): Hand Secrets: Questions You Will Be Asked—On Rounds—In the Clinic—On Oral Exams. Hanley & Belfus, Philadelphia, 1998

45. Sarmiento A: The brachioradialis as a deforming force in Colles' fractures. Clin Orthop 38:86, 1965

46. Beasley R: Hand Injuries. WB Saunders, Philadelphia, 1981

47. Clyburn TA: Dynamic external fixation for comminuted intra-articular fractures of the distal end of the radius. J Bone Joint Surg 69(A):248, 1987

48. Boyes JH: Bunnell's Surgery of the Hand. JB Lippincott, Philadelphia, 1964

49. Sorenson MK: Fractures of the wrist and hand. p. 197. In Moran CA (ed): Hand Rehabilitation. Clinics in Physical Therapy. Churchill Livingstone, New York, 1986

50. Sorenson MK: Pulse galvanic stimulation for post-op edema in the hand. Pain Control 37:1, 1983

51. Paris SV: Extremity Dysfunction and Mobilization. Institute of Graduate Health Sciences, Atlanta, GA, 1980

52. Byron TM, Muntzer EM: Therapist's management of the mutilated hand. In Mackin EJ (ed): Hand Clinics. Vol. 2, No. 1. WB Saunders, Philadelphia, 1986

53. Hunter JM, Mackin EJ: Management of edema. p. 77. In Hunter JM, Schneider LH, Mackin EJ, et al (eds): Rehabilitation of the Hand. Surgery and Therapy. 4th Ed. CV Mosby, St. Louis, 1995

54. Szabo RM: Carpal tunnel syndrome as a repetitive motion disorder. Clin Orthop 351:78–89, 1998

55. Novak CB, Mackinnon SE: Nerve injury in repetitive motion disorders. Clin Orthop 351:10–20, 1998

56. Stock SR: Workplace ergonomic factors and the development of musculoskeletal disorders of the neck and upper limbs: a meta-analysis. Am J Ind Med 19:87–107, 1991

57. Vender MI, Kasdam NL, Truppa KL: Upper extremity disorders: a literature review to determine work-relatedness. J Hand Surg 20A:541–543, 1995

58. Phalen GS: The carpal tunnel syndrome: seventeen years experience in diagnosis and treatment of six hundred and fifty-four hands. J Bone Joint Surg 48(A):211, 1966

59. Taylor N: Carpal tunnel syndrome. Am J Phys Med 4:192, 1971

60. Schuind F, Ventura M, Pasteels JL: Idiopathic carpal tunnel syndrome: histologic study of flexor tendon synovium. J Hand Surg 15A:497–503, 1990

61. Detmars DM, Housin HP: Carpal tunnel syndrome. Hand Clin 2:525, 1986

62. Gelberman RH, Hergenroeder PT, Hargens AR, et al: The carpal tunnel syndrome: a study of carpal tunnel pressures. J Bone Joint Surg 63A:380–383, 1981

63. Hunter JM, Davlin LB, Fedus LM: Major neuropathies of the upper extremity: the median nerve. p. 910. In Hunter JM, Mackin EJ, Callahan AD (eds): Rehabilitation of the Hand. Surgery and Therapy, 4th Ed. CV Mosby, St. Louis, 1995

64. Silverstein BA, Fine LJ, Armstrong TJ: Occupational factors and carpal tunnel syndrome. Am J Ind Med 11:343–358, 1987

65. Rosenbaum RB, Ochoa JL: Carpal tunnel syndrome: clinical presentation, p. 35. In Carpal Tunnel Syndrome and Other Disorders of the Median Nerve. Butterworth-Heinemann, Boston, 1993

66. Johnson EW: Diagnosis of carpal tunnel syndrome. The gold standard. Editorial. Am J Phys Med Rehabil 72:1, 1993

67. Gerr F, Letz R: The sensitivity and specificity of tests for carpal tunnel syndrome vary with the comparison subjects. J Hand Surg (British and European volume) 23B(2):151–155, 1998

68. Jablecki CK, Andary MT, So YT, et al: Literature review of the usefulness of nerve conduction studies and electromyography for the evaluation of patients with carpal tunnel syndrome. AAEM Quality Assurance Committee. Muscle Nerve 16:1392–1414, 1993

69. Kimura J: The carpal tunnel syndrome: localization of conduction abnormalities within the distal segment of the median nerve. Brain 102:619–635, 1979

70. MacDermid J: Accuracy of clinical tests used in the detection of carpal tunnel syndrome: a literature review. J Hand Ther 4:169–175, 1991

71. Koris M, Gelberman RH, Duncan K, et al: Carpal tunnel syndrome: evaluation of a quantitative provocation diagnostic test. Clin Orthop 251:157–161, 1990

72. Clinical Assessment Recommendations. 2nd Ed. American Society of Hand Therapists, Chicago, 1992

73. Rempel D, Manojlovie R, Levinsohn DG, et al: The effects of wearing a flexible wrist splint on carpal tunnel pressure during repetitive hand activity. J Hand Surg 19A:106–110, 1994

74. Rozmaryn L, Dovelle S, Rothman ER, et al: Nerve and tendon gliding exercises and the conservative management of carpal tunnel syndrome. J Hand Ther 11:171–179, 1998

75. Hunter J, Belkin J: Therapist's management of carpal tunnel syndrome. p. 644. In Hunter JM, Schneider LH, Mackin EJ, et al (eds): Rehabilitation of the Hand. Surgery and Therapy. 3rd Ed. CV Mosby, St. Louis, 1990

76. Katz BE: Silasticgel sheeting: effective in scar surgery. Cosm Derm 32:1–3, 1992

77. Doyle JR: Extensor tendons—acute injuries. p. 1941. In Green DP (ed): Operative Hand Surgery, 3rd Ed. Churchill Livingstone, New York, 1993

78. Burton RI: The hand. p. 137. In Goldstein LA, Dickerson RC (eds): Atlas of Orthopaedic Surgery, 2nd Ed. CV Mosby, St. Louis, 1981

79. Zancolli E: Structural and Dynamic Bases of Hand Surgery. p. 105. JB Lippincott, Philadelphia, 1968

80. Burton RI: Extensor tendons—late reconstruction. p. 1976. In Green DP (ed): Operative Hand Surgery. 3rd Ed. Churchill Livingstone, New York, 1993

81. Hermann Wright H, Rettig AC: Management of common sports injuries. p. 1830. In Hunter JM, Schneider LH, Mackin EJ, et al (eds): Rehabilitation of the Hand: Surgery and Therapy. 4th Ed. CV Mosby, St. Louis, 1995

82. Valdata Eddinton L: Boutonniere deformity. p. 143. In Clark GL, Wilgis EF, Aillo B, et al (eds): Hand Rehabilitation: A Practical Guide. Churchill Livingstone, New York, 1993

83. Carducci AT: Potential boutonniere deformity. Its recognition and treatment. Orthop Rev 10:121–123, 1981

84. Evans RB: An update on extensor tendon management. p. 577. In Hunter JM, Schneider LH, Mackin EJ, et al (eds): Rehabilitation of the Hand. Surgery and Therapy. 4th Ed. CV Mosby, St. Louis, 1995

85. Evans RB: Therapeutic management of extensor tendon injuries. Hand Clin 2:157, 1986

86. Small JO, Brennen MD, Colville J: Early active mobilization following flexor tendon repair in zone II. J Hand Surg 14B:383–391, 1989

87. Rosenthal EA: The extensor tendons: anatomy and management. p. 536. In Hunter JM, Schneider LH, Mackin EJ, et al (eds): Rehabilitation of the Hand: Surgery and Therapy. 4th Ed. CV Mosby, St. Louis, 1995

88. Littler JW: The digital extensor-flexor system. p. 3166. In Converse JM (ed): Reconstructive Plastic Surgery. Vol. 6. WB Saunders, Philadelphia, 1977

89. McDiarmid T, Ziskin MC, Michlovitz SL: Therapeutic ultrasound. p. 169. In Michlovitz SL (ed): Thermal Agents in Rehabilitation. 3rd Ed. FA Davis, Philadelphia, 1996

90. Rennie GA, Michlovitz SL: Biophysical principles of heating and superficial heating agents. p. 119. In Michlovitz SL (ed.): Thermal Agents in Rehabilitation, 3rd Ed. FA Davis, Philadelphia, 1996

91. Jupiter JR: Flynn's Hand Surgery. 4th Ed. Williams & Wilkins, Baltimore, 1991

92. Cannon NM, Foltz RW, Koepfer JN, et al: Manual of Hand Splinting. Churchill Livingstone, New York, 1985

93. Travell JG, Simons DG: Myofascial Pain and Dysfunction. Williams & Wilkins, Baltimore, 1983

94. Green DP: Operative Hand Surgery, 2nd Ed. Churchill Livingstone, New York, 1982

■ Suggested Readings

Cole IC: Fractures and ligament injuries of the wrist and hand. p. . In Bearrie (ed): Home Study Course 95-2 Topic: The Wrist and Hand. Orthopaedic Section, American Physical Therapy Association, La Crosse, WI, 1995

Gilliam J, Barstow IK: Joint range of motion. p. 49. In Van Deusen J, Brunt D (eds): Assessment in Occupational Therapy and Physical Therapy. WB Saunders, Philadelphia, 1997

Hicks PL: Evaluating a national outcomes data system: which one meets my needs? J Rehab Outcomes Measurement 1(2):38, 1997

Laseter GR, Carter PR: Management of distal radius fractures. J Hand Ther 9(2):114, 1996

Ramadan AM: Hand analysis. p. 78. In Van Deusen J, Brunt D (eds): Assessment in Occupational Therapy and Physical Therapy. WB Saunders, Philadelphia, 1997

Reiss B: Therapist's management of distal radial fractures. p. 337. In Hunter JM, Schneider LH, Mackin EJ, et al (eds): Rehabilitation of the Hand: Surgery and Therapy. 4th Ed. CV Mosby, St. Louis, 1995

Ross RG, LaStayo PC: Clinical assessment of pain. p. 123. In Van Deusen J, Brunt D (eds): Assessment in Occupational Therapy and Physical Therapy. WB Saunders, Philadelphia, 1997

Simmonds MJ: Muscle strength. p. 27. In Van Deusen J, Brunt D (eds): Assessment in Occupational Therapy and Physical Therapy. WB Saunders, Philadelphia, 1997

Skiren T, Fedorczyk J: Tendon and nerve injuries of the wrist and hand. p. 1. In Beattie P (ed): Home Study course 95-2 Topic: The Wrist and Hand. Orthopaedic Section, American Physical Therapy Association, La Crosse, WI, 1995

Stralka SW, Akin K: Reflex sympathetic dystrophy syndrome. p. 2. In Wadsworth C (ed): Home Study Course 97-2 Topic: The Elbow, Forearm and Wrist. Orthopaedic Section, American Physical Therapy Association, La Crosse, WI, 1997

Waggy C: Disorders of the wrist. p. 1. In Wadsworth C (ed): Home Study Course 97-2 Topic: The Elbow, Forearm, and Wrist. Orthopaedic Section, American Physical Therapy Association, La Crosse, WI, 1997.

CHAPTER 12
Reconstructive Surgery of the Wrist and Hand

Joseph S. Wilkes

The hand is the main manipulative organ of the human body and performs many different functions, ranging from lifting very heavy objects to repairing objects with microscopic instruments. Reconstructive surgical considerations for acquired and congenital problems of the hand and wrist pose considerable challenges for both the surgeon and the physical therapist. Attempts to correct these problems can be very satisfying to all involved; they can also prove frustrating if problems arise either in the surgical procedure or in the rehabilitation. To overcome these potential problems, a separate specialty dedicated to hand and wrist problems has been formed among both surgeons and therapists. These professionals are trained to examine all aspects of the hand, as well as to consider the lifestyle and occupation of the patient. Two patients with similar severe impairments but with different lifestyles may require different surgical procedures to restore function and to allow them to use the hand in their chosen lifestyle or occupation. Hand injuries alone, however slight, may render the patient completely unemployable in his or her normal occupation. Therefore, care of hand injuries, for patients and for workers' compensation boards, can be among the most costly areas of medical care in our modern technical world.[1]

■ Examination

A good history should accompany any physical examination, but especially one involving the hand. Specific areas to define are (1) the onset of the problem, whether acute or insidious; (2) the length of time the problem has been present; (3) the types of movements that exacerbate the problem, as well as what seems to reduce the problem; (4) the functional limitations that are caused by the problem; and (5) associated manifestations relating either to the arm or to other parts of the body. The examination itself should include both active and passive motion of all joints, along with palpation of the joints, as indicated by swelling or a history of pain.

Any deformity of the hand should be examined in detail. The tendons about the wrist as well as the fingers should be palpated through the skin and their excursion appreciated on active movement. The bony prominences that may be involved should be palpated, and the clinician should note whether they are in their normal position and whether there is any swelling or tenderness. The tendons and muscles should be tested separately for the wrist, as well as for each finger and each tendon or muscle for the fingers (Fig. 12–1). There can be some trick movements with intrinsic and extrinsic muscles, and therefore specific testing is necessary.[2] Specific testing for the radial, ulnar, and median nerves is necessary. These peripheral nerves innervate the hand; there is also occasional innervation of the dorsum of the wrist by the musculocutaneous nerve.

Once a thorough physical examination has been performed and a history has been taken, further studies may be necessary. Radiographs are valuable in evaluating the bony structures and joint spaces. Other tests for problems that are more difficult to diagnose may include bone scans, arthrograms, nerve conduction testing, tomograms, and electromyographic testing, as well as computed tomography and magnetic resonance imaging scans.

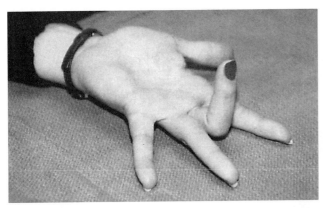

Figure 12–1. Inability to flex the DIP joint indicates that the flexor digitorum profundus to the finger is not functioning.

■ Traumatic Injuries

Traumatic injuries account for the largest number of problems of the hand and wrist.[3] The injuries can range from simple sprains or contusions to major disruptions of hand function, including amputation. Traumatic injuries can occur in any setting, including work, home, and recreational activities. Traumatic injuries frequently seen by the hand surgeon include fractures, tendon injuries, nerve injuries, and wrist sprains (Fig. 12–2).

Fractures

Fractures occur when the hand or wrist is struck by a force of such magnitude that the osseous structure is interrupted, causing a bone to separate into two or more fragments. Treatment of displaced fractures includes a general realignment of the part so that, when healing takes place, the part will function in an essentially normal manner. In the hand and fingers, close anatomic approximation of the fracture surfaces is generally required to achieve this level of function.

External support, such as a cast, is usually necessary for stable fractures for several weeks to allow bony union to occur. If the fracture is not immobilized long enough to allow healing to occur, nonunion may result, or malunion if the fracture is displaced during the healing process. The soft tissue structures should be tested at the time of initial examination to be sure that the neurovascular and muscular structures of the area are intact. If they are found to be involved, treatment of the fracture may be altered.

The distal radius fracture, or Colles' fracture, is one of the most common fractures of the wrist and hand. It can occur in any age group but appears to be more prevalent in older patients in whom osteoporosis is a factor. This injury generally occurs, as does a large proportion of hand injuries, when the patient falls on an outstretched hand. Depending on the magnitude of the force and the direction in which it is applied, the fracture pattern may vary, but most commonly the fracture occurs within 1 in. of the articular surface, causing dorsal angulation of the distal fragment in the metaphyseal area of the distal radius, with or without a fracture of the ulnar styloid (Fig. 12–3A). In most cases, this fracture can be treated by closed reduction with appropriate anesthesia to allow relaxation of the muscles. The type of cast varies from a short arm splint to a long arm cast, depending on the fracture pattern and whether there is comminution. In older individuals, the cast is retained for 3 to 4 weeks until early healing occurs. In younger patients, a longer period, closer to 6 to 8 weeks, is required for sufficient stability to start early motion. After the cast is removed, a removable splint is used to protect the fracture while early motion and strength of the healing bone are restored (Fig. 12–3B). If the fracture involves the articular surface or cannot be maintained by an external support such as a cast, some type of fixation of the fracture will be necessary.

There are many methods of fixation of a Colles' fracture. They include simple closed reduction, a pin or a rod across the fracture surface, plates and screws, or a metallic external fixator. The metallic external fixator is

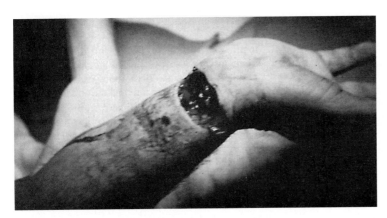

Figure 12–2. Severe laceration of the wrist disrupts the tendons and major nerves and arteries to the hand.

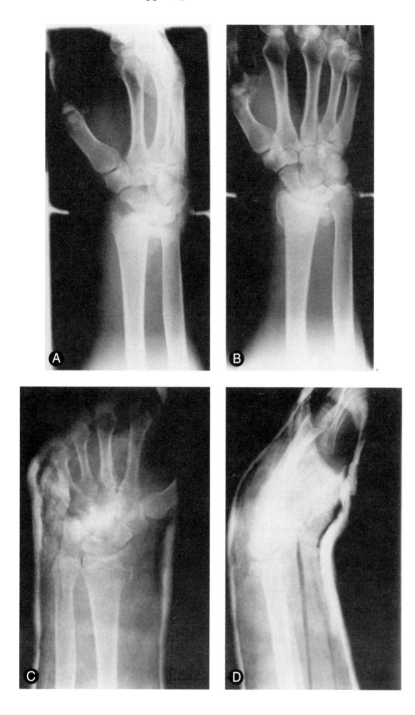

Figure 12–3. Distal radius fracture. (A,B) Radiographs show mild displacement; (C,D) after closed reduction and casting, acceptable alignment is seen.

held in place by pins placed in the bone proximal and distal to the fracture site, holding the fracture in a reduced position (Figs. 12–4 and 12–5). Generally, if this fracture can be reduced to even a marginally acceptable position in the older patient, good function will be regained after the fracture heals and appropriate therapy is concluded. Younger patients will require close anatomic reduction for long-term painless function.

Another very common fracture of the wrist and hand is navicular fracture (Fig. 12–6A). The navicular bone has an unusual blood supply, entering from the distal pole and proceeding retrograde into the proximal pole.[4] Fractures may occur at any level in the navicular, but the

more proximal the fracture, the greater the chance of avascular necrosis of the proximal fragment and nonunion of the fracture because of the loss of blood supply (Fig. 12–6B). Frequently, these fractures are hard to see on the initial radiograph because they have a hairline component. Also, because of the anatomy of the bone, it is very difficult to get straight anteroposterior and lateral views of the bone. The result is that these fractures are frequently missed. In this situation, when a patient has wrist trauma and pain in the anatomic snuffbox on the radial aspect of the wrist, the thumb, wrist, and forearm should be at least splinted for 10 to 14 days, after which a reexamination is performed to determine if a fracture has, in fact,

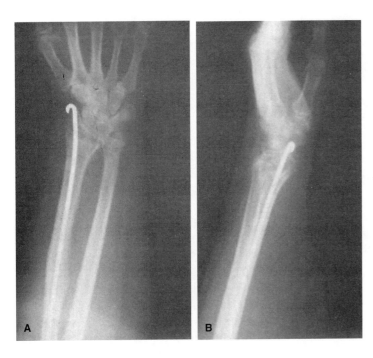

Figure 12–4. An unstable distal radius fracture is held with a Rush rod.

occurred. This protects the patient and should decrease the incidence of nonunion and avascular necrosis. Early immobilization is essential in this type of fracture to reduce the incidence of these problems. Displaced fractures of the navicular may require open reduction and internal fixation either with crossed Kirschner wires or with a special screw made particularly for the navicular called the *Herbert screw*.[5] Also, delayed union or nonunion of the fracture may require a subsequent surgical procedure for bone grafting and/or fixation of the fracture to stimulate healing.[6]

The length of time necessary for a navicular fracture to heal is variable, from a minimum of 6 weeks to as long as 9 months. This fracture is treated with a thumb spica cast, holding the thumb in the palmar abducted position.

The wrist is generally kept in a neutral position or in some other position that will maintain reduction of the fracture, and either a short or long arm cast is used, depending on the surgeon's preference.

Fractures or dislocations of the other carpal bones may occur, and a high index of suspicion is generally needed to diagnose these problems. A careful history and a physical examination are necessary to point the clinician to the appropriate area for consideration. Frequently, multiple radiographic views and/or follow-up studies with tomograms or bone scans may be necessary for a definitive diagnosis. Treatment of these fractures is by closed or open reduction as necessary, including the dislocations, and then splinting for an appropriate period of time to allow healing. Fractures of the nonarticular por-

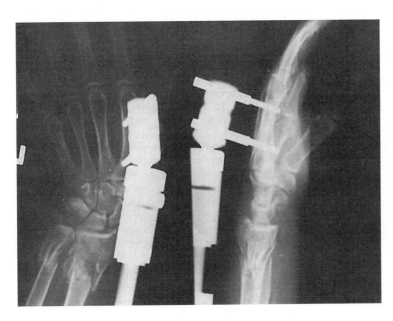

Figure 12–5. Extremely comminuted distal radius fracture held in alignment with an external fixator.

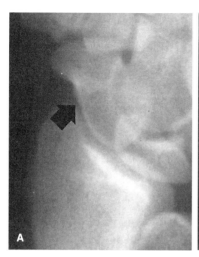
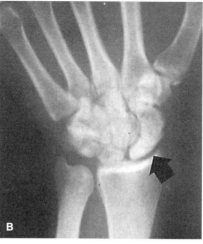

Figure 12–6. Navicular fracture. (A) A hairline navicular fracture; (B) a navicular fracture that progressed to avascular necrosis and nonunion.

tions of the metacarpals and phalanges most frequently are stable injuries, and close anatomic alignment with external support will generally suffice for these injuries.

Intra-articular fractures involving the wrist or hand require anatomic alignment of the articular surfaces. The articular surface is a smooth gliding surface on which movement occurs in the wrist and fingers. If there is a step-off or a significant gap in this smooth surface, deterioration of the joint can occur very quickly. If the fracture is displaced and cannot be reduced, open reduction and internal fixation must be considered to provide close to normal function when the fracture heals (Fig. 12–7). Also, fractures that are in close association with

the insertion of a tendon, whether in the wrist or the fingers, are frequently unstable because of the muscle pull, which cannot be completely neutralized. If the fractures cannot be brought into a stable, reduced position by closed technique, open reduction and internal fixation are frequently needed to immobilize the fracture against the pull of the muscle and tendon for alignment to be maintained.

Fractures associated with injuries to adjacent structures, such as tendon ruptures or nerve lacerations, may require more aggressive treatment, such as open reduction and internal fixation, to allow for appropriate repair and rehabilitation of the tendons and nerves.[7] This can allow for an earlier introduction of therapy for range of motion and gentle use of the hand for rehabilitation.

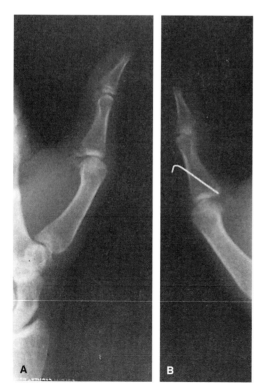

Figure 12–7. Intra-articular fracture. (A) Displaced intra-articular fracture of the thumb metacarpophalangeal joint; (B) after open reduction and pin fixation.

CASE STUDY

A 20-year-old man sustained an injury falling on his outstretched hand while playing rugby on the evening before evaluation. On evaluation, he was found to have swelling and deformity of the left wrist. On examination, his neurovascular function was found to be intact. The motors to the fingers appeared to be intact. Movement of the wrist was extremely painful and could not be tested. Radiographs showed a trans-scaphoid perilunate dislocation (Fig. 12–8A,B).

Immediately after evaluation with a xylocaine block in the area of injury, a closed reduction of the perilunate dislocation was accomplished without problems. Postreduction radiographs showed excellent relocation of the carpus, but the fracture of the navicular remained unacceptably displaced. The following day, the patient underwent an open reduction and internal fixation with a Herbert screw of the navicular fracture (Fig. 12–8C,D). He remained in a long-arm cast for 5 weeks and then in a short arm thumb spica cast for 4 weeks. At that time he was taken out of the cast, placed in a removable splint, and started on a physical therapy program for range of

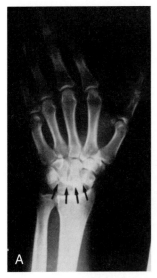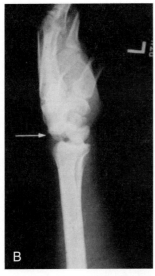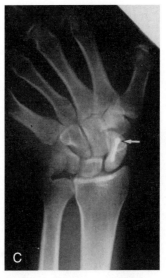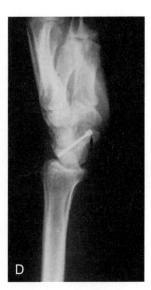

Figure 12–8. Radiographs showing (A) dorsal transscaphoid perilunate dislocation with overlapping of the carpal bones on the anteroposterior view (small arrows) and (B) dorsal displacement of the capitate from the lunate fossa on the lateral view (large arrow). (C,D) Anteroposterior and lateral views of the wrist after healing, with anatomic positioning of the carpal bones and healing of the fractured scaphoid with a retained Herbert screw fixation device.

motion of the wrist and thumb and muscle rehabilitation. His course was complicated by avascular necrosis of the proximal pole of the navicular. With only moderate use of his wrist, he regained full range of motion and strength in the hand and wrist. The avascular necrosis completely resolved spontaneously at 9 months postinjury.

Tendon Injuries

Tendinitis is an inflammation of the tendon unit. It can be associated with either an overuse syndrome or a sprain of the muscle-tendon unit resulting from a traumatic episode. Tendinitis can generally be treated with a period of immobilization to allow the initial inflammation to settle down, followed by gentle stretching and toning exercises with local therapy, such as ice, heat, and friction massage or other modalities as necessary to allow the tendinitis to subside.

More serious tendon injuries include ruptures and lacerations. These injuries generally are treated by open repair because approximation of the tendon ends is very difficult with closed methods of treatment, and therefore loss of function is likely. One condition in which rupture of a tendon can frequently be treated satisfactorily by closed methods is mallet finger.[8] In this injury, the extensor tendon is avulsed at the level of the distal interphalangeal joint, causing lack of extension of the joint (Fig. 12–9). Splinting in a hyperextended position generally allows healing of the tendon and excellent function subsequently.

Most other tendon injuries are approached surgically for open repair. A tendon that does not require significant excursion with motion, such as most extensor tendons, especially the wrist extensors or the abductor of the thumb, can be treated after open repair with casting for 4 to 6 weeks and then with gentle mobilization. Adhesions in extensor tendon areas generally are not severe, and near-normal function is usually achieved. In the flexor tendons of the fingers and thumb, the excursion is much greater, and therefore adhesions can significantly inhibit restoration of normal function. The repair of these tendons is very delicate, and an atraumatic method of repair is used to secure the tendon and ensure a smooth surface at the level of the cut (Fig. 12–10A). Repair of flexor tendons in "no-man's land," the area in the digits where the flexor superficialis and the flexor profundus glide

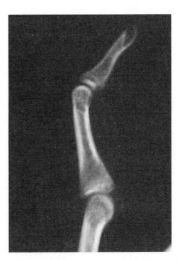

Figure 12–9. Abnormal flexion of the DIP joint after disruption of the extensor tendon distal to the PIP joint, typical of a mallet deformity.

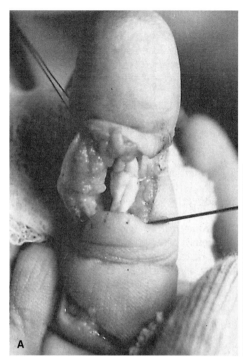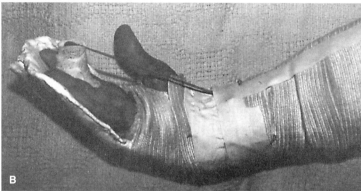

Figure 12–10. Tendon repair. (A) Suture of the flexor digitorum profundus after laceration;
(B) immediate dynamic splinting mobilization for early rehabilitation.

against one another in the fibro-osseous tunnel, is the hardest area in which to gain good function. Repair of both tendons at this level is generally recommended, as with all flexor tendon lacerations of the digits. Also, early motion with a dynamic splint as recommended by Lister et al.,[9] allows for early function and decreased problems with adhesions (Fig. 12–10B).

Repair of the pulley system of the fibro-osseous tunnel is very important in decreasing the incidence of serious adhesions to a lacerated flexor tendon.[10] If adhesions do limit the range of motion and function of the finger, tenolysis should be performed no earlier than 6 months after the original repair. This allows for settling down of the original scar tissue so that scarring is not reactivated and only the reaction to the new surgery becomes an inhibitor. With tenolysis, the fibro-osseous tunnel should be repaired if possible to allow for good nourishment of the tendon, decrease of adhesions, and better mechanical function of the tendon. After tenolysis, active and active-assisted range-of-motion exercises are initiated unless there has been a violation of the tendon itself. Late repairs of tendon ruptures may require insertion of a Silastic rod to reestablish the synovial space in the sheath and allow for reconstruction of the pulley system before introduction of a graft tendon. Once the pulley system has been established and full passive motion is achieved in all joints, a tendon graft can be inserted from the distal stump to the distal forearm.[11] Passive range of motion is performed over approximately 6 weeks to achieve full range. Again, early motion with a dynamic splint is recommended, with

a prolonged rehabilitation time to allow for vascularization of the grafted tendon.

CASE STUDY

A 47-year-old man who is active in karate sustained a kick to his left fifth finger, with subsequent loss of the ability to flex the distal interphalangeal (DIP) joint of the fifth finger. He was seen 10 days later with a history as noted and no symptoms of numbness or vascular compromise. Examination confirmed the absence of active flexion at the DIP joint of the fifth finger. The problem was complicated by the fact that the patient had sustained a fracture mallet deformity approximately 9 months previously, which was untreated. He was interested in regaining the function of flexion of the DIP joint and underwent advancement and repair of the flexor digitorum profundus, which had been disrupted at its insertion on the distal phalanx. Postoperatively, he was placed in a dynamic flexion splint with a mallet splint over the DIP joint to avoid overpull on the previously injured extensor mechanism. This splint was removed several times a day to allow for flexion of the DIP joint and pull-through of the flexor digitorum profundus. The patient was taken completely out of his splint in 5 weeks and started on phyiscal therapy. At the end of 3½ months, he had 0 to 35 degrees of motion in the DIP joint and 0 to 95 degrees in the proximal interphalangeal (PIP) joint. At the end of

4½ months, he still lacked 1 cm of closing the fifth finger to the distal palmar crease. He was continued on exercises but was satisfied with the result at that point. Because of work pressures, he was unable to undergo further physical therapy.

Nerve Injuries

Nerve injuries may occur anytime a nerve undergoes trauma. The injury may be a simple contusion, a stretch-type injury, or a disruption of nerve fibers secondary to a laceration. Nerve injuries are also frequently associated with fractures and particularly flexor tendon injuries, where the nerves run in close proximity to the flexor tendons, not only at the wrist but also in the fingers. Three types of nerve injury can cause nerve dysfunction. Neurapraxia occurs when an injury such as a contusion causes electrical interruption of nerve conduction, but without disruption of the nerve itself and without degeneration of the axons. Recovery is generally expected within days to several weeks. The next, more serious type of injury, axonotmesis, occurs when the nerve is injured to such an extent that, although the nerve appears intact when inspected, degeneration occurs from the point of injury distally. Healing requires regrowth of the axons from the point of injury to the area of innervation. This can cause a prolonged period of nonfunction of the nerve but generally results in excellent return of function once the axons have regenerated. The most serious type of injury to the nerve is neurotmesis, in which the nerve is actually severed. Because there is disruption of the nerve bundles, even with surgical repair these bundles are very crudely realigned and return of function is variable, although with microsurgical techniques the return of function is generally fair to good and occasionally excellent.[12]

In the rehabilitation of these nerve injuries, it is very important to educate the patient as to the type of nerve injury suspected or known and the length of time that dysfunction of the nerve is expected to persist. This allows the patient to adjust his or her daily lifestyle to the dysfunction and to protect any areas of lost sensation from injury.[13]

If nerves to muscle groups are involved, splinting may be necessary to avoid contractures of joints and loss of function secondary to the temporary loss of muscle function. Nerve regeneration from axonotmesis or neurotmesis occurs at a rate of approximately 1 mm/day; thus the length of time before return of function can be estimated by the distance from the nerve injury to the most proximal innervation site. Depending on the nature of the injury, the healing response of the particular individual, the amount of scarring in the area of injury, and the surgical technique used for repair, this return of sensation can range from only protective sensation (against sharp objects, heat, and cold) to almost normal sensation. Muscle groups are generally the most difficult to restore to function because of the time needed for return of the

axon to the muscle; during this time, atrophy and fibrosis can occur in the muscle.

Carpal tunnel syndrome is a very common acquired loss of nerve function which, if encountered and treated early, whether conservatively with splinting and medication or surgically with release of the transverse carpal ligament, results in early functional return of the nerve because the injury is only neurapraxic. Prolonged carpal tunnel disease with atrophy of the thenar muscles is associated with an axonotmesis, and occasionally scarring has already occurred in the area of compression. In these cases, functional return is sometimes incomplete even after release and neurolysis. With severe chronic carpal tunnel syndrome, some return of sensation is typically achieved, but motor return is poor. Both in carpal tunnel syndrome with atrophy of the thenar muscles and in neurotmesis injuries of motor nerves about the wrist, muscle transfers can be performed using muscles innervated by a different nerve to substitute for the muscles no longer functioning from the injured nerve. This naturally requires a period of rehabilitation for reeducation of the muscle tendon unit, as well as for mobilization of the joints that were immobilized to allow for healing of the transferred muscle-tendon unit. Loss of the nerve supply without full return can also cause hypersensitivity to cold weather. Therefore, repair of major nerves about the wrist and the fingers is indicated to restore satisfactory function of the hand.

Wrist Sprains

Sprains of the wrist are very common and generally mild. A sprained wrist that presents with moderate to large amounts of swelling or pain inappropriate to the level of suspected injury should indicate to the clinician that a more serious injury may have occurred.[14] One such injury is hairline fracture of the navicular bone, which frequently cannot be picked up on initial radiographs.

Other injuries associated with a wrist sprain that could be of clinical importance include tears of the intercarpal ligaments or of the triangular fibrocartilage complex. These injuries can be seriously debilitating and over time can cause degeneration of the wrist joints, further limiting function of the wrist and requiring more extensive and radical surgical correction. A tear of the scapholunate ligament is probably the most common symptomatic ligament tear of the wrist area. A tear of this ligament severs the connection between the proximal row of carpal bones, which includes the proximal half of the navicular, the lunate, and the triquetrum, from the distal row (Fig. 12–11). The scaphoid is the interconnecting link that coordinates not only flexion and extension movements but also radial and ulnar deviation between the two rows of carpal bones. When the scapholunate ligament is ruptured, the scaphoid generally falls into a plantar flexed position, and the proximal row is then an unconnected middle segment between the distal forearm and the more

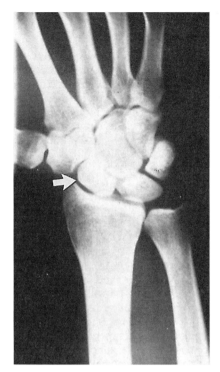

Figure 12–11. The space between the scaphoid and lunate (arrow) indicates scapholunate dissociation. Signet ring formation of the scaphoid indicates volar rotation of the scaphoid.

stable distal carpal row and the hand. This allows for subluxation in either a dorsal or a volar direction, depending on the forces transmitted, as well as any other ligamentous stretching that might have occurred at the time of the injury. The result is a painful, weak wrist which does not respond to conservative treatment. The wrist may get over the initial soreness, but when normal use is attempted, soreness and weakness are noted.

With a high index of suspicion, the ligament tear can be diagnosed by the history and physical examination, noting tenderness and swelling dorsally over the junction of the scaphoid and the lunate; on radiographic examination a widened space between the scaphoid and lunate is observed. On the anteroposterior radiograph, the scaphoid may have the appearance of a signet ring rather than its normal oblong shape. The ligament sometimes can be repaired acutely, but it is a very short ligament, and frequently it is difficult to get adequate sutures to repair it. In this situation or in the case of chronic scapholunate dissociation, a limited intercarpal fusion such as a tri-schaphi fusion can stabilize the carpus. This procedure fuses the scaphoid to the trapezium and the trapezoid so that it is maintained in a reduced position in its normal dorsiflexed attitude rather than the plantar flexed attitude associated with the ligament tear (Fig. 12–12). Minimal loss of motion in the wrist is associated with this limited fusion, but pain is generally relieved, advancement of degeneration can be slowed down or stopped, and strength returns.

On occasion, an intercarpal ligament tear or a tear of the triangular fibrocartilage cannot be diagnosed on clinical examination and plain radiography alone. In this situation, the patient generally presents with a prolonged

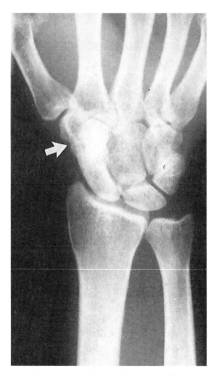

Figure 12–12. Treatment of scapholunate dissociation by tris-caphi fusion (arrow).

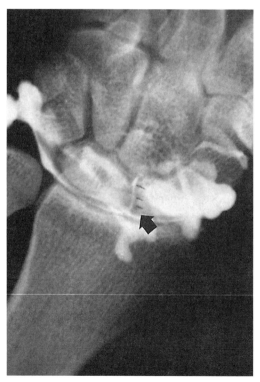

Figure 12–13. Arthrogram of the wrist showing dye leakage through the scapholunate space into the distal carpal row (arrow), indicating a disruption of the scapholunate ligament.

history, usually of several months' duration after a traumatic episode, complaining of persistent pain, occasional swelling, and popping or clicking in the wrist. A wrist arthrogram may be able to elucidate the torn ligament or triangular fibrocartilage (Fig. 12–13). Once the diagnosis of intercarpal ligament tear is made, a limited intercarpal fusion may solve the problem, and if a torn triangular fibrocartilage is found, it should be repaired if possible. Arthroscopic partial debridement of the triangular fibrocartilage may be sufficient. With advanced degenerative changes from old trauma, either Silastic replacement with limited intercarpal fusion to unload the Silastic prosthesis or a wrist fusion, may be necessary to restore satisfactory function of the hand.

After repair of an intercarpal ligament or an intercarpal fusion, immobilization is necessary for a sufficient length of time to allow the ligament to heal or the fusion to become solid. Immobilization frequently will need to include one or several fingers besides the wrist and forearm. The time in the cast is usually no less than 6 weeks, and the wrist and hand can be very stiff once the cast is removed. Physical therapy is generally indicated to increase the range of motion both passively and actively, as well as to strengthen the wrist. Methods for reduction of swelling along with heat and ultrasound can be useful to decrease the likelihood of tendinitis associated with the prolonged immobilization.

■ Wrist Arthroscopy

Wrist arthroscopy has become available in recent years and is being perfected. Currently, the indications for wrist arthroscopy are identification of problems that may be associated with unresolved wrist pain; removal of loose bodies; debridement of the triangular fibrocartilage, as mentioned above; synovectomy for a chronic synovitis or associated with rheumatoid arthritis; and visualization of depressed intra-articular wrist fractures during limited open reduction and internal fixation. This approach can limit the amount of scarring associated with this procedure and allow for more normal return of function and a more adequate reduction of the fracture under visualization.

Technique

Wrist arthroscopy is a surgical procedure that is performed in the surgical suite. The patient is given either a regional or a general anesthetic, and the shoulder is abducted 90 degrees and the elbow flexed 90 degrees with the fingers suspended, usually from a finger-trap device, to distract the wrist. The wrist and hand are then prepared for surgery. Arthroscopic visualization with an arthroscope of 3 mm or smaller provides the best overall view and is the least traumatic to the wrist (Fig. 12–14). The arthroscope

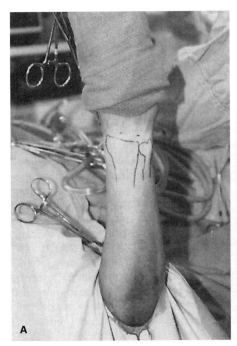
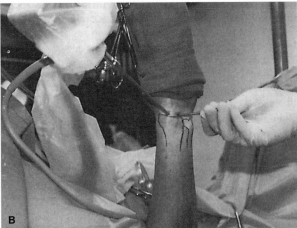

Figure 12–14. Technique of wrist arthroscopy. (A) Primary portals for the arthroscope and working instruments are between dorsal compartments 3 and 4 and compartments 4 and 5; (B) setup for wrist arthroscopy, with the arthroscope placed in the entrance portal between the third and fourth extensor groups.

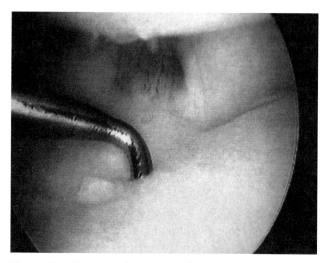

Figure 12–15. Intra-articular view of the wrist. The junction of the radial articular surface with the triangular fibrocartilage is visible. The anterior radio-carpal ligaments are in the middle, and the lunate articular surface is superior.

is introduced between the third and fourth extensor compartments after insufflation of the wrist joint with normal saline by injection needle.

Working instruments can be introduced either between the first and second dorsal compartment groups, more laterally between the fourth and fifth compartments, or just lateral to the sixth compartment. Visualization of the articular surfaces is usually very good, and the intercarpal ligaments between the scapholunate and lunotriquetral articulations can be evaluated (Fig. 12–15). The triangular fibrocartilage and the fossa of the ulnar styloid are also visualized through the arthroscope. The midcarpal joint can also be entered between the lunate and the capitate, visualizing these surfaces for occult chondromalacia and loose bodies.

Assuming that no open procedure is necessary in association with the arthroscopy, the patient is usually allowed to go home the same day with a light dressing on the wrist, and gentle range-of-motion exercises are started immediately. After the initial soreness disappears in 2 to 5 days, physical therapy can be started to increase mobility and regain strength about the wrist. When the procedure is performed under appropriate conditions, patients generally function at a normal level within at least a few weeks, and return to normal activities is much faster than when an open procedure is used.

■ Overuse Syndromes

Overuse syndromes of the wrist and hand are very common in modern work conditions. Work that requires repetitive use of the hand, especially assembly-line activities or clerical tasks such as key punching or invoice rectification, can produce these overuse syndromes. Heavier work such as the use of air hammers and power equipment can

also cause overuse syndromes. The most common overuse entity is carpal tunnel syndrome. It is usually related to either repetitive microtrauma to the wrist that causes inflammation of the tissues about the median nerve in the carpal canal or inflammation secondary to flexor tendon overuse. Other overuse syndromes include wrist or digital flexor and extensor tendinitis. All of these problems can result in time lost from work and should be treated aggressively with splinting, anti-inflammatory medication, and therapy as well as evaluation of the workplace to try to decrease the recurrence of repetitive use trauma.

■ Arthritis

Arthritis by definition means inflammation of a joint, but the term generally refers to a pathologic process involving inflammation that causes destruction of the joint. Many processes can cause cause arthritis, such as general wear and tear producing osteoarthritis; metabolic abnormalities, such as that which causes gouty arthritis; immune abnormalities resulting in rheumatoid arthritis or lupus arthritis; infections that can cause septic arthritis; and traumatic injuries that result in damage or unevenness of the joint surfaces, causing traumatic arthritis.

Osteoarthritis of the wrist and hand occurs mostly in the wrist, the DIP joints of the fingers, and the carpometacarpal joint of the thumb. The inflammation may be controlled conservatively by using nonsteroidal anti-inflammatory medications, heat, and maintenance of motion in the joints. Developing deformities may be controlled by intermittent splinting, although this is necessary only in a small proportion of patients with osteoarthritis. Surgical procedures for severe arthritis, in which there is uncontrolled pain, destruction of the joint on x-ray evaluation, or deformity with loss of function, may include simple debridement of the joint with removal of osteophytes or bone spurs and debridement of abnormal cartilage in the joint. Capsular reinforcement may also be necessary to control deformities. For more involved destruction, fusion of the joint may be necessary or, specifically in the case of the basilar thumb joint and wrist, a Silastic prosthesis may be useful to retain function after removing the abnormal joint. Physical therapy is occasionally necessary with conservative treatment for maintenance of range of motion in acutely inflamed joints by the use of gentle range-of-motion exercises, as well as heat, paraffin baths, and massage. Again, intermittent splinting may be necessary for some patients. After surgical procedures, immobilization is usually needed for a period of time, after which return of function is achieved through exercise and strengthening.

Rheumatoid arthritis is particularly debilitating to the hand, and treatment can be very involved (Fig. 12–16A–C). Briefly, rheumatoid arthritis not only affects the articular surfaces but also involves the soft tissues to a large extent, including the ligamentous structures as well as

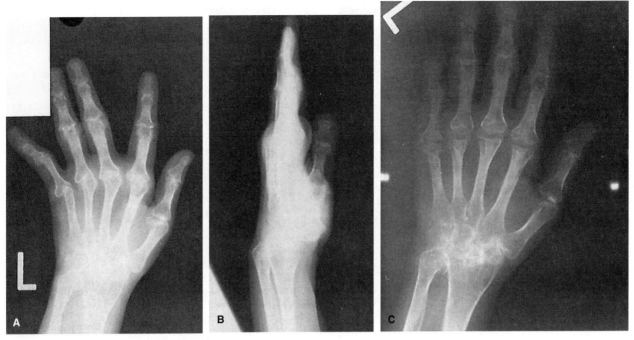

Figure 12–16. Rheumatoid arthritis. (A,B) Severely degenerative rheumatoid hand showing degeneration and subluxation of the metacarpophalangeal joints as well as severe degeneration of the wrist. (C) Postoperative view with Silastic metacarpophalangeal joints in place.

the tendinous structures about the wrist and hand. The cartilage surfaces are destroyed, and the soft tissue structures are weakened by degradation of the collagen and infiltration by the rheumatoid process. The joints most often involved are the wrist, the carpometacarpal joint of the thumb, and the metacarpophalangeal joints of the fingers. Deformity can occur simply by collapse of the joint surfaces or in combination with laxity of the surrounding capsular and ligamentous structures, causing subluxation and subsequent abnormal pull of the muscle-tendon units, resulting in grossly abnormal function of the hand. The tendons can also become involved, particularly the flexor tendons, and chronic uncontrolled inflammation can cause rupture of the tendons.

Treatment consists of controlling the disease process with medication, splinting to prevent stretching of the soft tissue structures and subsequent subluxation of the joints, and vigorous therapy to maintain strength and motion in the digits and the wrist. Surgical treatment in cases of minimal involvement of the articular surfaces can be accomplished by synovectomy and soft tissue reconstruction as necessary and then rehabilitation once healing of the reconstruction has occurred. In cases of more advanced destruction of the joints along with subluxation, soft tissue releases of the tight structures and reinforcement and reconstruction of the loose structures are necessary. Silastic joint replacement of the metacarpophalangeal joints and fascial arthroplasty of the basilar joint of the thumb and the wrist may be indicated (Fig. 12–16C). Fusion of the joints may be required for stability if there

is severe involvement of the soft tissues. Reconstruction of ruptured tendons is necessary to regain function, but it will fail if control of the disease by medication or synovectomy is not achieved. Prolonged dynamic splinting after reconstruction is generally necessary, with slow return of function, but because of the severe deformities, reconstructions of rheumatoid hands are generally very satisfying.

Septic arthritis can occur either through direct introduction of bacteria into the joint from a puncture wound or surgical procedure or via the bloodstream through hematogenous seeding of the joint with bacteria. Sepsis in a joint that is not treated early will result in destruction of the articular surfaces of the joint and cause septic arthritis.[15] Initially, control of the infection is necessary. If arthritis sets in from the septic process, a fusion or resection arthroplasty may be indicated, depending on the joint involved. It is only with hesitation that a Silastic or artificial joint would be placed in a previously septic joint.

Traumatic arthritis can occur when any traumatic episode results in injury to the articular surface and damage to the cartilaginous covering or to the ligamentous stability of the joint that causes abnormal mechanics and motion about the joint. Once the arthritis has set in, it is approached much like osteoarthritis, with control by nonsteroidal anti-inflammatory medications. Maintenance of joint mobility and function is important. Once the disease process had advanced past the point of control by conservative methods, arthrodesis or replacement of the joint may be indicated.

CASE STUDY

A 60-year-old woman who worked in a cafeteria had ongoing limitation of motion and pain in both hands, but it became acutely severe in the right index and long fingers, for which she came in for consultation. She was found to have a severely swollen index finger DIP joint and long finger proximal interphalangeal (PIP) joint. On examination, she was found to have limitation of motion of the index DIP joint and a large cystic mass on the long finger PIP joint with ulnar deviation at the joint. Radiographs confirmed severe degeneration of the index DIP joint and moderate degeneration with ulnar deviation at the long finger PIP joint (Fig. 12–17A,B). After examination assuring function of the neurovascular structures and all tendons, the patient underwent excision of the cyst and radial collateral ligament reconstruction of the long finger PIP joint and fusion of the DIP joint of the index finger with a Herbert Screw technique (Fig. 12–17C,D).

The patient was treated with a splint for the index finger and early range of motion for the long finger, with buddy taping to the index finger. At 4 months, she had excellent fusion of the DIP joint but still lacked some motion in the PIP joint of the index finger as well as the long finger. The index finger had excellent range of motion at the end of 6 months except for the DIP joint, which was fused. The patient was able to gain motion in the long finger PIP joint to approximately 10 to 90 degrees, with good function in the hand. She returned to work and was satisfied with her result.

■ Amputation

Amputations may occur for many reasons; trauma, vascular disease, surgical resection of tumors, and uncontrolled infections are some of the possible causes. Traumatic amputations or near-amputations that have, because of the mechanism of injury, maintained satisfactory tissue on either side of the amputation may lend themselves to reimplantation. This has become a specialized area within hand surgery. The reimplantation surgeon must consider many complex problems when anticipating reimplantation of a digit or hand. The length of the period of ischemia and the temperature of the divided part during that time can play a very important role in determining whether the tissue of the amputated part will survive. Also, with longer periods of ischemia, the arterial and venous anastomoses have a lower incidence of patency after repair. The coordination of several procedures—fixation of the skeletal structure, repair of the muscle-tendon units, as well as repair of the arteries, veins, and nerves that supply the part—must be taken into account. This is very tedious work, and frequently failure of one or more of these areas can cause subsequent loss of the digit. Reimplantation of digits distal to the DIP joint is rarely considered except on the thumb, and reimplantation of amputated tissue proximal to the wrist becomes much more complicated because of the amount of muscle tissue involved and the amount of myoglobin produced because of muscle necrosis, which can cause systemic complications, particularly in the kidneys.[16]

After loss of a part of the hand, if digits remain, it is very important to provide some type of pincer mechanism

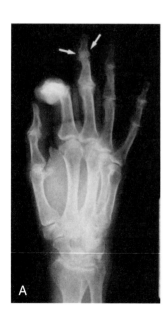
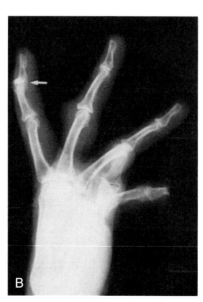
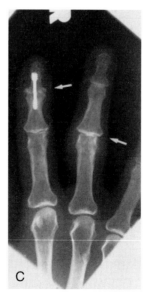
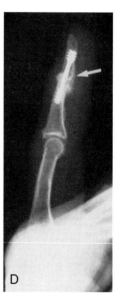

Figure 12–17. (A,B) Anteroposterior and lateral views of the right hand showing a severely degenerative index finger DIP joint and a large cystic mass with ulnar deviation of the PIP joint of the long finger. (C,D) Anteroposterior and lateral views of the index finger showing fusion of the DIP joint with a retained Herbert screw device, decreased soft tissue swelling about the PIP joint of the long finger, and decreased ulnar deviation.

for grasping. Therefore, if the thumb has been lost, one of the other digits will need to be transferred into an opposing position to the other one or two digits to produce the pincer motion.

Loss of a single digit distal to the DIP joint from a sharp amputation can neccessitate replantation for good function.[17] Loss of a single digit proximal to the PIP joint, particularly the long or ring finger, can cause dysfunction when trying to hold fairly small objects such as coins, which can fall through the gap in the fingers.[18] In these patients, ray amputation is frequently indicated to allow for more normal hand function. A hand with three fingers and one thumb seems to work very satisfactorily, almost as well as a regular hand. Occasionally, in a heavy laborer, maintenance of the partially amputated digit rather than ray amputation may be desirable to maintain the breadth of the hand and allow for greater grip strength. When the thumb has been amputated or when all the digits have been amputated with maintenance of some function of the thumb, a toe-to-hand transfer using free tissue technique can restore the former pincer movement of the hand.[19] Amputation proximal to the base of the metacarpals is very difficult to reconstruct, and a prosthetic replacement may provide satisfactory function.

Rehabilitation when only a single digit is involved can be as simple as reeducating the individual in the use of the hand without the amputated digit. If a transfer of digits within the same hand or toe-to-hand transfer of digits is performed to replace the thumb, the rehabilitation and reeducation in use of the hand can be very complex. Therapy after reimplantation is very prolonged because of scarring through the area of the amputation and repair. Consideration must be given to bone healing, the sliding and gliding motions of the tendons, and protection of the digit until sensation returns.

■ References

1. Flynn JE: Disability evaluations. p. 635. In Flynn JE (ed): Hand Surgery. 2nd Ed. Williams & Wilkins, Baltimore, 1975

2. Lee M: Tendon injuries. p. 150. In Crenshaw AH (ed): Campbell's Operative Orthopaedics. 7th Ed. Vol. 1. CV Mosby, St. Louis, 1987

3. Nichols HM: Manual of Hand Injuries. Year Book Medical Publishers, Chicago, 1957

4. Taleisnik J, Kelly PJ: The extraosseous and intraosseous blood supply of the scaphoid bone. J Bone Joint Surg 48(A):125, 1966.

5. Herbert TJ: Use of the Herbert bone screw in surgery of the wrist. Clin Orthop 202:79, 1986

6. Cooney WP, Dobyns JH, Linscheid RL: Fractures of the scaphoid: a rational approach to management. Clin Orthop 149:90, 1980

7. Lee M: Fractures. p. 186. In Crenshaw AH (ed): Campbell's Operative Orthopaedics. 7th Ed. Vol. 1. CV Mosby, St. Louis, 1987

8. Abouna JM, Brown H: The treatment of mallet finger: the results in a series of 148 consecutive cases and a review of the literature. Br J Surg 55:653, 1968

9. Lister GD, Kleinert HE, Kutz JE, et al: Primary flexor tendon repair followed by immediate controlled mobilization. J Hand Surg 2:441, 1977

10. Pennington DG: The influence of tendon sheath integrity and vincular blood supply on adhesion formation following tendon repair in hens. Br J Plast Surg 32:302, 1979

11. Schneider LH, Hunter JM: Flexor tendons—late reconstruction. p. 1969. In Green DP (ed): Operative Hand Surgery. 2nd Ed. Vol. 3. Churchill Livingstone, New York, 1988

12. Poppen NK: Recovery of sensibility after suture of digital nerves. J Hand Surg 4:212, 1979

13. Frykman GK, Waylet J: Rehabilitation of peripheral nerve injuries. Orthop Clin North Am 12:361, 1981

14. Johnson RP: The acutely injured wrist and its residuals. Clin Orthop 149:33, 1980

15. Neviaser RJ: Infections. p. 1027. In Green DP (ed): Operative Hand Surgery. 2nd Ed. Vol. 2. Churchill Livingstone, New York, 1988

16. Urbaniak JR: Replantation of amputated parts—technique, results, and indications. p. 64. In AAOS Surgical Symposium on Microsurgery: Practical Use in Orthopaedics. CV Mosby, St. Louis, 1979

17. Soucacos PN, Beris AE, Touliatos AS, et al: Current indications for single digit replantation. Acta Orthop Scand suppl 264:12, 1995

18. Chow SP, Ng C: Hand function after digital amputation. J Hand Surg (Br) 18:125, 1993

19. Wei FC, el-Gammal TA: Toe-to-hand transfer. Current concepts, techniques, and research. Clin Plast Surg 23:103, 1996

CHAPTER 13
Mobilization of the Upper Extremity

Michael J. Wooden

Joint mobilization has become an increasingly popular and important physical therapy tool. As recently as 25 years ago, manipulation was a controversial topic, considered off-limits to any practitioners other than chiropractors or osteopaths. Thanks, however, to the dedication of many pioneers in this field, peripheral and vertebral joint mobilization has become standard fare in most physical therapy curricula.

In particular, the profession is indebted to such teachers as Paris, Maitland, and Kaltenborn, themselves physical therapists, and to such physicians as Mennell, Cyriax, and Stoddard, who were willing to share their knowledge. Their efforts have mushroomed into such developments as continuing education courses as well as graduate programs in manual therapy and orthopaedics. These programs have stimulated an increase in graduate-level research, both basic and clinical. Indeed, interest in joint mobilization was the main factor leading to creation of the American Physical Therapy Association's Orthopedic Section, which has paved the way for specialization in physical therapy.

An additional benefit has been the publication of some excellent books dealing with assessment and treatment including joint mobilization. Many are cited in the references and suggested readings of this chapter and Chapter 27. The purpose of these two chapters is to summarize briefly the information contained in the various textbooks and to describe the peripheral joint techniques with which I have had the most success.

General Principles

In general terms, mobilization is defined as restoration of joint motion,[1] which can be accomplished by different forms of active or passive exercise or by such mechanical means as continuous passive motion (CPM) machines.

In the context of manual therapy, however, mobilization is passive range-of-motion exercise applied to the joint *surfaces*, as opposed to the physiologic, cardinal plane movement of the joint as a whole. Passive movement of the joint surfaces requires a knowledge of arthrokinematics, first described by Basmajian and MacConail,[2] such as intimate movements of roll, spin, glide, compression, and distraction. These movements occur between the joint surfaces (hence the term *arthrokinematic*) and are necessary for normal, physiologic, or *osteokinematic* movement of bones.

To illustrate, Basmajian and MacConail described movement of a convex joint surface on a concave surface (e.g., the head of the humerus in the glenoid cavity). As the convex bone rolls in any direction, it must simultaneously slide (minutely) in the opposite direction on the concave bone to keep the two surfaces approximated. Conversely, when a concave bone surface moves on a convex one (e.g., the tibia on the femur), the glide of the concave surface will occur in the same direction.

Mennell[3] elaborated on these arthrokinematic movements, labeling them "joint play": movements which are small but precise, which cannot be reproduced by voluntary muscle control, but which are necessary for full, painless range of motion. An example is the downward movement of the humeral head in the glenoid cavity during shoulder flexion and abduction. Similarly, Paris[4] classified these movements as *accessory* movements, either joint play or component. He stressed that these movements occur not only during physiologic movement but also at end-range to protect the joint from external forces. End-range joint play is assessed by applying overpressure at end-range to determine end-feel and the presence of pain. Kaltenborn's[5] system uses similar arthrokinematic principles.

The techniques described later in this chapter are based on accessory motion concepts and are primarily osteopathic. Where possible, they are linked with the physiologic movements that they theoretically enhance.

■ Theories of Mobilization

In the periphery, mobilization is used either for its effect on reducing joint restrictions (mechanical) or to relieve pain or muscle guarding (neurophysiologic). This section reviews the theoretic bases for each.

Joint Restrictions

Loss of range of motion can be caused by trauma or immobilization or, most often, a combination of the two. Picture a contracted elbow joint that has been immobilized for 6 to 8 weeks after a supracondylar fracture. Experience tells us that this elbow, despite weeks of aggressive therapy, may never regain full mobility. What are the reasons for this? The effects of trauma and immobilization on joint-related structures are discussed in detail in Chapter 1. To summarize, the most significant range-limiting effects are as follows:

1. Loss of extensibility of periarticular connective tissue structures: ligaments, capsule, fascia, and tendons[6-9]
2. Deposition of fibrofatty infiltrates acting as intra-articular "glue"[10]
3. Adaptive shortening of muscles[11,12]
4. Breakdown of articular cartilage[13]

All the above could contribute to abnormal limitation of movement and must be dealt with in treatment.

Muscle has been shown to be an incredibly plastic tissue, with the ability to regenerate and return to normal length even after prolonged immobilization.[11,12] However, there is little research to show the direct effects of mobilization techniques per se on immobilized connective tissue. It has been demonstrated that passive movement does seem to maintain distance, lubrication and mobility between collagen fibers.[6,14] During the healing of traumatized connective tissue, passive movement restores the ability of collagen fibers to glide on one another as scar tissue matures.[15] Stress to this healing connective tissue, applied as early as 3 weeks but no later than 3 to 4 months after injury appears to reduce the formation of cross-links between and within collagen fibers.[16,17] Therefore, the scar is allowed to lengthen in the direction of the stress applied as its tensile strength increases. Thus, joint contracturing is reduced.[16,17] Finally, forceful passive movement has been shown to rupture intra-articular adhesions that form during immobilization.[10,18]

Pain and Muscle Guarding

Wyke[19] has identified receptor nerve endings in various periarticular structures. These nerve endings have been shown to influence pain, proprioception, and muscle relaxation.

Type I (postural) and type II (dynamic) mechanoreceptors are located in joint capsules. They have a low threshold and are excited by repetitive movements including oscillations. Type III mechanoreceptors are found in joint capsules and extracapsular ligaments; they are similar to Golgi tendon organs in that they are excited by stretching and perhaps thrusting maneuvers. Pain receptors, or type IV nociceptors, are found in capsules, ligaments, fat pads, and blood vessel walls. These receptors are fired by noxious stimuli, as in trauma, and have a relatively high threshold.

Pain impulses from type IV nociceptors are conducted slowly. Impulses from type I and II mechanoreceptors are fast, conducting at a much lower threshold. The differences between types I and II and type IV conductivity may explain why oscillating a joint relieves pain. Theoretically, the faster mechanical impulses overwhelm the slower pain impulses. Whether this is achieved by "closing the gate"[20] or perhaps by release of endorphins in the central nervous system is still under investigation.

Muscle relaxation is an additional benefit of passive movement. One theory is that causing type III joint receptors and Golgi tendon organs to fire by stretching or thrusting a joint results in temporary inhibition or relaxation of muscles crossing the joint.[4,19] This in itself may cause an increase in range of motion and helps prepare the joint for further stretching and mobilization.

■ Application

There are many schools of thought regarding the hands-on approach to manual therapy. Mobilization can be applied with osteopathic articulations, distraction of joint surfaces, oscillations, stretching, and thrust manipulations. When using stretching and oscillations, I favor those techniques that stress accessory motion based on arthrokinematics. These are primarily glides, distractions, and capsular stretches. Except for gentle stretching, one should avoid mobilizing, especially thrusting, in physiologic movements. Ultimately, which techniques are chosen should not matter as long as the therapist is well trained and follows a few guidelines. Most importantly, the therapist should follow Paris'[4] simple but critical rules *before* mobilizing:

1. Identify the location and direction of the limitation; for example, in a stiff ankle, is it posterior glide of the talus that is restricted?
2. Prepare the soft tissues (i.e., first decrease swelling, pain, muscle guarding or tightness, and so on).
3. Protect neighboring hypermobilities. This is particularly important in spinal mobilization but could apply, for example, to a shoulder dislocation that has resulted in anterior capsule laxity. In mobilizing to increase

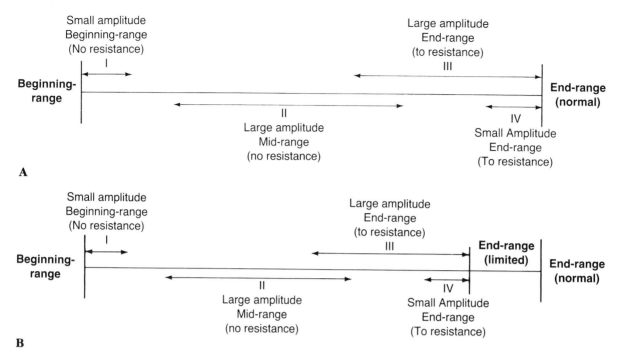

Figure 13–1. Grades of movement. (A) In a normal joint; (B) in a stiff joint. (Adapted from Maitland,[21] with permission.)

abduction and rotation, one would want to avoid anterior glide or other maneuvers that would stress the anterior capsule.

A fourth rule, really an extension of the above, applies to postsurgical cases.

4. Communicate with the surgeon. Find out which tissues have been cut or sacrificed and what motions to avoid at least initially.

Maitland's[21] description of the grades of joint movement has been a major contribution to manual therapy. He uses oscillatory movements of different amplitudes applied at different parts of the range of motion, either accessory or physiologic. Grade I oscillations are of very small amplitude at the beginning of the range, whereas grade II oscillations are large-amplitude oscillations from near the beginning to midrange. No tissue resistance is encountered with grade I or II movements, and so they do not "mobilize" to increase range. However, they do reduce pain and induce relaxation through the mechanoreceptor mechanisms already described. The actual mobilization movements, those that are taken into tissue resistance, are grades III, IV, and V. A grade III movement uses large amplitudes from mid- to end-range, hitting at end-range rather abruptly. A grade IV movement also goes to end-range but is of very small amplitude. Because they may be less painful and less likely to traumatize a joint, grade IV movements should be used before grade IIIs, the latter being more useful as the joint becomes less acute. A grade V movement is a small-amplitude thrust beyond end-range, a so-called manipulation.

Figure 13–1A depicts Maitland's grades of movement in a normal joint, whereas Figure 13–1B shows movements are applied to a restricted joint. Note that in the latter the end-range (limited) will gradually approach end-range (normal) as treatment progresses.

Often a restricted joint is also painful, and the therapist must decide whether to treat the pain or the stiffness. One advantage of the Maitland system is that grades of movement provide the tools for either form of therapy.

To generalize, grades I and II oscillation are used for pain; grades III, IV, and V are for stiffness. The therapist must now decide when to use them.

▪ Indications for Mobilization

After trauma, surgery, and immobilization, there are no predetermined schedules that state when mobilization can begin. The severity of trauma, extent of surgery, complications, and length of time since onset all need to be considered. Even when the patient has been cleared for rehabilitation, including passive exercise, experience tells us that there is great variability regarding safety and tolerance.

To reduce the chances of being too aggressive, the therapist should try to determine what stage of the healing process the injured joint is in: acute with extravasation, fibroplasia, or scar maturation (see Chapter 1). At best, this is an educated guess, but certain steps in the subjective and objective evaluation will increase accuracy.

Subjectively, one must determine the irritability[21] of the joint, that is, how much of a particular activity increases the pain and to what extent. Consider, for example, a posttraumatic knee. At one extreme is the patient

□□□□□ □ □ □

Table 13–1. Objective Reactivity Levels

Reactivity Level	Sequence	Stage of Healing	Treatment
High	Pain before resistance	Acute, inflammatory	Immobilize Grade I oscillations for pain
Moderate	Pain and resistance simultaneous	Fibroblastic activity	Active range of motion Grade II oscillations for pain
Low	Resistance before pain	Scar maturation and remodeling	Passive range of motion Grade III, IV, and V movements as indicated

who experiences severe pain and effusion for several days after mowing the lawn. Compare this patient to the patient who reports moderate soreness for a few hours after playing two sets of tennis. Obviously, the first patient's joint is highly irritable, whereas that of the tennis player is much less so.

Subjective responses can be reinforced by assessing objectively the level of reactivity.[4] By carefully taking the joint through its passive range, the therapist monitors the sequence of pain versus resistance.[4,22] If the patient reports pain before tissue resistance (not muscle guarding) is felt by the therapist, the joint is highly reactive and, theoretically, is in an acute inflammatory stage. Therefore, the joint should remain protected and splinted. If necessary, the therapist can apply grade I oscillations to reduce pain.

Moderate reactivity is assumed when pain and tissue resistance are simultaneous. The joint injury is now subacute, perhaps indicating that fibroplasia and early scar formation are underway. The patient will tolerate careful active range-of-motion exercises as well as grade I and II oscillations to decrease pain. Actual mobilization (grades III and IV) should be delayed, however, to avoid disturbing the immature scar.

If significant tissue resistance is felt before (or in the absence of) pain, low reactivity is assumed. By now the collagen matrix has matured, and mobilization is needed to stress and remodel the scar. At this time grade III, IV, and V movements are indicated (Table 13–1). If these more aggressive maneuvers induce soreness, the therapist can fall back on grade I and II movements to ease the pain.[21] The key to preventing overaggressiveness is to assess the patient's response to treatment and reactivity for each restriction at every session.

Some conditions that require precautions before mobilization in the periphery are moderate reactivity, osteoporosis, and recent fractures. Choose techniques that will minimize stress to a fracture site while mobilizing an adjacent joint. Also beware of the patient with poor tolerance of treatment (i.e., when mobilization sessions consistently increase pain and reactivity).

A few contraindications should also be considered: high reactivity, indicating the presence of acute inflammation; active inflammatory disease; malignancy; and hypermobility from trauma or disease (e.g., rheumatoid arthritis).[4,21]

■ Techniques

It is always difficult to determine which techniques are most effective. The References and Suggested Readings sections list volumes in which literally hundreds of techniques are described. One cannot state which ones are best for every clinician, but those discussed here are, in my experience, safe, easy to apply, and effective. Each technique is either an accessory motion or a specific capsular stretch and can be applied with any grade of movement. However, grade V thrust maneuvers are not discussed and should not be used without appropriate hands-on training.

The reader must realize that these are also evaluative techniques. They should first be used to determine reactivity and the need for mobilization. Besides goniometric measurement of physiologic range of motion, accessory movement testing is performed using the mobilization positions. To assess the quality and quantity of movement, the accessory motions are usually compared with those in the contralateral limb. This passive movement testing is somewhat out of context in this chapter because it is actually part of the evaluation process. The reader is referred to Chapters 8 to 12, which review other evaluation procedures for each joint. These chapters also contain information pertaining to anatomy, mechanics, and pathology.

Mobilization is difficult to teach on paper without the benefit of laboratory sessions. However, those experienced in basic manual therapy will be able to follow the figures. For each technique, the patient's position, the therapist's hand contacts, and the direction of movement are described. Table 13–2 is for reference, listing each technique with the physiologic movement it theoretically enhances.

□□□□□ □ □ □

Table 13–2. Summary of Upper Extremity Techniques

Joint	Mobilization Technique	Movement Promoted	Figure
Sternoclavicular	Superior glide	Elevation	13–2
	Inferior glide	Depression	13–3
	Posterior glide	General	13–4
Acromioclavicular	Anteroposterior glides	General	13–5, 13–6
Scapulothoracic	Distraction	General	13–7, 13–8, 13–9
	Superior glide	Elevation	13–10B
	Inferior glide	Depression	13–10C
	Upward and downward rotation	Rotation	13–11A,B
Glenohumeral	Anteroposterior glides in neutral, flexion, abduction	Flexion, abduction	13–12, 13–13, 13–14, 13–15
	Inferior glide	Flexion, abduction	13–16, 13–17
	Lateral glide	General	13–18
	Long axis distraction	General	13–19
	Distraction with rotation	Internal and external rotation	13–20
	Distraction in flexion	Flexion	13–21
	Anterior capsule stretch	External rotation	13–22
	Anterior capsule stretch	Horizontal abduction	13–23, 13–24
	Inferior capsule stretch	Abduction	13–25
	Inferior capsule stretch	Flexion	13–26
	Posterior capsule stretch	Horizontal adduction	13–27
Humeroulnar	Abduction	Extension	13–28
	Adduction	Flexion	13–29
	Distraction	General	13–30
Radiohumeral and radioulnar	Distraction	General	13–31
	Upward and downward glides	Radial and ulnar deviation	13–32
Distal radio-ulnar	Inward and outward roll	Pronation, supination	13–33
	Anteroposterior glides	General	13–34
Radiocarpal	Glides	Flexion, extension, deviation	13–35A,B
	Distraction	General	13–36
	Scaphoid glide	General	13–37
	Lunate glide	General	13–38
Ulnomeniscotriquetral	Glide	General	13–39
Intercarpal and carpometacarpal	Specific carpal movements	Hand and wrist mobility	13–40, 13–41, 13–42, 13–43, Table 13–3
Metacarpophalangeal	Distraction	General	13–44
	Anteroposterior glide	Flexion, extension	13–45
	Mediolateral glide	Adduction, abduction	13–46
	Mediolateral tilt	Adduction, abduction	13–47
	Rotations	Rotation, grasp	13–48
Interphalangeal	Distraction	General	13–49
	Anteroposterior glides	Flexion, extension	13–49
	Mediolateral glide and tilt	Adduction, abduction	13–50

■ The Shoulder

The Sternoclavicular Joint

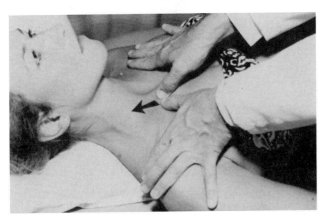

Figure 13–2. Superior glide.
Patient position: supine.
Contacts: both thumbs inferior to the proximal end of the clavicle.
Direction of movement: push cephalad.

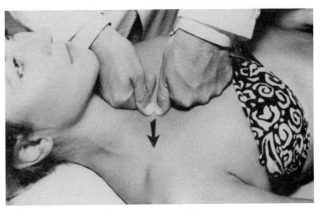

Figure 13–4. Posterior glide.
Patient position: supine.
Contacts: both thumbs anterior to the proximal end of the clavicle.
Direction of movement: push posteriorly.

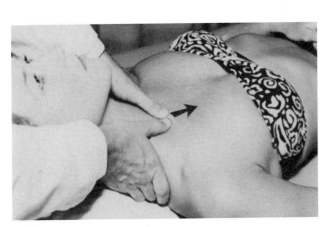

Figure 13–3. Inferior glide.
Patient position: supine.
Contacts: both thumbs superior to the proximal end of the clavicle.
Direction of movement: push caudally and slightly laterally.

The Acromioclavicular Joint

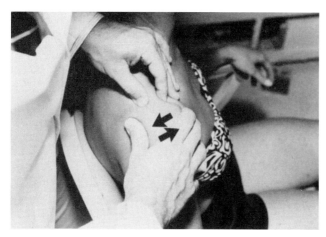

Figure 13–5. Anteroposterior glide.
Patient position: sitting.
Contacts: grasp the distal end of the clavicle with the thumb and forefinger of one hand; the other hand grasps the acromion process.
Direction of movement: glide the acromion anteriorly and posteriorly.

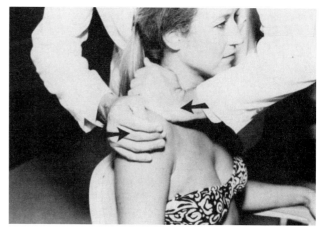

Figure 13–6. Anteroposterior glide.
Patient position: sitting
Contacts: the pisiform of one hand contacts the anterior aspect of the distal end of the clavicle; the carpal tunnel of the other hand contacts the posterior aspect of the acromion.
Direction of movement: hands push in opposite directions.

The Scapulothoracic Joint

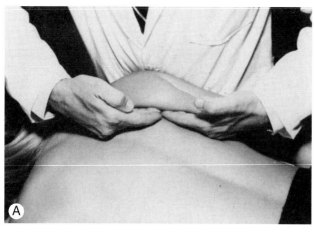

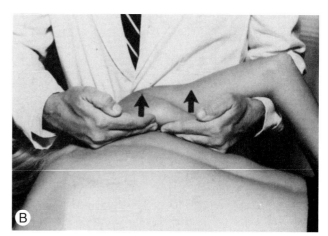

Figure 13–7. Scapular distraction.
Patient position: prone, arm at side.
Contacts: (A) ulnar fingers of both hands under the medial scapular border.
Direction of movement: (B) the scapula is distracted or "lifted" away from the thorax.

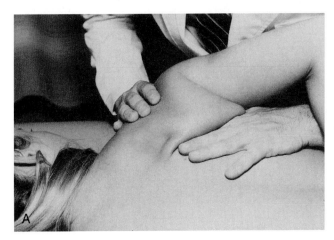
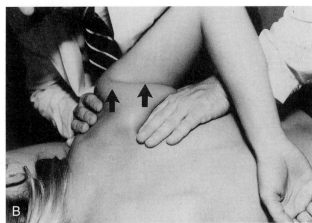

Figure 13–8. Scapular distraction.
Patient position: prone, forearm behind back (if patient is able).
Contacts: (A) index finger of one hand under the medial scapular border; the other hand grasps the superior border.
Direction of movement: (B) the scapula is distracted from the thorax.

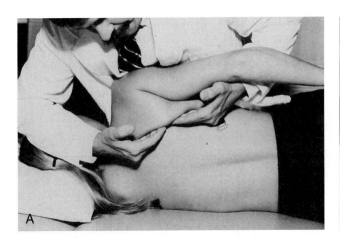
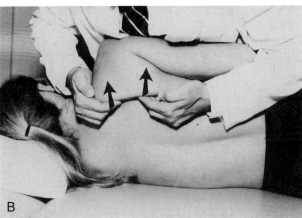

Figure 13–9. Scapular distraction.
Patient position: side-lying, arm at side.
Contacts: (A) ulnar fingers under the medial scapular border.
Direction of movement: (B) the scapula is distracted from the thorax.

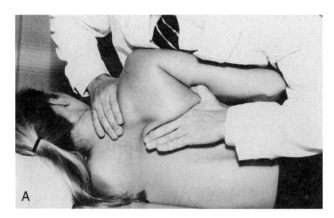

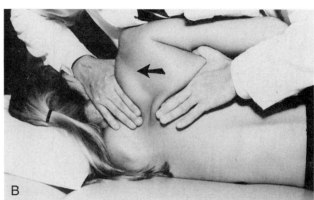

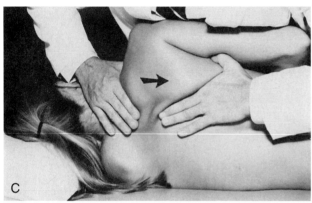

Figure 13–10. Superior and inferior glide.
Patient position: side-lying, arm at side.
Contacts: (A) index finger of one hand under the medial scapular border; the other hand grasps the superior border.
Direction of movement: under slight distraction, the scapula is moved (B) superiorly and (C) inferiorly.

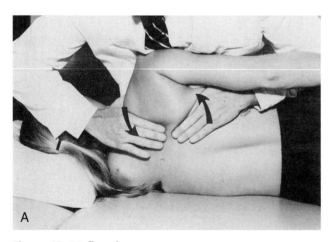

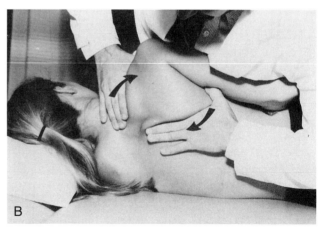

Figure 13–11. Rotation.
Patient position: side-lying, arm at side.
Contacts: same as in figure 13.20A.
Direction of movement: (A) under slight distraction, rotate the scapula upward and (B) downward.

The Glenohumeral Joint

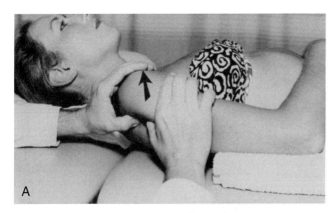
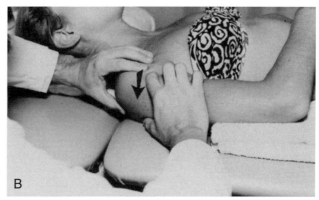

Figure 13-12. Anteroposterior glide.
Patient position: supine, arm at side, elbow propped.
Contacts: hands grasp the humeral head; thumbs posterior, fingers anterior.
Direction of movement: (A) glide the humeral head anteriorly and (B) posteriorly.

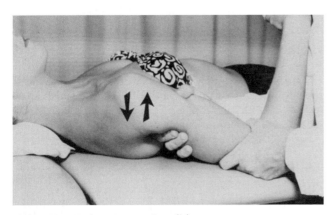
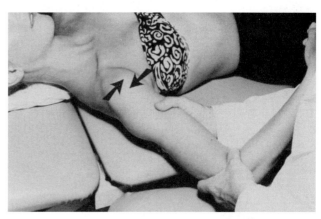

Figure 13-13. Anteroposterior glide.
Patient position: supine, arm at side.
Contacts: one hand stabilizes at the lateral aspect of the elbow; the other hand grasps the humerus near the axilla.
Direction of movement: glide the humeral head anteriorly and posteriorly.

Figure 13-14. Anteroposterior glide at 45 degrees.
Patient position: supine, arm in 45 degrees of abduction.
Contacts: one hand stabilizes the lateral aspect of the elbow; the other hand grasps the humerus near the axilla.
Direction of movement: glide anteriorly and posteriorly while maintaining abduction.

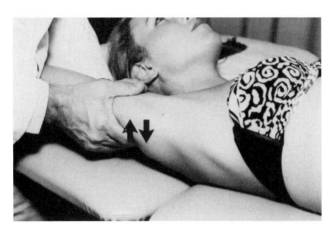

Figure 13–15. Anteroposterior glide in full flexion.
Patient position: supine, arm at end-range flexion.
Contacts: both hands grasp the proximal humerus, with the thumbs near the axilla.
Direction of movement: glide anteriorly and posteriorly.

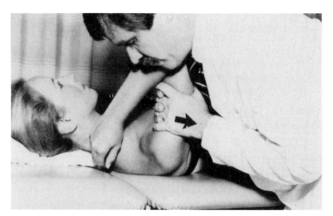

Figure 13–16. Inferior glide (depression) in flexion.
Patient position: supine, shoulder flexed to 90 degrees.
Contacts: the patient's elbow is stabilized by the therapist's shoulder; hands grasp the proximal humerus, with fingers interlocked.
Direction of movement: pull the humeral head inferiorly.

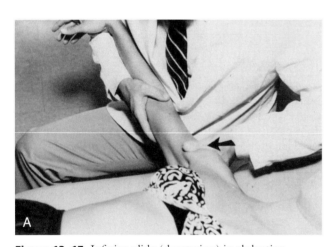

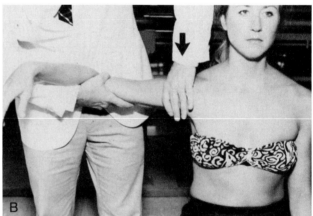

Figure 13–17. Inferior glide (depression) in abduction.
Patient position: (A) supine or (B) sitting.
Contacts: grasp the arm near the elbow to stabilize in 90 degrees of abduction; the first web space of the other hand contacts the head of the humerus.
Direction of movement: depress the head of the humerus (inferiorly).

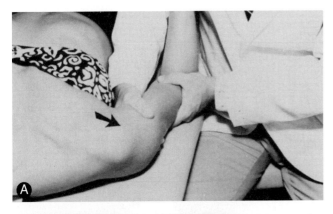

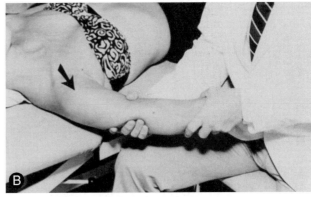

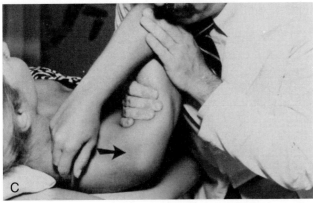

Figure 13–18. Lateral glide (distraction).
Patient position: (A) supine, arm at side; (B) supine, arm in 45 degrees of abduction; (C) supine, arm in 90 degrees flexion.
Contacts: grasp near the elbow to stabilize; the other hand grasps the proximal humerus at the axilla.
Direction of movement: distract the humeral head laterally.

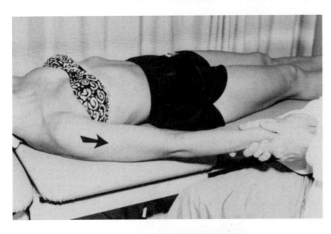

Figure 13–19. Long axis distraction.
Patient position: supine.
Contacts: hands grasp the forearm above the wrist.
Direction of movement: pull along the long axis of the arm.

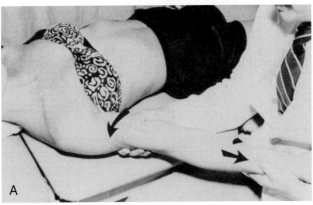

Figure 13–20. Long axis distraction with rotation.
Patient position: supine.
Contacts: one hand grasps the forearm to distract; the other hand grasps the proximal humerus medially.
Direction movement: (A) while distracting, rotate externally or (B) internally.

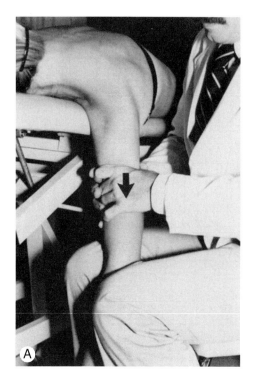

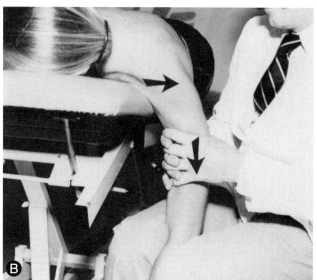

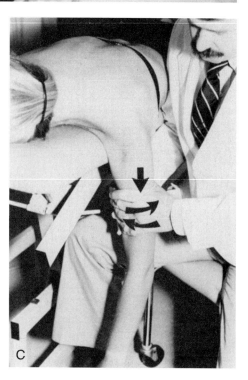

Figure 13–21. Distraction in flexion.

Patient position: Prone, arm in 90 degrees of flexion off the edge of the table.

Contacts: hands grasp the midshaft of the humerus, with fingers interlocked.

Direction of movement: (A) distract along the long axis of the arm; while distracting, glide (B) laterally or (C) rotate.

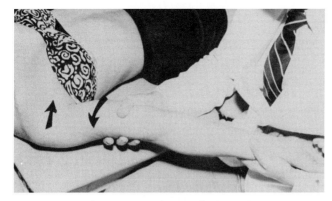

Figure 13-22. Anterior capsule stretch.
Patient position: supine, arm abducted.
Contacts: one hand grasps the forearm to stabilize; the other hand grasps the proximal humerus medially.
Direction of movement: externally rotate while gliding anteriorly.

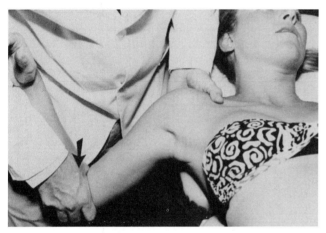

Figure 13-23. Anterior capsule stretch.
Patient position: supine, near the edge of the table.
Contacts: one hand stabilizes the posterior aspect of the shoulder; the other hand grasps the humerus above the elbow.
Direction of movement: stretch into horizontal abduction.

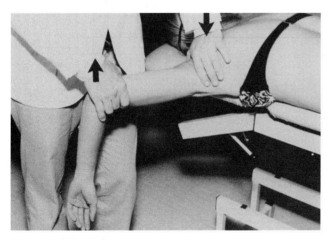

Figure 13-24. Anterior capsule stretch.
Patient position: prone, near the edge of the table.
Contacts: the palm of one hand stabilizes the posterior aspect of the shoulder; the other hand grasps the humerus above the elbow.
Direction of movement: stretch into horizontal abduction.

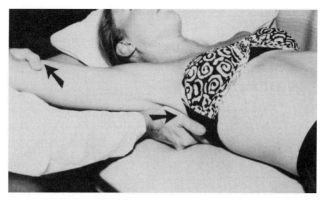

Figure 13-25. Inferior capsule stretch.
Patient position: supine, arm in end-range abduction.
Contacts: carpal tunnel contact of one hand stabilizes the lateral border of the scapula; the other hand grasps the humerus above the elbow.
Direction of movement: stretch into abduction.

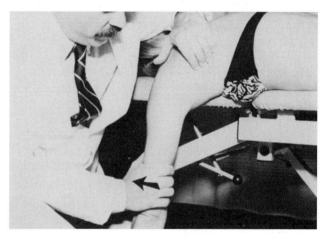

Figure 13-26. Inferior capsule stretch.
Patient position: prone, arm in flexion off the edge of the table.
Contacts: the fingertips of one hand stabilize the lateral scapular border; the other hand grasps the humerus above the elbow.
Direction of movement: stretch into flexion.

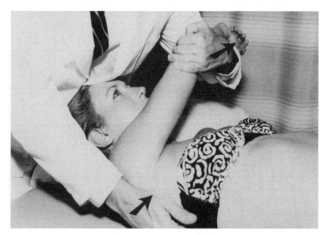

Figure 13-27. Posterior capsule stretch.
Patient position: supine, arm in 90 degrees of flexion, elbow flexed.
Contacts: stabilize the lateral scapular border with carpal tunnel contact; the other hand grasps the elbow and cradles the forearm.
Direction of movement: stretch into horizontal adduction.

■ The Elbow

The Humeroulnar Joint

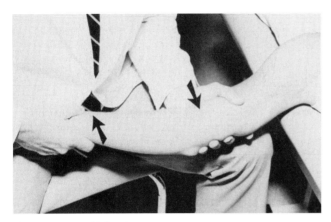

Figure 13–28. Abduction.
Patient position: supine.
Contacts: stabilize the distal humerus laterally; the other hand grasps the ulnar aspect of the forearm above the wrist.
Direction of movement: the forearm is abducted on the humerus.

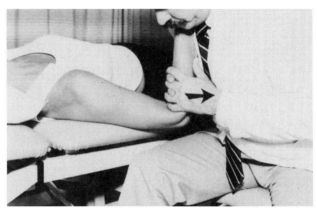

Figure 13–30. Distraction.
Patient position: supine, elbow flexed to 90 degrees.
Contacts: the patient's forearm is stabilized against the therapist's shoulder; the therapist's hands grasp the proximal aspect of the forearm, with fingers interlocked.
Direction of movement: distract the forearm from the humerus.

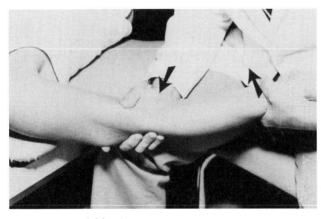

Figure 13–29. Adduction.
Patient position: supine.
Contacts: stabilize the distal humerus medially; the other hand grasps the radial aspect of the forearm above the wrist.
Direction of movement: the forearm is adducted on the humerus.

The Radiohumeral and Proximal Radioulnar Joints

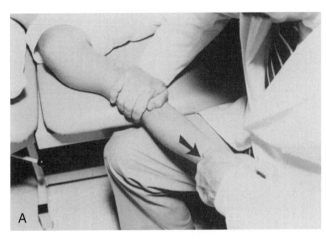
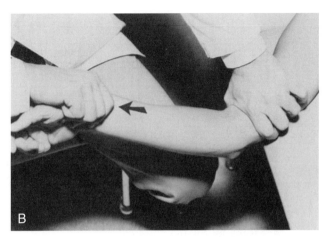

Figure 13–31. Radial distraction.
Patient position: supine, arm abducted.
Contacts: stabilize by holding the elbow on the treatment table; the other hand grasps the radius above the wrist.
Direction of movement: (A,B) pull the radius distally.

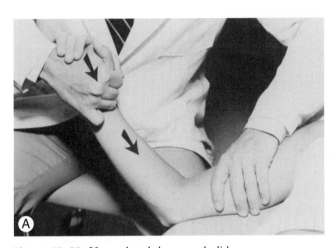
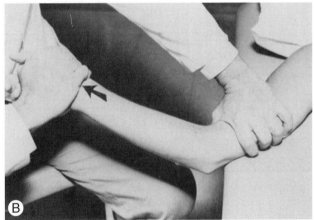

Figure 13–32. Upward and downward glide.
Patient position: supine.
Contacts: stabilize by holding the arm on the table; grasp the thenar eminence with a "hand-shake" grip.
Direction of movement: (A) glide the radius upward by pushing the wrist into radial deviation; (B) glide the radium downward by pulling the wrist into ulnar deviation.

■ The Wrist and Hand

The Distal Radioulnar Joint

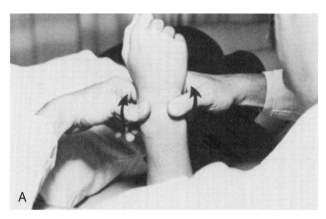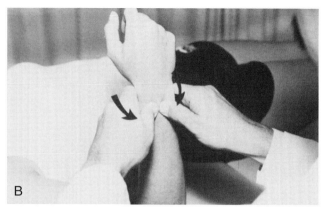

Figure 13–33. Inward and outward roll.
Patient position: supine or sitting.
Contacts: grasp the distal aspects of the radius and ulna, with thumbs dorsal and fingertips volar.
Direction of movement: roll the radius and ulna (A) inward and (B) outward on one another.

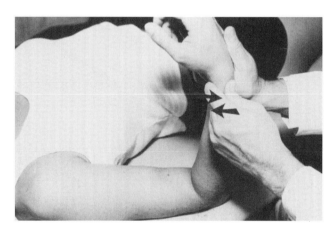

Figure 13–34. Anteroposterior glide.
Patient position: sitting or supine, elbow flexed.
Contacts: stabilize the ulna with thenar grasp; the other hand grasps the radius with the thumb and forefinger.
Direction of movement: glide the radius anteriorly and posteriorly.

The Radiocarpal Joints

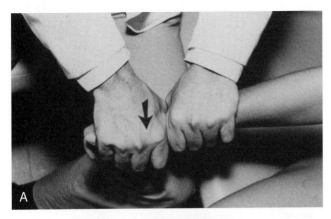

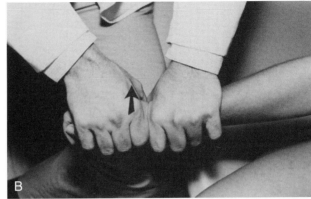

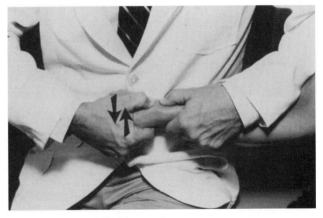

Figure 13–35. Radiocarpal glides.
Patient position: supine or sitting.
Contacts: with the thumb, index finger, and first web space, stabilize the radius and ulna dorsally; the other hand grasps the proximal row of carpal bones.
Direction of movement: glide the carpal bones (A) anteriorly, (B) posteriorly, medially, and (C) laterally.

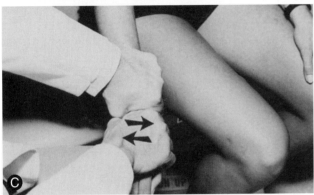

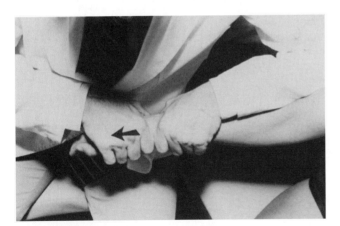

Figure 13–36. Distraction.
Patient position: supine or sitting.
Contacts: same as in Figure 13–35.
Direction of movement: distract the carpal bones distally.

Figure 13–37. Scaphoid on radius.
Patient position: supine or sitting.
Contacts: using the thumbs and forefingers, stabilize the radius and grasp the scaphoid.
Direction of movement: glide the scaphoid anteriorly and posteriorly on the radius.

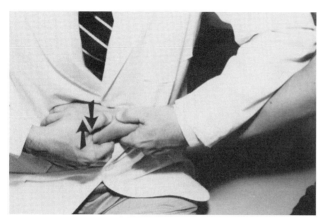

Figure 13–38. Lunate on radius.
Patient position: supine or sitting.
Contacts: stabilize the radius; grasp the lunate.
Direction of movement: glide the lunate anteriorly and posteriorly on the radius.

The Ulnomeniscotriquetral Joint

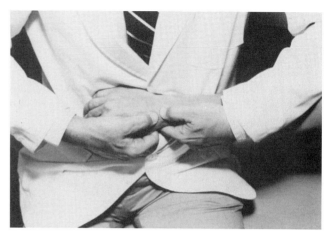

Figure 13–39. Ulnomeniscotriquetral glide.
Patient position: supine or sitting.
Contacts: stabilize the ulna and grasp the triquetrum.
Direction of movement: glide the triquetrum anteriorly and posteriorly on the ulna.

The Intercarpal Joints

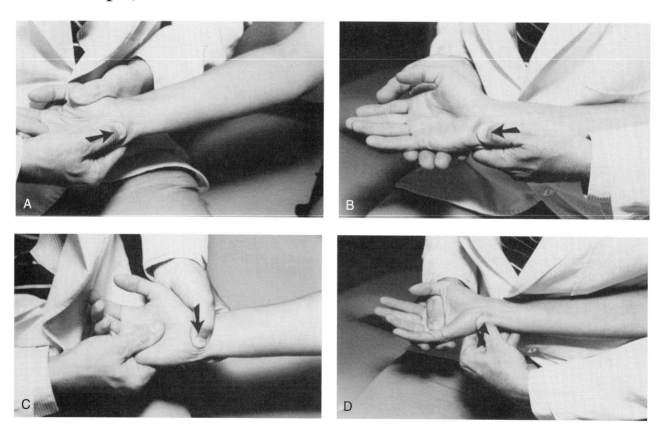

Figure 13–40. Pisiform glides.
Patient position: supine or sitting.
Contacts: grasp the patient's hand firmly to stabilize; contact the thumbtip against the pisiform bone.
Direction of movement: glide the pisiform (A) cephalad, (B) caudally, (C) medially, and (D) laterally.

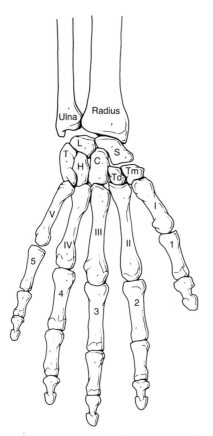

Figure 13–41. The bones of the wrist, hand, and fingers (dorsal view of the right wrist). S, scaphoid; L, lunate; T, triquetrum; Tm, trapezium; Td, trapezoid; C, capitate; H, hamate; I–V, metatarsals; 1–5, proximal phalanges.

□□□□□□ □ □
Table 13–3. Specific Intercarpal and Carpometacarpal Glides

Stabilize	Mobilize
Scaphoid	Lunate
	Capitate
	Trapezium
	Trapezoid
Lunate	Capitate
	Triquetrum
	Hamate
Triquetrum	Hamate
Hamate	Capitate
	Base of 5th metacarpal
	Base of 4th metacarpal
Capitate	Base of 3rd metacarpal
	Trapezoid
Trapezium	Base of 1st metacarpal
Trapezoid	Base of 2nd metacarpal

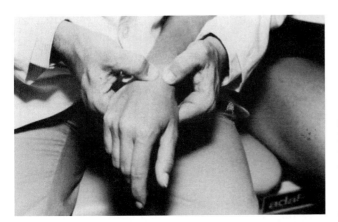

Figure 13–42. Intercarpal and carpometacarpal glides.
Patient position: supine or sitting.
Contacts: use the thumbs and forefingers of both hands, with the thumbs on the dorsal aspect; grasp the adjacent carpal bones (see Table 13–3).
Direction of movement: glide the carpals anteriorly and posteriorly.

The Intermetacarpal Joints

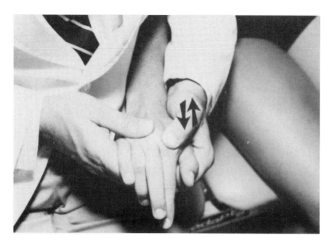

Figure 13–43. Intermetacarpal glide.
Patient position: supine or sitting.
Contacts: stabilize the head of the third metacarpal with the thumb and forefinger; the other hand grasps the head of the second metacarpal.
Direction of movement: glide the second metacarpal anteriorly and posteriorly; repeat for the third, fourth, and fifth metacarpals.

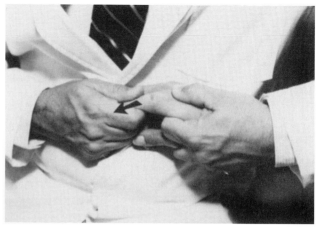

Figure 13–44. Metacarpophalangeal distraction.
Patient position: supine or sitting.
Contacts: stabilize the shaft of the second metacarpal; the other hand grasps the shaft of the proximal phalanx.
Direction of movement: distract the phalanx from the metacarpal; repeat at each metacarpophalangeal joint.

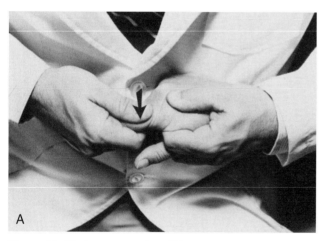

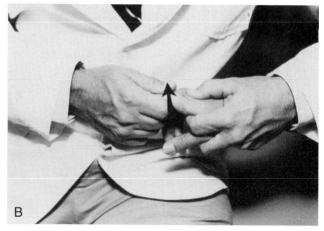

Figure 13–45. Anteroposterior glide.
Patient position: supine or sitting.
Contacts: same as for metacarpophalangeal distraction.
Direction of movement: glide the proximal phalanx (A) anteriorly and (B) posteriorly; repeat at each joint.

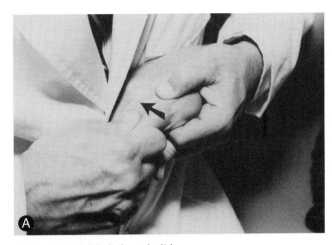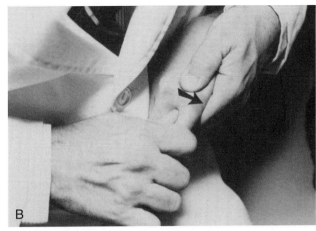

Figure 13–46. Mediolateral glide.
Patient position: supine or sitting.
Contacts: stabilize the shaft of second metacarpal as above; the proximal phalanx is grasped on the medial and lateral aspects of the shaft.
Direction of movement: glide the phalanx (A) medially and (B) laterally; repeat at each metacarpophalangeal joint.

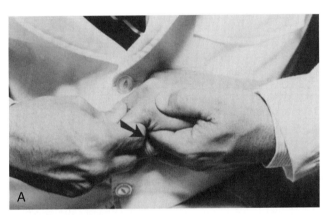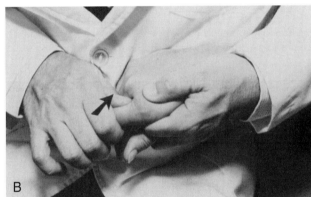

Figure 13–47. Mediolateral tilt.
Patient position: supine or sitting.
Contacts: stabilize the shaft of the second metacarpal; the proximal shaft is grasped the same way as for mediolateral glide.
Direction of movement: tilt the phalanx medially (A) and laterally (B) by using the forefinger or thumb as a fulcrum; repeat at each metacarpophalangeal joint.

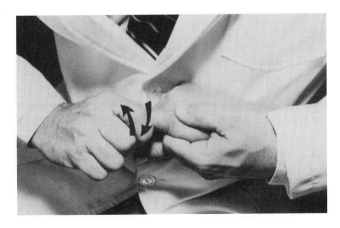

Figure 13–48. Rotation.
Patient position: supine or sitting.
Contacts: same as for mediolateral tilt.
Direction of movement: rotate the phalanx medially and laterally; repeat at each metacarpophalangeal joint.

The Interphalangeal Joints

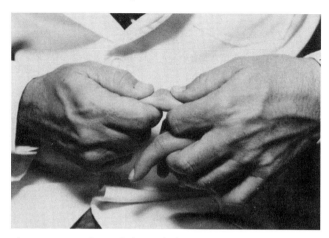

Figure 13–49. Interphalangeal distraction and anteroposterior glide.

Patient position: supine or sitting.

Contacts: stabilize the shaft of the proximal phalanx; the other hand grasps the anterior and posterior aspects of the middle phalanx.

Direction of movement: the middle phalanx can be distracted or glided in an anterior or posterior direction; repeat for all proximal and distal interphalangeal joints.

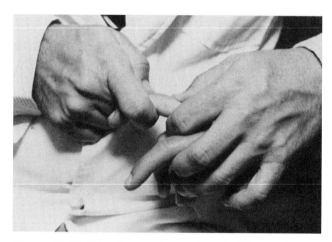

Figure 13–50. Interphalangeal mediolateral glide and tilt.

Patient position: supine or sitting.

Contacts: stabilize the shaft of the proximal humerus; the other hand grasps the medial and lateral aspects of the shaft of the middle phalanx.

Direction of movement: glide or tilt the middle phalanx in a medial or lateral direction; repeat for all proximal and distal interphalangeal joints.

■ Acknowledgments

The author thanks Janie Wise, MMSc, PT (the photographer), Amelia Haselden, PT (the model), and the Physical Therapy Department at Emory University Hospital for their valuable assistance.

■ References

1. Clayton L (ed): Taber's Cyclopedic Medical Dictionary. FA Davis, Philadelphia, 1977
2. Basmajian JV, MacConail C: Arthrology. p. 237. In Warwick R, Williams P (eds): Gray's Anatomy. 35th Br. Ed. WB Saunders, Philadelphia, 1973
3. Mennell JM: Joint Pain: Diagnosis and Treatment Using Manipulative Techniques. Little, Brown, Boston, 1964
4. Paris SV: Extremity Dysfunction and Mobilization. Institute Press, Atlanta, GA, 1980
5. Kaltenborn F: Manual Therapy of the Extremity Joints. Olaf Norlis Borkhandel, Olso, 1973
6. Akeson WH, Amiel D, Woo S: Immobility effects of synovial joints: the pathomechanics of joint contractures. Biorheology 17:95, 1980
7. Woo S, Mathews JV, Akeson WH, et al: Connective tissue response to immobility: correlative study of biomechanical and biochemical measurements of normal and immobilized rabbit knees. Arthritis Rheum 18:257, 1975
8. Akeson WH, Amiel D, LaViolette D, et al: The connective tissue response to immobility: an accelerated aging response. Exp Gerontol 3:289, 1968
9. LaVigne A, Watkins R: Preliminary results on immobilization: induced stiffness of monkey knee joints and posterior capsules. In Proceedings of a Symposium of the Biological Engineering Society, University of Strathclyde. University Park Press, Baltimore, 1973
10. Enneking W, Horowitz M: The intra-articular effects of immobilization on the human knee. J Bone Joint Surg 54(A):973, 1972
11. Tabary JC, Tabary C, Tardieu C, et al: Physiological and structural changes in cat soleus muscle due to immobilization at different lengths by plaster cast. J Physiol (Lond) 224:231, 1972
12. Cooper R: Alterations during immobilization and regeneration of skeletal muscle in cats. J Bone Joint Surg 54(A):919, 1972
13. Ham A, Cormack D: Histology. 8th Ed. JB Lippincott, Philadelphia, 1979
14. Akeson WH, Amiel D, Mechanic GL, et al: Collagen crosslinking alterations in joint contractures: changes in reducible crosslinks in periarticular connective tissue collagen after 9 weeks of immobilization. Connect Tissue Res 5:5, 1977
15. Peacock E: Wound Repair. 3rd Ed. WB Saunders, Philadelphia, 1984
16. Arem AJ, Madden JW: Effects of stress on healing wounds: intermittent non-cyclical tension. J Surg Res 20:93, 1976
17. Kelly M, Madden JW: Hand surgery and wound healing. p. 237. In Wolfort FG (ed): Acute Hand Injuries: A Multidisciplinary Approach. Little, Brown, Boston, 1980
18. Evans E, Eggers G, Butler J, et al: Immobilization and remobilization of rats' knee joints. J Bone Joint Surg 42(A):737, 1960

19. Wyke B: Articular neurology—a review. Physiotherapy 58:94, 1972

20. Melzack R, Torgerson WS: On the language of pain. Anesthesiology 34:50, 1971

21. Maitland G: Peripheral Manipulation. 2nd Ed. Butterworths, London, 1978

22. Magarey ME: The first treatment session. p. 503. In Grieve G (ed): Modern Manual Therapy of the Vertebral Column. Churchill Livingstone, Edinburgh, 1986

■ Suggested Readings

Basmajian JV, MacConail C: Arthrology. p. 237. In Warwick R, Williams P (eds.): Gray's Anatomy, 35th Br. Ed. WB Saunders, Philadelphia, 1973

Brooks-Scott J: Handbook of Mobilization in the Management of Children with Neurologic Disorders. Butterworth-Heineman, London, 1998

Butler D: Mobilization of the Nervous System. Churchill Livingstone, Melbourne, 1991.

Corrigan B, Maitland GD: Practical Orthopaedic Medicine. Butterworths, London, 1985

Cyriax J: Textbook of Orthopaedic Medicine. Vol. 1: Diagnosis of Soft Tissue Lesions. Balliere Tindall, London, 1978

Cyriax J, Cyriax PL: Illustrated Manual of Orthopaedic Medicine. Butterworths, London, 1983

D'Ambrogio KJ, Roth GB: Positional Release Therapy: Assessment and Treatment of Musculoskeletal Dysfunction. CV Mosby, St. Louis, 1997

Donatelli RA (ed): Physical Therapy of the Shoulder. 3rd Ed. Churchill Livingstone, New York, 1997

Glasgow EF, Twomey L (eds): Aspects of Manipulative Therapy. Churchill Livingstone, Melbourne, 1986

Hoppenfeld S: Physical Examination of the Spine and Extremities. Appleton-Century-Crofts, East Norwalk, CT, 1976

Konin JG, Wiksten DL, Isear JA: Special Tests for Orthopaedic Examination. Slack, Inc., Thorofare NJ, 1997

Loudon J, Bell S, Johnston J: The Clinical Orthopedic Assessment Guide. Human Kinetics, Champaign, IL, 1998

Magee DJ: Orthopedic Physical Assessment. WB Saunders, Philadelphia, 1987

Maitland GD: Peripheral Manipulation. Butterworths, London, 1978

Mennell JM: Joint Pain: Diagnosis and Treatment Using Manipulative Techniques. Little, Brown, Boston, 1964

■ CHAPTER 14
Lower Quarter Evaluation: Structural Relationships and Interdependence

David A. Schiff, Robert A. Donatelli, and Randy Walker

The interrelationships and interdependence of the lower quarter segments are best described by Dempster,[1] who said that "integrated and harmonious roles of all links are necessary for full normal mobility." The lower quarter is a series of bony segments interconnected and interrelated by soft tissue and muscle. Movement at one segment within the lower quarter influences and is dependent on movement of the other segments. The lower quarter segments include the lumbar spine, sacrum, pelvis, femur, tibia, and foot and ankle complex. These segments make up what is commonly referred to as the *lower kinetic chain*.

The lower extremity is frequently defined as a closed kinetic chain during the stance phase of gait. Steindler[2] defined a closed kinetic chain as "a combination of several successively arranged joints constituting a complex motor unit, where movement at one joint influences movement at other joints in the chain." The lower quarter functions as a complex organ during ambulation. Proper arthrokinematic and osteokinematic movement influences the ability of the lower quarter to distribute and dissipate forces such as compression, extension, and shear during the gait cycle.[2] Inadequate distribution of forces can lead to abnormal stress and the eventual breakdown of connective tissue and muscle. The harmonious effect of muscle, bone, ligaments, and normal mechanics will result in the most efficient force attenuation.

Besides normal arthrokinematic and osteokinematic movement, the proper relative arrangement and relationship of each segment to the others is essential for coordinated intersegmental function. Proper arrangement of the lower quarter segments is referred to as *normal posture*. By definition, normal posture is the state of muscular and skeletal balance that protects the supporting structures of the body against injury or progressive deformity.[3] Faulty posture may cause prolonged mechanical deformation of soft tissue and length adaptations of muscle.[3] The maintenance of an erect upright posture and the performance of voluntary movements are highly integrated harmonious functions of muscle, soft tissue, and the central and peripheral nervous systems.[2,3]

This chapter discusses the normal interrelationships and interdependence of the lower quarter structures. The connecting tissues are described in terms of their anatomic relationships and function. The interdependence of the structural links during active movement is emphasized. The functional components of gait are reviewed to demonstrate how the links are interrelated during functional movement. Pathomechanical changes resulting in joint dysfunction and a comprehensive treatment approach are examined in a case study.

■ Applied Anatomy and Mechanics of the Lower Quarter

The lower quarter structures are anatomically and functionally interrelated and interdependent. Muscles and connective tissue connect the segments of the lower kinetic chain and rely upon the central nervous system to create smooth, efficient actions.

During normal body motions, muscles act in groups, promoting integrated movements. Single-joint muscles allow for segmental motion of the lumbar spine, pelvis, and lower extremities.[4] Two-joint muscles synergize the functions of these structures, in particular at the hips, knees, and feet. For example, the sartorius flexes the hip and knee in initiating the forward swing of the lower extremity after push-off.[4] This dual action produces an important coordinated movement of the lower extremity during gait. Without it, much more energy would be expended during this phase of the gait cycle.

Fourteen muscle groups in the lower quarter are classified as two-joint muscles. They are the iliacus, psoas major and minor, gluteus maximus, piriformis, rectus femoris, semitendinosus, semimembranosus, biceps femoris, sartorius, gracilis, gastrocnemius, plantaris, and tensor fasciae latae. The psoas minor and plantaris are not present in most individuals,[5] and their role as connecting links in the lower quarter is insignificant.

Ligaments and fascia further connect the lumbar spine and pelvic region. Mechanoreceptors in these and muscular structures allow for constant feedback to the central nervous system. Motor centers, especially the voluntary movement center in the cerebral cortex, are organized not just anatomically, on the basis of muscles, but physiologically, on the basis of movements.[6] These centers and reflex arcs provide servo-control over movements in the lower quarter.

Two-Joint Muscles of the Lower Quarter

The *psoas* muscle requires special consideration as providing a connection of the lumbar spine and each innominate bone of the pelvis to the femur. It originates from the anterior and inferior surfaces of the lumbar transverse processes, as well as the sides of the lumbar vertebral bodies and their corresponding intervertebral discs. It then courses downward into the pelvis, where it unites with the iliacus to form the iliopsoas tendon. The iliopsoas tendon passes beneath the inguinal ligament and in front of the hip capsule, inserting on the lesser trochanter of the femur. In an open kinetic chain system, the iliopsoas complex typically functions as the prime flexor of the hip. In certain circumstances, the iliopsoas may become a hyperextensor of the lumbar spine. This reversed function is called the *psoas paradox*.[4] Contraction or simply tightness of the iliopsoas flexes the hip but also pulls the lumbar vertebrae in an anterior and inferior direction.[4] Sufficiently strong abdominal muscles counteract this anterior pelvic tilt and ensure pelvic stability. Weak abdominals, by contrast, lead to an anterior pelvic tilt, thus increasing the normal lumbar lordosis. It is important to note that tightness of the latissimus dorsi muscles, typically considered upper quarter muscles, can mimic psoas dysfunction by producing increased lumbar lordosis.[7] Secondary functions of the iliopsoas include weak external rotation of the hip and lateral bending of the lumbar spine.[5]

The iliac fascia covers the psoas and iliacus. It is connected to the origins of both of these muscles as well as the upper part of the sacrum. It is continuous with the inguinal ligament and the transversalis fascia (the part of the fascia between the peritoneum and the abdominal walls).[5]

The lumbar spine, pelvis, and femur are interconnected by ligamentous and fascial tissue. The iliolumbar ligament is one ligament of the pelvic region that connects the pelvis to the lumbar spine. It establishes a strong attachment of the transverse processes and bodies of the fourth and fifth lumbar vertebrae to the iliac crest.[5,8] Part of the ligament also passes downward into the pelvis to blend with the anterior sacroiliac ligament. The upper part of the iliolumbar ligament attaches to the quadratus lumborum and the lower portion to the lumbodorsal fascia.

The lumbodorsal fascia is an extensive connective tissue organ joining many tissues within the pelvic region. This massive structure attaches to the transverse processes of the lumbar vertebrae, iliac crest and iliolumbar ligament, 12th rib, quadratus lumborum, lateral portion of the psoas major, and the aponeurotic origin of the transversus abdominus.[5]

The *gluteus maximus* is not traditionally described as a two-joint muscle. However, it clearly crosses over not only the hip but also the sacroiliac joint. The muscle originates from the posterior gluteal line of the ilium and the posterior portion of the lower part of the sacrum. The upper half of the muscle inserts entirely into the strong lateral portion of the fascia lata, also called the *iliotibial band*. The lower half divides such that half of its fibers insert into the iliotibial tract, and the remaining half insert on the gluteal tuberosity of the femur.[6] Because of this extensive insertion into the iliotibial tract, the gluteus maximus is able to attain greater leverage than by its insertion on the gluteal tuberosity alone. It is an important extensor of the hip but is also an external rotator. When the hip is flexed, the gluteus maximus aids in abduction. When the hip is extended, it assists in adduction.[6]

The *piriformis* is the most prominent lateral rotator of the hip. It arises from anterior sacral segments 2 and 3 and attaches to the greater trochanter of the femur. From extension to 60 degrees of hip flexion, it acts as a lateral rotator and abductor of the hip. Beyond 60 degrees of hip flexion it still acts as an abductor, but it becomes a medial rotator.[9] The piriformis is one of 10 muscles of the gluteal region that function collectively to stabilize the pelvis, on which the body is supported and balanced.[10] Seven of these muscles are lateral rotators of the thigh (the sartorius, obturator externus and internus, superior and inferior gemelli, piriformis, and quadratus femoris), and three are medial rotators (the gluteus medius and minimus and tensor fasciae latae).[2,10]

Balancing the pull of the pirifomis on the sacrum is believed to be important when treating sacroiliac joint dysfunction. Since the muscle has two distinctly different actions, there is no singular exercise that adequately addresses this muscle.[7]

The sciatic nerve crosses under the belly of the piriformis. In 15 percent of anatomic dissections studied, the piriformis has two muscle bellies, with the sciatic nerve passing between them.[6,11,12] Hollinshead noted that in more than 10 percent of cases, the pirifomis is perforated by the sciatic nerve.[12] Because of this anatomic variant, dysfunction of the piriformis can lead to sciatic nerve entrapment, with resultant pain and sometimes impairment of the lower extremity.[11,13]

The *sartorius,* as noted previously, is an important muscle, initiating forward movement of the lower extremity after push-off. It flexes the hip and knee. The muscle originates from the anterior superior iliac spine and inserts on the proximal part of the medial surface of the tibia.[3,4]

The *rectus femoris* is the only two-joint muscle of the quadriceps group. It crosses the hip joint and functions as a hip flexor, in addition to joining the vastus medialis, lateralis, and intermedius to serve as a powerful knee extensor.[6]

The *gracilis* is a long, thin muscle arising from the inferior ramus of the pubis and inserting into the medial tibia. It is a good adductor of the thigh but can also flex the knee. If the knee is kept extended, it will help flex the thigh at the hip.[6]

The fascia of the thigh is continuous with the fascia of the gluteal region and the leg. It crosses the knee joint, attaching to the patella and the fibular head.[14] A portion of the thigh fascia overlying the vastus lateralis forms the *iliotibial band.* The band is attached above to the gluteus maximus posteriorly and to the tensor fascia latae anteriorly.[5,8] Together they form a Y-shaped structure designed to act as a lateral stabilizer of the hip and pelvis.[8]

The hamstrings are composed of the *semitendinosis, semimembranosis,* and *biceps femoris.* This two-joint muscle group extends the hip and flexes the knee. The biceps femoris has the greatest clinical interest. Although the long head of the biceps attaches to the ischial tuberosity, many of its fibers are continuous with the sacrotuberous ligament.[15] Tightness of the hamstrings may lead to increased tension of the sacrotuberous ligament and contribute to pelvic imbalances and pain.

Finally, the *gastrocnemius* is the only significant two-joint muscle below the knee. The primary actions of the gastrocnemius include knee flexion, plantarflexion of the talocrural joint, and supination of the subtalar joint.[16] In a closed kinetic chain system, it helps maintain extension at the knee.[6]

Action of Two-Joint Muscles

The actions of two-joint muscles are complex. During normal movement, muscles tend to act in groups to produce a coordinated action of several joints. The muscles are selected according to the type of motion desired.[4] The combination of tendinous action and Lombard's paradox reveals the teamwork and versatility of the muscular system. For example, hip flexion is caused by contraction of the iliopsoas. Simultaneously, the rectus femoris is slackened, allowing the tightness of the hamstrings to flex the knee by tendinous action. Knee flexion allows the gastrocnemius to slacken, which in turn permits contraction of the tibialis anterior to dorsiflex the ankle.[4] If the hip, knee, and ankle joint are in a position of flexion, the muscle action changes. The gluteus maximus contracts,

extending the hip and removing the tension on the hamstrings while stretching the rectus femoris. Knee extension is facilitated by this action of the gluteus maximus. Knee extension takes up the slack in the gastrocnemius, causing plantar flexion at the ankle.[4]

The functional activity of rising up from a sitting position describes Lombard's paradox. Palpation of the rectus femoris and the hamstrings reveals a cocontraction of both muscle groups. It may seem contradictory to find both muscle groups active, since the rectus femoris tends to extend the knee and flex the hip, whereas the hamstrings extend the hip and flex the knee.[4] Studies of the action of two-joint muscles in dogs seem to indicate that one end of a two-joint muscle may shorten while the other end lengthens.[4] In humans, the action of two-joint muscles occurs at both ends at the same time.

Kinematics of Functional Movement

Functional activities of the lower quarter mainly involve walking and running. The mechanics of the lower quarter during gait, described in Chapter 15, exemplify the interdependence and interrelationship of function.

Inman et al.[17] described six determinants of gait: pelvic rotation, pelvic list, knee flexion in the stance phase, foot and knee mechanisms, and the lateral displacement of the pelvis. Inman et al.[17] described intersegmental rotation as an important component of the six determinants of gait. Rotation is defined as movement of a body in a circular motion about its center of mass.[17] The axis of rotation is perpendicular to the plane of movement.[17] For example, rotation in the sagittal plane is accomplished by the movements of flexion and extension.

The interrelated movements of the body segments during walking are best exemplified by intersegmental rotations. Inman et al.[17] described rotation in three body planes—coronal, sagittal, and transverse—during walking.

Coronal Plane Rotations

Coronal or frontal plane rotations begin at the hip joint. Hip joint rotation is nearly the same as thigh rotation.[17] In the coronal plane it is influenced by side-to-side motion of the trunk and rotation of the pelvis.[17] Coronal plane rotation of the hip and knee depends on the amount of abduction and adduction or the side-to-side movement of the trunk. At toe-off, the pelvis is centrally positioned and is moving toward the side of the weightbearing foot.[17,18] The total excursion of hip adduction is approximately 2 cm. Maximum hip adduction is reached shortly after midstance.[17] After midstance, the pelvis starts to deviate toward the opposite side. The foot remains stationary on the ground while this side-to-side motion is occurring. The leg segments between the foot and the pelvis accommodate this motion by rotating in the coronal plane.[17,18]

At the knee, apparent adduction and abduction movements occur during the first half of the swing phase and the middle of stance, respectively.[17] The coronal plane movement at the knee is measured by observing the combined effect of flexion, extension, adduction, and abduction.[17]

The foot and ankle also accommodate the side-to-side movement of the pelvis by movement in the coronal plane. The long axis of the foot is perpendicular to the long axis of the leg. Therefore, when describing abduction and adduction between the lower leg and the heel, the terms *inversion* and *eversion* apply.[17] Immediately after heel-strike, the subtalar joint pronates, producing an everted calcaneus.[16,19] From midstance to toe-off, the subtalar joint is supinating, producing inversion of the calcaneus.[16,19] The coronal plane movements of inversion and eversion at the subtalar joint correspond to the side-to-side movements of the pelvis. From heel-strike to toe-off, the ankle joint is also moving from adduction to abduction, attempting to accommodate the side-to-side movement of the pelvis. This movement can be observed by movement of the talus. Directly after heel-strike, talus adduction occurs in conjunction with calcaneal eversion. From midstance to toe-off, abduction of the talus coincides with inversion of the calcaneus. The movements of the talus and the calcaneus correspond to the transverse rotations of the tibia during the stance phase. Tibial internal rotation, talar adduction, and calcaneal eversion occur simultaneously directly after heel-strike.[16,17] Tibial external rotation, talar abduction, and calcaneal inversion occur from midstance to toe-off.[16,17] Clinically, movement at the ankle joint in the coronal plane can best be observed by the combined movement of the tibia and the talus.

In summary, the side-to-side movement of the pelvis is accommodated throughout the lower quarter during the stance phase of gait. The greater part of this accommodation takes place at the hip, knee, ankle, and subtalar joint. Hip adduction, knee adduction, tibial internal rotation, talus adduction, and calcaneal eversion occur simultaneously to allow proper intersegmental movement and lower extremity function.

Sagittal Plane Rotations

Hip, knee, and ankle movements in the sagittal plane are coordinated throughout the gait cycle. Hip flexion, knee flexion, and ankle joint dorsiflexion are sagittal plane rotations. They occur synchronously for clearance of the non-weightbearing limb as it swings past the weightbearing limb. At the beginning of stance, the hip extends and the knee straightens, reaching maximal extension shortly before heel-strike, and the ankle is dorsiflexed.[17] At heel contract, the foot rapidly descends to the ground with plantar flexion at the ankle, the knee is immediately flexed, and the hip is maintained in flexion.[17] The shock-absorbing mechanism of hip and knee flexion coincides with ankle plantar flexion and subtalar pronation. The

ankle joint dorsiflexion continues into the stance phase. As toe-off begins, there is a rapid plantar flexion movement that continues until shortly after toe-off.[17] Maximum knee flexion is achieved directly after heel contact. The knee then starts to straighten, reaching maximum extension at midstance.[17] The hip joint is extending through most of the stance phase, supplying the power at push-off.[20]

In summary, the sagittal plane rotations at the hip, knee, and ankle are coordinated to allow for foot clearance and propulsion.

Transverse Plane Rotations

Finally, transverse rotations are the most extensive interconnecting movements in the lower quarter. Gregerson and Lucas[21] studied the transverse rotations of the spine during walking. Their studies, conducted on seven men walking at the rate of 73 m/min on a treadmill, indicate that rotation in the transverse plane occurred as high as the first thoracic vertebra.[21] The vertebrae below T7 rotated forward, with the pelvis on the side of the swinging leg. Above T7 rotation occurred forward, with the shoulder girdle on the side opposite the swinging leg.[21] Maximum rotation occurred between T6 and T7 (Fig. 14–1). Lumbar vertebral rotation was minimal and coincided with pelvic rotations.[21]

From heel-strike to foot-flat, the whole lower limb rotates internally. From midstance to push-off, the lower limb rotates externally.[19] As noted previously, the rotations of the lower limb coincide with the foot's triplane movements of pronation and supination.

The talus, an important component of the subtalar joint, has been described as the torque convertor of the lower limb. Movement of the talus is dictated by the rota-

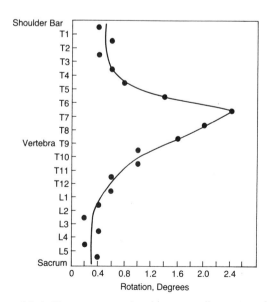

Figure 14–1. Transverse rotation between adjacent vertebrae. Seven adult men walking at 73 m/min. (From Inman et al,[17] with permission.)

tion of the tibia. The talus is often referred to as the extension of the tibia into the foot.[17,19] The transverse rotations of the lower limb are converted at the subtalar joint into sagittal plane and transverse plane movements of the talus. Plantar flexion of the talus occurs during pronation, and dorsiflexion occurs during supination[19] (Fig. 14–2).

In conclusion, the kinematics of the lower quarter have been described in terms of the interrelationship of movements throughout the lower kinetic chain. The rotational components of normal ambulation occur in the coronal, sagittal, and transverse planes. The segmental rotations are interdependent and interrelated with each other. Movement at one joint in the chain influences and to some degree dictates movement at other joints within the lower kinetic chain. This interdependence of movement is established by connective tissue and muscle function. In the evaluation of the lower quarter, it is important to understand the significance of the integrated and harmonious roles of all its links.

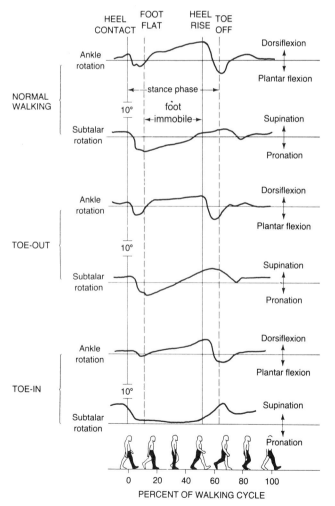

Figure 14–2. Synchronous motions in the ankle and subtalar joints. Variations in toe-out and toe-in cause variations in the magnitude, phasic action, and angular movement of both ankle and subtalar joints. (From Inman et al,[17] with permission.)

Motor Control

Motor control of muscles occurs on several different levels, including the cerebral cortex, brain stem, spinal cord, and ultimately the final common pathway, the alpha motor neuron, which stimulates muscle fibers to contract. Feedback loops to the spinal cord constantly modulate central control of the alpha motor neuron. One of the important reflex pathways to consider is the one governing reciprocal innervation and inhibition.[22] During joint flexion, the flexor contracts and, by reciprocal inhibition, the extensor group relaxes, allowing controlled flexion activity. For joint extension, the reverse holds true: when the extensor contracts, the flexor is inhibited and then relaxes. This reciprocal inhibition occurs not only ipsilaterally but also contralaterally. When the ipsilateral flexor contracts, the contralateral flexor relaxes due to inhibition. The harder a muscle contracts, the more it inhibits its antagonist. Thus, a muscle that is tight and in a shortened position can inhibit its antagonist, which may become weakened.[22] This can have both diagnostic and therapeutic implications.

Muscle Fiber Type

Muscle is often classified on the basis of its fiber type, either slow or fast twitch. Slow-twitch muscle utilizes oxidative metabolism and has a high capillary density, thus imparting a red color. These muscles are considered tonic or postural muscles. They respond to functional disturbance by shortening and tightening. Fast-twitch muscle, by contrast, utilizes glycolytic metabolism, has a lower capillary density, and appears white. Muscles of this type are called *phasic* or *dynamic* muscles. They react to functional disturbance by weakening.

Muscles in the hip and pelvic region with a preponderance of slow-twitch fibers that have a postural or tonic function include the hamstrings, iliopsoas, rectus femoris, tensor fascia lata, thigh adductors, and piriformis. The corresponding phasic muscles in the hip and pelvis region include the vastus medialis and lateralis anteriorly, as well as the gluteus maximus, medius, and minimis posteriorly. In the lower extremity the gastrocnemius and soleus are tonic, whereas the tibialis anterior and peroneal muscles are phasic.

Muscle Imbalances

Muscle balance is the body's constant postural adaptation to gravity. It is a complex process requiring regulation by the spinal cord and higher neural centers. Janda has determined that muscle dysfunction is not a random occurrence, but that muscles respond in characteristic patterns.[23] Postural-tonic muscles respond to dysfunction by facilitation, hypertonicity, and shortening, whereas dynamic-phasic muscles respond to dysfunction by inhibition, hypotonicity, and weakness. Janda referred to this weakness as "pseudoparesis." The affected muscle is not intrinsically weak but rather inhibited. Janda has described patterns of muscle dysfunction in which certain muscles become inhibited and weak, while others become facilitated and tight. In the hip region, the inhibited weak muscles are the gluteus medius and maximus, while the facilitated tight muscles are the iliopsoas, piriformis, adductors, and tensor fascia lata.

Muscle dysfunction can be manifested not only by facilitation and inhibition but also by altered sequential firing patterns. The normal firing pattern of prone hip extension is hamstring, gluteus maximus, contralateral lumbar erector spinae, and then ipsilateral erector spinae. Failure of activation with weakness of the gluteus maximus is the most common deviation, and is manifested as substitution by the hamstrings and erector spinae. The normal firing sequence for hip abduction in the sidelying position is gluteus medius, tensor fascia lata, ipsilateral quadratus lumborum, and erector spinae muscles. The substitution pattern for weakness of the gluteus medius is early firing of the tensor fascia lata or quadratus lumborum. Early firing of the tensor fascia lata results in internal rotation and flexion of the hip during hip abduction. In an even worse scenario, hip abduction is initiated by the quadratus lumborum.

Janda also described three different syndromes that result from muscle imbalance. One of these syndromes, called the *lower crossed syndrome*, occurs in the pelvic girdle. It includes weakness of the gluteus maximus and tightness of the hip flexors, weak abdominals and short erector spinae, weak gluteus medius and minimis with short tensor fascia lata and quadratus lumborum, increased lumbar lordosis, and anterior pelvic tilt, with hypermobility of the lower lumbar levels and altered functional activities that include curling up and sitting up from a supine and forward-bent posture.[22] The evaluation of these muscle imbalances will be addressed later in this chapter.

■ Evaluation of the Lower Quarter

Evaluation of the lower quarter should include a combined assessment of muscle and soft tissue flexibility, neurologic impairment and pain, and lower quarter function. This section presents an overview of evaluation of the lower quarter.

Static Posture

The screening examination should be initiated with observation of static posture. Skeletal alignment and soft tissue deviations are assessed by comparing the left half of the body with the right half. The individual should be observed from three points of view: anteriorly, posteriorly, and laterally. A suggested order is either to begin with the head and progress in an orderly fashion down to the feet or to begin at the feet and progress up to the head. The individual should be dressed in such a manner that the trunk and lower extremities can be easily observed, and the feet should be bare. The subject is instructed to stand erect, with the weight evenly distributed on each foot and the upper extremities relaxed at the sides. Each area of the trunk and lower extremity should be inspected for soft tissue deformity, joint effusion, and skeletal alignment.

From an anterior viewpoint (Fig. 14–3), the head should be held erect and oriented straight ahead with respect to the trunk. The shoulders should be level, with the upper extremities evenly positioned. The trunk should not be rotated to either side, and the pelvis should be level. The lower extremities should be positioned directly under the pelvis, the patellae facing directly ahead, the knee joints in a slight valgus position, and the feet not pronated or supinated. The toes should not be gripping the floor. Such gripping, if present, indicates that the individual has too much weight shifted forward onto the forefoot. The toes also should be evaluated for the presence of deformities.[24]

From a lateral viewpoint (Fig. 14–4), the head and upper trunk should be evaluated for the presence of a foreward head and protracted shoulders. The thoracic and lumbar spine should be observed for excessive or diminished kyphosis or lordosis. If the knee joints extend

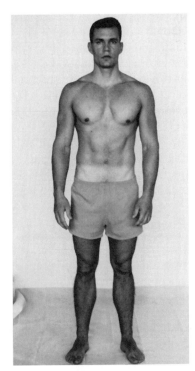

Figure 14–3. Postural alignment as viewed from the anterior perspective. Check for right to left symmetry.

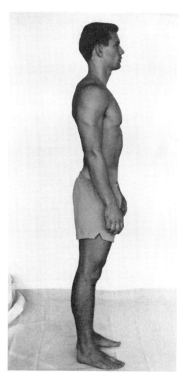

Figure 14–4. Postural alignment as viewed from the lateral perspective. Check head, neck, trunk, pelvis, and lower extremity relationships.

beyond neutral, they should be further evaluated for instability.[24]

When observing static posture from a posterior viewpoint (Fig. 14–5), the spine should be vertical, with the head centered between the shoulders. The shoulders, along with the inferior angles of the scapulae, should be level. There should not be any lateral curvature of the vertebral column, and the ribs should be symmetric. The soft tissues of the trunk should also be observed for any asymmetric skin folds or apparent restrictions. When observing the lower kinetic chain, the iliac crests, posterior superior iliac spines, greater trochanters, gluteal folds, popliteal lines, and medial malleoli all should be level. The knee joints should appear to be in a slightly valgus position, with females exhibiting a greater degree of valgus than males. The Achilles tendon should be straight in alignment with the posterior calcaneus.[24]

Dynamic Posture

A visual gait analysis should be performed to observe whether the individual has any gait deviations, such as an antalgic gait or a positive Trendelenburg sign. Gait should be observed as the patient is walking away from and toward the therapist. The patient should also be observed in the process of standing up and sitting down.[25] If a dysfunction is observed during one of these activities, the therapist should perform a more definitive evaluation to determine the probable cause(s) of the dysfunction. Refer to Chapter 23 for a description of gait.

Active Movements

Active movements of synovial joints are performed with the intent of reproducing the patient's chief complaint. If a joint can be actively moved through the normal extent of all its ranges of motion and a passive overpressure or a stretch at end-feel can be applied without reproducing the complaint, the joint and associated soft tissues probably are not contributing significantly to the problem. Maitland[26] calls this evaluative tool "clearing the joint."

A quick test of the active movements of all joints in the closed lower kinetic chain is to have the individual squat. Although it is not appropriate to have all individuals who are undergoing a screening of the lower kinetic chain perform this activity, it is an excellent method to assess mild musculoskeletal compaints.

Each joint of the lower kinetic chain should be screened for pain and dysfunction. The screening consists of asking the individual to move each joint actively against gravity through each of the available movements of that joint.

Six movements should be performed for the lumbar spine: flexion, extension, right and left lateral flexion, and right and left rotation. Facet joint loading should also be assessed by passively introducing right and left rotation with extension. These motions are best performed in the standing position, with the therapist observing from the posterior position. Gravity is not a significant factor in performing several of these movements in the erect posi-

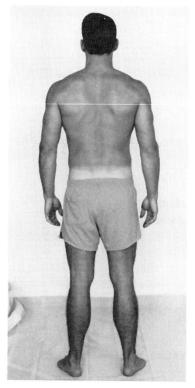

Figure 14–5. Postural alignment as viewed from the lateral perspective. Check position of the shoulders, scapulae, and upper extremities as well as the pelvis for symmetry.

☐☐☐☐☐ ☐ ☐

Table 14–1. Segmental Innervation Levels for the Lower Extremity

Spinal Cord Level	Muscle	Dermatome (skin over the following)	Reflex
L1		Inguinal ligament	
L2	Psoas major	Medial proximal thigh	
L3	Quadriceps femoris	Medial femoral epicondyle	Knee jerk
L4	Quadriceps femoris	Medial malleolus	Knee jerk
L4	Tibialis anterior		
L5	Extensor hallicis longus	Great toe	
S1	Gastrocnemius	Fifth toe	Ankle jerk
S2	Flexor digitorum	Inferior surface, heel	Ankle jerk

tion, and they frequently demonstrate the presence of spinal or sacroiliac joint dysfunction.

Likewise, the hip joint has six basic movements. Flexion, extension, abduction, and adduction are typically performed in the standing position. Internal and external rotation are more easily accomplished and isolated while sitting on a plinth. Knee flexion and extension, ankle dorsiflexion, plantar flexion, inversion, and eversion should be performed in this position.

The patient is repeatedly asked to report whether any movement at each of the joints tested is painful. If a movement is painful or uncomfortable or the joint active movement is not within a normal range of motion, the joint should be evaluated more completely. When the patient can actively move a joint through a full range of motion for all available motions without pain and a passive stretch can be applied without reproducing any symptoms, that joint is not likely to be contributing to the patient's problem.

Neurologic Assessment

If the individual reports or appears to demonstrate some dysfunction of the neurologic system while performing the active movements, a brief neurologic examination should be performed. Gross muscle strength, light touch, and deep tendon reflexes should be evaluated. Table 14–1 lists the segmental innervation levels for the lower extremity—L1 to S2.

Each muscle should be tested bilaterally, using an isometric break test to compare for weakness. Strength assessment is best performed in the sitting position. While in this position, the patient is instructed to flex the hip as resistance is applied to the distal femur (Fig. 14–6) (psoas major, L2), extend the knee with resistance applied to the distal tibia (Fig. 14–7) (quadriceps femoris, L3-L4), dorsiflex the foot with resistance applied to the dorsum of the foot (Fig. 14–8) (tibialis anterior, L4), extend the great toe with resistance applied across the interpha-

langeal joint (Fig. 14–9) (extensor hallucis longus, L5), and evert the forefoot with resistance applied at the distal forefoot (Fig. 14–10) (peroneal muscles, S1-S2). An alternate test for S1-S2 nerve roots is to instruct the patient to stand on one foot and perform heel raises to test the strength of the gastrocnemius-soleus muscle group. Ten heel raises is considered to indicate normal strength. The testing of S2 can be performed more precisely by asking

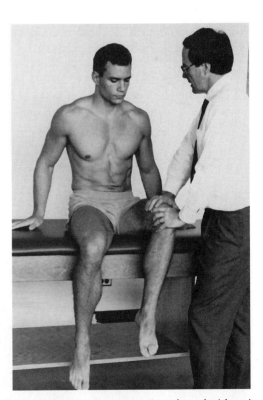

Figure 14–6. The L1-L2 myotome is evaluated with an isometric contraction of the iliopsoas muscle group. The pelvis should be positioned in a slight anterior tilt to minimize lumbar spine stress.

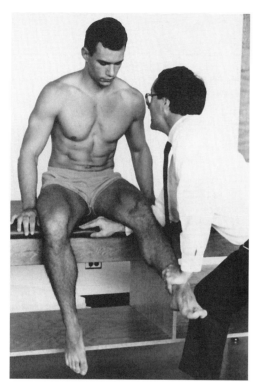

Figure 14–7. The L3-L4 myotome is evaluated with an isometric contraction of the quadriceps femoris. Care should be taken to make certain that the knee is not locked in full extension.

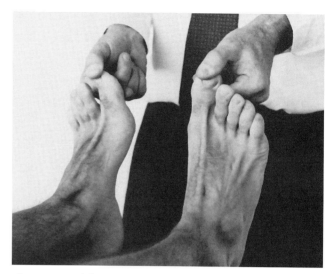

Figure 14–9. The extensor hallucis longus is primarily innervated by L5 and is tested by applying an isometric resistance across the interphalangeal joint of the first digit.

the patient to flex the great toe, with resistance applied to movement at the interphalangeal joint (flexor hallucis longus and brevis).

Sensation can be quickly tested by lightly touching specific areas within each dermatome (Fig. 14–11). The appropriate areas of skin on each lower extremity should be touched simultaneously, and the patient should be

asked whether the sensation is the same in both areas. To test the integrity of the L1 dermatome, lightly touch the skin located over the inguinal ligament. To test the remaining dermatomes, touch the medial thigh midway between the hip and knee (L2), medial femoral epicondyle (L3), medial malleolus (L4), great toe (L5), fifth toe (S1), and inferior aspect of the heel (S2). If the patient reports that there is a difference between the two limbs, more definitive testing should be implemented.[27]

Two deep tendon reflexes can be tested in the lower quarter, the knee jerk and the Achilles tendon or ankle

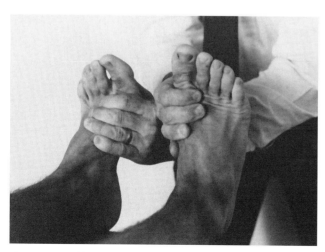

Figure 14–8. Isometric testing of the tibialis anterior tests the L4-L5 myotome.

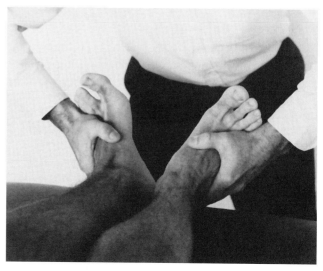

Figure 14–10. The peronius longus and brevis (S1-S2) are tested bilaterally as the subject everts both feet against resistance. Note the stabilization at the heels.

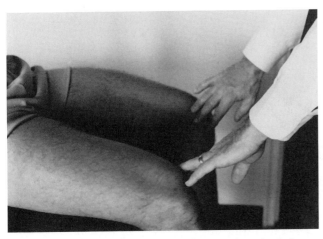

Figure 14–11. Dermatomes should be tested on both lower extremities simultaneously. The dermatome for L3 is pictured.

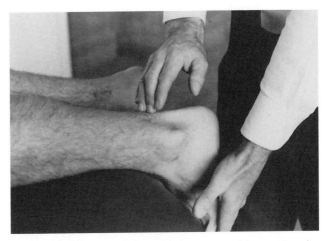

Figure 14–13. The ankle jerk (S1-S2) is tested by tapping the Achilles tendon while a mild dorsiflexon stretch is applied to the sole of the foot.

jerk. With the other neurologic tests, both reflexes should be tested and compared bilaterally. The knee jerk (L3) should be tested with the patient positioned either supine or sitting on a plinth, with the knee joint flexed and the quadriceps femoris muscle relaxed. The patella ligament should be briskly tapped, observing the response of the quadriceps femoris muscle (Fig. 14–12). The ankle jerk reflex should be tested with the patient positioned either prone or sitting on a plinth. A slight stretch to the gastrocnemius muscle should be applied by placing the foot in a minimal degree of dorsiflexion. The Achilles tendon should be briskly tapped, observing the response of the muscle (Fig. 14–13). Deep tendon reflexes are considered to be abnormal if the response between the two limbs is unequal.

Muscle and Soft Tissue Flexibility

It is important to assess the flexibility and function of the interconnecting soft tissue structures and muscles of the lower quarter. There are several tests to determine the flexibility of the two-joint muscles throughout this area.

The Thomas test assesses the flexibility of the iliopsoas[24] (Fig. 14–14). Care must be taken to prevent hyperextension of the lumbar spine during the test. The opposite hip is flexed, and pillows are placed under the head and upper trunk area to flex the lumbar spine. The test is traditionally performed on a hard surface such as a treatment table. A modification of the test is to perform it over the edge of a treatment table, with the opposite hip flexed and held against the side of the examiner (Fig.

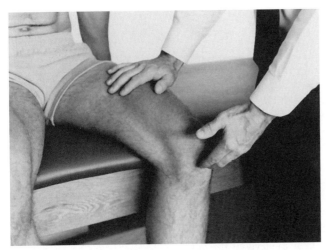

Figure 14–12. Deep tendon reflexes for the lower extremities should be assessed for quality and symmetry. The test for the knee jerk (L3-L4) is pictured.

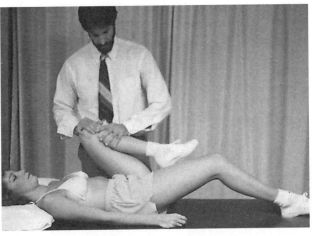

Figure 14–14. Thomas test. Positive test for hip flexion contracture on the right. The hip is at approximately 20 degrees of flexion.

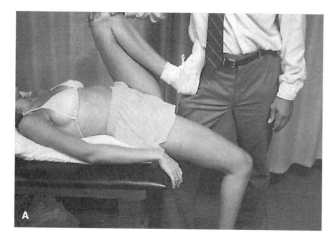

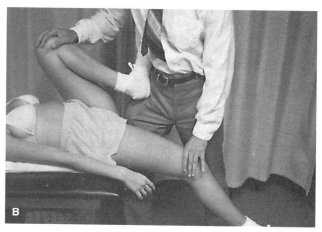

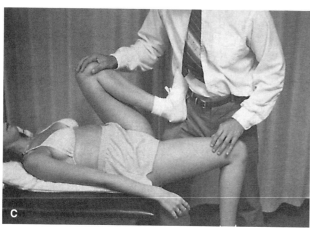

Figure 14–15. (A) Modified Thomas test. The left hip is held in flexion with the foot against the examiner's hip. Pillows are used to reduce the lumbar lordosis. The hip is in extension and the knee is flexed to 90 degrees, demonstrating normal flexibility of the hip flexors and the rectus femoris. (B) Modified Thomas test positive for tight rectus femoris. The knee does not fall into 90 degrees of flexion. (C) Modified Thomas test positive for tight hip flexors. The hip is flexed approximately 15 degrees.

14–15A). This modified test can determine rectus femoris flexibility (Fig. 14–15B,C).

The Ober test is used to determine flexibility of the fasciae latae and the iliotibial band. The test is performed with the patient in a side-lying position, with the hip held in extension and the knee flexed (Fig. 14–16). Stretching of a tight fascia lata or iliotibial band from this test position can produce pain at the lateral aspect of the hip or the knee, respectively Reid et al.[28] demonstrated that iliotibial band tightness is a contributing factor in lateral hip and knee

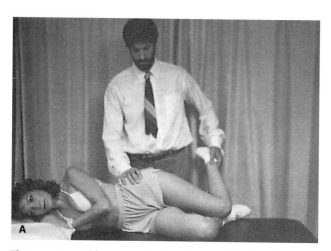

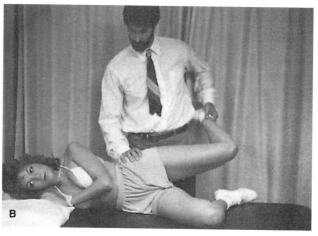

Figure 14–16. Ober test. The hip is extended while the ankle is held at the level of the hip. (A) Negative test: The knee falls to the table. (B) Positive sign for tightness of the iliotibial band: The knee does not drop to the table. The lack of flexibility causes the thigh to be held in abduction without the assistance of the examiner.

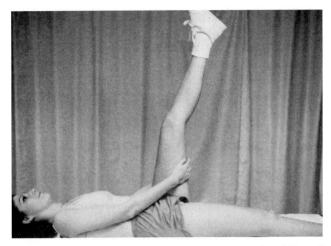

Figure 14–17. Hamstring flexibility test assesses the ability of the patient to extend the knee with the hip flexed to 90 degrees.

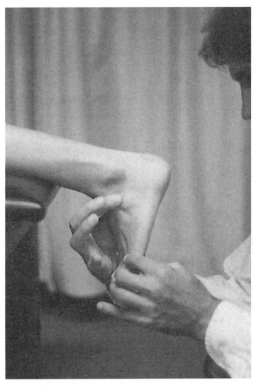

Figure 14–19. Dorsiflexion of the ankle with the subtalar joint held in the neutral position. The examiner is palpating the head of the talus while loading the lateral border of the forefoot. Passive dorsiflexion is performed, not allowing the forefoot to evert.

pain. Iliotibial band syndrome, external snapping hip syndrome, and greater trochanteric bursitis are several "friction syndromes" associated with a tight iliotibial band.

Hamstring flexibility is also important to determine in lower quarter assessment. Hamstring flexibility should be tested in the supine position, preventing the contralateral hip from moving into flexion. First flex the hip to 90 degrees and then straighten the knee (Fig. 14–17). Knee extension will be limited by a tight hamstring muscle group.

To isolate the two-joint hip adductor, the gracilis, from the one-joint hip adductors, the leg is abducted with the knee in extension and with the knee flexed (Fig. 14–18). By maintaining knee extension, the gracilis is put on maximum stretch. The gracilis is a primary hip adductor and secondary knee flexor and internal rotator. Knee flexion places the gracilis on slack, isolating the one-

joint hip adductors (pectineus, adductor longus, adductor brevis, and adductor magnus).

Gastrocnemius tightness can be masked by pronation of the foot in the nonweightbearing and weightbearing positions. Open kinetic chain pronation includes dorsi-

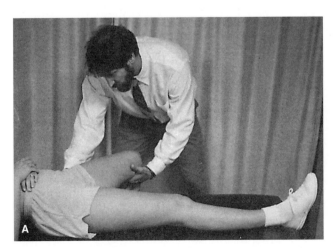

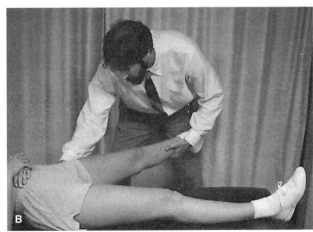

Figure 14–18. (A) Test for flexibility of the one-joint hip adductors. The knee is flexed to 90 degrees. (B) Test for flexibility of the two-joint hip adductors (gracilis). The knee is extended.

flexion, eversion, and abduction of the foot.[16] If the gastrocnemius muscle group is tight, the patient can compensate by pronating the foot. Dorsiflexion of the ankle joint should be isolated by holding the subtalar joint in a neutral position (Fig. 14–19; Chapter 21 describes the neutral position). The gastrocnemius should also be differentiated from the soleus muscle group by maintaining the knee in extension (Fig. 14–20).

Muscle Balances and Postural Control

There are six diagnostic tests to assess if there is muscle imbalance and faulty postural control.[22] The first test examines pelvic control in three dimensions by performing pelvic clock maneuvers in the supine position. The patient initially tilts the pelvis posteriorly and anteriorly to the 12 o'clock and 6 o'clock positions, respectively, while the examiner monitors the movement with the thumbs under the anterior superior iliac spines (ASIS). With good pelvic control, the ASIS stay positionally symmetric from neutral to 12 o'clock and 6 o'clock. With poor pelvic control, the ASIS are not symmetric at the 12 o'clock and/or 6 o'clock positions. For example, with attempted posterior pelvic tilt, the right ASIS does not travel as far cephalically as the left ASIS at the 12 o'clock position, and the left ASIS does not travel as far caudally as the right ASIS at the 6 o'clock position. Similarly, pelvic control is evaluated by monitoring the ASIS as the pelvis moves to the 3 o'clock and 9 o'clock positions. With good pelvic control, the pelvis rolls smoothly and symmetrically from 3 o'clock to 9 o'clock and vice versa. Poor pelvic control is identified when there is elevation of one ASIS by hip hiking and substitution by lumbar spine extension.

The second test evaluates passive hip abduction and external rotation in the supine position. The patient is asked to perform a posterior pelvic tilt while the examiner places the thumbs under the ASIS. While holding the 12 o'clock position, the patient is asked to drop the knees apart. The inability to maintain the posterior pelvic tilt is indicative of muscle imbalance, especially tightness of the short hip adductors. One thus observes the ASIS drop caudally when hip adduction and external rotation are introduced.

The third test evaluates posterior pelvic tilt and heel slide in the supine position. In the supine position with the knees flexed, the patient is asked to maintain a posterior pelvic tilt and then slowly to extend one leg and then the other by eccentrically lengthening the iliopsoas. If the iliopsoas is tight or if the abdominals are weak, the patient will not be able to keep the lumbar spine flat on the exam table.

The fourth test is active trunk rotation in the supine position. With the hips and knees flexed and the knees and feet together, the patient is asked to drop the knees first to one side and then to the other. Once the trunk is fully rotated, the patient is asked to rotate the knees slowly back to the midline using abdominal control rather than hip rotation. With good abdominal oblique and short deep lumbar muscular control, the patient will be able to rotate the lumbar spine back to the table from above downward without any arching of the lower thoracic or lumbar spine. Loss of segmental control of the lumbar spine is often associated with nonneutral lumbar spine dysfunctions.

The fifth and sixth tests are the muscle firing sequences of hip extension and hip abduction mentioned earlier in this chapter.

Pain Assessment in the Lower Quarter

The assessment of pain is important in the evaluation of the lower quarter. The clinician must differentiate between local pain and referred pain from the lumbar spine.

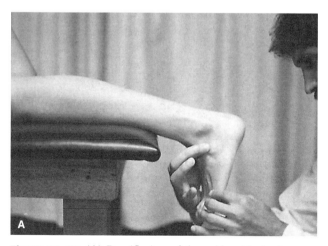
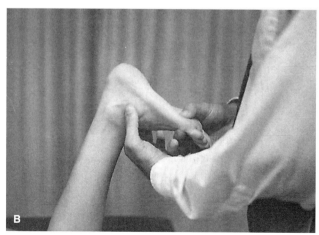

Figure 14–20. (A) Dorsiflexion of the ankle with the knee extended. (B) Dorsiflexion of the ankle with the knee flexed.

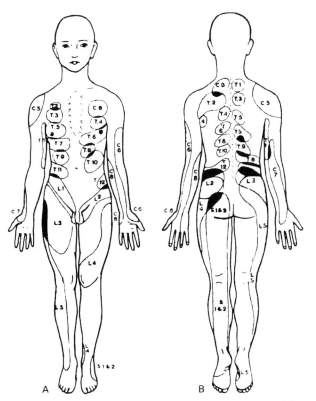

Figure 14–21. (A & B) Referral pain pattern may extend from the lumbar spine into the foot.

terns may be very misleading. The patient's complaint of pain can be unrelated to the location of the trauma.

Besides musculoskeletal pain within the lower quarter, spinal pain must be assessed. Spinal pain may originate from the vertebral column and its related tissues. O'Brien[31] classified three distinct anatomic areas, each with different sensations of pain. The first area, the motion segment, includes the disks, the vertebrae, the facet joints, and their connecting ligaments and muscles. The second anatomic area consists of the superficial tissues surrounding the vertebral column, including the skin, the fascia, the superficial ligaments and muscles, and the tips of the spinous processes. The third category involves the spinal nerve and the sympathetic trunk.

Pain from spinal sources can also be referred into the lower extremity. The referral pain pattern usually follows a dermatome, sclerotome, or myotome (Fig. 14–23). The greater the intensity of the pain, the more distally it is perceived.[29] However, anatomically identifying the source of the pain is difficult because of the overlap of innervation at each level and the overlap of pain patterns.[31] For example, pain arising from root compression or from soft tissue injuries can be felt superficially within the affected dermatome. The referred pain is felt not only

Pain following trauma to the musculoskeletal system may be local or referred, immediate or delayed.[29] Local pain of immediate onset may be a result of distortion of the subcutaneous, perivascular, and periarticular nerve plexuses.[29] Delayed local pain usually results from distention of the joint capsule or fascial compartments by blood or tissue fluid transudate.[29] The persistence of pain after the effects of the injury have subsided indicates a continued inflammatory reaction.[29]

Referred pain may be deep or superficial and shows a segmental pattern following the existing sclerotomes, myotomes, or dermatomes. The transference of pain away from the injured area represents an interconnection of the lower quarter structure. Referral pain patterns may extend from the lumbar spine into the foot (Fig. 14–21).

Referred pain patterns may result from myofascial pain. Myofascial pain is associated with trigger points or fibrositis nodules. A trigger point is a hyperirritability in a muscle or its fascia.[30] Compression of the trigger point area gives rise to local tenderness and may also refer pain away from the local trigger point area (Fig. 14–22). For example, pain from a trigger point in the adductor muscle group may refer pain distally into the ankle. A gluteus minimus trigger point may refer pain anteriorly and posteriorly into the thigh, calf, and ankle. Referred pain pat-

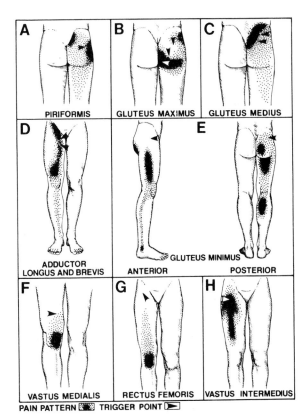

Figure 14–22. (A-H) Myofascial referral pain patterns into the lower extremity. (From Simons and Travel,[30] with permission.)

within the skin but also within the deeper tissues. The deeper pain will follow sclerotome patterns of the affected tissue.[29]

The initial assessment of pain is made by taking a thorough patient history. A careful clinical history will give the examiner useful information about the lesion. The mechanism of injury will often help to determine the general location of the involved tissues and the extent of damage. The immediate response to injury is a useful index of severity. For example, rapid swelling indicates bleeding within the joint. Slow swelling suggests a traumatic synovitis.[29]

The following key questions should be asked as part of the pain assessment and history[32]:

1. Was the onset of pain insidious or sudden?
2. How long have the symptoms persisted?
3. What was the mechanism of injury (twist or strain, lifting or pushing)?
4. Is this the first occurrence of the pain?
5. Is there a history of previous injuries?
6. Where is the location of the worst pain?
7. Where does the pain radiate to?
8. Is there numbness or paresthesia?
9. Is the pain constant or intermittent?
10. What reduces the pain or increases it?

In summary, assessment of the soft tissues of the lower quarter should follow a sequential examination to determine the source of pain and injury. The sequence should include a history, inspection, palpation of soft tissue structures, active and passive range-of-motion testing of the joints, and resisted testing of the surrounding muscles.[33] The active and passive testing will help to distinguish normal from abnormal tissue end-feels,

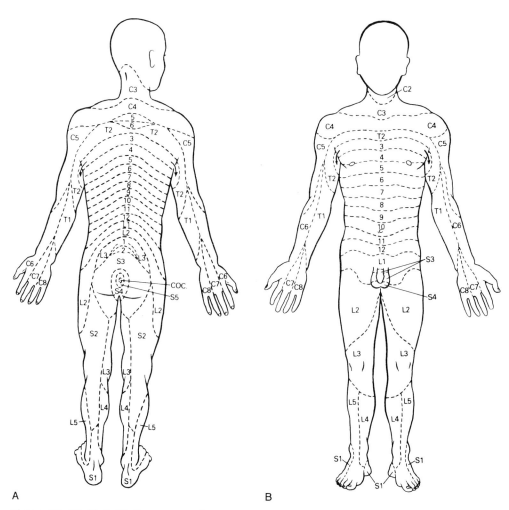

A   B

Figure 14–23. (A & B) Dermatome charts.

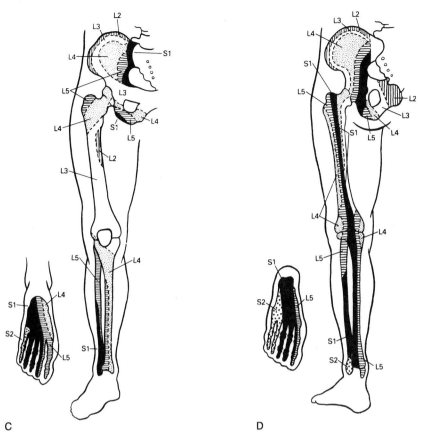

Figure 14–23. *Continued.* (C & D) Sclerotome charts. (From Devinsky and Feldmann,[37] with permission.)

■ Dysfunction of the Lower Quarter

Dysfunction is defined as abnormal, inadequate, or impaired function of an organ or part.[34] Dysfunction in the lower quarter can result from changes in the muscle and connective tissue structures surrounding synovial joints. These changes in soft tissue structures can result from immobilization or trauma. The trauma can be macrotrauma, such as a compound fracture, or microtrauma, in which the persistent irritation of periarticular tissue produces an inflammatory response. Continued irritation can cause scarring, tendinitis, bursitis, capsulitis, and muscular trigger points.[35] The pain associated with microtrauma is insidious. Usually the patient is unaware of the exact cause of the pain. A sequential evaluation of the soft tissue will assist the clinician in determining the location and cause of the microtrauma.

the sequence of pain and limitation, capsular versus noncapsular patterns, ligamentous adhesions, internal derangement, and extra-articular lesions.

The following section presents a hypothetical sequence of events leading to dysfunction in the lower quarter. It demonstrates how a change in the normal mechanics and function of one segment can alter the mechanics of other segments in the chain.

CASE STUDIES

Dysfunction and pain in the lower quarter can also originate from dysfunction in the lumbar spine and sacroiliac joints. The problem may be as straightforward as an acute strain of the erector spinae muscles from a hyperflexion injury or as complex as an overuse syndrome with a history of repeated injury to structures about the lumbar spine. Patients may simply complain of localized low back pain or they may complain of bilateral weakness and paresthesias in the lower extremities. The primary task of the clinician is to perform a thorough patient examination, including a relevant history, to identify the tissues involved, and to develop and implement a treatment program to manage the problems identified. The treatment program should not only address the patient's chief complaint, but should also include a total approach to management of dysfunction in the lower quarter. The following case is an example of how low back dysfunction can have an impact on function in the kinetic chain.

CASE STUDY 1

Orthopaedic Assessment

A 35-year-old male office worker with a diagnosis of muscle strain recently presented with a complaint of right hip and buttock pain, which occasionally radiated down into his calf. The patient's pain was localized to an area extending from the iliac crest superiorly to just above the gluteal fold inferiorly. Anteriorly, the pain extended to within 1 in. of the greater trochanter; the pain did not cross the midline posteriorly. The patient reported that his pain was not constant, but was brought about by standing without walking for approximately 15 minutes. The pain was relieved by walking about for a couple of minutes or by rest in the supine position. The pain felt deep and muscular in origin.

The history revealed that the patient had not experienced any traumatic injury to the area or to his low back. He experienced this pain about four times per year, usually after some outdoor activity such as golf or after playing several games of softball. Previous treatment consisted of muscle relaxers, which gave temporary relief, and ultrasound and stretching exercises, which usually helped relieve the symptoms. The patient now complained that the repetitive episodes of pain were increasing in frequency.

The objective examination revealed that the patient stood erect, with a slightly increased lordotic curve at the lumbar spine, and his pelvis was rotated to the left and anteriorly tilted on the right. These signs were consistent with adaptively shortened iliopsoas muscles, with the right side being tighter than the left, and restrictions of the fascia iliaca, which covers the psoas major and iliacus. The patient could bend forward to a point where his fingertips reached midtibia, whereupon he complained of both buttock pain and posterior leg discomfort bilaterally. Forward bending of the trunk is commonly limited by a combination of adaptively shortened erector spinae and hamstring muscles and restricted thoracolumbar fascia and deep fascia of the thigh.

Kendall et al.[3] pointed out that shortened gastrocsoleus muscles also contribute to limitations in forward bending when the knees are extended. Extension in this patient was limited to approximately 40 degrees; sidebending to the left was approximately 30 degrees and caused pain in the right buttock; sidebending and trunk rotation to the right were moderately limited and did not reproduce any symptoms. The neurologic examination was negative for muscular weakness and altered sensations.

Passive testing of the lumbar spine (central posterior/ anterior glides and sidebending) showed mild restrictions throughout the entire lumbar area, with sidebending to the left having a greater restriction than that to the right. Passive straight leg raising was restricted to approximately 60 degrees on the left and 50 degrees on the right, both limited by tight hamstring muscles. Neither the buttock pain nor the radiating leg pain was reproduced during straight leg raising. The Ober test of the tensor fasciate latae was positive only on the right. This positive test was consistent with the continuation of the fascial restrictions located about the right pelvis. The fascia lata is continuous with the pectineal fascia and fascia iliaca. The Thomas test for the iliopsoas was minimally positive bilaterally. Dorsiflexion of the ankle was within the normal range, both passively and actively.

Palpation of the right buttock revealed a tender and tight piriformis; the left side was tight but not tender. A trigger point was present in the right piriformis, which reproduced the referred pain down into the calf. The right iliopsoas muscle was tender and tight to palpation. The erector spinae muscles along the lumbar spine and the thoracolumbar fascia were restricted in mobility and minimally tender to deep palpation.

Treatment Program

Because the patient's primary goal was to be able to participate in sports occasionally without pain and to reduce the episodic periods of pain, the initial treatment program consisted of ultrasound, parallel and perpendicular soft tissue mobilization, and stretching exercises of the right piriformis muscle and bilateral iliopsoas muscles. The patient was also treated with grade III central posterior/ anterior glides for his lumbar spine hypomobility.

After six treatments, the patient's goal was achieved, and he could have been discharged with a positive end result. However, because of the generalized restrictions in the muscles of the lower quarter and because the symptoms were recurrent, this patient was treated further with soft tissue mobilization, joint mobilization, and a home exercise program intended to diminish the restrictions in his soft tissues and reverse the adaptive shortening of the involved muscles. The soft tissue techniques used to treat the muscle restrictions included strumming, perpendicular strokes, and parallel strokes to the hamstrings and erector spinae muscles and parallel stroking of the iliotibial band. The joint hypomobility in the lumbar spine was treated with accessory and physiologic grade III central posterior/anterior glides, as described by Maitland.[36] The patient's home exercise program consisted of sustained stretching and functional activities to encourage lengthening of the back and thigh muscles. After an additional 2-week period of three treatments per week, the patient was discharged with his home program pain-free, and his flexibility was greatly improved.

A 33-year-old man was referred by his family physician with a diagnosis of low back pain. He had been experiencing repeated exacerbations for the past year, with each occurrence becoming more intense and frequent. He worked as a newspaper reporter and writer, which required him to walk several blocks, drive about the city, and sit in front of a computer terminal for extended periods of time, all of which caused him to have low back pain. He also complained of occasional left foot and medial knee pain, occurring mostly after walking two blocks. He liked to jog, and his goal was to be able to jog for up to 3 miles without experiencing any pain in his back or leg.

The patient reported that radiographs of his spine showed that he had a thoracolumbar scoliosis. He was taking Flexeril as prescribed, with limited, short-term relief. Previous physical therapy treatments consisted of moist heat, ultrasound, and flexibility exercises for his low back pain. This treatment approach provided temporary relief.

A screening examination was performed to determine whether the patient's low back pain was causing his leg pain or whether he had two related problems. Static observation revealed that his right shoulder was high and his left pelvis was low. He stood with more weight on his left lower extremity than on the right. Also, he had an uncompensated S-curve scoliosis, with the apex of the primary curve located at the level of the first lumbar vertebra. This curve was convex to the left, and the midthoracic curve was convex to the right. Closer observation revealed that his left forefoot was pronated.

During walking, the patient demonstrated a mild limp over his left lower extremity, and the step length of his left leg was shorter than that of the right.

Forward flexion of the trunk from the erect position revealed that the patient could only reach the midshaft of his tibia with his fingertips before he experienced the pain in his low back plus a pulling sensation down the posterior aspects of his thighs. Trunk extension was limited to approximately 10 degrees by pain. Lateral flexion to the left increased his lumbar scoliotic curve, while lateral flexion to the right decreased it; however, motion in both directions was limited. All active movements in both of his hip, knee, and ankle joints were within functional limits of range of motion except for a loss of 5 degrees of active dorsiflexion in the left ankle joint.

A quick check of the dermatomes and myotomes of the lower extremities revealed that the patient did not have any neurologic deficits.

Performance of the special tests revealed that the patient's left leg was ½ in. shorter than the right, he had bilaterally shortened hamstrings, and his left gastrocnemius was shortened hamstrings, and his left gastrocnemius was shortened. More definitive testing indicated that he has a sacroiliac dysfunction along with hypomobility of his lower lumbar spine and paraspinal muscle tenderness. Although the muscles and joints of his upper lumbar and lower thoracic spine were hypomobile, he did not exhibit any muscle spasm or pain during testing of these structures.

Treatment Program

In the ensuing 3 weeks, the patient was treated with joint mobilization and a flexibility exercise program for the lumbar and sacroiliac joint dysfunction. Also, a temporary orthotic device with medial forefoot posting was fabricated, which he wore along with a ¼-in. shoe insert to compensate partially for fore-foot pronation and the short left lower extremity. After the first week of care, he was instructed to begin stretching his hamstring and gastrocnemius muscle groups to improve their functional length. After 3 weeks of an intensive stretching and exercise program, the patient was able to walk six blocks without any low back or leg pain, and he was able to begin jogging for short distances. In an effort to bring his pelvis up closer to level, a ⅜-in. shoe insert was substituted for the ¼-in. lift in his left shoe. The patient immediately complained that he experienced low back pain after walking one block, so the old insert was replaced. At discharge, he was able to forward bend to his ankles without any pain, but there was no significant change in his extension and lateral flexion range of motion. He was discharged with instructions to begin increasing his activities within his comfort level and to return to the clinic if needed.

■ Summary

Evaluation of the lower quarter requires examination of all sort tissues and synovial joints in the lower kinetic chain. This chapter has emphasized the importance of performing a thorough screening examination to determine which structures are contributing to an individual's lower quarter dysfunction.

It is important for the clinician to recognize the interdependence of the structures and movements of the lower kinetic chain. Dysfunction of one link of the chain can produce muscle imbalances, altered alignment, and abnormal mechanics throughout the lower quarter. Evaluation and treatment of all the links in the chain are necessary to restore normal function.

■ References

1. Dempster WT: Mechanism of shoulder movement. Arch Phys Med Rehabil 46(A):49, 1965
2. Steindler A: Kinesiology of the Human Body. Charles C Thomas, Springfield, IL, 1966
3. Kendall HO, Kendal FP, Boynton DA: Posture and Pain. Robert E Krieger, Huntington, NY, 1977

4. Rasch PJ, Burke RK: Kinesiology and Applied Anatomy. Lea & Febiger, Philadelphia, 1974

5. Warwick R, Williams PL (eds): Gray's Anatomy. 35th Ed. (B) WB Saunders, Philadelphia, 1973

6. Hollinshead WH: Functional Anatomy of the Limbs and Back. WB Saunders, Philadelphia, 1988

7. Bourdillon JF: Spinal Manipulation. Butterworth-Heinemann, Oxford, 1998

8. Pratt WA: The lumbopelvic torsion syndrome. JAOA 51:335, 1952

9. Kapandji IA: The Physiology of the Joints, Vol 11. Churchill Livingstone, Edinburgh, 1970

10. Tepoorten BA: The piriformis muscle. JAOA 69:126, 1969

11. Pace JB, Nagle D: Piriform syndrome. West J Med 124:435, 1976

12. Hollinshead WH: Buttock, hip joint and thigh. p. 108. In Hollinshead WH (ed): Anatomy for Surgeons: The Back and Limbs. Hoeber Medical Division, Harper & Row, New York, 1969

13. Retzlaff EW, Berry AH, Haight AS, et al: The piriformis muscle syndrome. JAOA 73:55, 1974

14. Gardner E, Gray D, O'Rahilly R: Anatomy: A Regional Study of Human Structure. WB Saunders, Philadelphia, 1967

15. Cathie AG: The influence of the lower extremities upon the structural integrity of the body. JAOA 49:443, 1950

16. Root ML, Orien WP, Weed JN: Clinical Biomechanics. Vol. 11. Normal and Abnormal Function of the Foot. Clinical Biomechanics, Los Angeles, 1977

17. Inman VT, Ralston JH, Todd F: Human Walking. Williams & Wilkins, Baltimore, 1981

18. Saunders M, Inman VT, Eberhart HD: The major determinants in normal and pathological gait. J Bone Joint Surg 35(A):543, 1953

19. Subotnick SI: Podiatric Sports Medicine. Futura, New York, 1979

20. Cavanagh PP: The biomechanics of lower extremity action in distance running. Foot Ankle 7:197, 1987

21. Gregerson GG, Lucas DB: An in vivo study of the axial rotation of the human thoracolumbar spine. J Bone Joint Surg 57(A):759, 1975

22. Greenman PE: Principles of Manual Medicine, Williams & Wilkins, Baltimore, 1996

23. Janda V: Muscle Function Testing. Butterworths, London, 1983

24. Kendall FP, McCreary EK: Muscles: Testing and Function. Williams & Wilkins, Baltimore, 1983

25. Whittle MW: Gait Analysis, An Introduction. Butterworth-Heinemann, London, 1991

26. Maitland GD: Peripheral Manipulation. 3rd Ed. Butterworth-Heinemann, London, 1991

27. Maitland GS: Musculo-skeletal Examination and Recording Guide. 3rd Ed. Lauderdale Press, Glen Osmond, Australia, 1981

28. Reid DC, Burnham RC, Saboe LA, et al: Lower extremity flexibility patterns in classical ballet dancers and their correlation to lateral hip and knee injuries. Am J Sports Med 15:347, 1987

29. Yates A, Smith MA: Musculo-skeletal pain after trauma. p. 234. In Wall PD, Melzack R (eds): Textbook of Pain. Churchill Livingstone, Edinburgh, 1984

30. Simons DG, Travell FG: Myofascial pain syndrome. p. 263. In Wall PD, Melzack R (eds): Textbook of Pain. Churchill Livingstone, Edinburgh, 1984

31. O'Brien JP: Mechanisms of spinal pain. p. 240. In Wall PD, Melzack R (eds): Textbook of Pain. Churchill Livingstone, Edinburgh, 1984

32. McRae R: Clinical Orthopaedic Examination. Churchill Livingstone, Edinburgh, 1983

33. Cyriax J: Textbook of Orthopaedic Medicine. Vol. I. Diagnosis of Soft Tissue Lesions. Williams & Wilkins, Baltimore, 1976

34. Clayton L. (ed): Taber's Cyclopedic Medical Dictionary. FA Davis, Philadelphia, 1977

35. Travell JG, Simons DG: Myofascial Pain and Dysfunction. The Trigger Point Manual. Williams & Wilkins, Baltimore, 1983

36. Maitland GD: Vertebral Manipulation. 5th Ed. Butterworths, London, 1986

37. Devinsky O, Feldmann E: Examination of the Cranial and Peripheral Nerves. Churchill Livingstone, New York, 1988

CHAPTER 15
Dysfunction, Evaluation, and Treatment of the Lumbar Spine

Peter I. Edgelow

This chapter discusses the consequences of dysfunction of the lumbar spine in a manner that will help the physical therapist effectively treat and manage patients with these disorders. The proper role of the physical therapist is to mobilize all positive forces that can improve function. These forces consist of the body's ability to heal itself and the practitioner's ability to identify through examination the signs and symptoms of dysfunction, to apply effective treatment methods, and to teach patients to become their own therapists by participating in and enhancing the healing process through positive expectations and constructive actions.

The *mobile segment* is the structure that forms the basic anatomic unit of the lumbar spine.[1-4] A brief review of the anatomy of the mobile segment is presented in this chapter, emphasizing those aspects that are relevant to the patient's understanding of the mechanisms of injury to the system and as a rationale for treatment. Methods that can assist the therapist in training the patient to understand the nature of the injury and to assist the healing process are presented throughout this chapter.

Next, the value and limitations of diagnostic labels are discussed. Traditionally, the pathology of a particular body region involves the study of structural and functional changes that occur in disease. Many textbooks effectively describe the pathologic symptoms in the lumbar spine that indicate specific diagnoses.[5-10]

The discussion of pathology here has two purposes. The first is to present some of the features of musculoskeletal disorders of the lumbar spine that a clinician can discuss with patients to assist them in approaching the problem from a position of real knowledge. This will assist patients in establishing a positive belief system about getting well.[11] The second purpose is to distinguish between two types of diagnostic labels in physical treatment: those that either contraindicate or indicate the need for caution in applying physical treatment, and those in which

the signs and symptoms are what must guide the therapist in treatment, not the labels themselves.

In the discussion of dysfunction, the practitioner is encouraged to look closely at the history of specific signs and symptoms and then to develop appropriate treatment plans. These treatment plans, in turn, are modified as the patient responds during the healing process.

In treatment as it relates to the diagnostic label, the approach in this chapter is guided by the history of signs and symptoms of the disorder as much as by the knowledge implied in the disorder's diagnostic label. For purposes of this discussion, theories of medical treatment are separated into two broad categories: those that are "pathology focused" and those that are "signs, symptoms, and patient focused." Before Hippocrates, the Cnidian school of medicine rested on the notion that for every illness there existed one specific cause and one specific treatment.[12] Present-day medicine, or at least one aspect of it, is very Cnidian in approach. For every infection, there is a specific antibiotic for treatment, and for every injury, a specific routine of exercises. One can view this Cnidian approach as a pathology-focused treatment in which the medical practitioner focuses on the diagnosis that the patient's condition has been given and offers the standard treatment for this diagnosis.

The problem with the pathology-focused, or one-cause, one-treatment approach is that it fails to appreciate the broader picture of the disorder. This approach also ignores the fact that the physical body that houses the ailment also houses an emotional and intellectual being, the human patient. The injury invariably affects the person intellectually and emotionally as well as physically, and an essential aspect of effective treatment is that the whole person must be acknowledged and ministered to for treatment to progress optimally. In short, the foundation of treatment should rest on the signs, symptoms and patient-focused treatment model of medicine, the roots of which can be traced to Hippocrates. In this approach, the practitioner looks at the total wellness of the patient and how to strengthen the body's own defenses against illness or injury, as well as treating the signs and symptoms with a foreign agent or set of physical treatments.[13]

Because Chapters 16 and 17 discuss surgical and mobilization treatment methods in detail, this chapter focuses on patient handling and home care, paying special attention to the role of walking in the treatment process. The chapter closes with a case study which illustrates the important concepts presented.

■ Anatomy

This section discusses those aspects of the anatomy of the lumbar region that should be communicated to patients so they can take an active role in the treatment process. The characteristics of the anatomy of the mobile segment that affect treatment procedures are also highlighted.

The vertebral mobile segment is a more complex structure than a peripheral joint, and this complexity and the interrelationships of anatomic, biomechanical, and neurophysiologic factors in the lumbar region have crucial implications for treating injuries or disease in this area. One aspect of the complexity of injuries to the mobile segment is that they almost invariably bring the sympathetic nervous system into play. The sympathetic nervous system, the main vasomotor controlling system in the body, tends to exaggerate the disturbance. This results in an impeding of blood flow; normalizing the sympathetic nervous system thus has a beneficial effect on the circulation. When you control the blood flow to a given area, you control its life, its capacity for recovery, and its ability to survive, resist further injury, and maintain its integrity as a tissue.[14]

Another aspect of the complexity of the mobile segment is illustrated by contrasting pathology in a mobile segment with pathology in a peripheral joint such as the hip. When the hip joint becomes osteoarthritic and symptomatic, the muscles that move that joint undergo characteristic changes. In general, one group of muscles becomes tight, with the antagonistic group becoming weak and undergoing atrophy. In the case of the hip, the flexors become tight and the extensors weak.[15] Further, a loss in proprioception in the joint coupled with weakness and poor motor control sets up a perpetuating cycle of further microtrauma.

In injuries of the mobile segment, it is more difficult to maximize healing throughout all stages of recovery than with a peripheral structure such as the hip. To promote healing of an injured body part, one must control the amount of stress placed on the injury. During stages when the hip is acutely inflamed, the patient can still remain functional by using crutches to reduce stress. During subsequent stages in recovery, when passive motion of the hip in a nonweightbearing position will promote

further healing,[16] this can again be accomplished fairly easily while still allowing function. Peripheral structures are easier to treat than mobile segments because we have more control over the stresses placed on them. However, because the spine is central to virtually everything we do mechanically, it is much more difficult to isolate and protect any one mobile segment from stresses that do not promote healing or lead to further damage. Once the body part has recovered sufficiently to allow loaded activity to promote healing, resolution of the condition is much more rapid.

The discussion of anatomy in this chapter is divided into the following three topics:

1. A brief description of the mobile segment, as a base for comparison or analogy to a hinge
2. A description of the structures that act as pain generators in the mobile segment (Table 15–1)
3. Discussion of the circulation to the mobile segment and the factors that might interfere with nutrition to the system and lead to degeneration of the segment or interfere with maximum healing of injuries

All these topics are covered within the context of how the information can be conveyed to the patient to empower the patient to assist in the healing process. What follows is a description of the mobile segment that the therapist can use to assist the patient in gaining a better picture of those factors that contribute to an understanding of the injury. It can be helpful for the therapist to draw a picture of the motion segment for the patient, diagrammatically emphasizing its features (Figs. 15–1 and 15–2).

The mobile segment consists of two vertebrae with an intervening disk. A bridge of bone connects the left and right sides of the vertebrae. Projections of bone, the facets, jut inferiorly from this bridge to join the other facets from below, overlapping one another like the shingles of a roof. These zygapophyseal joints have ligamentous and capsular support and a synovial membrane lining that provides synovial fluid for lubrication and nutrition.

□ □ □ □ □   □   □   □

Table 15–1. Structures That Act as Pain Generators in the Mobile Segment

Vertebral body and epidural veins

Intervertebral disk and supporting ligaments

Zygapophyseal joints, surrounding capsule, and supporting ligaments

Dorsal and ventral ramus and mixed spinal nerve

Dorsal root ganglion

Muscles

Dura mater

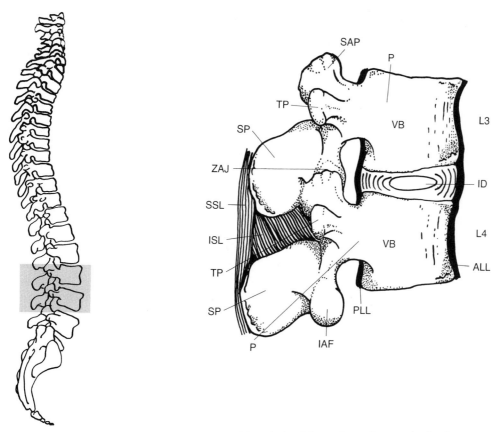

Figure 15–1. Lumbar 3-4 mobile segment and its relationship to the entire vertebral column. P, pedicle; SAP, superior articular process; VB, vertebral body; ID, intervertebral disk; ALL, anterior longitudinal ligament; PLL, posterior longitudinal ligament; IAF, inferior articulate facet; SP, spinous process; TP, transverse process; ISL, interspinous ligament; SSL, supraspinous ligament; ZAJ, zagapophyseal joint. (Adapted from Bogduk and Twomey,[4] with permission.)

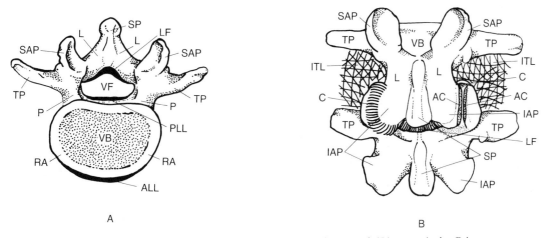

Figure 15–2. Lumbar 3-4 mobile segment viewed from (A) above and (B) posteriorly. RA, ring apophysis; P, pedicle; TP, transverse process; SAP, superior articular process; L, lamina; SP, spinous process; LF, ligamentum flavum; VF, vertebral foramen; PLL, posterior longitudinal ligament; VB, vertebral body; ALL, anterior longitudinal ligament; IAP, inferior articular process; C, capsule of the joint; ITL, intertransverse ligament; AC, articular cartilages. (Adapted from Bogduk and Twomey,[4] with permission.)

Other projections of bone, the right and left transverse processes and the spinous process, act as outriggers for the attachment of ligaments and muscles. The ligamentous attachments provide static support, the muscular attachments provide dynamic stability, and together they control and guide movement. As the therapist describes the mobile segment to the patient, it is useful to draw an analogy with the hinges on a door. A hinge consists of the following components: two flanges, a connecting pin, and screws to connect the flange to the frame of the doorway and to the door. Problems in function can be described, such as the door squeaking when moved. The patient can be led through the problem-solving process by considering whether the squeak is due to "loose screws" (problems of instability) or "need for oil" (problems of quality of movement). To carry the hinge analogy further, the therapist can compare a patient's problem involving a mobile segment that is both unstable and lacking in mobility to a hinge that has loose screws and cannot be fully opened or closed. Proper treatment would be to use gentle oscillating midrange movements (oil the hinge) to reduce friction and then carefully use gentle end-range oscillating movements (open or close the door). A change in pain behavior is used as a guide to whether the structure can withstand the stress of the motion. If the structure cannot withstand the end-range motion, bracing or surgery (tightening up the screws of the hinge) might be necessary. Such analogies are important methods of translating anatomic knowledge into more familiar language to ensure that the patient's understanding will be a guide in treatment and not a source of confusion.

In discussing the ligaments of the mobile segment with the patient, it can be of value to name the ligaments (Table 15–2) and briefly describe their function in providing stability. The ligaments function like the screws that support the hinge. If they are too loose, they will allow excess movement to occur during function (opening the door). If they are too tight, they restrict motion in certain directions.

Function of the Muscles of the Lumbar Spine

The function of the muscles of the lumbar spine is well described by Macintosh and Bogduk.[17] Of particular im-

portance is their hypothesis that the inter-transversarii mediales may act as large proprioceptive transducers. These muscles, together with the multifidus, are innervated by the lumbar dorsal rami of the nerve of that segment. Therefore, injury to that segment can interfere with the muscle activity of the prime proprioceptive muscle and the prime stabilizing muscle of the segment. However, such injuries do not necessarily interfere with the innervation to the multisegmental muscles of the spine such as the latissimus dorsi and the gluteus maximus, which initiate and control movement and function of the extremities, and also the erector spinae, which provides both power and control of movement of the spine as a whole.

Pain arising from one or more of the structures listed in Table 15–1 remains poorly understood, and over time, many "stories" have developed to account for pain arising from the back. Bogduk and Twomey[4] discuss two types of classical lumbar pain: (1) pain generated from structures 1, 2, 3, 6, or 7 in Table 15–1, termed *somatic pain,* and (2) pain from disorders of structures 4 or 5 in Table 15.1, termed *radicular pain.*

Bogduk and Twomey cite studies that have clearly incriminated the zygapophyseal joints,[18,19] disks,[20–26] and dura mater[27,28] as possible sources of pain, with only the epidural blood vessels and the vertebral bodies not having been studied experimentally to prove that they can also be a source of pain. Circumstantial evidence points to the epidural blood vessels as a possible source of pain.[29] Only the bone of the vertebral bodies has not been proved to be a pain generator, although it could, wisely or unwisely, be assumed that the pain of osteoporosis is an example of bone as a pain generator.[4] The possible causes, then, of pain arising from any one of the somatic structures are any pathologic processes that stimulate nociceptive nerve endings in any one of the structures named. This stimulation may be due to either chemical or mechanical irritation. The methods by which these processes can cause stimulation are well described,[4,30] and this detailed knowledge is not essential for patients' understanding of why they hurt, although this information can help therapists assist patients in viewing pain as a guide rather than a curse.

To paraphrase Bogduk and Twomey,[4] the somatic referred pain mechanism appears to be the activation by afferent impulses from the mobile segment of neurons in the central nervous system, which also happen to receive afferents from the lower limbs, buttocks, or groin. Stimulation of central system neurons by messages from the mobile segment may cause the perception of pain arising from all the other tissues innervated by these neurons. Therefore, pain is perceived as arising from a structure in the limbs, even though there is no signal actually coming from this structure. There is some evidence that the distance of referral into the limb is proportional to the intensity of the stimulus of the mobile segment.[4]

□□□□ □ □ □ □

Table 15–2. Ligaments of the Mobile Segment

Anterior longitudinal ligament

Posterior longitudinal ligament

Ligamentum flavum

Interspinous and supraspinous ligaments

Intertransverse ligament

Anterior and posterior facet capsular ligaments

The pathology of nerve root compression is a complex issue, and there are conflicting and erroneous explanations in the literature. The reader is encouraged to explore the explanation advanced by Bogduk and Twomey as the most interesting one currently available.[4]

The pain generator is unlikely to be one structure. A much more common scenario is the nerve root compression syndrome. In the presence of neurologic changes (e.g., weakness, numbness, decreased reflexes) together with the characteristic lancinating pain of radicular origins, there may be concomitant somatic and somatic referred pain from the structures adjacent to and surrounding the nerve root.

For patients to have some understanding of the origin of their complaints, the following factors can be discussed with them: pain generators, somatic as well as radicular referral of pain, and central nervous system modulation of pain.

Circulation and Nutrition of the Mobile Segment

Six circulatory systems are involved in nutrition within the mobile segment: (1) the arterial/venous system, (2) the internal intervertebral disk system, (3) the cerebrospinal fluid system, (4) the lymphatic system, (5) the synovial fluid system, and (6) the interneuronal transport system. Optimum functioning of all of these systems is essential for health. Any factor that interferes with this optimum function will affect the process of injury repair.

It is not the purpose of this chapter to consider the function of these systems in detail. The reader can obtain this information from many sources,[4,31–36] although a great deal is not yet fully understood. However, from the patient's point of view, the important factors are those that interfere with circulation and nutrition. The disk appears to live and thrive on movement, and to change and die slowly through lack of it.[37] The same is true of all structures of the mobile segment. If one considers the negative effects of immobilization on all structures and systems, the clinician's job in treatment is to convince the patient of the need to move the injured parts.[38–41]

A useful metaphor in making the patient aware of the importance of adequate circulation is that of a lake. When the flow of water (circulation) in and out of the lake (the mobile segment) is impeded by damming of the exiting tributary (injury), the lake may turn into a swamp (inflammation). Increasing the water flow by removing the dam (mobility) drains the swamp and restores life to the lake.

The normal healing response to injury is as follows: Injury results in an inflammatory process, set off by the enzymes released by the damaged tissue in dead cells. Inflammation is a change in the local network of capillaries that leads to an outpouring of inflammatory exudate, a fluid rich in antibodies that lays down a network of fibrin. Within the exudate, vast numbers of cells enter and begin to clear up the dead cells. The inflammatory exudate may still be growing by the third or fourth day after injury, especially if there is a large amount of damage or more damage from continuous use.[42]

The general method of healing of tissue is by fibrous repair. Repeated damage to fibrous connective tissue will not only mean a thickened and contracted tissue but will also result in extensive loss of proprioceptive nerve endings. The repair process that follows results in an initial consolidation of the injured tissue. This consolidation period is followed by scarring. If the tissue being healed is kept absolutely immobile, the resultant fibrous scarring is weak.

When there are no natural forces on the healing tissue, collagen is laid down haphazardly and, although it may be plentiful, it is poorly engineered. Fibrous healing is stronger if natural movements are encouraged. The stress of the natural movements determines the manner in which the collagen fibers are laid down. Gentle, normal movements provide natural tensions in the healing tissue, resulting in much stronger healing. However, if there is continued inflammation, fibrous healing will be poor.

Healing also requires a good blood supply to support the phagocytes by supplying oxygen and nutrients to the worker cells, carrying off waste, and preventing further cell death secondary to anoxia and other factors. No injury can be made to heal faster than its natural speed. The tools of healing, the cells getting on with their job, cannot be improved. All that can be done is to make sure that no contrary influences are allowed and that all possible favorable conditions are encouraged.

The important factor that is often forgotten, or at least not stressed in repair, is that there is a remodeling period after scar formation that results in a strengthening and realignment of the scar to the point where the opportunities for reinjury are minimized. It is this remodeling stage that is of critical importance in repair of injury to the mobile segment, and in particular the disk.

After an injury, the healed tissue is never the same as it was before. Fibrous connective tissue, such as the ligament or joint capsule, will be repaired, but it will not have exactly the same structure or properties as the original. Moreover, the nerve end organs do not regenerate. Damaged muscles do not regenerate. They heal with a scar of fibrous tissue.[42]

■ Consequences of Dysfunction in the Lumbar Region

Pathology is the study of the structural and functional changes that occur in disease. This section expresses some philosophical views on the value of pathologic knowledge and the risks and drawbacks of this knowledge as it relates to treatment. It lists disorders under three broad categories: those in which physical therapy treatment is contraindicated, those that call for certain precautions in treatment, and those in which physical therapy is indicated, guided by the signs and symptoms. Finally, this section presents a method of looking at disorders of the musculoskeletal system that is functionally oriented and designed to assist the therapist in explaining to the patient what is wrong in a manner that facilitates treatment. It is important to stress that when the clinician collects the data, a methodical, orderly method of establishing a necessary minimum of information is used. These data are then used to arrive at a presumptive diagnosis, or treatment diagnosis. Tables 15–3 and 15–4 show what types of information gathered in the examination process are associated with a particular pathology and should alert the examiner to the potential risks in treatment. The tables are organized according to the method of examination taught by Maitland.[43,44]

Effective treatment of low back injuries should include a careful neuromusculoskeletal evaluation and careful instructions on which movements risk further injury and which movements enhance healing. The common sense that the patient uses instinctively to reduce stress to an injury to a peripheral joint is simply not as useful in the lumbar spine, with its immense backup system of mobile segments. Also, the patient's knowledge of this region is not as clear as his or her knowledge of peripheral joints such as the knee or hip.

Thus, the therapist must isolate the particular injured segment through careful methodical examination and then determine which is the appropriate resting position as well as the best functional movement. Because the biomechanics of the spine changes from level to level, the resting positions and positions of stability also change. This helps to explain why in upper lumbar injuries the patient is more comfortable in a semireclined than a fully reclined position. Conversely, in injuries to the lower lumbar region, the patient is more comfortable either fully reclined, with the hips and knees flexed to allow lumbar flexion, or with a rolled towel to support the low lumbar spine in some degree of extension. After these determinations, the therapist explains to the patient how to best assist the healing process through an appropriate combination of rest and activity.

The pathologic label, or diagnosis, provides the therapist with information that may contraindicate certain treatments or indicate caution in treatment. An example of a diagnosis that contraindicates treatment is that of a spinal tumor. In this instance, physical treatment would be useless in correcting the problem. Another example is cauda equina symptoms, such as difficulty in initiating urination and numbness in the perineum. These symptoms indicate the possibility of compression of the sacral nerve roots or cauda equina, which innervates the bladder and provides sensory distribution to the perineum. Any lesion that is gross enough to produce these symptoms requires immediate referral to a physician for emergency evaluation and treatment (Table 15–3).

An example of a disorder that indicates the need for caution in treatment is osteoporosis. (See Table 15–4 for a more detailed account of disorders that indicate the need for caution in treatment.) The diagnostic label itself indicates that there is at least a 35 percent demineralization of the bone, which may be responsible in part for the patient's problem.[31] It is important to understand, however, that there may be a mechanical component besides the demineralization. In treatment of the mechanical component, one should be careful not to apply forces that might fracture a bone weakened by demineralization. Still, the therapist should guide the treatment by assessing changes in the patient's signs and symptoms that may be caused by mechanical problems within the system rather than by the weakened bone structure. Because the diagnosis of osteoporosis is not always clear-cut, the therapist should be particularly careful in the treatment of injuries of postmenopausal women in which a minor back injury has produced a severe response, particularly in the presence of involuntary muscle spasm. Routine radiography may miss a minor compression fracture.

Once the clinician has excluded those disorders that contraindicate or indicate caution in physical treatment, treatment of the pathologies that remain should be guided more by the history, signs, and symptoms than by the information inherent in the diagnostic label alone. There is a tendency in some treatment situations to stop once one has a diagnostic label and carry on with treatment based strictly on this label. This practice should be guarded against because it is the signs, symptoms, and stage of the pathology that require treatment, not the label.

Some pieces of information are pathognomonic, or so specific to one pathologic condition that by themselves they can guide one in treatment. For example, the knowledge that a patient has spondylolisthesis tells the practitioner that a structural weakness exists with both extension movements of the spine and posteroanterior forces on the spine. This does not imply that all extension movements or posteroanterior mobilizations are contraindicated, but rather that the signs and symptoms must be read carefully, as the therapist uses these movements to ensure that functional extension for the patient is restored while respecting the structural weakness.

In contrast, other patients present constellations of signs and symptoms that point in certain treatment directions but are not as clear-cut. In these more vague cases, the therapist must carefully observe changes in signs and symptoms as the patient responds to a particular treatment plan, refining and altering the treatment plan in response to these changes.

■ Examination of the Thoracolumbar Spine

To make the most use of the signs and symptoms of a disorder or injury, a detailed examination is essential.

Table 15-3. Disorders in Which Physical Treatment Is Contraindicated

	Subjective Symptoms						Objective Signs			
Disorder	Area	Description	Behavior	History	Special Questions	Radiographic Evidence	Observation	Active and Passive Movements	Neurologic Examination	Other Tests
Malignancy (primary or secondary)	Nonspecific	Severe intractable pain	Not always altered by rest or activity Worse at night; patient wakes and must get up and move around	Onset slow and insidious; patient may have past history of illness or surgery	General health poor, recent weight loss	Early in disease no changes; later may show loss of spinous process, transverse process, or pedicle				
Inflammatory conditions Tuberculosis Osteomyelitis Paget's disease		Constant and severe pain	Unaltered by rest or activity Night sweats		General health poor, possible weight loss					
Spinal cord compression	Bilateral paresthesia of hands and/or feet, stocking/glove, nearly always bilateral						Unsteadiness of gait		Hyperreflexive, hypertonic, ankle clonus, positive plantar response (Babinski)	Incoordination, muscle weakness in lower extremities
Cauda equina disorder	Saddle paresthesia or anesthesia				Bladder retention; possible overflow, incontinence, or bowel retention			Protective spasm	Hyperreflexive, hypertonic, ankle clonus, positive plantar response (Babinski)	

(Data from Grieve.[31])

Table 15-4. Disorders in Which Caution Is Indicated in Applying Physical Treatment

Disorder	Subjective Symptoms					Objective Signs				
	Area	Description	Behavior	History	Special Questions	Radiographic Evidence	Observation	Active and Passive Movements	Neurologic Examination	Other Tests
Recent fracture		Pain may be intermittent, sharp, and severe	Severe catches of pain with minimal movement	History indicates possible compression fracture, sudden loading of spine, severe coughing, fall on buttocks		May not be evident on standard radiograph and may require CT scan		Protective spasm		
Osteoporosis	General ache	Persistent pain	Relieved by lying, aggravated by prolonged standing, sitting, or walking	Age—postmenopausal, Sex—female > male; Prolonged immobilization, onset may be insidious or sudden and severe from minimal incident	Prolonged steroid therapy	Will require at least 35–50% demineralization before radiologic appearance	May have a degree of kyphosis	Severe protective spasm		
Ankylosing spondylitis, active stage		Severe intractable pain	Worse at night, morning stiffness takes longer than 30 minutes to loosen (generally 1 hour)		Signs of systemic illness, weight loss			If tests positive, reduces sidebending bilaterally and equal early in disease; reduced chest expansion	General weakness secondary to disease	Sacroiliac tests often positive, raised erythrocyte sedimentation rate

Condition								
Spondylolisthesis	Pain increases with standing and walking, decreases with sitting				Characteristic "scotty dog" appearance		Extension decreased and painful, passive testing (posterior/anterior) produces pain easily. Palpations of "step"; PP-MT test* positive for instability	
Juvenile disk			Often onset associated with trauma (e.g., in sports)	Often complaints are minimal and yet patient may have difficulty walking		Loss of lordosis	Considerable spasm	Pronounced tension signs
Scheuermann's disease	May be described as "like growing pains"	Often vague pain in lower extremities, nondermatomal	Present in adolescents (boys more than girls); onset insidious	Pain is stress- and time-dependent	Often severe changes, fuzziness of disk/vertebral body interface; vertebral wedging may occur	May have thoracic kyphosis		

* PP-MT, passive physiological movement test.
(Data from Grieve.[31])

Once the data have been gathered by examination, they can be used in assessment and as a guide to treatment, one of the cornerstones of the Maitland concept of examination, treatment,and assessment as a continuous loop.[43–46]

The examination process is divided into two sections: the subjective examination, or what the patient reveals about the complaint in response to questioning, and the objective examination, or what the examiner determines based on certain tests and measures.

The subjective examination can be divided into four sections:

1. The area of the symptoms, in which one clarifies the location of the complaint and its distribution and obtains a description of the complaint.
2. The behavior of the symptoms, in which one traces the aggravating and easing characteristics of the complaint, based on a functional evaluation over the previous 24-hour period.
3. The history of the onset of the complaint and the progress of symptoms and signs from onset until the present, as well as its present stability and any past history of similar complaints that might relate to this problem.
4. The patient's response to certain specific questions as they may relate to an understanding of the disorder or of its cause. These questions relate to such factors as general health, relevant change in the patient's weight, whether radiographs have been taken and the findings, and any medically prescribed drugs the patient is using. Of specific significance in the low lumbar spine is the possibility of cauda equina symptoms (numbness in the perineum and difficulty in initiating urination). In the upper lumbar spine, the possibility of a cord lesion with symptoms of bilateral numbness of the feet and unsteadiness of gait is also significant.

The objective examination covers the following factors:

1. Observation of posture and gait
2. Active movements of the spine
3. Passive movements of the spine
4. Accessory movements of the spine
5. Tests for muscle function (e.g., weakness, lack of coordination, or muscle pain)
6. Tests of other joints (e.g., sacroiliac, hip, knee, and ankle)
7. Neurologic tests (e.g., reflexes, sensation, and motor power)
8. Dural tension signs tested singly or in combination (e.g., passive neck flexion, straight leg raise, prone knee flexion, and slumped sitting)

The purpose of testing movements is to determine the quantity and quality of the range of motion, the effect of movement on the patient's resting symptoms or on production of symptoms, and the presence of spasm or lack of symmetry during movement. Abnormal movement is a fact to be assessed for relevance to the complaint and to try to determine why the complaint exists. It is also a piece of data to be used in assessing changes during treatment. For example, suppose that a patient presents with constant right-sided lumbar pain and intermittent right calf pain. Trunk flexion is limited such that the patient's finger tips reach only to the upper border of the patella, with an increase in lumbar pain and production of calf pain. On returning to the erect position, there is a further increase in lumbar pain, and the patient has to assist him- or herself by pushing on the thighs. In this example, the quantity of motion is measured by the position of the finger tips, the quality is characterized by the pain on attempted extension from the flexed position, and the abnormal movement is relevant to the complaint because it alters the symptoms. The quantity and quality of this range of flexion motion will provide useful benchmarks in assessing the patient's progress.

Data from the objective examination are very seldom pathognomonic. It is not one piece of information that indicates a specific direction in treatment but rather how the pieces fall into a pattern. An effective examination process involves gathering one piece of data, interpreting its meaning or relevance, and then reassessing that interpretation as new data are added. It is not poor technique to jump to a conclusion based on one piece of information, provided that the therapist confirms this interpretation through other supportive data or forms a new interpretation if additional data so indicate. For example, a flattened lumbar spine might indicate a loss of extension mobility, requiring increased extension to restore maximum function. Similarly, a lateral shift with a flattened lumbar spine in the standing position might require restoration of lateral movement and then restoration of extension before the patient can regain maximum function. However, the critical point is that, by itself, lack of extension on observation does not indicate a need for extension. The observed posture together with the effect of movements on the symptoms are the factors that direct treatment.

The objective examination is divided into those tests performed in standing, sitting, and lying positions to minimize patient movement (Table 15–5). A methodical examination allows for development of the intuitive process, which Erik Berne describes as "knowledge based on experience." Berne believes that the beginning clinician must "resort to a method of data collection which is additive in nature in order to reach the advanced skills seen in the experienced clinician."[47] As the beginner gains experience through a systematic approach to making diagnoses, he or she gradually rises to a level where diagnostic processes begin to occur at an earlier stage of the examination and on a more subconscious level.

After completing the objective examination, the therapist should ideally have found the specific joint or struc-

□ □ □ □ □ □ □   □

Table 15–5. Movements Tested in Standing, Sitting, and Lying Positions

Movements tested in the standing position
  Observation of static posture
  Observation of gait
  Functional test—squatting
  Trunk flexion—single and repeated movements
  Trunk extension—single and repeated movements
  Lateral shift—left and right
  Sidebending—left and right
  Neurologic tests in standing—gastrocnemius power
  Combination of movement—i.e., extension, sidebending,
    and rotation

Movements tested in the sitting position
  Trunk rotation—left and right
  Spinal canal movements—slump tests

Movements tested in the supine position
  Passive neck flexion to assess spinal cord mobility
  Passive straight leg raising test to assess sacral plexus
    mobility
  Resisted isometric muscle tests for pain production
  Neurologic tests when indicated, tested in the supine
    position
  Sacroiliac joint tests
  Other tests—leg length, circumferential tests for muscle
    wasting

Movements tested in the prone position
  Prone knee flexion to assess lumbar plexus mobility
  Palpation for
    Temperature and sweating changes
    Soft tissue tenderness and thickening
    Position and alignment of the vertebrae
    Intervertebral accessory movements
  Passive accessory intervertebral movement test

Movements tested in the side-lying position
  Passive physiologic intervertebral movement tests
  Passive posteroanterior stability tests

tures causing the symptoms and should have clarified the type of movement disorder present. The type of disorder may be hypermobility or hypomobility and must be verified by performing a passive physiologic movement test in the side-lying position or a stability test.[48]

After using the data collection process outlined here, the therapist should

1. Understand the area of pain and be able to "live" the patient's symptoms over a period of 24 hours.
2. Know at least two activities that aggravate or ease the symptoms and that are measurable enough to allow assessment of small increments of change.
3. Have identified at least two objective measures that will cause an increase in the patient's symptoms and can be used to assess small increments of change. Where there is both spinal and dural movement ab-

normality, an objective measure of each component is required.

With this information, treatment becomes a logical process of action and reaction. As the patient is affected by a treatment technique, the above information is used to measure the change that occurs. The therapist who examines and treats in this manner can only improve as experience teaches him or her how to proceed in assisting the patient to restore maximal function to the musculoskeletal system. In the more acute stage of the condition, if the therapist finds both limitation and pain when examining the tension sign (straight leg raise), this sign may be used to assess the effect of the treatment technique, whereas the distance and frequency of walking can be used to assess progress over time. As the condition improves, other objective factors may be more appropriate to use in assessment, such as trunk mobility, repetitive bending, and lifting of weight.

Assessment

After gathering the data about physical signs and symptoms, the therapist should make a judgment as to whether the intellectual and emotibral responses of the patient are interfering with the patient's problem or are a main component of the problem. One simple way to characterize this judgment is through the use of the PIE notation, which expresses the relationship between the physical (P), intellectual (I), and emotional (E) factors.

If the condition is primarily physical, with intellectual and emotional characteristics not affecting accurate assessment of the physical findings, this is noted as "Pie," with the capital "P" indicating the primacy of the physical factors. However, if it is the practitioner's judgment that the intellectual and emotional factors have equal importance with the physical findings, this can be indicated by the notation "PIE."

In the "PIE" notation, the term *intellectual* applies to the patient's problem-solving or cognitive abilities, whereas *emotional* applies to the patient's feelings. Thus, if a patient is particularly disorganized and unable to follow a treatment routine, the patient's primary obstacle to progress is intellectual, and this is noted as "pIe." If a patient is well organized but prone to assume the worst, the negative emotions that accompany the injury can be an obstacle to effective treatment; this situation is noted as "E."

The following example illustrates the use of this notation: Assume that during the subjective examination of a patient's complaint, the patient describes the symptoms with general statements such as "I can't do anything" and "I feel terrible." At this point, it would be realistic to note that the intellectual and emotional components of the patient's response to the injury are likely to be important considerations in treating the problem. The clinician's notation of the physical, intellectual, and emotional relationship would be "pIE" to indicate that the intellectual and emotional factors may be interfering with accurate assessment of the physical problem. However, if during the objective examination the patient presents consistent objective data that clarify the physical complaint, the notation at the end of the objective examination would be "PIE," indicating that the physical, intellectual, and emotional characteristics all require consideration in treatment. On the second visit, if the patient responds to the question "How are you?" with "I'm feeling better" and to "How much better?" with "I slept better, only waking up once instead of three or four times," the assessment would be "Pie," indicating that the intellectual and emotional factors of this patient's condition are not interfering with the patient's understanding of the physical problem.

One indication of intellectual or emotional interference is an inability to express clearly what aggravates and what eases the problem. A patient who is unable to give a clear picture of what has happened from the onset of the disorder to the present tends to have intellectual and emotional factors that, although they may not be responsible for the problem, often interfere with adequate recovery and need to be addressed in treating that problem.

The physical, intellectual, and emotional factors form a circle of interrelationships (Fig. 15–3). For example, a physical stimulus (e.g., a slap in the face) elicits a physical response (red face and pain), an intellectual response (wondering why it was done and how to respond), and an emotional response (anger). Similarly, an emotional stimulus such as being ridiculed produces an emotional response (embarrassment), a physical response (blushing), and an intellectual response (why?). To harness the full power of the patient in the recovery process, one wants to have P, I, and E working in concert with one another. One way to assist patients in doing this is to share with them information that will help them grasp

the problem cognitively while gathering data during the examination process. As patients become involved intellectually in understanding their problems, they feel more in control, and emotional reactions are diffused.

Recent medical studies scientifically demonstrate what has long been common wisdom, namely, that positive emotions maximize the body's healing abilities.[11,49] These studies demonstrate a relationship between positive emotions and increased pituitary gland secretion. The pituitary hormones released in turn stimulate the adrenal cortex to release steroids, which have an anti-inflammatory effect. Positive thinking has also been shown to be related to hypothalamic release of endorphins.[50] Negative emotions, such as fear and anxiety, will not result in production of the same high levels of endorphins and steroids. Therefore, in assessing the intellectual and emotional components of the injury and teaching the patient to have greater access to the positive emotions, the therapist can actually have a constructive impact on the patient's biochemistry.[51]

"No-Name" Disorders and Dysfunctions

The problem with classifying the more common disorders of the lumbar spine is that the injuries are not always severe enough to clearly incriminate one structure rather than another. In a patient with low back injury, although it is clear that the mobile segment is not functioning properly and is responsible for symptoms, what is not as clear is what aspect or part of the mobile segment is the pain generator. Whether it is a simple problem with one structure or a link in a series of interrelated problems requires further clarification. Even in conditions that present with radiographic changes, such as spondylolisthesis, in which one might be led to blame the mechanical fault seen on the film for the symptoms, it is not always the spondylolisthesis that is responsible for the symptoms. It may be a segment above or below that segment, and the radiographic findings may, in fact, be of no value in indicating which level is responsible for the patient's complaint.

Therefore, in discussing the more common disorders that are not illuminated by radiographic findings, electromyographic findings, computed tomography (CT) scans, and other standard tests, the term *no-name disorders* will be used. In theory, the skilled diagnostician considers the initial diagnostic label a treatment diagnosis and one step in a total process. The final step in this process is a definitive differential diagnostic label. In practice, the treatment diagnosis often is the first and last label. Physical therapists are very familiar with diagnoses that do not clearly define what the pathology is, but rather speak in terms of symptoms (e.g., low back strain, low back sprain, lumbosacral strain, low back strain with sciatica, sacroilitis, muscle spasm, muscle strain, degenerative disk disease, spondylitis).

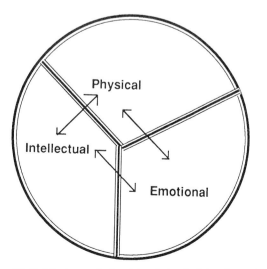

Figure 15–3. The interrelationship of physical, intellectual, and emotional factors in treatment.

The difficulty in using these diagnostic labels in treatment is that they never clearly indicate how to treat the problem because there is no basis for equating two patients with the same diagnostic label. They may, in fact, have the same label, but the severity and presentation of the problem can differ, and hence the signs and symptoms they present will differ. Similarly, even the same patient during different stages of the condition can present with a different picture of pain, spasm, and disability. Therefore, the signs and symptoms and the functional limitations produced by the disorder have more meaning in terms of understanding the problem and knowing how to treat it than does the label itself.

In short, diagnostic labels in mechanical injuries do more to interfere with effective treatment than to assist it. Hence, in the no-name disorder there is no textbook for patients to use to compare with how their no-name disorder behaved. The only textbooks are the patients themselves, and as each patient understands his or her own textbook—that is, his or her own signs and symptoms—and the aggravating and easing factors of the problem, the patient will have a more positive experience in recovering. As the severity of the disorder becomes apparent through CT scans, magnetic resonance imaging (MRI) scans, and the like, the clinician can be aided in treatment by this kind of knowledge. But those aids only provide assistance in directing treatment; they do not provide a rigid set of directives for a treatment plan.

It has been demonstrated that abnormal CT scans can be found in asymptomatic individuals.[52] Hence, it is imperative to relate these test results with other relevant data such as those provided by movement tests. The findings of passive movement tests indicating a symptomatic motion segment may assist in determining whether the abnormal CT findings are, in fact, associated with the patient's symptoms. Similarly, other objective tests such as thermograms may also assist in determining whether abnormal CT and MRI scans indicate disorder. Studies that have compared abnormal thermograms and abnormal movement tests before and after treatment have indicated that treatment resulted in normalized thermograms and normalized movements[53] (P. Goodley, personal communication). There is a real need for further clinical research to show the relationship among CT scans, MRI scans, movement tests, and thermograms.

A more accurate diagnostic label for all the conditions listed under the no-name disorder category is "somatic dysfunction of a specific mobile segment."[54] For example, picture a 33-year-old man who has never had symptoms of back pain other than minor stiffness from sitting too long or not getting enough exercise. He now develops acute low back pain after working in the garden over the weekend, lifting, bending, hoeing, and raking. The patient walks into the physician's office with a flattened lumbar spine, obvious muscle spasm, and pain in the low back that is greater on the right than on the left. After the initial examination, the physician might come up with one of five or more different diagnostic labels for the condition, depending on the physician's experience and expertise. Thus, diagnostic labels are not only relatively useless in forming a treatment plan, they are also highly subjective.

If on examining this hypothetical patient one were to find that the L5-S1 mobile segment had the most abnormal movement and was most responsible for the patient's pain, one could hypothesize that during the activity described the patient injured that mobile segment, resulting in abnormal movement of that segment. If radiographs, CT scans, MRI scans, and neurologic findings are all within normal limits, then the label "somatic dysfunction of the L5-S1 mobile segment secondary to a strain" makes total sense. Such a description has no negative connotations. One would expect the patient to heal quite well if it is a first injury and if the patient is an otherwise healthy individual who knows how to deal with the problem. Also, given the knowledge gained in the treatment process, the patient should be able to prevent a similar occurrence.

If the patient has habits that need to be changed to prevent a problem from developing or recurring, these habits will change only if the patient is self-motivated. These patients, who can be looked on as accidents waiting to happen, will not be motivated to make these changes in habits based on theory. They will be motivated by compelling emotional forces such as fear, and fear is what they experience when they begin to develop symptoms and signs of a disabling problem.

The signs and symptoms that are found in patients with somatic dysfunction of a specific mobile segment are illustrated in Tables 15–6 and 15–7. Table 15–6 lists those symptoms that indicate the need to be gentle in applying physical treatment. Table 15–7 lists the symptoms that would not limit treatment before its application. In the final analysis, these tables are only an aid in the therapist's learning process. The ultimate guide is the patient and the manner in which the signs and symptoms change as treatment is applied.

■ Treatment

Since Chapters 16 and 17 discuss surgical treatment and mobilization methods of the thoracolumbar spine area in detail, comments here will emphasize approaches to patient handling and home care, paying special attention to the role of walking in the healing process.

In treatment, the teaching of the patient is crucial. Many people, even very academically intelligent people, are what one might think of as "physical illiterates." These patients often ignore bodily symptoms and stoically go on about their business. Such patients must be taught to pay attention to the signals from the body to maximize recovery. However, hypochondriac patients will be so overwhelmed by symptoms as to not know how to cope.

□ □ □ □ □

Table 15–6. Symptoms and Signs Indicating the Need for Gentleness in Treatment

| | Subjective Symptoms | | | | Objective Signs | | |
Area	*Description*	*Behavior*	*History*	*Special Questions*	*Observation*	*During Testing of Active or Passive Movements*	*Neurologic Examination*
Distal symptoms more severe than proximal symptoms	Constant pain with difficulty finding relief	Irritable: small amount of movement produces severe increase of symptoms, requiring a long time to settle	Acute	Frequent medication	Patient appears to be in acute distress, with severe pain and very ill	Pain alters markedly with movement	Positive tension signs
Dermatomal distribution suggesting nerve root compression	Latent pain	All movements hurt severely	Severity of the incident and degree of disability are not comparable	Anti-inflammatories	Postural spasm or deformity protecting joint	Pain severe	Any evidence of conduction loss
	Paresthesia or anesthesia	All postures and positions painful; pain difficult to ease	Easily provoked	Steroids for a prolonged period		Pain occurs early in range	Muscle weakness
	Severe pain		Condition is getting worse	Potent analgesics required		Pain builds quickly	Sensory deficit
	Shooting or lancinating pain		Suggests a neurologic deficit (nerve root, cord, cauda equina)	Poor general health		Pain felt earlier than stiffness	Lost or diminished reflex
	Intractable pain			Recent weight loss or suggestion of systemic illness		Area: spinal movements provoke distal symptoms	

Pain at rest

Unable to bear weight or lie on affected side

Unable to sleep well

Unable to find comfortable position

Wakes with severe pain, forcing patient to move from bed

Wakes frequently, requires a long time to return to sleep

Coughing and sneezing provoke distal symptoms related to vertebral column

Positive response to questions about the cord, cauda equina, vertebral artery

Spread: buildup of pain or spread distally with sustained midrange position

Latent pain

Pain through range that builds to an "ache" and may require an extended period to settle

Spasm provoked with slow, gentle handling

Abrupt spasm limits further movement

Nature of limit is pain, empty end-feel and boggy

(Data from Grieve.[61])

□ □ □ □ □

Table 15-7. Symptoms and Signs That Allow Progressive Vigor in Physical Treatment

| | Subjective Symptoms | | | | | Objective Signs | |
Area	Description	Behavior	History	Special Questions	Observation	During Testing of Active or Passive Movements	Neurologic Examination
Proximal symptoms more severe than distal symptoms Nondermatomal distribution suggesting somatic referral pain	Not severe Intermittent Occasional Momentary symptoms	Not irritable Pain not severe Moderate pain, when provoked, settles immediately One or two provoking movements Eased with rest Symptoms present only with prolonged activity or sustained position at limit of range Sleep not disturbed, or wakes but pain is eased with change of position; patient returns to sleep immediately	Subacute Chronic bouts require initial prolonged, vigorous activity Condition static or improving	Infrequent use of mild analgesics as needed	No acute distress Patient looks well Patient moves easily Minimal functional loss	Minimal change in pain on movement Pain not severe Pain only at limit of range Pain builds or spreads only with sustained positions at the limit "Ache" during testing which settles immediately on cessation of movement or subsides quickly Soft tissue approximation on stretch with elastic, capsular end-feel	No evidence of neurologic deficit; or, where deficit is present, is most likely related to previous episodes

(Data from Grieve.[61])

316

In either case, the treatment process becomes more effective as the patient understands which specific mobile segment is injured and how that segment needs to be protected yet still used to promote healing. Also, we no longer live in a society in which people will blindly follow the suggestions of an authority.[55] Many people will become engaged in their own treatment only if they have a thorough understanding of why they should follow a certain regimen and only if this knowledge fits with their personal knowledge and beliefs.

Another important aspect of treatment is the role the therapist plays in increasing the patient's commitment to the healing process. A person with a basically healthy mobile segment that is traumatized has a much better chance of recovery than someone with an initially unwell mobile segment. Frequently, however, one is not only treating the injury, but also attempting to catalyze a change in the patient's lifestyle, which is often a lifestyle that led to the injury in the first place. The essential problem in treating such a patient is determining what changes in lifestyle need to occur. This process involves problem solving by both the patient and the therapist, although the ultimate responsibility for change rests with the patient. Still, by acting as an educator and a coach, the therapist can encourage the patient to make the necessary lifestyle changes.

Therefore, the beginning of treatment is the time to discuss the need for prevention with the patient. Although the patient has not been able to prevent the first occurrence, preventing recurrence and progressive deterioration of a system is a realistic goal. It is important, then, to recognize the first signs of deterioration of a system and to understand the pattern of behavior that led up to it. At that point, the therapist can assist the patient in making changes that will aim at reestablishing a healthy system and maintaining that system throughout life. It is important not to impose advice on the patient because this advice comes from the therapist's reality, not the patient's. If you ask the patient, "How can you change?" and leave the patient to come up with the correct answer, you will get a better result. For example, if a patient says he or she cannot remember to exercise and uses this as an excuse for not following a home exercise program, one solution would be to advise the patient to use a timer on the kitchen stove as a reminder to exercise. If the therapist instead asks questions so that the patient can arrive at the correct answer independently, the patient's mind is involved in the process of problem solving, and the solution is the patient's and will be better adhered to and remembered.

Communication Style

The communication style of the therapist is an essential element in promoting the patient's healing process. To get along with and make changes in the patient, the therapist must understand the patient's point of view as it relates to the problem. Then, from the patient's reality, the therapist is better able to assist the patient in the direction of health. A classic story involving Milton Erickson, the founder of modern hypnotherapy, illustrates this. Erickson went to work at a certain mental hospital, and within his first few weeks there, he came across a patient who introduced himself as Jesus Christ. Erickson's response was, "Oh, you are a carpenter." He then told the man that he needed help with some carpentry and asked if he would help build some bookshelves in his new office. Erickson got the equipment, the man built some shelves, and from then on Erickson used carpentry as his way of treating that person. Eventually, the man left the hospital, went out into the community, and became a carpenter. He still believed he was Jesus Christ, so that aspect of his belief system was not changed, but he had become a functional member of the community as a carpenter.[56]

If one looked at only the negative aspects of this story, one would focus on the patient's delusion. This is not wrong, any more than looking at a half-full bottle of milk and saying that it is half empty is wrong. The facts can be viewed from many perspectives. In Erickson's example, if one is concerned with improving function rather than breaking the patient's delusional mode, one can do so by focusing the patient's thinking on a realistic function, in this case carpentry, that is consistent with his or her delusion. When we as therapists are confronted by patients who state that they are in pain and have certain functional limits, we should accept what they say as truth. There may be symptom magnification, but practitioners should not allow that possibility to interfere with getting a real feeling of what the patient is experiencing. If we as therapists take what a patient says as the truth, because whatever we are told at that moment is true to the patient, we can communicate that we believe the patient. Then the patient is more likely to regard us as allies in the healing process. We can then go on to use what we know about pain generators, pain behavior, and natural healing to move the patient in the direction of recovery.

Walking as Treatment

One of the most effective methods for treating injuries to the lumbar area is walking. Part of the therapist's job is to convince the patient that walking is the right thing to do. By showing the patient, through the use of visualization techniques, the segment that has been injured and what effect walking will have on it, the patient will get a graphic sense of the nature of the problem and the value of the treatment. This approach not only enlists patients in "becoming their own therapists" but also gives them a tool for visualization while walking. Briefly, have the patient place his or her hands on his or her own back and feel the contraction and relaxation of the muscles during walking so that the patient can visualize the pumping action of the muscles assisting in "lubricating" the injured area. This has the effect of enlisting the patient's positive energy in the healing process and creates a psychological advantage by helping the patient feel less powerless while relieving negative emotions such as fear and anxiety.

In our sedentary culture, there is a high incidence of degenerative changes in the low lumbar segments in persons aged 50 years and older compared with people of age 20 years, even when they have not sustained an obvious injury to this area. In primitive cultures, in which people are physically active, the incidence of degeneration in the mobile segment from aging is less pronounced. In one study, 450 radiographs were taken of a group of 15- to 44-year-old members of the Bihl tribe in India and compared with radiographs of individuals from similar age groups in Sweden and the United States. The results indicated disk narrowing in 80 percent of a Swedish group of heavy laborers by age 55 years, 35 percent narrowing in a group of light workers in San Francisco, and only 9 percent narrowing in the Bihl tribe members at age 55 years. The incidence of disk narrowing was about 5 percent in all three series equally in the youngest age group studied.[57]

From this study, one could conclude that the incidence of disk degeneration is not coincident with age but has some correlation with such factors as activity, diet, and heredity. Therefore, one hypothesis would be that disk degeneration is not natural to the human body between the ages of 20 and 50 years but rather is a response to the stress placed on it. One might also hypothesize that maximizing nutrition of the mobile segment through positive activity would limit some of the aging changes that lead to low back disorders.

The job of the practitioner then becomes one of improving the nutrition of the mobile segment. This can be done through walking. In attempting to motivate patients to make behavioral changes, it can be helpful to use the following reasoning: State that walking is an effective treatment for lumbar injuries because it stimulates movement of cells, nutrients, and waste products directly from the blood supply of the vertebrae into the disk via imbibition and pumping action. Continue by telling patients that when they are sedentary, nutrition to the disk and other structures is impeded, but that if they walk for 15 to 20 minutes regularly over a period of several months, circulation will be stimulated, facilitating recovery.

Besides providing nutrition through the blood supply, synovial fluids function both as a lubricant and as a medium for nutrition of the cartilage of the zygapophyseal joints. Studies have demonstrated a rapid degeneration of the joint cartilage after immobility.[58] It has been hypothesized that this degenerative change is partly due to a decrease in nourishment of the cartilage secondary to a decrease in synovial fluid movement.[38] Therefore, when muscle spasm and decreasing activity immobilize the joints of a mobile segment for more than 48 hours, the cartilage can be expected to begin to undergo degenerative changes. The synovial fluids then begin to demonstrate chemical and physiologic changes, starting a process

that is difficult and time-consuming to reverse. Walking produces repetitive movement of the joints, which mechanically increases the fluid lubrication and stimulates the secretion of normal synovial fluid by the synovial lining of the joint, aiding in regeneration and restoration of normal cartilage.[40,41]

In normal gait, the arms swing in alternation with the legs, imparting a cyclical motion to the spine. Spinal motions occurring in walking are flexion, lateral bending, and rotation, followed by extension, lateral bending, and rotation in the opposite direction. There are also small-magnitude strain deflection movements when the joints are subjected to the stress of weightbearing.[59] This strain deflection may stimulate the body to make the bone even stronger, because bone is living tissue and can adapt to stress, and careful training can increase its strength. Muscle contractions increase blood flow, and tiny electric voltages that stimulate growth are generated within the bone. However, a mild stress repeated thousands of times can cause the bone to develop minute fractures that can grow into full-scale fractures. These so-called stress fractures result from an attempt by the body to make the bone even stronger, but before new bone can be set in place, old bone must be removed by special demolition cells. Therefore, there is a moment in time when the bone is weaker than before and vulnerable to fracture. Hence, an important treatment principle—subjective though it may be—is derived from this theory. A brief period of rest will give the bone a chance to fill in, and then training can be resumed.[60] This conceptual framework is necessary in approaching a progressive walking program for back injuries.

The impact of walking is much broader than merely its effect on the mobile segment and muscles and nerves of the spinal column. It also does the following:

1. Stimulates circulation of the blood, the cerebrospinal fluid, and the lymphatics.
2. Benefits cardiovascular and cardiopulmonary fitness and stimulates the endocrine system.
3. Reduces the vicosity of the nucleus of the disk, allowing for a better fluid exchange within the nucleus itself.
4. Assists mechanically in the exchange of fluid between the vertebrae and the nucleus by increasing and decreasing the pressure on portions of the disk. In other words, walking on the left leg increases pressure on the left side of the disk and decreases pressure on the right side. When one then puts weight on the right leg, that pressure gradient is changed so that it is greater on the right side and less on the left. This reciprocal motion creates a pump-like action that increases pressure on one side of the disk and moves fluid into the vertebral body. Conversely, when the area is under decreased pressure, a sucking effect pulls fluid from the vertebra back into that area.

5. Stimulates the mechanoreceptors, facilitating the normal neurophysiologic status of the whole mobile segment.[30]

6. Improves coordination and strength of the muscles necessary to control the movement of the mobile segment. This is accomplished through the reciprocal contraction and relaxation of the muscles engaged in walking.

7. Impacts positively on the patient psychologically, maximizing the placebo effect.[49] It has been clinically observed that patients who have lost the ability to function after injury of the musculoskeletal system will heal more rapidly when their treatment plan consists of a repetitious activity with which they are already familiar. In contrast, if you ask the patient to learn a new motor skill such as the pelvic tilt, the patient not only must deal with the difficulties resulting from the injury but also must struggle with the stress involved in learning a new motor skill.

8. Moves the patient from the role of passive victim to one of active healer—a crucially important psychological shift in the promotion of wellness.

The amount of walking that is indicated depends on the stage of the pathology. One must first establish a base of activity that does not aggravate the underlying symptoms. For example, if what aggravates a patient's symptoms is sitting or standing for more than half an hour, lifting more than 10 lb from waist to shoulder level, lifting from the floor to the waist and from the shoulders to above the head, and walking for more than 10 minutes, then this level of activity becomes the base. From this base, the patient slowly increases the amount of walking until an optimum level is reached, which should be maintained until the patient is well.

A moderate walking program is most effective in enhancing recovery. If the base level of the patient's walking activity is 10 minutes, the walking program then must be to walk four times a day for a 10-minute period, provided that this does not increase the pain. Activity should be increased on alternate days, and as a general rule, the patient should not increase the activity by more than 10 percent of the previous level. Slow increases in activity are preferable to sudden quick increases, and the body must be given less stress on alternate days. The stress of the activity on one day will cause the body to make adjustments that will weaken it the next day, but the body will then recover and be stronger because of this stress. Clinical experience suggests that it may be helpful to increase the walking to a total of 5 to 8 miles a day to achieve maximum benefit.

As the clinician assists the patient from the most acute stage of the injury through progressive improvement, the need for walking is critical at all levels except when strict bed rest is called for. At the acute stages, the patient may walk for only 2 minutes at a time, but the patient should walk as often as several times an hour. As the patient's condition improves, walking should increase to 5 minutes every hour, then 10 minutes every 2 hours, up to 15 minutes four times a day. The goal in walking is to have the patient do a brisk half-hour to 40-minute walk four times a day without discomfort. This amounts to anywhere from 6 to 8 miles a day. Once patients can walk that amount without aggravating symptoms, they need to stay at that level for anywhere from several weeks to a lifetime in order to maintain a healthy condition.

As the patient is recovering, the therapist can often relate the decrease in pain to the degree of healing that occurs. However, just because pain has been reduced to zero does not mean that there is 100 percent recovery. As the disk and other structures in the mobile segment heal, there is a point at which the patient will become asymptomatic. The therapist knows from clinical experience that this patient can be reinjured with excessive activity, even at this essentially asymptomatic stage.

By stressing the joint during the examination, the therapist can determine its integrity. The structure can be considered recovered only when the segment is asymptomatic to all examination movements including end-range overpressure and combined movements. Further assessment of repetitive functional activity may be necessary to determine the endurance of the segment.

When teaching patients to become their own therapists, therapists must give them an understanding of the healing process so that they can prevent recurrence of injury. Patients may need to be taught to think in a commonsense manner about injury and repair. These are not areas in which people are commonly instructed, and people frequently fear injury and do not understand the physiologic process of repair. To clarify the injury process and the normal repair process is to remove fear and give the patient more conscious control over what is going on. In a case of obvious injury to a mobile segment, even after reaching an asymptomatic level, the patient must continue to maximize disk nutrition. This process should continue for as long as is necessary for all the supportive structures in that segment to gain sufficient endurance to minimize the chance of reinjury.

CASE STUDY

The following case study illustrates many of the concepts presented in this chapter.

History

The patient, a 46-year-old man, 5 ft 10 in. tall and weighing 190 lb, sustained a low back injury at age 19 years when as a lifeguard he was carrying an accident victim from the water. He developed severe right sciatica with bladder paralysis and weakness of his right lower extremity. He was hospitalized for 3 weeks with total bladder paralysis but recovered approximately 30 percent of function by use of massage, hot and cold compresses, and whirlpool. He was able to improve his condition an additional 25 percent by adhering for 5 months to a program that included swimming 5 hours a day and walking. For 20 years after that severe episode, he had minor incidents of low backache and occasional feelings of weakness in the right leg. Otherwise, he led an active life, which included expert skiing and playing racketball regularly.

Four years ago, while moving some heavy furniture from a warehouse to his office, the patient developed a severe recurrence of his right sciatica. His right foot began to drag, and he noted that the bladder weakness had returned. The symptoms gradually improved during the following year so that he could lie down and walk comfortably. But he had more problems walking uphill than on level ground, and prolonged sitting of more than 8 hours, such as was required on long plane flights, resulted in increasing pain.

At the time of the recurrence, the patient had a CT scan, which identified a calcified disk at the L5-S1 level, with possible foraminal stenosis on the right at the L4-L5 level. His neurologic examination revealed a decreased reflex in the right calf, with 90 degrees of straight leg raise on the left and 80 degrees on the right. His standing posture was symmetric, with a slightly flattened lordosis. He had a limitation of full extension with a slight increase in low back pain. His flexion was 50 percent, and a left deviation accompanied the flexion. Lateral flexion left and right was within normal limits. Muscular strength tested as normal.

Treatment

At that time, physical therapy treatment was initiated. It included end-range mobilization in rotation bilaterally and inversion gravity traction in flexion. This treatment resulted in a rapid resolution of the patient's sciatica, and within 1 month he had returned to his pre-exacerbation level of activity. He had remained well until he sustained a further injury after lifting 150 lb from waist level to overhead. He resorted to his home treatment program, which involved swimming for a half hour each morning and walking 2 miles a day, combined with inversion traction and repeated flexion in the lying position. He felt 40 percent relief following this program. However, for the next 4 months, despite cutting back on his activity level and avoiding lifting and sitting, he was unable to achieve a feeling of stability in his spine.

Physical therapy involving gentle oscillatory transverse movements at the L4-L5 mobile segment was then initiated. After these treatments the patient felt significant relief of his pain, but he was unable to get sufficient relief to be able to resume his strengthening exercises without suffering exacerbation. He sought further medical advice and had another CT scan. The surgeon's opinion was that he had an unstable L5-S1 segment and a disk bulge

at L4-L5. He recommended microsurgery at that disk and fusion of the L5-S1 motion segment. The patient was scheduled to have a myelogram to add further to this diagnostic and treatment decision, but before the scheduled myelogram, autotraction treatment was initiated. The autotraction treatment resulted in further improvement, and within six treatments he felt 70 percent recovered and was feeling better than he had since the exacerbation 9 months before.

This patient's current functional level is such that he is walking 5 to 7 miles a day without pain. He stands and works 11 to 12 hours a day with minimal discomfort, avoids sitting except when driving, and stands for a maximum of 30 minutes at a time. Treatment progression will consist of adding spine-strengthening exercises to the autotraction program to teach protective body mechanics, allowing the patient to maintain an optimum neutral spinal posture for his condition at the same time as he performs stretching exercises of his lower extremity musculature.

Discussion

Even before considering treatment, the therapist must understand the patient as a human being. In this case study, the therapist sensed that the patient was a stoic and someone who had to be in control of his life. He was also someone who had to learn to limit himself in order not to exacerbate his condition.

To put this awareness to work, the therapist had to verify with the patient that he was, in fact, this type of person. This was accomplished by asking him if he considered himself a stoic who needed to be in control of his treatment to get better. When the patient agreed, the therapist added that he needed to learn to live within certain limits. The patient agreed here also. The important aspect of this question-and-affirmation process is that it enlists the patient's participation. It would be of little value for the therapist's assessment to be "right" if the patient did not agree. Because the patient has to make the changes, it is the patient's reality that matters, not the practitioner's.

It was then necessary for the therapist to understand what the patient was willing to live with. The patient wanted to be able to ski on the expert slopes, to play racketball, to lift weights, and to be relatively comfortable doing all this. Therefore, in educating this patient, it was necessary for the therapist to emphasize to him that his injury was real, not emotional, and not something that would go away if he ignored it. At the same time, the therapist stated that the injury could be healed if the patient did the right things in selectively stressing his low back to stimulate body repair to stabilize that injured mobile segment.

The next point the therapist emphasized was that as the patient increased his activity level and felt better, he could not ignore the fact that he still had a back problem.

He therefore had to increase his activity level by no more than 10 percent at a time. If even that 10 percent was, in fact, too much, he would find that out by an increase in his symptoms, and he would then need to reduce his activity level. Through this trial-and-assessment process, the patient was able to monitor his level of discomfort and achieve the necessary stress to activate recovery without causing further injury to the mobile segment.

In this case, the surgeon's recommendation for surgery was based on objective signs such as CT scans and MRI findings, which are not fully meaningful unless correlated clearly with the signs and symptoms. It can be a mistake to interpret those findings as completely explaining the patient's problem. Findings on CT and MRI scans explained the symptoms of spinal instability and the pain the patient experienced, but they did not indicate that the only means of resolution of this problem was surgery.

The patient's case history indicated that the injury to the L5-S1 segment 25 years earlier was a major injury. Yet the body was able to stabilize that injury through calcification of the disk. Thereafter the patient was able to lead a normal life, at least as normal as one could have expected had he had surgical intervention. In short, the physician from within (the body's natural healing process) did as good a job as one could have expected of any physician from without.

The patient's injury 9 months earlier might have stabilized in the same way as the prior injury did, or it might have reached a stage at which surgical stabilization was necessary. To make this decision entirely on the basis of the CT and MRI scans, myelography, and other standard tests would be to risk unnecessary surgery. Instead, all conservative approaches should be attempted first, including maximizing the positive psychological benefit of involving the patient in his own care and modifying any behavior that is detrimental to the resolution of the problem. Only if these approaches fail should one proceed with surgery.

The clinician must also be methodical in making decisions about what treatment to use. Three years earlier, mobilization at end-range had resulted in rapid resolution of signs and symptoms and a return to optimum functioning, making that treatment the correct one at that time. More recently, the same approach to treatment did not result in the same rapid improvement. This necessitated a change in approach, even though the aims were the same. Had the autotraction not been effective, another approach would have been used until all conservative approaches were exhausted. At that point, surgical intervention to stabilize that mobile segment would have been the logical next step.

Throughout this patient's history, he consistently responded positively to movement, so long as it was performed repetitively and over an extended period of time in a way that did not increase the symptoms. For example, when he was initially injured, he spent 5 months swimming in addition to his other activities. This could well have contributed to his initial recovery. The one thing the patient was able to do 3 years ago that would consistently relieve his symptoms was walk. The more he walked, the better he felt, provided that he did not go beyond his limits. As he got stronger and stronger, his limits became greater, until he was able to walk 5 to 6 miles a day.

The patient found that by getting up first thing in the morning and going for a 2- to 3-mile walk, he was far more comfortable during the day than if he got up and rushed off to work without walking. If he tried to do spinal stabilization exercises, play racketball, or ski before walking 5 to 6 miles a day, he exacerbated his symptoms. Even when he could walk 5 to 6 miles a day, he needed to do that over an extended period of time before he became stable enough to be able to progress to the next stage of activity.

One approach to the treatment of the problem would be to categorize the patient as having a calcified disk, a disk bulge at L4-L5 with bladder paresis that indicates cauda equina involvement, a decreased gastrocnemius reflex, and weakness of the gastrocnemius muscle. Based on that list of signs, the treatment could be surgery or pelvic traction and a corset.

Another approach is to make the same statements about the facts but to recognize that there are many different resolutions, many different ways to accomplish return to function. Also, the "history, signs, symptoms, and patient-focused" treatment approach recognizes the need to harness the power of patients to maximize their own progress and to let the signs and symptoms of the injury guide the treatment process.

This case study illustrates the following main principles:

1. The importance of the patient's taking an active role in treatment
2. The need for the therapist to see the injury from the perspective of the patient
3. The need to activate the body's built-in healing methods through activities such as walking
4. The importance of the home treatment program being one of gradual and monitored increases in activity
5. The need for the patient to recognize and work within a necessary set of realistic limits
6. The need for the therapist to guide the treatment by the signs and symptoms and by focusing on the patient rather than on a diagnostic label
7. The need to teach the patient to become his or her own therapist
8. The need to allow time for the body's natural healing process, the physician from within, to work.

■ Conclusion

In physical therapy, patients often ask, "What's wrong with me?" Trying to explain what is wrong in terms of a diagnostic label often leads to more problems than it solves. The essence of the medical model in Western medicine today is to examine several people with similar conditions and to study those conditions to try to come up with a general view of the etiology, pathology, and prognosis.

The diagnostic label is usually unclear to patients and gives them either a confused picture of the problem or one in which their knowledge of the negative aspects of the diagnosis dominates their awareness. We must give patients confidence so that they can assume an active role in freeing themselves from pain as they learn to be their own doctors.

It is a natural human response to look at the worst-case scenario to be prepared for the worst. The problem with this manner of thinking is that it can lead the patient to look only at the medical prognosis. But prognoses are based on statistical analyses of group means, not specific individual patients. Therefore, patients who focus on the diagnostic label will be looking at a broad range of prognostic data that may or may not relate to them directly. This can lead the patient to self-program a negative outcome that may not be applicable. Patients create their own reality through their sets of expectations and beliefs. If a patient sees a negative outcome as reality, then that is often the reality the patient will experience.

Positive thinking maximizes the body's healing processes, whereas negative thinking is counterproductive.[11,49–51] Therefore, to focus a patient's thinking and understanding of the problem on specific factors that relate to his or her problem rather than on the universe of people with that problem is to focus the patient in a constructive direction.

By clarifying the signs and symptoms that patients have in a manner that is understandable, the therapist can assist patients in personalizing the problem as it relates to their own condition. Through this increased understanding, patients will be better able to understand the problem and be in control of the condition rather than the victim of it.

There also is no clear relationship between the diagnostic label and the treatment. The therapist must attempt to clarify the diagnostic label for the patient by explaining it not as a pathology in the sense of a sickness or a disease, which is the common perception of pathology, but rather as a strain or sprain of a specific structure in the musculoskeletal system. When the diagnostic label does not specifically incriminate a structure, the injury should be explained as occurring within a specific mobile segment. A further description of the movement's characteristics can clarify the biomechanical nature of the disorder. One can describe that dysfunctioning mobile segment in terms of pain and pain patterns or in terms of aggravation and easing of the pain with activity or rest.

A functional profile of the disorder is far more meaningful to the patient than any diagnostic label. It is also more meaningful to those who have to deal with the problem, such as insurance carriers and employers. People will better understand a problem if they can experience that problem in their own minds rather than try to understand a set of medical labels that have little relationship to their personal experience.

As clinicians, it is also important for us to remember that we cannot hasten the natural healing process. When we involve ourselves in treating the patient who has a problem that is solvable by the patient's inner physician, we need to be very careful that we do not get in the way and interfere with the body's natural healing. Effective treatment consists of minimizing those factors that interfere with the natural healing process and simultaneously encourage that process through our art and science.

■ References

1. Warwick R, Williams P (ed): Gray's Anatomy. 35th Br. Ed. WB Saunders, Philadelphia, 1973
2. McMinn RMH, Hutchins RT: Color Atlas of Human Anatomy. Year Book Medical Publishers, Chicago, 1977
3. Netter F: The CIBA Collection of Medical Illustrations, Vol. 1. Part 1. CIBA, West Caldwell, NJ, 1983
4. Bogduk N, Twomey L: Clinical Anatomy of the Lumbar Spine. Churchill Livingstone, Edinburgh, 1987
5. McNab I: Backache. Williams & Wilkins, Baltimore, 1977
6. Dixon ASJ: Diagnosis of low back pain—sorting the complainers. p. 77. In Jayson M (ed): The Lumbar Spine and Back Pain. Sector Publishing, London, 1976
7. Dvorak J, Dvorak V: Manual Medicine: Diagnostics. Thieme-Stratton, New York, 1984
8. Corrigan B, Maitland BD: Practical Orthopaedic Medicine. Butterworth-Heinemann, London, 1983
9. Yong-Hing K, Kirkaldy-Willis WH: The pathophysiology of degenerative disease of the lumbar spine. Orthop Clin North Am 14:491, 1983
10. Cyriax J: Textbook of orthopaedic medicine. 6th Ed. Vol. 1. Bailliere Tindall, London, 1975
11. Simonton O, Creighton J: Getting Well Again. Bantam, New York, 1980
12. Arey BL, Burrows W, Greenhill JP, et al (eds): Dorland's Illustrated Medical Dictionary. 23rd Ed. WB Saunders, Philadelphia, 1959
13. Feinstein A: Clinical Judgement. Robert E. Krieger, Malabar, FL, 1967
14. Korr IM: The facilitated segment: a factor in injury to the body framework. p. 27. In Stark EH (ed): Clinical Review Series: Osteopathic Medicine. Publishing Sciences Group, Acton, MA, 1975
15. Jull G, Janda V: Muscle and motor control in low back pain: assessment and management. p. 257. In Twomey L, Taylor J (eds): Physical Therapy of the Low Back. Churchill Livingstone, New York, 1987
16. Frank C, Akeson WH, Woo SL-Y, et al: Physiology and therapeutic value of passive joint motion. Clin Orthop 185:113, 1984
17. Macintosh J, Bogduk N: The anatomy and function of the lumbar back muscles and their fascia. p. 103. In Twomey L, Taylor J (eds): Physical Therapy of the Low Back. Churchill Livingstone, New York, 1987

18. McCall IW, Park WM, O'Brien JP: Induced pain referral from posterior lumbar elements in normal subjects. Spine 4:441, 1979

19. Mooney V, Robertson J: The facet syndrome. Clin Orthop 115:149, 1976

20. Wiberg G: Back pain in relation to the nerve supply of the intervertebral disc. Acta Orthop Scand 19:211, 1947

21. Hirsch C: An attempt to diagnose the level of a disc lesion clinically by disc puncture. Acta Orthop Scand 18:1132, 1949

22. Lindblom K: Technique and results in myelography and disc puncture. Acta Radiol 34:321, 1950

23. Perey O: Contrast medium examination of the intervertebral discs of the lower lumbar spine. Acta Orthop Scand 20:327, 1951

24. Collis JS, Gardner WJ: Lumbar discography—an analysis of 1,000 cases. J Neurosurg 19:452, 1962

25. Simmons EH, Segil CM: An evaluation of discography in the localization of symptomatic levels in discogenic disease of the spine. Clin Orthop 108:57, 1975

26. Wiley JJ, MacNab I, Wortzman G: Lumbar discography and its clinical applications. Can J Surg 11:280, 1968

27. Smyth MJ, Wright V: Sciatica and the intervertebral disc. An experimental study. J Bone Joint Surg 40(A):1401, 1959

28. El Mahdi MA, Latif FYA, Janko M: The spinal nerve root innervation, and a new concept of the clinicopathological interrelations in back pain and sciatica. Neurochirurgia 24:137, 1981

29. Boas RA: Post-surgical low back pain. p. 188. In Peck C, Wallace M (eds): Problems in Pain. Pergamon, Sydney, 1980

30. Wyke B: Neurological aspects of low back pain. p. 189. In Jayson M (ed): The Lumbar Spine and Back Pain. Sector Publishing, London, 1976.

31. Grieve GP: Common Vertebral Joint Problems. Churchill Livingstone, Edinburgh, 1981

32. Dommisse GF: The blood supply of the spinal cord. p. 37. In Grieve GP (ed): Modern Manual Therapy of the Vertebral Column. Churchill Livingstone, Edinburgh, 1986

33. Aki T, Toya S: Experimental study on the circulatory dynamics of the spinal cord by serial fluorescence and geography. Spine 9:262, 1984

34. Crock H, Goldwasser M: Anatomic studies of the circulation in the region of the vertebral end-plate in adult greyhound dogs. Spine 9:702, 1984

35. Butler D: Axoplasmic flow and manipulative physical therapy. Manipulative Therapist Association of Australia Proceedings, Adelaide, South Australia 1991

36. Butler D: Mobilization of the Nervous System. Churchill Livingstone, Melbourne, 1991

37. Hansen HJ: Comparative views of the pathology of disc degeneration in animals. Lab Invest 8:1242, 1959

38. Kahanovitz N: The effects of internal fixation on the articular cartilage of unfused canine facet joint cartilage. Spine 9:268, 1984

39. Wyke B: Neurological aspects of low back pain. In Jayson M (ed): The Lumbar Spine and Back Pain. Sector Publishing, London, 1976

40. Hunter L, Braunstein E, Bailey RW: Radiographic changes following anterior cervical fusion. Spine 5:399, 1980

41. Tredwell SJ, O'Brien JP: Apophyseal joint degeneration in the cervical spine following halo pelvic distraction. Spine 6:497, 1980

42. Evans P: The healing process at cellular level: a review. Physiotherapy 66:256, 1980

43. Maitland GD: Vertebral Manipulation. 5th Ed. Butterworth-Heinemann, London, 1986

44. Maitland GD: Examination and Recording Guide. 4th Ed. Lauderdale Press, Glen Osmond, South Australia, 1986

45. Margarey ME: Examination and assessment in spinal joint dysfunction. p. 481. In Grieve GP (ed): Modern Manual Therapy of the Vertebral Column. Churchill Livingstone, Edinburgh, 1986

46. Maitland GD: The Maitland concept: assessment, examination, and treatment by passive movements. p. 135. In Twomey LT, Taylor JR (eds): Physical Therapy of the Low Back. Churchill Livingstone, New York, 1987

47. Berne E: Intuition and Ego States. Harper & Row, San Francisco, 1977

48. Grieve GP: Lumbar Instability. p. 416. In Grieve GP (ed): Modern Manual Therapy of the Vertebral Column. Churchill Livingstone, Edinburgh, 1986

49. Borysenko J: Minding the Body, Mending the Mind. Addison-Wesley, Menlo Park, CA, 1987

50. Benson H, Proctor W: Beyond the Relaxation Response. Berkley, New York, 1985

51. Pelletier K: Mind as Healer, Mind as Slayer. Dell Books, New York, 1977

52. Wiesel S, Tsourmas N, Feffer H, et al: A study of computer-assisted tomography: the incidence of positive CAT scans in an asymptomatic group of patients. Spine 9:6, 1984

53. Gillstrom P: A Clinical and Objective Analysis of Autotraction as a Form for Therapy in Lumbago and Sciatica. Unpublished thesis, University of Stockholm, Sweden, 1985

54. Rumney I: The relevance of somatic dysfunction. Am Orthop Assoc 74:723, 1975

55. Schön DA: The Reflective Practitioner. Basic Books, New York, 1983

56. Haley J: Uncommon Therapy: The Psychiatric Technique of Milton Erickson. WW Norton, New York, 1973

57. Fahrni WH: Back Ache: Assessment and Treatment. Evergreen Press, Vancouver, 1978

58. Holm S, Nachemson A: Nutritional changes in the canine intervertebral disc after spinal fusion. Clin Orthop 169: 243, 1982

59. Farfan H: Mechanical Disorders of the Low Back. Lea & Febiger, Philadelphia, 1973

60. Padmore T: Limp in, jog out: sports medicine up and running. Chronicle, p. 22. University of British Columbia, Vancouver, Spring 1982

61. Grieve GP: Mobilization of the Spine. 4th Ed. Churchill Livingstone, Edinburgh, 1984

■ Suggested Readings

Boissannault W: Examination in Physical Therapy Practice. Churchill Livingstone, New York, 1991

CHAPTER 16

New Advances in Lumbar Spine Surgery

Lee A. Kelley

Lumbar spinal surgery is much more commonly performed in the United States than it is in other countries. The most common lumbar spinal surgery in America is surgical treatment of lumbar disk herniation, and it is performed far more frequently than it is in most European countries. In most afflictions of the lumbar spine, surgical treatment should be seen as the final phase of treatment when all other forms of treatment have not been effective in relieving pain or restoring normal neurologic or physiologic function. There is, however, a common misconception that there is an ultimate surgical treatment for every painful condition of the lumbar spine. The unfortunate truth is that many chronically painful conditions of the lumbar spine are not amenable to surgical treatment. The failure rate of many lumbar surgeries can be attributed to poor patient selection and to attempts to fashion a surgical treatment for a condition that will not respond to surgery.

If one were to reduce the treatment of lumbar disk disease to a very simple mantra, it would be that surgical treatment for leg pain related to lumbar disk disease is successful in most instances and surgical treatment for lower back pain related to lumbar disk disease is unsuccessful in most instances. It should be noted, of course, that there are conditions related to the lumbar disk that can cause lower back pain which can be successfully treated surgically and some causes of leg pain that do not respond to surgical treatment. However, the concept that radicular pain or leg pain related to lumbar nerve root compression is the problem with the highest success rate after surgical treatment remains part of current surgical thinking.

As this chapter will demonstrate, there are several conditions other than disk problems which lend themselves to surgical treatment of the lumbar spine. This chapter will review the general indications for surgical treatment and will discuss the standard techniques that

have been established for surgical treatment of these lumbar conditions. New techniques which have been recently developed will be discussed. Some of these new techniques are still in the experimental stages. It will remain to be seen if they turn out to be better than the standard techniques now in use.

■ General Indications for Surgical Treatment of the Lumbar Spine

Lumbar Disk Herniation

Lumbar disk herniation remains the lumbar problem most commonly treated by surgery in the United States. Lumbar disk herniation results from preceding degenerative changes within the lumbar disk. These degenerative changes cause the posterior annular fibers of the lumbar disk to become incompetent and subsequently allow nuclear material from within the disk to extend into the area of the spinal canal, causing nerve compression. Lumbar disk herniations may occur in relation to traumatic injury, but they do not necessarily require traumatic injury to occur. Lumbar disk herniations may occur with various degrees of severity. Smaller herniations are often referred to as "bulges of the disk." These frequently do not cause nerve compression, but they may be a source of back pain. Larger disk herniations frequently cause compression of spinal nerves or the cauda equina in the lumbar spinal canal and may be the source of significant leg pain. The term *extruded fragment* refers to lumbar disk nuclear material which herniates beyond the limits of the annulus fibrosis and frequently beyond the limits of the posterior longitudinal ligament to cause direct compression of nerve elements at a distance from the area of the disk itself (Fig. 16–1).[1]

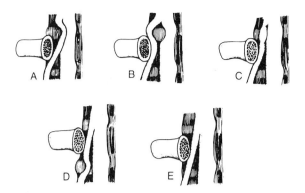

Figure 16–1. Disk herniation may occur in one of several positions. Always identify the nerve root before incising the presumed herniation. (From Yong-Hing,[1] with permission.)

The typical evolution of lumbar disk herniation is an initial episode of back pain which then leads to a radiating leg pain. As the leg pain becomes more prominent, the back pain may lessen or resolve altogether. The typical pattern of radiating leg pain is dermatomal pain. This means that the pain follows a well-known distribution in the leg which is a dermatome related to one of the lumbar nerve roots. There are occasional disk herniations such as central disk herniations which cause primarily back and/or upper buttock pain rather than radiating leg pain. The hallmark of pain related to lumbar disk herniation is that it is mechanical in nature; in other words, the provocation of pain is closely related to activity and is generally relieved with rest. The most common activities which lead to this pain are bending, twisting, standing for prolonged periods of time, lifting, and prolonged sitting. Lying supine will frequently provide some relief of this pain.

Physical findings generally include pain and limitation in bending, a positive straight leg raise, a decreased patel-lar or Achilles reflex, decreased sensation in a dermatomal area of the leg, and possibly muscle weakness. It is not common for all of these physical findings to be present in a given individual, but generally two or three of them will be present. Commonly, the primary presentation is one of radiating leg pain with no specific physical findings. The diagnosis of lumbar disk herniation is ultimately confirmed by an imaging study such as a computed tomography (CT) scan, a magnetic resonance imaging (MRI) scan, or a CT myelogram (Fig. 16–2).[2]

The treatment of lumbar disk herniation is generally approached in stages. Oral anti-inflammatory medications, activity modification, and physical therapy are the first line of treatment. The second line of treatment involves epidural steroid injections. If these measures are not effective in relieving pain or restoring neurologic function, surgery can be considered. However, it is generally accepted that a period of nonoperative treatment should be instituted for at least 6 to 8 weeks and preferably 12 weeks prior to considering surgical treatment. In approximately 80 percent of patients with lumbar disk herniations, the symptoms related to the herniation will resolve within 3 months.

Lumbar Spondylolisthesis

Lumbar spondylolisthesis refers to the forward slippage of a cephalad vertebra onto a caudal vertebra. There are different types of lumbar spondylolisthesis. These types were described in a classic article by Wiltse et al. in 1976.[3] The two most common forms of spondylolisthesis are isthmic and degenerative spondylolisthesis. Degenerative spondylolisthesis refers to the anterior slippage of a vertebra related to degenerative changes within the facet joint and will be covered in the section on Lumbar Spinal Stenosis. Isthmic spondylolisthesis is an entirely different

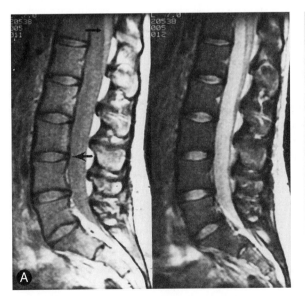

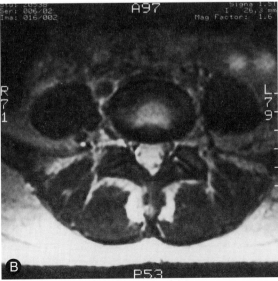

Figure 16–2. Lumbar spine MRI scan. (A) Sagittal view showing disk protrusion at L4-L5. (B) Image through the L4-L5 intervertebral disk showing a normal posterior disk margin. (From Gundry and Heithoff,[2] with permission.)

entity. It occurs in relation to a defect in a portion of the bone known as the *pars interarticularis*. The defect itself is known as a *spondylolytic defect*. It may occur at any level in the lumbar spine but is most common at L5-S1. The spondylolytic defect generally is present by the age of 5 or 6 years. The slip or spondylolisthesis generally occurs during adolescence. The majority of isthmic spondylolistheses that become symptomatic do so during the adult years, generally in the fourth and fifth decades. A minority of isthmic spondylolistheses become symptomatic during the teen years and very occasionally require surgical treatment during this period. It is fairly common for isthmic spondylolisthesis to become symptomatic in adults following an injury when no symptoms existed prior to the adult years.

The typical symptoms associated with isthmic spondylolisthesis are radicular leg pain in an L5 dermatomal distribution. At L5-S1 the spondylolysis involves the L5 pars interarticularis and may ultimately lead to compression of the L5 nerve root. An L4-L5 isthmic spondylolisthesis most commonly involves the L4 nerve root and causes dermatomal pain in the leg following the L4 dermatome. In adolescence, isthmic spondylolisthesis may present as primarily back pain. In adults, there may be a combination of back and leg pain; whether axial back pain without leg pain in an adult with spondylolisthesis is entirely attributable to the spondylolisthesis has not been determined.

Treatment of symptomatic spondylolisthesis is much the same as treatment of lumbar disk herniation. An initial period of activity modification, physical therapy, and oral anti-inflammatory medication is the first level of treatment. Epidural steroid injections can be helpful in treating the radicular leg pain (Fig. 16–3).[4] If after a course of

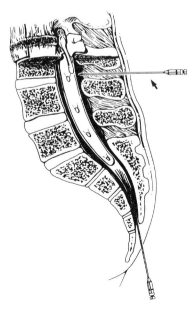

Figure 16–3. Epidural injection may be performed through the sacral hiatus or by the interlaminar technique. (From Bernard Jr,[4] with permission.)

conservative treatment there is still a persisting leg pain or, in the adolescent, a persistent back pain, surgical treatment can be considered. The most widely accepted surgical treatment for isthmic spondylolisthesis at this time is laminectomy and decompression of the effected nerve roots (Gill procedure) along with posterolateral fusion.

Lumbar Spinal Stenosis

The word *stenosis* refers to narrowing of a tube. In lumbar spinal stenosis, the spinal canal or the space where the dural sac is transmitted through the spine to the pelvis and lower extremities is the structure which is narrowed. Spinal stenosis is generally an end-stage process whereby the arthritic involvement of facet joints, as well as the progressive degenerative collapse of the lumbar disk and the thickening and infolding of the ligamentum flavum and other supportive ligaments, concentrically narrow the spinal canal. In contrast to a disk herniation, which is an acute nerve compression, lumbar spinal stenosis is a gradual compression of the lumbar nerve roots and/or the cauda equina. The classic symptoms associated with lumbar spinal stenosis are radicular leg pain, frequently involving both legs and almost always becoming more severe with ambulation. The term *neurogenic claudication* has been applied to the progressive radicular pain in the legs which occurs with ambulating distances of less than 100–200 feet. Most commonly, the patient indicates that the amount of walking that it takes to provoke the radicular leg pains has steadily decreased over time. The patient frequently walks with a forward list and must sit and bend forward to relieve the leg pain.

Physical findings may be very sparse, and in most instances there is no pain with lumbosacral bending and no neurologic findings in the legs. Perhaps the hallmark of spinal stenosis is the absence of a straight leg raise. In some long-standing cases, a motor deficit is noted; in some cases, there is a sensory deficit as well. Many elderly patients are areflexic, so that the absence of a reflex is very seldom helpful in the diagnosis of this problem.

Plain film x-rays may show diffuse arthritic changes and degenerative disk changes throughout the lumbar spine (Fig. 16–4). Associated degenerative spondylolisthesis is fairly common in spinal stenosis and often contributes to the canal compromise at the level of the spondylolisthesis. The definitive diagnosis is provided by imaging studies such as CT and MRI scans. In spinal stenosis, lumbar myelography is extremely helpful. It is much more accurate in determining the integrity of the spinal canal than an MRI scan.

The treatment of lumbar spinal stenosis follows the same stages as the above-mentioned lumbar conditions, with oral anti-inflammatory medications being instituted initially, followed by epidural steroid injections. Surgical decompression is frequently the ultimate treatment in spinal stenosis with progressive symptoms. Surgical treat-

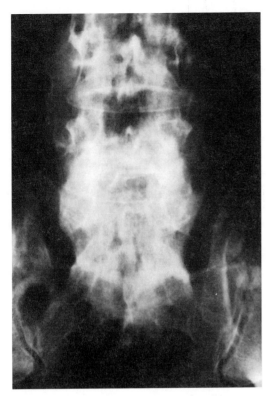

Figure 16–4. Severe degenerative arthritis of L5 with spinal canal stenosis. The actual canal stenosis is imaged with CT or MRI.

ment is almost always the preferred treatment of spinal stenosis with neurogenic claudication.

Lumbar Fracture

Fractures of the lumbar spine may occur in response to multiple forms of trauma. Osteoporotic fractures frequently occur without any trauma. Osteoporotic fractures of the lumbar spine are almost never treated surgically. Other types of fractures are treated surgically when these fractures compromise the stability of the lumbar spine or lead to nerve compression in the lumbar spine. The majority of lumbar fractures, however, are treated nonoperatively. A detailed discussion of instability related to fracture and the fine points of surgical indications for fracture are beyond the scope of this chapter. But when fractures of the lumbar spine are treated surgically, they are almost always stabilized with some form of fixation device, and a fusion is performed.

Lumbar Scoliosis

Lumbar scoliosis is a common condition in both adolescents and adults. Although lumbar scoliosis frequently occurs with an associated thoracic scoliosis, it may also occur as an isolated entity. In adolescence, lumbar scoliosis of certain magnitudes may require surgical treatment. Progressive lumbar scoliosis in adults may require surgical

treatment as well. At this time, scoliosis is treated with instrumentation, for both correction and stabilization, and with a fusion.

Degenerative Disk Disease

Degenerative disk disease is a fairly common problem in the majority of the adult population. It is an extremely common source of lower back pain. It is almost always treated nonoperatively. However, there are rare cases of degenerative disk disease which may be considered for surgical treatment.

The primary symptom associated with degenerative disk disease is lower back pain. This generally occurs as an episodic recurrence of lower back pain which is frequently accompanied by trunk listing and muscle spasm. The typical cycle of degenerative disk pain is one of a sudden, severe back pain which may be related to bending or lifting activities or any other form of injury. The initial severe pain may render the patient bedridden for 1 or 2 days. This severe pain then improves, to be followed by a lesser degree of pain, again related to activity, which lasts for a few weeks and then resolves. Between episodes of severe pain, the patient is frequently pain-free and able to perform all activities. In rare instances this type of pain persists for long periods of time, and there are reports in the literature of some patients who required up to 12 months to resolve the pain. In the rare individual with a persisting degenerative disk pain that lasts for more than 12 months and who is disabled by the pain, fusion of the degenerative disk may be considered.

The physical findings suggestive of degenerative disk disease include muscle spasm, trunk listing, and pain with bending. The examination of the lower extremities, particularly as it pertains to neurologic findings, is normal. There may be back pain with a straight leg raise, but there is no radiating leg pain with the straight leg raise. The MRI scan will show degenerative disk changes. However, the MRI scan does not indicate which disk is symptomatic in a lumbar spine that has more than one degenerative disk. Lumbar diskography may be used to help determine the symptomatic degenerative disk. This method is commonly used to select patients for fusion on the basis of degenerative disk disease. However, the results of fusion for degenerative disk disease continue to be disappointing.

Infection

Infection or septic spondylitis can occur spontaneously in the lumbar spine. There may be hematogenous seeding of blood-borne bacteria into the lumbar disk, which may then spread into the lumbar vertebral bodies. Recent studies have indicated hematogenous seeding directly into the vertebral body and development of spontaneous osteomyelitis of the lumbar vertebral bodies. The symptom of spontaneous infection of the lumbar spine is a progressive

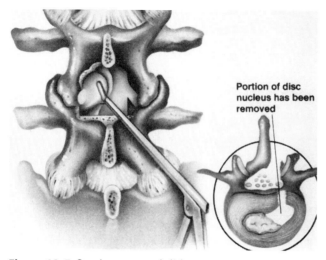

Portion of disc nucleus has been removed

Figure 16–5. Laminotomy and diskectomy.

and unrelenting back pain. Signs of systemic sepsis are frequently absent. Patients often present with severe pain with any type of lumbosacral motion and may have some leg symptoms in the buttocks and the posterior or anterior thigh. The diagnosis of diskitis or lumbar vertebral osteomyelitis may be made on plain films. There is generally a significant elevation of the erythrocyte sedimentation rate on blood studies. The MRI scan is the definitive study in diagnosing this problem. In order to obtain specific bacterial cultures for treatment, CT-directed needle biopsy is frequently required. Spontaneous diskitis is often successfully treated with antibiotics alone, although in some instances surgical treatment is required. Vertebral osteomyelitis is more commonly treated with surgical debridement and a prolonged course of intravenous antibiotics. Fusion is frequently indicated in the treatment of infection in the lumbar spine.

Pseudoarthrosis of a Previous Fusion

Lower back pain related to a previous fusion which did not heal is a common problem, but it must be distinguished from other sources of back pain which could also cause similar symptoms. In this era of spinal fixation, the typical history of a lumbar pseudoarthrosis involves a patient who underwent a fusion procedure with spinal fixation and for a period of time (often measured in months postoperatively) did have relief of preoperative pain but then experienced recurrent back pain that increased over time, particularly with activity. Plain film x-rays will often show signs of loosening of the fixation device. Often the only way to confirm the presence of a pseudoarthrosis is to remove the fixation device and explore the fusion area. If a pseudoarthrosis is identified, repeat fixation and bone grafting is often indicated. Postoperative symptoms of leg pain, however, are rarely related to a pseudoarthrosis. If leg pain is the primary postoperative complaint, other sources of this pain should be investigated.

■ Standard Techniques for Surgical Treatment

Laminotomy and Microdiskectomy

The standard technique for lumbar disk excision is a laminotomy through a technique that is currently known as *microdiskectomy*. This involves a limited exposure of the hemilamina on the right or left side, depending on the location of the disk. A small amount of hemilamina on the cephalad and caudal sides of the ligamentum flavum is removed along with the ligamentum flavum (Fig. 16–5). A small portion of the medial aspect of the facet joint is also removed. The underlying nerve root is identified and retracted toward the midline with a small retractor, and the underlying disk material is removed (Fig. 16–6). The technique may involve division of the lumbodorsal fascia at the tips of the spinous processes and lateral retraction of the unilateral paraspinal muscle or it may involve splitting the muscle overlying the lamina area, with less muscular retraction. Magnification is not required in order for this technique to be a microdiskectomy. Some surgeons prefer to use loupes. Others prefer to use an actual operating microscope, and still others may use no magnification at all. But some type of accessory light such as a headlight is often used to illuminate the small area of exposure. The advantages of this procedure involve minimal disruption of the important stabilizing structures. Specifically, the interspinous and supraspinous ligaments are left intact. The facet joint and its capsule are largely undisturbed. There is essentially no destabilizing effect from removal of small portions of the lamina and unilateral ligamentum flavum, which is often left partially intact in the midline. This technique may be performed at one level or at more than one level, depending on the needs of the individual patient. This procedure generally

Figure 16–6. Disk removal. Avoid damaging the nerve by inserting the pituitary forceps with its jaws closed. Avoid damaging great vessels by referring to the depth mark scored on the forceps. (From Yong-Hing,[1] with permission.)

lasts for approximately 1 hour for a unilateral diskectomy. Patients may be discharged on the same day or the day following surgery.

Laminectomy

Laminectomy technically refers to removal of an entire lamina. It involves bilateral exposure of the hemilamina, generally by splitting the lumbodorsal fascia in the midline and then performing subperiosteal dissection to expose the entire lamina. In a true complete laminectomy, the entire lamina, along with the spinous process and the ligamentum flavum caudal and cephalad to the lamina, are removed. This allows access to the entire spinal canal at a given laminar level, as well as to four nerve roots, two cephalad and two caudal. The facet joints are generally preserved, but when this technique is used—and it is often used in spinal stenosis—the facets are undercut. This procedure involves removal of inferior osteophytes underneath the facet by reaching from within the spinal canal rather than removing the entire facet, which causes significant destabilization of the motion segment. Complete laminectomy produces a destabilizing effect. However, this procedure is generally performed in older individuals with degenerative disk settling and degenerative facet joints, and these areas are generally stable due to the degenerative changes. It is not necessary to perform a fusion whenever a complete laminectomy is performed. In spinal stenosis it is common to perform laminectomy at multiple levels, as symptomatic spinal stenosis is often a multilevel disease. When a complete laminectomy is performed to decompress a spondylolisthesis, it is often referred to as a *Gill procedure*.

Fusion

The standard technique for lumbar spinal fusion is a posterolateral fusion. This is also called an *intertransverse process fusion* (Fig. 16–7). The original fusion technique involves harvesting of an iliac crest bone graft, which is currently performed through the same midline incision by dissecting subcutaneously to the iliac crest and then harvesting the bone graft either from the outer table of the iliac crest or from between the inner and outer tables of the iliac crest. The bone graft is then placed in the area between two transverse processes which are being fused together. Transverse processes are decorticated using an osteotome or a burr. Generally, the facet joint that is involved in the area to be fused is denuded of its capsular structures. It is frequently partially resected with either an osteotome or a burr. Current concepts in lumbar posterolateral fusion almost always involve the use of spinal instrumentation, specifically pedicle screw instrumentation. Isolated L5-S1 fusions are often performed without instrumentation. This is also the procedure used when grade I and grade II spondylolisthesis is being fused as an isolated L5-S1 fusion. However, fusions above the

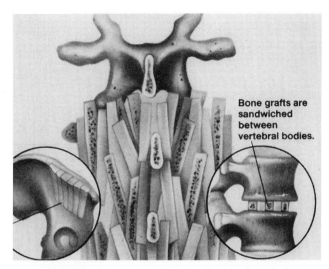

Figure 16–7. Lumbar spine fusion. Bone is rarely placed in the midline in a posterolateral fusion, as depicted here. The majority of the bone is placed in the posterolateral position between the transverse processes and in the area of the facets.

L5-S1 level and multilevel fusions most commonly involve pedicle screw devices, which obtain a higher rate of fusion (Fig. 16–8). A review of the literature reveals a wide variety of fusion rates in both instrumented and uninstrumented fusion. However, the literature of the 1990s indicates that pedicle screw fixation has increased the success rate of posterolateral fusion.[5]

■ New Techniques in Lumbar Surgery

Indirect Discectomy

There are basically three different techniques of indirect diskectomy. This procedure involves placing a laser heat device, a chemical, or a mechanical device into the disk itself through an anterior or anterolateral approach. Central disk material is either dissolved chemically, burned with a laser, or removed mechanically with a device called a *nucleotome* or a *rongeur* in order to allow prolapsed disk to fall out of the spinal canal and back inward toward the disk (Fig. 16–9). The prerequisite for an indirect diskectomy is a contained disk herniation, which means that disk material is still within the annulus fibrosus and has not become free within the spinal canal or sequestered at a distance from the disk. Chymopapain is the most thoroughly studied of the three techniques, and it has been shown to be highly effective in indirect diskectomy. There have been some anaphylactic reactions with the use of chymopapain which have resulted in death, and at the time of this writing, chymopapain has been temporarily removed from the market by the U.S. Food and Drug Administration. Laser diskectomy and mechanical anterior diskectomy have been less well studied than chymopapain, but neither technique has yielded a success rate high

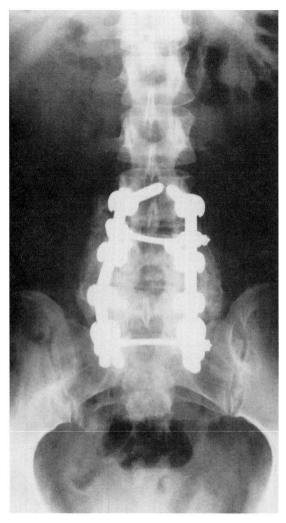

Figure 16–8. Lumbar spinal fusion with internal fixation by pedicle screws.

enough to promote their popularity. Neither form of indirect diskectomy is widely used at the time of this writing.

Microendoscopic Diskectomy

Microendoscopic diskectomy is a newer technique of microdiskectomy which is performed through a tubular structure known as a *cannula*. The lumbar paraspinal muscle is split, and a cannula is placed at the intralaminar area. Small portions of the lamina are removed along with a portion of the ligamentum flavum. The technique involves the use of an endoscope fixed to the cannula, which directs the procedure on a television screen in much the same way that arthroscopic surgery of the knee or shoulder is performed (Fig. 16–10).[6] The original technique involved the use of local or spinal anesthetic, but the procedure is most commonly performed under general anesthetic, as it sometimes requires more time than a standard microdiskectomy. This is basically the same technique as a microdiskectomy with a smaller exposure and a smaller area of decompression. It is much more like the original microdiskectomy, in which only the ligamentum flavum was excised and a true laminotomy was not performed. The original microdiskectomy technique was abandoned due to a high failure rate secondary to missed disk fragments and persisting lateral stenosis which was not decompressed during the procedure. At this time, microendoscopic diskectomy represents the initial phase of a coming trend which will involve endoscopic techniques for disk removal. This will almost certainly involve smaller exposures and perhaps a local anesthetic and a shorter operative time, which will speed recovery and postoperative rehabilitation. At this time, however, microendoscopic diskectomy is being used on a limited basis, and its future usefulness is still to be determined.

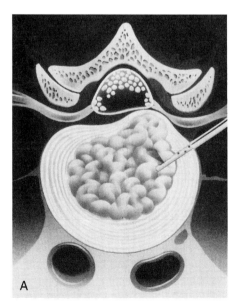
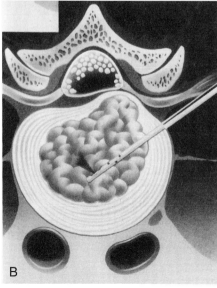

Figure 16–9. Laser diskectomy.

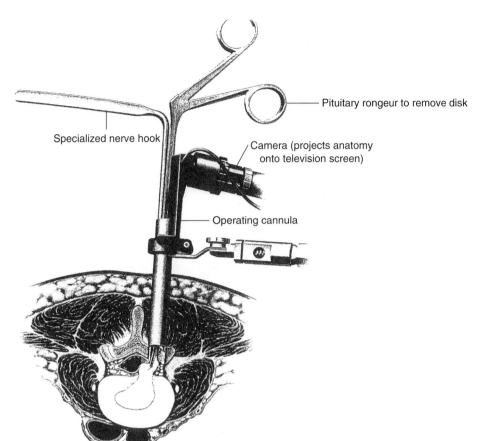

Pituitary rongeur to remove disk

Specialized nerve hook

Camera (projects anatomy onto television screen)

Operating cannula

Figure 16–10. Lumbar diskectomy by the microendoscopic technique. (From Medtronic Sofamor Danek,[6] with permission.)

New Techniques for Interbody Fusion

Perhaps the most exciting and intense area of research in orthopaedics has been in the area of bone morphogenetic proteins. Some years ago, it was discovered that demineralized bone matrix induced bone formation. A group of proteins known as *bone morphogenetic proteins* (*BMP*) were isolated and cloned from demineralized bone matrix. Initial studies of BMP involved its use in fracture repair, but this soon spread to evaluation of its use as a potential bone graft substitute in fusions. BMP has been placed in interbody devices for use in interbody fusion. It has also been used experimentally in posterolateral fusion and is an extremely promising innovation in increasing the rate of bone fusion in both of these techniques. At the time of this writing, BMP has not yet been released for general use, but it is being used for fusion in humans on a trial basis in pilot study centers. It is likely that some form of BMP will be employed more generally for lumbar spinal fusions in the near future.

Interbody fusion is a fusion technique in which all or part of the disk is removed and bone graft is placed in the area between the vertebral bodies previously occupied by the disk. This procedure may be performed from an anterior approach and is then called *anterior lumbar interbody fusion* (*ALIF*). It may also be performed from a posterior approach through the spinal canal and is then referred to as *posterior lumbar interbody fusion* (*PLIF*).

The original techniques for both ALIF and PLIF involved the use of bone graft, either autogenous bone graft from the patient's iliac crest or allograft from a bone bank. These techniques are still being used; however, some new variations have been developed.

In recent years, laparoscopy has been used as an aid in performing ALIF.[7] A general surgeon works with a spinal surgeon in performing the laparoscopic portion of the procedure, and the interbody fusion is performed entirely through a laparoscope rather than through an open abdominal or retroperitoneal procedure. At this time, laparoscopic techniques are being used primarily for L5-S1 interbody fusions and occasionally for L4-L5 interbody fusions. The location of the great vessels has limited the use of this technique above the L4-L5 level, although some retroperitoneal techniques are being developed for laparoscopic interbody fusion at levels above L4-L5.

The use of threaded interbody fusion devices has increased along with the development of laparoscopic fusion techniques. Allograft bone has been machine threaded so that it has screw threads. It is subsequently "screwed into" the interbody area, which has been reamed with a mechanical reamer and then threaded with a tap. Titanium "cage" implants have also been developed. These are threaded titanium screw devices which are hollow and are filled with bone graft. The interbody area is reamed and threaded with a tap, and the titanium cage is screwed into the interbody space after a reamer is used to create the channel. The theoretical advantage of the titanium cage is immediate stabilization without the use of other forms of fixation such as a pedicle screw device (Figs. 16–11 and 16–12).[8] Both titanium cage devices and threaded allograft bone can be used as a PLIF as well as an ALIF, with or without a laparoscope. Recent data indicate, however, that the healing rate of the titanium screw-in cages is not as good as the initial studies indicated. These devices are still in widespread use, but the future popularity of the titanium implants will be determined after further studies of healing have been completed. There is also growing evidence that other forms of fixation, such as pedicle screw fixation, are needed to stabilize these devices, thereby removing the theoretical advantage of using a titanium implant rather than allograft or autograft bone.

A "carbon fiber cage" has been developed as a carrier of autogenous bone which can be placed in an interbody position.[9] It has the advantage of giving structural support that a bone graft may not be able to give, especially an autogenous bone graft. It eventually becomes incorporated into the fusion mass, and therefore the radiographic appearance is one of incorporated bone without a metallic

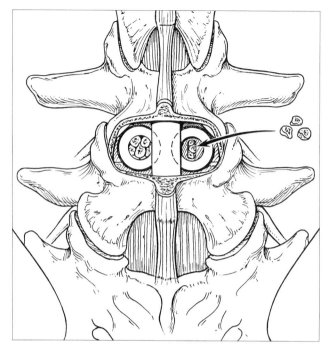

Figure 16–12. Posteroanterior view of the posterior lumbar spine with two BAK cages in place from a PLIF. A bone graft is inserted in the cage prior to seating the cage in the interbody position. (From Spine-Tech,[8] with permission.)

implant. This technique is currently being used in various centers in the United States.

A titanium mesh cage developed by Dr. Jurgen Harms in Germany has been used for several years for interbody fusion in the United States. This mesh cylinder is filled with autograft and may be used as an anterior or a posterior interbody spacer. It can also be used as a strut graft for vertebral body replacement in the lumbar and thoracolumbar spine and is used as a strut graft after corpectomy in the cervical spine. Unlike the carbon fiber cage, the titanium mesh cage remains radiographically apparent. This cage does require additional fixation, generally posteriorly or anteriorly, but it has been used successfully for several years and is currently in widespread use.

Anterior Surgery for Scoliosis

Various devices have been used for anterior correction of lumbar scoliosis. The original device was a cable-and-screw device which linked screws in the anterior vertebral bodies to a cable. The cable was subsequently replaced by a threaded rod, which was found to be too weak for the forces of the lumbar spine. Stainless steel rods were then used for correction of the lumbar curve anteriorly, and they have become popular for the treatment of lumbar scoliosis. Newer techniques involve treating both thoracic and lumbar scoliosis with an anterior rod. Dr. Brasil H. Kaneda in Japan introduced a technique for scoliosis correction using double anterior rods. Randall Betz in

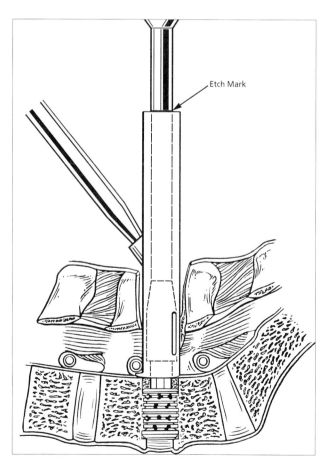

Figure 16–11. Posterior surgical technique. (From Spine-Tech,[8] with permission.)

the United States has popularized the use of a single rod for anterior correction of thoracic, thoracolumbar, and lumbar scoliosis.[10] It is likely that the future will see more anterior lumbar instrumentation for scoliosis, as it has the advantage of a more complete correction of the curve. There is a biomechanical advantage to anterior fixation, and the interbody technique used in this form of treatment has a higher rate of healing. The procedure is technically demanding, but it is gaining acceptance in many centers in the United States.

Electrothermal Treatment for Degenerative Disk Disease

A recent pilot study by Saal et al.[11] indicates that an electrothermal coil may be used to treat degenerative disk pain. This technique was borrowed from the electrothermal treatment of anterior shoulder capsular disorders. The anterior capsule of the shoulder was electrothermally treated with a heated coil in order to cause contraction of the structure to provide stability for the shoulder. The theory in the electrothermal treatment of degenerative disk disease is that an electrothermal coil can be used to coagulate the internal portions of the annulus fibrosis where innervation is received from the sinuvertebral nerve. Theoretically, this could eliminate the innervation to the internal annulus fibrosis and thus eliminate the pain created in degenerative disk with annular tears and other internal annular disorders. Preliminary studies indicate that this may be an effective treatment, and electrothermal treatment has been expanded to numerous centers in the United States. A considerable amount of study will be necessary to determine whether or not this treatment is truly effective for degenerative disk-related pain in the lumbar spine. There are some theoretical problems with this treatment, one of which is the poor success of surgical treatment, which involves complete extirpation of the disk and the interbody graft. If complete removal of the disk is not effective in relieving pain, it is difficult to understand how electrothermal treatment of the annulus fibrosis will cause relief of pain for a prolonged period of time. There is also a problem with patient selection because discography is the only diagnostic test that is currently available to identify painful disks. Recent studies have pointed out the shortcomings of discography as a patient selection technique.

■ Postoperative Rehabilitation

It is difficult to fashion a single rehabilitation program for any given postoperative setting after lumbar spine surgery. Following are general guidelines for postoperative rehabilitation after lumbar laminotomy and laminectomy with lumbar fusion.

In a patient who has undergone a microdiscectomy, rehabilitation may begin immediately after surgery. In some current protocols therapy begins on postoperative day 1, with gentle stretching and strengthening exercises of the lower extremities and gentle motion exercises of the lumbosacral spine. The author prefers to allow patient ambulation, increasing the rate and distance of ambulation over the first 2 postoperative weeks. At the end of the second postoperative week the wound is checked. At this point more involved physical therapy commences, with stretching and strengthening of the hip and leg muscles as well as gentle range-of-motion exercises of the lumbosacral spine. Lumbar strengthening exercises are usually started at around the fourth postoperative week, along with conditioning exercises that include riding a stationary cycle, using a stair stepper, and swimming in a pool. All of these are low-impact cardiovascular exercises which allow the patient to begin postoperative reconditioning. At the 6th postoperative week in a patient with minimal pain, straight-ahead jogging is allowed as well as activities such as golf, but more involved running and rotation activities such as tennis or racquet ball are generally contraindicated until the 8th postoperative week and high-impact contact activities such as basketball, football, and soccer are generally not allowed until the 12th postoperative week. Occasionally in elite athletes with excellent postoperative results, these activities are allowed at around the 8th postoperative week. Some physical therapy protocols have certain restrictions, such as one against sitting for prolonged periods of time after surgery. There is little basis for such restriction and, in general, postoperative patients are allowed to sit for as long as they are comfortable, beginning immediately after surgery. Patients are encouraged to either sit up straight or in slight extension and to use a chair with a back support and arm rests.

Postoperative rehabilitation in fusion patients is generally confined to ambulation for the first 6 weeks, with lower extremity exercises such as stretching and strengthening without trunk motion exercises being allowed prior to the 6th week. With spinal fixation, if a brace is used postoperatively, it is generally discontinued at 6 weeks. At this point, stretching and strengthening exercises of the trunk may begin. In a patient who is progressing slowly after surgery, these exercises may be delayed until approximately 8 weeks postoperatively. Trunk and lower extremity exercises are gradually progressed from the 8th to the 12th week. At 12 weeks, if the patient is doing well clinically and x-rays show progression of healing, more involved activities such as running may begin. Golf and tennis may be allowed after 12 weeks in these patients. Patients can begin low-impact exercises such as stationary cycling and stair stepping at approximately 4 weeks postoperatively, as neither of these requires significant trunk motion. These activities are predicated on the patient's postoperative response. Obviously, a patient who is still having considerable back and muscular pain is progressed much more slowly than a patient with minimal pain. Once again, there is no restriction against sitting for periods of time in the postoperative rehabilitation of fusion patients. The use of braces in general has declined, and therefore physical therapy regimens are starting earlier in the postoperative course of fusion patients than they have in past years.

■ References

1. Yong-Hing K: Surgical Techniques. p. 315. In Kirkaldy-Willis WH (ed): Managing Low Back Pain. 2nd Ed. Churchill Livingstone, New York, 1988
2. Gundry CR, Heithoff KB: Lumbar spine imaging. p. 171. In Kirkaldy-Willis WH, Burton CV (eds): Managing Low Back Pain. 3rd Ed. Churchill Livingstone, New York, 1992
3. Wiltse LL, Newman PH, and McNab I: Classification of spondylolysis and spondylolisthesis, Clin Orthop 117:23–24, 1976
4. Bernard Jr, TN: Diagnostic and therapeutic techniques. p. 149. In Kirkaldy-Willis WH, Burton CV (eds): Managing Low Back Pain. 3rd Ed. Churchill Livingstone, New York, 1992
5. Masferrer R, Gomez CH, Karahalios DG, et al: Efficacy of pedicle screw fixation and the treatment of spinal instability and failed back surgery: a five year review. J Neurosurg 89(3):371–377, 1998
6. MED Surgical Technique booklet, part number LIT.MED. ST97. Medtronic Sofamor Danek, Memphis, TN, 1997
7. Olsen D, McCord D, Law M: Laparoscopic discectomy with anterior interbody fusion of L5-S1. Surg Endosc 10(12):1158–1163, 1996
8. Posterior Surgical Technique: BAK Interbody Fusion System. Spine-Tech, Minneapolis, MN, 1996
9. Brantigan JW, Steffee AD: A carbon fiber implant to aid interbody lumbar fusion. Spine 18(14):2106–2107, 1993
10. Betz RR, Harms J, Clements DH III, et al: Comparison of anterior and posterior instrumentation for correction of adolescent thoracic idiopathic scoliosis. Spine 24(3):225–239, 1999
11. Saal JA, Saal JS: Intradiscal Electrothermal Treatment (IDET) for chronic discogenic low back pain: A prospective outcome study with minimum two year follow-up, North American Spine Society meeting, New Orleans, LA, October 2000

■ Suggested Reading

Bolender NF: The role of computed tomography and myelography and the diagnosis of central spine stenosis. J Bone Joint Surg 67(A):240, 1985

Bostrom MP, Camacho NP: Potential role of bone morphogenetic proteins in fracture healing. Clin Orthop 255 (suppl):S274–S282, 1990

Bradford DS, Lonstein JE, Moe JH, et al: Moe's Textbook of Scoliosis and other Spinal Deformities. 2nd Ed. WB Saunders, Philadelphia, 1987

Brown CA, Eismont FJ: Complications in spinal fusion. Orthop Clin North Am 29(4):679–699, 1998

Eismont FJ: Lumbosacral spine. Maine Orthop Rev 151:101, 1985

Frymoyer JW (ed): The Adult Spine: Principles and Practice. Raven Press, New York, 1991

Karahalios DG, Apostolides PJ, Sonntag VK: Degenerative lumbar spinal instability: technical aspects of operative treatment. Clin Neurosurg 44:109–135, 1997

MacNab I: Back Ache. Williams & Wilkins, Baltimore, 1977

Niggemeyer O, Strauss JM, Schulitz KP: Comparison of surgical procedures for degenerative lumbar spinal stenosis: a meta-analysis of the literature from 1975 to 1995. Eur Spine J 6(6):423–429, 1997

Reddi AH: Initiation of fracture repair by bone morphogenetic proteins. Clin Orthop 355(suppl):S66–S72, 1998

Rosen C, Kahanovita N, Viola K: A retrospective analysis of the efficacy of epidural steroid injections. Clin Orthop 228:270, 1988

Sakou T: Bone morphogenetic proteins: from basic studies to clinical approaches. Bone 22(6):591–603, 1998

Schneiderman G, Flannigan B, Kingston S: Magnetic resonance imaging in the diagnosis of disc degeneration: correlation with discography. Spine 12:276, 1987

Waddell G: A new clinical model for the treatment of low back pain. Spine 12:632, 1987

Watkins RG, Collis JS: Lumbar Discectomy and Laminectomy. Aspen, Rockville, MD, 1987

Weinstein JN, Wiesel SW (eds for The International Society for the Study of the Lumbar Spine): The Lumbar Spine. WB Saunders, Philadelphia, 1990

White AA, Punjabi MM: Clinical Biomechanics of the Spine. 2nd Ed. JB Lippincott, Philadelphia, 1990

White AA, Rothman RH, Rey CD (eds): Lumbar Spine Surgery: Techniques and Complications, CV Mosby, St. Louis, 1987

Williams RW, McCullouch JA, Young PH: Microsurgery of the Lumbar Spine: Principles and Techniques in Spine Surgery. Aspen, Rockville, MD, 1990

Young-Hing K: Surgical techniques. p. 315. In Kirkaldy-Willis WH (ed): Managing Low Back Pain. 2nd Ed. Churchill Livingstone, New York, 1988

CHAPTER 17

Manual Therapy Techniques for the Thoracolumbar Spine

Robert W. Sydenham

Spinal mobilization and manipulation are arts that have been practiced since ancient times. Early recordings of such treatments were made by Hippocrates, Galen, Pare, Pott, Paget, and many others.[1,2] The literature indicates that primitive forms of manipulation were used by the ancient Greeks and Romans, by the Japanese, by South American civilizations, and in India, Egypt, China, and Europe.[1-4] In 1876, the renowned British surgeon Sir James Paget (1814–1899) published his famous lecture "Cases That Bonesetters Cure" in the *British Medical Journal*. However, orthodox medicine at that time found the rationale behind bonesetting untenable, despite support from patients.[5] Today these services are provided by osteopaths, chiropractors, allopathic physicians, physical therapists, and various other specialists.

Osteopathy owes its origin and development to Andrew Taylor Still (1828–1917), who founded the American School of Osteopathy in 1892 at Kirksville, Missouri.[5] The practice of chiropractic had its origin with Daniel David Palmer, who after reading some of Still's works founded the first chiropractic school in Davenport, Iowa, in 1897.[5] Although only a few allopathic physicians use mobilization or manipulative techniques, some have been paramount in the development and integration of mobilization and manipulation techniques that are in use today. James Mennell, his son John, and James Cyriax have contributed immensely by their individual efforts and their publications, with which most therapists are familiar.[6,7]

Therapists today are able to credit their own colleagues, such as Grieve, Maitland, Paris, Kaltenborn, and McKenzie, for the significant change during the past 20 years in the manner in which manual therapy is practiced by physical therapists.[5,8-11] The increasing interest in the interrelationship between the biomechanical effects of mobilization and manipulation and the neurophysiologic mechanisms that come into play has resulted in investigations into the efficiency of mobilization and manipulation in an effort to determine their mechanisms of action.

A significant step in this direction was taken by the National Institutes of Health. The National Institute of Neurological and Communicative Disorders and Stroke held a conference, which resulted in the publication edited by Goldstein[12] in 1975 on "The Research Status of Spinal Manipulative Therapy." Of special interest is the work by Sato[13] and Perl[14] in that publication. This conference was followed by another in Italy in 1978, at which Granit and Pompeiano[15] presented additional research applicable to manual therapy. Freeman and Wyke[16] in 1967 coined the term *articular neurology*. Additional research by Wyke and Polacek,[21] and others, further explained the neurophysiologic ramifications of manual therapy.[17-22] Research by Polacek[23] and Halata[24] also contributed to our understanding of articular neurology.

Another meeting of the clinical and scientific worlds took place in Melbourne, Australia, in 1979 at a conference sponsored by the Lincoln Institute of Health Sciences on "Manipulative Therapy in the Management of Musculo-Skeletal Disorders."[25] This conference was significant in that it brought together clinicians, researchers, and scientists from many different schools of thought from all over the world.

Until recently, manipulation and mobilization have been considered empirical treatment procedures. However, researchers have put forth theories to explain why mobilization and manipulation play an important part in treating somatic dysfunction. Unfortunately, the saving of lives and the accurate diagnosis of a broad spectrum of medical conditions have a prior claim on the time and effort of the medical profession. The time spent in medical school studying the assessment and treatment of musculoskeletal disorders is not in proportion to the number of patients who attend a medical or especially a physical therapy practice. However, there is an increased awareness in the undergraduate programs that manual therapy is a vital part of our skills, and many postgraduate courses are available, with specialization in many areas in preparation or in place. The more time spent raising the level of expertise in the diagnosis and treatment of musculoskeletal disorders, the better off our patients will be.[25]

■ Terminology

Mobilization

Mobilization has been described by Grieve[8] as the attempt to restore full, painless joint function by rhythmic, repetitive, passive movements within the patient's tolerance and within the voluntary and accessory range and graded according to examination findings. The patient is at all times able to stop the movement if he or she so wishes. Mobilization may affect the whole vertebral region or may be localized to a single segment.[8] The term *mobilization* thus applies to a wide variety of techniques.

Kaltenborn[26] advocates different mobilization techniques such as translating or gliding movements, and angular or rolling movements, in addition to different degrees of traction, all of which form part of some very exacting, specific techniques.

Maitland's[9,27] approach to mobilization is strongly based on assessment of range of motion, pain, stiffness, and spasm, with alterations in signs and symptoms used as indicators for modification of further treatment. Maitland's techniques are quite gentle, are easily controlled by the patient, and vary in intensity from grades I to IV.

Mennell's[7,28] approach to mobilization is based on the restoration of joint play or accessory joint movements, with techniques aimed at restoration of joint dysfunction, followed by exercises to maintain the newly restored range.

Although not known for his mobilization techniques per se, James Cyriax[6] developed a detailed, comprehensive examination involving contractile and noncontractile tissue, normal and abnormal end-feels of joint movement, and classification of joint restrictions into capsular and noncapsular patterns.

Articulation

Articulation is an osteopathic term that refers to the same type of movement that occurs in mobilization; however, the effects are intended to be localized to a single spinal segment in an attempt to improve the restricted range of a single movement of that segment.[8] Osteopaths believe that these articulatory techniques gradually stretch contracted muscles, ligaments, or joint capsules, besides restoring the normal movements of which the joint is capable. Articulatory techniques also attempt to ensure that the movements that normally are not under voluntary control of the joint are also free. Besides the mechanical aspects of articulatory techniques, reference is made to the nutritional and circulatory factors that influence the joint. Articulatory techniques are frequently used in preparation for specific manipulations, as there may be less reactive tissue response and the benefit may be more lasting.[29]

Articulation differs from simple passive movement in that the operator should be constantly sensing the feedback from the tissue under his or her hand and measuring the intensity of pressure or stretch that the operator feels is necessary, according to what he or she is feeling. Articulation is often combined with a small "bounce" at the end of the range of motion to test tissue reactivity.[30] Localized mobilizations or articulations are often distinguished by the use of direct contact through soft tissues with the bony apophyses of a single vertebral body.[27]

Manipulation

Manipulation is often described as an accurately localized, single, quick, and decisive movement of small amplitude after careful positioning of the patient. It is not necessarily energetic and is completed before the patient can stop it. Manipulation may have a regional or a more localized effect, depending on the technique of the therapist and the positioning of the patient.[8]

Manipulation has also been defined as a passive manual maneuver during which the three-joint complex is suddenly carried beyond its normal physiologic range of movement without exceeding the boundaries of anatomic integrity. The usual characteristic is a brief, sudden, and carefully administered "impulsion" given at the end of the normal passive range of movement. Usually it is accompanied by a cracking noise.[31,32]

Many forms of manipulation involve variations of leverage, thrust, and momentum. The effectiveness of one group of techniques over another is probably due more to the skill of the clinician than to the superiority of a particular procedural technique.

Manipulation has also been referred to as *spinal manipulative therapy*[12] and *high-velocity thrust*.[33]

Soft Tissue Techniques

Soft tissue techniques involve stretching of connective and/or muscle tissue in an abnormal state that generally crosses joints (e.g., spasm, weakness, wasting, tightness, and ultimately some degree of fibrosis), which prohibits normal painless joint range of motion.[8] Stretching techniques, both specific and general, have proven to be most effective and are illustrated and described in great detail by Olaf Evjenth and Jern Hamberg.[34] Their most common use, however, is to prepare the tissue for and reduce the stress of articulatory techniques. A few such techniques are illustrated in Figures 17–1 to 17–10.

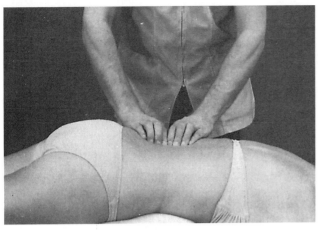

Figure 17–1. The patient is prone, with the lumbar spine in a neutral position. The therapist, with finger tips in a row lateral to the spinous process, uses a pulling motion to stretch the erector spinae muscle mass at right angles to the spine.

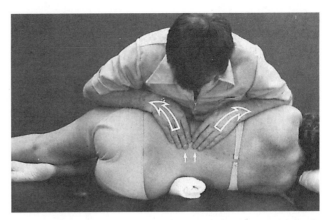

Figure 17–4. The therapist applies outward pressure with both forearms, causing the lumbar spine to arch and stretching the quadratus lumborum and erector spinae muscles. Arching is assisted by placing a roll under the patient's lumbar spine and flexing the patient's bottom hip, and by the therapist pulling up with the fingers on the erector spinae mass.

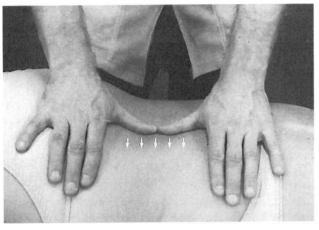

Figure 17–2. This technique uses the same principles as in Figure 17–1. The therapist's thumbs push the opposite erector spinae laterally, at right angles to the spinous processes. A scooping motion of the thumb assists the lateral movement of the muscle.

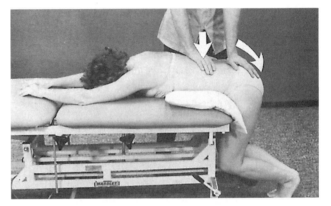

Figure 17–5. While increasing the flexion of the lumbar spine in the prone position, the therapist stabilizes the T12–L1 segment and presses against the patient's sacrum. Further stretch may be achieved by the therapist pushing downward along the patient's thighs.

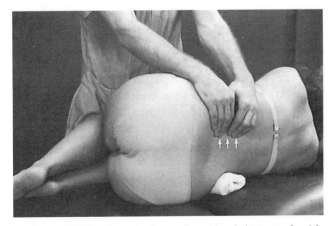

Figure 17–3. The therapist flexes the patient's knees and, with the thighs, pushes against the patient's knees, causing the lumbar spine to flex. With the erector spinae in some degree of stretch, the therapist pulls the erector spinae mass in a transverse direction. Altering pressure on the knees varies the tension on the erector spinae muscle.

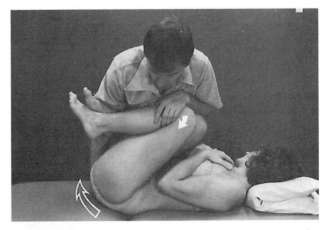

Figure 17–6. The therapist stretches the lumbar extensors by pressing on the patient's knees while simultaneously lifting the patient's sacrum. Further stretch may be achieved by pushing downward along the patient's thighs.

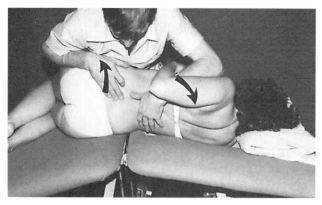

Figure 17–7. Technique to increase extension, left rotation, and right sidebending. A cushion under the waist may be used to produce right sidebending if the bed does not elevate in the middle. As the patient exhales, the therapist pushes the left shoulder and thorax posteriorly and cranially while pulling the left ilium forward and caudally.

Traction

Traction is a combination of distraction and gliding movements between two joints or surfaces. Different types of traction can be applied to the lumbar spine. Often, for the therapist's benefit, a mechanical apparatus is used to achieve the effects of traction. Continuous traction is generally applied for several hours at a time, with minimal weight, and is not considered very effective in causing mechanical separation of the vertebrae.[35] Sustained traction involves shorter periods of constant pull, varying in time for up to one-half hour.[35] A variation is intermittent mechanical traction, in which pressure is applied and released in a rhythmic fashion. Efficiency is increased with the use of a traction table, the caudal half of which is on rollers, thus reducing friction. Manual traction can be

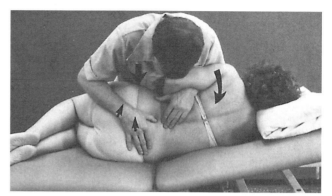

Figure 17–9. Technique to increase flexion and left rotation and sidebending at the L2–L3 level. The pelvis may be stabilized with a belt. As the patient exhales, the therapist pushes the patient's left shoulder and thorax backward. The head of the bed is progressively elevated to sidebend the lumbar spine to the left. Rotation may be enhanced by pulling the right arm and shoulder forward. The pelvis is stabilized between the therapist's chest and forearm and by the therapist's hand over the sacrum. The patient's upper leg may be extended, and a roll may be put under the lower lumbar spine.

used as a treatment technique or in determining the patient's tolerance to traction or finding the most comfortable position in which to apply a traction force (Figs. 17–11 through 17–13).

An alternative method of applying manual traction is vertical adjustive traction[29] (Fig. 17–14).

Three-dimensional traction allows the patient's position to be precisely adjusted by means of pillows, foam wedges, sand bags, or, if available, a three-dimensional mobilization table (Fig. 17–15). Autotraction uses a two-segment traction table that can be individually angled

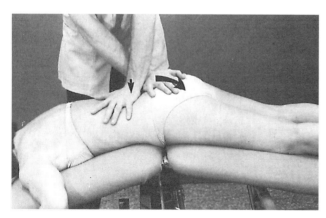

Figure 17–8. Technique to increase the flexion of L5 on S1. The middle of the couch is elevated. A roll may be placed under the abdomen. As the patient exhales, the therapist pushes the sacrum caudally and ventrally. This technique may be used for all the lumbar segments. The therapist's hypothenar eminence stabilizes the proximal lumbar segment.

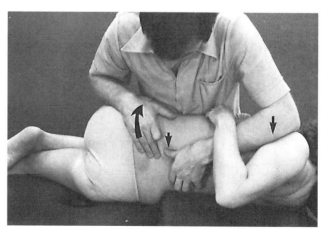

Figure 17–10. Technique to increase flexion and left rotation and sidebending of L5 on S1. The upper lumbar spine is flexed and right sidebent, causing right rotation, thus locking the upper lumbar segments. If the midsection of the bed will not lift, use a roll. As the patient exhales, the therapist pulls the pelvis forward and cranially.

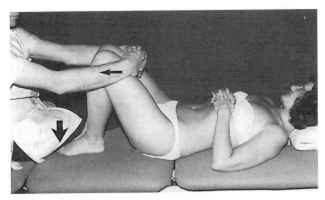

Figure 17–11. Surprisingly effective manual traction may be applied in crook lying through the patient's hips when the therapist leans back. The therapist's thighs fix the patient's feet. The angle of pull may be guided by the patient's response.

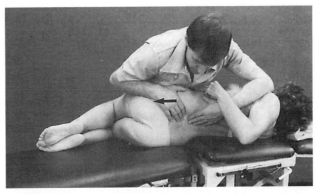

Figure 17–13. Specific distraction in lumbar extension. The patient's pelvis may also be stabilized with a belt. Sidebending of the lumbar spine may be prevented by a pillow if the bed does not lift.

and rotated according to the patient's response as treatment progresses.

Gravity lumbar traction is applied in a variety of ways. In one technique, the patient is tilted up on a circular or elevating bed into an approximately vertical position while at the same time being suspended by a vest around the chest. In this position, the free weight of the legs and hips exerts a traction force on the lumbar spine equal to approximately 40 percent of body weight.[36,37]

Probably the most prevalent type of gravity traction uses inversion boots worn in conjunction with a gravity guider.[38] A variation of this technique uses another apparatus in which the patient bends forward at the waist and is able to hang inverted while being supported on the anterior thighs, with the hips and knees flexed approximately 90 degrees. However, the patients who would benefit the most from this type of treatment are usually in too much pain even to get on the machine.

Strain and Counterstrain

Strain and counterstrain techniques involve putting the joint into the position of greatest comfort, thus relieving pain by reduction and arrest of the continuing inappropriate proprioceptor activity. The tender point is shut off by

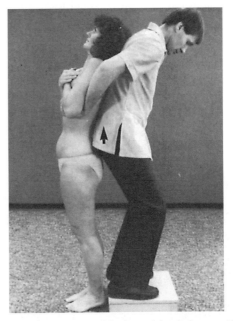

Figure 17–14. The patient is lifted up with relative ease if patient and therapist are of the same height. A small platform may be used to position the therapist's sacral base at the desired level of the patient's lumbar spine. Straightening of the therapist's knees and forward flexion lift the patient off the floor. Traction is exerted by the therapist coming up onto the balls of the feet, then rapidly dropping onto the heels. Different degrees of sidebending or rotation may be used. The patient should be able to extend the lumbar spine; otherwise, the technique may cause discomfort.

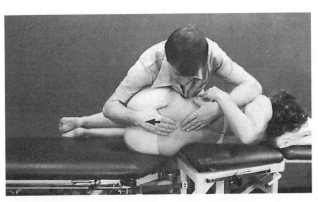

Figure 17–12. Specific distraction in lumbar flexion is facilitated by the use of a mobilization bed to sidebend and by the use of accessories to assist with distraction. The patient's pelvis is stabilized by the therapist's shoulder, chest, forearm, and hand.

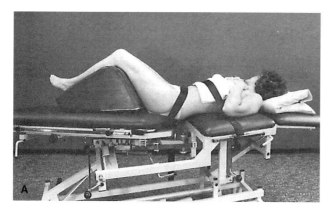

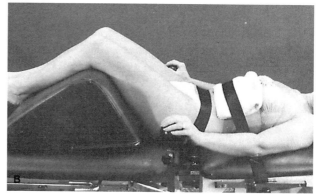

Figure 17–15. (A,B) Different degrees of rotation and sidebending may be incorporated to reduce discomfort. Traction may be applied by the therapist or the patient with the use of appropriate accessories.

markedly shortening the muscle that contains a malfunctioning muscle spindle by applying mild strain to its antagonist[39] (Figs. 17–16 and 17–17).

Strain in this context refers to overstretching of muscles, tendons, ligaments, or fascia, along with the associated altered neuromuscular reflex. Treatment is directed at the neuromuscular reflexes rather than tissue stretching. Generally, the position in which there is spontaneous release of tissue tension assumes that the disorder is unilateral and moves to the position of greatest ease on the abnormally tense side. The position of the patient in the treatment position often mimics the position in which the original strain was experienced. Selected anterior and posterior lumbar dysfunction techniques are illustrated in Figures 17–18 to 17–22.

Functional Techniques

Functional technique is a method of treating joints in which the direction of movement of the joint is that of least resistance and greatest comfort. The technique thus reduces exaggerated spindle responses from facilitated segments of spinal muscles and restores normal joint mobility. The end position is that in which the tensions of tissues around the joint are equal; this position is known as *dynamic neutral.*[40] This technique is similar to that of strain and counterstrain in that the position of spontaneous release is the same, and the direction of movement is toward immediate ease and comfort. However, functional technique differs in that the dynamic neutral concept seeks a balance of tissue tension fairly near the anatomic neutral position (Fig. 17–23). This reduction in tissue

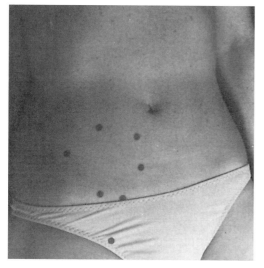

Figure 17–16. Tender points for anterior lower thoracic and lumbar dysfunctions.

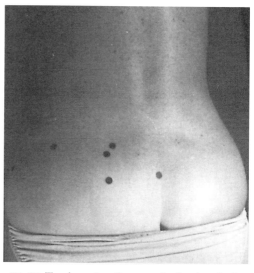

Figure 17–17. Tender points for posterior lumbar dysfunctions.

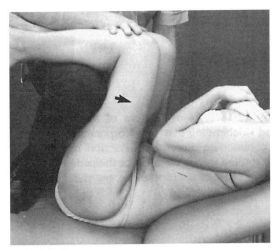

Figure 17–18. Treatment for a forward-bending dysfunction of L1. Flexion of the thoracolumbar junction is assisted by lifting the end of the bed. Further flexion is produced by the therapist's knees against the back of the patient's thigh, with slight rotation of the patient's knee toward the side of tenderness. The position is one of marked flexion, rotation away, and sidebending toward the restriction. The position is held and the tender spot monitored for 90 seconds.

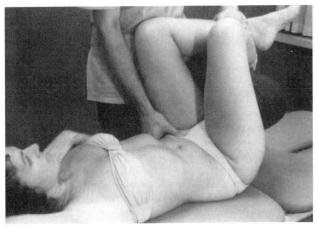

Figure 17–20. Treatment for iliacus dysfunction. A tender point is located in the iliac fossa. The hips are flexed, the ankles crossed, and the thighs externally rotated.

tension is obtained when the spinal segment is put through different physiologic motions that relax or reduce tissue tension. The process of finding the easy physiologic motion, following it until tissue tension starts to decrease, and rechecking may go through one or two directions until a state of equilibrium is found in which tissue texture indicates relaxation or ease of movement. Neurophysiologically, Korr postulated that the segmental resistance to motion may be due to high discharge of the gamma fibers, causing sustained contraction of the intrafusal fi-

bers, which keep the annulospiral endings firing continuously. In the muscle, this maintains high resistance to stretching, and perhaps this is the tension or the bind that is encountered as a segment is moved in a specific direction.[41] The functional technique involves positioning the joint such that the facilitated muscle spindle is shortened, thus reducing its apparent discharge from the primary annulospiral ending. The central nervous system subsequently decreases the gamma motor neuron discharge.[42] The patient's palpable muscular tension provides information to the practitioner regarding what movement is required.[41] In functional techniques, all the possible parameters of movement and direction are used, and the movements that cause and result in the greatest ease are summed and combined to maximize the relaxation of a particular segmental level[30] (Fig. 17–24).

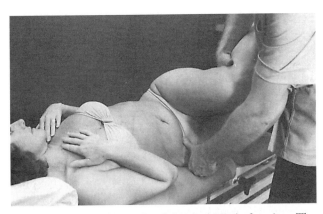

Figure 17–19. Treatment for abdominal L2 dysfunction. The hips are flexed and the pelvis is rotated to the right, and the patient's feet are lifted to the left to sidebend the lumbar spine. Adductor strain can be reduced by slightly lifting behind the upper knee.

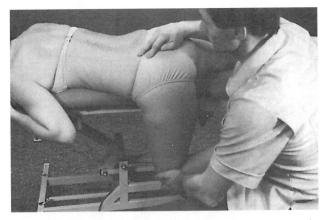

Figure 17–21. Treatment for L5 dysfunction. Approximately 20 degrees of pelvic rotation plus adduction of the thigh reduces the tender spot under the index finger. The third finger marks the posterior superior iliac spine.

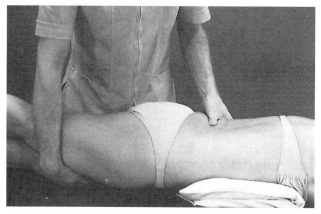

Figure 17–22. Treatment for L3, L4, and L5 dysfunctions. Adduction of the thigh is necessary at all levels. More rotation is needed for L3, whereas L5 requires more extension.

Muscle Energy

The muscle energy technique developed by Fred Mitchell, Sr., involves active, distinct, controlled muscle contraction in a precisely controlled position, in a specific direction, against a distinct counterforce.[43] The aim of muscle energy techniques is to restore the normal neurophysiology of the segment. The guiding principle is that the joint is taken up to the sense of a barrier in the three

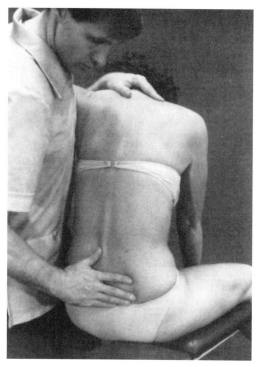

Figure 17–24. End position of a functional treatment technique. The point of greatest tissue relaxation determines the movement and position of the patient.

separate cardinal planes. The therapist resists the isometric contractions of the patient and prevents any actual movement from taking place. Only minimal pressure is necessary, as it is the neurophysiologic effect that is of primary importance in the reduction of abnormal tissue tension in the segment. The position is held momentarily, and after a few seconds, the tension relaxes and the therapist then moves the joint further toward the barrier, which should be found to have moved. When the new barrier has been located, the therapist asks the patient to perform an isometric contraction again while the therapist resists any movement. This procedure is repeated three or four times while the therapist monitors any increase in range of motion and alteration of tissue tension.[44] Selected muscle energy techniques are illustrated in Figures 17–25 to 17–29.

Cranial Techniques

Cranial osteopathy, originally developed by William Sutherland in the early 1900s, embraces the concept that there is mobility between the cranial bones. The rhythmic movement of 6 to 12 cycles per minute is very small but is a measurable 10 to 25 m.[45] Sutherland suggests that distortions in the movement pattern of the cranium, the sacrum, and the dural membrane system can be responsible for signs and symptoms locally and elsewhere.[46] The

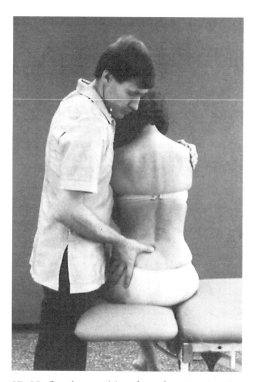

Figure 17–23. Starting position for a functional technique for lumbar dysfunction. The therapist palpates changes in tissue tension with the right thumb.

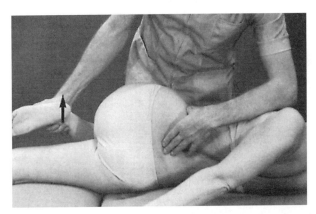

Figure 17–25. Technique for correcting an L5 that is flexed, rotated right, and sidebent right (FRSR). The aim of treatment is to extend, rotate, and sidebend left (ERSL). The patient resists lifting up of the left ankle. The patient may look over the left shoulder to reduce stress on the upper thoracic spine.

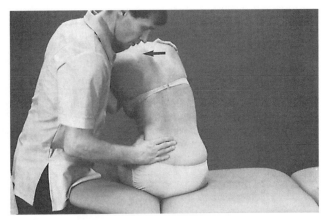

Figure 17–27. Technique for correcting an L4 that is extended, rotated right, and sidebent right in a sitting position. The therapist flexes and rotates the patient to the segment involved; the patient resists sidebending further to the left. The aim of treatment is to flex, rotate, and sidebend left L4.

guiding principles of craniosacral therapy can be listed under five headings:

1. The existence of inherent mobility of the central nervous system (i.e., the brain and spinal cord)
2. Production, resorption, and pulsatility of the cerebrospinal fluid
3. The existence of reciprocal tension membranes, namely, the dura, which forms the periosteum of the cranial vault, attaching to the foramen magnum (C2–C3) and the sacrum (S2); the vertical membranes, the falx cerebri and cerebelli; and a horizontal membrane, the tentorium cerebelli
4. The mobility of the cranial bones around articular axes

5. Mobility of the sacrum between the ilia

To those not familiar with this concept, these principles may seem rather unusual. However, they are palpable phenomena, and documented evidence supports their existence.

The craniosacral rhythmic impulses can be felt throughout the body but are strongest when contact is with the cranial bones, which are the vehicle through which cranial techniques are classically performed. A whole series of holds designed to influence different aspects of the above-listed points has been worked

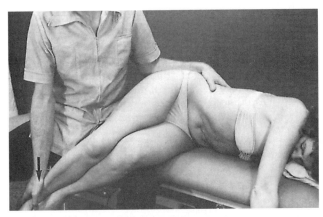

Figure 17–26. Technique for correcting an L5 that is extended, rotated right, and sidebent right (ERSR). The aim of treatment is to flex, rotate, and sidebend left (FRSL). The patient resists pushing down of both feet. The therapist protects the patient's left thigh from the edge of the bed by supporting it with his or her own left thigh.

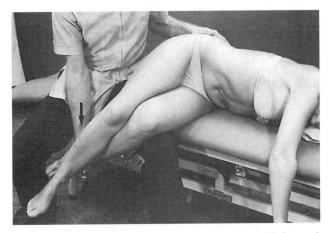

Figure 17–28. Technique for correcting a forward left sacral torsion (L/L). This is an often forgotten technique to restore full function of the L5–S1 segment. The aim of treatment is to restore symmetry and motion to the sacrum by reciprocally inhibiting the right piriformis by contracting the left. The patient resists pushing down with the left leg but allows the right leg to fall in the relaxation phase or to be gently stretched.

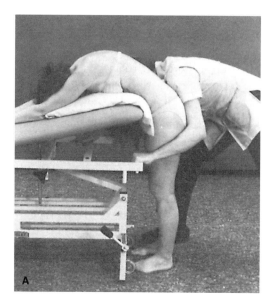

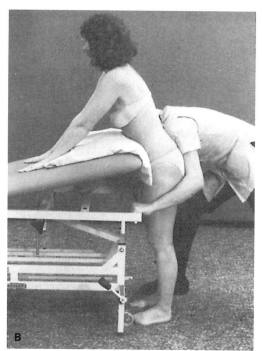

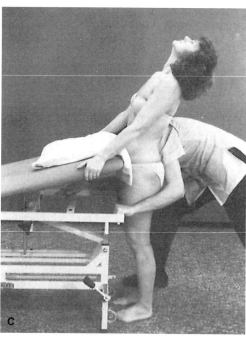

Figure 17–29. An acute sacral torsion is often termed a *bilateral flexed L5*. The patient presents with a significantly kyphotic lumbar spine. Correction is provided by (A) stabilizing the patient's sacrum against the end of the bed and (B) having the patient walk the hands up the bed until (C) an upright position of the lumbar spine is achieved. Two or three attempts may be required. Caution is warranted, as the symptoms are similar to those of an acute lumbar disk prolapse. Clinical examination should differentiate the two conditions.

out.[47] These techniques use fine palpation skills and the specific direction of minute forces to alter osseous or membrane restrictions.[48] They can produce quite specific and sometimes dramatic results in many cases, and they form a very useful addition to the categories of reflex techniques. Adept practitioners can successfully treat many seemingly remote symptoms, such as headaches caused by a lumbar sacral lesion or restriction, as well as local symptoms originating from a craniosacral dysfunction.[30]

■ Indications for Treatment

After the history taking and the usual review of medical information such as medication and radiographic reports, a decision must be made concerning what approach or direction should be taken with respect to treatment. In some situations, such as joint hypomobility caused by sprains or surgery in which some form of splinting or casting is involved, the choice and direction of treatment may seem fairly obvious.

□□□□□ □ □ □

Table 17–1. Common Nonradicular Spondylogenic Reflex Syndromes

Syndrome	References
Referred pain	Kellgren,[70,71] Sinclair et al.,[72] Hockaday and Whitty[73]
Myofascial trigger points	Melzack,[74,75] Reynolds,[76] Rubin,[77] Simons,[56,57] Travell and Rinzler,[78] Travell[79,80]
Pseudoradicular	Brugger[58,59,81,82]
Tender points	Mitchell et al.,[44] Jones,[39] Hoover,[40] Lewit[83]
Spondylogenic reflexes	Sutter,[62] Maigne,[69] Caviezel,[84,85] Sell,[86] Jones[39]

(Data from Dvorak and Dvorak.[68])

Neurophysiologic Indications

In some situations, however, no specific pathology can be identified. Often the term *syndrome* is used, implying a certain diagnostic vagueness, and frequently is characterized by several approaches to treatment.[49] It is well known that it is extremely difficult, if not impossible, to make a precise diagnosis in many cases of low back pain.[50-54]

Empirical observations of the nonradicular pain syndromes have been gaining more importance through the experimental neurophysiologic work of Korr, Simons, and Wyke.[17,19,55-57] Different authors, with their own language and terminology reflecting their own opinion or school of thought, often describe the same somatic phenomenon (e.g., Brugger,[58,59] Feinstein et al.,[60] Hohermuth,[61] Jones,[39] Mitchell et al.,[44] Hoover,[40] Sutter,[62] Sutter and Frohlich,[63] and Waller[64] (Table 17–1). The result of this diversity of terminology and theories is that these valuable clinical observations have found limited diagnostic use in mainstream medicine.[65-68] However, these observations together indicate that the reflex is mediated through the reflexogenic pathways of the central nervous system and is the reproducible, causative factor linking the skeletal segmental dysfunction and the soft tissue changes. These have been described by Maigne[69] as "derangements intervertebrales mineurs." Causes of the segmental dysfunction with its consequential soft tissue changes include trauma, muscle imbalance, uncoordinated or sudden movement, chronic strain, and degenerative joint changes.[87]

However, not all syndromes with respect to low back pain are so controversial. Experience plus awareness of the literature facilitates the therapist's choice of approach in managing somatic dysfunction. Often the neurophysiologic approach seemingly may be less appropriate in light of a more direct or mechanical means of treatment.

Mechanical Indications

McKenzie[11] describes "three syndromes that have characteristics, definition, causes of development, clinic presentation, and specific treatment procedures." He proposes that uncomplicated mechanical spinal pain is caused by mechanical deformation of soft tissues containing nociceptive receptors.

Postural Syndrome

Patients are usually younger than the age of 30 years, have sedentary occupations, and often do not exercise regularly. Pain is never produced by movement and is never referred or constant. There is no loss of range of motion and no pathology, and there are no signs on examination. The pain is due to the mechanical deformation or prolonged stretching of normal spinal tissue, probably ligamentous, causing stimulation of the nociceptors.

Dysfunction Syndrome

The patient is usually older than 30 years of age (unless trauma is the cause), generally exhibits poor posture, and frequently lacks exercise. Pain is always felt at the end range of motion, never during motion, and unless there is an adherent nerve root, pain is never referred. Loss of range of motion—loss of extension is the most frequent—is generally due to long-standing poor posture causing adaptive shortening or contracture of fibrous tissue, which forms an inextensible scar. Pain results immediately from the stretching of the inextensible but unidentifiable shortened tissue, causing deformation of the nociceptors. Selected techniques to increase extension of the lumbar spine are illustrated in Figures 17–30 to 17–36.

Derangement Syndrome

Patients are usually 30 to 50 years of age, have poor sitting posture, and often experience an acute onset of

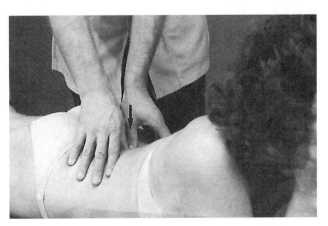

Figure 17–30. Specific posteroanterior central pressure to increase extension.

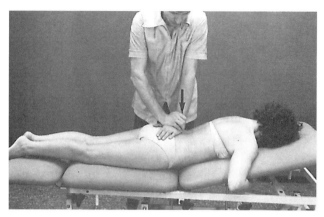

Figure 17–31. Specific extension mobilization with the pisiform. As mobility increases, the end of the bed may be elevated farther.

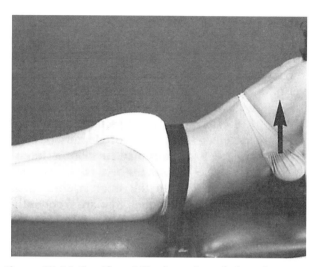

Figure 17–34. Specific stabilization using a belt as the patient attempts extension.

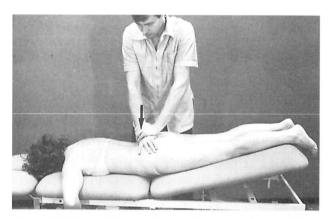

Figure 17–32. Specific extension mobilization with the pisiform as a contact. The caudal end of the bed is elevated as much as mobility allows.

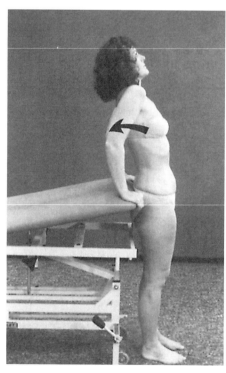

Figure 17–35. Nonspecific extension over the end of the bed. Be sure that the patient's knees do not flex.

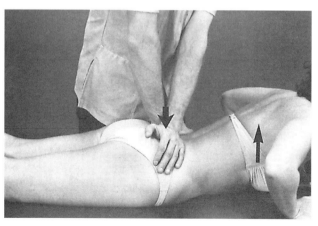

Figure 17–33. Specific stabilization over the transverse processes as the patient attempts extension.

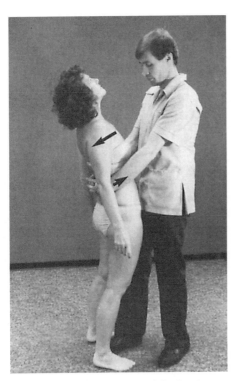

Figure 17–36. Specific stabilization of the lumbar segment by the therapist's hypothenar eminences. Extension may be assisted by pulling forward with the hands as the patient leans back. The patient's pelvis is stabilized by the therapist's thigh.

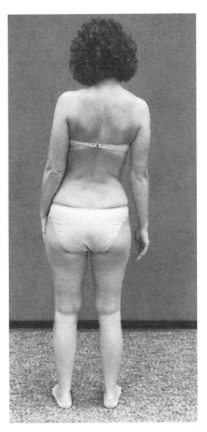

Figure 17–37. Typical presentation in which the lumbar spine is shifted slightly to the right.

pain for no apparent reason. Symptoms may be painful and localized or may be referred in the form of pain, paresthesia, or numbness. The symptoms usually are directly affected by certain movements and postures; therefore, a discogenic origin must be considered. Although the pain may fluctuate in intensity, it is usually fairly constant because of the anatomic disturbance within the intervertebral disk complex. Selected techniques that are frequently successful in treating derangement syndrome in the clinic are illustrated in Figures 17–37 to 17–46.

Mobilization

A joint is usually suitable for treatment if the symptoms are aggravated by certain movements or postures and relieved by rest or other movements or positions.[88] The patient may not always present with true articulatory signs; however, the symptoms generally respond to mobilization techniques.

Visceral pathology may cause spinal pain, but this pain is not typically aggravated by spinal movement. Manual therapy techniques are either contraindicated or of no value.

The degree of intensity of mobilization depends on the examination findings and has an almost direct relationship to the number of factors assessed. Observation of the patient and the history will indicate the necessity of a gentle approach. Such findings, as indicated by Grieve,[88] are the following:

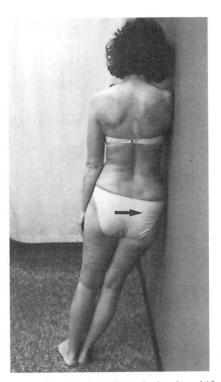

Figure 17–38. Self-correction of a right lumbar shift. Alternatively, the patient may stand in a doorway and let the pelvis sag to the right.

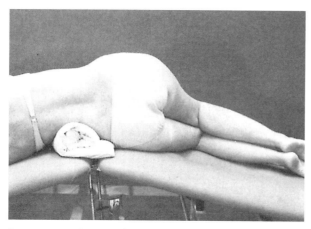

Figure 17–39. Positional traction in the side-lying position to correct a right lumbar shift to the left.

Much joint irritability

Severe pain accompanying all movements

Severe pain in certain postures

Severe limb pain

Interruption of sleep

Protective spasm

Long-standing severe pain

Distal pain produced by coughing and sneezing.

The examination reveals the following:

Facial distortion caused by increased pain on movement

Distal limb pain on spinal movement

Increased pain or paresthesia after testing

Increased spasm

Distal pain or paresthesia with gentle pressure

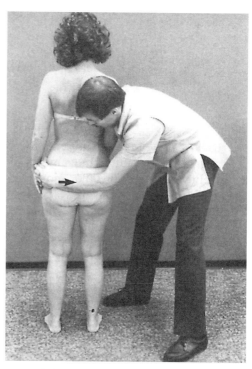

Figure 17–41. The therapist assists in correcting a right-deviated lumbar spine. This technique is not recommended because it involves poor body mechanics by the therapist, and frequently the stabilization provided by the therapist's shoulder is too high.

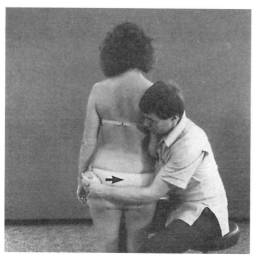

Figure 17–40. The therapist assists in correcting a right-deviated spine. The therapist stabilizes with the shoulder while pulling on the patient's pelvis. A slow, constant pull is most beneficial. A slight overcorrection may be needed.

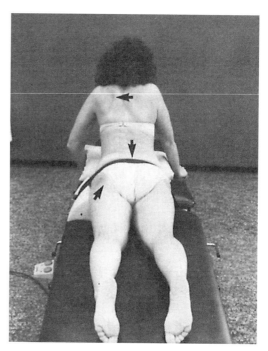

Figure 17–42. Correction of a right-deviated lumbar spine in the prone position. The technique is assisted by belt stabilization, a foam wedge under the hip opposite the deviation, and extending to the left when pressing up. If a three-dimensional mobilization bed is used instead, it may be adjusted accordingly.

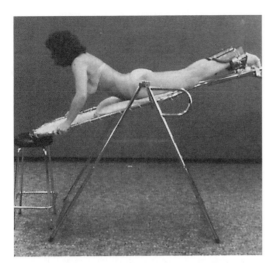

Figure 17–43. Extension exercises with the assistance of progressive inversion for reducing persistent pain.

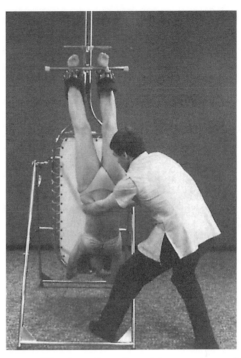

Figure 17–45. The therapist assists with extension and correction for a right-deviated lumbar spine with persisting referred pain to the left.

Presence of a neurologic deficit

Increased pain after minimal examination

Obviously, more vigorous mobilization may commence on reassessment when there is reduced or minimal spasm, pain, paresthesia, or distal symptoms as a result of previous examination and treatments. The indications and steps for progression of treatment have been meticulously set out by Grieve.[88] The importance of a thorough and efficient examination cannot be overemphasized.

Manipulation

Manipulation is a natural progression from a grade IV mobilization if the maximum improvement in signs and symptoms has not been achieved. Manipulation is of benefit if there are no articular signs but only hypomobility

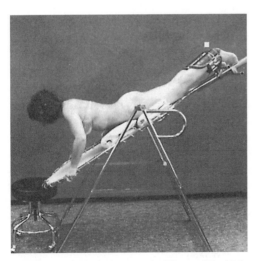

Figure 17–44. Same technique as in Figure 17–43 but with more inversion. If the pain is to one side, extension exercises accommodating for unilateral pain may be helpful.

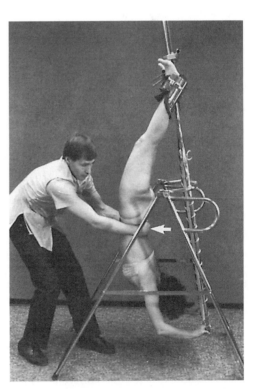

Figure 17–46. The therapist assists with extension of the lumbar spine with persisting central pain.

of the segment and if minimal pain does not appear until near the end of the range of motion.

The clinical difficulty in the selection of patients for manipulation is partly due to a lack of clear understanding of pathogenesis and of objective examination techniques, as well as differing intentions with regard to manipulation. There appear to be five different philosophies regarding the effects of manipulation and thus five differing purposes. These consist of (1) the mobilizing or oscillating techniques, affecting soft tissue; (2) osteopathy, concerned with restoration of joint motion; (3) chiropractic, concerned with putting a vertebra that is "out" back in place; (4) the desire of laymen and bonesetters to cause a "click" in the joint when it is manipulated; and (5) Cyriax techniques, affecting the disk or a loose fragment of the disk. Although each school of thought has its degrees of success, a thorough examination with an understanding of anatomy will result in greater consistency of success than the blind following of a particular doctrine. Regardless of ideology, clinically certain conditions seem to benefit from the application of manipulative techniques.[89]

Uncomplicated Low Back Pain

Patients who develop uncomplicated low back pain of recent onset in the absence of radicular signs were found to be more responsive to manipulation than to a placebo treatment.[90] In a further study by Bergquist-Ullman and Larsson,[91] they were found to respond most favorably if their onset of symptoms was less than 9 days before treatment. Potter[92] also noted that patients with acute low back pain had the highest rate of improvement (93 percent) after manipulation.

Complicated Acute Low Back Pain

Patients with acute onset of low back pain complicated by leg pain or neurologic symptoms appeared to respond very well to spinal manipulation.[93,94] Both Potter[92] and Edwards[95] found that more than 75 percent of patients with pain radiating into the buttock or down into the leg recovered or improved considerably after spinal manipulation. Buerger,[96] in a blind clinical trial, showed that a painful limited straight leg raise was shown to improve after manipulation. Many practitioners, however, become very cautious when frank neurologic deficit or signs of such a deficit are present.[93,97] Research has indicated that patients with neurologic signs who have been subjected to spinal manipulation have not experienced rewarding results.[92,98]

Uncomplicated Chronic Low Back Pain

By definition, patients with uncomplicated chronic low back pain are not recovering spontaneously. Potter showed that although improvement in this group was less than in the group of patients with uncomplicated low back pain, 71 percent showed improvement of their symptoms.[92] A similar study by Riches[99] indicates that improvement occurs in as many as 86 percent. The results of another study by Kirkaldy-Willis and Cassidy[100] showed considerable variation, depending on the pathogenic diagnosis. However, 65 percent of patients showed some degree of improvement.[100]

Complicated Chronic Low Back Pain

Manipulation of patients with complicated chronic low back pain yielded results similar to those in patients with complicated acute pain, that is, the likelihood of a successful treatment decreased considerably when neurologic signs were present.[92] It was noted, however, that previous back surgery did not appear to play a significant role in the outcome of treatment and was not considered a contraindication to manipulation.

Disk Degeneration and Herniation

The causative effect of spinal manipulation on intervertebral disk dysfunction is very controversial. Such authors as Cyriax,[97] as well as Matthews and Yates,[101] claim that manipulation seems to have some beneficial effect on the intervertebral disk. Chrisman and associates,[98] as well as Kirkaldy-Willis and Cassidy,[100] were unable to achieve favorable results in patients who demonstrated lumbar disk protrusion. In light of this controversy, manipulation is often used on those patients diagnosed as having a degenerative disk without frank herniation or neurologic deficits.[29,97,102]

Facet Syndrome

Many practitioners believe that the primary effect of manipulation is on a fixated or blocked facet joint.[7,103,104] However, it appears that the basis for this belief is merely that there is an increase in mobility of the spine after manipulation.

Sacroiliac Syndromes

If the diagnosis is one of sacroiliac syndrome, manipulation appears to be a very effective treatment.[99,100] Many practitioners place a great deal of emphasis on the ability to analyze sacroiliac motion, or lack thereof, and choose an appropriate manipulative technique according to their findings.[105-107] Kirkaldy-Willis and Cassidy[100] and Riches[99] claim that more than 90 percent of patients with this diagnosis show improvement after manipulation.

Spondylolisthesis

Kirkaldy-Willis and Cassidy and associates found that they were able to reduce back pain in 85 percent of their cases.[100,108] However, they made it quite clear that spinal manipulation did not influence the spondylolisthesis itself but rather that spondylolisthesis was an incidental finding. In the study by Cassidy et al.,[108] great care was taken to ensure that manipulative forces were minimized at the level of instability and were aimed at the sacroiliac joints or the facet joints at a higher level.

Spinal Stenosis

Kirkaldy-Willis and Cassidy[100] and Potter[109] reported that a significant number of patients with lateral or central spinal stenosis experienced some improvement after manipulation. Very few of these patients ever became symptom-free, which is not surprising, and often relief was only temporary.[110]

Whatever the diagnosis or etiology, the objective remains the same: restoration of full, painless joint motion. Faulty mechanics prevent normal function, leading in turn to compensatory mechanisms. A functional diagnosis based on mechanical faults is more pertinent than a static positional evaluation.[111] When the body's adaptive potential both locally and regionally is exhausted, dysfunction ensues. Goldthwait et al.[112] were among the first to recognize a link between faulty mechanics and disease.

■ Principles and Rules of Mobilization and Manipulation

Regardless of the profession, nationality, or school of thought, all rational treatment must have a reasoned basis. The following list summarizes the principles and rules of procedures offered by such notable clinicians as Grieve, Maitland, Cyriax, Stoddard, and others.[8,9,26,97,113] The order of presentation is not an indication of relative significance.

Remember contraindications and conditions requiring extra care.

Do no harm to the patient—or to yourself.

A thorough, structured examination is fundamental.

Make as accurate a diagnosis as possible based on a solid knowledge of anatomy.

All pain arises from a lesion.

For treatment to be effective, it must reach the lesion.

Constantly reassess to determine the effect of the techniques being used.

Progress is governed by the response to previous treatment.

Discontinue techniques that are not productive.

Use the minimum amount of force consistent with achieving the objective.

If possible, use the patient's own weight to do the work.

Get the patient to relax; reduce the patient's anxiety and fear.

Timing is essential in the application of a technique so that the effects of its different components will be cumulative.

Do not force through a protective muscle spasm.

A slight alteration of joint position or angle of thrust often allows a technique to be much more effective.

In general, manipulate only if the expected degree of improvement is not being achieved with mobilization.

Warn patients of the potential for posttreatment soreness.

Do not overtreat; stop when symptoms abate.

Aim for restoration of normal, painless mobility.

■ Prevention of Complications

The main factors to consider with respect to prevention of complications are diagnostic assessment and procedural cautions that reduce the risk of complications from manipulation.

Assessment

The diagnostic assessment includes a patient history, physical examination, and radiologic examination.

History

The history is probably the most underrated portion of the examination. The significance and necessary detail of a case history have been discussed by Mennell,[7] Stoddard,[114] Maigne,[94] Matthews,[115] and many others.

Physical Examination

The importance of a complete physical examination is recognized when conditions such as abdominal aneurysms, occlusive vascular disease, hypertension, elevated temperature, prostatic enlargement, and abnormal lymph nodes are found.[116]

Radiologic Examination

Radiographs should always be obtained to rule out contraindications (e.g., underlying overt disease). The absence of either a thorough clinical examination or a radiologic examination is an overriding contraindication for manipulation.[116]

Procedures

The most common and important accident to prevent in the lumbar spine is the rupture of the intervertebral disk, with resultant cauda equina syndrome, characterized by paralysis, weakness, pain, reflex changes, and bowel and bladder disturbances.[116-118] Reports indicate that an uncomplicated herniated disk can be reduced by manipulation, possibly as a result of centripetal force.[97,101,119] Manipulation can, however, aggravate the symptoms when serious disk lesions are present.

The following screening tests, described in detail by Kleynhans and Terrett,[116] reduce the risk of disk rupture from lumbar spine manipulation:

> Straight leg raise (Laseque/buckling sign)
>
> Well leg raise (Laseque contralateral/crossed Laseque)
>
> Deyerle's sciatic tension test (bowstring test)
>
> Prone knee flexion test
>
> Dejerine's triad (coughing, sneezing, Valsalva's test)

■ Precautions

Although the following are not absolute contraindications, prudence and care must be observed in their presence.[119]

Mobilization

Mobilization procedures should be undertaken with caution in the presence of any of the following:

> Neurologic signs: avoid procedures that reduce the intervertebral foramen on the painful side.
>
> Rheumatoid arthritis: mobilization may be performed if there is no acute inflammation and if bone consistency is kept in mind.
>
> Osteoporosis: approximately 40 percent of bone structure is lost before osteoporosis becomes radiologically evident.
>
> Spondylolithesis: when treating adjacent levels, avoid stressing the level of instability.
>
> Previous malignant disease: if possible, rule out the presence of metastasis.
>
> Hypermobility.
>
> Pregnancy.

Manipulation

Some of the more common restricted indications for manipulation appear in Table 17–2.[116]

■ Causes of Complications

Complications resulting from manipulations may be related to either the practitioner or the patient.

Practitioner-Related Complications

Practitioner-related complications may result from diagnostic errors. Medical practitioners often do not have the diagnostic skills necessary to prescribe manipulations.[139] A thorough knowledge of tissue structure and of the conditions that cause signs and symptoms is necessary.[140] It must be remembered that referral by a physician does not necessarily mean that manipulation should be performed. The final decision concerning the indications, contraindications, technique, and execution of manipulation rests with the practitioner and cannot be made by referral.[122] A radiologic examination is a necessary part of the patient's assessment; diagnostic errors may result if it is omitted.[141]

Another possible cause of complications is the practitioner's lack of skill. A practitioner with excellent diagnostic ability but with inadequate training and inferior skills in mechanical diagnosis is just as great a threat to the safe practice of manipulation as are unqualified manipulators who lack diagnostic expertise.[82,142-144] The literature lists many cases of death or damage in which lack of skill and experience led to the use of brute force.[123,142,145,146]

The application of manipulation without any formal training is probably one of the greatest problems in manipulation. Reading a textbook or attending a weekend course does not make one a skilled practitioner of manipulation. As with any other skilled procedure, the results and complications depend on the ability of the clinician. Absence of manipulative skills on the practitioner's part should be a contraindication to manipulation.[89]

A third cause of practitioner-related complications is lack of interprofessional consultation. One situation in which this is especially important involves the patient on anticoagulant therapy because of the increased risk of hemorrhage.[147] Heparin, because of its anticoagulant and lipid-clearing characteristics, is widely used for the treatment of coronary artery disease, myocardial infarction, and venous thrombosis, in conjunction with vascular surgery, and as a prophylaxis against thromboembolism in pregnancy. Heparin-associated osteoporosis with resulting weakness, fracture, and pain is a well-documented entity.[148]

Patient-Related Complications

Other causes of complications stem from the patients themselves. Examples of patients in whom treatment is prone to complications include the following:

1. Patients with psychological intolerance of pain or discomfort.[94,114,149]
2. Patients in whom minimal stress causes a disproportionate vasoconstrictive response (this reaction can be enhanced in emotionally unstable individuals).[150]
3. Patients with an excessive pain response because of ethnic background or certain conditions that preclude manipulation.[94,149,151]

□□□□□□ □ □

Table 17–2. Relative Contraindications to Manipulation

Condition	References
Articular derangements	
Ankylosing spondylitis after the acute stage	Bollier,[120] Rinsky et al.,[121] Sandoz and Lorenz,[122] Stoddard[114]
Articular deformity	Cyriax[97]
Basilar impression	Kaiser[125]
Congenital anomalies	Grillo,[124] Janse,[125] Maigne,[94] Sandoz,[126] Valentini,[127] Yochum[128]
Hypertrophic spondyloarthritis	
Osteoarthritis	Sandoz and Lorenz[122]
Osteochondrosis with defective "holding apparatus"	Stoddard[114]
Bone weakening and modifying disease	
Hemangioma	Siehl[129]
Paget's disease	Sandoz and Lorenz,[122] Nwuga,[5] Lindner[130]
Scheuermann's disease	Beyeler,[131] Hauberg,[132] Janse,[125] Maigne,[94] Nwuga[5]
Spondylolisthesis, spondylolysis	Hauberg,[132] Sandoz and Lorenz[122]
Disk lesion	
Posterolateral and posteromedial disk protrusions	
Degenerative disease	Jaquet,[133] Odom,[134] Stoddard[114]
Neurologic dysfunction	
Myelopathy	Cyriax,[97] Stoddard[114]
Dysfunction of nonvertebral origin	Nwuga,[5] Stoddard[114]
Pyramidal tract involvement	Cyriax[97]
Radicular pain from disk lesion	Gutmann,[135] Stoddard[114]
Viscerosomatic reflex pain	Gutmann,[135] Nwuga,[5] Stoddard[114]
Unclassified	
Abdominal hernia	Sandoz and Lorenz[122]
Asthma	Beyeler,[131] Sandoz[136]
Basilar ischemia	Bourdillon,[137] Cyriax,[97] Nwuga[5]
Dysmenorrhea	Sandoz[136]
Epicondylitis	Droz[138]
Postspinal operations	Nwuga[5]
Peptic ulcer	Janse[125]
Pregnancy	Cyriax,[97] Nwuga,[5] Sandoz and Lorenz[122]
Scoliosis	Stoddard[114]
Lumbar spine	
Accessory sacroiliac joints	
Baastrup's disease	Maigne,[94] Grillo[124]
Cleft vertebra in the sagittal plane	Grillo[124]
Facet tropism	Grillo,[124] Janse[125]
Knife clasp syndrome	
Nuclear impression	Grillo[124]
Pseudosacralization	Grillo,[124] Janse[125]
Sacralization, lumbarization	Grillo,[124] Janse[125]
Spina bifida occulta	Janse[125]
Spondylolisthesis	Janse[125]

4. Patients in whom uncomplicated sciatica becomes a unilateral radiculopathy with distal paralysis of limbs, sensory loss in the sacral distribution, and sphincter paralysis; these patients do not respond to manipulation and should be considered a surgical emergency.[152]
5. Patients who develop a psychological dependence on manipulation. This is not uncommon, and the therapist must decide on the importance of the inevitable physical signs that any spine may produce, as treatments are doomed to failure if the patient is allowed to orient his or her neurosis around the spine.
6. Patients who have recently undergone treatments with another practitioner. Enough time must be allowed for latent symptoms to develop or reactions to settle down.
7. Patients in whom, on examination, the signs and symptoms do not match. Experienced practitioners often encounter situations in which there is no direct or obvious contraindication, but the practitioner develops an intuition that manipulation should not be attempted.
8. Patients involved in litigation.

■ Contraindications

Mobilization

Grieve[119] suggests the following contraindications to mobilization:

1. Malignancy involving the vertebral column
2. Cauda equina lesions producing disturbances of bladder and/or bowel function
3. Signs and symptoms of
   a. Spinal cord involvement
   b. Involvement of more than one spinal nerve root on one side or two adjacent roots in one lower limb alone
4. Rheumatoid collagen necrosis of vertebral ligaments; the cervical spine is especially vulnerable
5. Active inflammatory and infective arthritis
6. Bone disease of the spine

Manipulation

Besides the contraindications listed in Table 17–3, Grieve[88] also lists the following:

1. Evidence of involvement of more than two adjacent nerve roots in the lumbar spine
2. Lower limb neurologic symptoms caused by cervical or thoracic joint dysfunction
3. Undiagnosed pain
4. Protective joint spasm
5. Segments adjacent to the level being manipulated that are too irritable or hypermobile to allow stress to be applied for positioning before or during manipulation

6. Inability of the patient to relax
7. Rubbery end-feel of the joint

Inversion Therapy

The use of inversion therapy or gravity traction is not without risks. Certain conditions or situations must be addressed, and may restrict or preclude the use of inversion therapy in conjunction with manual techniques. Elevation of blood pressure, especially ophthalmic arterial pressure, increases the risk of subconjunctival and retinal hemorrhage.[155] Patients with a history of hypertension, cardiovascular disease, or stroke are at especially high risk.[155-158] Other pertinent factors include cardiac arrhythmias, heart murmurs, diabetes, thyroid problems, hiatal hernia, migraine headaches, glaucoma, asthma, sinusitis, recent surgery, and artificial joints.[159]

The same principles and rules promulgated for other manual procedures apply. A gradual increase in the degree of inversion, as well as its duration, will allow the patient to become familiar with and accommodate to the unusual feeling and the physiologic changes, thus reducing certain risks. Further study is required on the influence of gravitational stress on cardiovascular regulation during inversion therapy.[160]

■ Mobilization and Manipulation Techniques

Manual therapy is both a diagnostic and a treatment approach to somatic disorders. The choice of a treatment technique not only depends on the proper analysis of spinal mechanics, which involves exacting palpatory skills, but also must be suited to the patient's age, physical type, and general state of health, as well as the therapist's size, strength, weight, and manual dexterity.

It is impossible to illustrate every technique or even all the variations of a single basic technique. Many of the procedures selected are classic ones and are used by many disciplines. The variations of these techniques can be easily and successfully applied in the clinical situation.

There is an increasing awareness of the neurophysiologic component in addition to the mechanical effect of manual therapy. This awareness is reflected in Table 17–1 and by the recognition on the part of many clinicians of these seemingly unorthodox treatment approaches.

The use of arrows in Figures 17–47 to 17–69 gives a general indication of the direction of manipulation. Keep in mind individual anatomic variations and that most joint motion occurs in a curvilinear plane.

□□□□□□ □ □

Table 17-3. Contraindications for Manipulation

Condition	References
Articular derangements	
Arthritides	
Acute arthritis of any type	Hauberg,[132] Janse,[125] Maigne,[94] Maitland,[9] Stoddard,[114] Yochum,[128] Haldeman,[89] Grieve[88]
Rheumatoid arthritis	Bourdillon,[137] Janse,[125] Maigne,[94] Stoddard,[114] Yochum,[128] Grieve,[88] Haldeman[89]
Acute ankylosing spondylitis	Bollier,[120] Droz,[138] Hauberg,[132] Janse,[125] Nwuga,[5] Stoddard,[114] Haldeman,[89] Grieve[88]
Hypermobility	Gutmann,[135] Kaltenborn,[26] Maitland,[9] Stoddard,[114] Grieve,[88] Haldeman[89]
Bone weakening and destructive disease	
Calvé's disease	Lindner[130]
Fracture	Gutmann,[135] Heilig,[153] Maigne,[94] Nwuga,[5] Rinsky et al.,[121] Siehl,[129] Stoddard,[114] Haldeman[89]
Malignancy (primary or secondary)	Bourdillon,[137] Gutmann,[135] Maigne,[94] Maitland,[9] Nwuga,[5] Timbrell-Fisher,[154] Stoddard,[114] Grieve,[88] Haldeman[89]
Osteomalacia	Lindner[130]
Osteoporosis	Bollier,[120] Bourdillon,[137] Maigne,[94] Nwuga,[5] Siehl,[129] Stoddard,[114] Grieve,[88] Haldeman[89]
Osteomyelitis	Hauberg,[132] Nwuga,[5] Sandoz and Lorenz,[122] Stoddard[114]
Tuberculosis (Pott's disease)	Bourdillon,[137] Hauberg,[132] Maigne,[94] Siehl,[129] Stoddard,[114] Timbrell-Fisher[154]
Disk lesions	
Prolapse with serious neurologic changes (including cauda equina syndrome)	Bourdillon,[137] Cyriax,[97] Hooper,[118] Jaquet,[133] Jennett,[152] Nwuga,[5] Odom,[134] Stoddard,[114] Haldeman,[89] Grieve[88]
Neurologic dysfunction	
Micturition with sacral root involvement	Cyriax,[97] Stoddard,[114] Haldeman,[89] Grieve[88]
Painful movement in all directions	Maigne[24]
Unclassified	
Infectious disease	Maigne,[94] Nwuga[5]
Patient intolerance	Maigne,[94] Lescure[148]

(Modified from Haldeman,[161] with permission.)

Mobilization Techniques: Flexion

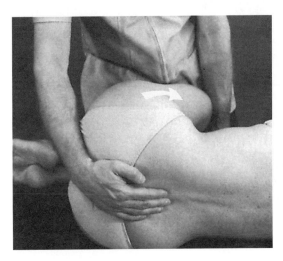

Figure 17–47. One of the basic positions for applying lumbar flexion. The patient's knees rest on the therapist's abdomen, and the therapist's left hand guides the knees into flexion as the therapist sidebends or sways at the hips. The fingers of the therapist's right hand palpate the interspaces for movement.

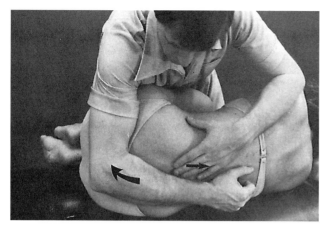

Figure 17–48. Very strong flexion is applied by a combination of full hip flexion and a strong pull with the therapist's right forearm against a firm pull by the therapist's left hand on a spinous process. Strain on the therapist's back is reduced by leaning on the patient's left hip, which assists in stabilization. The therapist must adopt a wide stance.

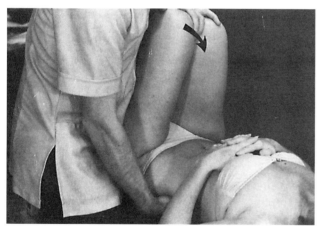

Figure 17–49. Suitable techniques for thin subjects. The therapist flexes the patient's hips with the left hand. The therapist's right hand may palpate the intraspinous process or stabilize the spinous process.

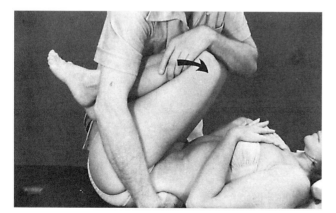

Figure 17–50. Fairly forceful flexion may be applied by the therapist leaning on the patient's knees. The therapist guides with the left hand and palpates or stabilizes with the right.

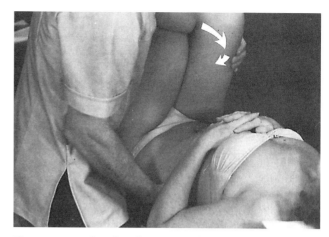

Figure 17–51. Crossing the patient's knees induces slight side-bending; the therapist's left hand adds flexion. The right hand palpates or stabilizes the spinous process.

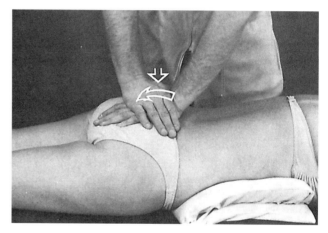

Figure 17–52. The therapist applies firm ventral pressure over the sacrum and then applies a rocking motion caudally to flex the lumbosacral joint. A pillow under the patient's abdomen is recommended.

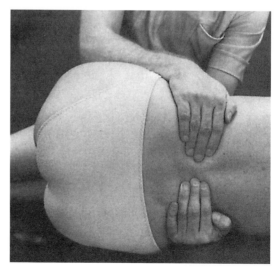

Figure 17–53. The patient's knees are pushed toward the pelvis as the therapist pulls ventrally on the lumbar segment, causing extension.

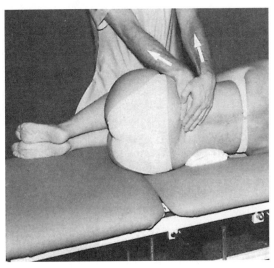

Figure 17–54. An alternative method for extending the lumbar spine. This method is not as forceful or localized as that shown in Figure 17–53.

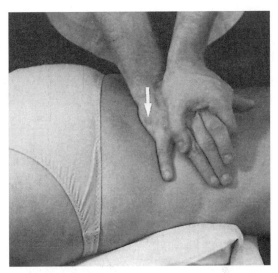

Figure 17–56. Specific extension over the spinous process with the pisiform bone of one hand, reinforced by the other hand. The therapist's arms are straight. Note the quality and quantity of movement of each lumbar segment.

Selected Sidebending Techniques

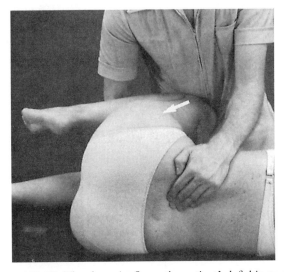

Figure 17–55. The therapist flexes the patient's left hip to approximately a right angle and supports the patient's knee with the abdomen and right forearm. The therapist pushes along the patient's thigh, pushing the left side of the pelvis back and causing extension and left rotation of the lumbar vertebrae. Stabilization can be provided by placing the thumb against the side of the spinous process, or the fingers may palpate for mobility.

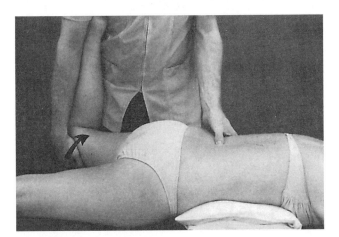

Figure 17–57. Specific technique to assess or increase left side-bending of the lumbar segment with the patient prone. The therapist's thumb palpates the lateral aspect of the interspinous space. Lumbar spine extension may be increased without the use of a pillow. The therapist steadies the patient's leg and knee with a firm grip while abducting the patient's hip beyond its physiologic barrier.

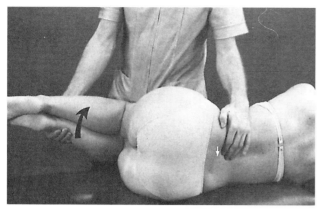

Figure 17–58. Specific technique to assess or increase left side-bending in the side-lying position. The patient's knees are supported by the therapist's abdomen or groin. The therapist palpates the lateral aspect of the interspinous space while lifting up on the patient's leg above the ankle.

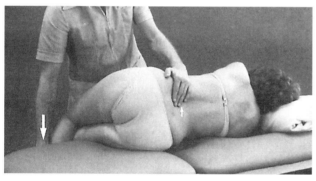

Figure 17–59. Specific technique to assess or increase right side-bending. While pushing down on the patient's legs, the therapist palpates for interspinous movement or stabilizes the lateral aspect of the spinous process. Note the degree of sidebending that can be produced by increased downward movement of the patient's legs. The edge of the bed on the patient's lower thigh may be uncomfortable.

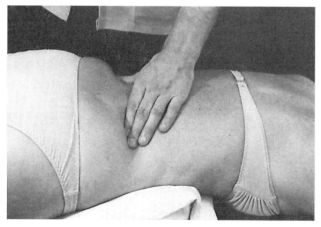

Figure 17–60. Basic hand position used to apply side-to-side rocking of a lumbar segment. The thumb and index finger are over the transverse process of the vertebrae.

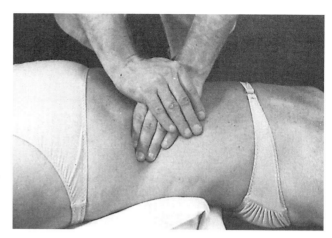

Figure 17–61. With support from the other hand, the therapist rocks the lumbar segment from side to side. Pressure is applied to attempt a lateral shift motion rather than sidebending.

Selected Rotation Techniques

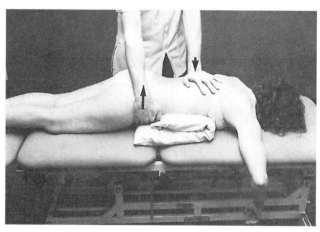

Figure 17–62. Nonspecific technique to increase left rotation of the lumbar spine. A pillow may be used to reduce lumbar extension. The therapist fixes the thoracolumbar junction and lifts with a comfortable but firm grip of the ilium over the anterior superior iliac spine.

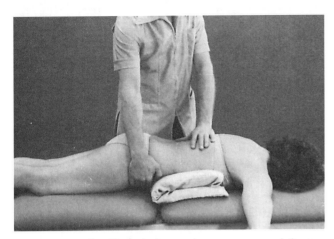

Figure 17–63. Specific technique to increase or assess left rotation of a lumbar segment. The therapist stabilizes the cranial vertebrae by applying pressure against the lateral aspect of the spinous process and lifts with a comfortable grip over the anterior superior iliac spine.

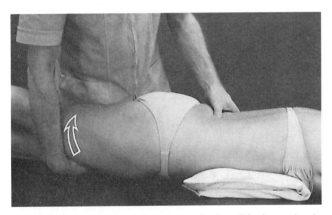

Figure 17–64. Minimal effort is required to lift the patient's crossed right thigh with the right forearm, causing rotation of the pelvis to the right. The therapist's right hand grasps the patient's anterior left thigh. The patient's thighs are stabilized at the edge of the bed by the therapist's right thigh.

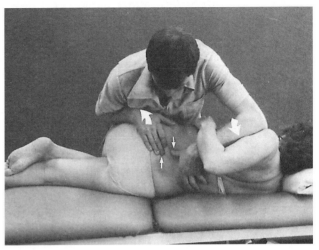

Figure 17–65. Probably the most common basic position for treating a rotation restriction of the lumbar spine. The patient's left knee is flexed until movement is palpated at a specific lumbar level. The patient's right shoulder is then pulled forward, and the left shoulder is rotated backward to lock the thoracolumbar spine at the desired level. This is further assisted by pressure of the left thumb on the lateral aspect of the cranial spinous process. Gapping of the left apophyseal joint is accomplished by (1) simultaneous opposing thrusts of the therapist's left and right forearms; (2) the therapist pulling forward with the right hand; and (3) the therapist lifting up with the index or middle finger of the right hand on the underside of the caudal spinous process.

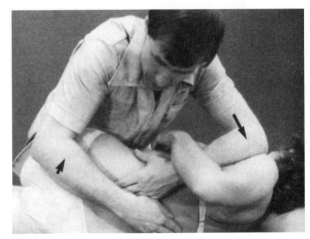

Figure 17–66. A variation of a nonspecific basic position in which the therapist uses the inner aspect of the forearm against the posterior ilium, allowing for more extension. The therapist palpates with the fingers of the left hand and stabilizes the patient's left shoulder with the left forearm.

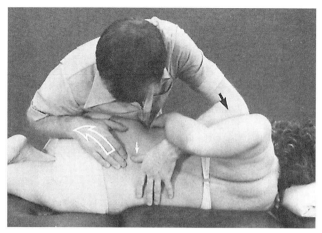

Figure 17–67. A variation of a specific position in which the patient's left shoulder as well as the cranial lumbar segment are stabilized by the therapist's left thumb. The fingers of the therapist's right hand pull up on the underside of the spinous process. The patient's left knee lies over the edge of the table, with the left foot hooked comfortably behind the right knee. If the edge of the midsection of the bed does not lift up, a cushion may be placed under the patient's side. Additional distraction may be applied by the therapist's right hand and forearm.

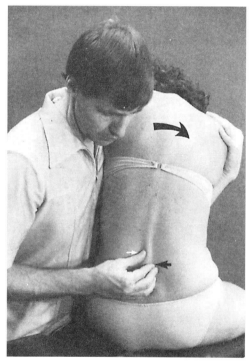

Figure 17–68. The therapist's left arm is placed under the patient's folded arms, and the therapist reaches across the patient's chest while firmly holding the right shoulder. The patient leans forward as the therapist rotates the patient to the left. The therapist assists the rotation with the right thumb pushing on the lateral aspect of the spinous process while stabilizing the caudal spinous process with the second finger, reinforced by the third. Alternatively, the therapist may resist rotation of the caudal spinous process by stabilizing with the thumb instead of the fingers.

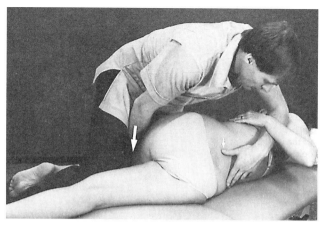

Figure 17–69. Specific technique to gap the left lumbosacral facet joint. With the patient lying close to the edge of the bed, the left knee is flexed and allowed to hang over the edge of the bed. If the patient cannot comfortably keep the left foot behind the right knee, the therapist can place his or her own flexed right knee on the bed, allowing the patient's left ankle to rest on the posterior aspect of the therapist's right leg. The therapist places the thumb and index finger on either side of the patient's left knee, with the popliteal space covered by the web of the hand. The therapist's right forearm is along the posterior aspect of the patient's left thigh. Leaning well forward, the therapist thrusts through the popliteal space. Stabilization of L5 is provided by the therapist's left forearm and thumb, which are on the lateral aspect of the spinous process of L5. As there is a wide range of angles for the lumbosacral facets, the degree of left hip flexion will vary to accommodate the sagittal or more coronal joint plane.

CASE STUDY

A 44-year-old woman was referred for a second opinion regarding persisting and increasing lower left thoracic rib cage pain. The patient was initially referred to physical therapy with a diagnosis of back and chest wall pain. The physical therapist was concerned about the possibility of a bulging thoracic disk or a tumor. Initially, treatments with transcutaneous electrical nerve stimulation and traction reduced discomfort; however, after 10 treatments, the symptoms were exacerbated. Medications consisting of muscle relaxants and nonsteroidal anti-inflammatory drugs provided no relief from pain. Symptoms had been present for 8 months, increasing during the last 3 months, and exacerbated by most movements, sneezing, and breathing. The severity of symptoms increased as the day progressed. Lying down reduced the severity of symptoms; however, the patient was subject to pain during the night.

The past history included surgery for removal of a tissue mass in the left breast 5 years earlier and subsequent use of tomoxifin. Radiation therapy for 6 weeks and chemotherapy for 6 months were undertaken again 2 years later. Chiropractic treatment for recurrent low back pain as a result of a tobogganing accident 30 years earlier was sought on an intermittent basis.

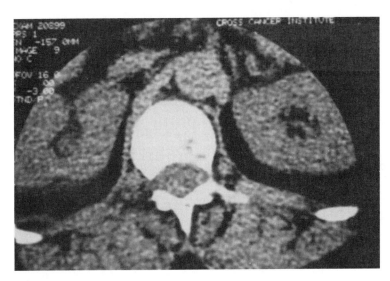

Figure 17–70. CT scan of a metastatic lesion of L1.

Current mammograms were unchanged from previous reports. Chest view reports were unremarkable, thoracic, lumbar, sacroiliac, and pelvic view reports were unremarkable, and the dimensions were within normal limits. There was no evidence of osseous metastases.

A bone scan 2 weeks before consultation revealed increased uptake at L1, the intensity of which had increased since the time of studies performed 6 and 12 months earlier.

Clinical examination revealed normal reflexes of the upper and lower limbs, hypothesia on the posterior aspect of the left upper arm (since the breast surgery 5 years previously), painful hyperthesia at the left lateral costal area (T10–T12), increased thoracic spine pain with cervical spine flexion, a positive dural or slump test, a straight leg raise of 30 degrees on the right and 70 degrees on the left with pain produced at the thoracolumbar junction, and increased lower thoracic spine pain with manual thoracic spine traction.

The patient was instructed to return to her physician to request a computed tomography (CT) scan. No treatment was provided.

The results of the CT scan revealed a spinal metastasis at L1 (Figs. 17–70 and 17–71).

Follow-up indicated that the patient received five treatments of radiation therapy for the problem. She experienced increased pain at the thoracolumbar junction; with treatment, however, this pain subsided. The radiologist indicated that this pain was caused by aggravation of the disk. The potential risk of a pathologic fracture should be kept in mind.

■ Summary

Metastatic tumors involve the vertebral column more often than any other segment of the bony skeleton[162]; in one study, 122 of 176 cases (70 percent) of patients were affected.[163] Bone metastases occur more frequently from tumors that do not kill quickly, and the more silent the primary tumor, the more probable the bone secondaries.[164] The patients are usually female, with the primary tumor usually having occurred in the breast (74 percent).[165,166]

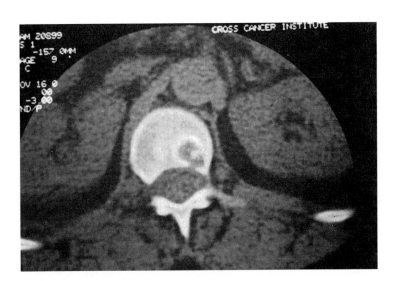

Figure 17–71. CT scan of a metastatic lesion of L1, enhanced view.

The history and pain pattern characteristics are significant in the clinical examination. Patients who complain of spinal pain and who have a past history of malignancy should be considered to have spinal metastases despite a negative x-ray examination until proven otherwise.[162,167] Bone destruction of 30 to 50 percent is necessary for a lesion to appear on x-ray films,[168] thus the need for alternative forms of imaging.

The above case is presented to remind those providing patient care that all spinal symptoms must be evaluated thoroughly and that in some patients, symptoms contraindicate manual therapy. The significance of this knowledge increases as the physical therapist achieves the right of direct access to patient care.

■ Acknowledgment

I express my thanks to Jennie Turner for her expert photographic assistance.

■ References

1. Lomax E: Manipulative therapy: a historical perspective from ancient times to the modern era. In Goldstein M (ed): The Research Status of Spinal Manipulative Therapy. NINCDS Monograph No. 15. DHEW Publication No. (NIH) 76-998. National Institute of Neurological and Communicative Disorders and Stroke, Bethesda, MD, 1975

2. Schiotz EH: Manipulation treatment of the spinal column from the medical-historical viewpoint. Tidsskr Nor Laegeforen 78:359, 372 (NIH library translation, 1958)

3. Gibbons RW: Chiropractic in America. The historical conflicts of cultism and science. Presented at the 10th Annual History Forum of Duquesne University, Pittsburgh, 1976

4. Schaefer RD: Chiropractic Health Care. 2nd Ed. Foundation for Chiropractic Education and Research, Des Moines, IA, 1976

5. Nwuga V: Manipulation of the Spine. Williams & Wilkins, Baltimore, 1976

6. Cyriax J: Textbook of Orthopaedic Medicine. 6th Ed. Vol. 1. Bailliere Tindall, London, 1975

7. Mennell JM: Back Pain—Diagnosis and Treatment Using Manipulative Techniques. Little, Brown, Boston, 1960

8. Grieve GP: Common Vertebral Joint Problems. Churchill Livingstone, Edinburgh, 1981

9. Maitland GD: Vertebral Manipulation. 4th Ed. Butterworths, London, 1977

10. Paris SV: The Spinal Lesion. Pegasus, Christchurch, New Zealand, 1965

11. McKenzie RA: The Lumbar Spine. Mechanical Diagnosis and Therapy. Spinal Publications, Waikanae, New Zealand, 1981

12. Goldstein M: The Research Status of Spinal Manipulative Therapy. NINCDS Monograph No. 15. DHEW Publication No. (NIH) 76-998. National Institute of Neurological and Communicative Disorders and Stroke, Bethesda, MD, 1975

13. Sato A: The somato-sympathetic reflexes: their physiological and clinical significance. p. 163. In Goldstein M (ed): The Research Status of Spinal Manipulative Therapy. NINCDS Monograph No. 15. DHEW Publication No. (NIH) 76-998. National Institute of Neurological and Communicative Disorders and Stroke, Bethesda, MD, 1975

14. Perl E: Pain, spinal and peripheral nerve factors. In Goldstein M (ed): The Research Status of Spinal Manipulative Therapy. NINCDS Monograph No. 15. DHEW Publication No. (NIH) 76-998. National Institute of Neurological and Communicative Disorders and Stroke, Bethesda, MD, 1975

15. Granit R, Pompeiano O: Reflex control of posture and movement. Prog Brain Res 50:1, 1979

16. Freeman MAR, Wyke BD: The innervation of the knee joint. An anatomical and histological study in the cat. J Anat 101:505, 1967

17. Wyke BD: The neurological basis of thoracic spinal pain. Rheumatol Phys Med 10:356, 1967

18. Wyke BD: Neurological mechanisms in the experience of pain. Acupuncture Electrother Res 4:27, 1979

19. Wyke BD: Neurology of the cervical spinal joints. Physiotherapy 65:72, 1979

20. Wyke BD: Perspectives in physiotherapy. Physiotherapy 32:261, 1980

21. Wyke BD, Polacek P: Structural and functional characteristics of the joint receptor apparatus. Acta Chir Orthop Traumatol Cech 40:489, 1973

22. Jayson MIV: The Lumbar Spine and Back Pain. 2nd Ed. Pitman, London, 1980

23. Polacek P: Receptors of the joints: their structure, variability and classification. Acta Fac Med Univ Brunensis 23:1, 1966

24. Halata Z: The ultrastructure of the sensory nerve endings in the articular capsule of the knee joint of the domestic cat (Ruffini corpuscles and Pacinian corpuscles). J Anat 124:717, 1977

25. Maitland GDL: Foreword. In Glasgow EF, Twomey LT, Scull ER, Kleynhans AM (eds): Aspects of Manipulative Therapy. 2nd Ed. Churchill Livingstone, Melbourne, 1985

26. Kaltenborn FM: Mobilization of the Extremity Joints. Olaf Norlis Bokhandel, Oslo, 1980

27. Maitland GD: Peripheral Manipulation. 2nd Ed. Butterworths, London, 1977

28. Mennell JM: Joint Pain—Diagnosis and Treatment Using Manipulative Techniques. Little, Brown, Boston, 1964

29. Stoddard A: Manual of Osteopathic Technique. Hutchinson of London, London, 1974

30. Hartman LD: Handbook of Osteopathic Technique. N.M.K. Publishers, Herts, England, 1983.

31. Sandoz R: Some physical mechanisms and effects of spinal adjustments. Ann Swiss Chiropract Assoc 6:91, 1976

32. Sandoz R: Some reflex phenomena associated with spinal derangements and adjustments. Ann Swiss Chiropract Assoc 7:45, 1981

33. Gainsbury JH: High velocity thrust and pathophysiology of segmental dysfunction. In Glasgow EF, Twomey LT, Scull ER, et al. (eds): Aspects of Manipulative Therapy. 2nd Ed. Churchill Livingstone, Melbourne, 1985

34. Evjenth O, Hamberg J: Muscle Stretching in Manual Therapy—A Clinical Manual—The Spinal Column and the TM Joint. Vol. 2. Alfta Rehab, Alfta, Sweden, 1984

35. Judovich B: Lumbar traction therapy. JAMA 159:549, 1955

36. Burton C: Low Back Pain. 2nd Ed. Philadelphia, JB Lippincott, 1980

37. Burton D, Nida G: The Sister Kenny Institute Gravity Lumbar Reduction Therapy Program. Publication No. 731. Sister Kenny Institute, Minneapolis, 1982

38. Martin RM: The Gravity Guiding System. Essential Publishing, San Marino, CA, 1981

39. Jones LH: Strain and Counterstrain. American Academy of Osteopathy, Colorado Springs, CO, 1981
40. Hoover HV: Functional technic. In 1958 Yearbook. Academy of Applied Osteopathy, Carmel, CA, 1958
41. Korr I: Muscle spindle and the lesioned segment. p. 45. In Proceedings of the International Federation of Orthopaedic Manipulative Therapists, Vail, CO, 1977
42. Lee D: Principles and practices of muscle energy and functional techniques. p. 640. In Grieve GP (ed): Modern Manual Therapy of the Vertebral Column. Churchill Livingstone, New York, 1986
43. Goodridge JP: Muscle energy techniques: definition, explanation, methods of procedure. Osteopath Assoc 81:249, 1981
44. Mitchell FL, Moran PS, Pruzzo NA: An Evaluation and Treatment Manual of Osteopathic Muscle Energy Procedures. Mitchell, Moran and Pruzzo, Valley Park, MO, 1979
45. Upledger JE, Vredevoogd JD: Craniosacral Therapy. Eastland Press, Chicago, 1983
46. Magoun HI: Osteopathy in the Cranial Field. 3rd Ed. Sutherland Cranial Teaching Foundation, Meridian, ID, 1976
47. Gehin A: Atlas of Manipulative Techniques for the Cranium and Face. Eastland Press, Seattle, 1985
48. Brookes D: Lectures on Cranial Osteopathy. A Manual for Practitioners and Students. Thorsons Publishers, Wellingborough, England, 1981
49. Anderson JAD: Problems of classification of low back pain. Rheum Rehabil 16:34, 1977
50. Cailliet R: Low Back Pain Syndrome. 3rd Ed. FA Davis, Philadelphia, 1983
51. Jayson MIV: Preface. In Jayson MIV (ed): The Lumbar Spine and Back Pain. 2nd Ed. Pitman Medical, Tunbridge Wells, England, 1980
52. Nachemson A: A critical look at conservative treatment for low back pain. In Jayson MIV (ed): The Lumbar Spine and Back Pain. 2nd Ed. Pitman Medical, Tunbridge Wells, England, 1980
53. Yates DAH: Treatment of back pain. In Jayson MIV (ed): The Lumbar Spine and Back Pain. 2nd Ed. Pitman Medical, Tunbridge Wells, England, 1980
54. Dixon AS: Diagnosis of low back pain—sorting the complainers. In Jayson MIV (ed): The Lumbar Spine and Back Pain. 2nd Ed. Pitman Medical, Tunbridge Wells, England, 1980
55. Korr IM: Proprioceptors and somatic dysfunction. J Am Osteopath Assoc 74:638, 1975
56. Simons DG: Electrogenic nature of palpable bands and local twitch response associated with myofascial trigger points. In Bonica JJ, Albe-Fessard D (eds): Advances in Pain Research and Therapy. Vol I. Raven Press, New York, 1976
57. Simons DG: Muscle pain syndromes. Am Phys Med 54:289, 1975; 55:15, 1976
58. Brugger A: Pseudoradikulare syndrome. Acta Rheumatol 19:1, 1962
59. Brugger A: Die Erkrankungen des Bewegungsapparatus und seines Nervensystems. Fisher, Stuttgart, 1977
60. Feinstein F, Langton JNK, Jameson RM, et al: Experiments on pain referred from deep somatic tissues. J Bone Joint Surg 36(A):981, 1954
61. Hohermuth HJ: Spondylogene Kniebeschwerden. Vortrag anlablich der 4. Deutsch-schweizerischen Forbildungstagung fur Angiologie und Rheumatologie, Rheinfelden, Switzerland, May 1981
62. Sutter M: Wesen, Klinik und Bedeutung spondylogener Reflexsyndrome. Schweiz Rundsch Med Prax 64:42, 1975
63. Sutter M, Frohlich R: Spondylogene Zusammenhange im Bereich der oberen Thorax-Apparatus. Report of the Annual Meeting of the Swiss Society for Manual Medicine, 1981
64. Waller U: Pathogenese des spondylogenen Reflexsyndroms. Scweiz Rundsch Med Prax 64:42, 1975
65. Dvorak J: Manuelle Medizin in USA in 1981. Manuelle Med 20:1, 1982
66. Gibson RW: The evolution of chiropractic. In Haldeman S (ed): Modern Developments in the Principles and Practice of Chiropractic. Appleton-Century-Crofts, East Norwalk, CT, 1980
67. Wardwell WI: The present and future role of the chiropractor. In Haldeman S (ed): Modern Developments in the Principles and Practice of Chiropractic. Appleton-Century-Crofts, East Norwalk, CT, 1980
68. Dvorak J, Dvorak V: Manual Medicine Diagnostics. Georg Thieme Verlag, Stuttgart, 1984
69. Maigne R: Wirbelsaulenbedingte Schmerzen. Hippokrates, Stuttgart, 1970
70. Kellgren HL: Observation of referred pain arising from muscles. Clin Sci 3:175, 1938
71. Kellgren HJ: On the distribution of pain arising from deep somatic structures with charts of segmental pain areas. Clin Sci 4:35, 1939
72. Sinclair DC, Feindel WH, Weddell G, et al: The intervertebral ligaments as a source of segmental pain. J Bone Joint Surg 30(B):515, 1948
73. Hockaday JM, Whitty CWM: Patterns of referred pain in normal subjects. Brain 90:481, 1967
74. Melzack R: Phantom body pain in paraplegics: evidence for central "pattern generating mechanisms" for pain. Pain 4:195, 1978
75. Melzack R: Myofascial trigger points: relation to acupuncture and mechanisms of pain. Arch Phys Med 62:114, 1981
76. Reynolds MD: Myofascial trigger point syndromes in the practice of rheumatology. Arch Phys Med 62:111, 1981
77. Rubin D: Myofascial trigger point syndromes: an approach to management. Arch Phys Med 62:107, 1981
78. Travell J, Rinzler SH: The myofascial genesis of pain. Postgrad Med 2:425, 1952
79. Travell J: Myofascial trigger points: clinical view. In Bonica JJ, Albe-Fessard DG (eds): Advances in Pain Research and Therapy. Vol. 1. Raven Press, New York
80. Travell J: Identification of myofascial trigger point syndromes: a case of atypical facial neuralgia. Arch Phys Med 62:100, 1981
81. Brugger A: Uber die tendonomyse. Dtsch Med Wochenschr 83:1048, 1958
82. Brugger A: Pseudoradikulare Syndrome des Stommes. Huber, Bern, 1965
83. Lewit K: Muskelfazilitations und Inhibitionstechniken in der manuellen Medizin. Manuelle Med 10:12, 1981
84. Caviezel H: Beitrag zur Kenntnis der Rippenlasionen. Manuelle Med 5:110, 1974
85. Caviezel H: Klinisch Diagnostik der Funktionsstorung an den Kopfgelenken. Schweiz Rundsch Med Prax 65:1037, 1976
86. Sell K: Spezielle manuelle Segment-Technik als Mittel zur Abklarung spondylogener Zusammenhangsfragen. Manuelle Med 7:99, 1969
87. Northup GWL: Osteopathic Medicine: An American Reformation. American Osteopathic Association, Chicago, 1966
88. Grieve GP: Mobilization of the Spine. 3rd Ed. Churchill Livingstone, Edinburgh, 1979

89. Haldeman S: Spinal manipulative therapy in the management of low back pain. In Finneson BE (ed): Low Back Pain. 2nd Ed. JB Lippincott, Philadelphia, 1981

90. Glover JR, Morr JG, Khosia T: Back pain: a randomized clinical trial of rotational manipulation of the trunk. Br J Ind Med 31:59, 1974

91. Bergquist-Ullman M, Larsson U: Acute low back pain in industry. Acta Orthop Scand (suppl) 170:1, 1977

92. Potter GE: A study of 744 cases of neck and back pain treated with spinal manipulation. J Can Chiropract Assoc 21(4):154, 1977

93. Fisk JW: A Practical Guide to Management of the Painful Neck and Back. Charles C Thomas, Springfield, IL, 1977

94. Maigne R: Orthopaedic Medicine. A New Approach to Vertebral Manipulations (translated by WT Liberson). Charles C Thomas, Springfield, IL, 1972

95. Edwards BC: Low back pain and pain resulting from lumbar spine conditions: a comparison of treatment results. Aust J Physiother 15:104, 1969

96. Buerger AA: A clinical trial of rotational manipulation. Pain Abstracts 1:248. Second World Congress on Pain. International Association for the Study of Pain, Montreal, 1978

97. Cyriax J: Textbook of Orthopaedic Medicine. 8th Ed. Vol. 2. Bailliere-Tindall, London, 1971

98. Chrisman OD, Mittnacht A, Snook GA: A study of the results following rotatory manipulation in the lumbar intervertebral disc syndrome. J Bone Joint Surg 46(A):517, 1964

99. Riches EW: End results of manipulation of the back. Lancet 957, 1930

100. Kirkaldy-Willis WH, Cassidy JO: Effects of manipulation on chronic low back pain. Presented at a conference on Manipulative Medicine in the Management of Low Back Pain. Sponsored by the University of Southern California and the North American Academy of Manipulative Medicine, Los Angeles, October 1978.

101. Matthews JA, Yates DAH: Reduction of lumbar disc prolapse by manipulation. Br Med J 20:696, 1969

102. White AA, Panjabi MM: Clinical Biomechanics of the Spine. JB Lippincott, Philadelphia, 1979

103. Gillet H, Liekens M: Belgian Chiropractic Research Notes. 10th Ed. Belgium Chiropractic Association, Brussels, 1973

104. Lewit D: Manuelle Medizin. Im Rahmen der Medizinischen Rehabilitation. 2nd Ed. Johann Ambrosius, Leipzig, 1977

105. Gitelman R: A chiropractic approach to biomechanical disorders of the lumbar spine and pelvis. In Haldeman S (ed): Modern Developments in the Principles and Practice of Chiropractic. Appleton-Century-Crofts, East Norwalk, CT, 1980

106. Gonstead CS: Gonstead Chiropractic Science and Art. Sci-Chi Publications, 1968

107. Logan VF, Murray FM (eds): Textbook of Logan Basic Methods. LBM, St. Louis, 1950

108. Cassidy JD, Potter GE, Kirkaldy-Willis WH: Manipulative management of back pain in patients with spondylolisthesis. J Can Chiropract Assoc 22:15, 1978

109. Potter GE: Chiropractors (letter). Can Med Assoc J 121:705, 1979

110. Henderson DJ: Intermittent claudication with special reference to its neurogenic form as a diagnostic and management challenge. J Can Chiropract Assoc 23:9, 1979

111. Bowles CH: Functional orientation for technique. In 1957 Year Book. Academy of Applied Osteopathy, Carmel, CA, 1957

112. Goldthwait JE, Brown LT, Swain LT, et al: Essentials of Body Mechanics in Health and Disease. JB Lippincott, Philadelphia, 1945

113. Fryette HH: Principles of Osteopathic Technique. Academy of Applied Osteopathy, Carmel, CA, 1954

114. Stoddard A: Manual of Osteopathic Practice. Hutchinson of London, London, 1969

115. Matthews JA: The scope of manipulation in the management of rheumatic disease. Practitioner 208:107, 1972

116. Kleynhans AM, Terrett AG: The prevention of complications from spinal manipulative therapy. In Glasgow EF, Twomey LT, Scull ER, et al (eds): Aspects of Manipulative Therapy. 2nd Ed. Churchill Livingstone, Edinburgh, 1985

117. DePalma AF, Rothman RH: The Intervertebral Disc. WB Saunders, Philadelphia, 1970

118. Hooper J: Low back pain and manipulation paraparesis after treatment of low back pain by physical methods. Med J Aust 1:549, 1973

119. Grieve GP: Common Vertebral Joint Problems. Churchill Livingstone, Edinburgh, 1981

120. Bollier W: Inflammatory infections and neoplastic disease of the lumbar spine. Ann Swiss Chiropract Assoc 1960

121. Rinsky LA, Reynolds GG, Jameson RM, et al: Cervical spine cord injury after chiropractic adjustment. Paraplegia 13: 233, 1976

122. Sandoz R, Lorenz E: Presentation of an original lumbar technic. Ann Swiss Chiropract Assoc 1:43, 1960

123. Kaiser G: Orthopedics and traumatology (translated from the German). Beitr Orthop 20:581, 1973

124. Grillo G: Anomalies of the lumbar spine. Ann Swiss Chiropract Assoc 1:56, 1960

125. Janse J: Principles and practice of chiropractic: an anthology. In R Hildebrandt (ed): National College of Chiropractic, Lombard, IL, 1976

126. Sandoz R: Newer trends in the pathogenesis of spinal disorders. Ann Swiss Chiropract Assoc 5, 1971

127. Valentini E: The occipito-cervical region. Ann Swiss Chiropract Assoc 4:225, 1969

128. Yochum TR: Radiology of the Arthritides (lecture notes). International College of Chiropractic, Melbourne, 1978

129. Siehl D: Manipulation of the spine under anaesthesia. In 1967 Yearbook. Academy of Applied Osteopathy, Carmel, CA, 1967

130. Lindner H: A synopsis of the dystrophies of the lumbar spine. Ann Swiss Chiropract Assoc 1:143, 1960

131. Beyeler W: Scheuermann's disease and its chiropractic management. Ann Swiss Chiropract Assoc 1:170, 1960

132. Hauberg GV: Contraindications of the Manual Therapy of the Spine (translated from the German). Hippokrates, Stuttgart, 1967

133. Jaquet P: Clinical Chiropractic—A Study of Cases. Chrounauer, Geneva, 1978

134. Odom GL: Neck ache and back ache. In Proceedings of the NINCDS Conference on Neck Ache and Back Ache. Charles C Thomas, Springfield, IL, 1970

135. Gutmann G: Chirotherapie, Grundlagen, Indikationen, Geneninidikationen and objektivier Barkeit. Med. Welf. Bd. 1978

136. Sandoz R: About some problems pertaining to the choice of indications for chiropractic therapy. Ann Swiss Chiropract Assoc 3:201, 1965

137. Bourdillon JF: Spinal Manipulation. W Heinemann, London, 1973

138. Droz JM: Indications and contraindications of vertebral manipulations. Ann Swiss Chiropract Assoc 5:81, 1971

139. Wolff HD: Remarks on the present situation and further development of manual medicine with special regard to chi-

rotherapy. Presented to the Deutsche Gesellschaft fur Manuelle Medizin, February 1972

140. Smart M: Manipulation. Arch Phys Med 730, 1946

141. Robertson AHM: Manipulation in cervical syndromes. Practitioner 200:396, 1968

142. Bollier W: Chiropractic and medicine—editorial. Ann Swiss Chiropract Assoc 1960

143. Lewit K: Complications following chiropractic manipulations. Deutsch Med Wochenshr 97:784, 1972

144. Livingston M: Spinal manipulation causing injury. Br Columbia Med J 14:78, 1971

145. Oger J: 1966 The dangers and accidents of vertebral manipulations (translated from the French). Rev Rhum 33:493, 1966

146. Kuhlendahl H, Hansell V: Nil nocere. Shaden bei Wirbelsaulenreposition (translated from the German). Med Wochenschr 100:1738, 1958

147. Dabbert O, Freeman DG, Weis W: Spinal meningeal hematoma, warfarin therapy and chiropractic adjustment. JAMA 214:11, 1970

148. Lescure R: Incidents, accidents, contreindications des manipulations de la colonne vertebrae. (translated from the French). Med Hyg 12:456, 1954

149. Ladermann JP: Accidents of spinal manipulations. Ann Swiss Chiropract Assoc 7:161, 1981

150. Janse J: Unpublished lecture notes. National College of Chiropractic, Lombard, IL, 1961

151. Peters RE: Heparin Therapy—Contraindications to Manipulation. Charter House Publishing, Wagga Wagga, Australia, 1983

152. Jennett WB: A study of 25 cases of compression of the cauda equina by prolapsed IVD. J Neurol Neurosurg Psychiatry 8:19, 1956

153. Heilig D: Whiplash—mechanics of injury, management of cervical and dorsal involvement. In 1965 Yearbook. Academy of Applied Osteopathy, Carmel, CA, 1965

154. Timbrell-Fisher AG: Treatment by Manipulation. HK Lewis, London, 1948

155. Klatz RM, Goldman RM, Pinchuk BG, et al: The effects of gravity inversion on hypertensive subjects. Phys Sports Med 13:85, 1985

156. Goldman RM, Tarr RS, Pinchuk BG, et al: The effects of oscillating inversion on systemic blood pressure, pulse, intraocular pressure and central retinal arterial pressure. Phys Sports Med 13:93, 1985

157. Klatz RM, Goldman RM, Pinchuk BG, et al: The effects of gravity inversion procedures on systemic blood pressure and central retinal arterial pressure. J Am Osteopath Assoc 82:853, 1983

158. Lemarr JD, Golding LA, Crehan KD: Cardiorespiratory responses to inversion. Phys Sports Med 11:51, 1983

159. Cooperman J, Scheid D: Guidelines for the use of inversion therapy. Clinical Management 4:6, 1984 (In Physical Therapy, published by American Physical Therapy Association, Alexandria, VA)

160. Zito M: Effects of two gravity inversion methods on heart rate, systolic brachial pressure, and ophthalmic artery pressure. Phys Ther 68:20, 1988

161. Haldeman S (ed): Modern Developments in the Principles and Practice of Chiropractic. Appleton-Century-Crofts, East Norwalk, CT, 1980

162. Bhalla SK: Metastatic disease of the spine. Clin Orthop 73:52, 1970

163. Turek SL: Orthopaedics. JB Lippincott, Philadelphia, 1984

164. Grieve GP: Common Vertebral Joint Problems. Churchill Livingstone, Edinburgh, 1981

165. Wong PA, Fornosier VL, McNabb I: Spinal metastases: the obvious, the ocult and the imposters. Spine 15:1, 1990

166. Spjat HJ et al: Tumours of bone and cartilage. In Atlas of Tumour Pathology. 2nd Series, Fascicle 5. Armed Forces Institute of Pathology, Washington, DC, 1971

167. Harrington KD: The use of methylmethacrylate for vertebral body replacement and anterior stabilization of pathologic fracture dislocations of the spine due to metastatic disease. J Bone Joint Surg 63(A):36, 1981

168. Boland P, Lane J, Sundareson N: Metastatic disease of the spine. Clin Orthop 169:95, 1982

CHAPTER 18

Use of Lumbar Rotations in the Treatment of Low Back Pain and Lumbopelvic Dysfunction

David A. McCune and Robert B. Sprague

Conservative treatment of pain and dysfunction in the lumbopelvic region has traditionally relied heavily on the use of passive techniques, active exercise, and postural management as a primary form of treatment. Although many authors advocate the use of rotation techniques,[1-19] few offer guidelines for their application or a rationale for their clinical effectiveness. This chapter presents guidelines for the use of rotation techniques in lumbopelvic dysfunction and suggests a scientific rationale for their application and apparent effectiveness.

Lumbopelvic dysfunction can present clinically as pain in the low back or lower extremity. The term *lumbopelvic dysfunction* is preferred to *low back pain,* as many patients do not present exclusively with low back pain, but rather pain in the lumbopelvic region, with or without associated lower extremity pain.

Clinicians have long found active and passive rotational movements to be useful in the treatment of lumbopelvic dysfunction. Rotational movements are used to (1) normalize movement in lumbar motion segments, (2) reduce lateral lumbar shifts, (3) centralize peripheral symptoms of neural origin, (4) facilitate trunk motor control, proprioception, and strength, (5) reduce and eliminate local nociceptive pain, and (6) reduce and eliminate neurogenic pain.

Conservative Management

The current trends in management of lumbopelvic pain and dysfunction advocate nonsurgical intervention. The growing realization that few patients need surgery has placed the responsibility for effective management of these conditions on physical therapists and other practitioners who employ conservative measures in treatment. Reports by Saal et al.[15,16] advocate conservative management through active and passive exercises even for some patients with documented herniated nucleus pulposus. Aggressive nonoperative care includes therapeutic exercises, traction, walking, and swimming. Reported success rates are more than 90 percent in patients with disc extrusions and radiculopathy. O'Sullivan et al.[17] reported not only pain relief but, more significantly, reduction in the recurrence rate with application of a very specific exercise regimen in patients with documented spondylolisthesis. Alaranta et al.[18] observed that conservative therapy was successful for sciatica patients with pathologic findings if the symptoms were mild. One hundred twenty-two patients were treated conservatively using rest, physical exercise, traction, injection, and corseting.

When applying manual therapy techniques of passive movements and exercise to patients with lumbopelvic dysfunction, it appears that the specific medical diagnosis is of less concern in the choice of management method than the actual movement dysfunction present.

Biomechanical Considerations

Rotation is defined as the movement of all points on a bone around a fixed point or axis. The actual axis of rotation of any motion segment is determined by both the bony architecture of the moving structures and the external forces acting on them to produce torque. Rotation of the lumbar intervertebral joint normally occurs around an axis located in the posterior third of the intervertebral bodies and intervertebral disc.[20] Segmental lumbar rotation is limited by impaction of the zygapophyseal joints and tension within the anulus fibrosus secondary to lateral shear of the intervertebral disc.[21-23] Lumbar segmental range of rotation does not exceed 1–2 degrees at any segment and will cause injury of the anular fibers if the motion exceeds 3 degrees.[22,24-26] Range of motion in lumbar axial rotation varies by age and sex. Twomey and

Taylor[27] reported that adolescent girls were more mobile than boys of the same age, while both sexes demonstrated a decline in range of motion with increasing age. In a normal lumbar intervertebral joint, the zygapophyseal joints, posterior ligaments, and muscles of stability all work together to protect the intervertebral disc from excessive torsion. Tension, compression, and translation, when imposed on lumbar motion segments during rotation, allow complex movement within each lumbar segment.

Lateral flexion and rotational movements in the lumbar spine do not occur individually, but rather as coupled movements.[24,25] Though there is ongoing controversy on this topic, coupled movements in the lumbar spine appear to be variable and dependent on the vertebral level. Pearcy et al.[24,25] state in radiologic studies that lateral flexion and rotation occur to the same side at L5–S1 and opposite sides at and above L3–L4. Coupled movements at the L4–L5 segment are variable and transitional.

The zygapophyseal joints possess intracapsular fat deposits and meniscoids, which may become entrapped or extrapped with flexion and rotational movement. These internal derangements of the zygapophyseal joints result in pain and disruption of normal movement at the involved motion segment.[28,29] During both lateral flexion and rotation, it is suggested that compressive forces are applied unilaterally to the ipsilateral zygapophyseal joint and the intervertebral disc. Simultaneously, distraction forces are applied to these structures on the contralateral side. Rotational movements applied to the lumbar spine motion segment can therefore produce favorable therapeutic effects on both the zygapophyseal joints and the intervertebral disc.

The intervertebral disc is an integral component of the lumbar motion segment and, for maintenance of optimum health, requires movement.[30] It consists of two components, the nucleus pulposis and the anulus fibrosis. In typical young individuals, the nucleus pulposis is a viscous semifluid material which contains 70–90 percent water, proteoglycans, irregular collagen fibers, and free-floating cartilage cells.[31–35] The biomechanical significance of the nucleus pulposis lies in its function as a hydraulic shock absorber when it is contained within the intact anulus fibrous. When external force is applied, the nucleus is capable of deformation in all directions.

The anulus fibroses is principally 50–60 percent water, with the balance containing collagen cells. The arrangement of collagen within the anulus typically contains between 10 and 20 circumferentially arranged lamellae.[36] These lamellae are generally thicker centrally and thinner posterolaterally.[37,38] Though all lamellae within each layer are parallel and connect adjacent vertebral bodies, alternate layers possess opposite directional orientations and range from 65 to 75 degrees from the horizontal.[26,39] Rotation of the intervertebral segment therefore creates simultaneous tension and approximation in alternate layers of the anulus.

Farfan et al.[23] and Vernon-Roberts and Pirie[40] state that anular tears of the disc are the result of torsional rather than compressive failure. Excessive rotational forces allegedly produce failure of the intervertebral junction, characterized by separation of the peripheral layers and resulting in circumferential tears of the anulus. It has been proposed that torsion and bending are likely to cause anular failure and protrusion.[26,27,41] This failure is most likely to occur posterolaterally as a result of the combined effects of forward bending and rotation. Prolonged positioning of the lumbar intervertebral segment has also been determined to cause deformation as a result of creep and hysteresis.[42]

In the clinical situation, we may use biomechanical theories to guide our thinking, but other factors, such as symptom behavior, patient irritability, movement palpation, muscle reactivity, and neural involvement, also contribute to the selection of the technique. Biomechanical theories therefore can be utilized both to assist in the choice of treatment techniques and to clarify the underlying causes of the dysfunction. For example, if right lateral flexion of the L3–L4 motion segment is found to demonstrate restricted mobility on passive intervertebral motion (PIVM) testing, similar restrictions in left rotation may also be demonstrated. However, if a complementary restriction is not noted on PIVM testing of rotation at L3–L4, then the clinician may need to rethink the source of the dysfunction as not purely mechanical but rather muscle spasm or neural irritation. Application of biomechanical principles is also important, as often the patient may not tolerate positioning for or application of lateral flexion techniques, while techniques utilizing rotation are better tolerated. In such an instance, treatment employing a rotational technique, which is better tolerated by the patient, may be used to improve mobility in lateral flexion. For the astute manual therapist, application of the biomechanical principles of coupled motions can provide greater flexibility in determining the source of the underlying dysfunction, treatment options, and appropriate treatment techniques.

■ Neurophysiologic Considerations

The lumbar intervertebral motion segment integrates afferent and efferent information from associated muscles, joints, the intervertebral disc, and neural tissue. These neurologic impulses combine with descending information from higher centers and interneurons from levels above and below the motion segment in question.[43–46] Articular nerves carry information from several spinal segments. This information includes autonomic, motor, and sensory stimuli. The larger myelinated Ia sensory fibers act as primary proprioceptive endings that are sensitive to both position and movement. The smaller C fibers serve as pain endings and terminate in the joint capsule, ligaments, and adventitia of blood vessels. These smaller free nerve endings are particularly sensitive to twisting and stretching, both of which occur during rotation.[47]

The zygapophyseal joints have a dual innervation. Primary innervation occurs through the dorsal rami of the segmental nerve at the specific level as well as the level above, with secondary innervation supplied by branches of nerves to the deep paravertebral muscles.[42,48–52] These fibers contain both mechanoreceptors (types I and II) and nociceptive free nerve endings (type IV).[49] Mechanical deformation of segmental joint and soft tissue nociceptors provides the nervous system with proprioceptive information as well as facilitory and inhibitory stimuli and can potentially produce pain. Active and passive movements such as rotation can neurophysiologically modulate a patient's perceived level of pain, kinesthetic awareness, and motor control, as capsular and surrounding structures are particularly sensitive to stretch.[53,54]

The intervertebral disc has nociceptive free nerve endings only in the outer one-half to one-third fibers of the anulus.[44,55] These free nerve endings, when deformed mechanically, may be a source of significant low back pain. The intervertebral disc does contain encapsulated receptors which have been postulated by Malinsky to be a source of proprioception.[54]

Innervation of the lumbar musculature is through the dorsal rami.[43] These nerve fibers are mixed and include mechanoreceptors as well as nociceptive fibers which reside within the lumen of the arteriole. These structures within the musculature can serve as sources of pain and proprioceptive information for the involved motion segment. Additionally, Amonoo-Kuofi[56] reported a high density of muscle spindles in the erector spinae, hypothesizing a significant role for these structures in postural control and proprioception.

Of particular interest in the lumbar spine are the multifidi. These muscles are innervated by the medial branch of the dorsal rami and have been found to supply information concerning proprioception and zygapophyseal joint coordination during movement. Hides et al.[57] have demonstrated that these muscles are adversely affected in their motor control of the lumbar spine following first-time injury. Histologic changes in these muscles from type I to type II have been noted in patients with "failed back syndrome," further emphasizing their importance in the maintenance of optimum lumbopelvic function.[58,59] The lumbar multifidi have also been found to work in conjunction with the transversus abdominis, diaphragm, and pelvic floor muscles to provide crucial dynamic segmental stabilization to the lumbar spine.[60] As a result of these findings, the motor control of the lumbar multifidi, transverse abdominis, diaphragm, and pelvic floor have been found to play a crucial role in the effective treatment of lumbopelvic dysfunction.

Consideration of the neural components is essential in the determination of appropriate active or passive movements to decrease pain, improve motor coordination, or improve kinesthetic awareness in the lumbopelvic segments. This is accomplished by developing treatment goals that encompass the neural, muscular, and articular systems. As these systems are integrally connected, treatment of one system will often create positive changes within the others. For example, if the therapist is treating a painful, hypermobile motion segment with instability and neural irritation, the application of a midrange oscillatory rotational technique designed to stimulate type II mechanoreceptors and reduce pain and reactive muscle spasm may also reduce the associated neural irritation. This active technique might then facilitate isometric midrange rotations, stressing low-load, high-repetition contractions to improve dynamic segmental stability and proprioception in the involved joints while minimizing neural irritation.

Therapeutic Uses of Rotational Techniques

Therapeutic rotational movements may be performed both passively by the therapist and actively in the form of patient exercise. Prescribed movements may range from very gentle midrange movements to more vigorous full-range or end-range movements. These movements can also be performed as neural interface movements in different positions or degrees of neural loading and provocation. It should be stressed that the key to successful treatment is the performance of a thorough subjective and objective clinical assessment, not strict adherence to hypothetical theories or approaches to treatment. Therapeutic rotational techniques may be successfully performed in prone, side-lying, supine, sitting, and standing positions. The versatility of these techniques allows the clinician almost unlimited options in devising an acceptable and effective treatment approach.

Use of Rotation to Restore Normal Spinal Movement

In the presence of reduced segmental motion, the purpose of rotational techniques is to impart specific motion to the involved articular and periarticular structures and surrounding muscles that may be restricting normal movement. Much has been written about movements designed to open or gap the zygapophyseal joints, physical movement of joint menisci, and stretching of the joint capsule.[28,61–65] Ongoing debate persists over the actual joint arthrokinematics when having a patient rotate with the painful side up or down.[66–69] Whether the therapist chooses to treat the motion segment via neurophysiologic or biomechanical means, selection of the appropriate technique is ultimately dictated by the patient's response to the technique.

Use of Rotation to Correct a Lateral Shift

A *lateral list* or *shift*[13,14,70-72] is defined as a temporary deformity related to a recent bout of low back pain and/or sciatica in which the upper trunk is leaning either away from (contralateral) or toward (ipsilateral) the painful side. The shift may present as a static condition or may be noted as a lateral deviation through an arc of movement. A lateral shift may be noted in up to 6 percent of patients and can associated with no pain, central pain, or bilateral pain.[73,74] The actual cause of a lateral shift can be difficult to ascertain. It can be caused by discogenic pathology, zygapophyseal joint dysfunction, localized segmental muscle spasm, protective positioning of neural tissue, and sacroiliac dysfunction.[13,14,28,75,76]

The shift is often visible, but occasionally it may be recognized only on lateral glide testing while standing, as described by McKenzie.[13] Standing lateral glide testing may be used both to detect and, frequently, to correct a lateral shift. In the normal spine, standing lateral glide movements are theoretically coupled movements of lateral flexion and rotation at all levels of the lumbar spine. As previously mentioned, coupled motions of lateral flexion and rotation occur differently at different levels of the lumbar spine. As a result of this coupling, rotational techniques may be used effectively to correct the lateral shift at each level, regardless of the underlying pathology.

Rotation may be utilized with the lumbar spine in neutral, flexion, or extension through techniques performed in side-lying, supine, or prone positions. The theoretical basis for application of rotational techniques for dysfunction of discal origin is varied. Structurally, when torque is applied in the form of rotation to the lumbar motion segment, the collagenous structure, particularly the alternate layers of the anulus, are stretched. Reversal of the motion would thus relax the same fibers, and fibers in the other layers become stretched.[77,78] Further, if rotation of the intervertebral segment reduces the mechanical deformation of injured anular collagen fibers and their associated nociceptive endings, symptom reduction should follow. McKenzie[13] states that lateral shifts in the lumbar region result from disc pathology and offers hypotheses concerning the possible mechanics involved. Others[74] have found no correlation between the side of the shift and the location of the disc bulge at surgery.

Bogduk and Engel[28] have outlined the pathologic entrapment or extrapment of intracapsular meniscoids and fat deposits in the lumbar zygapophyseal joints. The presence of such mechanical deformation within the joint may present as a lateral shift away from, or a restriction in, lateral flexion toward the painful side. Rotation in these joints is hypothesized to cause the involved joint to gap, allowing normalization of the internal derangement and correction of the movement dysfunction.

Unilateral localized spasm of the lumbar paraspinals or iliopsoas can also be the source of a lateral shift. The erector spinae, multifidus, and iliopsoas have the potential to create a lateral shift, whether in response to underlying pathology elsewhere within the motion segment and sacroiliac joint or from intrinsic muscle pathology or injury. The use of rotational movements for the treatment of spasm can be effective through direct mechanical stretching of the involved musculature, as well as neurophysiologically through the inhibition of motor tone within the affected motion segment.[19]

Individuals with lateral flexion motion restrictions within the sacroiliac joint, whether from articular dysfunction or reactive muscle spasm, may also present with a lateral shift as well as asymmetries with unilateral weight-bearing.[76] Rotation, though less effective in treating the articular components of these problems, can be effective in treating the resulting muscular hypertonicity using the neurophysiologic methods mentioned previously.

Use of Rotation to Centralize Pain

The centralization of lumbar origin peripheral pain was allegedly first described by McKenzie in 1956.[79] This centralization phenomenon has also been described further by numerous authors.[30,80-83] Centralization of peripheral symptoms is described as the reduction of peripheral symptoms, often associated with a temporary increase in central symptoms, followed by a reduction and/or elimination of the centralized symptoms. It is often, if not always, associated with a theoretical decrease in the mechanical deformation and restoration of normal movement (e.g., restoration of lateral flexion and extension movement). McKenzie states that centralization takes place only in the "derangement" syndrome. Rotations may be used to enhance or achieve centralization of symptoms. Theoretically, the mechanical deformation in the lateral aspects of the lumbar spine is being reduced either by stretching or by compressing deformed soft tissue. The decision concerning which side to have the patient lie on is based on the clinical assessment before, during, and after the procedure or technique is applied. If symptoms centralize as a result of the rotational movements, the correct technique has been selected. Conversely, if symptoms peripheralize, the correct procedure has not been selected.

If the symptoms are, for example, right-sided and consistent with symptoms that are associated with dysfunction at the level of L4–L5, with right lateral flexion being restricted and painful, a left rotation technique will frequently be successful in centralizing these symptoms.

Use of Rotation to Improve Coordination and Strength

Until recently, the role of muscular stabilization of the lumbar spine was thought to be equally shared by all trunk muscles. New evidence has better defined the specific roles of the muscles in stabilization of the trunk. The muscles particularly identified as segmental stabilizers are the transversus abdominis, multifidus, diaphragm, and the muscles of the pelvic floor.[57,60,84,85] Specific training of these muscles has been outlined by Richardson et al.[86] The activity of the obliquely orientated multifidus in rotation and segmental stabilization[87,89] warrants special attention when the treatment goal is restoration of localized segmental stabilization of the lumbar spine and sacroiliac joint. The lumbar multifidus muscles provide stability to these regions both through direct attachment to the vertebrae and sacrum and through attachments to the deep layers of the thoracolumbar fascia.[88–90] Early-stage training involves specific exercises that facilitate isometric, low-load contractions stressing cocontraction of the transversus abdominis, and multifidus muscles, pelvic floor, and diaphragm. Following successful restoration of these muscles in their role as isometric stabilizers, rotational exercises are added to restore functional dynamic stability to the lumbar spine. These rotational movements are performed in both the caudocephalad and cephalocaudad directions to mirror actual functional activities. Progression from isometric exercise while lying down to more complex movements while standing should occur as rapidly as possible to better restore functional stability to the spine.

Use of Rotation for Pain Reduction

Reduction of both local nociceptive and peripheral neurogenic pain will often occur in conjunction with restoration of movement, correction of a lateral shift deformity, symptom centralization, and restoration of segmental stability and motor control. However, there are rare circumstances in which pain is present in the absence of the above deficits or deformities. In these instances, pain reduction through the use of rotational techniques is thought to be achieved through the effects of manipulation-induced analgesia and mechanoreceptor stimulation.[91] Early work by Wyke[92,93] revealed that pain reduction is greatly enhanced by appropriate stimulation of joint mechanoreceptors. In general, relief of pain is perceived both through prolonged end-range stretch stimulating type I mechanoreceptors and through midrange oscillatory movement, which works by stimulating type II receptors. Stimulation of each of these receptors through passive movement and exercise has been found to inhibit pain. The importance of proprioceptive and kinesthetic information in pain reduction and treatment is emphasized by Porterfield and DeRosa.[69] More recent work has emphasized the role that passive movement can play in the production of analgesia in affected regions.[91,94–96] Even simple exercises such as swimming and walking have components of rotation that reduce pain. The positive impact of walking on the lumbar spine is thoroughly discussed by Edgelow,[97] though these activities alone are insufficient for complete rehabilitation of lumbar spine dysfunctions.

■ Clinical Applications for Lumbar Rotation

Rotation of the lumbar spine may be performed in side-lying, supine, prone, sitting, and standing positions. Here we have chosen to illustrate a few of the many techniques that can be utilized to treat lumbopelvic dysfunction. The techniques described can be used, with minor modifications, to achieve many different treatment goals. A rationale for clinical application is offered for each technique. The movements described are both midrange and end-range techniques, with the direction of rotation movement being defined by the movement of the cephalad segment on the caudad segment.

Rotation in the Side-Lying Position

The patient is comfortably positioned in the side-lying position, with both knees flexed, while the therapist positions the lumbar spine into flexion or extension as necessary for the chosen technique. For flexion/rotation techniques, the lower leg is extended while the upper hip remains flexed and is allowed to rotate gently toward the supporting surface (Fig. 18–1). Extension/rotation techniques require the lower leg to be extended up to the desired level, with the upper hip gently flexed, using care not to impart flexion to the lumbar spine. Grasping the patient's arm which is toward the bed, the therapist rotates the lumbar spine down to the level to be mobilized, being careful not to change the desired flexion or extension position. The patient's downside hand is placed under the head while the upside elbow is flexed and placed on the lateral torso with the hand lying on the stomach.

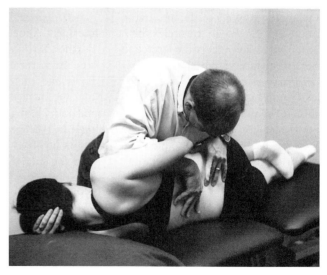

Figure 18–1. Utilization of rotation in the side-lying position allows the therapist many variations of technique application. In this position, the therapist may stabilize the torso while imparting movement at the pelvis or stabilize the pelvis while moving the torso. Flexion and extension are varied through lower extremity positioning.

The therapist fixes the patient's upside arm by placing the cephalad arm through the space between the patient's ribs and elbow and leaning on the patient's torso, thus fixing the torso. Care must be taken not to overly compress the ribs. The therapist's torso should be used to provide localized counterrotation through the abdomen to the cephalad segment mobilized. The cepalad thumb is placed on the upside aspect of the spinous process of the upper level to be mobilized. The index finger of the caudad hand is placed on the downside aspect of the spinous process of the lower vertebral level (Fig. 18–2). The caudad forearm is placed on a part of the pelvis that is comfortable for the patient. Try to avoid pressure in the area of the sciatic notch. The area between the iliac crest and the greater trochanter is usually the most comfortable area. The therapist mobilizes the spine by imparting movement either through the pelvis or through the shoulder and torso. When caudocephalad rotation is performed, motion is directed through the pelvis, either by drawing it forward (opening technique) or away (closing technique) as desired. Force through the pelvis varies, depending on the desired level of treatment, and is provided by rotating the pelvis forward in a curvilinear fashion while simultaneously stabilizing the thorax and shoulder. Cephalocaudad rotation is performed in a similar fashion, with the pelvis being stabilized while the rotational forces are directed through the shoulder and thorax, allowing rotation to proceed from cephalad to caudad. Positioning in this fashion can provide the basis for performance of both midrange and end-range techniques.

This technique can be performed as an interface technique between the articular and neural structures in the spine by tensioning the neural elements of the lower extremity during mobilization. This is performed as above, though the involved extremity is gradually and gently extended until the therapist notes motion restrictions at the involved motion segment. With the leg maintained in this position of neural tension, the therapist imparts

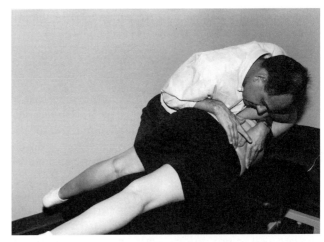

Figure 18–3. Side-lying rotation performed in conjunction with loading of the neural system allows for simultaneous treatment of the neural and articular systems. Left hip flexion and knee extension provide the neural provocation while the therapist imparts the desired movement at the motion segment.

the rotational motions to the involved motion segment. As with all techniques involving provocation of the neural system, care must be taken not to be too aggressive when utilizing this technique (Fig. 18–3).

Uses

Side-lying rotation techniques can be useful in the treatment of restrictions within the motion segment secondary to mechanical disc pathology, zygapophyseal dysfunction, neural adherence, and muscle spasm. Midrange movements may be used to reduce the treatment soreness created by end-range movements, as well as to decrease reactive segmental muscle spasm and the resulting pain. End-range motions can be utilized as both sustained passive stretches and oscillatory motions. We have found sustained passive motions to be helpful in conditions where there appears to be a local nociceptive source of pain in the presence of segmental motion restrictions within the motion segment. Oscillatory end-range techniques are often useful in the treatment of conditions which present with peripheral neurogenic pain. When performed as an interface neural technique, the desired treatment approach entails utilizing a very slow oscillatory technique.

Rotation in the Supine Position

The patient is supine near the side of the treatment table. The therapist guides the patient's lower extremities into hip and knee flexion bilaterally. While stabilizing the patient's opposite shoulder, the therapist rotates the lumbar spine in flexion by moving the patient's knees over the edge of the treatment table. The extent of the rotation

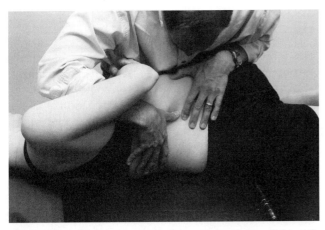

Figure 18–2. Optimal control of rotation is obtained through stabilization of the torso and pelvis by means of the forearms while specific motion is imparted and palpated through accurate hand placement.

and the depth of the flexion are determined by clinical assessment of the patient's symptoms (Fig. 18–4).

Uses

Rotation in the supine position is often used to reduce pain by theoretically closing down the painful lateral compartment or through neurophysiologic inhibition in patients who do not tolerate neutral or extension positioning of the spine. Application of rotation in this manner is often successful in reducing pain when side-lying rotations performed in extension or in slight flexion fail to reduce symptoms. This technique is particularly helpful when sustained at the end of range for patients with far lateral disc protrusions, with or without peripheral neurogenic pain. The versatility of this technique allows both mid- and end-range oscillatory and end-range sustained applications.

Active Rotation in the Prone (Cephalocaudad Left) Position

The patient is prone and lifts the desired shoulder off the treatment table using the posterior global trunk muscles in an asymmetrical fashion. The exercise is performed slowly, through the full range of motion, until the pelvis begins to rotate off of the treatment surface. The degree of resistance can be modified by asking the patient to place his or her arm down at the side and progress to overhead as greater difficulty is desired (Fig. 18–5).

Uses

This movement is used to facilitate active cephalocaudad rotation in individuals who exhibit generally poor global

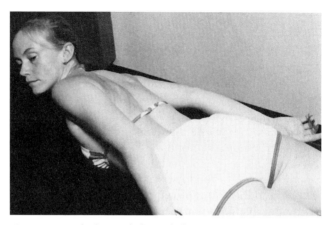

Figure 18–5. Active cephalocaudad rotation in the prone position is performed with the patient initiating the rotation from the cephalad segments, being careful to keep the pelvis stable on the supporting surface.

trunk control. As segmental control improves, the patient should quickly be progressed to more upright, functional activities.

Active Rotation in the Prone (Caudocephalad Left) Position

The patient is prone and attempts to lift the desired side of the pelvis and knee off the treatment table using the superficial multifidus muscle fibers. In the initial stages of training for segmental stabilization using the deep fibers of the multifidus, this activity is performed as an isometric, low-load contraction, with the therapist being cautious not to allow motion in the spine. Once segmental stabilization is achieved, the exercise is performed slowly through the full available range of motion. Care must be taken to ensure that the patient's feet and knees stay positioned together to prevent substitution of hip rotation for true lumbar rotation (Fig. 18–6).

Uses

This movement is used initially to train the multifidus in cocontraction with the other local segmental stabilizers of the trunk. As the patient's motor control progresses, this movement is useful in training coordination of caudocephalad rotation. Often the unilateral wasting of the multifidus which occurs segmentally can be reduced using this exercise.

Rotation in the Sitting Position

This activity can be performed for both cephalocaudad and caudocephalad training. If the desired motion is cephalocaudad rotation, the patient sits on the treatment table or stool with the feet shoulder width apart while firmly planted on the floor. The upper trunk is moved slowly

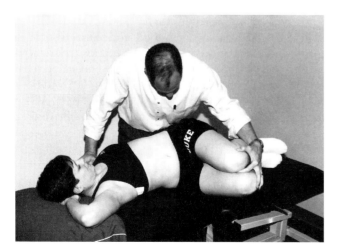

Figure 18–4. Rotation in the supine position can be performed in various ways, altering the degree of flexion, type of motion (sustained vs. oscillatory), point in range of motion, and grade of movement (midrange vs. end-range).

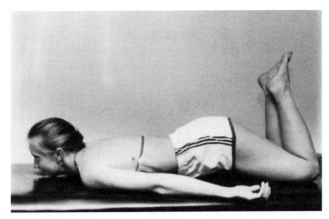

Figure 18–6. Active caudocephalad rotation in the prone position is performed with the knees and hips moving together. The patient is performing this movement correctly when the ipsilateral ASIS and knee are lifted off the supporting surface simultaneously.

in the desired position. This exercise can be performed both without resistance and with resistance through the use of pulleys and weights (Fig. 18–7).

In caudocephalad rotation, the patient sits on a rotation surface (swivel chair or stool) and stabilizes the upper torso by holding on to a solid object. The activity is performed by rotating the pelvis under the fixed torso, facilitating rotation in a caudocephalad direction (Fig. 18–8).

Uses

This movement is used to increase range of motion, improve rotational motor control, and restore the strength of functional rotational activities in sitting. It should be performed as a progression of prone rotation in either the cephalocaudad or caudocephalad direction.

Rotation Stabilization in the Standing Position

The patient stands in a stable stride-length position and either pulls or pushes an object that allows arm movement in an isotonic mode. While performing the desired upper extremity motion, the patient cocontracts the segmental stabilizers while isometrically resisting the flexion, extension, and rotational movements placed on the spine. This activity is most helpful in preparing the patient for functional tasks (Fig. 18–9).

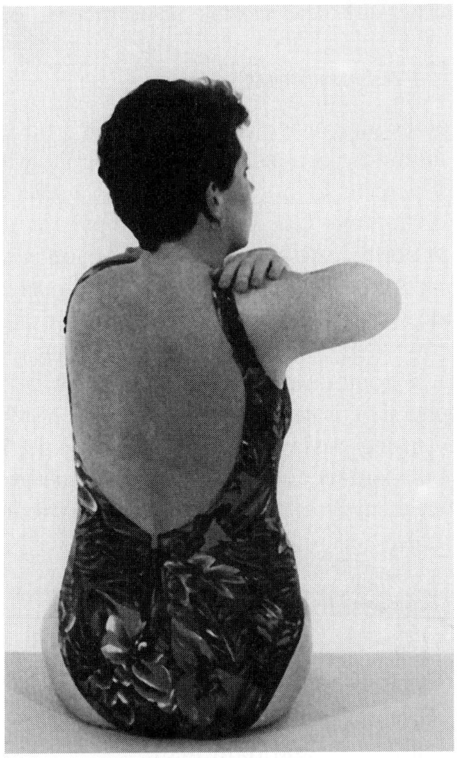

Figure 18–7. Cephalocaudad rotation in the sitting position is performed with the patient initiating the rotation sequentially from cephalad to caudad. Minimal resistance is utilized initially and can be increased through the use of pulleys or resistive apparatus.

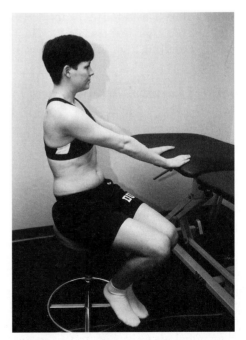

Figure 18–8. Caudocephalad rotation in the sitting position is performed with the patient initiating the desired rotation from the pelvis while keeping the superior segments stable through arm fixation on a solid object. Verbal cues to utilize either the anterior or posterior musculature will preferentially facilitate the desired trunk stabilizers.

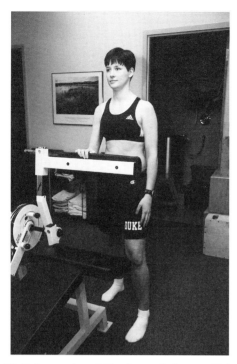

Figure 18–9. Isometric stabilization techniques utilizing traditional exercise apparatus (here a Cybex leg curl machine) can provide patients with rotational spinal forces that mirror functional activities.

Uses

This movement is used for dynamic and functional stabilization of the trunk. This exercise, performed with very light weights, is often the first resisted exercise tolerated by the patient recovering from all forms of low back pain.

Summary of Clinical Applications

Rotational movements, both passive and active, are effective in treating the lumbar spine, especially if mechanical symptoms are unilateral. Rotations may be used to restore normal motion, correct a lateral shift, eliminate or centralize pain, and restore coordination and control of lumbopelvic musculature.

If the intent of the treatment is to centralize, reduce, and eliminate pain, then the rotations, when repeated sufficiently in either the mid- or end-range, will normally be successful. If the intent of the treatment is to restore motion, then the rotations must reproduce the pain of the restricted range with the least amount of rotational force. Stretching into rotation will often improve movements not only in the frontal plane (lateral flexion) but also in the sagittal plane (flexion and extension). Thus, rotational techniques are successful in the treatment of mechanical low back pain as a bridge to other exercises. For example, if extension range of motion (active and passive) is restricted, restoration of rotation may improve extension secondarily.

In the author's experience, rotations are a very useful clinical tool in the treatment of low back pain. It is also obvious that there is a lack of agreement in the literature regarding not only the effectiveness of rotation but also the underlying mechanisms, whether physiologic, neurologic, biomechanical, or psychological.

CASE STUDY

Subjective Assessment

A 77-year-old retired woman presented with intermittent right-sided low back pain and intermittent right leg pain extending into the foot. Onset was 6 months prior to presentation for no apparent reason. She reported an identical attack of the same low back and leg pain 5 years previously that lasted for about 2 months.

The patient's back and lower extremity pain were produced or made worse by bending, sitting in a soft chair, and lying on her right (involved) side. Her symptoms were better, and at times eliminated, when she sat in a hard chair with a lordosis and when she was walking. Her sleep was disturbed, requiring her to change positions, on average, two or three times each night. Coughing and sneezing signs were both negative. Radiograph reports described degenerative disc disease at L2–L3 and L3–L4. The patient's general health was very good for a person of her age. She was taking no medications.

Objective Assessment

Flexion of the lumbar spine while standing produced end-range pain at the patient's pathologic limit, which was about 50 percent of normal. Extension while standing produced the same type of end-range pain at about 75 percent of normal. Active right lateral flexion was limited when compared with active left lateral flexion, and passive right glide was also limited compared with passive left glide. Active right lateral flexion, passive right glide, and passive right rotation reproduced the patient's low back and peripheral neurogenic leg pain. Palpation of her lumbar spine, using passive accessory movements, revealed hypomobility only centrally at L4 and L5, but right unilateral posterior anterior pressures at L5–S1 reproduced her low back pain and right leg pain.

General Assessment

Mechanical low back pain and peripheral neurogenic pain were relatively stable at the time of examination, with hypomobility of the lumbar spine in flexion, extension, right lateral flexion, and right glide.

Treatment Plan

The treatment plan was to eliminate the peripheral neurogenic pain, to restore normal movement to the lumbar spine, and to complete the rehabilitation program through motor control training as needed.

WEEK 1

The patient was seen three times during week 1. The proper sitting posture was established with a lumbar roll. Active right glide and repeated extension while standing were performed as home exercises every 2 hours, as tolerated and with precautions. Midrange oscillatory passive right rotation reproduced the low back pain and produced partial reduction of the peripheral neurogenic pain. Left passive rotation did not affect the symptoms in any way. Training of the transversus abdominis and multifidus was begun, but it did not reduce the patient's subjective complaints.

RESULTS. The patient complained of soreness from both the passive and active exercises, but that was expected because hypomobile joints were being stretched. The peripheral neurogenic component of her pain was unchanged. The patient was capable of a mild isolated contraction of the transversus abdominis only.

WEEK 2

The patient was seen three times during week 2. Both active and passive exercises were combined as before, except that passive right rotation was increased from midrange to end-range mobilizations. The patient was doing her home exercises correctly, and she understood the reason for doing them. Her compliance was improving. She was able to do active right rotation exercises in the side-lying position at home.

RESULTS. The low back pain and leg pain were decreasing slowly in intensity, frequency, and duration. Flexibility in physiologic movements was also improving, and passive accessory movements were less restricted. Passive accessory movements had not been used as treatment because active exercises and passive physiologic rotations had been sufficient. Good isolated transversus abdominis contraction was achieved in supine.

WEEK 3

The patient was seen twice, and the exercises were unchanged. Both the passive and active exercises were performed more vigorously and/or for a longer period of time. Training of lumbar multifidus was initiated.

RESULTS. At the patient's second visit during week 3, she reported spontaneously that she was "the best she had been in 5 years." The patient stated that she had very infrequent sciatica, and she was able to function effectively in her daily activities.

WEEK 4

The patient was seen twice during week 4. One visit was devoted to localizing a foot problem, and the second visit was devoted to further motor control training of the segmental stabilizers, as well as strength testing of her low back and hips. Right hip abduction was weak, and appropriate home exercises were progressed accordingly for both trunk stabilization, using co-contraction of transversus abdominis and multifidus, and hip strengthening.

RESULTS. The patient's local foot problem was corrected, and she was progressing nicely in her rehabilitation program. She was seen once about 2 weeks later for a final recheck.

WEEK 5

This one appointment took place 2 weeks later. All home exercises were rechecked. The patient's lumbar spine movements were deemed acceptable for a person of her age and were painless at her limits. She was instructed to continue her stabilization and strengthening program, incorporating it into her functional activities while performing flexibility exercises a minimum of twice daily or more frequently as needed.

RESULTS. The patient was discharged on an appropriate home exercise program.

■ Summary

The theory and rationale for the use of lumbar rotation in the treatment of low back pain have been discussed. Theoretical considerations, clinical models, and application suggestions have been described. Regardless of the underlying pathology, it is likely that the neurophysiologic effects of mechanoreceptor stimulation, mechanical deformation of the disc and surrounding soft tissue, biomechanical restoration of zygapophyseal joint movement, and restoration of optimum muscular coordination and control all occur through the judicious application of rotational techniques. Though only a few of the available techniques have been described here, the reader is encouraged to apply the principles outlined to any rotational technique, in any patient position, to achieve the desired treatment outcome.

■ References

1. Maitland G: Vertebral Manipulation. 5th Ed. Sydney: Butterworths, 1986
2. Edwards B: Combined movements in the lumbar spine: their use in examination and treatment. p. 561. In Grieve G (ed): Modern Manual Therapy of the Vertebral Column. Churchill Livingstone, Edinburgh, 1986
3. Van Hoesen L: Mobilization and manipulation techniques for the lumbar spine. p. 736. In Grieve G (ed): Modern Manual Therapy of the Vertebral Column. Churchill Livingstone, Edinburgh, 1986
4. Trott P, Grant R, Maitland G: Manipulative therapy for the low lumbar spine: technique selection and application to some syndromes. p 199. In Twomey L, Taylor J (eds): Physical

Therapy of the Low Back. Churchill Livingstone, New York, 1987

5. Cyriax J: Textbook of Orthopaedic Medicine. Vol. 2. Balliere Tindall, London, 1971

6. Cyriax J: Textbook of Orthopaedic Medicine. Vol. 1. Williams & Wilkins, Baltimore, 1975

7. Grieve G: Common Vertebral Joint Problems. Churchill Livingstone, Edinburgh, 1981

8. Sydenham R: Manual therapy techniques for the thoracolumbar spine. p 421. In Donatelli R, Wooden M (eds): Orthopedic Physical Therapy. Churchill Livingstone, New York, 1989

9. McCune D, Sprague R: Exercises for low back pain. p 299. In Basmajian J (ed): Therapeutic Exercise. Williams & Wilkins, Baltimore, 1990

10. Woodman R: Cyriax approach to lumbar dysfunction. p 48. In Postgraduate Advances in the Evaluation and Treatment of Low Back Dysfunction. Forum Medicum, Berryville, VA, 1989

11. Saunders H: Evaluation, Treatment and Prevention of Musculoskeletal Disorders. Educational Opportunities, Eden Prairie, MN, 1985

12. Lee D, Walsh M: A Workbook of Manual Techniques for the Vertebral Column and Pelvic Girdle. Nascent Publishers, Delta, British Columbia, 1985

13. McKenzie R: The Lumbar Spine. Mechanical Diagnosis and Therapy. Spinal Publications, Lower Hut, New Zealand, 1981

14. Paris S: The Paris approach. p 58. In Postgraduate Advances in the Evaluation and Treatment of Low Back Dysfunction. Forum Medicum, Berryville, VA, 1989

15. Saal J, Saal J, Herzog R: The natural history of lumbar intervertebral disc extrusions treated nonoperatively. Spine 15:683, 1990

16. Saal J, Saal J: Nonoperative treatment of herniated lumbar intervertebral disc with radiculopathy, an outcome study. Spine 14:431, 1989

17. O'Sullivan P, Twomey L, Allison G: Evaluation of specific stabilizing exercise in the treatment of chronic low back pain with radiologic diagnosis of spondylosis or spondylolisthesis. Spine 22:2959, 1997

18. Alaranta H, Hurme M, Einola S: A prospective study of patients with sciatica, a comparison between conservatively treated patients and patients who have undergone operations, part II: results after one year followup. Spine 15:1345, 1990

19. Hartman L: An osteopathic approach to manipulation. Orth Phys Ther Clin North Am 7(4):565, 1998

20. Cossette JW, Farfan HF, Robertson GW, et al: The instantaneous center of rotation of the third lumbar intervertebral joint. J Biomechanics 4:149, 1971

21. Farfan H, Gracovetsky S: The nature of instability. Spine 9:714, 1984

22. Farfan HF, Cossette JW, Robertson GW, et al: The effects of torsion on the lumbar intervertebral joints: the role of torsion in the production of disc degeneration. J Bone Joint Surg 52A:468, 1970

23. Farfan H, Huberdeau R, Dubpw H: Lumbar intervertebral disc degeneration. The influence of geometrical features on the pattern of disc degeneration—a postmortem study. J Bone Joint Surg 54A:492, 1972

24. Pearcy M, Portek I, Shepherd J: Three-dimensional X-ray analysis of normal movement in the lumbar spine. Spine 9:294, 1984

25. Pearcy M, Tibrewwal S: Axial rotation and lateral bending in the normal lumbar spine measured by three-dimensional radiography. Spine 9:582, 1984

26. Hickey D, Hukins S: Relation between the structure of the annulus fibrosus and the function and failure of the intervertebral disc. Spine 5:100, 1980

27. Twomey L, Taylor J: Factors influencing ranges of movement in the lumbar spine. p. 289. In Grieve G (ed): Modern Manual Therapy. Churchill Livingstone, Edinburgh, 1986

28. Bogduk N, Engel R: The menisci of the lumbar zygapophyseal joints. Spine 9:454, 1984

29. Engel R, Bogduk N: The menisci of the lumbar zygapophyseal joints. J Anat 135:795, 1982

30. Mooney V: Where is the pain coming from? Presidential address, International Society for the Study of the Lumbar Spine, Dallas, 1986. Spine 12:757, 1987

31. Maroudas A, Nachemson A, Stockwell R, et al: Some factors involved in the nutrition of the intervertebral disc. J Anat 120:113, 1975

32. Beard H, Stevens R: Biochemical changes in the intervertebral disc. p. 407. In Jayson M (ed): The Lumbar Spine and Backache. Pitman, London, 1980

33. Gower W, Pedrini V: Age related variation in protein polysaccharides from human nucleus pulposis, annulus fibrosis and costal cartilage. J Bone Joint Surg 51A:1154, 1969

34. Naylor A: Intervertebral disc prolapse and degeneration. The biochemical and biophysical approach. Spine 1:108, 1971

35. Schmorl G, Junghanns H: The Human Spine in Health and Disease. Grune & Stratton, New York, 1971

36. Taylor J: The development and adult structure of lumbar intervertebral discs. J Man Med 5:43, 1990

37. Marchand F, Ahmed A: Investigation of the laminate structure of lumbar disc anulus fibrosus. Spine 15:402, 1990

38. Jayson M, Barks J: Structural changes in the intervertebral disc. Ann Rheum Dis 32:10, 1973

39. Hickey D, Hukins S: X-ray diffraction studies of the arrangement of collagen fibres in human fetal intervertebral discs. J Anat 131:81, 1980

40. Vernon-Roberts B, Pirie C: Degenerative changes in the intervertebral discs of the lumbar spine and their sequelae. Rheumatol Rehab 16:13, 1977

41. Twomey L, Taylor J: Age changes in lumbar intervertebral discs. Acta Orthop Scand 56:496, 1985

42. Twomey L, Taylor J: Flexion creep deformation and hysteresis in the lumbar vertebral column. Spine 7:116, 1982

43. Bogduk N, Wilson A, Tynan W: The human dorsal rami. J Anat 134(2):383, 1982

44. Bogduk N, Tynan W, Wilson A: The nerve supply of the human lumbar intervertebral discs. J Anat 132:39, 1881

45. Bogduk N: The innervation of the intervertebral discs. p. 135. In Ghosh P (ed): The Biology of the Intervertebral Disc. Vol. 1. CRC Press, Boca Raton, FL, 1988

46. Kimmel D: Innervation of spinal dura mater and dura mater of the posterior cranial fossa. Neurology 10:800, 1960

47. American Rheumatism Association: Primer on rheumatic disease. JAMA 224:669, 1973

48. Stillwell D: The nerve supply of the verebral column and its associated structures in the monkey. Anat Rec 125:139, 1956

49. Wyke B: Articular neurology and manipulative therapy. p. 75. In Glasgow EEA (ed): Aspects of Manipulative Therapy. Churchill Livingstone, New York, 1985

50. Edgar M, Ghadially J: Innervation of the lumbar spine. Clin Orthop 15:35, 1976

51. Bogduk N: The innervation of the lumbar spine. Spine 8:286, 1983

52. Bradley K: The anatomy of backache. Aust NZ J Surg 44:227, 1974

53. Radin E: The physiology and degeneration of joints. Semin Arthritis Rheum 2:245, 1972–1973

54. Malinsky J: The ontogenic development of nerve terminations in the intervertebral discs of man. Acta Anat 38:96, 1959

55. O'Brien J: Neuropathology of intervertebral discs removed for low back pain. J Pathol 132:95, 1980

56. Amonoo-Kuofi H: The density of muscle spindles in the medial, intermediate, and lateral columns of human intrinsic postvertebral muscles. J Anat 136(3):509, 1983

57. Hides J, Richardson C, Jull G: Multifidus recovery is not automatic following resolution of acute first episode low back pain. Spine 21(23):2763, 1996

58. Rantanen J, Hurme M, Falck H: The lumbar multifidus muscle five years after surgery for a lumbar intervertebral disc herniation. Spine 18:568, 1993

59. Sihvonen T, Herno A, Paljavri L, et al: Local denervation atrophy of paraspinal muscles in postoperative failed back syndrome. Spine 18:575, 1993

60. Hodges P, Richardson C: Inefficient muscular stabilization of the lumbar spine associated with low back pain: a motor control evaluation of transversus abdominis. Spine 21:2640, 1996

61. Panjabi M, Goel V, Takata K: Physiologic strains in the lumbar spinal ligaments. Spine 7:192, 1982

62. Ahmed A, Duncan N, Burke D: The effect of gacet geometry on the axial torque—rotation response of lumbar motion segments. Spine 15:391, 1990

63. Gunzburg R, Hutton W, Fraser R: Axial rotation of the lumbar spine and the effect of flexion. Spine 16:22, 1991

64. Shirazi-Adl A, Ahmed A, Shrivastava S: Mechanical response of a lumbar motion segment in axial torque alone and combined with compression. Spine 11:914, 1986

65. McFadden K, Taylor J: Axial rotation in the lumbar spine and gaping of the zygapophyseal joints. Spine 15:295, 1990

66. Edwards B: Manual of Combined Movements. Churchill Livingstone, Melbourne, 1992

67. Siemon L: Treatment of acute locked back by spinal manipulation. J Bone Joint Surg 67B:500, 1985

68. Cyriax J: Dural pain. Lancet, April 29, 1(8070):919, 1978

69. Porterfield J, De Rosa C: Perspectives in Functional Anatomy. WB Saunders, Philadelphia, 1991

70. Arangio G, Hartzell S, Reed J: Significance of lumbosacral list and low-back pain. Spine 15:208, 1990

71. Tenhula J, Rose S, Delitto A: Association between direction of lateral shift, movement tests, and side of symptoms in patients with low back pain syndrome. Phys Ther 70:480, 1990

72. Fernando C: Use of lateral shift questioned. Letter to the editor. Phys Ther 71:167, 1991

73. Porter R, Miller C: Back pain and trunk list. Spine 11(6):597, 1986

74. Khuffash B, Porter R: Cross leg pain and trunk list. Spine 12:602, 1989

75. Elvey R: Physical evaluation and treatment of neural tissue. Course Manual. Curtin University of Technology, Perth, 1990

76. Lee D: Treatment of pelvic instability. p. 445. In Vleeming AEA (ed): Movement, Stability and Low Back Pain. Churchill Livingstone, New York, 1997

77. Jensen G: Biomechanics of the lumbar intervertebral disc: a review. Phys Ther 60:765, 1980

78. Gracovetsky S, Farfan H: The optimum spine. Spine 11:543, 1986

79. McKenzie R: The Cervical and Thoracic spine, Mechanical Diagnosis and Therapy. Spinal Publications, Waikanae, New Zealand, 1990

80. Donelson R, Silva G, Murphy K: Centralization phenomenon, its usefulness in evaluating and treating referred pain. Spine 15:211, 1990

81. Long A: The centralization phenomenon: its usefulness as a predictor of outcome in conservative treatment of chronic low back pain. Spine 20(23):2513, 1995

82. Donelson R, Aprill C, Medcalf R, et al: A prospective study of centralization: lumbar and referred pain. Spine 22(10):1115, 1997

83. Di Fabio R: Toward understanding centralisation of low back symptoms. JOSPT 29(4):206, 1999

84. Hodges P, Richardson CA: Contraction of the human diaphragm during postural adjustments. J Physiol 505:239, 1997

85. Sapsford R, Hodges P, Richardson C: Activation of the abdominal muscles is a normal response to contraction of the pelvic floor muscles. In International Continence Society Conference, Japan, 1997

86. Richardson CA, Jull GA, Hodges PW, Hales J: Therapeutic exercise for spinal segmental stabilization in low back pain. Churchill Livingstone, Sydney, 1999

87. Taylor J, Twomey L: Age changes in the lumbar zygapophyseal joints: observation on structure and function. Spine 11:739, 1986

88. McGill S: Electromyographic activity of the abdominal and low back musculature during the generation of isometric and dynamic axial trunk torque: Implications for lumbar mechanics. J Ortho Res 9:91, 1991

89. Wilke HJ, Wolf S, Claes LE, et al: Stability increase of the lumbar spine with different muscle groups. A biomechanical in vitro study. Spine 20:192, 1995

90. Vleeming A, Pod-Gondgwaard AL, Stoeckart R, et al: The posterior layer of the thoracolumbar fascia: its function in load transfer from spine to legs. Spine 20:753, 1995

91. Wright A: Manipulation induced analgesia. p. 27. In Jull GA (ed): Clinical Solutions. MPAA Proceedings. St. Kilda, Australia, 1995

92. Wyke B: Articular neurology and manipulative therapy. In Glasgow EEA (ed): Aspects of Manipulative Therapy. Lincoln Institute of Health Sciences, Melbourne, 1980

93. Wyke B: The neurology of low back pain. p. 56. In Jayson M (ed): The Lumbar Spine and Back Pain. Churchill Livingstone, Edinburgh, 1987

94. Wright A, Vicenzino B: Cervical mobilization techniques, sympathetic nervous system effects and their relationship to analgesia. p. 164. In Butler D (ed): Moving in on Pain. Butterworth-Heinemann, Melbourne, 1995

95. Zusman M, Edwards B, Donaghy A: Investigation of a proposed mechanism for the relief of spinal pain with passive joint movement. J Man Med 4:58, 1989

96. Wright A: Hypoalgesia post manipulative therapy: A review of a potential neurophysiological mechanism. Man Ther 1(1):11, 1995

97. Edgelow P: Dysfunction, evaluation, and treatment of the lumbar spine. p. 321. In Donatelli REA (ed): Orthopaedic Physical Therapy. Churchill Livingstone, New York, 1989

CHAPTER 19

Evaluation and Treatment of Dysfunction in the Lumbar-Pelvic-Hip Complex

Allyn L. Woerman

This chapter emphasizes the interrelatedness of the main components of the lumbar-pelvic-hip complex, especially the pelvis. The lumbar spine is discussed in Chapters 15, 16, and 17, so in this chapter only those aspects that are directly involved with pelvic and/or hip function are discussed. By establishing the relationship among these three functional components of the kinetic chain, the clinician can better evaluate the patient and formulate more effective treatment programs.

Many textbooks offer detailed anatomic and kinesiologic descriptions of the lumbar spine, hip, and pelvis, as well as a plethora of evaluative and treatment techniques for these areas. This chapter gives the reader sufficient information to be able to render accurate assessment and treatment for the syndromes described. For simplicity's sake and for continuity, most illustrations and anatomic descriptions are taken or adapted from Kapandji.[1] The reader must keep in mind the possible effects and influences of other components of the kinetic chain such as the foot, the ankle, and the knee to complete the picture of dysfunction. The assessment and treatment techniques described are primarily osteopathic in nature and use the so-called muscle energy techniques popularized by Fred Mitchell, Sr.

■ Functional Anatomy and Mechanics of the Hip

Osteology of the Hip

The hip joint is formed by the articulation of the head of the femur with the acetabulum of the pelvis. This joint is a classic example of a ball-and-socket joint and has three degrees of freedom of motion.[1]

The head of the femur is ellipsoid in shape, forming roughly two-thirds of a sphere approximately 4 to 5 cm in diameter. It is covered with hyaline cartilage, which is thicker centrally and thinner at the periphery. Two basic functional adaptations have been identified in the structure of the femoral head (Fig. 19–1). In the first (type I), the femoral head is greater than two-thirds of a sphere with maximal angles. Its shaft is slender, and the associated pelvis is small and high-slung. This adaptation is suited for speed and movement. The type II adaptation has a femoral head that is nearly a full hemisphere and has minimal angles. Its shaft is thick, and its associated pelvis is broad. This adaptation is for power and strength.

The femoral neck projects laterally from the head and fans out. This projection is usually between 120 and 125 degrees in adults and is known as the *angle of inclination* (Fig. 19–1). In infants, this head-to-neck angle can be as much as 150 degrees. The decrease in this angle from infancy to adulthood is the result of compression and bending forces acting on the head during weightbearing. From a mechanical standpoint, this head–neck relationship may be likened to a gibbet and strut. The gibbet is an over-hang. Vertical forces exerted on it are transmitted to the shaft by means of a horizontal lever. Shear forces are produced near the junction of the horizontal and vertical beams, and so a strut must be interposed to counteract the shear. The struts in the hip are the trabecular systems.

There are two main trabecular systems and one accessory system in the femoral head and neck, and these systems correspond to the lines of force (Fig. 19–2). The medial system begins in the cortical layer of the lateral femoral shaft and ends on the inferior aspect of the cortical layer of the femoral head (arcuate bundle of Gallois). The lateral system arises from the internal aspect of the shaft and the inferior part of the neck and ends in the superior cortical bone of the head (supporting bundle). The accessory system has two bundles, which arise in the trochanter and fan out from there. The intersection of these systems

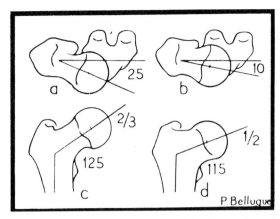

Figure 19–1. Functional adaptations of the femoral head and neck. Type I (A and C) has a head equal to two-thirds of a sphere and maximal angles; type II (B and D) has a head greater than half of a hemisphere and minimal angles. The angle of inclination is shown in parts C and D, and the angle of declination is shown in parts A and B. (From Kapandji,[1] with permission.)

forms a structure similar to gothic arches with keystones, one of the strongest architectural forms known. One gothic arch is formed by the intersection of the trochanteric bundle of the accessory system and the lateral set of the main system. Its inner pillar is less dense and weakens with age. The other gothic arch is formed by the intersection of the medial and lateral systems and forms very dense bone (nucleus of the head). It rests on extremely strong cortical bone at the inferior spur of the neck known as the *vault of Adams*. Between these two arches is a zone of weakness; this weakness increases with age and is the site of basal neck fractures.

The femoral head and neck project anteriorly in relation to the femoral condyles. The angle formed is known as the *angle of declination* (Fig. 19–1) and is usually 23 to 26 degrees in the adult. If this angle is significantly increased, the condition known as *anteversion* (toe-in) occurs. If the angle is significantly decreased, the condition known as *retroversion* (toe-out) occurs.

A 5 to 7 degree angle exists in the shaft of the femur with respect to the vertical plane, thus causing an anteroposterior bend. This bend produces strength to withstand ground reaction forces.

The acetabulum or socket portion of the hip joint is formed by the junction of the ilium, ischium, and pubic bones of the pelvis (Fig. 19–3A). It is ellipsoidal and not quite hemispheric. Its orientation is directed laterally, inferiorly, and anteriorly 30 to 40 degrees with the horizontal. A fibrocartilaginous ring called the *labrum* inserts into the acetabular rim. The labrum is triangular in shape and serves to deepen the acetabulum. It bridges the acetabular notch along with the transverse acetabular ligament (Fig. 19–3B). Within the acetabulum is a horseshoe-shaped hyaline cartilage lining, which is thicker and broader at the roof and thinner and narrower at the floor. No cartilage exists in the central fossa. Instead, a

fat pad covers the floor because there is no compression or contact by the head there.

The ligamentum teres, comprising three bundles, is a flattened fibrous band 3 to 3.5 cm long that arises from the acetabular notch and inserts into the fovea capitis. It lies in the floor of the acetabulum and has minimal if any mechanical function in the hip joint, as it comes under tension only in adduction. Its main function is to protect the delicate posterior branch of the obturator artery, which supplies the head of the femur (Fig. 19–4).

The osteology of the pelvis is described in greater detail in the discussion of the sacroiliac joints. For now, the pelvis can be described as a closed ring composed of the two innominate bones, which are conjoined anteriorly by the pubic symphysis and posteriorly by the interposed sacrum and the resulting two sacroiliac joints. The pelvis functions to transmit vertical forces from the vertebral column to the hips via the sacroiliac joints and to transmit ground reaction forces from the legs and hips to the vertebral column, also via the sacroiliac joints. These force transmissions and dissipations are accomplished through two trabecular systems, the sacroacetabular system and the sacroischial system. The sacroacetabular system resists

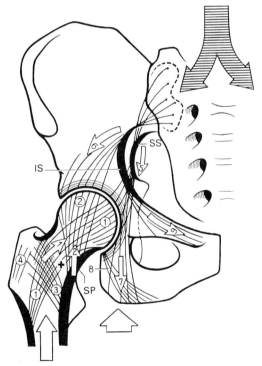

Figure 19–2. Trabecular systems of the hip and pelvis. Main system: (1) arcuate and (2) supporting bundles. Accessory system: (3) and (4). The intersections of (1) with (3) and (1) with (2) form the main gothic arches of the hip. A third arch, of less importance, is formed by the intersection of (3) and (4). Sacroacetabular trabeculae (5) and (6) take stress away from the sacroiliac joint. Set (5) converges with set (1) from the femur, while set (6) converges with set (2). Sacroischial trabeculae (7) and (8) intersect to bear the body weight in sitting (Adapted from Kapandji,[1] with permission.)

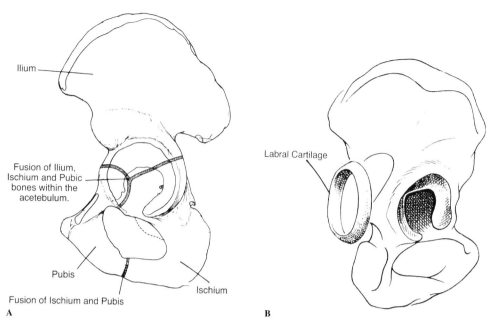

Ilium

Fusion of Ilium, Ischium and Pubic bones within the acetebulum.

Pubis

Ischium

Fusion of Ischium and Pubis

A

Labral Cartilage

B

Figure 19–3. The innominate, acetabulum, and labrum. (A) Left innominate, lateral view. Note the junction of the ischium, ilium, and pubic bones in the fossa of the acetabulum. (Adapted from Warwick and Williams,[3] with permission.) (B) Acetabulum and three-sided circular labral cartilage (Adapted from Kapandji,[1] with permission.)

the forces of compression and traction through the kinetic chain, whereas the sacroischial system resists the forces of compression applied to the pelvis. The sacroischial system especially bears the weight of the trunk when the individual is seated (Fig. 19–2).

Arthrology of the Hip

Maximal joint congruence of the hip is achieved only in 90 degrees of flexion, slight abduction, and slight external

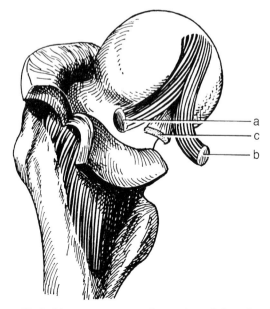

Figure 19–4. Ligamentum teres. It consists of three bundles: (a) posterior ischial bundle; (b) anterior pubic bundle; (c) intermediate bundle. (Adapted from Kapandji,[1] with permission.)

rotation.[1] In the erect posture, the femoral head is not completely covered by the acetabulum but is exposed superiorly and anteriorly. It is only in the "all-fours" position that the two joint surfaces come into true physiologic congruence.

The capsule of the hip comprises four sets of fibers: longitudinal, oblique, arcuate, and circular (Fig. 19–5). The circular fibers form the zona orbicularis around the neck of the femur and divide the joint cavity into two spaces, medial and lateral. The medial capsule inserts into the acetabular rim and the transverse ligament and is intimate with the rectus femoris tendon. The lateral capsule inserts into the base of the femoral neck along the trochanteric line and posteriorly just above the groove and into the trochanteric fossa. The frenulum (pectinofoveal fold of Amantini) is the longest part of the inferior capsule and unpleats itself, especially in abduction, thereby lengthening the capsule and increasing range of motion.

The closed-packed position of the hip is at 0 to 15 degrees of extension, 30 degrees of abduction, and slight internal rotation.[2] This is the position of greatest joint stability because of the combination of ligamentous tightness and joint congruity. The capsular pattern of restriction of motion is limitation of internal rotation and abduction *more than* flexion and extension *more than* external rotation and adduction.

The anterior ligaments of the hip form a Z-shaped pattern and are analogous to the glenohumeral ligaments of the shoulder (Fig. 19–6). The iliofemoral ligament (the Y-shaped ligament of Bigelow) is made up of two bands: the iliotrochanteric (superior) band and the infe-

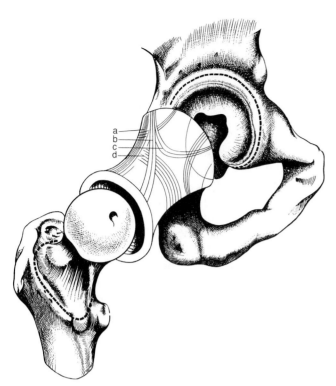

Figure 19–5. Hip capsule fibers. The directions in which the fibers of the hip capsule are oriented resist stresses placed on the hip: (a) longitudinal; (b) oblique; (c) arcuate; (d) circular. (Adapted from Kapandji,[1] with permission.)

rior band. The superior band is the stronger of the two and is 8 to 10 mm thick; it is strengthened by the iliotendinotrochanteric ligament. The inferior band inserts into the lower trochanteric line. The other anterior ligament, the pubofemoral, blends medially with the pectineus muscle and attaches anteriorly into the trochanteric fossa. Between the arms of the Z, the capsule is thinner. The

iliofemoral bursa lies over this area beneath the iliopsoas tendon.

The posterior ligament of the hip, the ischiofemoral ligament (Fig. 19–7), arises from the posterior acetabular rim and the labrum and attaches into the trochanteric fossa and tendon of the obturator externus muscle. Both the anterior and posterior ligaments are coiled in the same direction around the hip as a result of bipedal stance. In the erect posture, all ligaments are under modest tension. In extension, all ligaments tighten, especially the inferior band of the iliofemoral ligament, which checks posterior tilting of the pelvis. In flexion, all ligaments relax. In external rotation, all anterior ligaments tighten and the posterior relaxes. Just the reverse occurs with internal rotation. With adduction, the iliotrochanteric band tightens, the pubofemoral ligament slackens, and the ischiofemoral ligament relaxes. In abduction, the pubofemoral ligament tightens, the iliotrochanteric band slackens, and the ischiofemoral band tightens.

Neurovascular Supply of the Hip

The nerve supply of the hip joint is derived from the L3 somite with basic spinal cord connections from L2, L3, and L4.[3] The nerve supply is derived directly from the femoral nerve through its muscular branches: the obturator, the accessory obturator, the nerve to the quadratus femoris, and the superior gluteal nerve.

The arterial supply is derived from the obturator artery, the medial and lateral circumflex femoral arteries, and the superior and inferior gluteal arteries. The venous supply comes from the femoral vein and the medial and lateral circumflex femoral veins.

Lymphatic drainage is accomplished primarily by the deep inguinal lymphatic chain, especially the upper and

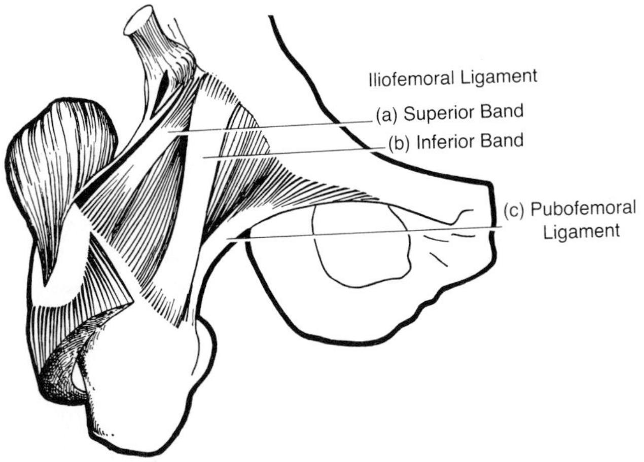

Iliofemoral Ligament
(a) Superior Band
(b) Inferior Band
(c) Pubofemoral Ligament

Figure 19–6. Anterior capsular ligaments of the hip. Capsular ligaments are thickenings that reinforce the capsule. The iliofemoral ligament has two bands: (a) superior and (b) inferior. The pubofemoral ligament (c) blends with the pectineus muscle. (Adapted from Kapandji,[1] with permission.)

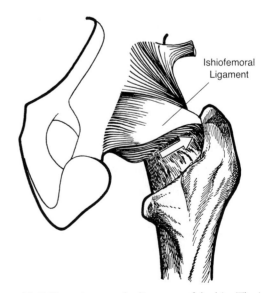

Ishiofemoral Ligament

Figure 19–7. Posterior capsular ligament of the hip. The ischiofemoral ligament is coiled in the same direction as the anterior capsular ligaments. (Adapted from Kapandji,[1] with permission.)

middle nodes in the femoral canal and the lateral part of the femoral ring and the extrailiac lymph nodes.

Myology of the Hip

Posterior Musculature

Gluteus Maximus

The gluteus maximus is innervated by the inferior gluteal nerve, L5, S1, and S2.[1,3–5] This muscle is primarily an extensor of the hip and assists in pelvic stability at heel-strike during the gait cycle. It is a phasic muscle and tends to weaken with dysfunction.

Gluteus Medius

The gluteus medius is innervated by the superior gluteal nerve, L5–S1. It is primarily an abductor, but its anterior fibers can flex and internally rotate the hip while the posterior fibers externally rotate. It is the main lateral stabilizer of the pelvis. Its fibers run parallel to the femoral shaft. It is not a very strong muscle until the femur is abducted 30 degrees or more, bringing its fibers more perpendicular to the shaft. It is a phasic muscle and tends to weaken with dysfunction, producing the Trendelenburg gait pattern.

Gluteus Minimus

The gluteus minimus lies deep to the medius and is likewise innervated by the superior gluteal nerve, L5–S1. It functions as a medial-lateral stabilizer of the hip. It is a phasic muscle and tends to weaken with dysfunction.

Piriformis

The piriformis muscle arises on the anterior surface of the sacrum (S2–S4), the sacroiliac capsule, and the ilium, and its tendon passes through the greater sciatic foramen to the greater trochanter of the femur. It is a two-joint muscle, acting on both the sacrum and the femur. External rotation of the femur, especially when the hip is flexed, is its primary action, although it may also extend and abduct. When acting on the sacrum, it will produce torsion of the sacrum to the opposite side. The piriformis derives its innervation from the L5–S2 nerve roots. The nerves of the sciatic plexus and the inferior gluteal vessels run intimately together. In 90 percent of individuals, these nerves and vessels pass under the piriformis. In 10 percent of the population, the nerves and vessels pierce the body of the muscle, passing through it. Dysfunction can compress the sciatic nerve against the foramen. The piriformis is a postural muscle and tends to tighten with dysfunction, producing external rotation of the femur and restriction of internal rotation. Dysfunction of the piriformis can thus cause problems with both the sacroiliac joint and the hip.

Superior and Inferior Gemelli, Obturator Externus and Internus, Quadratus Femoris

All these muscles are external rotators of the hip and function best when the hip is in extension. They run close to the capsule and help reinforce it. They are postural muscles and tend to tighten with dysfunction. The obturator externus is innervated by the posterior obturator nerve, L3–L4, and the obturator internus is innervated by the nerve to the obturator internus, L5–S1. All the others are innervated by nerve roots L5 and S1.

Hamstrings

The hamstrings are two-joint muscles acting at both the knee and the hip. They are most effective in extension of the hip when the knee is extended. They are postural muscles and tend to tighten with dysfunction. Bilateral tightness or contracture produces a posterior pelvic tilt. The semitendinosus is innervated by the tibial division of the sciatic nerve, L5–S2, as is the semimembranosus. The biceps femoris has its long head innervated by the tibial division of the sciatic nerve, L5–S2, whereas the short head is innervated by the peroneal division.

Medial Musculature

The medial muscles as a group arise from the pubis and insert on the posterior and posteromedial aspects of the femur. They are postural muscles and tend to tighten with dysfunction. Tightness unilaterally produces a lateral pelvic tilt high to the involved side, giving the appearance of a long leg.

Adductors

The adductor longus is innervated by the anterior obturator nerve, L2–L4; the adductor magnus is innervated by the obturator nerve and the tibial division of the sciatic nerve, L2–L4; the adductor brevis is innervated by the obturator nerve, L2–L4.

Pectineus

The pectineus muscle, along with the iliopsoas and the adductor longus, forms the floor of the femoral triangle. It is innervated by the accessory obturator nerve, L2–L3, and the femoral nerve, L2–L3.

Gracilis

The gracilis is the only two-joint adductor and is innervated by the obturator nerve, L2–L3.

Anterior Musculature

Iliopsoas

The iliopsoas is formed as the iliacus from the iliac fossa unites with the psoas major, which arises from the transverse processes of L1 through L5, inserting by a common tendon into the lesser trochanter of the femur. The iliopsoas is a two-joint muscle: When the spine is stable, it flexes the hip (and adducts and externally rotates it to some degree); when the femur is stable, it extends the lumbosacral spine. Unilateral contraction sidebends the spine to the same side and rotates the spine to the opposite side. The iliopsoas is a primary stabilizer of the hip in erect posture. Being a postural muscle, it tightens with dysfunction, producing hip flexion and increased lumbar lordosis. The iliopsoas is innervated by the femoral nerve, L2–L3, and the lumbar nerves, L1–L3.

Rectus Femoris

The rectus femoris has two heads. The straight head arises from the anterior superior iliac spine (ASIS); the reflected head arises from the margins of the hip joint capsule. The rectus femoris inserts into the common quadriceps tendon and into the tibial tubercle. It is a hip flexor when the knee is extended and tends to tighten with dysfunction. It is innervated by the femoral nerve, L2–L4.

Sartorius

The sartorius obliquely crosses the thigh from the ASIS to the superomedial tibia. It flexes, abducts, and externally rotates the hip. It forms the lateral border of the femoral triangle (the superior border is the inguinal ligament, and the medial border is the adductor longus). It tightens with dysfunction and is innervated by the femoral nerve, L2–L3.

Musculature

Tensor Fasciae Latae

The tensor fasciae latae arises from the iliac crest, the ASIS, and the fascia and inserts into the iliotibial band along with the superior fibers of the gluteus maximus to form the "deltoid" of the hip. It is primarily an abductor, but it can also flex and internally rotate the hip. It has a very long lever arm, as the iliotibial band crosses the knee. It tightens with dysfunction. Unilateral tightness produces a lateral pelvic tilt low to that side. Bilateral tightness produces an anterior pelvic tilt. The tensor fasciae latae is innervated by the superior gluteal nerve, L4–L5.

Entrapment Syndromes of the Hip and Pelvis

Several peripheral nerve entrapment syndromes that can occur in and around the hip and pelvis[6] are briefly mentioned here, not only to alert the clinician to the possibility of neurogenic pain in this region but to emphasize their anatomic considerations as well.

Femoral Nerve

The femoral nerve, L2–L4, descends through the psoas and travels on top of the iliacus. It exits the pelvis behind the inguinal ligament. It lies close to the femoral head, from which it is separated only by a small amount of muscle and capsule. Trauma or hematoma here may cause entrapment, producing pain and muscle weakness in the

iliopsoas, sartorius, pectineus, and quadriceps muscles. The main complaint is pain that starts below the inguinal ligament and can encompass the anteromedial surface of the thigh and the medial surface of the leg down to the medial surface of the foot. Local tenderness in the groin is almost always present. Muscle stretch reflexes of the knee will be diminished.

Sciatic Nerve

The sciatic nerve, L4–S2, usually passes deep to the piriformis muscle. If the nerve pierces the piriformis, it is usually the lateral division that does so. The lateral division forms the peroneal trunk. It is postulated by some that the basis for the piriformis syndrome is a hip flexion posture with a compensatory lordosis, which tightens the sciatic nerve against the notch. A true neuropathy will result in a flail leg and foot, but neuropathy secondary to direct external trauma at the sciatic notch is rare. The sciatic nerve innervates the hamstrings, the adductor magnus, and all the muscles of the leg and foot. It provides sensory innervation to the posterolateral leg and the plantar and dorsal aspects of the foot (see the section on the piriformis under "Myology of the Hip").

Obturator Nerve

The two most common causes of obturator nerve (L2–L4) entrapment are obturator hernia and osteitis pubis. Both conditions entrap the nerve in the obturator foramen. Obturator nerve entrapment is characterized by groin pain to the inner thigh, increasing during Valsalva maneuver and not relieved with rest. True neuropathy will cause pain and weakness in its distribution. The obturator nerve provides motor innervation to the adductors, the gracilis, the obturator externus, and occasionally the pectineus. Its pain reference is the medial thigh from the groin. Motion of the hip in a neuropathy will cause pain. Patients may exhibit a waddling gait pattern due to pain and adductor weakness and in an attempt to restrict hip motion.

Ilioinguinal Nerve

The ilioinguinal nerve, L1–L2, is vulnerable to entrapment in the region of the ASIS. This nerve follows the pattern of an intercostal nerve and arrives in the region of the ASIS. Here it turns medically and traverses the abdominal muscles in a step-wise fashion, piercing the transversus abdominis and internal oblique to reach the spermatic cord under the external oblique muscle. Entrapment of this nerve will cause pain into the groin, with some radiation to the proximal inner surface of the thigh. It is aggravated by increasing tension in the abdominal wall on standing erect and by hip motion, especially extension. There is a high incidence of lower back difficulties associated with this condition. Pressure over a point medial to the ASIS will cause pain to radiate into the area of innervation.

Lateral Femoral Cutaneous Nerve

The lateral femoral cutaneous nerve, L2–L3, is vulnerable to entrapment in the region of the ASIS where the nerve passes through the lateral end of the inguinal ligament. This condition is known as *meralgia paresthetica*. It is characterized by a burning pain in the anterior and lateral portions of the thigh. Pressure over the ASIS should aggravate the pain. The mechanism of onset may be traumatic, but very often the condition is without known cause. Pelvic tilt or a short leg resulting in postural alterations may be associated with this condition.

■ Functional Anatomy and Mechanics of the Pelvis

Bernhard Siegfried Albinus (1697–1770) and William Hunter were the first anatomists to demonstrate that the sacroiliac joint was a true synovial joint. Other researchers such as Meckel in 1816 and Von Luschka in 1854, who first classified the joint as diarthrodial, confirmed the earlier findings. Later investigators, including Albee in 1909 and Brooke in 1924, confirmed a synovial membrane and articular cartilage within the joint.[7] Solonen,[8] in 1957, conducted a comprehensive study on the osteology and arthrology of the pelvic girdle.

The pelvis is considered to be a closed ring composed of three functional pieces: the two pelvic halves (innominates) and the sacrum. The two innominates are conjoined anteriorly by the pubic symphysis and posteriorly by the interposed sacrum and the resulting two sacroiliac joints. The pelvis functions to attach the spine and the lower limbs, transmitting vertical forces between them as part of the kinetic chain, and also to protect the viscera. Many practitioners are mistakenly taught that the articulations of the pelvis (the pubic symphysis and the sacroiliac joints) have no functional movements except in childbirth and therefore do not contribute to complaints of pain or dysfunction except in rare instances such as disease and trauma. However, the pelvic joints do indeed move[3] and are probably involved directly or indirectly in the majority of mechanical low back problems.[9,10]

Osteology of the Pelvis

Innominate Bones

The innominate bones (left and right pelvic halves) are each formed by the fusion of the ilium, ischium, and pubic bones. This fusion is complete, with no movement between them whatsoever. Their common junction is in the acetabulum. As there is no functional movement between the bones of the innominates, each half is a functional unit by itself (Fig. 19–3A).

The left and right innominate bones are joined anteriorly in the midline by the pubic symphysis (Fig. 19–8). This articulation is bound together by the superior pubic ligament and inferiorly by thick arcuate fibers. Between the two halves is a fibrocartilaginous disk. A cavity (nonsynovial) may often be found in the disk, especially in women, and may extend the length of the disk. The pubic symphysis receives muscle attachments from the external oblique abdominal and the rectus abdominis muscles.

Sacrum

The iliac portions of the posterior innominate bones are joined together through the sacrum. The articulations here form the sacroiliac joints. The sacrum is formed by the fusion of the five sacral vertebrae and sits as a wedge between the innominates. The base of the sacrum (S1) forms the lumbosacral junction with the fifth lumbar vertebra. Its anterior projecting edge is known as the *sacral promontory*. The sacral apex (S5) articulates with the coccyx. The sacrum is curved ventrally, increasing the capacity of the true pelvis for visceral contents and childbearing. Posteriorly, the sacrum encases the spinal canal and the end of the cauda equina.

The sacroiliac joints are synovial articulations. Some classify the sacroiliac joint as a syndesmosis because of its synovial nature,[3] whereas others consider it to be a synchondrosis because of its fibrous articulation.[11] In the adult, the joint has an auricular shape and is characterized by irregularities (elevations and depressions) in the joint surfaces. These irregularities fit reciprocally with one another, lending strength to the joint, but also tend to restrict its movements. The sacral surface is fibrocartilaginous, whereas the iliac surface consists of hyaline cartilage.

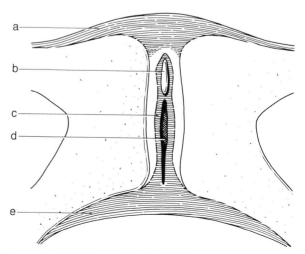

Figure 19–8. Pubic symphysis. (a) Superior pubic ligament; (b) hyaline cartilage; (c) fibrocartilaginous disk; (d) nonsynovial cavity; (e) inferior pubic ligament. (Adapted from Kapandji,[1] with permission.)

Sacroiliac Ligaments

The ligaments surrounding the sacroiliac joint are the strongest in the body and serve as attachments and origins for some of the strongest muscles in the body.[8] The strength of these ligaments has led some authorities to the belief that the sacroiliac joint is relatively immobile and consequently is rarely the source of pain or pathology,[12,13] or that the sacrum moves only as a unit with the innominates.[14] However, the fact that the sacroiliac joints do move has been convincingly proved as experimental methods have improved. For example, Frigerio, Stowe, and Howe,[15] using stereoradiography and computer vector analysis, demonstrated movement of up to 26 mm between the sacrum and the innominates in vivo. Others[16,17] have documented similar findings. Turek[18] stated that the sacroiliac joints have motion of 3 to 5 degrees until late middle age. For simplicity, the sacroiliac ligaments are presented here in two groups: intrinsic and extrinsic.

Intrinsic Ligaments

The anterior sacroiliac (capsular) ligament is a thickening of the capsule and is relatively weak compared with its other supporting structures. It is considered with its other supporting structures. It is considered by some[3] to be continuous with the iliopsoas and occasionally the piriformis, having origins from each muscle. It surrounds the joint surfaces completely and is continuous with the periosteum caudally, where it is about 1 mm thick, becoming better developed at the level of the arcuate line (Fig. 19–9). The interosseous ligaments are massive and form the chief bond between the two joint surfaces. The deep cranial and caudal bands blend with a more superficial sheet, which also has cranial and caudal portions that form

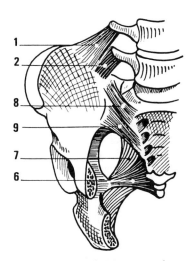

Figure 19–9. Anterior sacral joint capsule and ligaments. (1) and (2) are the iliolumbar ligaments; (8) and (9) are anterior sacroiliac ligaments, consisting of a superior and an inferior band; (6) sacrospinous ligament; (7) sacrotuberous ligament. (From Kapandji,[1] with permission.)

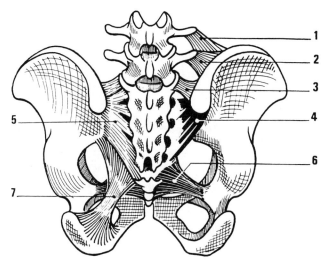

Figure 19–10. Posterior view of the pelvis showing the ligamentous support of the sacroiliac joint. (1) and (2) iliolumbar ligaments; (3) intermediate plane ligament from the iliac crest to the transverse process of S1; (4) posterior fibers of the interosseous ligaments; (5) anterior plane of the sacroiliac ligaments (deep fibers of the interosseous ligaments); (6) sacrospinous ligament; (7) sacrotuberous ligament. (From Kapandji,[1] with permission.)

the short posterior sacroiliac ligaments (Fig. 19–10). The dorsal ligaments overlie the interosseous ligaments. Their lower fibers may form a separate fasciculus known as the *long posterior sacroiliac ligament*. This ligament blends with the sacrotuberous ligament and the thoracolumbar fascia. Because of the directions of fiber arrangements of the anterior and posterior sacroiliac ligaments, some authors tend to group them into caudal and cranial groups, indicating their functional capacities.[1,19]

Extrinsic Ligaments

The sacrotuberous and sacrospinous ligaments bind the sacrum to the ischium. The lower fibers of the sacrotuberous ligament blend with the gluteus maximus and the biceps femoris. This ligament functions to resist the upward tilting of the lower sacrum under the downward thrust of the weight of the trunk imparted to the sacral base from above. The sacrospinous ligament connects the spine of the ischium to the lateral margins of the sacrum and coccyx.

The iliolumbar ligaments have two bands: a superior band, which connects the tip of the L4 transverse process to the iliac crest, and an inferior band, which connects the tip of the L5 transverse process to the iliac crest anteromedially to the superior band (Fig. 19–11). Sometimes the inferior band displays two distinct divisions: one strictly iliac portion and one portion that is strictly sacral. The influence of the iliolumbar ligaments on lumbosacral motion is discussed later (see the section "Lumbopelvic Rhythm").

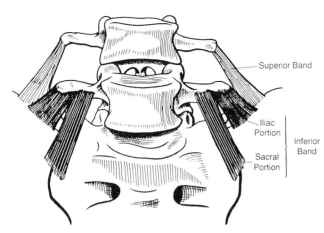

Figure 19–11. Iliolumbar ligaments. (From Kapandji,[1] with permission.)

Pelvic Types

Four types of pelves are described in *Gray's Anatomy*[3]: anthropoid, android, gynaecoid, and platypelloid. The differences among them depend mainly on the sex of the individual. These pelvic types differ in the dimensions of the superior and inferior apertures, the greater sciatic notch, and the subpubic arches. There are also proportional differences between the fore and hind pelves, as well as between the anterior and posterior transverse diameters of the inlets.

Sexual differences between male and female pelves have to do with function. Although the primary function in both pelves is locomotion, the major difference is in the female role in childbirth. The male pelvis is more heavily built, and the general architecture, being more angular in orientation, is more for power and strength. The female pelvis is broader and deeper, with its iliac wings more vertically set but shallower than in the male pelvis.

The pelvis functions to transmit vertical forces from the vertebral column to the hips via the sacroiliac joints or to transmit ground reaction forces from the legs and hips to the vertebral column via the sacroiliac joints. These force transmissions and dissipations are accomplished through two trabecular systems previously mentioned, the sacroacetabular system and the sacroischial system (see the section "Osteology of the Hip").

Innervation

The innervation of the sacroiliac joint is not always symmetric.[3] The joint is most consistently found to be innervated by segments S1 and S2 dorsally and segments L3 to S2 ventrally. Participation of the obturator nerve in the innervation of the sacroiliac joint is not confirmed.[8]

Muscular Influences

Solonen[8] noted that the sacroiliac joint is normally in a state of stable equilibrium and that much force is required

to disturb this equilibrium. He further pointed out that the strongest muscles in the body surround the sacroiliac joint but that none have the primary function of moving it. Thus, he concluded, there are no voluntary movements of the sacroiliac joint, and what movements do occur are produced by other movements of the body, especially weight changes and postural influences. Such movements are referred to by some as *joint play motions*[20,21] or *accessory joint motions*.[3]

Some authorities[11,22–25] believe that the following muscle or muscle groups can indirectly impart force on the sacroiliac joint, either through their primary actions or by their reverse actions, depending on the points of fixation: the iliopsoas, rectus femoris, hip abductors and adductors, sartorius, external rotators and piriformis, gluteus maximus, hamstrings, abdominals, quadratus lumborum, and multifidus. Rather than give a detailed synopsis of each muscle in terms of its morphology, each muscle or group is presented according to its action.

Iliopsoas

With the femur and pelvis fixed, the iliopsoas produces powerful ipsilateral flexion of the lumbar spine with rotation contralaterally. It flexes the lumbar spine relative to the pelvis, increasing lordosis. If the lumbar spine and pelvis are fixed, the iliopsoas produces flexion of the hip as well as some lateral rotation of the hip and may have some adduction function. Some fibers, especially from the iliacus, blend with the anterior sacroiliac ligament and joint capsule. Bilateral contraction of the iliopsoas produces an anterior force on the pelvis, causing anterior motion of the innominate as well as an anterior force on the sacrum because of its attachment on the sacral ala. Unilateral contraction may cause an anterior force ipsilaterally, resulting in anterior rotation of the innominate, and may produce anterior movement of the sacrum on that side. Simultaneously, it may produce a torsion of the sacrum to the opposite side.

Rectus Femoris

The rectus femoris can simultaneously flex the hip and extend the knee. If the pelvis is fixed, it will flex the thigh on the pelvis. If the thigh is fixed, it will flex the pelvis on the thigh. If the thigh and the lumbar spine are both fixed, with the pelvis free to move, the rectus femoris has the potential to cause anterior rotation of the innominate.

Sartorius

The sartorius can simultaneously flex the knee and the hip. It assists with hip abduction and external rotation. It may exert an anterior influence on the innominate when the knee is fixed in some flexion and the hip is extended.

Hip Abductors

The hip abductors indirectly influence the sacroiliac joints through the public symphysis (see the sections "Myology of the Hip," "Evaluation," and "Treatment").

Tensor Fasciae Latae

See the section "Myology of the Hip."

Gluteus Maximus

The gluteus maximus extends a flexed thigh and prevents the forward momentum of the trunk from causing flexion of the hip during the gait cycle. It is inactive in standing but powerfully rotates the pelvis backward in raising the trunk from a forward bent position. It can be a strong lateral rotator of the thigh and abductor as it exerts influence on the iliotibial tract. Bilateral contraction may assist in trunk extension if the femur is fixed. Bilateral contraction produces posterior movement of the innominates through the sacrotuberous and posterior sacroiliac ligaments. Unilateral contraction produces a posterior force on the innominate ipsilaterally, causing posterior rotation on that side.

Hip Adductors

The hip adductors exert indirect action on the sacroiliac joints through the pubis (see the sections "Evaluation" and "Treatment"). Tightness or weakness of the adductors may influence hip position, which in turn influences the sacroiliac joints.

Hamstrings

The hamstrings as a group are the primary knee flexors, but they can extend the hip when the hip is flexed and the knee is in extension (see the section "Myology of the Hip"). They work to convert the posterior ligaments, especially the sacrotuberous ligament, into dynamic movers. Tightness or weakness of the hamstrings can cause either an anterior or a posterior rotation of the pelvis on the hip (see the section "Lumbopelvic Rhythm").

External Rotators and Piriformis

Bilateral contraction of the piriformis will produce an anterior force on the sacrum and cause it to flex forward. Unilateral contraction may produce an anterior force on the side of contraction, causing rotation to occur to the opposite side. Tightness or spasm of the piriformis may have significant influence on the sacroiliac joint (see the sections "Myology of the Hip," "Gait and Body Position," "Sacral Torsions," "Evaluation," and "Treatment").

Quadratus Lumborum

The quadratus lumborum fixes the 12th rib and can be an accessory muscle of inspiration. Bilateral contraction results in stabilization of the lumbar spine, preventing deviation from the midline. Unilateral contraction produces ipsilateral sidebending when the pelvis is fixed. Some elevation and rotation anteriorly occur with unilateral contraction. Bilateral contraction may produce an anterior flexion of the sacrum through its attachments onto the base and ala. A unilateral contraction may produce an ipsilateral sacral flexion, with rotation to the side opposite the contraction.

Multifidus

Along with the rotators (transversospinalis group), the multifidus is primarily a postural muscle and stabilizes the lumbar spinal joints. A bilateral contraction extends the vertebral column from the prone or the forward bent position and, conversely, performs in controlled forward bending (eccentric contraction). In the lumbar spine during rotation, the contralateral group is more active. A bilateral contraction may produce a posterior force on the pelvis through its attachments with the erector spinae, the posterior superior iliac spine (PSIS), and the posterior sacroiliac ligaments. A unilateral contraction may produce a posterior rotation of the vertebrae on that side.

Abdominals

The importance of the abdominals in relation to the lumbar spine and the pelvis is in lifting. By exerting pressure internally (Valsalva), the abdominals significantly reduce axial compressive forces. The abdominals resist the shear forces. The abdominals resist the shear forces produced by the multifidus and the psoas on the lumbar facets.[26] A bilateral contraction, especially of the rectus abdominis, produces a posterior rotation of the pelvis when the vertebral column and the sternum are fixed. Lack of abdominal tone will result in increased lumbar lordosis and an increased sacral flexion position.

Anatomic Considerations for Sacroiliac Dysfunction

According to Cyriax,[13] sacroiliac joint problems are more common in females than in males. The following anatomic factors may explain why the occurrence of sacroiliac dysfunctions in the general population is six times greater in females than in males (see the section "Functional Anatomy and Mechanics of the Pelvis").

1. The lateral dimension of the pelvic foramen is greater in females than in males.
2. The bone density of the male pelvis is greater.
3. The sacroiliac joint surfaces are smaller in females.
4. The sacroiliac joint surfaces are flatter in females.

5. The sacroiliac joints are located farther from the hips in females than in males.
6. The iliac crests are set farther apart in the female pelvis than in the male pelvis.
7. The vertical dimension of the pelvis is greater in the male pelvis.
8. The more rectangular the shape of the sacrum, the more stable it is within the innominates.
9. The more vertical the orientation of the sacrum within the innominates, the flatter or less lordotic is the lumbar spine; this increases compressive forces on the lumbar spine.
10. The more horizontal the orientation of the sacrum within the innominates, the greater will be the lumbar lordosis; this increases the shear forces across the lumbosacral angle.
11. Three types of sacral articular surfaces have been classified according to shape:
    a. Average or normal auricular surface
    b. Smooth and convex anteroposteriorly (this is the type of articular surface in which the rare inflare and outflare dysfunctional lesions of the innominates occur)
    c. Extremely irregular and concave auricular surfaces (these are very stable and usually uniform bilaterally but occasionally may be asymmetric in shape)

Orientation Planes of the Pelvis

To understand the relationships of the structure and movements of the sacrum, lumbar spine, and lower extremities to one another, one must understand and be able to relate the reference planes of the pelvis to the cardinal planes of the body. Knowing these planes, one is then able to describe the direction and degree of motion of any given pelvic landmark in relation to any other specified landmark.

The cardinal planes of the body are (1) the transverse plane, which bisects the body through the center of gravity into upper and lower halves; (2) the sagittal plane, which bisects the body in the midline through the center of gravity into right and left halves; and (3) the frontal plane, which bisects the body through the shoulders anteroposteriorly into ventral and dorsal halves.

The orientation planes of the pelvis are (1) the pelvic frontal plane, which is parallel to the frontal plane, running through the anterior edge of the symphysis pubis to the ASIS; (2) the pelvic transverse plane, which is parallel to the transverse plane and runs through the ASIS to the PSIS; and (3) the pelvic dorsal plane, which is parallel to the pelvic frontal plane and runs through the PSIS. These reference planes are shown in Figure 19–12.

Principal Pelvic Axes of Motion

The movements of the pelvic joints can be somewhat confusing if one does not understand the axes about

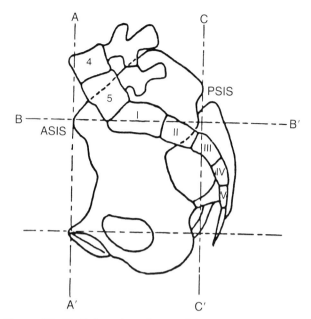

Figure 19–12. Orientation planes of the pelvis. A–A′, pelvic frontal plane; B–B′, pelvic transverse plane; C–C′, pelvic dorsal plane. (Adapted from Mitchell,[27] with permission.)

which these movements occur. It is important to realize that these movements are conjoined and do not occur as pure movements in pure planes (Fig. 19–13).

Pubis

The pubis has its axis in the frontal plane, which allows anteroposterior rotation of the one innominate against the other. Movement in any other plane at this joint is pathologic. The greatest functional movements of the pubis occur in the gait cycle (see the section "Gait and Body Position").

Sacroiliac Joint

The sacroiliac joint can be considered as two joints: the iliosacral and the sacroiliac. The term *iliosacral* implies the innominates moving on the sacrum. Conversely, the term *sacroiliac* implies the sacrum moving within the innominates. Functionally and from a treatment standpoint, these designations are correct because they are based on the recruitment of motion and the transmission of forces from the spine or lower members through the pelvis even though it is one and the same joint.

Iliosacral motion occurs primarily in the sagittal plane about the inferior transverse axis (anterior and posterior rotation of the innominates; see "Gait and Body Position"). Iliosacral motion is conjoined with rotation at the pubis and through the sacrum at the contralateral oblique axis.

Sacroiliac motions occur about multiple axes, two transverse and two oblique. The principal axis of regular sacroiliac movement (nutation/counternutation) is the

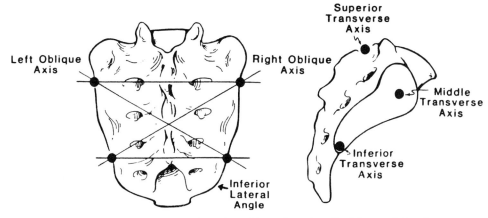

Figure 19–13. Principle axes of sacral motion. (From Saunders,[28] with permission.)

middle transverse axis. However, because iliosacral motion is conjoined with the pubis, the sacrum must make adaptive movements about the two oblique axes alternately (see the sections "Gait and Body Position" and "Sacral Torsions"). The superior transverse axis is often referred to as the *respiratory axis*. This axis is actually a fulcrum formed by the attachments of the posterior sacroiliac ligaments and the thoracodorsal fascia. As one inhales, the sacrum extends (counternutates), and as one exhales, the sacrum flexes (nutates).

Functional Integration of Related Areas

The transmission of vertical forces from the spine to the lower members, and of ground reaction forces from the lower limbs to the spine (Fig. 19–14), occurs through

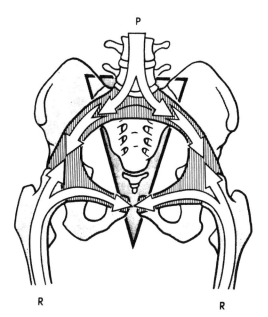

Figure 19–14. Transmission of ground reaction forces and vertical compression forces from the upper body through the sacroiliac joints and pubic rami. P, compression forces; R, ground reaction forces. (From Kapandji,[1] with permission.)

trabecular lines (see the section "Osteology of the Hip"). The manner in which these forces are transmitted and dispersed (i.e., from the top down versus from the bottom up) helps explain why certain dysfunctional lesions of the pelvis occur regularly with certain actions or activities as are discussed later.

Lumbopelvic Rhythm

The concept of normal functional integration among the lumbar spine, pelvis, and hip joints is basic to the understanding of dysfunction in this region. In the total forward bending of the spine, there is synchronous movement in a rhythmic rotation of the lumbar spine to that of pelvic rotation about the hips.[14,28]

As one bends forward, the lumbar lordosis reverses itself from concave to flat to convex. At the same time, there is a proportionate amount of pelvic rotation about the hips. The amount of movement between lumbar levels will vary, with the most movement occurring at L5–S1 and lesser amounts at successively higher levels. Nonetheless, the rhythm between levels should be smooth and precise, rendering a balance between lumbar reversal and pelvic rotation (Fig. 19–15). Obviously, the ability of a person to bend forward will be influenced by this rhythmic balance or lack of it. Many factors can influence this rhythm, such as facet restriction, degenerative joint disease, or tight hamstring muscles. Thus, to achieve full forward bending, the lumbar spine must fully reverse itself, and the pelvis must rotate to its fullest extent. During these movements, the sacrum is also moving within the ilia. Initially, the sacrum nutates (flexes), but as motion in the lumbar spine is recruited and the hamstrings begin to tether the pelvis in its rotation around the hips, the sacrum begins to counternutate (extend) within the ilia.

At the same time as these movements are occurring in the sagittal plane, there is a backward translation of the pelvis and the hips in the horizontal plane. This represents a shift in the pelvic fulcrum so that the center of

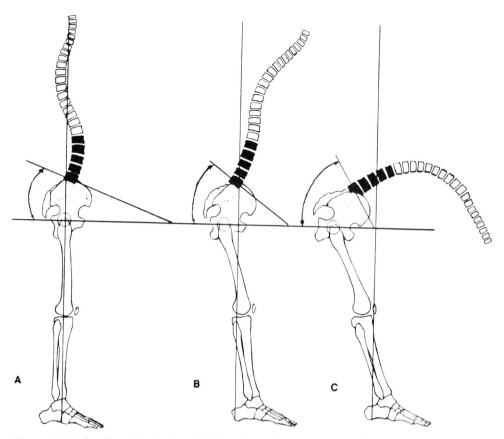

Figure 19–15. Lumbopelvic rhythm. (A) Normal standing posture with lumbar concavity; body weight superimposed directly over the hip joints; normal pelvic inclination with respect to horizontal. (B) Flattening of the lumbar spine; the pelvis begins to rotate anteriorly around the hips; the hips and pelvis move posteriorly in the horizontal plane. (C) Reversal of the lumbar spine into lumbar convexity; the pelvis rotates anteriorly to the fullest extent; the hips and pelvis are posteriorly displaced in the horizontal plane. (From Saunders,[28] with permission.)

gravity is maintained over the feet. If this did not occur, the person would fall forward.

As the person returns to the standing position, the reverse process should occur in an equally smooth manner. It is a fallacy to think that just because a person can bend forward and touch the toes, he or she has full range of motion of the lumbosacral spine. Such an individual may very well have loose hamstrings, which never engage the pelvis to tether it. Thus, the lumbar spine is allowed to remain relatively concave or flat and the sacrum in relative nutation. Conversely, the hamstrings may be tight and can markedly restrict pelvic rotation about the hips. Should this person try to force flexion of the trunk, as in lifting, a strain may occur in the lumbosacral area. The point is made to encourage the clinician to assess closely the integration of motion between the lumbar spine and pelvic components.

Sacroiliac movement in forward bending occurs first at the middle transverse axis. As one approaches the middle of forward bending, a small amount of sacral extension occurs. This is followed by the base moving slightly anterior and the apex to the middle transverse axis. In forced forward bending, the movement shifts more to the superior transverse axis, and the base of the sacrum moves posteriorly and superiorly and the apex anteriorly.

The iliolumbar ligaments directly influence the integration of movement between the lumbar and pelvic components of the complex. The superior and inferior bands are selectively stretched during different movements and serve to greatly limit motion and stabilize the lumbosacral junction. In sidebending, the iliolumbar ligaments become taut contralaterally and relax ipsilaterally. They allow only 8 degrees of movement of L4 relative to the sacrum.[1] In flexion, the inferior band is relaxed and the superior band tightens. In extension, the inferior band tightens and the superior band relaxes.

To reiterate, certain motions in the pelvic complex must be differentiated from each other. Although the joint is called the sacroiliac joint, and although the motion occurring at this joint can rightly be called sacroiliac motion, the term must be narrowed somewhat. In certain contexts, *sacroiliac motion* will be viewed as motion of the sacrum within the two innominates. Motion of the innominates on a fixed sacrum will be termed *iliosacral motion.* These two categories of movement comprise sacroiliac motion in the broader sense (see the section "Principal Pelvic Axes of Motion").

■ Mechanics of Dysfunction

The following descriptions fit a model for sacroiliac dysfunction as taught by osteopathic practitioners[11,22–24] It must be remembered that very few if any motions in the human body occur in a single plane about a single axis. So it is in the sacroiliac joint. The models described present concepts of motion about the principal axes and form a basis for examination and a rationale for treatment. The seven most common dysfunctions will be presented in some detail. The other less common ones will be briefly mentioned (see the section "Signs of Sacroiliac Problems").

Innominate Rotations

There are two principal rotatory dysfunctions of the innominates: anterior (forward) and posterior (backward). The axis through which these rotations occur in the transverse axis through the pubic symphysis in the horizontal plane. To visualize this, form an open ring with your hands between the tips of the long fingers. The space between the thumbs represents where the sacrum would be placed to complete the ring. The pubic symphysis is represented by the touching of the fingertips. Rotating one hand up or down in relation to the other represents the motion of one innominate in relation to the other (Fig. 19–16). Dysfunctional innominates are thus described as either anterior or posterior according to the side of involvement (e.g., left posterior, right anterior). By far the most common of these dysfunctional rotations is the left posterior innominate, and the next most common is the right anterior innominate.[22] Some practitioners believe that left anterior and right posterior dysfunctions

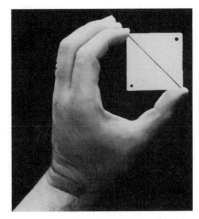

Figure 19–17. Left oblique axis.

almost never occur,[22] whereas others believe that their incidence is related to the type of population being treated and the types of stresses sustained in working situations (military, mining, business, industrial, etc.; S.A. Stratton, personal communication).[29]

Posterior innominate dysfunctions occur most frequently in the following situations: (1) repeated unilateral standing; (2) a fall onto an ischial tuberosity; (3) a vertical thrust onto an extended leg; (4) lifting in a forward bent position with the knees locked; and (5) intercourse positions in females (hyperflexion and abduction of the hips). Anterior innominates occur most frequently in the following situations: (1) golf or baseball swing; (2) horizontal thrust of the knee (dashboard injury); and (3) any forceful movement on a diagonal (ventral proprioceptive neuromuscular facilitation [PNF]) pattern.

Sacral Torsions

Sacral torsions are perhaps the hardest dysfunctions to conceptualize. They occur as fixations on either of the oblique axes, usually during the gait cycle, and are held in this dysfunctional position by the piriformis (see the section "Gait and Body Position"). Torsions might be thought of as half the sacrum flexing and the other half extending on one of the two oblique axes.[30] Torsions do not occur purely on the oblique axes but have a sidebending component as well as a flexion component. To visualize the concept of sacral torsion, take a matchbook cover to represent the sacrum in three-dimensional space. Holding the top left corner and the bottom right corner between the thumb and long finger (the diagonal between them representing the left oblique axis [LOA]); [Fig. 19–17]), push forward on the top right corner, and allow the "sacrum" to rotate between the fingers; the effect approximates that of a sacral torsion to the left on the left oblique axis (Fig. 19–18). It must be remembered that all anatomic referencing is from the standard anatomic model, and what is considered to be forward or backward must be in relation to this position. Clinically,

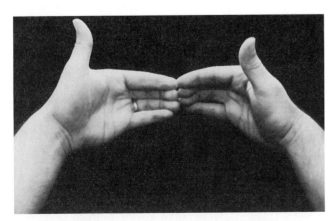

Figure 19–16. Demonstration of the principle of innominate rotation. (For explanation of Figs. 19–16 to 19–22, see text.)

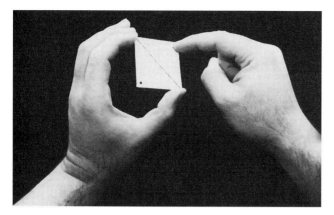

Figure 19–18. Left-on-left forward sacral torsion.

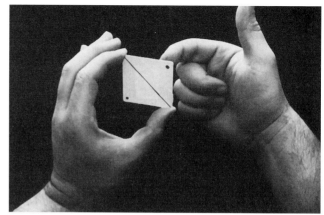

Figure 19–20. Right-on-left backward sacral torsion.

however, patients with back problems are viewed from the posterior aspect, and sometimes confusion arises as to what is forward and backward with regard to sacral torsions. Thus, in the model described, the dysfunction is labeled according to the *direction* of motion of the sacrum and the *axis* on which the motion occurred: left forward torsion *on* the left oblique axis, or a left-on-left forward torsion (L on L).

By simply changing the finger holds on the matchbook to the opposite diagonal corners and pushing forward on the top left corner (Fig. 19–19), one now approximates a right forward torsion on the right oblique, axis of a right-on-right forward torsion (R on R). (Note: Forward torsions are *only* left-on-left or right-on-right.)

Backward torsions positionally in space appear to be identical to forward torsions. They are, however, quite different. To visualize this concept, take the matchbook and, while holding it on the left oblique axis (top left and bottom right corners), pull the top right corner backward (Fig. 19–20). This approximates a right backward torsion on the left oblique axis, or a right-on-left backward torsion (R on L). Grasping the opposite diagonal corners (top right and bottom left) and pulling the top left corner backward approximates a left backward torsion on the right oblique axis (L on R). (Note: Backward torsions are *only* left-on-right or right-on-left.)

Unilateral Sacral Flexions

Sacral flexion lesions might be thought of as failure of one side of the sacrum to extend (counternutate) from the flexed (nutated) position.[29] In this situation, the sacrum has flexed on the middle transverse axis. As the dysfunction occurs, the sacrum is forced down the long arm of the joint, where it becomes restricted. Thus, there is a large sidebending component in this dysfunction as well as a flexion component. Because of this restriction, the sacrum is unable to extend on that side. Sacral flexion lesions tend to be traumatic and usually do not occur as the result of everyday stresses and strains.

Again using the matchbook cover, holding the cover about one-third of the way down on either side simulates the middle transverse axis. Turning the cover forward between the fingertips simulates nutation. Now, by turning forward with one hand and turning backward with the other, adding a little bending to the side that is turning backward, the sacral flexion lesion is approximated (Fig. 19–21).

Pubic Shear Lesions

Pubic shears are, as the name implies, a sliding of one joint surface in relation to the other in either a superior

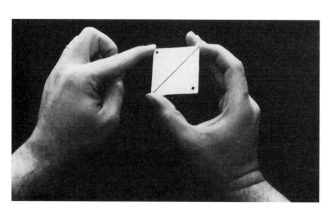

Figure 19–19. Right-on-right forward sacral torsion.

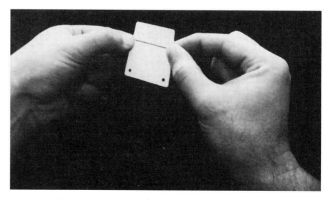

Figure 19–21. Unilateral sacral flexion lesion.

or an inferior direction. To visualize this dysfunction, place the knuckles of your two fists together and slide one fist superiorly one knuckle width (Fig. 19–22).

Pubic shears are probably the most commonly overlooked pelvic dysfunction. However, their recognition and proper treatment are mandatory for success in treating pelvic dysfunctions. Pubic shears very frequently occur with innominate rotations and upslips and are often the cause of groin pain as a presenting symptom (see the section "Evaluation").

Superior Innominate Shear (Upslip)

Innominate shears, either superior or inferior, were once usually thought of as rather rare. However, Greenman[31] indicated that their occurrence is much more common than was previously thought. As the name suggests, an innominate shear is a sliding of one entire innominate superiorly (upslip) or inferiorly (downslip) in relation to the other. These shears are usually traumatic and result from a fall onto an ischial tuberosity or from unexpected vertical thrust onto an extended leg.

Etiology of Sacroiliac Joint Dysfunction

Sacroiliac joint dysfunctions, whether mechanical or disease related, are usually characterized by localized pain in the sulcus. Diseases such as ankylosing spondylitis, Paget's disease, or tuberculosis all may give rise to sacroiliac pain as an initial complaint.[15,32] In the general population, acute strains with joint involvement are actually rare. This may not be true in certain populations such as athletes and the military.[33] Far more common in terms of mechanical dysfunction are structural and muscular imbalances and joint hypermobilities that give rise to sacroiliac complaints.

Signs of Sacroiliac Problems

The types of pain that can occur with sacroiliac dysfunction are variable.[9–11,22,24,34] The pain may be sharp or dull,

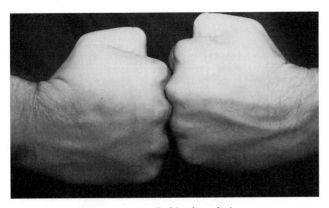

Figure 19–22. Pubic shear lesion.

aching or tingling, and so on. The pain is most often unilateral and local to the joint (sulcus) itself, but it may refer down the leg (usually posterolaterally and not below the knee) because of innervation from the L2 through S2 segments. There are no associated neurologic symptoms with sacroiliac dysfunction. A straight leg raise test may be positive but only for pain, and usually in the higher are above 60 degrees. The pain is usually worse with walking and stair climbing, and the patient usually limps (with a Trendelenburg or similar gait pattern). The intensity of pain usually does not increase with prolonged sitting; however, when the condition is acute, the patient may sit shifted onto one ischium. The patient often maintains lumbar lordosis in forward bending, recruiting motion around the acetabuli (see the section "Lumbopelvic Rhythm"), and may also complain of some lumbar pain. The clinician may note ipsilateral tension over the erector spinae muscles and may see a slight swelling over the dorsal aspect of the sacrum. Pain may often arise from the nonblocked side (i.e., the dysfunctional side may be nonpainful, but it causes the opposite side to become hypermobile and painful). Finally, sacroiliac pain is more common in females in the general population (see the section "Anatomic Considerations for Sacroiliac Dysfunction").

Gait and Body Position

A patient with sacroiliac joint dysfunction will often complain of pain during walking or stair climbing. An understanding of the relative positions and movements of the sacrum, innominates, and other body parts will help account for the pain produced during locomotion. The following is a synthesis of an article by Mitchell on this topic.[11,22,27] The cycle of movement of the pelvis in walking is described in sequence as though the patient were starting to walk by advancing the right foot first:

1. Trunk rotation in the thoracic region occurs to the left, accompanied by left sidebending of the lumbar spine, forming a convexity to the right.
2. The body of the sacrum begins a torsional movement to the left, locking the lumbosacral junction and shifting the body weight to the left sacroiliac. This locking mechanism establishes movement of the sacrum on the left oblique axis. As the sacrum can now turn torsionally to the left, the sacral base must also move down on the right to conform to the lumbar convexity that has formed on the right.
3. As the right leg accelerates forward through action of the quadriceps, tension accumulates at the junction of the left oblique axis and the inferior transverse axis and eventually locks. As the body weight swings forward, slight anterior movement is increased by the backward thrust of the restraining left leg as the right heel strikes the ground.
4. Tension in the right hamstrings begins with heelstrike. As the body weight moves forward and up-

ward toward the right crest of femoral support, there is a slight posterior movement of the right innominate on the inferior transverse axis. This movement is also increased by the forward thrust of the propelling leg action. This ilial rotational movement is also influenced, directed, and stabilized by the torsional movement of the pubic symphysis on its transverse axis. Also at heel-strike, the right piriformis contracts to fixate the left oblique axis at the inferior lateral angle, thus allowing for a left forward torsion of the sacrum on the left oblique axis (left-on-left forward torsion). From the standpoint of total pelvic movement, one might consider the transverse pubic symphyseal axis as the postural axis of rotation for the entire pelvis.

5. As the right heel strikes the ground, trunk rotation and accommodation begin to reverse themselves. At midstance, as the left foot passes the right and the body weight passes over the crest of femoral support, the accumulating forces move to the right. At this point, the sacrum changes its axis to the right oblique axis, which then allows the left sacral base to move forward and torsionally to the right. The cycle of movements is then repeated in identical fashion on the left.

Vertebral Motion

Frequently, in attempting to describe the motion of a vertebral segment, terms become confused. Sometimes terms describing motion are inappropriately interchanged with terms that describe position. This section defines the terms for both vertebral segment motion and vertebral segment positioning. These must be clearly differentiated to ensure accurate communication.

A vertebral motion segment consists of two adjacent vertebrae, specifically, the inferior half of the superior vertebra and the superior half of the inferior vertebra, which includes the posterior intervertebral facet joints and the intervertebral disk anteriorly.[1] Vertebral motion

Table 19–1. Standard Vertebral
Motion Terminology

Term	Definition
Flexion	Forward bending of the trunk in the sagittal plane about a transverse axis
Extension	Backward bending of the trunk in the sagittal plane about a transverse axis
Sidebending	Movement (left or right) in the coronal plane about an anteroposterior axis
Rotation	Movement (left or right) in the transverse plane about a vertical axis

Table 19–2. Laws of Physiologic Spinal
Motion (Fryette's Laws)

Law I	If the vertebral segments are in the neutral (or easy normal) position without locking of the facets, rotation and sidebending are in opposite directions (type I motion) (Fig. 19–23)
Law II	If the vertebral segments are in full flexion or extension with the facets locked or engaged, rotation and sidebending are to the same side (type II motion) (Fig. 19–24)
Law III	If motion is introduced into a vertebral segment in any plane, motion in all other planes is reduced.

occurs in a plane around an axis and is named for the superior segment moving on the inferior segment. Table 19–1 defines the standard motion terms with regard to anatomic planes and axes.

In the early 1900s, Fryette described the coupling of the various spinal motions with one another.[35] His observations have, with certain clarifications, remained substantially valid over the years. These "laws" of spinal motion are summarized in Table 19–2 and Figures 19–23 and 19–24.

The range of vertebral motion may be considered either active or passive. Active vertebral motion is the result of the patient's voluntary activity. It involves multiple segmental activity and is frequently compound in nature. Passive vertebral motion is the result of clinician activity or an external force. It may involve one or multiple segments and may be simple or compound. Vertebral segment dysfunction may be compensatory as a result of long-standing postural imbalance, inequality of muscle

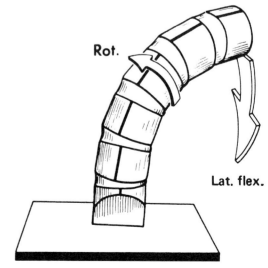

Figure 19–23. First law of physiologic spinal motion: sidebending and rotation are in opposite directions when the spine is in a neutral posture. (From Kapandji,[1] with permission.)

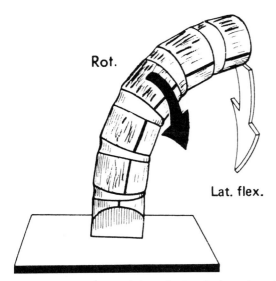

Figure 19–24. Second law of physiologic spinal motion: side-bending and rotation are in the same direction when the spine is in flexion or extension. (Adapted from Kapandji,[1] with permission.)

tone, or single-segment dysfunction above or below. It may also be traumatic.

Quality of Vertebral Motion

The ease with which a patient moves through a range of motion is as significant as the total range of motion itself. With careful palpation, the clinician can assess subtle aberrations in the freedom of motion within a segment or group of segments that appear to have a normal range of motion. Thus, the clinician must be able to evaluate quality as well as quantity of motion for diagnostic as well as therapeutic considerations. Segments with restricted range of motion (usually symmetric) may have normal degrees of freedom or ease. Hypermobility is increased range and freedom (laxity) of joint motion. Hypermobile segments are frequently symptomatic, and thrust mobilizations are generally contraindicated. Hypermobile joints are most frequently the result of compensatory change caused by restricted motion (above or below the joint) or are traumatic in origin.[22]

Barrier Concept of Vertebral Motion Restriction

Not every object moving in space has 6 degrees of freedom of motion; however, the vertebral segment does.[28] A normal functional range of motion exists in or across the three planes of motion for each segment. If, for whatever reason, motion becomes restricted in one plane, motion in the other two planes is also reduced (Fryette's third law). This may be perceived as a restriction in overall movement during an analysis of spinal movement.

Somatic dysfunction has been described as impaired or altered function of related components of the somatic

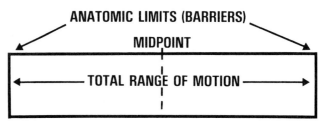

Figure 19–25. Total range of motion for any joint. (Adapted from Kimberly,[24] with permission.)

(body framework) system. Somatic dysfunction is characterized by impaired mobility, which may or may not occur with positional alteration.[11,22,23,36] Figure 19–25 illustrates the total range of motion for any given joint. It is bounded at its extremes by its anatomic limits (barriers). A barrier is an obstruction or a restriction to movement. Anatomic barriers include the bone contours and/or soft tissues, especially the ligaments, that serve as the final limit to motion in an articulation beyond which tissue damage will occur. Physiologic barriers are the soft tissue tension accumulations that limit the voluntary motion of an articulation. Further motion toward the anatomic barrier can be induced passively.

Figure 19–26 illustrates the divisions of active and passive motion within the total range of motion of a given joint. Active motion is movement of an articulation by the individual between the physiologic barriers. Passive motion is movement induced in an articulation by the clinician. It includes the range of active motion, as well as the movement between the physiologic and anatomic barriers permitted by soft tissue resilience that the individual cannot initiate voluntarily. Soft tissue tension accumulates as the joint is passively moved from its active range through physiologic barriers toward anatomic barriers. Thus, when the clinician tests a joint for end-feel or joint play, it is these barriers that are being tested and compared.

In somatic dysfunction, minor motion loss sometimes occurs, implying that a restrictive barrier has formed somewhere within the normal active range of motion, thus limiting the ability of the joint to complete its full, pain-free range of motion. A minor motion loss is one

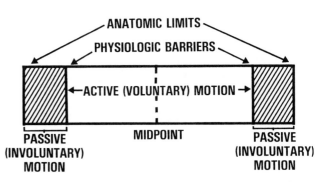

Figure 19–26. Active and passive divisions in somatic dysfunction. (Adapted from Kimberly,[24] with permission.)

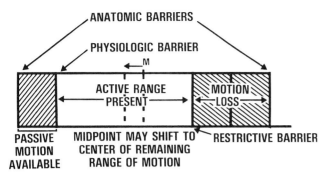

Figure 19–27. Minor motion loss in somatic dysfunction. M, midpoint. (Adapted from Kimberly,[24] with permission.)

in which the barrier does not cross the midpoint of the joint's normal range of motion. This concept is illustrated in Figure 19–27.

A major motion loss occurs when the motion barrier crosses the normal midpoint of the active range of motion of the joint. This is illustrated in Figure 19–28. Motion loss, whether major or minor, is maintained until something occurs to change the barrier. Different factors influence these restrictions, such as taut joint capsules, shortened ligaments and fascias, muscles shortened due to spasm or fibrosis, or a shift in the gamma gain mechanism.[37] Long-standing lesions lead to changes in the adjacent tissues (adnexae), especially in circulatory (edema with dilation or vasoconstriction), neural (pain, tenderness, hyperesthesia, itching), and myofascial components (muscle contraction, fibrosis). These can lead to changes in segmentally related tissues, especially circulatory (usually vasoconstriction) and neural (altered efferent or afferent flow).

Nomenclature for Vertebral Segment Dysfunction

Asymmetry in position and restriction in motion of the vertebral segment(s) (superior segment on inferior seg-

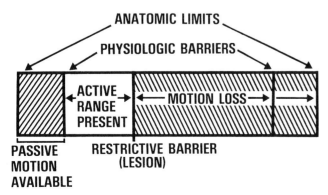

Figure 19–28. Major motion loss in somatic dysfunction. (Adapted from Kimberly,[24] with permission.)

Table 19–3. Differentiation Between Vertebral Motion Position and Restriction

Motion Segment	Position	Motion Restriction
L3 on L4	Flexed	Extension
	Left rotated	Right rotation
	Left sidebent	Right sidebending

ment) must be differentiated.[22,38] Table 19–3 illustrates this point. The example given is of the L3 vertebra, which has been found to be in a flexed, left rotated, and left sidebent position. The motion restriction of this segment (what it cannot do) is just the opposite of the dysfunctional position: The segment cannot extend, right rotate, or right sidebend. Note that the main difference between the terms describing position and motion is in the suffixes used. The positional terms use the past participle, whereas the motion terms are in the present tense (Table 19–4).

The intervertebral facet joints function primarily to guide motion of the spinal segment. Table 19–5 depicts facet function in relation to trunk motion. Factors that restrict vertebral motion may be interpreted as interfering with the ability of the facets to open or close.

The clinician must be able to accurately assess mechanical problems of the spine by differentiating between the positions that the vertebral segments assume or fail to assume during active motion.[11,22,24] The following examples typify why this concept is important. To the casual observer, the two schematics in Figure 19–29 of a right sidebent vertebral segment may look the same. In reality, they represent two different lesions and must be treated differently if the clinician hopes to be successful in caring for this patient.

In Figure 19–29A, the left facet will not close (extend). Thus, when the patient is asked to perform backward bending, the right transverse process becomes more prominent. The reason is that, as motion is recruited through the segment from top to bottom, the right facet, which is already in a relatively closed (extended) position,

Table 19–4. Suffixes for Vertebral Segment Positioning and Corresponding Motion Restriction

Position	Motion
Flex*ed*	Exten*sion*
Extend*ed*	Flex*ion*
Right rotat*ed*	Left rotat*ion*
Left side*bent*	Right sidebend*ing*

□ □ □ □ □ □ □ □ □

Table 19–5. Control of Vertebral Motion by Facet Function

Trunk Motion	Facet Function
Forward bending (flexion)	Facets open
Backward bending (extension)	Facets close
Sidebending right	Right facet closes, left facet opens
Sidebending left	Left facet closes, right facet opens

is carried along into more extension as a part of the whole spinal movement. In forward bending, both transverse processes become more equal. This occurs because as motion is recruited, the right facet opens from its relatively extended position to become equal to the left facet in its blocked (flexed) position. Knowing this, the clinician can now make a *positional diagnosis* of this dysfunctional vertebral segment in three-dimensional space: The segment is *flexed, right sidebent,* and *right rotated* (FRS right). Therefore, the *motion restriction* of the segment (what it cannot do) is just the opposite of the positional diagnosis: *extension, left sidebending,* and *left rotation.* The clinician will thus select a technique that will facilitate motion in the directions of the restriction (see the section "Treatment").

In Figure 19–29B, the right facet will not open (flex). Thus, when the patient is asked to forward bend, the right transverse process becomes more prominent. This occurs because as motion is recruited from the top down through the spinal segment, the right facet (which is in a relatively extended position) is carried along by the overall spinal movement in this extended position. There is no restriction to the left facet, which is already in a relatively opened position. Thus, the right transverse process becomes more prominent. When the patient is asked to backward bend, both transverse processes become more equal, because the left facet is able to close, bringing its transverse process into line with the right one. Know-

ing this, the clinician can now state the *positional diagnosis* of the affected segment: *extended, right sidebent,* and *right rotated* (ERS right). The motion restriction of the segment is *flexion, left sidebending,* and *left rotation.* A treatment technique appropriate to the motion restriction is then selected (see the section "Treatment").

The reader should now be able to appreciate that, in the neutral position, the two lesions described would appear to be the same. However, through the use of positional diagnosis and assessment of motion restriction, they are found to be quite different. Thus, they must be treated by different techniques.

The value of using the transverse processes through a flexion–extension arc of spinal motion is that it clearly distinguishes normal vertebral motion from dysfunctional motion. Use of the transverse processes gives the clinician the ability to discern structural from functional asymmetry and has been shown to be a consistently accurate method among examiners and with the same examiner over time.[11,22,24]

Palpation of the transverse processes is performed through the fascial planes of the paravertebral muscles (erector spinae) (Fig. 19–30). Indirect contact is made with the tips of the transverse processes with the clinician's thumbs. Even pressure is applied to appreciate the relative anteroposterior position of the left transverse process to the right one (see the sections "Evaluation" and "Treatment").

Adaptation

The lumbar spine must make certain adaptations to the position of the sacrum.[11,22,24,30] It has already been noted that L5 and S1 are coupled through the iliolumbar ligaments and that the sacrum nutates and counternutates in response to lumbar flexion and extension (lumbopelvic rhythm). It has also been noted that certain spinal movements are coupled together consistently and have been defined as Fryette's laws (type I = neutral and type II = nonneutral). *Neutral mechanics* refers to the situation in which vertebral weightbearing is on the vertebral bodies, and the introduction of sidebending results in the vertebral bodies twisting out from under the load (in the

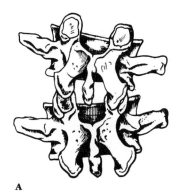

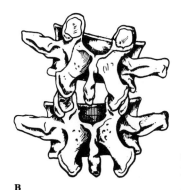

A B

Figure 19–29. Lumbar facet restrictions. (A) The left facet will not *close* (extend); (B) the right facet will not *open* (flex). (From Kapandji,[1] with permission.)

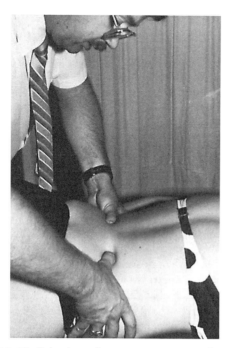

Figure 19–30. Palpation of transverse processes through fascial planes.

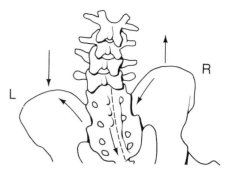

Figure 19–32. Posterior view of the lumbar spine and pelvis showing a left-on-left forward sacral torsion lesion. The fourth and fifth lumbar vertebrae are nonadapting into right rotation and right sidebending following type II mechanics. (Adapted from Pratt,[30] with permission.)

opposite direction of the sidebending). *Nonneutral mechanics* of the spine refers to the situation in which there has been sufficient sagittal plane motion that the vertebral arches (facets), either through stretch or compression, influence motion so that the introduction of sidebending results in a vertebral body twisting into the intended concavity, thus permitting sidebending to occur. Neutral mechanics are usually grouped (three to five segments), and nonneutral mechanics are usually single segment.

It may be easier to think of the sacrum as behaving like a sixth lumbar vertebra when considering the functional integration of total spinal motion. Normally, if the sacrum sidebends left, L5 sidebends right. In neutral (type I) spinal mechanics, if the L5 segment is sidebent right, rotation to the left is coupled to it. Thus, if the sacrum

is left sidebent and the L5 vertebra is found to be left rotated, one can presume, according to type I mechanics, that the spine has made a normal adaptation to the dysfunctional sacral position (Fig. 19–31). When attempting to assess the presence of neutral adaptations in the lumbar spine, the clinician should start at the bottom and work up to the first segment with dysfunction. Then everything relates to the last segment that was found to be normal.

Normal neutral adaptive lumbar spinal behavior occurs over three to five segments and produces a minimal flexion or extension restriction to overall spinal movement. The principal restriction to motion is sidebending. The sacrum should *always* face the concavity of the lumbar spinal curve if the lumbar spine is normally adaptive. This is the usual situation in forward sacral torsion lesions.

Nonneutral or type II restrictions are coupled with sidebending and rotation to the same side. Here the facets influence the motion to a greater extent, and the flexion or extension component is part of the restriction. In the L4 and L5 segments, the iliolumbar ligaments greatly influence these mechanics if flexion or extension is great enough to produce tension in them. A nonneutral restriction will restrict the segment above and below it. Thus, if the sacrum is left sidebent and it is found that the L5 vertebra is right rotated and right sidebent, one can presume, according to type II mechanics, that the lumbar spine has not made a normal adaptation to the sacral dysfunction (Fig. 19–32). Nonadaptive lumbar responses to sacral positioning are highly significant in patients who do not get better or have chronic recurrences. These responses must be treated before the underlying sacral lesion. Nonadaptive lumbar responses are very common in backward sacral torsion lesions.

■ Evaluation

Development of the Tactile Sense

The clinician specializing in musculoskeletal disorders must hone his or her palpatory skills to a fine degree.

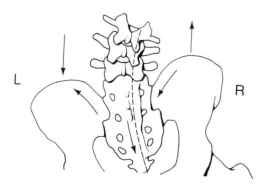

Figure 19–31. Posterior view of the lumbar spine and pelvis showing a left-on-left forward sacral torsion lesion. The lumbar vertebrae are normally adapting into right sidebending and left rotation following type I mechanics. (Adapted from Pratt,[30] with permission.)

Through palpation, the clinician should be able to (1) detect a tissue texture abnormality; (2) detect asymmetry of position of comparable body parts visually and tactilely; (3) detect differences in the quality as well as the range of joint movement; (4) sense position in space, both the patient's and his or her own; and (5) detect changes in the palpatory findings from one examination to the next.

Development of palpatory skills involves three components within the neurophysiologic makeup of the clinician: reception of information through the fingertips and eyes, transmission of this information to the brain, and interpretation of the information.

The sensitivity or tactile discriminatory power of the fingertips is extremely fine. A good exercise for practicing palpatory skills is to take a 25-cent piece, close one's eyes, and then try to palpate George Washington's nose on the coin.[21] Another exercise is to pluck a single hair from one's head and, without looking, place it on a hard surface under a piece of paper, locate the hair, and trace its length with the fingertip.[39]

The clinician's palpatory examination should begin with light touching over the area under observation. This allows a sort of scanning examination of the area and will reveal the presence of any large abnormalities in the superficial or deep layers of tissue. The clinician can then identify the structures or planes as the compression increases. The clinician may use shear movements across the tissues to determine the different structures, planes, or extent or size of a lesion. The palpatory examination takes concentration, and errors in reception result from too much pressure and too much movement of the palpating fingertips.

Layer Palpation

Somatic dysfunction is the impaired or altered function of related components of the somatic (body framework) system: skeletal, arthrodial, and myofascial structures and related vascular, lymphatic, and neural elements.[22,24] The discussion in this section is based on work by Philip Greeman.[40]

The goal of palpatory diagnosis is to identify and define areas of somatic dysfunction. Once such an area is defined, the goal of manual therapy is to improve function in that area, that is, to improve the mobility of tissues (bone, joint, muscle, ligament, fascia, fluid) and to restore normal physiologic motion, if and as much as possible.

The diagnostic criteria for the palpatory examination may be easily remembered through the simple mnemonic "PART" (Table 19–6).

Differentiation of Structural and Functional Asymmetry

Structural asymmetry is the rule, not the exception, particularly in the lower lumbar and sacral spine. If the relative

□□□□□ □ □ □

Table 19–6. Diagnostic Criteria for the Palpatory Examination ("PART")

P	Pain
A	Asymmetry of related parts of the musculoskeletal system either structurally or functionally (e.g., shoulder height by observation, height or iliac crest by palpation, contour and function of thoracic area).
R	Range of motion abnormality of one joint, several joints, or a region of the musculoskeletal system by either hypomobility (restriction) or hypermobility. This is ascertained by observation and palpation using both active and passive patient cooperation.
T	Tissue texture abnormality of the soft tissues of the musculoskeletal system (skin, muscle, or ligament). This is ascertained by observation and palpation.

position of comparable anatomic parts (right and left transverse processes, right and left inferior lateral angles of the sacrum, etc.) is observed to remain constant throughout the full flexion–extension range of motion, then the perceived positional asymmetry is due to *structural variation* of the anatomic part. If, however, the relative position of the comparable anatomic parts changes within the full flexion–extension range of motion, then the perceived asymmetry is due to *functional alteration* of the anatomic parts.

Key Landmarks for Pelvic Girdle Evaluation

The clinician must be able to palpate accurately and consistently the following anatomic landmarks and be able to relate their relative positions to the pelvic and cardinal planes of motion already discussed. Only then will the clinician be able to assess dysfunction and be able to test, retest, and evaluate the effects of treatment.

Iliac Crest

The iliac crests are compared with the patient in the standing and prone positions. Soft tissue must be moved out of the way by pushing it superiorly and medially above the crests. The crests are evaluated for their superoinferior relationship (Fig. 19–33).

Anterior Superior Iliac Spine

The clinician must be able to locate the anterior-medial aspect of the inferior slope of the ASIS with the patient standing and in the supine position and assess their relative positions (superoinferior and/or mediolateral) (Fig. 19–34).

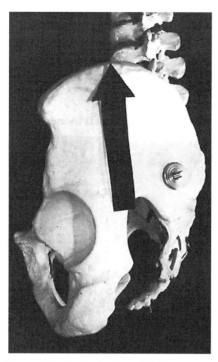

Figure 19–33. Skeletal model, iliac crests.

Pubic Tubercles

With the patient supine, the anterior aspects of the pubic tubercles are palpated for their relative anteroposterior position. Then the superior aspects of the tubercles are examined by pushing the soft tissue out of the way cephalically to assess their relative cephalocaudal position (Fig. 19–35).

Posterior Superior Iliac Spine

The PSIS is a most important landmark and must be assessed in the standing, seated, and prone positions by locating the inferior slope of the posterior aspect of the

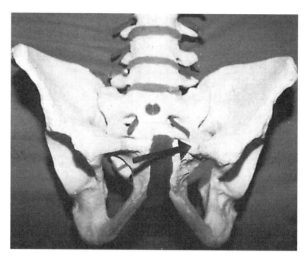

Figure 19–35. Skeletal model, pubic tubercles.

prominence. Its relative position must be assessed as superoinferior and/or mediolateral (Fig. 19–36).

Inferior Lateral Angle

Another very important landmark, the inferior lateral angle (ILA), is found by palpating laterally approximately 1 to 1½ in. from the sacral cornua. Its posterior aspects must be assessed for their anteroposterior relationship, and its inferior aspects must be assessed for their superoinferior relationship (Fig. 19–37).

Sacrotuberous Ligament

The sacrotuberous ligament is located between the ILA and the ischial tuberosity and needs to be compared for equality of tension and tenderness (Fig. 19–38).

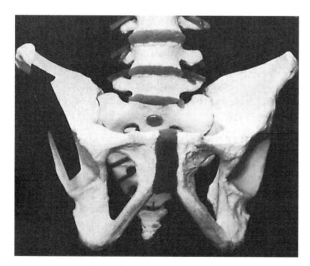

Figure 19–34. Skeletal model, anterior superior iliac spine.

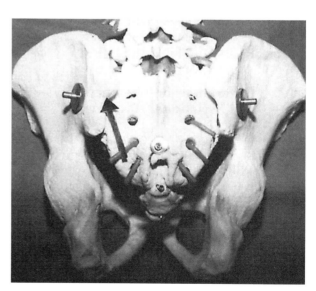

Figure 19–36. Skeletal model, posterior inferior iliac spine.

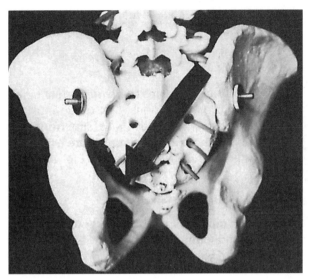

Figure 19–37. Skeletal model, inferior lateral angle of the sacrum.

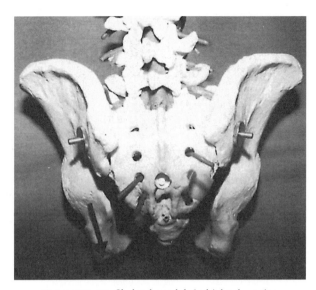

Figure 19–39. Skeletal model, ischial tuberosity.

Ischial Tuberosity

The ischial tuberosities are palpated at their inferior aspects in the prone position and are assessed for their relative superoinferior position (Fig. 19–39).

Medial Malleolus

The inferior slopes of the medial malleoli must be located in both the supine and prone positions. They are then compared for their relative superoinferior positions (see Fig. 19–40).

Lower Quarter Screening Examination

The patient positions used in the examination of pelvic girdle dysfunction are standing, seated, supine, and prone.

To avoid unnecessary movement of the patient from one position to the other, which wastes time and may exacerbate the patient's condition, as many relevant tests should be performed in one patient position as possible. The lower quarter screening examination is included here for completeness since aspects of it might be needed in a pelvic dysfunction examination for the purpose of ruling out certain diagnoses. The advantage of this examination sequence is that the clinician can rapidly evaluate many areas and functions and be assured of not missing any major dysfunction (see appropriate chapters for related tests and their meanings).

The areas included in the examination are the thoracic spine (T6–T12), the lumbar spine, the sacroiliac joint, the pubic symphysis, the hip, the knee, the ankle, and the foot.

The examination begins with an inspection of the patient's posture, with attention to the following:

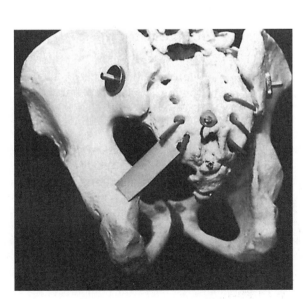

Figure 19–38. Location of the sacrotuberous ligament.

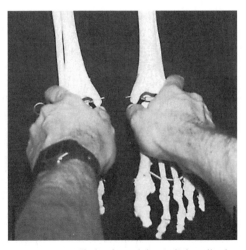

Figure 19–40. Skeletal model, medial malleolus.

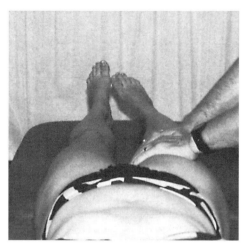

Figure 19–41. Log roll technique for capsular end-feel of the hip joint.

1. Feet
2. Knees
3. Pelvis
4. Thoracolumbar spine

   Next the following functional tests are performed:

1. Standing position
   a. Active range of motion in the lumbar spine, all planes
   b. Active clearing test for peripheral joints (full squat)
   c. Toe walking (S1, S2)
   d. Heel walking (L4, L5)
2. Sitting position
   a. Active and passive rotation of the thoracolumbar spine
   b. Knee jerk (L3, L4)
3. Supine position
   a. Straight leg raising (the Kernig, Lesague, and bowstring tests may also be included)
   b. Long sitting test for the sacroiliac joint (the patient must have a normal straight leg raising test)
   c. Range of motion of the hip, all planes (check for sign of the buttock[13])
   d. Resisted hip flexion (L1, L2); test for range of motion and pain
   e. Resisted knee extension (L3, L4); test for range of motion and pain
   f. Resisted ankle dorsiflexion (L4); test for range of motion and pain
   g. Resisted eversion of the foot (L5, S1); test for range of motion and pain
   h. Knee clearing tests (full extension, varus and valgus stress)
4. Prone position
   a. Femoral nerve stretch
   b. Ankle jerk (S1)
   c. Resisted knee flexion (S1); test for range of motion and pain

   d. Observation of gluteal mass
   e. Prone knee flexion to 90 degrees (SI)
   f. Spring testing (thoracolumbar spine and sacrum)
   g. Ankle clearing tests

Remember that the screening examination only indicates the area in which the lesion lies. Do a detailed examination of the area if a problem is detected. Do not persist in the examination if it is apparent that the condition is being exacerbated.

Clearing Tests for the Hip

Should the clinician need to clear the hip to differentiate between hip and lumbar or sacroiliac problems, the following special procedures are recommended for this purpose.

Log Roll

The log roll is a joint play movement for internal and external rotation of the hip in extension. The clinician simply rolls the thigh under his or her hands to get an end-feel of the joint in internal and external rotation. By watching the excursion of the feet, the clinician can estimate range of motion (Fig. 19–41).

Thomas Test

The Thomas test detects tightness of the long and short flexor muscles of the hip. While lying with one leg freely hanging over the edge of an examination table, the patient flexes the opposite hip toward the chest to a point where the lumbar spine flattens against the table. The freely hanging leg is then observed for its position in space. The knee should be flexed to 70 to 90 degrees, and the hip should be in 0 degrees of extension. If the knee is flexed sufficiently but the hip is found to be in flexion, this indicates tightness of the iliopsoas group. If the hip is in 0 degrees of extension but the knee lacks sufficient flexion, this indicates tightness of the rectus femoris (Fig. 19–42).

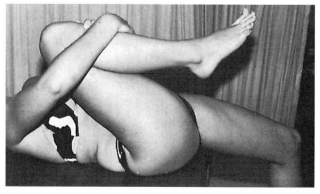

Figure 19–42. Thomas test for assessing tightness of the long and short hip flexor muscles.

Scour Test

The scour test is performed to "feel" the acetabular rim. The clinician literally scours the femoral head around the acetabular rim from the point of maximal flexion, adduction, and internal rotation to the point of maximal extension, abduction, and external rotation, with axial compression being applied to the hip through the knee. The clinician thus "palpates" for joint crepitation and for "bumps" in the smoothness of the range of motion that may indicate degenerative joint disease (Fig. 19–43).

FABERE Test

See the section "Objective Examination of the Sacroiliac Joint."

Piriformis Tightness

See the section "Objective Examination of the Sacroiliac Joint."

Femoral Nerve Stretch

With the patient in the prone position, the clinician passively flexes the knee in an attempt to bring the patient's heel to the buttock (Fig. 19–44). If the femoral nerve is entrapped, this movement should produce neurologic pain in the femoral nerve distribution of the anterior thigh. This test may also be used to test rectus femoris tightness. Normal muscle length should allow an individual to touch the heel to the buttock. If tightness exists, the clinician will observe the pelvis rising on that side as the hip flexes in response to the passive knee flexion (see "Entrapment Syndromes of the Hip and Pelvis").

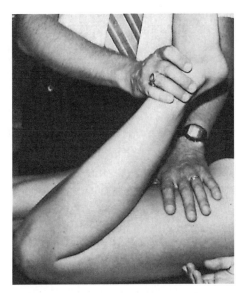

Figure 19–44. Femoral nerve stretch test.

Ober Test

The Ober test is used to determine the presence of tight hip abductor muscles, especially the gluteus medius and the tensor fasciae latae. The patient lies on the side, facing away from the clinician. The clinician asks the patient to raise (abduct) the leg toward the ceiling with the knee flexed to 90 degrees. This relaxes the iliotibial tract and fascia lata. Using his or her own body weight to stabilize the pelvis above the level of the hip joint, the clinician instructs the patient to lower the leg. Normal muscle length should allow the patient's thigh to cross the midline and touch the downside leg (Fig. 19–45).

Femoral Triangle Palpation

Palpation of the structures of the femoral triangle is important in distinguishing soft tissue problems in and around the hip. The borders of the femoral triangle are the inguinal ligament superiorly, the sartorius laterally,

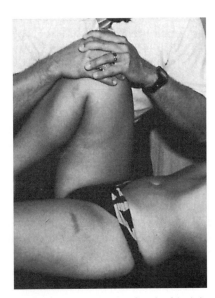

Figure 19–43. Scour test for the hip joint.

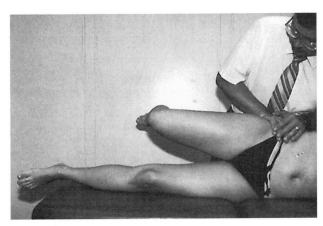

Figure 19–45. Ober test for tightness of the lateral hip musculature.

and the adductor longus medially. The floor of the femoral triangle is formed by portions of the adductor longus, the pectineus, and the iliopsoas muscles. Within the borders of the triangle may be found the femoral artery, the psoas bursa, and the hip joint. The inguinal ligament runs between the ASIS and the pubic tubercles and should be palpated for tenderness and tightness. The FABERE position is best for the examination of the femoral triangle (Fig. 19–46).

Common Hip Syndromes

Sacroiliac and pubic dysfunctions can give rise to pain, which is felt in the groin area. The clinician evaluating a patient with complaints in this area must be able to differentiate between complaints of hip origin and those of pelvic origin. The following discussion presents some of the signs and symptoms of several common hip problems that must be considered in any evaluation of this region.[18,32,41]

Degenerative Joint Disease (Osteoarthrosis)

Degenerative joint disease is the most common disease process affecting the hip. The degenerative tissue changes that occur with symptomatic degenerative joint disease are usually reactions to increased stress to the joint over time. Some predisposing factors include congenital hip dysplasia, osteochondrosis, slipped capital femoral epiphysis, leg length disparity, a tight hip capsule, and shock loading.

The patient is usually middle-aged or older, with an insidious onset of groin or trochanteric pain, which becomes more noticeable after use of the joint (walking, running, etc.). Typically, the pain is felt first in the groin and later in the L2 and L3 distributions (anterior thigh and knee). Later, it progresses to the lateral and posterior regions. The pain rarely extends below the knee. The usual complaints include morning stiffness and stiffness when arising from the sitting position, with pain by day's

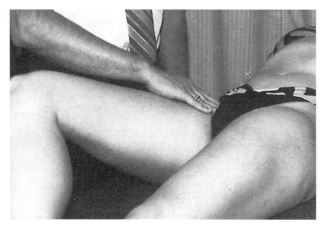

Figure 19–46. FABERE position and area of palpation for the femoral triangle.

end. This progresses to a constant ache at night and loss of functional abilities such as tying one's shoes and climbing stairs.

The clinician should assess range of motion of the hip, paying attention to loss of the motions of abduction and external rotation. The clinician should use the log roll test, the scour test, the Thomas test, and the FABERE test, as well as palpate the femoral triangle.

When early or even moderately advanced signs of degenerative joint disease of the hip are found, the clinician may elect to use capsular stretch techniques and long axis distraction techniques for pain control and improvement in function (see Chapter 25).

Iliopectineus Bursitis

The iliopectineal bursa lies anterior to the hip joint between the capsule and the iliopsoas tendon. Inflammation is fairly common and can be confused with degenerative joint disease of the hip and vice versa. The bursa can communicate with the hip.

The pain from an iliopectineal bursitis is insidious. It is felt in the groin, with some radiation into the L2 and L3 distributions. The clinician should check for a restriction in the capsular pattern of motion to rule out joint effusion or capsular involvement.

Pulsed ultrasound directed into the bursa may be beneficial in the treatment of iliopectineal bursitis, coupled with the use of nonsteroidal anti-inflammatory agents.

Trochanteric Bursitis

The onset of trochanteric bursitis is usually insidious. Occasionally, there is an acute history in which the patient heard a "snap" in the posterolateral region of the hip (e.g., when getting into a car). The pain is located in the lateral hip. There may be some radiation into the L5 distribution along the lateral thigh to the knee and lower leg. Occasionally, it may radiate proximally to the lumbar region and mimic an L5 spinal lesion. A tight tensor fasciae latae tendon may also produce a "snap" over the trochanter and result in a friction syndrome in this area.

The pain of a trochanteric bursitis is a deep, aching sclerotogenous pain rather than the sharp dermatomal L5 pain of nerve root involvement. Stair climbing and side-lying, both of which compress the bursa, will be painful. The patient may stand in a lateral pelvic shift away from the side of involvement, which also increases valgus stress at the knee.

The clinician tests the bursa by fully flexing the patient's hip passively and then moving it into adduction and internal rotation. This maneuver compresses the stretched bursa under the gluteus maximus. The clinician may also palpate the bursa, but it is located behind the trochanter rather than directly on top of it.

Ultrasound and the use of a hydrocortisone-based coupling agent (phonophoresis), iontophoresis, ice massage, and nonsteroidal anti-inflammatory agents may prove helpful in the treatment of trochanteric bursitis. If a tensor fasciae latae friction syndrome is suspected, stretching exercises may be indicated for it and the iliotibial tract.

Subjective Examination

Evaluation of the lumbopelvic unit begins with the subjective examination. A careful, detailed history is essential to proper diagnosis and management of these problems. The following outline by Maitland[42] gives a concise historical picture and tends to focus the clinician's attention on particular trouble spots.

Location of Pain

Use of a body chart is helpful. Note the length (proximal to distal), width (medial to lateral), depth (superficial to deep), type (burning, aching, etc.), and intensity (sharp, dull, etc.) of the pain. Also note any areas of paresthesia or anesthesia.

Present History

See Figure 19–47A.

Behavior of Symptoms

See Figure 19–47B.

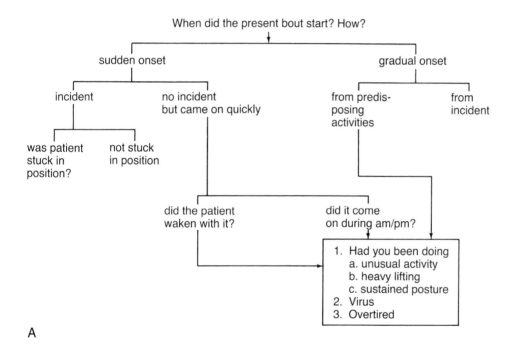

A

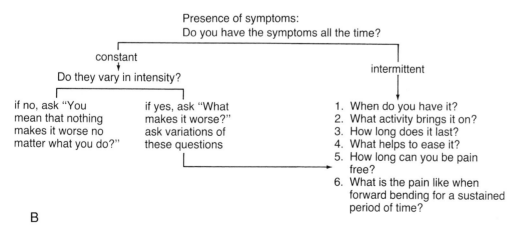

B

Figure 19–47. (A) Flowchart of the patient's present history; (B) flowchart for determining the presence of symptoms.

Previous History

The clinician should get a detailed account to the best of the patient's recollection of the first episode of similar lower back pain. Many times this is a vivid memory, and the patient will have no trouble in relating the episode. The clinician gathers information about subsequent episodes of the same problem including frequency of occurrence, the ease of the causation, what the patient did to lessen the pain, recovery time, and any previous treatments, whether successful or not.

Effect of Rest

The clinician then obtains answers to the following questions:

1. How does rest affect the pain? (Pain of musculoskeletal origin usually gets better with rest.)
2. Does the pain ever awaken the patient during the night? (Night pain that awakens an individual from a sound sleep may suggest neoplastic activity.)
3. What is the pain like in the morning? (Does the patient awaken pain-free and then experience worsening of symptoms as the day goes on, or does the patient awaken with the same pain, which remains at a constant level throughout the day?)
4. Is there any stiffness? (The clinician should suspect rheumatologic or degenerative processes.)

Particular Questions Concerning the Pelvic Joints

1. Have you experienced a sudden sharp jolt to the leg, for example, after unexpectedly stepping off a curb? (This is a very common mechanism for innominate rotations and shears.)
2. Have you recently experienced a fall directly onto your buttocks? (This is a very common mechanism for innominate rotations, shears, and sacral flexion lesions.)
3. What is the effect on the pain of sitting, standing, walking, or maintaining a sustained posture? (If pain, especially radicular pain, increases with sitting, then a discogenic etiology is more suspect; if pain increases with standing, then the sacroiliac joint may be implicated, especially if the patient habitually tends to stand with weight borne more unilaterally; if the pain increases with walking, then the sacroiliac joint is strongly implicated, and sacral torsion is especially likely.)
4. Have you recently experienced a sudden trunk flexion with rotation? (This is a common mechanism for sacroiliac strain.)

Special Questions Concerning Contraindications

1. How is your general health? (This is a very important question, especially if the clinician finds a history of carcinoma, chronic disease, or general malaise that indicates nonmusculoskeletal origin.)
2. Have you had a recent unexplained weight loss? (Recent unexplained weight loss implicates neoplastic activity.)
3. Are you currently taking any medications? (It is helpful to know what a patient may be taking and for what reasons.)
4. Have you had any recent radiographs of your spine? (In cases of trauma, radiographs are always mandatory. In cases of chronic back pain, radiographs should probably be no more than 1 year old.)

Objective Examination

As with any musculoskeletal complaint, the examination begins as the patient walks into the office. The clinician should observe how the patient walks, moves, sits, and so on, especially if the patient does not know that he or she is being observed.

The following outline for planning the objective examination is based on the work of Maitland.[42]

Cause of Pain

1. Name as the *possible* source of *any part* of the patient's pain every joint and muscle that must be examined:
   a. Joints that lie under the painful area
   b. Joints that refer pain into the area
   c. Muscles that lie under the painful area
2. Are you going to do a neurologic examination?
3. List the joints above and below that must be cleared.

Influence of Pain on the Examination

1. Is the pain severe?
2. Does the subjective examination suggest an easily irritable disorder?
3. Are the symptoms local or referred? Which is the dominant factor?
4. Give an example of
   a. An activity that causes increased pain
   b. The severity of the pain so caused
   c. Duration before the pain subsides
5. Does the nature of the pain indicate caution?
   a. Pathology (osteoporosis, rheumatoid arthritis, etc.)
   b. Episodes easily caused
   c. Imminent nerve root compression

Kind of Examination Indicated

1. Do you think you will need to be gentle or moderately vigorous with your examination of movements?
2. Do you expect a comparable sign to be easy or hard to find?

3. Do you think you will be treating pain, resistance, or weakness?

Cause of the Cause of the Pain (Other Factors)

1. What associated factors must be examined as reasons for the present symptoms that might cause recurrence? (Posture, muscle imbalance, muscle power, obesity, stiffness, hypermobility, instability, deformity in a proximal or distal joint, etc.)
2. In planning the treatment (after the examination), what patient education measures would you use to prevent or lessen recurrences?

Objective Examination of the Sacroiliac Joint

Evaluation of the lumbar-pelvic-hip complex by the osteopathic system of positional diagnosis uses a common-sense approach in the correlation of comparable signs. This means that a given dysfunctional lesion will reflect a fairly consistent pattern of findings, which when viewed together yield a diagnosis of the affected segment in three-dimensional space and in relation to adjoining segments. The clinician simply collects the raw data using his or her palpatory and observational skills, formulates a diagnosis, and then applies a specific technique to the affected segment based on that diagnosis. It should be kept in mind that each test viewed by itself does not make a diagnosis. Only when all data are gathered and correlated can the clinician make the diagnosis. The following outline of clinical testing procedures and their meanings is categorized according to patient position and follows a sequence that will minimize patient position changes.

Standing Position

Posture
Make sure that the feet are hip width apart and that the knees are fully extended. Assessment needs to be made from the anterior, posterior, and lateral aspects (Fig. 19–48) for the general postural conditions of the patient (e.g., scoliosis, kyphosis, lordosis, protracted shoulders, forward head, slope of waist, distances of arms from sides).

Gait
Observe the patient's gait pattern. Frequently, sacroiliac lesions may produce a Trendelenburg gait or a gluteus maximus gait, or they may sidebend the trunk away from the affected side. The patient may walk with difficulty or may limp.

Alignment and Symmetry
Observations of alignment and symmetry begin with the general postural assessment, but now the following are checked.

Iliac Crest Height. Iliac crest height is best observed by using the radial borders of the index fingers and the web spaces of the hands to push the soft tissue up and medially out of the way and then pushing down on each crest with equal pressure. The clinician's eyes must be level with his or her hands to assess whether one side is more caudad or

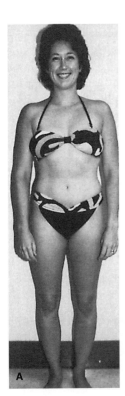
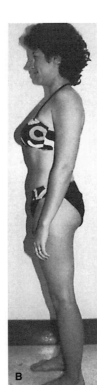
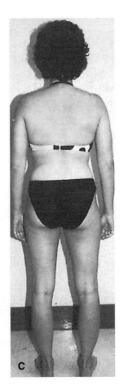

Figure 19–48. Postural assessment. (A) Anterior aspect; (B) lateral aspect; (C) posterior aspect.

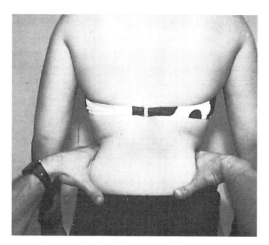

Figure 19–49. Palpation of iliac crests.

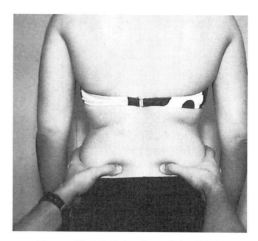

Figure 19–51. Palpation of the PSIS.

cephalad in relation to the other (Fig. 19–49). This method has been found to be quite accurate and precise in the detection of leg length discrepancies.[43] If an asymmetry is found, a lift of appropriate dimension should be placed under the short side before any of the other motion tests in the standing position are executed (Fig. 19–50). This is done to achieve symmetry of muscle tone and balance the pelvis in space before testing motion. Placing a lift under the foot does not imply that a determination has been made as to whether the asymmetry is due to a structural or functional leg length discrepancy.

Posterior Superior Iliac Spine. In the standing position, localization of the PSIS is very important (see the section

"Key Landmarks for Pelvic Girdle Evaluation"). An assessment needs to be made as to the relative superoinferior and mediolateral relationships in positions. This may be done with the ulnar borders of the thumbs or the tips of the index fingers, hooking them under the inferior aspect to the posterior spine. Again, the clinician must be at eye level with the PSISs to make an accurate assessment (Fig. 19–51). If the patient has an iliosacral dysfunction (anterior or posterior innominate), the iliac crests and the PSIS positions will be unlevel but in opposite directions.

Anterior Superior Iliac Spine. As with the PSIS, the superior/inferior and medial/lateral relationships of the ASISs must be assessed. This may be accomplished from behind the patient, with the clinician's arms extended (Fig. 19–52), or from the front by visual inspection and thumb palpation (Fig. 19–53).

Trochanteric Levels. Trochanteric levels are palpated by the same method as for the iliac crests, with the radial borders of the index fingers and the web spaces resting on the tops of the greater trochanters (Fig. 19–54). Levelness here and unlevelness at the iliacs indicate pelvic dysfunction, pro-

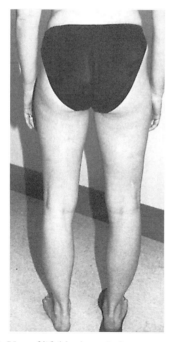

Figure 19–50. Use of lift blocks to induce symmetry of muscle tone and balance the pelvis for landmark palpation and motion testing.

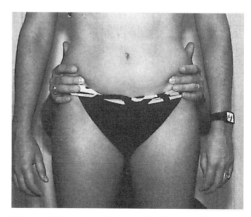

Figure 19–52. Palpation of the ASIS from behind the patient in the standing position.

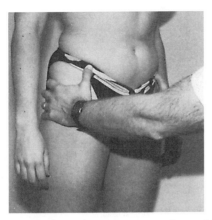

Figure 19–53. Palpation of the ASIS from in front of the patient in the standing position.

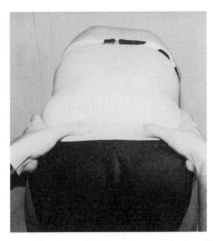

Figure 19–55. Palpation of PSIS movement during the standing flexion text.

ducing an apparent leg length discrepancy. Unlevelness here indicates a structural leg length discrepancy below the level of the femoral neck.

Standing Flexion Test (Forward Bending of the Trunk)

The standing flexion test of iliosacral motion is accomplished by localization of the PSISs, noting their relative position. The patient is asked to bend forward as if to touch the toes. The head and neck should be flexed, and the arms should hang loose from the shoulders. As the patient bends forward, the examiner should note the cranial movement of the PSISs (Fig. 19–55). The side that moves first or the farthest cranially is the blocked side. The standing flexion test may be thought of as iliosacral motion recruited from the top down.

Gillet's Test (Sacral Fixation Test)

Gillet's test is also a test of iliosacral motion, but recruitment here is from the bottom up. The PSISs are again localized. The patient is asked to stand first on one leg and then on the other while pulling the opposite knee up toward the chest (Fig. 19–56). The PSIS on the un-

blocked side will move farther inferiorly. The blocked side will move very little. An alternate method of assessment uses the S2 spinous process as a fixed reference point for the relative PSIS movement as the patient alternately pulls the knees toward the chest (Fig. 19–57). Hip flexion must reach at least 90 degrees.[9,44,45]

Active Lumbar Movements

Because lumbar lesions often occur along with iliosacral and sacroiliac dysfunctions, restrictions of lumbar movement must be assessed as well. Often when a sacroiliac dysfunction exists, sidebending of the lumbar spine toward the affected side will cause an exacerbation of pain (Fig. 19–58). Pain on backward bending may be indicative of a lumbar lesion as well (Fig. 19–59).

Sitting Position

The sitting position fixes the innominates to the chair or table and eliminates the influence of the hamstrings on

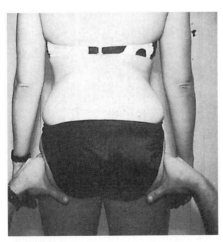

Figure 19–54. Palpation of the greater trochanters.

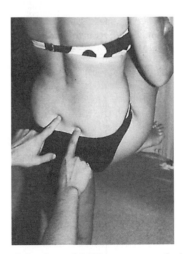

Figure 19–56. Palpation of PSIS movement during the sacral fixation (Gillet's) test. Here the examiner compares the inferior movement of one PSIS with the inferior movement of the other as the patient alternates the stance and the hip being flexed.

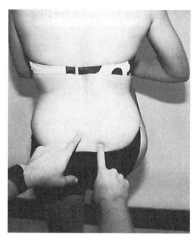

Figure 19–57. Palpation of PSIS movement during the sacral fixation (Gillet's) test. Here the examiner compares PSIS movement to the relatively fixed reference point of the S2 spinous process.

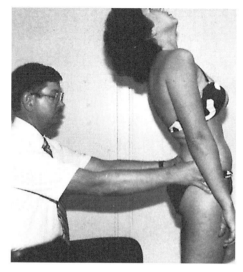

Figure 19–59. Active backward bending of the lumbar spine in the standing position. The patient's pelvis is stabilized by the examiner, who observes segmental deviations in the midline.

the pelvis. This allows for sacroiliac movement within the innominates when testing motion. Also, active trunk rotation can best be tested because hip and pelvic motions are stabilized. The clinician should also note the posture of the patient in this position; the patient with sacroiliac dysfunction often tends to sit on the unaffected buttock. The sitting position also facilitates the neurologic examination, which consists of testing muscle strength, sensation, and muscle stretch reflexes.

Neurologic Examination

The examiner tests the following:

1. Muscle stretch reflexes (deep tendon reflexes)
2. Sensation
3. Resistive muscle tests

Sitting Flexion Test (Forward Bending of the Trunk)

The clinician must again be at eye level after having localized the PSISs. The patient is asked to cross the arms across the chest and pass the elbows between the knees as if to touch the floor. The patient's feet should be in contact with the floor or resting on a stool if seated on the edge of an examination table (Fig. 19–60). The involved PSIS will move first or farther cranially (i.e., the blocked joint moves solidly as one, while the sacrum on the un-

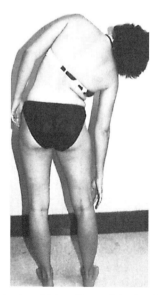

Figure 19–58. Active sidebending of the lumbar spine in the standing (neutral) position. The patient is asked to lean to the side as if to touch the knee until the opposite foot begins to come up off the floor.

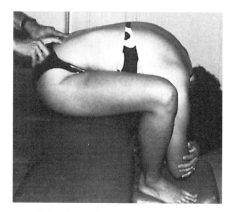

Figure 19–60. Palpation of PSIS movement during the sitting flexion test.

blocked side is free to move through its small range of motion with the lumbar spine). If a blockage is detected in this test and it is more positive (greater) than the restriction noted in the standing flexion test, the test is indicative of a sacral dysfunction. If the two PSISs move symmetrically, an innominate dysfunction is present (if the standing flexion or Gillet's test was positive). If the standing flexion test and the sitting flexion test are both equally positive, a soft tissue lesion is suspected.

Supine Position

Straight Leg Raising

The straight leg raising test is one of the most common clinical tests used in the evaluation of low back pain. It is perhaps one of the most commonly misinterpreted clinical tests as well.[46] The test applies stress to the sacroiliac joint in the higher ranges of the arc and can indicate the presence of a unilateral torsional dysfunction of the joint. It can also indicate a coexisting lumbar problem. The following guidelines are helpful in interpreting the results of the straight leg raising test:

> 0 to 30 degrees: hip pathology or severely inflamed nerve root
>
> 30 to 50 degrees: sciatic nerve involvement
>
> 50 to 70 degrees: probable hamstring involvement
>
> 70 to 90 degrees: sacroiliac joint is stressed

The patient is supine on the examining table. The clinician lifts one of the patient's legs by supporting the heel while palpating the opposite ASIS (Fig. 19–61). The leg is raised until the clinician can appreciate motion of the pelvis occurring under the fingertips of the palpating hand. This determines the hamstring length in the leg being raised.[4] The other side is then similarly tested.

Leg Lengthening and Shortening Test

The leg lengthening and shortening test assesses the ability of the sacroiliac joints to move in response to external forces that passively rotate the innominates. The rela-

tive levelness of the medial malleoli is assessed after the symmetrization maneuver described in Figure 19–62 (Wilson-Barstow maneuver).[11] One leg is then passively flexed on the abdomen, then abducted and externally rotated, and then extended (Fig. 19–63). The malleoli are then compared again for their relative levelness. The leg so moved should appear longer. The same leg is then flexed on the abdomen, adducted, internally rotated, and then extended (Fig. 19–64). The malleoli are again compared. This time, the leg should appear to have shortened. Failure of the leg to either lengthen or shorten may indicate pelvic dysfunction. The opposite leg is similarly tested.

Long Sitting Test

The long sitting test indicates an abnormal mechanical relationship of the innominates moving on the sacrum (iliosacral motion) and helps determine the presence of either an anterior innominate or a posterior innominate by a change in the relative length of the legs during the test. The levelness of the malleoli is assessed, as depicted in Figure 19–62. The patient is then asked to perform a sit-up, keeping the legs straight (Fig. 19–65). The clinician observes the change, if any, between the malleoli. The presence of a posterior innominate will make the leg in question (the side of the positive standing flexion test) appear to be getting longer from a position of relative shortness (short to long or equal to long). This phenomenon occurs because, in the posterior innominate, the posterior rotation of the innominate moves the acetabulum in a superior direction and carries the leg along with it. Thus, the leg appears shortened. Just the opposite occurs in the anterior innominate. When the long sitting test is performed, the leg in question will appear to move from long to short or from equal to short.[47] These mechanisms are shown in Figure 19–66.

Pelvic Rocking

The pelvic rocking test involves getting an end-feel for the relative ease or resistance to passive overpressure for each innominate. The clinician places his or her hands on the ASISs and gently springs the innominates alternately several times to assess the end-feel to this motion (Fig. 19–67). A relatively hard end-feel indicates a probable restriction of movement on that side.

Compression–Distraction Tests

Compression–distraction tests are used to ascertain the presence of joint irritability, hypermobility, or serious disease such as ankylosing spondylitis, Paget's disease, or infection. The clinician may leave his or her hands on the ASISs as in the pelvic rocking test or may cross them to opposite ASISs (Fig. 19–68). The clinician then applies pressure down on them to take up any slack and gives a sudden, sharp spring to the ASISs. This action compresses the sacroiliac joints posteriorly and gaps the joints anteriorly. The clinician then moves his or her hands to the

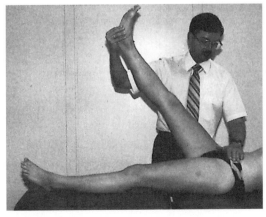

Figure 19–61. Performance of the straight leg raising test.

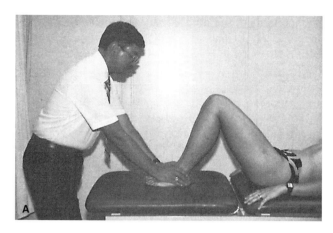

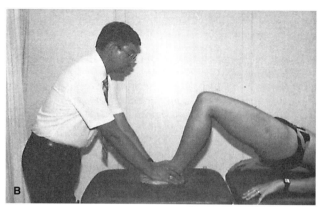

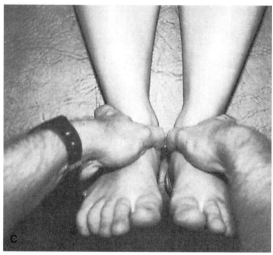

Figure 19–62. Wilson-Barstow maneuver for leg length symmetry.[11] (A) The examiner stands at the patient's feet and palpates the medial malleoli using the ulnar borders of the thumbs at the most distal prominence of the tibia. The patient is asked to bend the knees. (B) The patient is then asked to lift the pelvis from the examining table. (C) The patient returns the pelvis to the table, and the examiner *passively* extends the patient's legs toward him- or herself and compares the positions of the malleoli to one another using the borders of the thumbs.

lateral iliac wings and repeats the same maneuver (Fig. 19–69). In doing so, the clinician compresses the anterior and distracts the posterior sacroiliac joints. Pain as a result of either of these maneuvers is considered to be a positive sign.

FABERE (Patrick's) Test

The FABERE test is useful in differentiating between hip and sacroiliac pain. The hip is *f*lexed, *ab*ducted, and *e*xternally *r*otated, with the lateral malleolus being al-

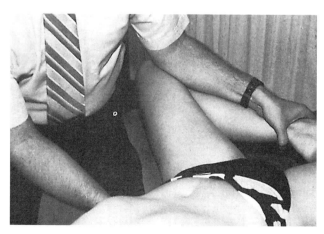

Figure 19–63. Lengthening maneuver for sacroiliac mobility.

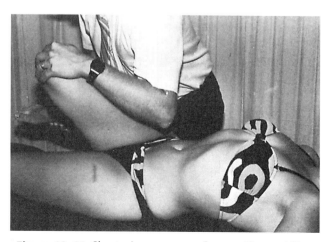

Figure 19–64. Shortening maneuver for sacroiliac mobility.

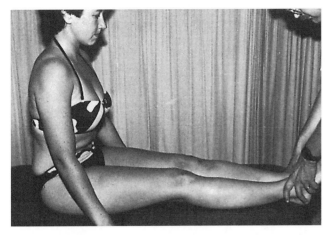

Figure 19–65. Comparison of the medial malleoli in the long sitting test.

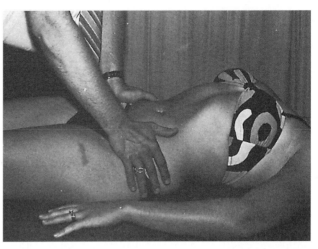

Figure 19–67. Pelvic rocking technique.

lowed to rest on the opposite thigh above the knee. The opposite ASIS is stabilized, and pressure is applied to the other externally rotated leg at the knee (Fig. 19–70). Pain caused in the groin or anterior thigh is indicative of hip pathology. Pain in the sacroiliac joint is indicative of sacroiliac involvement.

Piriformis Tightness

Tightness of the piriformis muscles is easily checked by flexing the hip and knee to 90 degrees and then passively rotating the hip into internal rotation through the lower leg (Fig. 19–71). Relative end-feel and range of motion can be assessed.

Pubic Tubercles

The pubic tubercles are assessed for their relative superior-inferior and anteroposterior relationships. If unlevelness is detected, the positive side is correlated to the side of the positive standing flexion and/or Gillet's test. To avoid embarrassment and unnecessary probing in this region, it is recommended that the clinician slide the heel of his or her hand down the abdomen until contact is made with the pubic bone (Fig. 19–72). The tubercles may then be easily located with the fingertips (Fig. 19–73). In most men and some women, because of the strength of the abdominal muscles, it is sometimes helpful to ask the patient to flex the knees a little to relax the muscles. Palpation is further facilitated by asking the patient to take a breath; on exhalation, the clinician slides his or her fingers over the top and presses down upon the tubercles (see the section "Key Landmarks for Pelvic Girdle Evaluation").

Anterior Superior Iliac Spine

Positioning of the ASISs must be assessed for any change from the standing position. In assessing the superoinferior

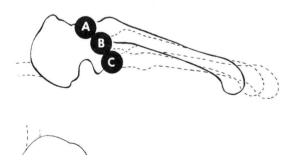

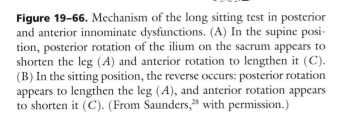

Figure 19–66. Mechanism of the long sitting test in posterior and anterior innominate dysfunctions. (A) In the supine position, posterior rotation of the ilium on the sacrum appears to shorten the leg (*A*) and anterior rotation to lengthen it (*C*). (B) In the sitting position, the reverse occurs: posterior rotation appears to lengthen the leg (*A*), and anterior rotation appears to shorten it (*C*). (From Saunders,[28] with permission.)

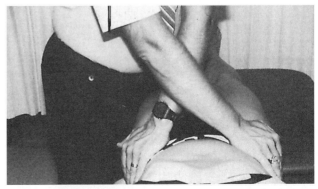

Figure 19–68. Compression–distraction test using the crossed hands method.

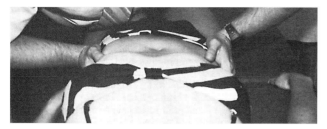

Figure 19–69. Compression–distraction test from the lateral aspect.

and mediolateral relationships, the clinician places his or her thumbs under the lip of the ASIS and sights in their plane from a position perpendicular to the midline (Fig. 19–74). To determine the anteroposterior relationship of the ASISs, the clinician places the fingertips on the tips of the ASISs and sights along the plane of the abdomen (Fig. 19–75). The umbilicus also becomes a reference point for the mediolateral positioning. A tape measure may be used from the umbilicus to the inside border of the ASIS to determine the presence of an iliac inflare or outflare (Fig. 19–76).

Prone Position

Palpation

Depth of the Sacral Sulci (Medial PSIS). The depth of the sacral sulci is best determined if the clinician uses the tips of the long fingers while curling his or her fingers around the posterior aspects of the iliac crests (Fig. 19–77). The clinician assesses not only the relative depth of each sulcus but the quality of the ligaments under the fingertips as well, for tightness and swelling. If one side is found to be deeper than the other, this could indicate the presence of a possible sacral torsion or an innominate rotation.

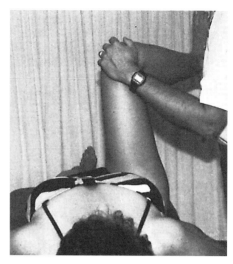

Figure 19–71. Piriformis tightness testing with the patient in the supine position.

Inferior Lateral Angles. The relative caudad/cephalad and anteroposterior positions of the ILAs are compared (Fig. 19–78). If one side is found to be more caudad and/or posterior than the other, a sacral lesion exists. If the ILAs are level and a deep sacral sulcus has been appreciated, the lesion is in one of the innominates (see the section "Key Landmarks for Pelvic Girdle Examination").

Symmetry of the Sacrotuberous and Sacrospinous Ligaments. These ligaments must be palpated through the gluteal mass (Fig. 19–79). The clinician must assess changes in tension and springiness from one side to the other. If such changes are noted, they are due to positional changes of the ilium.

Tenderness of the Sacral Sulcus. If a sacroiliac problem exists, tenderness in the sulcus is well localized. This can be elicited during the test for sacral sulcus depth.

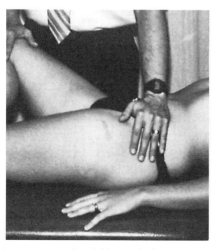

Figure 19–70. Patrick's test (FABERE test).

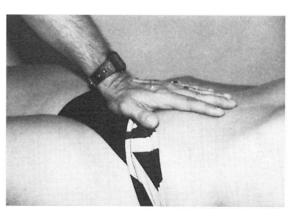

Figure 19–72. Locating the pubic tubercles by sliding the heel of the hand down the abdomen to make contact with the pubic bone.

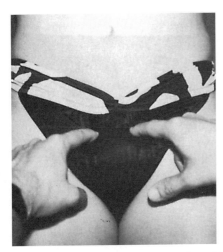

Figure 19–73. Palpation of the pubic tubercles with the fingertips.

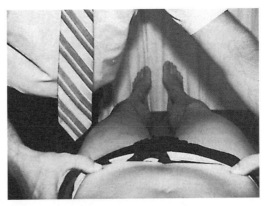

Figure 19–75. Palpation of the ASISs to determine their antero-posterior relationship.

Piriformis Tightness. The piriformis was tested in the supine position while on stretch. It is now tested while not on stretch by having the patient flex the knees to 90 degrees and internally rotate the hips by allowing the legs to move laterally (Fig. 19–80).

Ischial Tuberosities. The clinician checks for the relative anteroposterior and cephalad/caudad relationships of the ischial tuberosities by using the thumbs to push soft tissue out of the way (Fig. 19–81). A change in the anteroposterior relationship may indicate an innominate rotation, whereas a change in the cephalad/caudad relationship may indicate an ilium upslip or downslip (see the section "Key Landmarks for Pelvic Girdle Evaluation").

Rotation of L4 and L5. Testing for rotation of L4 and L5 is performed according to the method described in the section on the lumbar spine in this chapter (see the section "Nomenclature for Vertebral Segment Dysfunction"). Ro-

tation of these segments may indicate a compensated or noncompensated lumbar curve inresponse to a sacroiliac dysfunction.

Sphinx Test (Press-up or Backward Bending)

The patient is asked to come up from the prone position onto the elbows and rest the chin in the hands (Fig. 19–82). The clinician then palpates the following structures.

Sacral Sulci. The clinician now determines if there has been a change in the relative depth of the sacral sulci from that noted in the neutral prone position. If a sacroiliac dysfunction exists, the side that is blocked will remain shallow, and the side that is free to move will go deeper (remember that in backward bending of the lumbar spine there is relative nutation of the sacrum; see Fig. 19–77).

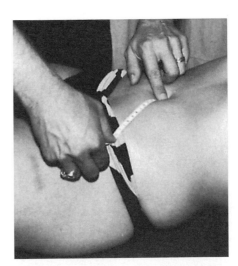

Figure 19–76. Use of a tape measure between the umbilicus and the ASIS to determine the possibility of iliac inflare or outflare dysfunction.

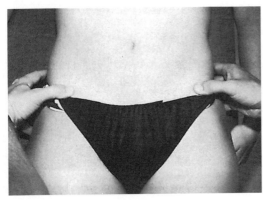

Figure 19–74. Palpation of the ASISs to determine superinferior and mediolateral relationships.

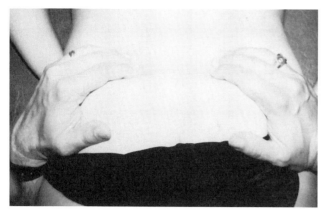

Figure 19–77. Palpation of the depth of the sacral sulci.

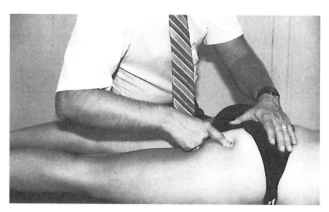

Figure 19–79. Palpation of symmetry in the sacrotuberous and sacrospinous ligaments. This is very difficult because of their depth within the gluteal mass.

Inferior Lateral Angles. The clinician now determines if there has been a change in the position of the ILAs. If the ILA opposite the deep sacral sulcus became more posterior by movement into the sphinx position, this indicates the presence of a forward sacral torsion. If the angle became more inferior on the same side as the deep sacral sulcus, it indicates the presence of a unilateral sacral flexion (Fig. 19–78).

Mobility Test

To test the passive mobility of the sacrum within the innominates, the clinician palpates the sacral sulci while applying negative posteroanterior pressure on the sacrum (Fig. 19–83). Hypermobility or hypomobility is assessed by the relative amount of movement that occurs between the PSIS and the dorsal aspect of the sacrum.

Spring Test

The standard spring test is applied to the lumbar spine to rule out the possibility of a lumbar lesion (Fig. 19–84).

Prone Knee Flexion to 90 Degrees

The clinician stands at the foot of the examination table and holds the patients's feet in a symmetric position, with the thumbs placed transversely across the soles of the feet just forward of the heel pad. Sighting through the plane of the heel with the eyes perpendicular to the malleoli (Fig. 19–85), the clinician assesses the relative length of the legs in the prone position (the short side may not be the same as in the supine or standing position). If one leg appears shorter, it is the positive side. The knees are then simultaneously flexed to 90 degrees (Fig. 19–86). Care must be taken to maintain the feet in the neutral position and to bring the feet up in the midline. Deviation to either side will cause a false impression (Fig. 19–87). If the leg still appears short, an anterior innominate should be suspected. If the leg that seemed short now appears longer, a posterior innominate should be suspected.

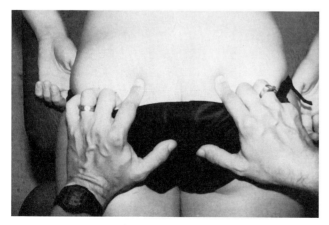

Figure 19–78. Palpation of the ILAs of the sacrum.

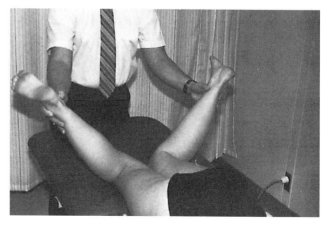

Figure 19–80. Bilateral test of piriformis tightness with the patient in the prone position.

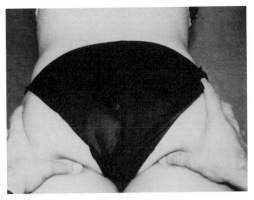

Figure 19–81. Palpation of the ischial tuberosities.

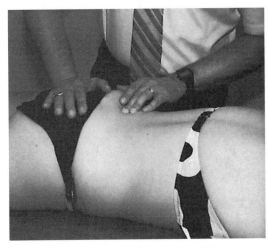

Figure 19–83. Passive mobility testing of the sacrum.

Sacral Provocation Tests

Sacral provocation tests should be performed only when applicable (i.e., when the above series of tests has not provided a clear picture of the dysfunction). These tests should not be performed if the previous tests have demonstrated a hypermobility. They are performed in a manner similar to the sacral mobility test (Fig. 19–83). In chronic sacroiliac pain, provocation should increase symptoms as a result of adaptive shortening of the soft tissues. The sacral provocation tests include the following:

1. Anteroposterior pressure on the sacrum at its base (this encourages sacral flexion).
2. Anteroposterior pressure on the sacrum at its apex (this encourages sacral extension).
3. Anteroposterior pressure on either side of the sacrum just medial to the PSISs (this encourages motion about the vertical axis).
4. Cephalad pressure on the sacrum applied near the apex (note pain or movement abnormalities).
5. Cephalad pressure on the sacrum applied near the base (note pain or movement abnormalities).

6. If a sulcus is found to be deep, pressure is applied on the opposite ILA to see if the sulcus comes up (this encourages torsional movement about an oblique axis).

Physical Findings and Diagnosis of Pelvic Girdle Dysfunctions

The following positive physical findings characterize the seven most common pelvic girdle dysfunctions.

Posterior Innominate

Posterior innominate is a unilateral iliosacral dysfunction. It is by far the most common pelvic dysfunction, whether iliosacral or sacroiliac. The following findings are those for a left posterior innominate:

1. Iliac crests: high on the left
2. PSIS: low and posterior on the left

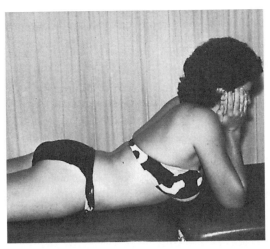

Figure 19–82. Sphinx position.

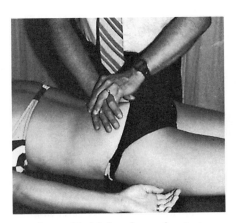

Figure 19–84. Lumbar spring test.

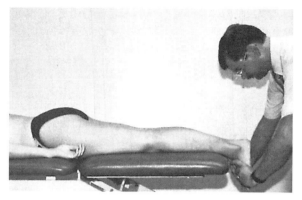

Figure 19–85. The prone knee flexion test begins with the examiner bringing the patient's feet into a neutral position and checking for a leg length difference at the level of the malleoli.

3. ASIS: high and anterior on the left
4. Standing flexion test: left PSIS moves first or farthest superiorly
5. Gillet's test: left PSIS moves inferiorly and laterally less than the right
6. Long sitting test: left malleolus moves short to long
7. Sitting flexion test: negative (unless a sacral lesion coexists)
8. Pubic symphysis: negative (may be superior if also involved)
9. Hip: may lie in some external rotation
10. Sulci: deep on the left
11. ILA: usually no change in position
12. Tensor fasciae latae: tight and/or tender on the right
13. Other findings: tense sacroiliac ligament; decreased lumbar lordosis; pain, usually well defined, in the sulcus and/or unilateral buttock pain

Anterior Innominate

Anterior innominate is also a unilateral iliosacral dysfunction and is essentially the reverse of the posterior innomi-

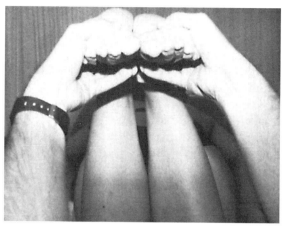

Figure 19–87. False-positive prone knee flexion test caused by the examiner allowing the legs to move away from the midline, thus shortening one leg in relation to the other.

nate. The following findings are those for a right anterior innominate:

1. Iliac crests: low on the right
2. PSIS: high and anterior on the right
3. ASIS: low and posterior on the right
4. Standing flexion test: right PSIS moves first and/or farther superiorly
5. Gillet's test: right PSIS moves less inferiorly and laterally compared with the left
6. Sitting flexion test: usually negative (unless a sacral lesion coexists)
7. Long sitting test: right medial malleolus moves long to short
8. Pubic symphysis: usually no change
9. Hip: right leg may lie in some internal rotation
10. Sulci: shallow on the right
11. ILA: usually no change in position
12. Tensor fasciae latae: may be tender on the left

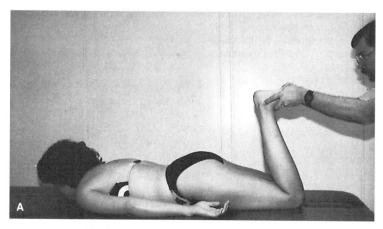

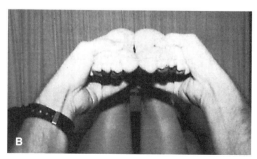

Figure 19–86. (A,B) The prone knee flexion test is completed as the examiner passively flexes the patient's knees to 90 degrees and sights through the plane of the heel pads to see whether a change in position has occurred.

13. Other findings: possibly increased lumbar lordosis; possible complaint of cervical and/or lumbar symptoms

Sacral Torsion (Left-on-Left Forward Torsion)

Left-on-left forward torsion is the most common sacroiliac lesion. The primary axis of dysfunction is the left oblique axis. The findings listed are the opposite of those for the less common right-on-right torsion:

1. Iliac crests: usually no change
2. PSIS: may be posteriorly situated in relation to the sacral dorsal plane on the right
3. ASIS: negative
4. Standing flexion test: may be negative
5. Gillet's test: may be negative
6. Sitting flexion test: blocked side moves first
7. Prone knee flexion test: left malleolus is short
8. Pubic symphysis: no change
9. Hip: left hip lies in external rotation in the supine position
10. Sulci: deep on the right, shallow on the left
11. ILA: posterior and inferior in the pelvic dorsal plane on the left
12. Piriformis and tensor fasciae latae: both are tender on the right
13. Other: usually a history of a pelvic twist injury

Sacral Torsion (Right-on-Left Backward Torsion)

Backward sacral torsion also occurs most often on the left oblique axis. The findings listed are the opposite of those for the much less common left-on-right backward torsion:

1. Iliac crests: usually no change
2. PSIS: posterior on the right in relation to the orientation planes but anterior to the sacral base
3. ASIS: may be carried posterior and superior on the right or anterior and inferior on the left in the supine position
4. Standing flexion test: may be negative
5. Sitting flexion test: blocked side moves first
6. Prone knee flexion: medial malleolus is short on the left
7. Pubic symphysis: no change
8. Hip: right leg may lie in slight external rotation
9. Sulci: shallow on the right, deep on the left
10. ILA: superior and anterior on the left in the pelvic dorsal plane
11. Piriformis: tender and tight on the right
12. Other: 90 percent of all sacroiliac torsions occur on the left oblique axis

Unilateral Sacral Flexion

Unilateral sacral flexion occurs primarily around the middle transverse axis of the sacroiliac joint. It might be thought of as failure of one side of the sacrum to counternutate from a fully nutated position. When this occurs, sidebending takes place, driving the sacrum down the long arm of the joint. Findings for a right unilateral sacral flexion are the following:

1. Iliac crests: usually no change
2. PSIS: posterior in relation to the sacral base on the right but not necessarily in relation to the orientation planes
3. ASIS: carried posterior and superior on the right
4. Standing flexion test: blocked side probably moves first
5. Sitting flexion test: blocked side probably moves first
6. Prone knee flexion test: long on the right
7. Pubic symphysis: no change
8. Hip: no change
9. Sulci: deep on the right
10. ILA: inferior and posterior on the right (the positional relationship of the left side is unchanged)
11. Tensor fasciae latae: left tensor is tight and tender

Superior Pubis

Dysfunctions of the pubic symphysis are probably the most commonly overlooked lesions of the pelvis. The lesions that usually occur at this joint are shear lesions, either in a superior or an inferior direction. Anterior and posterior shears are rare and, if present, are usually the result of trauma. Findings for a left superior pubis are the following:

1. Iliac crests: may be high on the left
2. PSIS: posterior in relation to the pelvic dorsal plane and anterior to the sacral base in the prone position
3. ASIS: superior on the left; may be slightly posterior
4. Standing flexion test: blocked side will move first; the side that is blocked (in this case the left) will indicate the type of pubic lesion (superior or inferior)
5. Sitting flexion test: probably negative
6. Long sitting test: may be equal or shorter on the left before becoming longer
7. Pubic symphysis: left pubic tubercle will be superior and tender
8. Hip: no change
9. Sulci: shallow on the left
10. ILA: no change
11. Other: almost all of these lesions occur simultaneously with the posterior innominate

Superior or Inferior Innominate Shear (Upslip/Downslip)

Usually considered uncommon, vertical shear lesions of an entire innominate have been shown to occur more frequently than was originally thought.[31] Signs of a left superior shear are the following (signs of an inferior shear are just the opposite):

1. Iliac crest: high on the left
2. PSIS: high on the left
3. ASIS: high on the left
4. Standing flexion test: positive on the left
5. Gillet's test: positive on the left
6. Long sitting test: positive on the left, short to long
7. Pubic symphysis: high on the left
8. Hip: no change
9. Sulci: left sulcus may be shallow
10. ILA: no change
11. Piriformis: no change
12. Other: high left ischial tuberosity

The following pelvic dysfunctions are quite rare. Their combined occurrence may represent fewer than 5 to 10 percent of all pelvic dysfunctions. For the sake of completeness, their findings are included.

Iliac Inflare

Use of a tape measure may be helpful in assessing inflare. Measure the relative distances between the ASISs and the umbilicus. An unequal measurement coupled with the findings below may indicate an iliac inflare (on the right):

1. Iliac crests: no change
2. PSIS: right moves away from the sagittal plane
3. ASIS: right moves medially toward the sagittal plane
4. Standing flexion test: blocked right side may move first if coupled with an anterior innominate
5. Gillet's test: may be positive if an anterior innominate exists
6. Long sitting test: no changes
7. Pubic symphysis: no change
8. Hip: may lie in some internal rotation on the right
9. Sulci: right sulcus widens
10. ILA: no change
11. Piriformis and tensor fasciae latae: no changes
12. Other: iliac inflare by itself is a rare finding; can be the result of muscle imbalance; occurs only with a convex sacral articulation; is best examined supine

Iliac Outflare

Iliac outflare is essentially the opposite of an iliac inflare. If a tape measure is used, a longer measurement (ASIS to umbilicus) coupled with the following findings may indicate the presence of an iliac outflare (on the right):

1. Iliac crests: no change
2. PSIS: right moves toward the sagittal plane
3. ASIS: right moves laterally away from the sagittal plane
4. Standing flexion test: blocked right side may move first when coupled with a posterior innominate

5. Gillet's test: may be positive if a posterior innominate also exists
6. Long sitting test: no change unless there is anterior or posterior innominate involvement
7. Pubic symphysis: no change
8. Hip: right leg may lie in some external rotation
9. Sulci: right sulcus is narrowed
10. ILA: no change
11. Piriformis and tensor fasciae latae: no change
12. Other: iliac outflare by itself is a rare finding; can be the result of muscle imbalance; occurs only with a convex sacral articulation and is best examined supine

Unilateral Sacral Extension

Unilateral sacral extension is essentially the opposite of unilateral sacral flexion. It might be thought of as the failure of one side of the sacrum to nutate (flex) from the fully counternutated position (extended). The following findings are those for a right unilateral sacral extension lesion:

1. Iliac crests: usually no change
2. PSIS: anterior in relation to the sacral base on the right
3. ASIS: carried anterior and inferior on the right
4. Standing flexion test: blocked side may move first
5. Sitting flexion test: blocked side may move first
6. Prone knee flexion test: short on the right
7. Pubic symphysis: no change
8. Hip: no change
9. Sulci: shallow on the right
10. ILA: superior and anterior on right
11. Piriformis and tensor fasciae latae: no change
12. Other: this lesion is very rare

Bilateral Sacral Flexion

Bilateral sacral flexion may be thought of as failure of the sacrum to return from a fully nutated position. The findings are as follows:

1. Iliac crests: no change
2. PSIS: equal bilaterally but approximated
3. ASIS: no change
4. Standing and sitting flexion tests: probably no difference
5. Long sitting and prone knee flexion tests: no change
6. Pubic symphysis: no change
7. Hip: no change
8. Sulci: deep bilaterally
9. ILA: posterior and inferior bilaterally
10. Tensor fasciae latae: possible tenderness and tightness bilaterally
11. Other: sacrotuberous and sacrospinous ligaments are under tension and are painful bilaterally

Bilateral Sacral Extension

Bilateral sacral extension is the opposite of bilateral sacral flexion and may be thought of as the failure of the sacrum to return from the fully counternutated position. The findings are as follows:

1. Iliac crests: no change
2. PSIS: equal in relation to each other bilaterally; both are anterior in relation to the sacral base
3. ASIS: no change
4. Standing and sitting flexion tests: probably no difference
5. Pubic symphysis: no change
6. Hip: no change
7. Sulci: shallow bilaterally
8. ILA: anterior and superior bilaterally
9. Tensor fasciae latae: possible tenderness and tightness bilaterally.
10. Other: individual is usually slouched, has a reversed or kyphotic lumbar curve, and often cannot straighten up

■ Treatment

Because of the conjoining of the different lumbar, pelvic, and hip components into an interrelated unit, the clinician should treat dysfunctions in a certain order when multiple lesions exist:

1. Pubic
2. Nonadapting lumbar compensations
3. Sacral lesions
4. Innominate lesions

This treatment order takes advantage of the axes of motion, so that unlocking a restriction in one area facilitates the unlocking of a restriction in another. For example, a very common combination of lumbopelvic dysfunctions consists of left superior pubic shear, left-on-left forward sacral torsion, and left posterior innominate. The lumbar spine is usually adaptive in response to these dysfunctions and does not need correction.

Muscle Energy Techniques

A muscle energy technique (MET) is any manipulative treatment procedure that uses a voluntary contraction of the patient's muscles against a distinctly controlled counterforce from a precise position and in a specific direction. MET is considered to be an active technique, as opposed to a passive technique in which the clinician does the work, and it requires direct positioning (where the motion restriction barrier is engaged but not stressed). MET may be used to lengthen shortened muscles, strengthen weakened muscles, reduce localized edema, and mobilize restricted joints.[11,22–24] The focus of this section is on the use of MET in mobilization of joint restrictions.

Types of Muscle Contraction

MET may use different forms of muscle contraction for the purposes outlined above. The contractions are usually isotonic and isometric but may also be isokinetic and isolytic.[22]

An *isotonic* muscular contraction is one in which the proximal and distal attachments approximate (i.e., a shortening or concentric contraction). An isotonic contraction may also occur when the proximal and distal attachments separate (i.e., a lengthening or eccentric contraction). An example is raising and lowering a weight.

An *isometric* muscular contraction is one exerted against an unyielding resistance in which the proximal and distal attachments neither separate nor approximate (i.e., no joint motion is produced).

An *isolytic* contraction is a contraction of modulated intensity against a force of greater intensity in the opposite direction, so that the joint motion produced is opposite that of the muscular contraction. Examples are certain PNF techniques.

An *isokinetic* contraction is one against a resistance in which speed is the controlled variable. Specialized equipment is usually required to produce this type of exercise contraction, but it may be performed manually as well.

Techniques[11,22,24,29,48]

Anterior Innominate

Pelvic examination: ASIS is low, PSIS is high

Positive standing flexion test

Positive long sitting test: long to short (on the side of the positive standing flexion test)

Positive prone knee flexion test: short to short

Check hip musculature for symmetry

Muscular correction of this positional fault uses muscles that can rotate the innominate in a posterior direction. In this case, the main mover is the gluteus maximus. The technique is as follows:

1. The patient is supine, with the opposite leg hanging free from the edge of the treatment table, supported at approximately the level of the ischium.
2. The hip and knee are flexed on the involved side until the freely hanging leg begins to come up.
3. The clinician may then stabilize the flexed knee with his or her shoulder or instruct the patient to hold the knee in that fixed position with his or her own hands (Fig. 19–88).
4. The patient is then instructed to push the knee (on the involved side) against his or her own hands (or

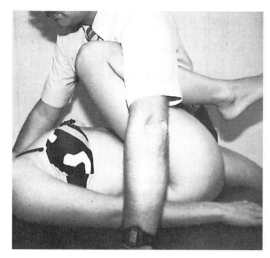

Figure 19–88. MET for anterior innominate.

the clinician's shoulder) with a submaximal sustained contraction (isometric) for about 7 to 10 seconds, all the while breathing in a smooth, relaxed manner. Note that the hip is not allowed to move into extension at any time, only flexion.

5. As soon as the contraction ends, the slack is taken up by further flexing the hip and knee toward the chest until the new barrier is reached. This occurs as the opposite, freely hanging leg begins to rise further. The contraction is repeated and then relaxed, and the slack is taken up. The procedure is repeated three or four times or until all slack is taken up.

6. The patient is now reexamined for any change, usually by the long sitting test or the standing flexion test. The treatment is repeated if necessary.

This treatment may be given to the patient to do as a home program two to three times per day for the next several days. This technique is a powerful rotator of the innominate and can be easily overdone unless specific guidelines are given.

Posterior Innominate

Pelvic examination: ASIS is high, PSIS is low

Positive standing flexion test

Positive long sitting test: short to long (on the side of the positive standing flexion test)

Positive prone knee flexion test: short to long

Check hip musculature for symmetry

Muscular correction of this positional fault uses muscles that can rotate the innominate in an anterior direction. In this case, the rectus femoris is the major mover:

1. The patient is supine, with the involved leg hanging free over the edge of the treatment table as described previously. The hip is extended and the knee is flexed.

2. The opposite hip and knee are flexed in a manner similar to that previously described until the freely hanging leg begins to come up. The patient is instructed to hold the flexed knee and the hip in that position with the hands. The clinician may assist this effort with a hand, arm, or shoulder.

3. The clinician places the other hand on the anterior supracondylar area of the freely hanging knee and gently pushes down to take up the slack (Fig. 19–89).

4. The patient is then instructed to push the freely hanging leg up against the clinician's hand with a submaximal force, holding it constant for 7 to 10 seconds while breathing in a relaxed, smooth manner. It is important for the clinician to give unyielding resistance to the contraction.

5. As the patient relaxes the contraction, the slack is taken up by the clinician, who pushes down on the freely hanging leg and assists the patient in pulling the flexed hip and knee up somewhat to the new barrier. The contraction is then again executed in the new position. This procedure is repeated three or four times.

6. The patient is now reexamined for any changes produced by these efforts, usually by the long sitting test. Treatment is repeated if necessary.

The patient can be instructed in a modification of this technique for home use by telling him or her to hang the uninvolved leg over the edge of the bed or another raised surface and flex the opposite hip and knee to the chest. The patient should then hold that position for 2 to 3 minutes and perform slow, relaxed breathing. The purpose of the breathing techniques used for both the anterior and the posterior innominate procedures is to take advantage of rotatory motion of the innominate around the superior transverse (respiratory) axis of the sacroiliac joints.

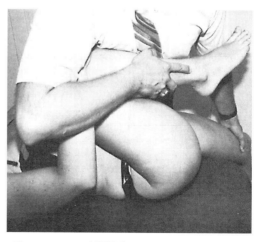

Figure 19–89. MET for posterior innominate.

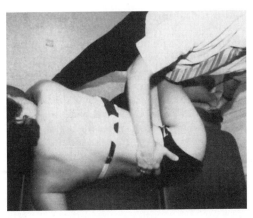

Figure 19–90. MET for left-on-left forward sacral torsion dysfunction.

Forward Sacral Torsion (Left-on-Left or Right-on-Right)

Forward sacral torsion is diagnosed by the following:

A deeper sacral sulcus on the *opposite* side

A more posterior and inferior ILA on the *same* side

Positive sitting flexion test usually on the *opposite* side (but may vary)

Positive prone knee flexion test short on the *same* side

Sphinx test: sulci become equal or less asymmetric

Muscular correction of forward sacral torsion uses muscles that will cause the sacrum to move backward on an oblique axis. This technique uses reciprocal inhibition of one piriformis by the opposite internal hip rotators (unlocks the axis) while the other piriformis moves the sacrum from the faulty position.

1. The patient lies on the side that corresponds to the axis of involvement. In other words, a patient with a left-on-left torsion would lie on the left side.
2. The clinician stands at the side of the table, facing the patient.
3. The patient should be as close to the edge of the table as possible. The downside arm should rest behind the trunk (the hand may be used to stabilize the patient by having the patient grip the edge of the treatment table behind him or her). The topside arm hangs over the edge of the table closest to the clinician as the trunk of the patient is rotated forward and the chest approximates the table.
4. The clinician's cephalad hand palpates the lumbosacral junction while the caudad hand flexes the patient's knees and hips to approximately 70 to 90 degrees or until the clinician can appreciate motion occurring at the lumbosacral junction. This is best achieved by grasping both legs together at the ankles

and moving the hips passively into flexion. The patient's knees should be resting in the hollow of the clinician's hip as the clinician translates his or her body laterally toward the patient's head, thus flexing the patient's hips and lumbar spine up to the lumbosacral junction (Fig. 19–90).

5. The clinician now moves his or her hand from the lumbosacral junction and places it on the patient's shoulder near the edge of the treatment table. The patient is instructed to "take a deep breath" and as he or she exhales to "reach toward the floor." As the patient does this, the clinician assists by pressing down on the patient's shoulder to help take up the slack. This is repeated two or three times.
6. The clinician now returns that hand to the lumbosacral junction and, using the hand holding the ankles, lowers the ankles toward the floor until resistance is met and/or motion is felt at the lumbosacral junction (Fig. 19–91).
7. The clinician now instructs the patient to "lift both ankles toward the ceiling." This is a submaximal contraction, and the clinician must be sure to give unyielding resistance (hold-relax contraction) to the patient's effort. The contraction is held for 7 to 10 seconds and is then relaxed.
8. As the contraction is relaxed, the clinician takes up the slack by translating his or her body cephalad (to increase flexion) and lowers the ankles toward the floor until resistance is met or motion felt at the lumbosacral junction (to increase side-bending), and the patient reaches toward the floor with the hanging arm (to increase rotation).
9. Steps 7 and 8 are repeated two or three times, and then the patient is retested to check for any changes

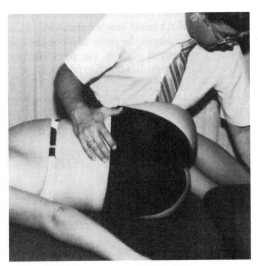

Figure 19–91. MET for left-on-left forward sacral torsion dysfunction.

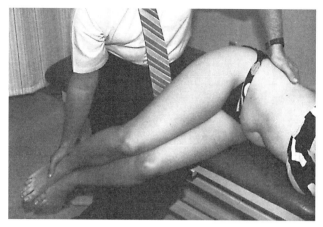

Figure 19–92. Alternate MET method for left-on-left forward sacral torsion dysfunction.

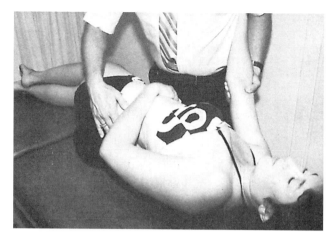

Figure 19–93. MET for left-on-right backward sacral torsion dysfunction.

in sacral position. The treatment is repeated if necessary.

In some instances, the edge of the treatment table is uncomfortable to the patient's downside thigh during performance of the contractions in step 7. The clinician must sometimes support the patient's knees with his or her own thigh or may sit on the treatment table and perform the technique from that position (Fig. 19–92).

Backward Sacral Torsion (Left-on-Right or Right-on-Left)

Backward sacral torsion is diagnosed by the following:

Deeper sacral sulcus on the *opposite* side

More posterior and inferior ILA on the *same* side

Positive sitting flexion test on the *same* side

Positive prone knee flexion test on the *opposite* side

Sphinx test: sacral sulci become *more* asymmetric

Muscular correction of backward sacral torsion uses muscles that will cause the sacrum to move forward on an oblique axis. The technique described uses the gluteus medius and the gluteus maximus for this purpose:

1. The patient lies on the side corresponding to the axis of involvement. This means that a patient with a left-on-right torsion would lie on the right side.
2. The patient lies as close to the edge of the table as possible, and the clinician stands at that edge facing the patient.
3. The patient's trunk is now rotated so that the back approximates the table surface. This is accomplished by the clinician grasping the patient's downside arm (usually above the elbow) and pulling it out from under the patient (Fig. 19–93). The clinician now flexes the patient's topmost leg somewhat at the hip and knee. The downside leg is allowed to remain straight for the moment.

4. The clinician now palpates the patient's lumbosacral junction with the cephalad hand. With the other hand, the clinician reaches behind the patient's top-side flexed knee and passively extends the patient's bottom hip by pushing the leg posteriorly. The clinician does this until motion is perceived occurring at the lumbosacral junction (Fig. 19–94).
5. The clinician now repositions his or her hands so that the caudal hand now palpates the lumbosacral junction and the cephalad hand is moved to the patient's shoulder.
6. The clinician now uses the forearm of his or her caudad arm to stabilize the pelvis and instructs the patient to "take a deep breath." As the patient exhales, the clinician presses down on the shoulder, causing greater trunk rotation, and further approximating the trunk to the table surface (Fig. 19–95). This maneuver is repeated two or three times to take up all the slack. The clinician must be careful not to allow the pelvis to move and change its alignment.

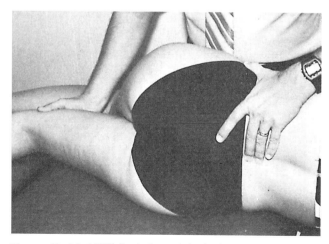

Figure 19–94. MET for left-on-right backward sacral torsion dysfunction.

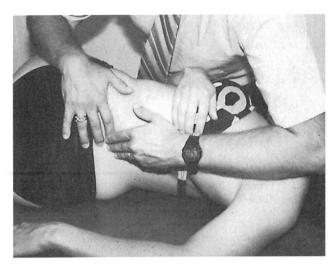

Figure 19–95. MET for left-on-right backward sacral torsion dysfunction.

7. Maintaining trunk rotation and pelvic alignment, the clinician instructs the patient to "straighten the top-side knee and allow the leg to hang freely" from the table. Being careful not to change pelvic alignment, the clinician slides the caudad hand down the thigh to the lateral supracondylar area of the patient's knee.

8. The patient is then instructed to "lift the knee toward the ceiling" while the clinician provides unyielding resistance to the effort. The contraction is held for 7 to 10 seconds and is then relaxed (Fig. 19–96).

9. Slack is taken up by the clinician moving the down-side leg back a little (to increase extension), rotating the trunk a little (to increase rotation), and pushing down on the hanging leg until resistance is met (to increase sidebending).

10. Steps 8 and 9 are repeated two or three times, and the patient is then retested to check for positional changes of the sacrum. Treatment is repeated if necessary.

Unilateral Sacral Flexion

Unilateral sacral flexion is diagnosed by the following:

Deep sacral sulcus on the *same* side

Inferior and posterior ILA on the *same* side

Positive prone knee flexion test *short* on the *opposite* side

Positive sitting flexion test on the *same* side

Sphinx test: no change

Muscular correction of this sacral positional fault takes advantage of the normal nutation–counternutation movement of the sacrum during respiration. By accentuating the breathing pattern and applying direct pressure to the sacrum, it can be made to move up the long arm of the joint axis to its normal resting position:

1. The patient is prone.
2. The clinician stands on the *same* side as the lesion.
3. The clinician palpates the sacral sulcus on the side of the lesion with a finger and abducts the patient's hip on the involved side approximately 15 degrees and then internally rotates that same hip. This hip position is maintained throughout the procedure (Fig. 19–97).
4. Using a straight arm force, the clinician places a constant downward pressure on the ILA on the side

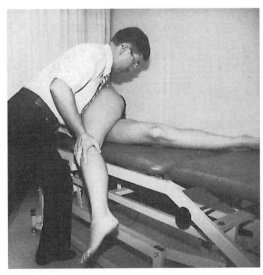

Figure 19–96. MET for left-on-right backward sacral torsion dysfunction.

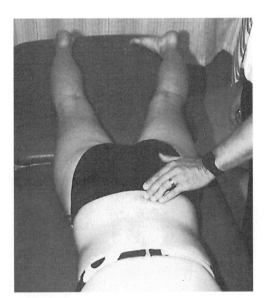

Figure 19–97. Palpation of the sacral sulcus and positioning of the hip for application of MET for a unilateral sacral flexion dysfunction.

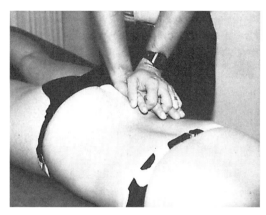

Figure 19–98. MET for unilateral sacral flexion dysfunction.

of the lesion with the heel of the hand in the direction of the navel (Fig. 19–98).

5. The clinician instructs the patient to take in his or her breath in "small sips" (as through a soda straw) until the patient can hold no more air, then hold his or her breath with the lungs maximally filled.

6. After several seconds, the clinician instructs the patient to release the air while the clinician maintains the constant downward pressure on the ILA.

7. Steps 5 and 6 are repeated three or four times, and then the patient is retested for positional changes of the sacrum. Treatment is repeated if necessary.

For a home self-treatment program, the patient may be instructed to sit in a chair with the legs abducted. The patient then takes a deep breath, holds it, and flexes the trunk between his or her spread knees, passing the elbows between the knees (Fig. 19–99). After several seconds, the patient releases the air and straightens the trunk. This procedure is repeated several times two or three times per day.

Superior Pubic Shear

Superior pubic shear is diagnosed by the following:

> Positive standing flexion test on one side
>
> Pubic tubercle *superior* on the *same* side as the positive standing flexion test
>
> Tense and/or tender inguinal ligament on the *same* side

Muscular correction of this very common pelvic dysfunction uses the combined forces of the rectus femoris and the hip adductor group to effect the mobilization:

1. The patient is supine, with the leg on the involved side freely hanging from the edge of the table (ischial contact).

2. The clinician stands on the same side as the lesion.

3. The lower portion of the freely hanging leg is passively extended at the knee and is held in this position, supported between the legs of the clinician (Fig. 19–100).

4. The clinician then reaches across the patient and places one hand on the ASIS opposite the side of involvement to stabilize it.

5. With the other hand, the clinician gently presses down on the supracondylar area of the freely hanging leg of the patient and takes up the available slack at the hip. The clinician does this while maintaining the position of the knee in passive extension between his or her own legs (Fig. 19–101).

6. The patient is then instructed to "squeeze your thigh against the table and push your leg up against my hand." The clinician offers unyielding resistance to the upward contraction, and the table offers unyielding resistance to adduction. The knee must be main-

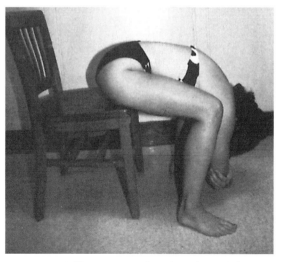

Figure 19–99. Self-treatment of unilateral sacral flexion dysfunction.

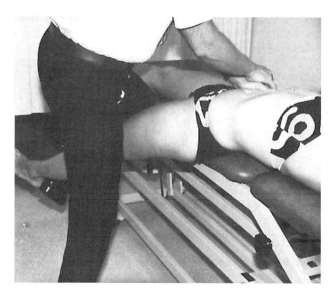

Figure 19–100. Support of the lower leg by the clinician's leg in positioning the patient for application of MET for a superior pubic shear dysfunction.

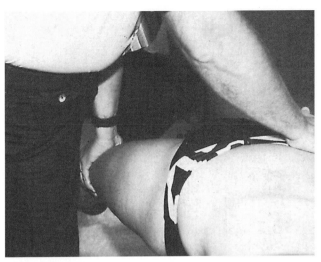

Figure 19–101. Taking up slack in the pelvic ligaments and the hip while supporting the patient's freely hanging lower leg before application of MET for a superior pubic shear dysfunction.

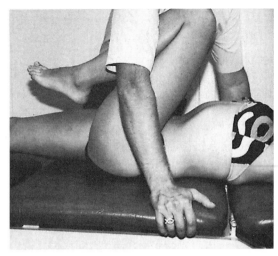

Figure 19–102. Positioning for application of MET for an inferior pubic shear dysfunction.

tained in passive extension as the patient tries to raise the leg. Note: The forces generated are to be submaximal—probably 10 lb is sufficient to accomplish the task. The contraction is held for 7 to 10 seconds, and the patient is then instructed to relax.

7. As the patient relaxes, the slack is taken up into hip extension. Stabilization of the opposite ASIS is important during this step. When the new barrier to motion is reached, step 6 is repeated (usually steps 5 and 6 are repeated a total of three or four times).

8. Retest. Repeat the treatment if needed.

Inferior Pubic Shear

Inferior pubic shear is diagnosed by the following:

Positive standing flexion test on one side

Pubic tubercle *inferior* on the *same* side as the positive standing flexion test

Possible tense and/or tender inguinal ligament on the same side

Muscular correction of this pelvic dysfunction is similar to the technique for the anterior innominate and uses the action of the gluteus maximus in combination with some direct pressure onto the ischium from the clinician. This allows the pubis to slide superiorly from the dysfunctional inferior position:

1. The patient is supine on the treatment table.
2. The clinician stands on the side of the patient *opposite* the side of involvement.
3. The patient is now instructed to flex the hip and knee completely on the involved side.
4. The clinician now reaches across the patient and grasps the edge of the treatment table on the oppo-

site side. The clinician allows the patient's flexed knee on the involved side to rest against the axilla of his or her shoulder (Fig. 19–102).

5. The clinician now makes a fist and brings it to bear against the ischial tuberosity, taking up all available slack, and then relaxes (Fig. 19–103).

6. The patient is then instructed to "attempt to straighten your leg" on the involved side as the clinician resists this motion. This effort by the patient should only be in the range of 5 to 10 lb of force and should be exerted for 7 to 10 seconds. The patient is then instructed to relax.

7. Step 5 is now repeated to take up the slack created by the muscular effort of step 6. Step 6 is then repeated. This sequence of steps 5 and 6 is repeated a total of three or four times each.

8. The patient is now retested and treatment repeated if necessary.

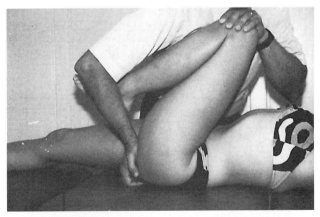

Figure 19–103. Taking up available slack before and between applications of MET for an inferior pubic shear dysfunction.

Combined Treatment for Superior and Inferior Pubic Subluxations

This technique is a powerful mover of the pubic symphysis. It first uses the hip abductors to "gap" the joint and then the hip adductors to "reset" the joint in its normal position.

1. The patient is supine, with the knees flexed and together. He or she should be positioned toward the end of the treatment table so that the toes are near the end of the table.
2. The clinician stands at the end of the table facing the patient.
3. The clinician places his or her hands on either side of the patient's knees and instructs the patient to "push your legs apart" (abduct the knees) (Fig. 19–104). This is performed with maximal force, and the clinician resists this effort by pushing against the lateral aspects of the patient's knees. This isometric contraction is held for 7 to 10 seconds. The patient is then instructed to relax.
4. The patient is then instructed to allow the legs to "fall apart" (abduct the knees). The clinician guides this action so that the feet are held together and the legs abduct 30 to 45 degrees. Step 3 is now repeated in this new position, with the patient giving a *maximal* contraction into abduction while the clinician resists this effort (Fig. 19–105).
5. As soon as the patient has ceased the contraction, the clinician quickly places his or her forearm between the patient's knees (the clinician's hand and elbow make contact with the medial aspects of the patient's knees), and the patient is instructed to "squeeze your knees together against my arm" (adduct the knees). This is also performed with a maximal contraction (Fig. 19–106).
6. The contraction is held for a few seconds and then relaxed. It may need to be repeated once or twice

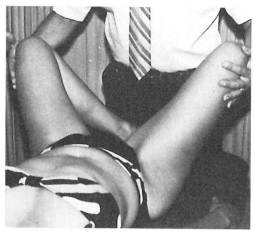

Figure 19–105. MET for combined pubic shear dysfunction: second step.

more before repositioning the patient on the table to retest. Treatment may be repeated if necessary.

Many times, an audible "pop" is heard during this treatment. This represents a separation of the pubic symphyses and allows them to reset themselves. This technique can be used separately or in combination with the specific pubic subluxation techniques previously described.

Superior Iliac Subluxation (Upslip)

Superior iliac subluxation is diagnosed by the following:

Superior iliac crest
Superior ASIS on the *same* side
Superior PSIS on the *same* side
Superior pubic tubercle on the *same* side
Superior ischial tuberosity on the *same* side

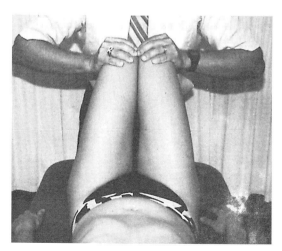

Figure 19–104. MET for combined pubic shear dysfunction: first step.

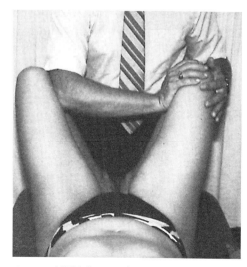

Figure 19–106. MET for combined pubic shear dysfunction: last step.

This technique is a direct action thrust technique but applies principles of "closed-packed" versus "loose-packed" joint mechanics to effect the mobilization.

1. The patient is prone, and the clinician stands at the foot of the treatment table on the side of the lesion.
2. The clinician grasps the patient's distal lower leg above the ankle and raises the entire leg into approximately 30 degrees of hip and lumbar extension, and abduction of 30 degrees, and then internally rotates the leg. This approximates the closed-packed position of the hip as much as possible.
3. The clinician then instructs the patient to grasp the top table edge with his or her hands. The clinician then proceeds to take up the slack by distracting the leg along its long axis until tightness is perceived along the kinetic chain (Fig. 19–107).
4. The clinician now applies a quick caudal jerk on the leg.
5. The patient is then retested, and treatment is repeated if necessary.

By using the closed-packed position of the hip, the effect of the distraction is applied to the innominate instead of the hip. Mobilization of the hip is performed supine in the loose-packed position.

Iliac Inflare

Iliac inflare is diagnosed by the following:

> Positive standing flexion test on the *same* side
>
> Wide sacral sulcus on the *same* side
>
> ASIS closer to the midline on the *same* side
>
> PSIS farther from the midline on the *same* side

Muscular correction of this positional fault primarily uses the hip adductors, but from extreme positions to generate an effect on the pelvis:

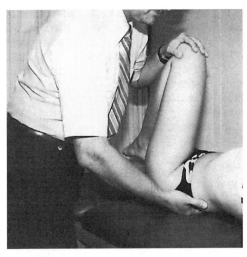

Figure 19–108. Palpation of the sacral sulcus and PSIS in positioning the patient for application of MET for correction of an iliac inflare dysfunction.

1. The patient is supine on the treatment table.
2. The clinician stands on the same side as the lesion. With the cephalad hand, the clinician reaches under the patient and palpates the sacral sulcus and the PSIS (Fig. 19–108).
3. With the other hand, the clinician now grasps the patient's knee on the involved side and flexes the hip until motion is perceived at the sacral sulcus by the palpating hand. At this point, the clinician then abducts the hip, moving it to its limit. This position must be maintained (Fig. 19–109).
4. The clinician now moves the palpating hand to the opposite ASIS to stabilize the pelvis, then shifts the other hand from the patient's knee to the medial aspect of the patient's ankle, grasping it. The clinician then produces external rotation of the hip by moving the foot medially to its limit while maintaining the

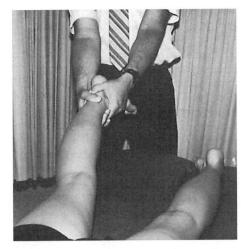

Figure 19–107. Long axis distraction technique for correction of superior iliac shear (upslip).

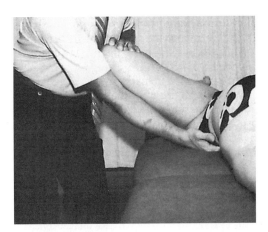

Figure 19–109. Positioning of the patient's hip into flexion and abduction while palpating the sacral sulcus in preparation for application of MET for an iliac inflare dysfunction.

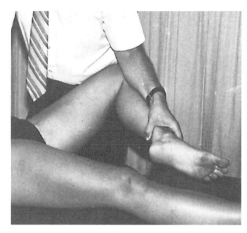

Figure 19–110. External rotation of the patient's hip in the flexed and abducted position before application of MET for an iliac inflare dysfunction.

flexed-abducted position achieved in step 3 (Fig. 19–110).

5. While holding the patient's ankle, the clinician places his or her elbow against the medial aspect of the patient's knee and then instructs the patient to adduct the leg against the unyielding resistance of the clinician (Fig. 19–111). Note that both of the clinician's hands are busy: One continues to support the opposite ASIS, while the other maintains the flexed, abducted, and externally rotated position of the hip on the involved side.

6. The patient maintains the isometric contraction for 5 to 7 seconds and is then told to relax. During the relaxation, slack is taken up into gaining additional abduction and external rotation of the hip.

7. Steps 5 and 6 are repeated three or four times. At the conclusion of the last contraction and relaxation, the clinician straightens the hip and knee to their

extended, neutral resting position while maintaining the abducted and externally rotated position through the hand and elbow on the involved side and stabilizing the pelvis on the opposite ASIS (Fig. 19–112).

8. The patient is retested, and the treatment is reapplied if necessary.

Iliac Outflare

Iliac outflare is diagnosed by the following:

Positive standing flexion test on the *same* side

Sacral sulcus narrowed on the *same* side

ASIS is moved away from the midline on the *same* side

PSIS is moved toward the midline on the *same* side

This technique is a combination of direct traction by the clinician coupled with the muscular effort generated primarily by the hip abductors.

1. The patient is supine on the treatment table, with the clinician standing on the same side as the lesion.

2. The clinician slips his or her cephalad hand under the patient until the fingertips come to rest in the sacral sulcus on that side. The clinician then exerts lateral traction on the PSIS, pulling toward him- or herself (Fig. 19–113).

3. With the other hand, the clinician grasps the patient's knee on that side and produces hip and knee flexion to 90 degrees.

4. The clinician now leans his or her shoulder against the lateral aspect of the patient's knee, causing adduction of the hip. While supporting the foot to maintain hip and knee flexion, the hip is moved into its limit of adduction.

5. The clinician now produces internal rotation of the hip by moving the foot laterally to its limit (the clinician's shoulder is the fulcrum). This position must be maintained (Fig. 19–114).

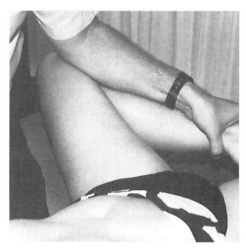

Figure 19–111. Application of MET for an iliac inflare dysfunction. The patient is instructed to adduct the thigh against the clinician's elbow from this position of flexion, abduction, and external rotation.

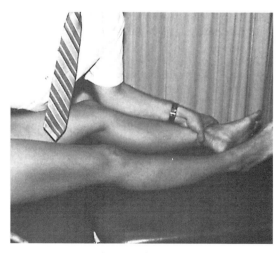

Figure 19–112. Completion of technique for an iliac inflare dysfunction. The clinician extends the patient's hip and knee from the flexed, abducted, and externally rotated position.

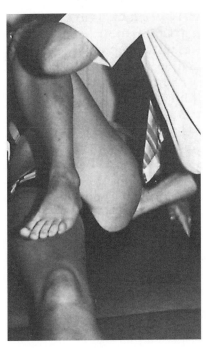

Figure 19–113. Palpation and application of lateral traction on the sacral sulcus and PSIS before application of MET for an iliac outflare dysfunction.

6. While maintaining the position obtained with the caudad hand and shoulder and the other hand applying lateral traction to the PSIS, the clinician instructs the patient to push the hip against the resistance.

7. The contraction is held for 5 to 7 seconds before the patient is instructed to relax. During the relaxation, slack is taken up into additional adduction and internal rotation.

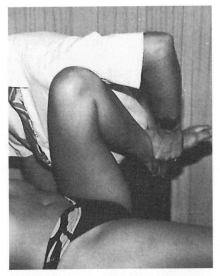

Figure 19–114. Positioning of the patient's hip into adduction and internal rotation with the clinician's shoulder as the fulcrum. Application of MET for an iliac outflare dysfunction is performed from this position.

8. Steps 6 and 7 are repeated two or three times. At the conclusion of the final contraction, the clinician returns the leg to its neutral resting position while maintaining the adducted and internally rotated position of the hip with the caudad hand and shoulder and lateral traction on the PSIS with the cephalad hand (Fig. 19–115).

9. The patient is then retested, and the treatment is reapplied if necessary.

Treatment Techniques for Lumbar Lesions

A description of the multiplicity of techniques that might be devised for the treatment of lumbar ERS and FRS lesions, as described in Figure 19–29, is beyond the scope of this chapter. The two techniques that are most simple and probably most often used are included as a starting point for the reader.

FRS Right: Lateral Recumbent Technique

Positional diagnosis: FRS right

Motion restriction: extension, left sidebending, left rotation

1. The patient is side-lying on the treatment table on the side of the more posterior transverse process (in this case, the right). The clinician stands facing the patient.

2. The patient's head is supported by a pillow, and the lower leg is straight. The upper leg is in some flexion of the knee and hip.

3. With the left hand, the clinician palpates the interspinous space of the involved segment. With the right hand, the clinician reaches behind the flexed upper knee to the thigh of the lower leg and passively

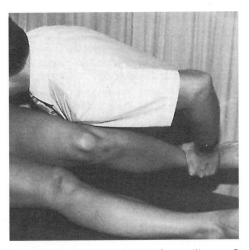

Figure 19–115. Completion of MET for an iliac outflare dysfunction. The clinician extends the patient's hip and knee from the flexed, adducted, and internally rotated position.

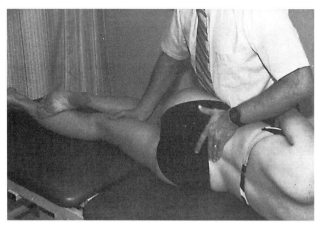

Figure 19–116. Positioning for application of MET for a right flexed, rotated, and sidebent (FRS right) lumbar facet restriction.

extends the patient's lower hip until motion is felt at the interspinous space (Fig. 19–116).

4. The clinician now repositions the hands so that the right hand is palpating the interspinous space and the left hand introduces trunk rotation by grasping the patient's upper arm and pulling it toward him or her. Thus, the patient's upper shoulder approximates the table surface. This movement is continued until the clinician perceives motion arriving at the interspinous space (Fig. 19–117).

5. The patient is instructed to grasp the edge of the table behind him or her with the upper hand. The patient is instructed to "take a deep breath and then let it out." As the patient does so, the clinician takes up any remaining slack.

6. The clinician now repositions the hands and palpates the interspinous space with the left hand. With the right hand, the clinician grasps the patient's uppermost leg at the ankle.

7. Using the crook of the hip as the pivot point and the elbow as the fulcrum, the clinician lifts the patient's leg up and introduces sidebending into the segment. The clinician then slowly extends the hip of the upper leg until extension is felt at the segment (Fig. 19–118).

8. At this point, the patient is instructed to "pull your ankle down toward the floor" and hold the contraction for 5 to 10 seconds and then relax.

9. The clinician then relocalizes movement to the segment by taking up the slack created by rotating the patient's trunk farther, sidebending the trunk by lifting the ankle a little higher and extending the trunk through the hip.

10. Steps 8 and 9 are repeated three or four times before retesting the patient. Treatment is repeated if necessary.

ERS Right: Lateral Recumbent Technique

Positional diagnosis: ERS right

Motion restriction: flexion, left rotation, left sidebending

1. The patient is side-lying on the treatment table, with the affected side up (the side of the most prominent transverse process). In this case, the patient will be lying on the left side.

2. The clinician stands facing the patient. The clinician palpates with the left hand the interspinous space at the level below the one to be treated while flexing the patient's hips with the other hand until he or she can appreciate motion being introduced into the segment being palpated (Fig. 19–119).

3. While supporting the patient's knees against the crook of his or her own hip or body, the clinician

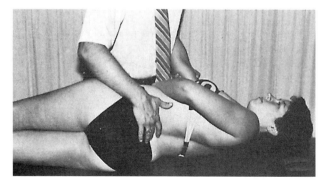

Figure 19–117. Positioning and taking up slack for application of MET for a right flexed, rotated, and sidebent (FRS right) lumbar facet restriction.

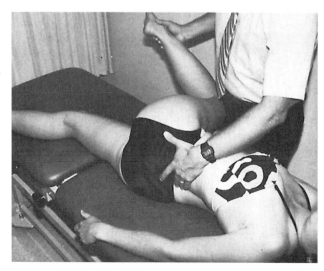

Figure 19–118. Positioning and application of MET for a right flexed, rotated, and sidebent (FRS right) lumbar facet restriction.

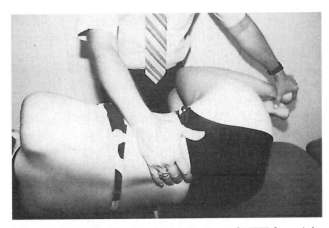

Figure 19–119. Positioning for application of MET for a right extended, rotated, and sidebent (ERS right) lumbar facet restriction.

lowers the patient's legs toward the floor until sidebending (left) can be perceived being introduced into the segment.

4. The patient is then instructed to "reach toward the floor with your uppermost arm." This introduces left rotation into the segment. Note: At times, this step can be omitted because rotation may be localized simultaneously with sidebending.
5. The clinician instructs the patient to "lift both ankles toward the ceiling." The clinician offers unyielding resistance to the patient's effort (right sidebending) for 5 to 10 seconds before the patient is told to relax. The force required is approximately 5 to 10 lb (Fig. 19–120).
6. The clinician takes up the slack created by increasing the sidebending, flexion, and rotational components until motion is relocalized to the segment.

7. Steps 5 and 6 are repeated three or four times before the patient is retested. Treatment is repeated if necessary.

Manipulation

The focus of the treatment techniques presented in this chapter has been on the "patient-active" METs. A variety of high-velocity thrust mobilizations for the sacroiliac joints exist. They primarily produce rotatory forces on the innominates and are thus more appropriate for the iliosacral lesions. One particularly effective thrust technique is included for completeness:

1. The patient is supine, with the hands locked behind the head (fingers interlaced).
2. The clinician stands opposite the affected side and makes hand contact on the patient's ASIS (on the affected side) with the caudad hand.
3. With the cephalad hand, the clinician reaches through the crook of the patient's elbow (on the affected side) from behind and allows the dorsum of his or her hand to contact the patient's chest (Fig. 19–121).
4. Using the dorsum of the hand as a fulcrum against the patient's chest, the clinician rolls the patient's torso toward him or her. The clinician instructs the patient to "relax, hang on to your head, and allow me to turn you."
5. The clinician takes up the slack through the pelvis using a stiff arm, with the direction of force applied down and away.
6. The clinician instructs the patient to "take in a deep breath and let it out." As the patient does so, the clinician takes up the remainder of the slack through

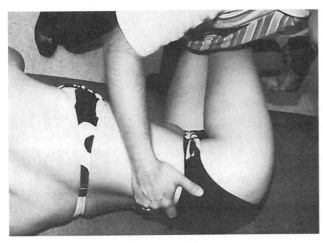

Figure 19–120. Positioning and application of MET for a right extended, rotated, and sidebent (ERS right) lumbar facet restriction.

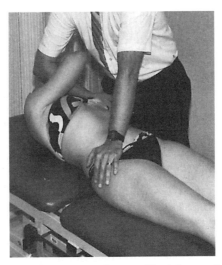

Figure 19–121. Positioning for sacroiliac joint manipulation.

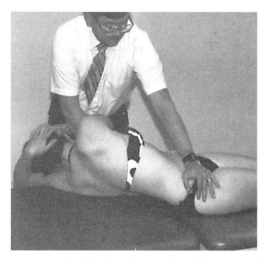

Figure 19–122. Positioning for sacroiliac joint manipulation and application of thrust to the ASIS.

the torso and pelvis and gives a quick thrust to the pelvis through the ASIS (Fig. 19–122).

CASE STUDY

The following case is an example of a lumbo-pelvic-hip dysfunction seen in our clinic. Variations of this scenario are commonly seen.

Subjective History

A 36-year-old woman presented for evaluation and treatment of a chronic left upper gluteal pain of several years' duration. She was experiencing occasional posterolateral thigh pain and inguinal pain, especially when climbing stairs. She had no complaints of distal paresthesias below the knee. She indicated that her problem began soon after the birth of her second child and that she had experienced much lower back pain during her last trimester of pregnancy. Within the previous year, she had begun a jogging routine that tended to aggravate the problem somewhat. Prolonged sitting did not seem to contribute to her complaint. Other than this discomfort, which she described as an "ache" with occasional "sharp twinges," her general health was excellent, with no significant history of disease or surgery.

Objective Examination

Posture: Normal kypho-lordosis but with a tendency toward a forward head and protraction of the shoulder girdles. No significant scoliosis was found, but a small left convex deviation was noted at the L4 and L5 levels from the midline.

Landmarks: Superior left iliac crest; superior left ASIS; inferior left PSIS; superior left pubic tubercle; trochanters levels; ischial tuberosities level; left foot pronated more than the right, with some internal tibial rotation.

Mobility examination: (+) Standing flexion test left; (+) Gillet's test left; nearly full recruitment of lumbosacral motion in forward bending without midline deviation except at L4 and L5; (−) paravertebral spasm/tightness; pain in upper gluteal region and lateral thigh noted with forward bending; limitation of motion into left sidebending at L4 and L5; limitation of motion into right rotation at L4 and L5; full backward bending without restriction; full squat-to-stand without difficulty; (+) sitting flexion test left but restriction was noted to be less than with the standing flexion test.

Special tests: (+) SLR left at 60 degrees for posterolateral thigh and buttock pain; (−) SLR right at 70 degrees with hamstring engagement; (+) long-sit test left short to equal; (+) pelvic rock left for harder end-feel and some discomfort in the left SI region; (+) Patrick's test left for left SI discomfort; (+) tenderness along the inguinal ligament; (+) tenderness over the tensor fascia latae (TFL) and iliotibial band; (−) hip scour; (+) posterior-anterior (PA) spring for discomfort at L5–S1; (−) sacral springing; deep right sacral sulcus in neutral; posterior left ILA in neutral; with sphinx testing, sulcus and ILA become more symmetric; piriformis noted to be tighter on the right than on the left.

Neurologic examination: Within normal limits.

Assessment

Assessment revealed the following: (1) Left superior pubic shear; (2) left posterior innominate; (3) possible left-on-left forward torsion; (4) possible TFL friction syndrome over the trochanter secondary to tightness; (5) kinetic chain influence secondary to overpronation and tibial torsion; and (6) probable type I lumbar dysfunction at L4 and L5 secondary to iliosacral and saroiliac dysfunctions noted.

Treatment Plan

METs were planned for this patient for (1) correction of left superior public shear; (2) correction of left-on-left forward torsion; (3) correction of left posterior innominate; (4) mobility exercises for the lumbar spine and stabilization exercises; (5) neutral subtalar orthotics; and (6) progression to an aerobic and conditioning program as tolerated.

Results

The patient's groin pain and upper gluteal discomfort were almost completely relieved after her first treatment. Her posterolateral thigh pain, although improved, persisted. However, with stretching of the TFL and the piriformis and the implementation of the lumbosacral mobility exercises and stabilization exercises, this complaint began to resolve. The combination of METs for the pelvis and lumbar mobility exercises resolved the type I lumbar dysfunction. The patient returned to jogging but began to reexperience some symptoms, with return of her groin and upper gluteal complaints. Reassessment noted a recurence of the pubic shear and posterior innominate. METs were reemployed, with resolution of the patient's pain. She did not run again until her neutral subtalar orthotics were received and fitted to her. This resolved her kinetic chain problem by balancing some biomechanical problems of the ankle and lower leg. Use of the orthotics also resolved the residual TFL complaints.

Discussion

The patient probably sustained an iliosacral and sacroiliac dysfunction secondary to her pregnancy and delivery. The pubic shear lesion may have also occurred with her pregnancy and delivery but may have been the result of her jogging program. It is possible that all these dysfunctions were the result of her biomechanical deficits in the lower kinetic chain and were magnified by her pregnancy and her later jogging program. A follow-up check 6 months after treatment revealed that she remained asymptomatic and was jogging 3 to 4 miles a day 3 to 5 days per week. She continued to perform her mobility and stabilization exercises before jogging or other exercise activities.

■ Acknowledgments

The author thanks Linda, Scott, and Sean for their understanding, patience, and encouragement along the way to completion of this work. Special thanks to Steve Stratton for his inspiration to excel and for his advice and to Barbara Springer for modeling.

■ References

1. Kapandji IA: The Physiology of the Joints. 2nd Ed. Vol. III. The Trunk and the Vertebral Column. Churchill Livingstone, Edinburgh, 1974
2. Kaltenbourn FM: Mobilization of Extremity Joints: Examination and Basic Treatment Techniques. 3rd Ed. Olaf Norlis Bokhandel, Oslo, 1980
3. Warwick R, Williams P (eds): Gray's Anatomy. 35th Br. Ed. Churchill Livingstone, Edinburgh, 1974
4. Kendall FP, Kendall-McCreary E: Muscles, Function and Testing. 3rd Ed. Williams & Wilkins, Baltimore, 1983
5. Janda V: Muscle Function Testing. Butterworth-Heinneman, London, 1983
6. Kopell HP, Thompson WAL: Peripheral Entrapment Neuropathies. Robert E Krieger, Huntington, NY, 1976
7. Lee D: The Pelvic Girdle. Churchill Livingstone, New York, 1989
8. Solonen KA: The sacroiliac joint in the light of anatomical, roentgenological and clinical studies. Acta Orthop Scand, suppl. 27:1, 1957
9. Kirkaldy-Willis WH: Managing Low Back Pain. Churchill Livingstone, New York, 1983
10. Stoddard A: Manual of Osteopathic Technique. Hutchinson, London, 1978
11. Mitchell FL Jr, Moran PS, Pruzzo NA: An Evaluation and Treatment Manual of Osteopathic Muscle Energy Procedures. Mitchell, Moran and Pruzzo Associates, Valley Park, MO, 1979
12. Hoppenfeld S: Physical Examination of the Spine and Extremities. Appleton-Century-Crofts, New York, 1976
13. Cyriax J: Textbook of Orthopaedic Medicine. 7th Ed. Vol 1. Diagnosis of Soft Tissue Lesions. Bailliere-Tindall, London, 1978
14. Cailliet R: Low Back pain Syndrome. 2nd Ed. FA Davis, Philadelphia, 1982
15. Frigerio NA, Stowe RR, Howe JW: Movement of the sacroiliac joint. Clin Orthop 100:370, 1974
16. Colachis SC, Werden C, Bechtol C, et al: Movement of the sacroiliac joints in the adult male. A preliminary report. Arch Phys Med Rehabil 44:490, 1963
17. Egund N, Olsson TH, Schmid H, et al: Movements in the sacroiliac joints demonstrated with roentgen stereophotogrammetry. Acta Radiol (Stockholm) 19:833, 1978
18. Turek SL: Orthopaedics: Principles and Their Applications. 4th Ed. JB Lippincott, Philadelphia, 1984
19. Weisl H: Movements of the sacro-iliac joint. Acta Anat 23:80, 1955
20. Mennell JM: Back Pain. Little, Brown, Boston, 1960
21. Paris SV: Course notes: the spine. Institute of Graduate Health Sciences, Atlanta, 1979
22. Course notes: tutorial on level I muscle energy techniques. Michigan State University College of Osteopathic Medicine, East Lansing, MI, 1986
23. Goodridge JP: Muscle energy technique: definition, explanation, methods of procedure. J Am Osteopath Assoc 82:249, 1981
24. Kimberly PE (ed): Somatic Dysfunction: Principles of Manipulative Treatment and Procedures, Kirksville College of Osteopathic Medicine, Kirksville, MO, 1980
25. Nyberg R: The lumbar and pelvic musculature. Unpublished manuscript, 1978
26. Farfan H: Muscular mechanism of the lumbar spine and the position of power and efficiency. Orthop Clin North Am 6:135, 1975
27. Mitchell FL Sr: Structural pelvic function. AAO Year-book II:178, 1965
28. Saunders HD: Evaluation, Treatment and Prevention of Musculoskeletal Disorders. 2nd Ed. H Duane Saunders, Minneapolis, 1985
29. Stratton SA: Course notes: muscle energy techniques. U.S. Army-Baylor University Program in Physical Therapy, Fort Sam Houston, TX, 1983–1984
30. Pratt WA: The lumbopelvic torsion syndrome. J Am Osteopath Assoc 51:335, 1952
31. Greenman PE: Innominate shear dysfunction in the sacroiliac syndrome. Manual Med 2:114, 1986
32. DiAmbrosia RD: Musculoskeletal Disorders. JB Lippincott, Philadelphia, 1977

33. Nitz PA, Woerman AL: Acute sacroiliac joint strain in young adult males as evidenced by bone scan. Preliminary research. 1988

34. Grieve GP: Common Vertebral Joint Problems. Churchill Livingstone, New York, 1981

35. Fryette HH: Principles of Osteopathic Technique. American Academy of Osteopathy, Carmel, CA, 1954

36. Greenman PE: The manipulative prescription. Mich Osteopath J 1982

37. Korr I: Proprioceptors and somatic dysfunction. J Am Osteopath Assoc 74:638, 1975

38. Greenman PE: Restricted vertebral motion. Mich Osteopath J 31, 1983

39. Clemente CD: Anatomy: A Regional Atlas of the Human Body. #376. Lea & Febiger, Philadelphia, 1975

40. Greenman PE: Motion sense. Mich Osteopath J January: 39, 1983

41. Kessler RM, Hertlig D: Management of Common Musculoskeletal Disorders. Harper & Row, Philadelphia, 1983

42. Maitland GD: Vertebral Manipulation. Butterworths, London, 1977

43. Woerman AL, Binder-MacLeod S: Leg length discrepancy assessment: accuracy and precision in five clinical methods of evaluation. J Orthop Sports Phys Ther 5:230, 1984

44. Kirkaldy-Willis WH, Hill RJ: A more precise diagnosis for low-back pain. Spine 4:102, 1979

45. Liekens M, Gillets H: Belgian Chiropractic Research Notes. 10th Ed. Brussels, 1973

46. Mooney V, Robertson J: The facet syndrome. Clin Orthop 115:149, 1976

47. Bemis T, Daniel M: Validation of the long sit test on subjects with iliosacral dysfunction. J Orthop Sports Phys Ther 8:336, 1987

48. Grieve GP: Mobilization of the Spine. 4th Ed. Churchill Livingstone, New York, 1984

■ Suggested Readings

Bachrach RM, Micelotta J, Winuk C: The relationship of low back pain to psoas insufficiency. J Orthop Med 13:34, 1991

Beal MC: The sacroiliac problem: review of anatomy, mechanics and diagnosis. J Am Osteopath Assoc 81:667, 1982

Bourdillon JF: Spinal Manipulation. 3rd Ed. Appleton-Century-Crofts, New York, 1982

Bowen V, Cassidy JD: Macroscopic and microscopic anatomy of the sacroiliac joint from embryonic life until the eighth decade. Spine 6:620, 1981

Erhard R, Bowling R: The recognition and management of the pelvic component of low back and sciatic pain. Bull Orthop Sect Am Phys Ther Assoc 2:4, 1977

Grieve GP: The sacroiliac joint. Physiotherapy 62:384, 1976

Johnston WL: Hip shift: testing a basic postural dysfunction. J Am Osteopath Assoc 63:923, 1964

Retzlaff EW, Berry AH, Haight AS, et al: The piriformis muscle syndrome. J Am Osteopath Assoc 73:799, 1974

Stoddard A: Conditions of the sacro-iliac joint and their treatment. Physiotherapy 44:97, 1958

Sutton SE: Postural imbalance: examination, and treatment using flexion tests. J Am Osteopath Assoc 77:456, 1978

Walheim G, Olerud S, Ribbe T: Mobility of the pubic symphysis. Acta Orthop Scand 55:203, 1984

Weismantel A: Evaluation and treatment of sacroiliac joint problems. Bull Orthop Sect Am Phys Ther Assoc 3:5, 1978

Wilder DG, Pope MH, Frymoyer JW: The functional topography of the sacroiliac joint. Spine 5:575, 1980

CHAPTER 20
Surgical Treatment of the Hip

William B. Haynes and David Paul Rouben

The differential diagnosis of pain in and around the pelvis, groin, and low back is a confusing and persistently perplexing problem. Pain in the anterior thigh and groin region can actually be referred from the knee. Disorders in and around the patellofemoral joint or degenerative inflammation of the knee can refer pain to the quadriceps musculature and to the groin. Pain perceived in the buttocks can be referred from the low back. Pain along the lateral aspect of the proximal femur is easily attributable to soft tissue bursitis or mechanical inflammation of the abductor musculature or fascia lata rubbing against the prominent greater trochanteric eminence of the proximal femur. Inflammation over the anterior aspect of the pelvic rim can refer pain to the anterior aspect of the groin and proximal thigh. A complete physical examination and assessment are needed to determine the source of the pain.

As a general guide, pain perceived in the buttocks is attributable to referred pain from the lumbosacral spine or to inflammation of the sacroiliac joint, the sciatic nerve, or the buttock muscles. Causes of anterior thigh pain can be an upper lumbar disk herniation, inflammation of the lumbar facet joints, referred pain from the knee, referred pain from the underlying thigh musculature or femur, soft tissue entrapment within the groin and inguinal ligament, or referred pain from inflammation at the anterior pelvic rim (i.e., the lateral femoral cutaneous nerve). As described earlier, pain to the proximal lateral femur is usually attributable to soft tissue inflammation at or over the prominence of the greater trochanter. In most cases, hip joint pain is perceived as anterior groin pain that worsens on weightbearing or on active and passive range of motion of the proximal femur during physical examination.

A careful history identifying where the pain comes from and when it is produced can often clarify these confusing issues. A careful examination of the joints and muscle groups in and around the area can also help to determine the origin of pain. Focal pain elicited when palpating the buttocks or the lower lumbosacral region usually emanates from the area in and around the bony or soft tissue aspects of the lumbosacral articulation or the sacroiliac joint. Firm palpation over the trochanteric prominence on the lateral aspect of the proximal femur usually reproduces pain originating from soft tissue irritation in that region. Gentle, passive internal and external rotation under no gravitational stress usually reproduces pain if it emanates from the hip joint itself.

Sometimes more complex examinations must be performed to confirm whether the pain is coming from the hip joint. If the patient is not particularly symptomatic, then the pain is often not elicited except in abduction or adduction positions when associated with internal and external rotation manipulation. Sometimes flexion must be added to elicit pain. Nevertheless, in most cases, reproducible hip joint pain is perceived in the anterior aspect of the proximal thigh articulation (the groin).

Appropriate to any discussion of the evaluation and treatment of pain in and around the hip joint is a consideration of the many causes of those conditions that may necessitate operative intervention.

Hip Joint Disorders

Trauma

Traumatic injuries to the hip joint can occur in every age group. Children as well as adults who are involved in motor vehicle accidents can have partial or total avascular necrosis and subsequent collapse of the femoral head despite early operative intervention. Femoral head dislocations and fracture dislocations of the femoral head and acetabulum can affect the vascular supply of the femoral head and cause irreparable acetabular incongruity necessitating extensive reconstructive surgery.

The acetabulum makes up the roof of the hip joint. It is a coalition of three pelvic bones: the pubis, ischium, and ilium. If traumatic disruption of the articular surface of the acetabulum exceeds 2 mm, open reduction and internal fixation of the articular surface of the acetabulum is often indicated. Open reduction is performed to avoid incongruence and posttraumatic osteoarthritis. Even after successful open reduction and internal fixation, damage to the articular surface may be so severe as to initiate cartilaginous necrosis and osteoarthritis. Hence, fractures necessitating open reduction and internal fixation of the acetabulum are often associated with traumatic dislocations of the femoral head. It is common to observe bony or cartilaginous fragments within the hip joint socket at the time of surgical reduction.

Surgical exposure of the acetabulum, whether by the anterior, lateral, posterior, or combined approach, involves several different techniques. Several exposures depend on the need for assessment and reduction of the anatomic surface. A thorough understanding of which exposure was used will be of value to anyone directly involved in the postoperative rehabilitative therapy of the patient. This information must be easily available to those directing postoperative ambulatory care. In general, passive range of motion should be initiated on day 2 or 3 after surgical stabilization. Toe-touch weightbearing with crutch or walker support can be initiated on the first or second postoperative day and can progress as pain allows. Weightbearing should be protected for the first 6 to 8 weeks after surgical intervention or as the surgeon instructs. Initiation of early postoperative range-of-motion exercise is important to prevent stiffness and may promote the healing of the cartilaginous surfaces. Abductor exercises can help to strengthen the hip and decrease the likelihood of a long-term limp or Trendelenburg gait.

Complications associated with open reduction and internal fixation of the acetabulum include infection, sciatic or common peroneal nerve palsy, loss of reduction, ectopic bone formation, and thromboembolic disease processes.[1]

Hip and fracture dislocations are the result of high-energy trauma to the bony structure of the femoral head or acetabulum, or both, as well as to the periarticular soft tissues. Most hip fracture dislocations are posterior. Some involve the anterior, central, and inferior aspects of the acetabulum. Traumatic disruption of the vascular supply to the femoral head and subsequent osteonecrosis of the femoral head can cause posttraumatic arthritis and necessitate total hip arthroplasty. Treatment for these traumatic maladies centers on early reduction and bone reconstruction and stabilization.

More than 275,000 fractures of the proximal femur involving the femoral neck and intertrochanteric region of the femur occur in the United States every year. Ninety-five percent of these patients are older than 50 years of age. The total annual cost of medical care for these frac-

tures will increase from approximately $7.2 billion currently to $16 billion in 2040.[1] Because of the overwhelming disability associated with these fractures, 10 percent of the patients die within the first 3 years. Another 10 percent die in the next 3 years; after 10 years, 77 percent of patients who have sustained fractures of the proximal femur have died.[2-6]

Fractures of the femoral neck should be reduced and stabilized as soon as possible. Nondisplaced fractures or fractures that have minimal displacement or angulation are most often treated by early structural stabilization with multiple screws placed by an open or percutaneous technique. Gradual, guarded toe-touch weightbearing is encouraged until fracture healing is ascertained by radiographic and clinical assessment—usually within 6 to 8 weeks. Displaced fractures are treated by removal of the femoral head and insertion of an endoprosthesis or hemiarthroplasty stabilized by cementing or by uncemented techniques. In younger patients who sustain displaced femoral neck fractures, open reduction and internal fixation may be indicated. Because of traumatic disruption of the blood supply to the femoral head, avascular necrosis can develop later. These patients may eventually require prosthetic replacement.

Intertrochanteric fractures of the proximal femur are usually treated by reduction and stabilization—most commonly by an extramedullary side plate and a sliding screw. Multiple intramedullary wires or rods have also been used, but they are seldom used today. A recently developed second-generation device that combines a short intramedullary device with a sliding hip screw shows promise as an alternative to the older methods. This technique allows the elderly, debilitated patient to bear more weight during the initial postoperative period.

The surgeon often recommends nonweightbearing or toe-touch status after fixation of an intertrochanteric fracture. However, few elderly patients can use a walker and remain nonweightbearing after hip surgery. Many of these patients have multiple medical problems and generalized upper extremity weakness. For this reason, secure intraoperative fixation that allows the patient to begin early weightbearing is very important.

Proximal femoral replacement is used when the entire medial bony structure or calcar is fractured down to or including the lesser trochanter. These patients can often be managed with weightbearing as tolerated, especially if the prosthesis is cemented. A calcar replacement device is also used after failure of a severe, unstable intertrochanteric fracture that was originally fixed with a side plate and sliding hip screw construct. It is important to coordinate the best rehabilitation plan with the surgeon before ambulation is allowed because some surgeons prefer toe-touch or partial weightbearing. If the prosthesis is a press fit or cementless type, full weightbearing might be delayed for up to 6 weeks.

Vascular Compromise

In addition to trauma, vascular compromise of the femoral head can be caused by Legg-Perthes disease in the young, in hereditary metabolic disorders such as Gaucher's disease, or in patients with chronic alcoholism, pancreatitis, overwhelming obesity, diabetes mellitus, polycythemia, chronic long-term corticosteroid use, sickle cell disease, nitrogen gas occlusion syndrome (diver's disease), or idiopathic disorders.[7,8]

The subsequent osteonecrosis may be partial (segmental) or complete. Early osteonecrosis, before any bony or articular surface collapse, is often treated by core decompression, and occasionally a vascularized bone graft is also inserted. Core decompression involves reaming of the head and neck to allow hemopoietic cells to reach the area. Patients are placed on protected weightbearing status for approximately 4 weeks, and then weightbearing as tolerated is allowed. If a vascular graft is added, a much longer period of protected weightbearing is required. Treatment of avascular necrosis is individualized and results vary, depending on its cause, stage of the disease, and the patient's activity level. Unfortunately, because most individuals do not present until after collapse of the femoral head, they require some type of reconstructive procedure.

Neoplastic Lesions

Several neoplastic lesions can afflict the femoral head, the acetabulum, or both. Among these are chondroblastoma and osteogenic sarcoma in young individuals. Giant cell tumor is seen in early adulthood and middle age. Paget's disease and metastatic cancers are seen in mature individuals.[7-9]

Collagen Vascular Disease

Rheumatoid arthritis in the young as well as the old can necessitate progressive reconstructive arthroplastic procedures in and around the hip joint. Collagen vascular diseases such as ankylosing spondylitis and rheumatoid arthritis have been shown to cause degenerative changes, if not ankylosis, necessitating operative reconstruction.[7,8]

Metabolic or Hormonal Disease

Chronic renal failure and treatments necessary to control this disease can cause avascular changes to the femoral head. Hyperparathyroidism, hyperthyroidism, and hypercortisolism can all lead to avascular changes in the femoral head. A slipped capital femoral epiphysis in the pubescent male seems to have some relationship to estrogen-testosterone homeostasis. Loss of estrogen has deleterious effects on the bony architecture of the hip joint in the older adult.[3]

Developmental Hip Disorders

Developmental disorders of the hip joint such as congenital dislocation and hip and acetabular dysplasia may make reconstructive procedures in and around the hip necessary as the patient matures into adulthood.

Infections

Acute septic hip infections in the young, if not diagnosed and treated quickly, can make joint reconstruction necessary as the child matures. Patients with sickle cell disease are prone to salmonella or staphylococcus infections, necessitating structural reconstruction of the hip joint. Chronic infections in and around the hip joint are prevalent in patients suffering from chronic tuberculous infection. These infections are most often seen in Third World countries.

■ Surgical Intervention

Each patient who requires reconstructive surgery in and around the hip joint must be evaluated and treated individually. The best treatment option for one patient is not necessarily optimal for another, even though the same pathoanatomy may be present in both. As orthopaedic research progresses, our treatment options grow as well. Each patient should be evaluated and provided with treatment options that offer the greatest chance of long-term, pain-free, ambulatory success. This is never a straightforward or easy decision. The surgeon must make a careful assessment, taking into account the patient's age and medical, emotional, physiologic, physical, and intellectual stability. The long-term goals and desires of each patient must always be respected.

Before modern metals made implantation and reconstruction of the hip joint anatomically feasible, many seemingly aggressive and definitive treatments were used routinely. Two of these procedures—resection arthroplasty and hip joint fusion—are still used today but for very limited indications.

Resection Arthroplasty

Resection arthroplasty, commonly known as the *Girdlestone resection,* involves surgical excision of the femoral head and neck, with purposeful soft tissue interposition. Indications for resection arthroplasty include incurable infection, postradiation necrosis of the proximal femur, and absence of any bone left to reconstruct. The procedure is also indicated for patients whose medical status is so compromised that a more definitive procedure to alleviate pain caused by developmental structural deformities would likely result in death.[10]

Historically, the patient was placed in skeletal traction for approximately 2 weeks after surgery and then was progressively taught ambulatory skills. Currently, early mobilization is begun as soon as the patient's pain allows. This is done initially with the patient in a nonweightbearing status, progressing to weightbearing as tolerated over a 2- to 3-month period. The procedure results in a 2- to 5-cm shortening of the limb. However, after the soft tissue has healed, the patient is able to walk with the use of an assistive device and a modified shoe. He or she may have a noticeable limp (Trendelenburg gait), but there is usually minimal disability and pain.[4,7,8,11]

Arthrodesis

Arthrodesis of the hip (hip fusion) is accomplished by a variety of techniques (Fig. 20–1). It is indicated for teenagers and young adults in whom total hip replacement is not appropriate because of premature age. The procedure is done more often in male patients than in female patients. Female patients in our culture are less likely to accept any visually obvious compromise in normal gait. The fusion is done by structurally stabilizing the proximal femur into the acetabular socket of the pelvis in neutral rotation, slight flexion, and neutral or slight adduction of the hip. Abduction and internal rotation are to be avoided. Postoperatively, these patients are taught to attain ambulatory skills that allow gait velocity at 40 percent of normal. They can attain the ambulatory skills needed to participate in aggressive athletics during their youth and can ambulate with a lift. As one might expect, they compensate for the loss of hip motion through increased motion of the lumbosacral region of the spine. These patients show evidence of early radiographic degenerative changes to the lumbosacral spine that may become symptomatic some 20 to 30 years later. If the technique used for hip fusion does not involve extensive amounts of hardware or large blocks of bone graft, a total hip arthroplasty may be possible at a later age.[4,13,14] Ar-

throplasty also requires preservation of the abductors. Nevertheless, reconstruction arthroplasty of hips that have previously undergone arthrodesis present the surgeon, therapist, and patient with unique rehabilitative hurdles to overcome postoperatively.

Fixed Head (Unipolar) Hemiarthroplasty

As our technical knowledge and skill with metal progressed, the first hemiarthroplasties were devised. They have been used successfully since the 1950s and 1960s. Complete transection and excision of the femoral head at the femoral neck with insertion of a metal stem into the cancellous aspect of the proximal shaft of the femur seems to offer patients with conditions that destroy the femoral head a chance to regain ambulatory skills. Today these prostheses are most often used in elderly patients whose fractures in and around the femoral neck preclude closed or open reduction and internal fixation of their femoral head fractures. Traditionally, the prostheses most often used were the Thompson and Austin-Moore types (Figs. 20–2 and 20–3). Currently, most orthopaedic implant companies provide a lower-demand cemented hemiarthroplasty (Fig. 20–4). These prostheses are inserted from an anterior, posterior, or anterolateral approach.

Bipolar Prostheses

A more complex proximal femoral replacement prosthesis is the bipolar type (Fig. 20–5). This prosthesis attempts to combine a rotating mobile acetabular bearing with a fixed femoral head. After insertion of a standard proximal femoral replacement into the femur, a plastic bearing is attached to the femoral ball and a metal cup is attached to the plastic bearing. The metal cup is free to move against the normal cartilaginous surface of the acetabu-

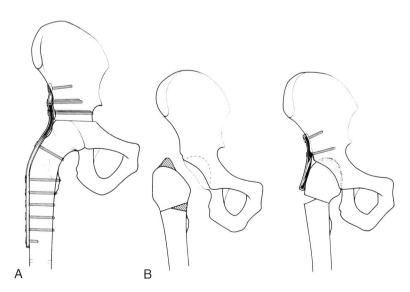

A   B

Figure 20–1. (A) Hip arthrodesis with rigid internal compression fixation (Schneider's cobra head plate, 1966). (B) Arthrodesis of a Girdlestone hip. (From Liechti,[12] with permission.)

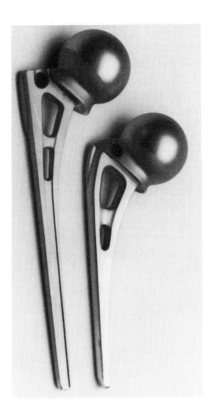

Figure 20–2. Austin-Moore prostheses with an early (right) and a later straight-stem design (left). These devices were designed for press-fit fixation in the femoral canal before methylmethacrylate was used to augment fixation. (From Stauffer,[15] with permission.)

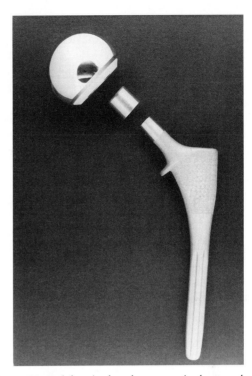

Figure 20–4. A hemiarthroplasty or unipolar prosthesis.

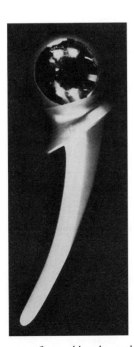

Figure 20–3. Thompson femoral head prosthesis. (From Stauffer,[15] with permission.)

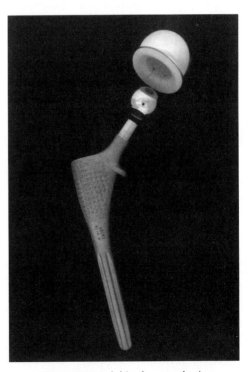

Figure 20–5. A bipolar prosthesis.

lum. It is hoped that this component will cause less acetabular pain than the single-ball proximal femoral prostheses (unipolar hemiarthroplasties). Nevertheless, a small number of patients eventually need acetabular replacement because of progressive destructive wear of the cartilaginous surface of the acetabulum.[16]

With a posterior approach, patients are protected postoperatively from adduction, internal rotation, and flexion maneuvers. Anterolateral approaches require protection from extreme extension and external rotation of the hip. After 6 to 8 weeks, these movement restrictions are reduced or eliminated. Regardless of the approach used, these patients are often allowed to ambulate with the support of a walker or crutches using toe-touch gait techniques. They progress to full weightbearing as tolerated.[17]

Proximal Femoral and Acetabular Osteotomy

In an attempt to postpone more aggressive joint reconstructive arthroplastic techniques, European orthopaedists have popularized periacetabular or transtrochanteric rotational osteotomies. Theoretically, these techniques are designed to redirect noninjured articular surfaces of either the acetabulum or the femoral head into directional alignment consistent with weightbearing. Prerequisites for osteotomy include subluxation, reasonable congruity, maintenance of at least one-half of normal cartilage thickness, and at least 60 percent of normal range of motion,

particularly in flexion and abduction. Good to excellent results are reported for the patient, and the clinician is afforded additional time to assess, evaluate, and suggest better long-term treatment options (Fig. 20–6).

The use of proximal femoral osteotomy or periacetabular osteotomy in young people with structural hip abnormalities plays an important role by prophylactically precluding early degenerative changes. Transtrochanteric rotational osteotomies are being used for the treatment of segmental osteonecrosis of the femoral head. Periacetabular osteotomies are used to place unaltered articular cartilage in juxtaposition to the femoral head. Periarticular osteotomies provide greater femoral head coverage to offset the pain associated with subluxation of the hip. Valgus osteotomy of the proximal femur is often used for patients with coxa magna.[11,18]

Total Hip Arthroplasty

John Charnley, in the early 1960s, popularized what is now known as *total hip arthroplasty*. Continued advances in the development of biologically compatible metals, surgical implantation techniques, and modifications to obtain the most biologically efficient structural shapes have made total hip arthroplasty the state-of-the-art treatment for patients with painful, incongruent hip joint disease.

In the past two decades, extensive research has yielded a very reliable, well-functioning artificial hip with both cemented and cementless implants. Current arthroplasty

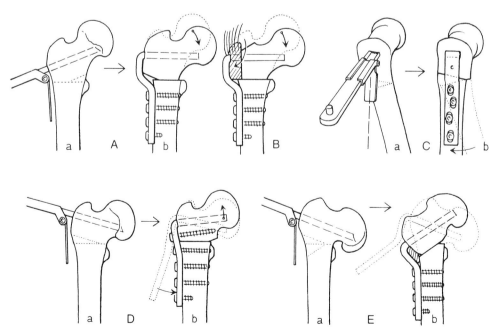

Figure 20–6. The five main types of intertrochanteric osteotomy. (A) Adduction osteotomy; (B) adduction osteotomy with distal displacement of the greater trochanter; (C) extension osteotomy before and after fixation; (D) abduction osteotomy of 50 degrees, fixed with a double-curved 120 degree blade plate; (E) abduction osteotomy with bone graft between the plate and the proximal fragment. (From Muller,[18] with permission.)

should allow the compliant patient approximately 15 years of good to excellent pain-free ambulatory function of the hip joint.

Although research and reevaluation of metals and component designs continue, titanium and cobalt chrome are the alloys generally used for total hip arthroplasty today. Both are used in cementless femoral and acetabular components. Cobalt chrome is currently the metal of choice for cemented femoral stems. Highly polished ceramic has also been used as a femoral head component that articulates with ultra-high-molecular-weight polyethylene (UHMWPE) plastic acetabular inserts.

Research efforts are focusing on total hip articulation and on efforts to minimize polyethylene particles, which can cause loosening with time. Metal on metal, ceramic on ceramic, and ceramic on polyethylene articulations are currently undergoing clinical trials. The results of these studies must be compared against the standard, which is cementing with methylmethacrylate cement for the femoral component and use of a cementless acetabular component—the so-called hybrid technique (Fig. 20–7). Contemporary techniques should give good to excellent results for a long period of time in more than 90 to 95 percent of patients, according to the National Institutes of Health Consensus Conference on Hip Replacements.[19]

Surgical Technique

The experience and technical expertise of the surgeon determine the surgeon's choice of approach to the hip. Some research supports the notion that posterior approaches are more inclined to result in dislocation posteriorly; however, this has never been consistently proved. The anterior and anterolateral approaches are considered to be more technically demanding and difficult[20,21] and can lead to a permanent limp secondary to hip abductor weakness.

The basic procedure for total hip arthroplasty is as follows. After exposure of the proximal femur and acetabulum, the femoral head and neck are resected. Although early total hip arthroplasty techniques provided for trochanteric osteotomies, these operations are no longer performed routinely. Trochanteric osteotomies are now used primarily for very complex reconstruction or for revision arthroplasty. The proximal femoral medullary canal is prepared, and the acetabular bony surface is prepared with appropriate rasping and articular cartilage debridement. If methylmethacrylate cement is used for acetabular fixation, it is mixed and inserted into the acetabular bed, and the all-polyethylene acetabular component is positioned in the acetabular bed until the cement hardens. If cement is not used, the bony acetabulum is prepared and reamed to a smaller size than the true acetabular component, thus affording a good, tight fit (press fit) when the noncemented acetabular component is hammered into the bony architecture of the pelvis. The acetabulum is usually placed at 15 to 20 degrees of anteversion and 45 degrees of abduction.[22–26]

After the proximal femur has been rasped and reamed properly, the surgeon must decide whether the patient will undergo cemented or noncemented proximal femoral fixation. If the cemented technique is used, a cement-restricting plug is inserted into the medullary canal approximately 2 cm distal to the most distal tip of the femoral component once it is inserted into the femur. This allows cement impregnation into the interstices of the proximal femur under pressure. The cement in a liquid stage is then pressure impregnated into the proximal fe-

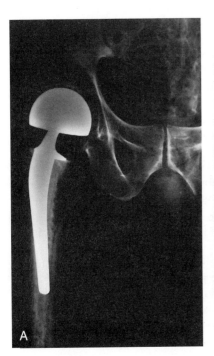
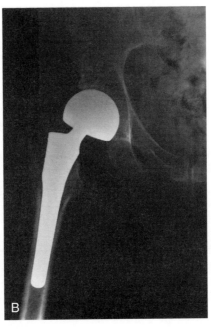

Figure 20–7. Radiographic appearance of (A) a bipolar hip device with a cemented femoral component and (B) a bipolar hip prosthesis with a noncemented, porous femoral component. (From Stauffer,[15] with permission.)

mur, and the femoral component is inserted into the cement mantle held in approximately 10 to 20 degrees of anteversion. If, however, no cement is desired, the proximal femur is underreamed so that a press fit can be achieved once the femoral component is impacted into the femur.

Reduction and testing of the structural stability of the hip is performed before soft tissue closure. The capsule may be resected or retained. The soft tissues are approximated in an anatomic fashion.

Postoperative care is as important as the decision concerning which prosthesis is to be used. The type of surgical exposure, the type of surgical implant fixation, and the physiologic ability of the patient involved determine the regimen. A close relationship between the patient and the physical therapist is necessary in these and all cases of ambulatory rehabilitation after surgery. It is very important that the physical therapist meet with the patient before surgery to establish this relationship and to begin to prepare the patient for the physical demands and expectations of ambulating after surgery. It is imperative that the therapist understand the anatomic approach used in the procedure so as to understand what muscles will be temporarily impaired structurally. If a posterior approach is used, there is a strong chance of posterior dislocation if the patient's hip joint is placed in adduction, flexion, and internal rotation. If an anterior approach is used, the most likely position to achieve anterior dislocation is adduction, extension, and external rotation. If the anterior or anterolateral approach is used, postoperative hip abduction exercises should be delayed for up to 6 weeks.

It is imperative that the therapist has a thorough understanding of the surgeon's goals in order not to confuse the patient during the ambulatory postoperative period. The patient may be toe-touch weightbearing, partial weightbearing, or weightbearing as tolerated, depending on the technique used, the intraoperative complications, or the surgeon's preference.

Revision Total Hip Surgery

Despite our attempts to develop better surgical techniques and to invent enhanced metals and structural designs to afford greater long-term acceptance, total hip arthroplasties intermittently continue to fail for a variety of reasons. The most common sources of failure are infection, component breakage or fragmentation, and loosening at the substrate–metal interface. The symptom of mechanical implant failure is quite simple—pain. Such failure is proven radiographically by understanding the subsidence of components within the bony construct of either the femur or the acetabulum. Visualization of a fracture of the component or its fixation substrate can also prove radiographic failure.[27] A significantly wide zone of radiographic lucency adjacent to certain areas of the prosthesis also indicates loosening. Osteolysis or focal bone resorption around an implant is often silent clinically. Regular follow-up examinations and early surgical intervention are usually required for progressive lesions.

Failure of component fixation necessitates reexploration of the hip joint through a more dramatic and more extensive approach, often using a trochanteric osteotomy. The failed component is removed, and all of its biologic and nonbiologic fixation tissue is completely excised[4,14,26,28–30] (Fig. 20–8).

The size and shape of replacement prostheses, as well as the type of fixation, continue to undergo development. Recently, more and more attempts to restore the damaged bony architecture to normal have been made by designing and modeling autologous and autogenous bone grafts to fit into the bony architectural defects. These unique attempts at reconstruction are proving to be successful. Whether revised components should be fixed with cement or with cementless fixation is still undecided.[19,31]

Postoperative care after revision must be planned and designed for the unique demands of the patient and the revision devices. A close working relationship and understanding of what has been done must be developed through direct communication between the treating therapist, operative surgeon, and patient.

Arthroscopy

Arthroscopy of the hip is a useful adjunct for treating some hip disorders. Technically, it is a relatively difficult procedure, and the results of hip arthroscopy are less rewarding than those of arthroscopy of other joints. Few orthopaedic surgeons treat hip disorders arthroscopically. It can be difficult to maneuver the arthroscope and operative instruments within the depths of the soft tissue of the proximal thigh.[32,33]

There are several indications for hip arthroscopy. Hip pain of unknown etiology is one of them. As noted earlier, hip pain can be perplexing for the physician. In one series of 200 hip arthroscopies, 40 patients who had normal studies underwent the procedure for undiagnosed hip pain.[32] Most were found to have hip dysplasia with degenerative labral tears.

Foreign bodies, such as those from gunshot or shrapnel wounds, and loose bodies can be removed arthroscopically.[34] It is also possible to remove broken screws or metal from previous surgery, such as those used for internal fixation of acetabular or femoral head fractures. Loose bodies from previous trauma can be present. Synovial chondromatosis also occurs in the hip. Hip infection can be treated arthroscopically with lavage and debridement, although it is traditionally treated with arthrotomy.

Other relative indications for hip arthroscopy are synovitis, degenerative joint disease, labral tears, and chondrolysis.[32] Arthroscopic surgery of the degenerative hip appears to produce results similar to those of arthroscopy of the knee. In moderate to advanced arthritis, it has unpredictable results. Relative contraindications are ad-

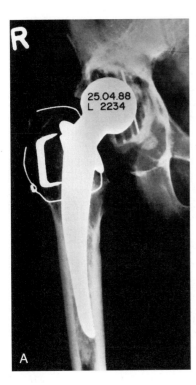
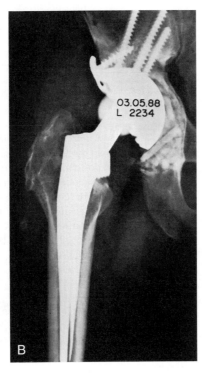

Figure 20–8. (A) Loosening of the socket, with bone loss and stem subsidence of 8 mm. Both components have to be revised. (B) Postoperative radiograph. (From Muller and Jaberg,[30] with permission.)

vanced arthritis, advanced avascular necrosis, and previous hip fusion.

Trochanteric bursoscopy has also been performed.[32] However, no reports of the results in long-term studies or large series are available. Arthroscopic treatment of snapping hip syndrome is also currently under investigation.

Rehabilitation of the hip in a patient who has had hip arthroscopy should be similar to that of other weight-bearing joints, such as the knee. In most instances, the patient can bear full or partial weight as tolerated soon after surgery. Postoperative hip abductor exercises are an important element of rehabilitation. Communication between the surgeon and the physical therapist is essential because one or two operative arthroscopic portals are established through the hip abductors.

CASE STUDIES

The following case studies offer the reader a chance to follow actual patient presentations and clinical plan. All the information in the preceding chapter offers a basis for analysis and a case plan.

CASE STUDY 1

A 13-year-old boy was involved in a motor vehicle accident. As a result, he sustained a fracture dislocation of his left hip. After clinical assessment and analysis of the structural competence of the femoral head and acetabu-lum, it was noted that the patient had sustained a displaced fracture of his femoral neck. He underwent open reduction and internal fixation of the femoral neck, using the most atraumatic surgical techniques available to avoid any further compromise of the vascular integrity of the femoral head. Nevertheless, within 6 months, radiographic evidence supported a complete avascular necrosis of the left femoral head and bony structural collapse. Arthrographic assessment of the left hip confirmed gross disruption of the articular surface of the femoral head as well as the acetabulum. Because the patient was 13 years old, at the end of puberty, and had many years of aggressive athletic potential, the decision was made to perform a left hip fusion. Anterior exposure of the left hip joint was achieved by exposing the anterior hip capsule after reflecting the head of the rectus femoris muscle off of its attachment to the pelvis. Decortication of the acetabulum was performed, and a trough was made into the anterior ridge of the acetabulum. The femoral head was decorticated, and a matching trough was made in the anterior edge of the femoral head and neck. The decorticated femoral head was placed into the decorticated acetabulum, fixed with autologous bone retrieved from the iliac crest, and fixed with three screws. Osteotomy of the proximal femur at the subtrochanteric level was achieved, and the patient was then placed into a 1 1/2 hip spica, holding the left lower extremity in 20 degrees of external rotation, 20 degrees of flexion, and neutral to 5 degrees of adduction. The patient healed properly. The spica cast was removed after 8 to 10 weeks, and its clinical integrity was assessed. Over the next 3 months, the patient underwent extensive physical therapy rehabilitation. Measured limb length inequality was corrected with a shoe lift, and the patient subsequently participated in activities of daily living including high school and extracurricular sports. Future plans and considerations with respect to this patient center on the probable onset of low back discomfort by 30 years of age and subsequent reconstruction or a total hip replacement at or about that time.

CASE STUDY 2

A 43-year-old man presented with right buttock and right thigh pain, having been referred by a family physician because of a suspected discogenic and lower back problem. Pain was accentuated when the patient walked, twisted, and bent at the lumbosacral spine. There was no history of trauma other than the fact that the patient had been an avid jogger but could no longer jog. Nonsteroidal anti-inflammatory medications seemed to be of no value in relieving the pain. Examination showed that the patient had no restricted range of motion to the lumbosacral spine, nor did the pain seem to be reproduced on examination of the lumbosacral spine. However, on flexion internal and external rotation maneuvers of the right hip, classic reproducible buttock and thigh pain occurred. Radiographic assessment of the lumbosacral spine was normal, but radiographic assessment of the pelvis revealed segmental collapse of the right femoral head, with concomitant sclerosis and irregular degeneration of the acetabulum on the right side. There was also evidence of segmental sclerosis of the left femoral head, with no overt collapse. A diagnosis of idiopathic bilaterally avascular necrosis of the femoral head was made and confirmed by technetium and magnetic resonance imaging scan techniques. There was no evidence of any history that would have produced this condition, hence the diagnosis of an idiopathic cause. Attempts to control the discomfort and pain through protected ambulation were made but failed. Thus, a right total hip arthroplasty was selected for this patient. Because the left hip was symptomatic at this time, a total hip replacement was not considered. The patient refused core decompression and autograft vascular supplementation. He subsequently underwent a right total hip replacement using noncemented techniques to the acetabulum and femur, with good results. Postoperatively, the patient underwent a course of protected ambulation for 6 weeks and progressive weightbearing as tolerated, associated with muscular strengthening and gait stabilization thereafter. At present, the patient is awaiting the onset of symptoms in the left hip.

■ Acknowledgment

Thanks go to Harold Cates, M.D., for his assistance with the revision of the section on total hip arthroplasty.

■ References

1. DeLee JC: Fractures and dislocations of the hip. p. 1211. In Rockwood CA, Green DP (eds): Fractures in Adults. Vol. II. JP Lippincott, Philadelphia, 1984
2. Elmerson S, Zetterberg C, Andersson G: Ten-year survival after fractures of the proximal end of the femur. Gerontology 34:186, 1988
3. Cummings SR, Rubin SM, Black D: The future of hip fractures in the United States. Numbers, costs, and potential effects of postmenopausal estrogen. Clin Orthop 252:163, 1990
4. American College of Orthopaedic Surgeons: Orthopaedic Knowledge Update III. American College of Orthopaedic Surgeons, Chicago, 1990
5. Letournel E, Judet R: Fractures of the acetabulum. Springer-Verlag, New York, 1981
6. Myo KA: Fractures of the acetabulum. Orthop Clin North Am 18:43, 1987
7. American College of Orthopaedic Surgeons: Orthopaedic Knowledge Update I. American College of Orthopaedic Surgeons, Chicago, 1984
8. American College of Orthopaedic Surgeons: Orthopaedic Knowledge Update II. American College of Orthopaedic Surgeons, Chicago, 1987
9. Enneking WF: Clinical Musculoskeletal Pathology. Storter Printing, Gainesville, FL, 1986
10. Crenshaw AH: Campbell's Operative Orthopaedics. Vol. II. CV Mosby, St. Louis, 1987
11. Evarts CM: The hip. p. 3. In Evarts CM (ed): Surgery of the Musculoskeletal System. Vol. 6. Churchill Livingstone, New York, 1983
12. Liechti R: Die Arthrodese des Huftgelentes und ihre Problematik. Springer-Verlag, Berlin, 1974
13. Liechti R: Hip arthrodesis. p. 99. In Evarts CM (ed): Surgery of the Musculoskeletal System. Churchill Livingstone, New York, 1983
14. Turner RH, Scheller AO (eds): Revision Total Hip Arthroplasty. Grune and Stratton, New York, 1982
15. Stauffer RN: Prosthetic hip replacement for femoral neck fractures. p. 2593. In Evarts CM (ed): Surgery of the Musculoskeletal System. 2nd Ed. Vol. 3. Churchill Livingstone, New York, 1990
16. Bochner RM: Bipolar hemi-arthroplasty for fracture of the femoral neck. J Bone Joint Surg 70(A):1001, 1988
17. Davy DT, Kotzar G, Brown RH: Telemetric force measurements across the after total arthroplasty. J Bone Joint Surg 70(A):45, 1988
18. Muller ME: Intertrochanteric osteotomies. p. 57. In Evarts CM (ed): Surgery of the Musculoskeletal System. Vol. 6. Churchill Livingstone, New York, 1983
19. NIH Consensus Conference: Total hip replacement. NIH consensus development panel on total hip replacement. JAMA 273:1950, 1995
20. Hoppenfeld S, de Boer P: Surgical Exposures in Orthopaedics. JB Lippincott, Philadelphia, 1984
21. Collis DK: Long-term followup of cemented total hip replacements in patients who were less than 50 years old. J Bone Joint Surg [Am] 73:593, 1991
22. Goldstein LA, Dickerson RC: Atlas of Orthopaedic Surgery. 2nd Ed. CV Mosby, St. Louis, 1981
23. Canen GH: Biologic Fixation of Porouscoat AML Hip. Depew, Wasau, IN, 1984

24. Canen GH: Biologic Fixation and Total Hip Arthroplasty. Slack, Inc., Thorofare, NJ, 1985

25. Canen GH: Porous coated hip replacement. J Bone Joint Surg 19(B):45, 1987

26. Rothman RH: Cemented vs. cementless total hip arthroplasty: a clinical review. Clin Orthop 254:153, 1990

27. Boullough PG: Pathologic studies of total joint replacement. Orthop Clin North Am 19:611, 1988

28. Harris WH: Replacement. J Bone Joint Surg 58(A):612, 1976

29. Maloney WJ: Endosteal erosion in association with stable uncemented femoral components. J Bone Joint Surg 72(A): 1025, 1990

30. Muller ME, Jaberg H: Total hip reconstruction. p. 2979. In Evarts CM (ed): Surgery of the Musculoskeletal System. 2nd Ed. Vol. 3. Churchill Livingstone, New York, 1990

31. Jasty M: Total hip reconstruction using femoral head allograft in patients with acetabular bone loss. Orthop Clin North Am 18:291, 1987

32. Sampson TG, Glick JM: Indications and surgical treatment of hip pathology. p. 1067. In McGinty JB, Caspari RB, Jackson RW, et al (eds): Operative Arthroscopy. 2nd Ed. Lippincott-Raven, Philadelphia, 1996

33. Glick JM, Sampson TG, Gordon RB, et al: Hip arthroscopy by the lateral approach. Arthroscopy 3:4, 1987

34. Cory JW, Ruch DS: Arthroscopic removal of a .44 caliber bullet from the hip. Arthroscopy 14:624, 1998

CHAPTER 21

Dysfunction, Evaluation, and Treatment of the Knee

Robert M. Poole and Turner A. Blackburn, Jr.

■ Anatomy of the Knee

The foundation for understanding the knee joint is comprehension of its anatomy. Although individual variations may occur, the functional components of knee anatomy remain unchanged.

Structural Foundation

The knee joint lies between the femur and the tibia, two of the largest and strongest levers in the human body. It is exposed to severe angular and torsion stresses, especially in athletes. The knee is basically a ligament-controlled joint, reinforced by the quadriceps, hamstring, and gastrocnemius muscle groups. These structures provide the main stabilizing influences for the knee joint.[1–3]

The distal end of the femur has an expanded medial and lateral condyle. The proximal end of the tibia is flared to create a plateau with medial and lateral sections to accommodate the medial and lateral femoral condyles (Fig. 21–1). These sections are divided by the tibial spine. Located in the medial and lateral sections are the menisci, which deepen the contour sections to ensure proper contact with the corresponding femoral condyle. The expanded femoral and tibial condyles are designed for weightbearing and to increase contact between the bones. The shape of the femoral condyles is also important in the movement of the tibia on the femur.

Besides the tibiofemoral joint, there is the patellofemoral joint, which consists of the patella and its articulating surface on the femur. The patella, the largest sesamoid bone in the body, is embedded in the quadriceps tendon. Its location allows greater mechanical advantage for the extension of the knee. The patellar groove on the distal end of the femur covers the anterior surfaces of both condyles and takes the shape of an inverted U (Fig. 21–2). The articular surface of the patella can be divided into a larger lateral part and a smaller medial part, which fit into the corresponding groove on the femur.[4]

Extensor Mechanism

The extensor mechanism of the knee consists of the quadriceps femoris muscle, which has four parts: the rectus femoris, the vastus intermedius, the vastus lateralis, and the vastus medialis. The vastus medialis muscle is further divided into the vastus medialis longus and the vastus medialis obliquus (Fig. 21–3A). These muscles come together to form a common tendon that continues from the quadriceps group to the tuberosity of the tibia and is called the *ligamentum patellae* or *patellar tendon*. The patella itself is used by the muscles to provide a greater mechanical advantage for the extension of the knee. The articularis genu muscle is also included in the extensor mechanism (Fig. 21–3B). This small muscle is attached to the suprapatellar bursa and synovial membrane of the knee and provides support for these structures during movements of the knee.

Other structures are included in the extensor mechanism. The patellar fat pad lies beneath the patellar tendon running from the inferior pole of the patella to the tibial tubercle. The patellofemoral and patellotibial ligaments, which are thickenings of the extensor retinaculum, also help to cover the anterior portion of the knee and stabilize the patella. The entire knee joint is surrounded by a synovial membrane that is one of the most extensive and complex in the human body (Fig. 21–3).

Medial Compartment

The medial compartment of the knee is supported by the extensor retinaculum and the muscles of the thigh. The pes anserinus group, composed of the sartorius, gracilis, and semitendinosus muscles (Fig. 21–4), crosses the pos-

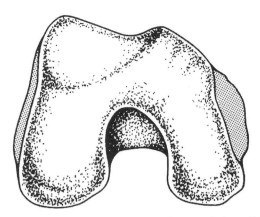

Figure 21-1. Distal end of femur with expanded medial and lateral condyles.

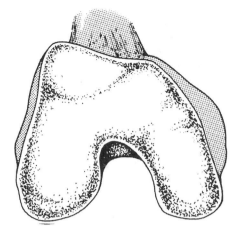

Figure 21-2. Distal end of femur showing patellar groove and anterior condylar surface.

teromedial aspect of the joint and attaches to the anteromedial part of the tibia at the level of the tibial tubercle. The adductor magnus muscle attaches to the medial femoral condyle at the adductor tubercle. The most important of these stabilizers is the semimembranosus muscle, which has five components; the principal component is attached to the tubercle on the posterior aspect of the medial tibial condyle. The semimembranosus is an important medial stabilizer of the knee; fibers from the other four slips of

this muscle support the posterior capsule and posterior medial capsule and also attach to the medial meniscus to pull it posteriorly from the joint as the knee flexes[5] (Fig. 21-5).

The C-shaped medial meniscus has an intimate attachment to the capsular ligament along its periphery. The capsular ligaments are divided into meniscofemoral and meniscotibial components.[6] The medial capsular liga-

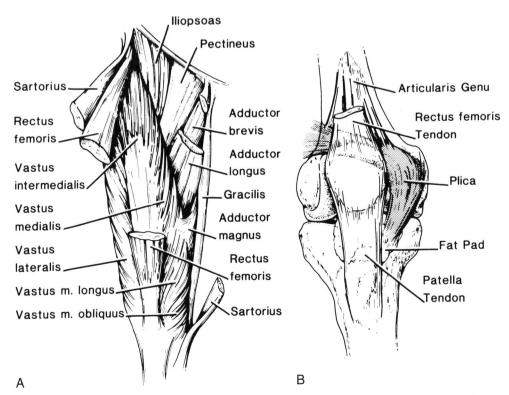

Figure 21-3. (A) Muscles of the extensor mechanism; (B) patellar tendon (ligament) and articularis genu muscle.

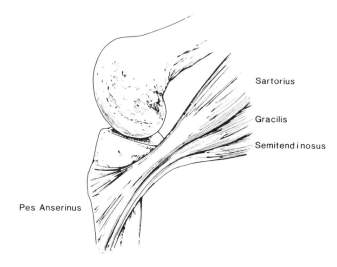

Figure 21–4. Muscles of the pes anserinus group, medial aspect of the knee.

ments can be further divided into anterior, middle, and posterior thirds (Fig. 21–6). The posterior third is often referred to as the *posterior oblique ligament* and is important in controlling anteromedial rotatory instability.[7] Lying superficial to these ligaments is the tibial collateral ligament. It originates at the medial condyle of the femur, medially below the adductor tubercle, and attaches distally to the medial condyle on the medial surface of the shaft of the tibia below the pes anserinus group.

The posterior cruciate ligament is also included in the medial compartment. It has often been referred to as the key to the stability of the knee.[8] It is attached to the posterior intercondylar area of the tibia and to the posterior extremity of the lateral meniscus, passing upward, forward, and medially as a broad band to attach to the lateral surface of the medial condyle of the femur.

The ligament is composed of the main posterolateral band and a smaller anteromedial band. Tension within each band varies as the knee moves from flexion to extension (Fig. 21–7).

Lateral Compartment

The structures of the lateral compartment of the knee are somewhat similar to those of the medial compartment. Muscular support for lateral structures is provided by the tensor fasciae latae, which can be separated into two functional components: the iliopatellar band and the iliotibial tract.[9] These structures attach anterolaterally to Gerdy's tubercle on the lateral aspect of the tibia (Fig. 21–8). Also providing support for the lateral side are the two heads of the biceps femoris. The long head and the

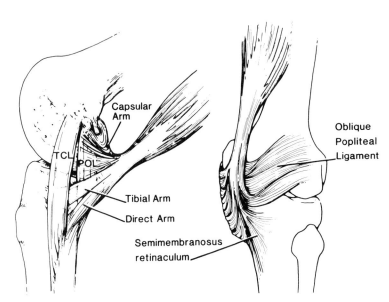

Figure 21–5. The five components of the semimembranosus muscle. TCL, tibial collateral ligament; POL, posterior oblique ligament.

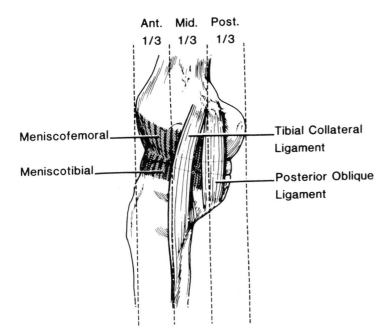

Ant. Mid. Post.
1/3   1/3   1/3

Meniscofemoral

Meniscotibial

Tibial Collateral
Ligament

Posterior Oblique
Ligament

Figure 21–6. Divisions of the medial capsular ligaments.

short head form a common tendon (lateral hamstring), which splits around the fibular collateral ligament and attaches to the head of the fibula.

The triangular and flat popliteus muscle forms the deep floor of the lower part of the popliteal fossa (Fig. 21–9). The larger part of the fossa arises on the lateral condyle of the femur and helps support the fibrous lateral capsule adjacent to the lateral meniscus. The popliteus muscle inserts in the posteromedial edge of the tibia and serves to reinforce the posterior third of the lateral capsu-

lar ligament. The fibular collateral ligament appears on the lateral aspect of the knee as a large rounded cord, which is attached to the lateral epicondyle of the femur and below to the head of the fibula; it has no attachment to the lateral meniscus (Fig. 21–10).

The lateral capsular ligaments attach to the lateral meniscus in much the same way that the medial capsular ligaments attach to the medial meniscus. The lateral capsular ligaments can also be divided into meniscofemoral and meniscotibial sections. These can be further subdi-

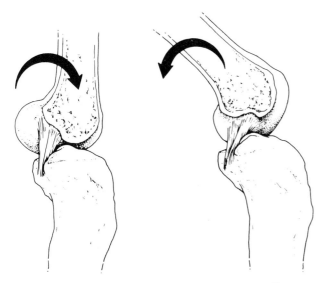

Figure 21–7. Attachment of the posterior cruciate ligament. The different bundles change in tension as the knee moves from extension to flexion.

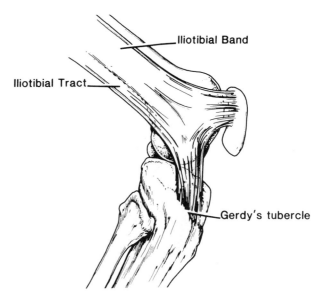

Iliotibial Band

Iliotibial Tract

Gerdy's tubercle

Figure 21–8. Iliotibial band and iliotibial tract and their attachment to Gerdy's tubercle.

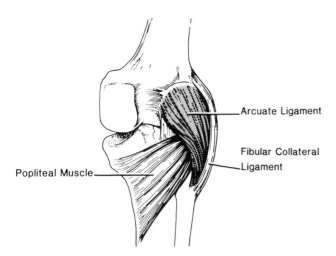

Figure 21-9. The popliteus muscle forms the deep floor of the popliteal fossa.

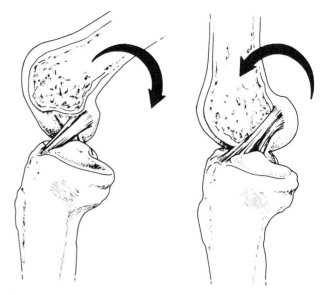

Figure 21-11. The attachments of the anterior cruciate ligament. The bundles change in tension as the knee moves from flexion to extension.

vided into anterior, medial, and posterior thirds. The middle third of the lateral capsular ligament provides support against anterior lateral rotatory instability. The posterolateral third of the lateral compartment is also supported by the arcuate ligament. The arcuate ligament consists of a Y-shaped system of capsular fibers, the stem of which is attached to the head of the fibula. The two branches of the upper portion extend medially to the posterior border of the intercondylar area of the tibia and anteriorly to the lateral epicondyle of the femur (Figs. 21-9 and 21-10). Collectively, the posterior third of the lateral capsular ligament, the fibular collateral ligament, the arcuate ligament, and the aponeurosis of the popliteus muscle are known as the *arcuate complex.* The arcuate complex provides lateral support for the knee joint.

The anterior cruciate ligament is also included in the lateral compartment. It consists of an anteromedial bundle, an intermediate bundle, and a posterolateral bundle. The anteromedial bundle originates on the posterior superior medial surface of the lateral femoral condyle and inserts on the medial aspect of the intercondylar eminence of the tibia. The posterolateral bundle lies more anterior and distal to the anteromedial bundle on the medial surface of the lateral femoral condyle and inserts laterally to the midline of the intercondylar eminence. The intermediate bundle lies between these two bundles. Tension on these bundles is altered as the knee moves from flexion to extension (Figs. 21-11, 21-12).

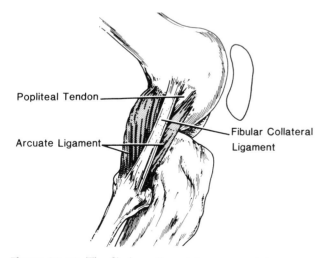

Figure 21-10. The fibular collateral ligament and the arcuate ligament. Components of the arcuate complex.

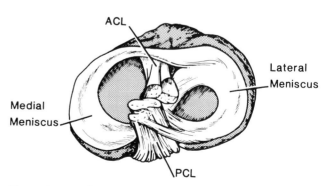

Figure 21-12. Cross-sectional view of the knee joint showing the medial and lateral menisci and bundles of the anterior and posterior cruciate ligaments. ACL, anterior cruciate ligaments; PCL, posterior cruciate ligament.

■ Evaluation of the Acutely Injured Knee

Evaluation of an acutely injured knee should be completed as soon as possible after injury.[8,10,11] A detailed history and description of the mechanism of injury are vital components of the initial evaluation. It is also very important to complete the evaluation before muscle spasm begins to determine accurately the extent of damage to the knee.

Pain parameters—the existence of pain, the onset of pain, and whether the patient can walk without pain—are good indicators of the extent of injury. Another important indicator is the extent of fluid accumulation in the joint. Fluid accumulation within 2 hours of injury indicates the possibility of a hemarthrosis, which could result from an anterior cruciate ligament tear, an osteochondral fracture, a peripheral meniscus tear, or an incomplete ligament sprain. Fluid accumulation that occurs 24 hours after injury is usually a synovial fluid buildup, which is indicative of meniscal tear, a tear of the capsular lining of the knee joint, or a subluxated fat pad. With a major tear of knee tissues, there is no fluid accumulation; instead, the fluid extravasates into the soft tissues. This is usually associated with extensive capsular tears or tears of the poste-

rior cruciate ligament. Palpation of the knee for areas of tenderness or local edema may help to isolate the site of injury. It is always important to establish pulses and the status of sensation around the joint because surrounding neurovascular structures may be damaged in any knee injury.

Diagnostic Tests

Once the history and mechanism of injury have been determined, along with the neurovascular status, several special tests should be performed to complete the examination (Table 21–1). All tests should be performed on the normal knee first. This helps to establish a baseline of stability in a normal joint and helps to gain the patient's confidence and promote relaxation. The patient should be positioned comfortably supine on the examining table, head down on a pillow and hands relaxed.

Abduction Stress Test

The extremity is slightly abducted at the hip and extended so that the thigh is resting on the surface of the examination table. The knee should be flexed to 30 degrees over the side of the table, with one of the examiner's hands

□ □ □ □ □ □ □   □

Table 21–1. Diagnostic Tests for Knee Instabilities

Instability	Tear	Test
Straight medial	Medial compartment and posterior cruciate ligament	Abduction stress in full extension
Straight lateral	Lateral compartment and posterior cruciate ligament	Adduction stress in full extension
Straight posterior	Posterior cruciate ligament, posterior oblique, arcuate complex	Posterior drawer
Straight anterior	Posterior cruciate ligament	Anterior drawer
AMRI	Medial compartment, posterior oblique, anterior cruciate ligament	Abduction stress test at 30 degrees, anterior drawer with external rotation
ALRI	Middle third lateral capsular, anterior cruciate ligament	Anterior drawer in neutral, adduction stress test at 30 degrees (may be normal or only mildly positive)
PLRI	Arcuate complex	Adduction stress test at 30 degrees, external rotation recurvatum test
Combined ALRI/PLRI	All lateral compartments (with or without iliotibial band)	Anterior and posterior drawer tests in neutral
Combined ALRI/AMRI	Medial and lateral capsular ligaments	Anterior drawer in neutral, abduction/adduction stress tests at 0 degrees, jerk test
Combined ALRI/AMRI/PLRI	Both medial and lateral capsular ligaments	Anterior drawer in neutral, posterior drawer, abduction/adduction stress test at 30 degrees

Abbreviations: AMRI, anteromedial rotatory instability; ALRI, anterolateral rotatory instability; PLRI, posterolateral rotatory instability.

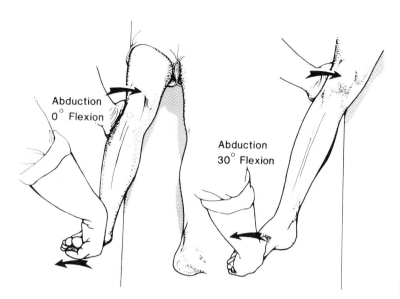

Figure 21–13. Abduction stress test.

placed on the lateral aspect of the knee while the other hand grasps the foot. A gentle abduction stress is applied to the knee while the examiner's hand on the foot provides gentle external rotation. By repeating this test in a consistent manner, the examiner can gradually increase the stress up to the point of pain and maximum laxity without producing a muscle spasm. The injured and uninjured knees are compared. The abduction stress test is always performed with each knee in full extension and in 30 degrees of flexion (Fig. 21–13).

A positive abduction stress test at full extension indicates injury to the posterior cruciate ligament and medial compartment; therefore, a rotatory instability cannot be classified. A negative test at full extension but a positive test at 30 degrees of flexion indicates a tear of the liga-

ments of the medial compartment, and a diagnosis of anteromedial rotatory instability can be made.

Adduction Stress Test

By simply changing hands, moving the hand to the medial aspect of the knee, and applying an adduction force at both 30 degrees and full extension, the examiner can perform the adduction stress test. A positive adduction stress test at 30 degrees indicates anterolateral rotatory instability (Fig. 21–14).

Anterior Drawer Test

In the anterior drawer test, the patient's actively raising his or her head produces hamstring tightening, which

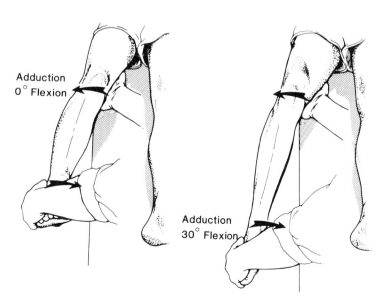

Figure 21–14. Adduction stress test.

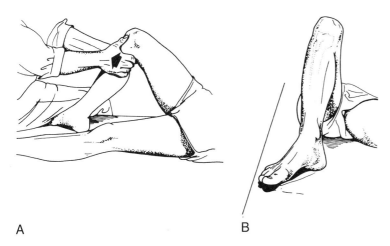

A   B

Figure 21–15. (A) Anterior drawer test with tibia in external rotation; (B) position of the lower extremity for anterior drawer test with tibia in external rotation.

can alter the results of the test. The lower extremity should be flexed at the hip to 45 degrees and the knee flexed to 80 or 90 degrees with the foot flat on the table. The examiner sits on the table, positioning his or her buttocks on the dorsum of the foot to fix it firmly. The examiner's hands are placed about the upper part of the tibia, with the forefingers positioned to palpate the hamstrings to ensure that they are relaxed. The thumbs are positioned at the anterior joint line both medially and laterally. The examiner provides a gentle pull repeatedly in an anterior direction. This test should be performed first with the foot and leg externally rotated beyond the neutral position (Fig. 21–15), then internally rotated as much as possible (Fig. 21–16), and finally in the neutral position (Fig. 21–17). Each lower extremity is tested, and results are compared.

A positive anterior drawer test with the foot in external rotation indicates anteromedial rotatory instability; with the foot in the neutral position, a positive test indi-

cates anterolateral rotatory instability; and with the foot in internal rotation, it indicates a posterior cruciate tear.

Posterior Drawer Test

In the posterior drawer test, the hip is flexed to 45 degrees, the knee is flexed to 90 degrees, and the foot is placed flat on the table. Again, the examiner sits on the dorsum of the foot to fix it firmly. The hands are positioned so that the middle fingers can palpate the hamstrings; the thumbs are placed along the tibia at the joint line. The examiner pushes straight back gently. Movement of the tibia on the femur is noted with a positive posterior drawer test (Fig. 21–18). A positive posterior drawer sign can often be misinterpreted as a positive anterior drawer sign. For additional clarification of the posterior instability test, a gravity test may be helpful. With the patient supine and the knees together and flexed to approximately 80 degrees and the feet planted together

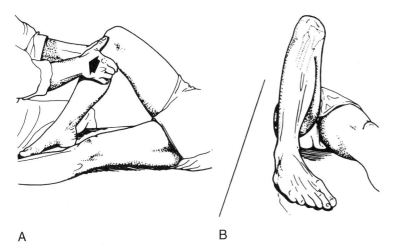

A   B

Figure 21–16. (A) Anterior drawer test with tibia in internal rotation; (B) position of lower extremity for anterior drawer test with tibia in internal rotation.

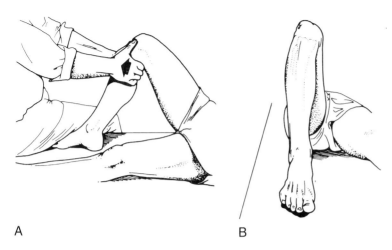

A   B

Figure 21–17. (A) Anterior drawer test with tibia in neutral position; (B) position of lower extremity for anterior drawer test with tibia in neutral position.

on the table, posterior displacement of the tibial tuberosity can be seen when viewed from the side (Fig. 21–19A). Another gravity test that may be helpful is the external rotation recurvatum test.[12] The patient's extended legs are lifted together by the toes, and an increase in recurvatum is noted in a positive test (Fig. 21–19B).

Jerk Test

The examiner supports the lower extremity and flexes the hip to about 45 degrees and the knee to 90 degrees while at the same time internally rotating the tibia. If the right knee is being examined, the foot should be in the examiner's right hand, internally rotating the tibia, while the left hand is placed over the proximal end of the tibia and fibula. The left hand is used to exert a valgus stress. The knee is gradually extended, maintaining the internal rotation and valgus stress. With a positive jerk test, a subluxation of the lateral femoral condyle on the tibia occurs at about 20 degrees of flexion. With further extension, a spontaneous relocation occurs. This relocation is described in engineering terms as a *jerk*, a sudden change in the rate of acceleration between surfaces. In this case, it is the change in the velocity of the tibia in relation to the femur (Fig. 21–20). A positive jerk test indicates anterolateral rotatory instability.

Anterior Drawer-in-Extension Test (Lachman-Ritchey)

The anterior drawer-in-extension test is performed with the patient's knee in approximately 20 degrees of flexion.

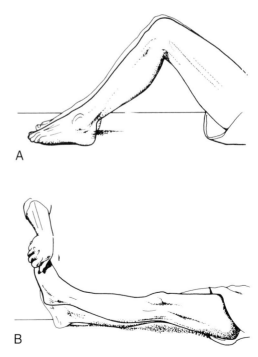

A

B

Figure 21–19. (A) Gravity test for posterolateral instability; (B) external rotation recurvatum test.

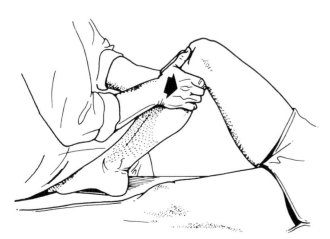

Figure 21–18. Posterior drawer test for posterolateral instability.

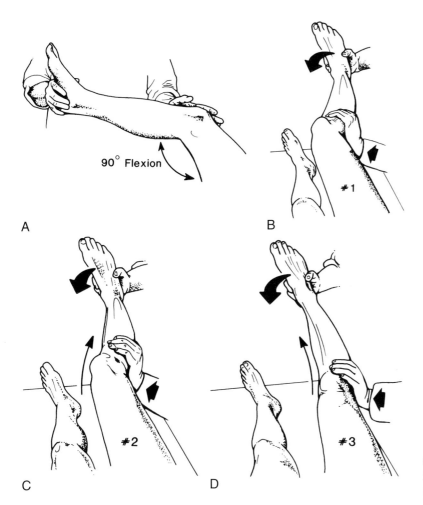

Figure 21–20. (A) Starting position for performing the jerk test; (B,C) jerk test sequence; (D) end position of jerk test.

The examiner uses one hand to stabilize the femur by grasping the distal thigh just proximal to the patella. With the other hand, the examiner grasps the tibia distal to the tibial tubercle. Firm pressure is applied to the posterior aspect of the tibia in an effort to produce anterior subluxation (Fig. 21–21). This test is one of the most sensitive methods of diagnosing anterior cruciate ligament injury.

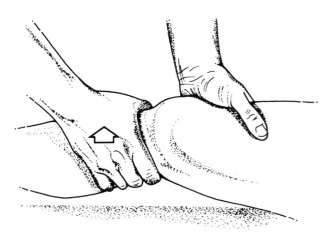

Figure 21–21. Anterior drawer in extension test.

■ Classification of Instability

Given the clinical findings of the tests just described and using the system of classification of knee ligament instabilities of Hughston et al.,[8,13] knee ligament instabilities can be classified as either straight (nonrotatory) or rotatory. Rotatory instabilities may be further subclassified as simple or combined.

Straight Instability

There are four types of instability that involve no rotation of the tibia on the femur. They are as follows:

1. Medial instability: a tear in the medial compartment ligaments with an associated tear of the posterior cruciate ligament. It is demonstrated by a positive abduction stress test with the knee in full extension.
2. Lateral instability: a tear in the lateral compartment ligaments and the posterior cruciate ligament. This is demonstrated by a positive adduction stress test with the knee in full extension.
3. Posterior instability: a tear in the posterior cruciate ligament and laxity in both the posterior oblique ligament and the arcuate complex. This is demon-

strated by a positive posterior drawer test in which both tibial condyles subluxate posteriorly by an equal amount with no rotation.

4. Anterior instability: a torn anterior cruciate ligament, torn medial and lateral capsular ligaments, and a torn posterior cruciate ligament. This is demonstrated by a positive anterior drawer sign in which both tibial condyles subluxate anteriorly by an equal amount with no rotation.

Simple Rotatory Instability

There are three types of simple rotatory instability. Each demonstrates a rotatory component of the tibia on the femur involving either the medial or the lateral tibial condyle.

1. Anteromedial rotatory instability: a tear of the medial compartment ligaments including the posterior oblique and/or the middle third of the medial capsular ligament. The anterior cruciate ligament may or may not be torn. The abduction stress test at 30 degrees of flexion is positive, as is the anterior drawer test with the tibia externally rotated.
2. Anterolateral rotatory instability: a tear of the middle third of the lateral capsular ligament and possibly the anterior cruciate ligament. It is demonstrated by a positive jerk test and a positive anterior drawer test with the tibia in the neutral position. The adduction stress test with the knee at 30 degrees of flexion may be normal or only mildly positive. The Lachman test is positive.
3. Posterolateral rotatory instability: a tear of the arcuate complex. The adduction stress test at 30 degrees of knee flexion is positive.

Combined Rotatory Instabilities

Three types of combined rotatory instability have been described.

1. Combined anterolateral and posterolateral instability: a tear of the lateral compartment capsular ligaments, which may or may not include a tear of the iliotibial band. The posterior cruciate ligament remains intact. The posterior drawer test, with the tibia in neutral position, shows that the lateral tibial plateau rotates forward and backward as stress is applied. An adduction stress test with the knee in full extension is positive. What seems to be a straight lateral opening is actually external rotation and posterolateral subluxation with a varus displacement of the knee. An adduction stress test with the knee at 30 degrees of flexion is only mildly positive because of migration of the iliotibial band posteriorly during flexion.
2. Combined anterolateral and anteromedial rotatory instabilities: tears of the medial and lateral capsular

ligaments in the middle third. The posterior cruciate ligament remains intact. The anterior drawer test with the tibia in the neutral position is positive, with both tibial condyles subluxating anteriorly. The anterior drawer test is also positive when performed with the tibia externally rotated. Both abduction and adduction stress tests are positive, although they may be only mildly so. The jerk test is also positive.

3. Combined posterolateral, anterolateral, and anteromedial rotatory instability: tears of the lateral capsular ligament, anterior cruciate ligament, arcuate complex, and medial capsular ligaments. In a knee with these lesions, anterior drawer tests with the tibia in the neutral position and in external rotation are positive. A posterolateral drawer test is positive and causes the tibia to rotate externally and backward. Adduction and abduction stress tests are positive with the knee at 30 degrees of flexion but negative with it at full extension. The jerk test is also positive.

■ Surgical Intervention for Rotatory Instabilities

Surgical treatment of rotatory instability should always be directed toward restoring the normal anatomy by correcting the pathologic anatomy. There are far too many surgical procedures to attempt to review them in this work. Understanding surgical procedures and surgical philosophy provides a starting point for restoring normal function through an effective rehabilitation program in the knee-injured patient.[14]

Basic surgical philosophy mandates the repair of acutely torn structures.[15,16] This may include a direct repair of the anterior cruciate ligament itself or a repair with augmentation. Acute repair of capsular ligaments may also be performed. In chronic situations, extra-articular reconstruction using capsular reefings, tendon transfers, and tenodesis as well as anterior cruciate intra-articular grafts is necessary. These materials may be composed of autografts (the body's own tissue, e.g., the patellar or semitendinosus tendon) or allografts (tissue from cadaver sources).

■ Rehabilitation for Knees with Rotatory Instability

With the refinement of diagnostic skills and the addition of complex new surgical techniques, the rehabilitation of knee injuries has become more complex. Rehabilitation programs should always be based on sound biomechanical principles and directed toward restoring a functionally stable knee that will meet the demands of the patient's sport or activity. Proper strength, flexibility, endurance, proprioception, agility, skill, and speed should be combined in an exercise program to meet this goal.[17,18] Maintenance of strength in the uninjured leg and upper extremity should also be included in any rehabilitation program.[19]

Paulos et al.[20,21] state two principles of rehabilitation: First, the effects of immobility must be minimized; second, healing tissues must never be overloaded. Immobility of a joint can lead to contracture, histochemical changes, and a decrease in ligamentous strength. Joint contracture is manifested mechanically in the amount of torque required to move the knee joint. The torque may have to be increased 10 times over the force normally required to move the joint. The ligament–bone complex also reacts to immobility. Not only is the ligament itself weakened, but its bony attachment has been found to be weakened by as much as 40 percent after only 8 weeks of immobility. Noyes and colleagues,[22] found that after 8 weeks of immobization, the joint required reconditioning for at least 1 year before 90 percent of its strength returned. Histochemically, selective atrophy of type I fibers, which are slow-twitch or red muscle fibers, has been shown to decrease total muscle mass by as much as 30 to 47 percent with immobilization.

The second principle concerns protecting the healing tissues from excessive overload. In the early phases of rehabilitation, healing tissues should be protected from abnormal joint displacement, such as twisting or falling on the knee. The second form of common mechanical failure is caused by subjecting the healing tissues to cyclic forces. This causes a fatigue-like failure. A third form of overload is induced by stretching the healing tissues past their elastic limit. Proper surgical technique is probably the most important means of preventing this type of ligamentous failure. However, high forces over an extended period of time can produce this type of failure; for example, when extending the knee rapidly from 30 degrees to full extension with high resistance, an anterior drawer effect creates a strain on the anterior cruciate ligament and weakens the repair if sufficient healing has not occurred. For this reason, it is vitally important to consider the surgical procedure used along with the other variables when formulating the rehabilitation program.

The patient who has just undergone an intra-articular anterior cruciate ligament reconstruction is placed in a splint in *full* extension for several days until quadriceps control is obtained and then no brace is used. Electrical stimulation may aid the patient in gaining quadriceps control. Ambulation is weightbearing as tolerated with crutches. At post-operative day 1 (POD1) flexion, range of motion (ROM) is begun and passive extension is emphasized to gain full extension (for that patient) as soon as possible. Quad sets, terminal knee extensions, straight leg raises, hip flexion, hip abduction, and hamstring curls with light resistance (0 to 5 lb) can be started as soon as possible. As noted earlier, the patient should be protected from overload of the healing structure. A slow progression is essential to produce a good end result with an intra-articular procedure. Therapeutic swimming may begin as

soon as the stitches are out. The patient may gradually increase weightbearing and wean him- or herself off the crutches over a period of several weeks. Stationary bicycling may begin as soon as tolerated.

Once the patient has worked off his or her crutches (3 to 6 weeks), closed-chain activities such as step-ups, mini-squats, and rubber tubing squats can begin. Leg press activities can also be started. By 12 weeks status postoperative (SPO), the patient is working up to 10 lb on straight leg raises, riding a bike for 30 minutes daily, walking 2 miles, and handling the closed-chain activities well. Isokinetic testing may be performed now. Isokinetic workouts at low intensity may start as soon as the patella femoral joint has calmed down, as well as mild running and other closed-chain activities. Once aggressive functional exercises are started, the patient may be placed in a functional brace.

The patient who has undergone an extra-articular reconstruction with iliotibial tract tenodesis may be in a cast for approximately 6 weeks. He or she is encouraged to do quadriceps setting and active-assisted straight leg raises. Hamstring contraction and ankle pumps are begun as tolerated. Gait is nonweightbearing.

Some patients are placed in a hinged immobilizer after extra-articular repair. Motion in the hinged immobilizer is limited to 40 to 70 degrees for the first 3 weeks. After 3 weeks, the flexion stop is eliminated, and the patient is allowed to gain as much flexion as possible. At 6 weeks, with the patient still non-weightbearing, active-assisted flexion ROM exercises are begun in an attempt to reach full flexion. The patient is encouraged to continue to work on quadriceps setting with the addition of hamstring curls and hip flexion strengthening exercises. The patient will actively work toward full extension with terminal knee extension and straight leg raise exercises in the period from 6 weeks to 12 weeks after surgery.

Twelve weeks after surgery, the patient gradually progresses from partial weightbearing to full weightbearing as tolerated. At full weightbearing, he or she is allowed to progress to advanced activities such as side step-ups and leg presses. The patient should use a toe-heel gait to encourage extension of the knee, but once full extension is reached, normal heel-toe gait is resumed. Bicycling and swimming may also start at this point. At 6 months postsurgery, the patient may begin agility and competitive preparation exercises. These are expected to help the patient progress back to his or her sport activities and should be designed to be the same types of activities the patient will use in his or her sport.

When prosthetic ligaments are used, the biomechanics and healing restraints that normally are a big factor in the postsurgical rehabilitation process are less important. The patient is again placed in a cast brace or a long leg brace, which is locked at 45 degrees for the first 3 days. The patient's gait is non-weightbearing. The patient is allowed to work on exercises out of the brace and work on active extension with straight leg raises, terminal knee extensions, and flexion-to-extension exercises as well as active-assisted flexion. Hamstring strengthening and hip strengthening begin during the first 3 weeks. After 1 week, the cast brace is reset to minus 15 degrees of extension, and partial weightbearing is allowed. At the end of 6 weeks, the brace is returned to full extension. At 12 weeks, the patient is allowed to progress off the crutches but must continue to wear the cast brace until 4 months after surgery. No running is allowed until after muscle strength has returned to 80 percent of normal. Isokinetic testing is again helpful in making this assessment.

For the patient who will return to athletic endeavors, the advanced rehabilitation program should contain functional and specific exercises that will imitate the motions demanded of the patient by his or her sport. Bicycling is a good means of building endurance and aerobic capacities for the patient who will be returning to an active sport. Straight leg raises should be continued until the patient can lift 10 lb. ROM activities should continue until the ROM in the operated leg is close to that of the normal extremity.

Once 10 lb of weight can be lifted with a high number of repetitions, different weight machines can be used to supplement the high repetition-low weight program. Hamstring curl and leg press machines are recommended for increasing the bulk of the leg. When an athlete can walk up and down stairs for 30 minutes, ride a bicycle for an hour, and has 80 percent of his or her quadriceps strength, as measured with isokinetic testing, and when proper healing has taken place, a running program can be initiated. When the patient can run 2 miles with no swelling, pain, or limp, he or she can begin to sprint. Once the athlete can sprint at nearly full speed, different cutting activities can be performed. These cutting activities promote agility and should be similar to the situations that the athlete would encounter in his or her sport.

Proprioception and balance are usually lost after major knee injury and/or surgery. Balancing activities such as standing on one foot with the eyes open and closed and standing on the toes with the eyes open and closed should be included in the advanced rehabilitation process.

One other factor is important in the advanced rehabilitation of the athlete. The athlete has to be psychologically ready to return to play. After any major knee injury and subsequent surgery, the rehabilitation process is never complete until the athlete is confident that he or she can again participate in his or her sport without being reinjured. A well-planned program of exercise with reasonably set goals will help the athlete return to the sport with the confidence needed to participate, without the lingering doubts caused by the previous injury.

The illustrations that follow the case studies (see Figs. 21–22 to 21–38) demonstrate the techniques discussed. As with any exercise program, a great deal depends on communication among the therapist, the surgeon, and the patient. Each must be aware of the biomechanical and healing restraints after an injury, and all must be willing to do their part to produce a good result after an injury.

CASE STUDIES

CASE STUDY 1

The following case study illustrates rehabilitation after reconstruction of the anterior cruciate ligament.

TW is a motorcycle policeman and an avid softball player who plays for several teams during the spring and summer seasons. During a late fall softball game, TW misjudged a fly ball, and as he was trying to change his direction of movement, he cut to the left and felt a pop, followed by a giving-way sensation in his left knee. It was quite uncomfortable, and he left the field limping. He applied ice to his knee, but it swelled immediately. Although he could still walk on it, he exhibited a severe limp.

He visited his orthopaedist the next day. With the examination and his history of cutting, the popping sound, the giving way, and the immediate swelling, it was obvious that he had torn his anterior cruciate ligament. He was diagnosed with an anterior lateral rotatory instability. Given the options that he could follow for the care of his knee, TW elected to have surgical correction of his problem. It was clear that he wanted to maintain an active lifestyle and was going to continue playing amateur sports in the future.

TW was then started on a conservative program of quadriceps sets, terminal knee extensions, straight leg raises, hamstring curls, and stationary biking as soon as he was comfortable. He was on crutches and partial weightbearing and elected not to use any type of immobilizer. He continued to use ice, compression, and elevation for his leg. In 1 week, his orthopaedist was able to complete a better examination because much of the swelling of the knee was gone. He was found to have a 2+ pivot shift, positive anterior drawer in extension, and 2+ anterior drawer at 90 degrees. The surgeon thought that the inflammatory process should calm down a bit before patella tendon graft surgery was performed. Six weeks after the injury, TW underwent patella tendon graft endoscopically performed anterior cruciate ligament surgery. His menisci were found to be in good shape at the time of surgery.

A straight immobilizer was used postoperatively and a point was made to ensure that the immobilizer was in an extremely straight position. Ice and elevation were used initially. On postoperative day 1, the patient was up on crutches, in a chair, and working diligently on ankle pumps to decrease the chance of phlebitis. Quadriceps setting exercises were begun to decrease swelling and maintain quadriceps tone. On postoperative day 2, the patient ambulated with partial weighbearing to the physical therapy department, where passive extension without immobilizer was begun with the heel propped up on pillows. Terminal knee extensions with electrical stimulation, hamstring stretching, and active-assisted flexion were also performed.

TW lived locally and was discharged late on postoperative day 3, leaving the hospital with 0 degrees of extension, 10 degrees of active extension, and 90 degrees of active-assisted flexion. He continued to work hard on a home exercise program as instructed by the hospital's physical therapist.

At postoperative week 2, TW continued his passive extension stretching many times throughout the day. Aggressive knee flexion, terminal knee extension, straight leg raises, hip abductors, hip flexors, and hamstring curls were performed, five sets of 10 twice a day to three times a day, working gradually up to 5 lb. Stationary bicycle exercise was started a couple of days later. Weightbearing was to tolerance, and the straight immobilizer was discarded at the 2-week mark because his quadriceps control was excellent.

At 1 month, crutches were discarded, as TW had good control of his quadriceps. ROM was 0 to 130 degrees. There was very little swelling about the knee and no limp when walking. He continued with his earlier exercises but began gentle closed-chain activities. These were performed using horizontal leg press machine, the Shuttle 2000, and rubber tubing mini-squats. Step-ups were added at the 6-week mark, and by 8 weeks he began mini-trampoline running and slide board activities. Isokinetic activities at mild to moderate intensity were begun at a variety of speeds.

At the 3-month mark, TW had a 20 to 25 percent deficit in his quadriceps when the two legs were compared, as shown with isokinetic testing. He was allowed to begin a month-long progressive running program, step-ups, and all activities in the weight room except heavy flexion-to-extension. He did work at heavier intensity in the 90 to 45 degree ROM. His patellofemoral joint was monitored closely. By the 4-month mark, he was performing these exercises quite aggressively. At 5 months, he began agility training, including figure-eight runs, hopping on one foot, and general plyometric jumping.

At 6 months, his isokinetic test showed equality between the two quadriceps. He was running, cutting with no problems, and was fitted with an anterior cruciate ligament brace to allow for his softball activities.

One-year postoperatively, the patient was having no problems whatsoever. ROM was 0 to 140 degrees.

CASE STUDY 2

The following case study illustrates rehabilitation after a surgical repair of a posterior lateral rotatory instability (PLRI).

SK is a 17-year-old defensive end on his high school football team. He is 6 ft 4 in. tall and weighs 265 lb.

During a first-round playoff game, SK sustained a non-contact posterior lateral injury to his knee. On the field he felt diffuse severe pain that did not allow full extension or flexion of the knee.

After being transported from the field, SK was thoroughly examined. There was little to no swelling, a positive anterior drawer-in-extension test, and adduction stress at 30 degrees. A compressive wrap was applied, and he was fitted with a hinged knee immobilizer locked at 45 degrees of flexion and allowed to ambulate without weightbearing with crutches.

SK was seen in the clinic by his orthopaedist the following morning. With his history and presentation, it was confirmed that SK has sustained a posterolateral injury that would require surgery to return him to function and sports. The following tests were positive during his physical exam: the reverse pivot shift test and the posterior drawer with external rotation test. Magnetic resonance imaging confirmed the results of the physical exam and also revealed no injury to the meniscus. SK's surgery was scheduled within 1 week of the initial injury.

During surgery the following damaged tissues were repaired: biceps femoris long and short heads, deep and capsulo-osseous layer of the iliotibial tract, arcuate ligament, head of the lateral gastrocnemius, and fibular collateral. Postoperatively, SK was placed in a hinged knee brace at 45 degrees with a pelvic band attached to prevent external rotation. Due to his postoperative positioning, SK was started on ankle pumps to aid in the prevention of phlebitis, and he was educated on the importance of maintaining neutral rotation of the femur with no external rotation.

On postoperative day 1, the precautions of femoral rotation were reviewed. SK was instructed in submaximal quad sets in the brace with the brace locked at 45 degrees. He was instructed in and practiced proper transfer techniques and gait mechanics on all surfaces and stairs with crutches without weightbearing. These activities were performed twice a day to develop proper lower extremity control.

On postoperative day 2, the dressing was changed to evaluate the wound. The wound consisted of a lateral "hockey stick" incision that was approximated with a subcutaneous stitch with surface closure using surgical staples. The wound was then redressed with 4/4's, secured with a white elastic wrap, and placed back in the brace. SK was then prepared for discharge from the hospital.

SK was scheduled for outpatient follow-up physical therapy during postoperative week 2. At this time, SK was instructed in the following exercises: active-assisted flexion, active extension over a bolster, quad sets and leg raises over a bolster, and pool activities to strengthen the hip. Extension was gained actively at a rate of 5–10 degrees per week, and the brace had to be adjusted accordingly. No hamstring stretches or passive extension were performed. Secondary to SK's strong quads, he was cautioned not to force extension and was reminded to gain extension of only 5–10 degrees per week to protect the repair.

The goals at this time were to gain ROM and increase quad strength for lower extremity control. During postoperative weeks 5–9, SK finally began to see major improvement. He was progressed to ambulation with crutches, with weightbearing as tolerated. The aim of weightbearing ambulation is to achieve full extension and lower extremity control through functional exercise. Closed-chain kinetic exercises such as hip shuttle, wall slides, and single leg stance were introduced. Use of the stationary bike was also initiated, with close attention to seat height. If the seat is too high, it can cause the patient to have an extension moment that is too forceful at the terminal end of the downstroke. This could stress the ACL repair. Aquatic therapy was continued.

On postoperative weeks 10–15, SK progressed to ambulation with one crutch and quickly advanced to no crutches for ambulation, with weightbearing as tolerated. The previous exercise program continued, and more function-oriented exercises were added. The single leg stance on firm and soft surfaces with perturbations for proprioceptive training was essential. Ankle strengthening with standing calf raises and posterior tibialis strengthening was added. Closed-chain kinetic exercises were also advanced to include the mini-trampoline, the stair climber, and elastic cord exercise backward and forward. Even though SK was advancing at the expected rate, constant counseling was provided to remind him of the final goals and of the need not to advance independently.

Postoperative months 5–7 began with careful assessment of strength, ROM, and functional testing. The functional test used in this case was the triple cross over hop test. SK was found to have full active ROM, 5/5 strength with the manual muscle test, and absolutely no pain or swelling. Once functional criteria had been established, more intense weight room activities were performed and a walking/jogging/running program was added. When SK's tolerance was established, functional and task (sport-specific and position-specific—in this case, defensive end-specific) training was also added.

On postoperative month 9, SK was prepared to return to full functional activities with the following presentation: 0/0/135 active ROM, within 95 percent of that on the contralateral side on his isokinetic test, and less than ¼ in. quad girth measurement difference when compared to the contralateral side. SK returned to two-a-day practice football camp that following summer without brace support and continued the season without limitations due to his injury.

Quadriceps Setting Exercise

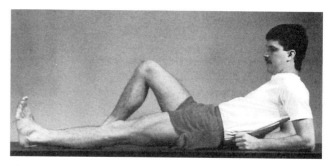

Figure 21–22. Quadriceps setting exercise. An isometric contraction of the quadriceps muscle. The leg should be straightened as much as possible, and the patella should track proximally. The patient should hold the contraction for at least five counts and perform about 50 times per hour.

Straight Leg Raise

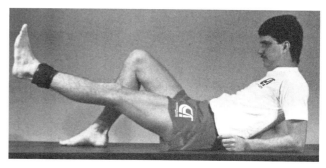

Figure 21–23. Straight leg raise. The patient is positioned supine, with the opposite leg flexed to 90 degrees and the foot planted flat next to the involved knee. The quadriceps muscle is contracted and the leg lifted to approximately 45 degrees and no higher than the thigh of the opposite leg. The leg is held there for at lease five counts and is then slowly lowered to the floor; relax for at lease two counts and repeat this exercise. Then sets of 10 lifts are completed, with a 1-minute rest between each set of 10. Straight leg raises are performed three times a day. Once the patient can complete 10 sets of 10, three times a day, ankle weights are added for resistance. Begin with a 1-lb weight and progress slowly to 5 lb, still maintaining 10 sets of 10 lifts. Weights are increased according to the patient's tolerance.

Terminal Knee Extension

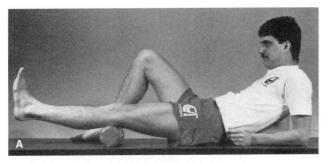

Figure 21–24. Terminal knee extension. (A) A support is placed beneath the knee to be exercised. The quadriceps muscle is again contracted, and the heel is lifted from the floor in a short arc range of motion. Five sets of 10 of this exercise are completed three times a day. (B) Resistance can be added as tolerated. The terminal knee extension can be incorporated with the straight leg raise to assist in bringing the knee out to full extension.

Hamstring Stretching

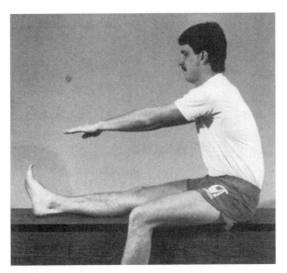

Figure 21–25. Hamstring stretching. The patient is in a sitting position, with one leg off the exercise table. The back is straight, and the leg to be stretched is straight. The patient reached forward slowly and holds for a count of 10. At least 5 minutes of stretching is performed three times a day. The patient should be cautioned not to bounce when stretching.

Hamstring Curls

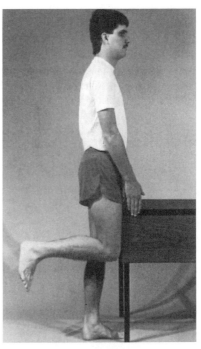

Figure 21–26. Hamstring curls. The patient stands with the thigh pressed against a wall or table to block hip flexion. The knee is flexed to its maximum position and held for a count of five. The foot is then lowered to the floor. Five sets of 10 of this exercise are performed three times a day. Resistance of 1 to 5 lb can be added progressively according to the patient's tolerance.

Active Range of Motion for Flexion

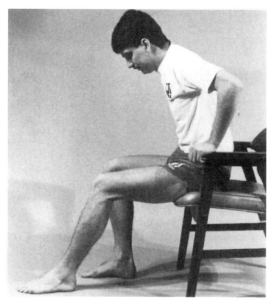

Figure 21–27. Active range of motion for flexion. The patient is seated, with the feet flat on the floor. The injured leg is allowed to slide back actively along the floor, keeping the foot flat on the floor. The foot is planted, and the hips are allowed to slide forward over the affected leg, providing some extra stretch. This exercise may be repeated 30 times three times a day. The stretch is held for at least a count of 10.

Hip Flexion Exercise

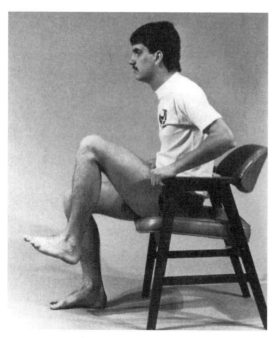

Figure 21–28. Hip flexion exercise. The patient is sitting, with the feet resting on the floor. The knee is lifted toward the chest at a 45 degree angle and held there for a count of five. The knee is lowered gently, and the foot is placed on the floor. Five sets of 10 repetitions of this exercise are performed three times a day, and resistance of 1 to 5 lb can be added at the knee as the patient tolerates it.

Flexion-to-Extension Exercise

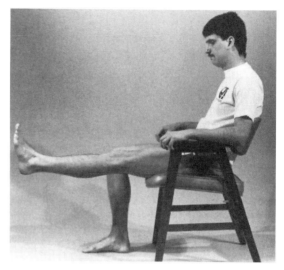

Figure 21–29. Flexion-to-extension exercise. In the starting position the patient sits, with the feet resting on the floor. The knee is then extended and held in as full extension as possible for a count of five and then gently lowered to the floor. This exercise can be repeated up to 10 sets of 10, three times a day. Resistance of 1 to 5 lb can be added as tolerated.

Hip Abduction Exercises

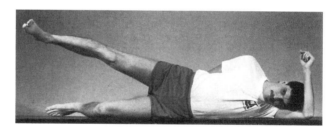

Figure 21–30. Hip abduction exercises. The patient is positioned side-lying, with the unaffected knee flexed at 90 degrees and the hip flexed at 45 degrees. The affected leg is straight, and the body weight is shifted forward. The leg is lifted, held for a count of five, and gently lowered back to the starting position. Resistance of 1 to 5 lb can be added at the ankle. This exercise should be performed in five sets of 10, three times a day.

Adductor Stretching

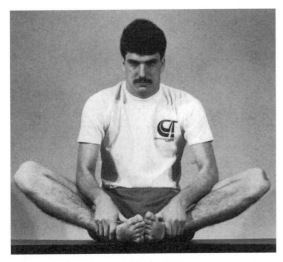

Figure 21–31. Adductor stretching. The patient should sit with the soles of the feet together and slide them back toward the buttocks as far as possible. With the elbows positioned on the leg, the patient pushes down toward the floor and holds for a count of 10. This should be repeated for approximately 5 minutes, three times a day.

Heel Cord Stretching

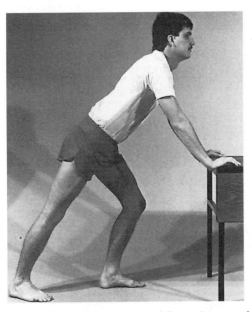

Figure 21–32. Heel cord stretching. The patient stands with the toes slightly pointed in and the heels on the floor. The knees are kept straight. The patient leans forward, stretching the muscles. The stretch should be held for a count of 10 and repeated for 5 minutes, three times a day. The soleus muscle can also be stretched in this position.

Adductor Leg Raise

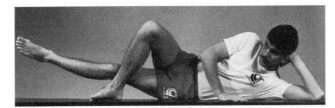

Figure 21–33. Adduction leg raise. The patient is again side-lying, with the affected leg against the table. The leg is lifted into adduction and held for a count of five. This exercise can be repeated in five sets of 10 and resistance of 1 to 5 lb added as tolerated.

Quadriceps Femoris Stretching

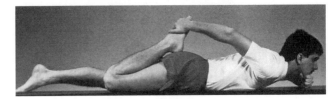

Figure 21–34. Quadriceps femoris stretching. The patient is positioned prone, and the heel is pulled toward the buttocks. The position is held for a count of 10 and then released. The patient should stretch for 5 minutes, three times a day.

Hip Flexor Stretching

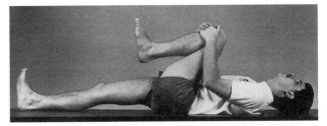

Figure 21–35. Hip flexor stretching. With the patient lying supine, one knee is pulled toward the chest while the opposite leg is held as straight as possible. The patient should hold this stretch for a count of 10 and then release; 5 minutes, three times a day is preferred.

Exercise Bicycling

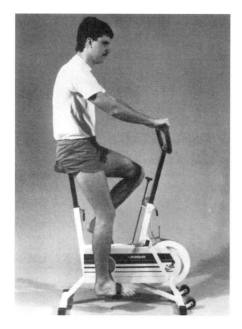

Figure 21–36. Use of the exercise bicycle is a good method to increase endurance, strength, and range of motion for knee-injured patients. The patient should be positioned on the bicycle with a high seat, with about a 15 degree bend in the knee when the foot is at the bottom of the pedal stroke. Toe slips can be used to help exercise both the quadriceps and the hamstring muscles. The patient should progress from 10 minutes at minimum resistance to 1 hour twice a day.

Side Step-up

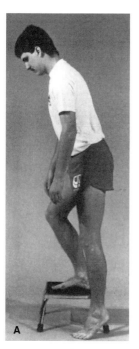
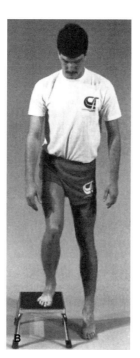

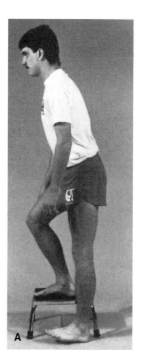
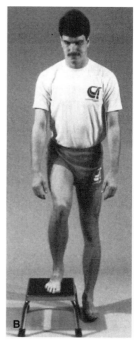

Figure 21–37. Side step-up. The patient should stand sideways, with the involved foot flat on a step. The body weight is lifted with the involved leg. The patient is allowed to push off with the uninvolved foot. Once the patient is able to complete this exercise 100 times once a day, the patient is progressed from a 4-in. step to a 7-in. step.

Figure 21–38. Side step-up. The progression of the side step-up exercise shows the patient again standing, with the involved leg on the step; however, in this exercise, the patient is now allowed to push off the uninvolved foot. The patient must push off with the uninvolved heel touching the floor only. Again, 100 of these exercises, or 10 sets of 10, should be performed once a day.

▪ Acknowledgments

The authors thank Mark Baker, PT (Hughston Sports Medicine Hospital, Columbus, GA), and Sammy Bonfim, SPT (North Georgia College and State University), for their assistance in revising this chapter.

▪ References

1. Blackburn T, Craig E: Knee anatomy: a brief review. Phys Ther 60:1556, 1980
2. Harty M, Joyce J: Surgical anatomy and exposure of the knee joint. p. 206. In AAOS Instructional Course Lectures. Vol. 20. CV Mosby, St. Louis, 1971
3. Kaplan E: Some aspects of functional anatomy of the human knee joint. Clin Orthop 23:18, 1962
4. Williams P, Warwick R (eds): Gray's Anatomy. 36th Ed. Churchill Livingstone, Edinburgh, 1980
5. Brantigan O, Voshell A: The mechanics of the ligaments and menisci of the knee joint. J Bone Joint Surg 23:1, 1941
6. Heller L, Langman J: The meniscofemoral ligaments of the human knee. J Bone Joint Surg 46:2, 1964
7. Hughston J, Eilers A: The role of the posterior oblique ligament in repairs of acute medial collateral ligament tears of the knee. J Bone Joint Surg 55:5, 1973
8. Hughston J, Andrews J, Cross M, et al: Classification of knee ligament instabilities. Part I. The medial compartment and cruciate ligaments. J Bone Joint Surg 58:2, 1976
9. Terry G, Hughston J, Norwood L: The anatomy of the iliopatellar band and iliotibial tract. Am J Sports Med 14:1, 1986
10. Bonnarens F, Drez D: Clinical examination of the knee for anterior cruciate ligament laxity. p. 72. In Jackson D, Drez D (eds): The Anterior Cruciate Deficient Knee. CV Mosby, St. Louis, 1987
11. Hughston J: Acute knee injuries in atheletes. Clin Orthop 23:114, 1962
12. Hughston J, Norwood L: The posterolateral drawer test and external rotational recurvation test for posterolateral rotatory instability of the knee. Clin Orthop 147:82, 1980
13. Hughston J, Andrews J, Cross M, et al: Classifications of knee ligament instabilities. Part II. The lateral compartment. J Bone Joint Surg 58:173, 1976
14. Hughston J: Knee surgery. A philosophy. Phys Ther 60:63, 1980
15. Hughston J, Barrett G: Acute anteromedial rotatory instability: long term results for surgical repair. J Bone Joint Surg 65:2, 1983
16. Hughston J, Bowden J, Andrews J, et al: Acute tears of the posterior cruciate ligament. Results of operative treatment. J Bone Joint Surg 62:438, 1980
17. Blackburn T: Rehabilitation of anterior cruciate ligament injuries. Orthop Clin North Am 16:241, 1985
18. Montgomery J, Steadman J: Rehabilitation of the injured knee. Clin Sports Med 4:333, 1985
19. Malone T, Blackburn T, Wallace L: Knee rehabilitation. Phys Ther 66:54, 1980
20. Paulos L, Noyes F, Grood E, et al: Knee rehabilitation after anterior cruciate ligament reconstruction and repair. Am J Sports Med 9:140, 1981
21. Paulos L, Payne F, Rosenburg T: Rehabilitation after anterior cruciate ligament surgery. p. 291. In Jackson D, Drez D (eds): The Anterior Cruciate Deficient Knee. CV Mosby, St. Louis, 1987
22. Noyes F, Torvik P, Hyde W, et al: Biomechanics of ligament failure. II. An analysis of immobilization, exercise, and reconditioning effects in primates. J Bone Joine Surg 56:1406, 1974

▪ Suggested Readings

Albert M: Eccentric Muscle Training in Sports and Orthopaedics. Churchill Livingstone, New York, 1991
Baker CI (Ed.): The Hughston Clinic Sports Medicine Book. Williams & Wilkins, Baltimore, 1995
Hughston J: Knee Ligaments: Injury and Repair. CV Mosby, St. Louis, 1993
Jackson DW (ed): The Anterior Cruciate Deficient Knee. CV Mosby, St. Louis, 1990
Jackson DW: The Anterior Ligament: Current and Future Concepts. Raven Press, New York, 1993
Kennedy JC: The Injured Adolescent Knee. Williams & Wilkins, Baltimore, 1979
Scott WN: Ligaments and Extensor Mechanism of the Knee: Diagnosis and Treatment. CV Mosby, St. Louis, 1991

CHAPTER 22
Surgery of the Knee: Rehabilitation Principles

Richard B. Johnston III

The surgical procedure used to treat a problem in the knee depends on the pathologic lesion, patient factors, and the surgeon's preference based on experience. Different surgical techniques can be used for the same problem. Similarly, physical therapy practices for the same problem can vary. Advances in physical therapy have closely followed advances in surgical technique and skill, and controversy over surgical and rehabilitation techniques does exist. Recent trends in postoperative rehabilitation of the knee include more rapid mobilization and early weight-bearing.[1-6]

The physical therapist should have an understanding of the principles of rehabilitation and follow the direction of the surgeon. Communication between the surgeon and therapist is important. The surgeon should make clear to the therapist what procedure was done and what the expectations for recovery are. While the outcome of surgery is ultimately the responsibility of the surgeon and patient, the therapist plays a critical role in the patient's recovery. The therapist guides the patient through rehabilitation to return satisfactory function to the knee. The objective of this chapter is to review basic principles in therapy for some frequently performed surgical procedures of the knee.

Clinical Anatomy

The therapist should have a fundamental understanding of knee anatomy. If the therapist knows the structures of the knee, he or she can easily identify problem areas or complications that can hinder or compromise rehabilitation and the outcome. This knowledge also helps the therapist understand what anatomic structure was injured and how it was treated surgically. Knee stability is provided primarily by four major ligamentous structures (Fig.

22–1). The medial collateral ligament (MCL) attaches to the medial femoral condyle and the medial tibial plateau and provides medial stability.[7-12] The lateral ligament complex includes the lateral collateral ligament and the posterolateral complex and provides lateral and posterolateral stability.[7,8,11-15] Attachment sites include the posterolateral tibial plateau, fibular head, and lateral femoral condyle. The anterior cruciate ligament (ACL) primarily provides anterior stability for the knee, preventing anterior translation of the tibia on the femur.[7,8,11,16] The posterior cruciate ligament (PCL) primarily provides posterior stability, preventing posterior translation of the tibia on the femur.[7,8,11,16,17] The ACL and PCL lie deep in the knee joint, attaching to the tibia and femur and crossing each other near their midpoint (Fig. 22–2).

Articular cartilage coats the surface of the articulating knee bones. Averaging 3 to 5 mm in thickness, articular cartilage provides a smooth surface for motion and acts as a cushion between the bones when force and weight-bearing are applied on the lower extremities.[7,18-21] The menisci are semicircular fibrocartilaginous structures attached to the tibia in the medial and lateral joint spaces of the knee. They help provide smooth tibiofemoral motion and act as shock absorbers[7,20-25] (Fig. 22–3).

Important tendons around the knee include the quadriceps, patellar, medial and lateral hamstring, and iliotibial band tendons. Any of these structures can be injured by trauma or overuse. Surgeons frequently use these tendons to help reconstruct an unstable knee (Fig. 22–4).

The popliteal vein and artery run next to each other in the posterior aspect of the knee (Fig. 22–5). Injury to these vessels can occur with trauma, such as with a knee dislocation or surgery, and can result in limb-threatening consequences.

The nerves surrounding the knee include the tibial, common peroneal, and saphenous nerves (Fig. 22–6).

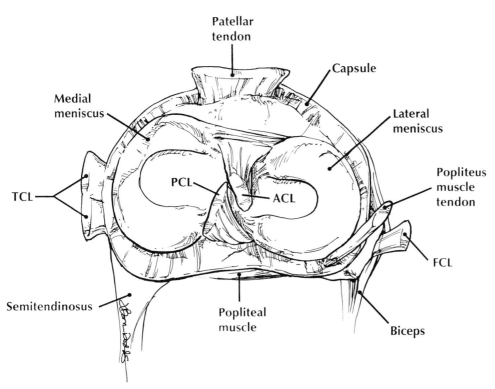

Figure 22-1. The anterior cruciate (ACL), posterior cruciate (PCL), tibial collateral (TCL), and fibular collateral (FCL) ligaments are the primary providers of knee stability.

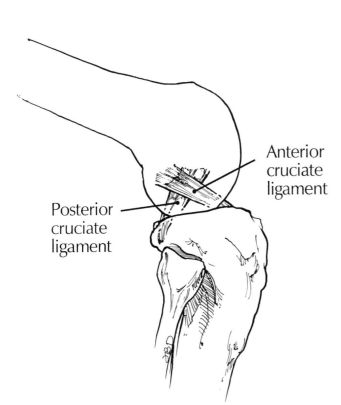

Figure 22-2. The anterior cruciate and posterior cruciate ligaments lie deep in the knee joint. Both ligaments attach to the tibia and femur, and they cross each other near their midpoints.

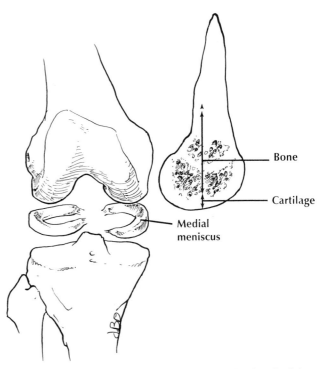

Figure 22-3. The articular cartilage coats the distal end of the femur. The semicircular fibrocartilaginous menisci attach to the tibia in the medial and lateral joint spaces of the knee. These structures provide a smooth surface for motion and a cushion between the bones for shock absorption.

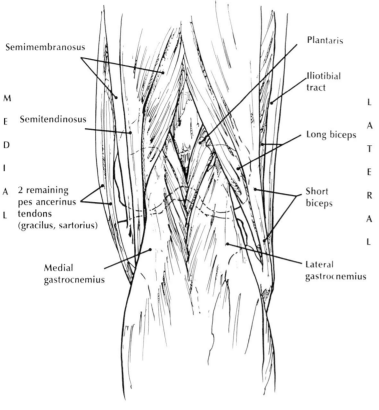

Semimembranosus

Semitendinosus

2 remaining
pes ancerinus
tendons
(gracilus, sartorius)

Medial
gastrocnemius

Plantaris

Iliotibial
tract

Long biceps

Short
biceps

Lateral
gastrocnemius

M
E
D
I
A
L

L
A
T
E
R
A
L

Figure 22–4. The medial and lateral hamstring and iliotibial band tendons are important tendons about the knee.

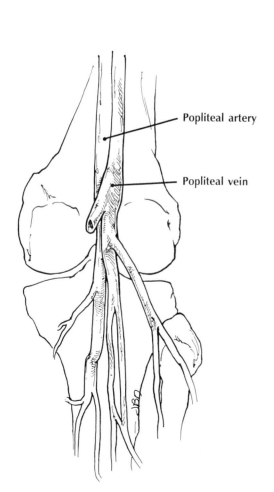

Popliteal artery

Popliteal vein

Figure 22–5. Injury to the popliteal vein and artery in the posterior aspect of the knee can occur with trauma or surgery.

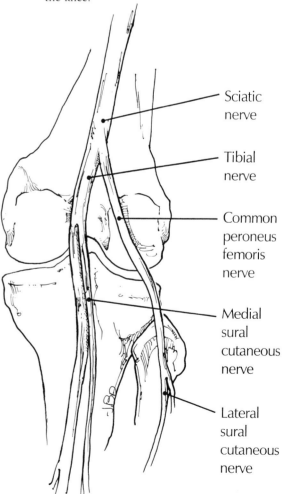

Sciatic
nerve

Tibial
nerve

Common
peroneus
femoris
nerve

Medial
sural
cutaneous
nerve

Lateral
sural
cutaneous
nerve

Figure 22–6. Injury to the tibial, common peroneal, and saphenous nerves that surround the knee can occur with trauma or surgery.

Nerve injury can occur with trauma or surgery. In addition, peroneal nerve palsy can result from prolonged cryotherapy because of the nerve's superficial location just below the fibular head.[26-28] Branches of the saphenous nerve are at risk for injury particularly with medial meniscal repair.[29,30]

■ Principles of Therapy for Knee Procedures

Arthroscopy

Arthroscopy is a well-established orthopaedic procedure for managing knee conditions.[31] It allows minimally invasive evaluation and treatment for many problems. I will review some of the most frequently performed arthroscopic procedures of the knee.

Patients undergoing an arthroscopic partial meniscectomy usually heal rapidly and recover quickly.[32,33] Rapid mobilization and immediate weightbearing after surgery usually are recommended. As needed, modalities are used to treat pain and swelling. The therapist needs to use more caution when rehabilitating a knee after a meniscal repair. For example, repair of a large bucket-handle meniscal tear can fail if the patient exerts significant shear forces across the knee before the tear heals (Fig. 22-7A & B). While some surgeons allow immediate full weightbearing, others prefer nonweightbearing for up to 6 weeks after surgery.[29,30,34] Follow the surgeon's guidance on whether the patient should bear weight immediately or after a period of nonweightbearing. I prefer to allow full weightbearing and range-of-motion exercises, with avoidance of squatting and strenuous weightbearing activities for 6 weeks. For simple chondroplasty (shaving of damaged articular cartilage), the surgeon usually prescribes rapid rehabilitation. For microfracture chondroplasty (in which exposed bone from damaged cartilage is punctured with an awl several times to encourage new

cartilage formation), weightbearing is usually limited for 6 weeks.[35-38] Typically, a continuous passive motion (CPM) device is used to encourage cartilage formation.[37,38]

The surgeon usually uses arthroscopic technique to reconstruct the ACL (Fig. 22-8A & B). The trend in rehabilitation after this procedure involves rapid mobilization and immediate weightbearing.[3-5,39,40-42] The surgeon decides the rehabilitation protocols, and the therapist should rely on the surgeon to provide guidance during rehabilitation. Some aspects of therapy after ACL reconstruction vary, depending on the graft used. Hamstring graft and allograft (cadaver) techniques generally lead to less postoperative pain and faster return of motion than patellar tendon autografts do. However, with early patellar mobilization and aggressive range of motion incorporated into the therapy plan, most patients with an ACL reconstruction using a patellar tendon do well.[3,4,6,43-49]

After a PCL reconstruction or after an MCL or lateral complex repair or reconstruction, the knee generally is moved less aggressively, and some surgeons immobilize the knee for a short period (2 to 4 weeks).[50-52] Follow the surgeon's guidance for therapy after these procedures.

Extensor Mechanism Injury

The surgeon uses open surgical technique to repair patellar or quadriceps ruptures. Some repairs are augmented by hamstring tendons or other tissue. Initially, the knee should be immobilized in extension or slight flexion. Electrical stimulation, straight leg raises, and full weightbearing with the knee in an extension brace can be initiated in the first week after surgery.[53] The patient works to gradually increase flexion, usually 3 to 4 weeks after surgery, depending on the stability of the repair. Knees with a transverse patellar fracture that must be treated surgically are rehabilitated in a similar fashion, with initial immobilization for a short period in extension and gradual progressive flexion, depending on the stability of the repair. Tension band techniques for patellar fractures gener-

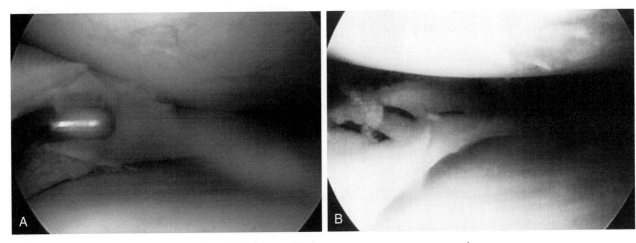

Figure 22-7. (A) Arthroscopic view of a meniscal tear; (B) the surgeon uses sutures to repair the tear.

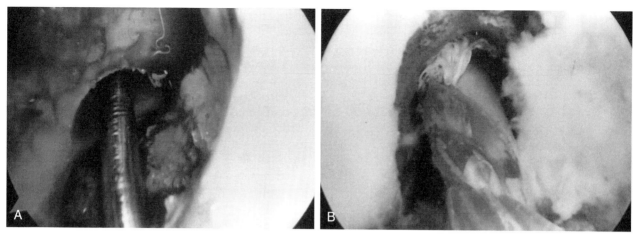

Figure 22–8. (A) Using arthroscopic technique, the surgeon drills the femur as part of reconstruction for the anterior cruciate ligament; (B) the surgeon pulls the anterior cruciate ligament graft into place and completes the reconstruction.

ally hold well, provide strong fixation, and enable the knee to be moved by 2 to 3 weeks after surgery[54–56] (Fig. 22–9). Extended immobilization (more than 4 to 6 weeks) for a patellar fracture can result in a stiff knee that must be manipulated to regain motion.

Realignment procedures for extensor mechanism problems including patellar instability range from a simple lateral release to proximal-distal bony realignment.[57,58] A short period of immobilization (1 to 2 weeks, depending on the procedure) and early initiation of range-of-motion exercises are recommended. Early quadriceps recruitment is encouraged. Immediate weightbearing with these procedures can be instituted with the knee locked in extension or slight flexion in a brace. As always, the surgeon

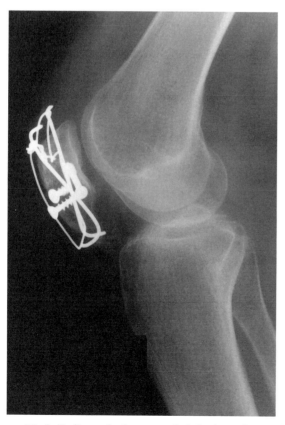

Figure 22–9. Radiograph shows surgical fixation of a patellar fracture.

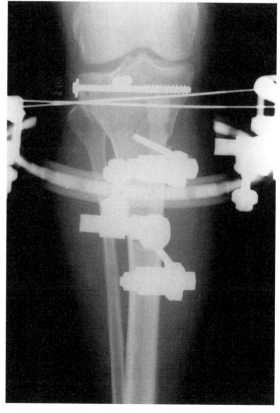

Figure 22–10. Radiograph shows repair of a tibial plateau fracture with screws and a plate.

rehabilitation. Fracture fixation and stability determine the aggressiveness of the therapy, and the surgeon should guide the physical therapist. For patellar fractures, follow the guidelines previously discussed.

Bony Realignment for Lower Extremity Deformity

Proximal tibial and distal femoral osteotomies are used to realign the bony structure of the knee to lessen degenerative wear.[63–66] The surgeon cuts and realigns the bone and then stabilizes the osteotomy with hardware (Fig. 22–11). Early initiation of range-of-motion exercises is recommended, but weightbearing usually is restricted until some healing is evident on radiographs.

Total Knee Replacement

Prosthetic replacement of the knee can be considered a salvage procedure for the painful, degenerated knee (Fig. 22–12). Early initiation of range-of-motion exercises and weightbearing is recommended. The surgeon initially may recommend partial weightbearing for the patient

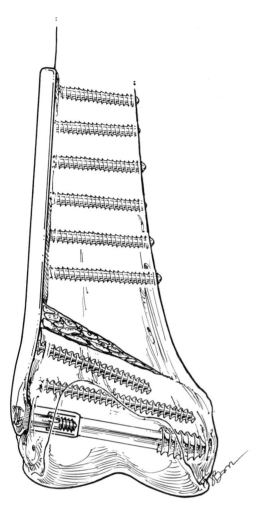

Figure 22–11. To lessen degenerative wear on the knee, the surgeon can perform a distal femoral osteotomy. The cut and realigned bone is stabilized with hardware.

should direct the therapist on when the patient can begin weightbearing and range-of-motion exercises after a realignment procedure.

Fractures

Fractures about the knee that typically are treated surgically include tibial plateau fractures and intra-articular distal femoral fractures (Fig. 22–10). These injuries can be severe, requiring extensive procedures and a prolonged recovery time. While weightbearing can be restricted for an extended period of time to prevent loss of fracture position, early initiation of range-of-motion exercises is recommended.[59–62] Recovery time may be shorter for patients who have a minimally invasive arthroscopic technique to treat an intra-articular fracture, such as an intercondylar, an osteochondral, or a minimally displaced tibial plateau fracture. Range-of-motion exercises and partial weightbearing can be initiated early. Continuous passive motion (CPM) can be useful during the early phases of

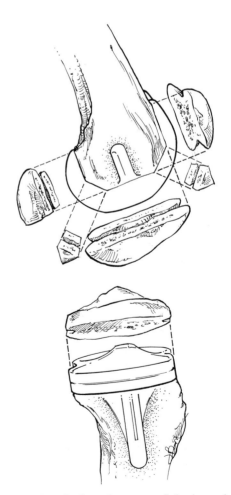

Figure 22–12. Prosthetic replacement of the knee should be used as a salvage procedure.

who has a noncemented knee replacement. CPM is used frequently; however, at 1 year after surgery, the results are about the same for patients who did and did not use CPM.[67] Many of these patients are elderly, and CPM probably helps them regain motion more quickly. Gait training is important after a knee replacement and should be initiated as soon as therapy begins.

Other Procedures

Although many other surgical procedures for knee problems exist, they cannot all be mentioned. Procedures including iliotibial band release, plica excision, and unicompartmental knee replacement require different rehabilitation. The surgeon needs to direct therapy.

■ Postoperative Bracing of the Knee

Postoperative bracing can help protect the surgically treated knee.[68-70] Bracing may be indicated to prevent excessive motion and to provide support and comfort in the immediate postoperative period. The decision to use bracing depends on the procedure done, patient factors, and the surgeon's preference. Braces are not necessary when the knee is stable and rapid mobilization is indicated.

The general trend is to brace the knee in fewer patients and for less time after surgery, particularly after minimally invasive procedures in which immediate weightbearing and rapid mobilization are prescribed.[2] Recent studies suggest that braces do not protect the knee in strenuous situations as well as was previously thought.[68,69] Some surgeons no longer brace the knee in patients after ACL reconstructive surgery, but others prefer some form of protection for up to 1 year after surgery.[2,69,70] However, long-term bracing, particularly after ACL surgery, is rarely necessary. If the operation was successful and if stability and function return, then the patient should not need a knee brace. After treatment for a patellar fracture, the patient's knee usually is placed in a brace locked in extension. The surgeon should make the decision on bracing and direct the patient and therapist accordingly.

■ Postoperative Problems

Many problems that can hinder rehabilitation can occur in the knee after surgery.[50,71-77] The physical therapist should be able to identify possible problems in order to address them expeditiously. Postoperative effusions are common and generally are treated with cryotherapy, compression, and aspiration if severe. If the therapist notes a rapidly increasing and painful effusion in the knee and if the patient has a fever, then the therapist should suspect infection and should refer the patient to the surgeon for evaluation as soon as possible. Superficial wound infec-

tions occasionally occur and should be treated with wound care techniques and antibiotics. The therapist initially can identify a wound problem and should promptly refer the patient to the surgeon.

Nerve injury can occur at the time of injury, surgery, or therapy, and an orthopaedist should evaluate it. Prolonged icing near the peroneal nerve should be avoided because neuropraxia and subsequent foot drop may result.[26]

Increasing calf swelling, pain, or erythema can suggest the formation of a deep venous thrombosis (DVT). If these findings are noted, they should be discussed with the surgeon. A radiologist can perform a Doppler venous ultrasound exam to confirm or rule out a diagnosis of DVT. Although uncommon, DVT can lead to a pulmonary embolus, which is a potentially life-threatening situation. DVT should be treated with anticoagulation.[78-80]

Stiffness after knee surgery is a relatively common problem. Early initiation of full range-of-motion exercises usually prevents this problem. However, manipulation and surgery are indicated when modalities, aggressive mobilization, and range-of-motion exercises fail to prevent stiffness and when true arthrofibrosis exists.[39,76,81-85]

Patellar tendinitis is a common problem seen in the aggressively rehabilitated knee. The rigorous quadriceps extension exercises that the patient does to regain strength put repetitive stress on the patellar tendon, resulting in tendinitis.[76,86-88] This problem occurs most frequently in knees that are being rehabilitated after simple arthroscopy. If tendinitis occurs, therapy should involve more straight leg lifts and terminal-extension exercises than full-extension exercises. Ice massage, anti-inflammatory medication, and a Cho-pat knee strap (Cho-pat, Inc., Hainesport, NJ) also can be helpful. If a problem is identified early, prompt, appropriate treatment can significantly decrease the risk of morbidity during rehabilitation. The therapist should notify the surgeon about any concerns.

■ Summary

The goal of surgery is to return normal function to the knee. With the surgeon, patient, and physical therapist working as a team, this goal should be achieved. Problems that can hinder rehabilitation should be identified early, and clear communication between the surgeon and therapist should always be present.[1] The patient plays a critical role in the recovery process and, with reasonable expectations and motivation, usually does well.

The general trend is for rapid mobilization and early weightbearing. Tissues appear to heal better and faster when motion and weightbearing are begun as soon as reasonably possible. As surgical technique advances and operations become less invasive, recovery time will continue to decrease. Development in functional therapy is likely to progress as patient expectations increase.

■ References

1. Buckwalter JA, Grodzinsky AJ: Loading of healing bone, fibrous tissue, and muscle: implications for orthopaedic practice. J Am Acad Orthop Surg 7:291–299, 1991

2. Howell SM, Taylor MA: Brace-free rehabilitation, with early return to activity, for knees reconstructed with a double-looped semitendinosus and gracilis graft. J Bone Joint Surg 78A:814–825, 1996

3. Shelbourne KD, Nitz P: Accelerated rehabilitation after anterior cruciate ligament reconstruction. Am J Sports Med 18:292–299, 1990

4. Gottlob CA, Gaunt BW: Principles of rehabilitation following anterior cruciate ligament reconstruction. Sports Med Arthroscopy Rev 4:350–360, 1996

5. Shelbourne KD, Klootwyk TE, DeCarlo MS: Rehabilitation program for anterior cruciate ligament reconstruction. Sports Med Arthroscopy Rev 5:77–82, 1997

6. Noyes FR, Mangine RE, Barber S: Early knee motion after open and arthroscopic anterior cruciate ligament reconstruction. Am J Sports Med 15:149–160, 1987

7. Pagnani MJ, Warren RF, Arnoczky SP, et al: Anatomy of the knee. pp. 581–614. In Nicholas JA, Hershman EB (eds): The Lower Extremity and Spine in Sports Medicine. 2nd Ed. CV Mosby, St. Louis, 1995

8. Fu FH, Harner CD, Johnson DL, et al: Biomechanics of knee ligaments. Basic concepts and clinical applications. Instr Course Lect 43:137–148, 1994

9. Hughston JC, Andrews JR, Cross MJ, et al: Classification of knee ligament instabilities. Part I. The medial compartment and cruciate ligaments. J Bone Joint Surg 58A:159–172, 1976

10. Warren LF, Marshall JL: The supporting structures and layers on the medial side of the knee. An anatomical analysis. J Bone Joint Surg 61A:56–62, 1979

11. Amiel D, Billings E Jr, Akeson WH: Ligament structure, chemistry; and physiology. pp. 77–91. In Daniel DM, Akeson WH, O'Connor JJ (eds). Knee Ligaments—Structure, Function, Injury, and Repair. Raven Press, New York, 1990

12. Grood ES, Noyes FR, Butler DL, et al: Ligamentous and capsular restraints preventing straight medial and lateral laxity in intact human cadaver knees. J Bone Joint Surg 63A:1257–1269, 1981

13. Hughston JC, Andrews JR, Cross MJ, et al: Classification of knee ligament instabilities. Part II. The lateral compartment. J Bone Joint Surg 58A:173–179, 1976

14. Gollehon DL, Torzilli PA, Warren RF: The role of the posterolateral and cruciate ligaments in the stability of the human knee. A biomechanical study. J Bone Joint Surg 69A:233–242, 1987

15. Grood ES, Stowers SF, Noyes FR: Limits of movement in the human knee. Effect of sectioning the posterior cruciate ligament and posterolateral structures. J Bone Joint Surg 70A:88–97, 1988

16. Fukubayashi T, Torzilli PA, Sherman MF, et al: An in vitro biomechanical evaluation of anterior-posterior motion of the knee. Tibial displacement, rotation, and torque. J Bone Joint Surg 64A:258–264, 1982

17. Van Dommelen BA, Fowler PJ: Anatomy of the posterior cruciate ligament. A review. Am J Sports Med 17:24–29, 1989

18. Ateshian GA, Soslowsky U, Mow VC: Quantitation of articular surface topography and cartilage thickness in knee joints using stereophotogrammetry. J Biomech 24:761–776, 1991

19. Mandelbaum BR, Browne J, Fu F, et al: Articular cartilage lesions: Current concepts and results. pp. 19–28. In Arendt EA (ed): Orthopaedic Knowledge Update: Sports Medicine 2. American Academy of Orthopaedic Surgeons, Rosemont, IL, 1999

20. Bullough PG. Cartilage. p. 21. In Owen R, Goodfellow J, Bullough PG (eds): Scientific Foundations of Orthopaedics and Traumatology. WB Saunders, Philadelphia, 1980

21. Kaplan EB: Some aspects of functional anatomy of the human knee joint. Clin Orthop 23:18–29, 1962

22. Seedhom BB, Hargreaves DJ: Transmission of the load in the knee joint with special reference to the role of the menisci: Part II. Experimental results, discussion and conclusions. Eng Med 4:220–228, 1979

23. Kettelkamp DB, Jacobs AW: Tibiofemoral contact area—determination and implications. J Bone Joint Surg 54A:349–356, 1972

24. Kurosawa H, Fukubayashi T, Nakajima H: Load-bearing mode of the knee joint: physical behavior of the knee joint with or without menisci. Clin Orthop 149:283–290, 1980

25. Brantigan OC, Voshell AF: The mechanics of the ligaments and menisci of the knee joint. J Bone Joint Surg 23:44–66, 1941

26. Dervin GF, Taylor DE, Keene GC: Effects of cold and compression dressings on early postoperative outcomes for the arthroscopic anterior cruciate ligament reconstruction patient. J Orthop Sports Phys Ther 27:403–441, 1998

27. Moeller JL, Monroe J, McKeag DB: Cryotherapy-induced common peroneal nerve palsy. Clin J Sport Med 7:212–216, 1997

28. Bassett FH III, Kirkpatrick JS, Engelhardt DL, et al: Cryotherapy-induced nerve injury. Am J Sports Med 20:516–518, 1992

29. Kale AA, Vangsness CT Jr: Technical pitfalls of meniscal surgery. Clin Sports Med 18(4):883–896, 1999

30. Van der Reis W, Cannon WD Jr: Arthroscopic meniscal repair using the inside-out technique. Sports Med Arthroscopy Rev 7:8–19, 1999

31. Di Giovine NM, Bradley JP: Arthroscopic equipment and setup. pp. 543–556. In Fu FH, Harner CD, Vince KG (eds): Knee Surgery. Williams & Wilkins, Baltimore, 1994

32. Gillquist J: Long-term results of partial meniscectomy. Sports Med Arthroscopy Rev 7:1–7, 1999

33. Burks RT, Metcalf MH, Metcalf RW: Fifteen-year follow-up of arthroscopic partial meniscectomy. Arthroscopy 13:673–679, 1997

34. Barber FA: Meniscus repair aftercare. Sports Med Arthroscopy Rev 7:43–47, 1999

35. Minas T, Nehrer S: Current concepts in the treatment of articular cartilage defects. Orthopedics 20:525–538, 1997

36. Rae PJ, Noble J: Arthroscopic drilling of osteochondral lesions of the knee. J Bone Joint Surg 71B:534, 1989

37. Salter RB, Simmonds DF, Malcolm BW, et al: The biological effect of continuous passive motion on the healing of full-thickness defects in articular cartilage: an experimental investigation in the rabbit. J Bone Joint Surg 62A:1232–1251, 1980

38. Steadman JR, Rodkey WG, Briggs KK, et al: The microfracture technique in the management of complete cartilage defects in the knee joint. Orthopade 28:26–32, 1999 (in German)

39. Cosgarea AJ, Sebastianelli WJ, DeHaven KE: Prevention of arthrofibrosis after anterior cruciate ligament reconstruction using the central third patellar tendon autograft. Am J Sports Med 23:87–92, 1995

40. Beynnon BD, Fleming BC, Johnson RJ, et al: Anterior cruciate ligament strain behavior during rehabilitation exercises in vivo. Am J Sports Med 23:24–34, 1995

41. Bynum EB, Barrack RL, Alexander AH: Open versus closed chain kinetic exercises after anterior cruciate ligament reconstruction: a prospective randomized study. Am J Sports Med 23:401–406, 1995

42. Yack HJ, Collins CE, Whieldon TJ: Comparison of closed and open kinetic chain exercise in the anterior cruciate ligament-deficient knee. Am J Sports Med 21:49–54, 1993

43. Shelbourne KD, Trumper RV: Preventing anterior knee pain after anterior cruciate ligament reconstruction. Am J Sports Med 25:41–47, 1997

44. Sachs RA, Daniel DM, Stone ML, et al: Patellofemoral problems after anterior cruciate ligament reconstruction. Am J Sports Med 17:760–765, 1989

45. O'Neill DB: Arthroscopically assisted reconstruction of the anterior cruciate ligament: a prospective randomized analysis of three techniques. J Bone Joint Surg 78A:803–813, 1996

46. Shelbourne KD, Foulk DA: Timing of surgery in acute anterior cruciate ligament tears on the return of quadriceps muscle strength after reconstruction using an autogenous patellar tendon graft. Am J Sports Med 23:686–689, 1995

47. DeMaio M, Noyes FR, Mangine RE: Principles for aggressive rehabilitation after reconstruction of the anterior cruciate ligament. Orthopedics 15:385–392, 1992

48. Shelbourne KD, Klootwyk TE, Wilckens JH, et al: Ligament stability two to six years after anterior cruciate ligament reconstruction with autogenous patellar tendon graft and participation in accelerated rehabilitation program. Am J Sports Med 23:575–579, 1995

49. Aglietti P, Buzzi R, Zaccherotti G, et al: Patellar tendon versus doubled semitendinosus and gracilis tendons for anterior cruciate ligament reconstruction. Am J Sports Med 22:211–218, 1994

50. Jacobson KE: Technical pitfalls of collateral ligament surgery. Clin Sports Med 18(4):847–882, 1999

51. Noyes FR, Barber-Westin SD: Treatment of complex injuries involving the posterior cruciate and posterolateral ligaments of the knee. Am J Knee Surg 9:200–214, 1996

52. Harner CD, Höher J: Evaluation and treatment of posterior cruciate ligament injuries. Am J Sports Med 26:471–482, 1998

53. Matava MJ: Patellar tendon ruptures. J Am Acad Orthop Surg 4:287–296, 1996

54. Cramer KE, Moed BR: Patellar fractures: contemporary approach to treatment. J Am Acad Orthop Surg 5:323–331, 1997

55. Carpenter JE, Kasman R, Matthews LS: Fractures of the patella. Instr Course Lect 43:97–108, 1994

56. Weber MJ, Janecki CJ, McLeod P, et al: Efficacy of various forms of fixation of transverse fractures of the patella. J Bone Joint Surg 62A:215–220, 1980

57. Boden BP, Pearsall AW, Garrett WE Jr, et al: Patellofemoral instability: evaluation and management. J Am Acad Orthop Surg 5:47–57, 1997

58. Halbrecht JL, Jackson DW: Acute dislocation of the patella. pp. 123–134. In Fox JM, Del Pizzo WJ (eds): The Patellofemoral Joint. McGraw-Hill, New York, 1993

59. Albert MJ: Supracondylar fractures of the femur. J Am Acad Orthop Surg 5:163–171, 1997

60. Duwelius PJ, Rangitsch MR, Colville MR, et al: Treatment of tibial plateau fractures by limited internal fixation. Clin Orthop 339:47–57, 1997

61. Marsh JL, Smith ST, Do TT: External fixation and limited internal fixation for complex fractures of the tibial plateau. J Bone Joint Surg 77A:661–673, 1995

62. Moore TM, Patzakis MJ, Harvey JP: Tibial plateau fractures: definition, demographics, treatment rationale, and long-term results of closed traction management or operative reduction. J Orthop Trauma 1:97–119, 1987

63. Grelsamer RP: Unicompartmental osteoarthrosis of the knee. J Bone Joint Surg 77A:278–292, 1995

64. Nagel A, Insall JN, Scuderi GR: Proximal tibial osteotomy: a subjective outcome study. J Bone Joint Surg 78A:1353–1358, 1996

65. Healy WL, Anglen JO, Wasilewski SA, et al: Distal femoral varus osteotomy. J Bone Joint Surg 70A:102–109, 1988

66. Hofmann AA, Wyatt RW, Beck SW: High tibial osteotomy: use of an osteotomy jig, rigid fixation, and early motion versus conventional surgical technique and cast immobilization. Clin Orthop 271:212–217, 1991

67. Ritter MA, Gandolf VS, Holston KS: Continuous passive motion versus physical therapy in total knee arthroplasty. Clin Orthop 244:239–243, 1989

68. Beynnon BD, Johnson RJ, Fleming BC, et al: The effect of functional knee bracing on the anterior cruciate ligament in the weightbearing and nonweightbearing knee. Am J Sports Med 25:353–359, 1997

69. Wojtys EM, Kothari SU, Huston LJ: Anterior cruciate ligament functional brace use in sports. Am J Sports Med 24:539–546, 1996

70. Cawley PW, France EP, Paulos LE: The current state of functional knee bracing research: a review of the literature. Am J Sports Med 19:226–233, 1991

71. Lonner JH, Lotke PA: Aseptic complications after total knee arthroplasty. J Am Acad Orthop Surg 7:311–324, 1999

72. Bealle D, Johnson DL: Technical pitfalls of anterior cruciate ligament surgery. Clin Sports Med 18(4):831–845, 1999

73. Nyland J: Rehabilitation complications following knee surgery. Clin Sports Med 18(4):905–925, 1999

74. Smith ST, Cramer KE, Karges DE, et al: Early complications in the operative treatment of patella fractures. J Orthop Trauma 11:183–187, 1997

75. Johnson DL, Fu FH: Anterior cruciate ligament reconstruction: why do failures occur? Instr Course Lect 44:391–406, 1995

76. Stapleton TR: Complications in anterior cruciate ligament reconstructions with patellar tendon grafts. Sports Med Arthroscopy Rev 5:156–162, 1997

77. Ayers DC, Dennis DA, Johanson NA, et al: Common complications of total knee arthroplasty. J Bone Joint Surg 79A:278–311, 1997

78. Robinson KS, Anderson DR, Gross M, et al: Ultrasonographic screening before hospital discharge for deep venous thrombosis after arthroplasty: the post-arthroplasty screening study. A randomized controlled trial. Ann Intern Med 127:439–445, 1997

79. Schulman S, Rhedin AS, Lindmarker P, et al: A comparison of six weeks with six months of oral anticoagulant therapy after a first episode of venous thromboembolism: duration of Anticoagulation Trial Study Group. N Engl J Med 332:1661–1665, 1995

80. Warwick DJ, Whitehouse S: Symptomatic venous thromboembolism after total knee replacement. J Bone Joint Surg 79B:780–786, 1997

81. Petsche TS, Hutchinson MR: Loss of extension after reconstruction of the anterior cruciate ligament. J Am Acad Orthop Surg 7:119–127, 1999

82. Harner CD, Irrgang JJ, Fu FH: Prevention and management

of loss of motion after arthroscopic anterior cruciate ligament reconstruction. Complications Orthop Spring:5–8, 1993

83. Rubinstein RA Jr, Shelbourne KD, VanMeter CD, et al: Effect on knee stability if full hyperextension is restored immediately after autogenous bone-patellar tendon-bone anterior cruciate ligament reconstruction. Am J Sports Med 23:365–368, 1995

84. Shelbourne KD, Wilckens JH, Mollabashy A, et al: Arthrofibrosis in acute anterior cruciate ligament reconstruction: the effect of timing of reconstruction and rehabilitation. Am J Sports Med 19:332–336, 1991

85. Klein W, Shah N, Gassen A: Arthroscopic management of postoperative arthrofibrosis of the knee joint: indication, technique, and results. Arthroscopy 10:591–597, 1994

86. Pellecchia GL, Hamel H, Behnke P: Treatment of infrapatellar tendinitis: a combination of modalities and transverse friction massage versus iontophoresis. J Sport Rehabil 3:135–145, 1994

87. King JB, Perry DJ, Mourad K, et al: Lesions of the patellar ligament. J Bone Joint Surg 72B:46–48, 1990

88. Aglietti P, Buzzi R, D'Andria S, et al: Patellofemoral problems after intraarticular anterior cruciate ligament reconstruction. Clin Orthop 288:195–204, 1993

CHAPTER 23
Kinematics and Kinetics During Gait

David Tiberio and Gary W. Graym

Human locomotion is an exquisite interaction of the body's neurologic, musculoskeletal, and cardiopulmonary systems. No one has to teach human beings how to walk or run. In fact, the ability to walk is considered by some authorities to be the product of programmed motor responses occurring at the spinal cord level.[1] Once acquired through the "practice" of normal development, human locomotion occurs at a subconscious level. During walking or running, there is no actual volitional activation of muscles. Even adjustments or alterations in our walking pattern, such as stepping off a curb, are responses to visual stimuli that we barely notice.

This lack of conscious learning, although quite amazing, works against the practitioner who tries to evaluate and rehabilitate patients with locomotor dysfunction. Walking is not a product of conscious practice that can be imparted to a patient in the way certain athletic skills can. To effectively evaluate and rehabilitate patients with locomotor dysfunction, practitioners must acquire knowledge regarding the joint motions (kinematics) and muscle forces (kinetics) during walking and running.

Energy Expenditure

Human locomotion is a very efficient activity. The main energy-expending activities of locomotion relate to the body's center of mass. As the body moves forward, the center of mass moves from side to side and up and down. Because of the force of gravity, most of the energy is spent lifting up the center of mass and catching it as it falls. Therefore, the efficiency of the human locomotor system lies in the body's abilities to minimize the vertical and horizontal displacements, to smooth the reversal of motion, and to translate as much energy as possible into forward motion.

In an effort to determine what factors contribute to locomotor efficiency, Saunders et al.[2] synthesized the major research findings of several studies. Their work identified the six "determinants" of gait: pelvic rotation, pelvic tilt, knee flexion in stance, the foot mechanism, the knee mechanism, and lateral displacement of the pelvis. Collectively, these determinants serve to decrease the arcs through which the center of mass must travel and to smooth the transition from one direction to another. They are not the only contributors to efficient locomotion, but the clinician should understand that abnormal function at any joint in the lower quarter will disrupt the normal locomotion pattern and increase energy expenditure.

Practitioners must gain knowledge of and recognize the difference between joint position and joint motion. Joint motion is the movement of the bones of a joint toward one extreme of the range of motion. For example, dorsiflex*ion* is movement of the dorsum of the foot toward the leg. The suffixes *-ion* and *-ing* denote motion. Position, however, refers to the alignment of the bones compared with a reference point. The reference point for the ankle is zero (90 degree position). If the bones are aligned on one side of this reference point, the ankle is dorsiflex*ed;* if on the other side, it is plantar flex*ed*. The suffix *-ed* (or *-us*) infers a joint position at a particular time.

The fact that motion and position are different concepts becomes crystallized when one considers that ankle motion can be one of dorsiflex*ion*, even though the joint at that instant may be in a plantar flex*ed* position. The difference is also important at the subtalar joint when considering the primary functions of the foot. Certain functions are dependent on subtalar joint position (supinat*ed*, or pronat*ed*), whereas other functions are dependent on motion (supinat*ion*, pronat*ion*).

Closed Chain Motion

Joint motion is usually described in the context of open chain motion. Open chain motion occurs when the proximal bone segment of a joint is fixed and the distal bone segment is free to move. Unfortunately, most clinically significant daily activities that involve the lower extremities occur when the foot is on the ground. Whenever the distal bone segment (in this case, the foot) is fixed, closed chain motion occurs. In closed chain motion, there is motion on both sides of the joint being evaluated. With open chain motion, the motion occurs distal to the joint being evaluated and studied. Closed chain motion alters the nature of muscle contractions as well as bone motion. An example of this is dorsiflexion of the ankle joint. During open chain dorsiflexion, the dorsum of the foot moves up toward the lower leg. Closed chain dorsiflexion of the ankle during gait occurs when the tibia moves forward while the foot remains stationary on the ground. This motion is not produced by contraction of the dorsiflexor muscles. Rather, the dorsiflexion results from forward movement of the lower leg over the foot. The muscles that produce plantar flexion (the calf group) are active during closed chain dorsiflexion to eccentrically control this motion.

An understanding of closed chain motion of the subtalar joint is particularly important because of its effect on the proximal bone segments of the lower quarter. In closed chain pronation, the calcaneus and the rest of the foot will still evert, abduct, and dorsiflex. As the calcaneus everts, the talus slides in a distal and medial direction; the head of the talus adducts and plantar flexes, with a resultant internal rotation of the body of the talus.[3] Because the ankle joint does not allow a significant amount of rotation in the transverse plane, the rotation of the body of the talus forces the ankle to rotate in the same direction. This creates an obligatory internal rotation of the lower leg whenever subtalar joint pronation occurs.[3–6] Closed chain supination of the subtalar joint produces an obligatory external rotation of the lower leg. These obligatory rotations will become important to appreciate during the discussion of knee motion and hip motion during gait.

It is also important to note the effect that closed chain pronation and supination at the subtalar joint have on arch height. The axis of the subtalar joint can vary significantly. Isman and Inman[10] found that the pitch of axes can range from 20 to 60 degrees up from the horizontal. These differences in the subtalar joint axis correlate with different inclination angles of the calcaneus and produce different arch heights. A higher pitch to the axis produces a high architecture to the foot, whereas a low inclination angle creates a lower architecture. Regardless of the arch height, motion of the subtalar joint creates a dynamic change in arch height. As the head of the talus adducts and plantar flexes during closed chain pronation, the arch height decreases. With closed chain supination, as the head of the talus abducts and dorsiflexes, the arch height relatively increases.[3,11] The practical implication of this motion is that the arch height is a response to motion at the subtalar joint as well as a response to motion at the midtarsal joint, which is influenced by the subtalar joint. Closed chain pronation not only lowers the arch but also lowers the pelvis by creating a functional decrease in leg length. If subtalar joint motion is asymmetric, then the motion of the pelvis will be asymmetric and must be assessed in all three planes of motion.

◼ Primary Foot Function

Joint motion and muscle function during human locomotion are much easier to understand in the context of the primary functions of the foot. The foot has three basic functions. First, it must adapt to ground surfaces that may not be level or smooth. The ability of the foot to perform this function comes from the significant amount of motion in all three body planes that is present in the joints of the rearfoot (ankle and subtalar joint) and the forefoot (oblique and longitudinal axes of the midtarsal joint).

The ability of the forefoot to adapt to the ground depends on the mobility of the midtarsal joint. For the midtarsal joint to be mobile, the subtalar joint must be in a pronated position. This pronated position alters the position of the talus and the calcaneus, thereby affecting the relative positions of the talonavicular and calcaneocuboid articulations. This pronated position allows increased mobility or "unlocking" of the midtarsal joint. Therefore the ability of the midtarsal joint and the foot to adapt adequately to their environment is provided by the pronated position of the subtalar joint.

A second major function of the foot is to act as a facilitator of shock absorption as the foot hits the ground. This occurs simultaneously with the surface adaptation. As the advancing leg begins to bear weight, the ground reaction force travels up the musculoskeletal system. To absorb a significant portion of this force, the knee must flex. It is this knee flexion, with the concurrent eccentric contraction of the quadriceps, that dampens the ground reaction force as it travels up the musculoskeletal system. The joint mechanics of the knee dictate that when the knee flexes, an internal rotation must occur at the tibia. This component motion of internal rotation with flexion is the reversal of the well-documented external rotation with extension (locking home mechanism). This obligatory rotation of the lower leg that occurs with knee flexion is present during the first 15 to 20 degrees of motion. As was mentioned in the section on closed chain motion, internal rotation occurs with subtalar joint pronation. Therefore, it is important for the subtalar joint to pronate when the knee is flexing in order for the lower leg to promote the necessary motion at both the knee and the subtalar joint. This will be discussed further in relation to human locomotion.

The third major function of the foot to act as a rigid lever for propulsion. For the heel to rise off the ground without the arch of the foot collapsing, the mobility of

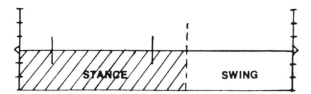

Figure 23–1. Gait cycle divided into the stance phase and the swing phase. (From Tiberio,[30] with permission.)

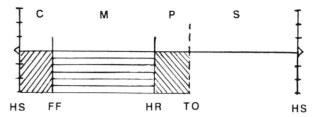

Figure 23–3. Division of the stance phase into contact, midstance, and propulsion. C, contact; M, midstance; P, pronation; S, supination; HS, heel-strike; HR, heel-rise; HF, heel-fall; FF, foot-flat; TO, toe-off. (From Tiberio,[30] with permission.)

the midtarsal joint must be reduced. This is described as *locking* of the midtarsal joint, and it occurs when the subtalar joint moves into a supinated position. This supinated position, by changing the relative alignment of the bones, reduces joint mobility and allows effective propulsion. A variety of structural changes have been postulated for this reduction in midtarsal joint mobility. When the subtalar joint is in the supinated position, there is more compression of the articular surfaces. There also appears to be capsular and ligamentous tightening, which reduces joint play. Finally, this increased stability has been attributed to alterations in the angle of muscle forces caused by increased arch height when the subtalar joint is in a supinated position. The reduction in midtarsal joint mobility, as a result of the supination of the subtalar joint, allows the foot to function as a rigid level and allows the propulsive mechanism off that rigid lever to be effective.

■ Kinematics of Locomotion

Gait Cycle

The basic unit of human locomotion is called the *gait cycle*. Repetition of this cycle allows the body to move from one place to another. A normal gait (or walking) cycle is defined as the period from heel-strike of one foot to heel-strike of that same foot again. Studying the components of the gait cycle facilitates an understanding of the practical aspects of human locomotion. Figure 23–1 depicts the cycle as divided into the time when the foot is in contact with the ground (stance) and when it is in the air (swing). The stance phase accounts for approximately 61 percent, whereas the swing phase lasts for 39 percent of the cycle.[9] To give some temporal refer-

ence to these two phases, it is advantageous to assume that the gait cycle lasts for 1 second. The stance phase then becomes slightly longer than 0.6 second, and the swing phase lasts just less than 0.4 second.

It is important to consider how the motion of the other leg affects the gait cycle. Figure 23–2 shows how the stance and swing phases of each leg overlap. Part of the time both feet are on the ground. This interval is called the *period of double limb support* and occurs twice in each cycle. Single limb support is created when the opposite leg swings forward to renew ground contact. Each period of double limb support lasts for only about 0.11 second, whereas each single limb support lasts for 0.39 second, which corresponds exactly to the swing time of the opposite leg.

The stance phase has three main subdivisions, which are determined by the manner in which the foot contacts the ground.[3,9] The stance phase of one leg is depicted in Figure 23–3. Four different events can be identified by analyzing the foot–ground interface. These four events—called *heel-strike, foot-flat, heel-rise,* and *toe-off*—divide the stance phase into three parts or phases. The period from heel-strike until the foot is flat on the surface is the contact phase. The midstance phase extends from foot-flat to heel-rise. The propulsion phase begins with heel-rise and ends with toe-off. By looking at the overlap of both legs (Fig. 23–4), it becomes apparent that as one leg propels the body forward, the other leg is receiving the body weight during contact.

Swing of one leg occurs simultaneously with midstance of the other leg. Swing can also be divided into

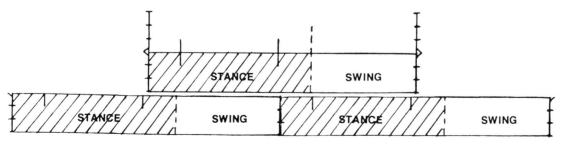

Figure 23–2. The relationship of the stance and swing phases of each leg. Overlap of stance produces double limb support, whereas swing produces single limb support. (From Tiberio,[30] with permission.)

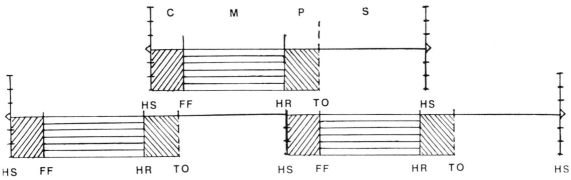

Figure 23–4. Overlap of two legs, indicating the transfer of body weight from the back leg (propulsion) to the front leg (contact). (For abbreviations, see Fig. 23–3.) (From Tiberio,[30] with permission.)

three sections, although the divisions are more arbitrary. These three sections are most commonly called *acceleration, midswing,* and *deceleration.* In addition to advancing the foot, the swing phase assists with propulsion of the stance leg. The forward movement of the mass of the lower extremity, along with the change in direction of the rotation of the pelvis in the transverse plane, work in concert with the muscles of the stance leg to accelerate the individual joint motions.

Individual Joint Motion

The patterns of limb rotation in all three planes are consistent with the primary functions of the foot and the phases of gait. By studying the joint motions separately and then detailing the kinematic links among the joints, the delicate synchronicity of human locomotion becomes evident.

The motion of the subtalar joint is shown in Figure 23–5. During the stance phase, the motion of the subtalar joint is directly related to the primary functions of the foot. The calcaneus strikes the ground on the lateral aspect, and the subtalar joint begins its pronation from a slightly supinated position. Once the subtalar joint is in a pronated position, midtarsal joint mobility is increased, and the foot is able to adapt to uneven ground surfaces during the contact phase. The closed chain pronation produces obligatory internal rotation of the tibia, which

facilitates the knee flexion that is necessary for shock attenuation and smooth weight acceptance.

When the foot is flat on the ground, surface adaptation and shock attenuation are complete. The subtalar joint now enters the midstance (transition) phase in changing from a mobile adaptor to a rigid lever. At foot-flat, the subtalar joint is maximally pronated. Subtalar joint supination begins to ensure that the joint reaches its neutral position before the heel rises from the ground. As the joint passes from a pronated to a supinated position, the mobility in the midtarsal joint decreases in preparation for propulsion.

Propulsion begins when the heel rises. The transition from mobile adaptor to rigid level has occurred. The foot is now an effective lever for propelling the body forward because of the stability of the midtarsal joint gained from the supinated position of the subtalar joint. The subtalar joint continues to supinate throughout propulsion as the center of mass is accelerated forward and the body's weight is transferred to the forward leg. During the swing phase, the subtalar joint moves from its maximally supinated position at toe-off to a position of slight supination just before heel-strike, at which time the cycle is repeated.[6]

Recent research has cast some doubt on the ability/necessity of the subtalar joint to pass into a supinated position prior to heel-rise.[10,11] These studies suggest that maximum pronation of the subtalar joint extends into the midstance phase. Additionally, while the subtalar joint is supinating during propulsion, the joint often does not reach a supinated position. It has been suggested that the subtalar joint functions within a range around the foot's relaxed standing position rather than subtalar neutral.[12]

Ankle

Ankle joint motion occurs primarily in the sagittal plane. At heel-strike, the ankle is close to the neutral (or 90 degree) position (Fig. 23–6). As the contact phase is initiated with heel-strike, the ankle plantar flexes until the foot is flat on the ground. During the midstance phase,

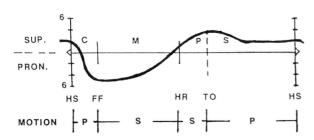

Figure 23–5. Motion of the subtalar joint. P, pronation; S, supination. (For other abbreviations, see Fig. 23–3.) (From Tiberio,[30] with permission.)

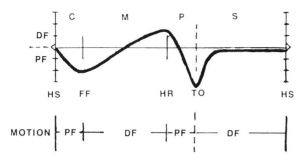

Figure 23-6. Motion of the ankle joint. PF, plantar flexion; DF, dorsiflexion. (For other abbreviations, see Fig. 23–3.) (From Tiberio,[30] with permission.)

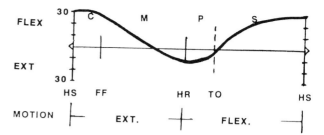

Figure 23-8. Hip flexion and extension during gait cycle. (For abbreviations, see Fig. 23–3.) (From Tiberio,[30] with permission.)

the lower leg moves forward over the foot. The average amount of dorsiflexion just before heel-rise is 10 degrees. The degree of dorsiflexion needed for normal ambulation will vary, depending on the surface inclination and heel height, as well as the forefoot structure.

Ankle dorsiflexion is quickly reversed during the propulsive phase. Plantar flexion reaches a peak at toe-off. Immediately on toe-off, the ankle dorsiflexes to prevent toe drag. The ankle returns to the neutral position, which it maintains until the heel strikes the ground again.[4,9]

Knee

Figure 23–7 depicts the motion of the knee joint during walking. The knee flexes to about 20 degrees during the contact phase. This flexion attenuates the shock caused by ground contact. Knee flexion and weight acceptance are complete at foot-flat. The knee then begins to extend as a result of the forward movement of the trunk over the foot. The knee almost attains full extension at the time of heel-rise. The knee flexes again during propulsion and continues to flex during the acceleration portion of swing. The knee then quickly extends to a minimally flexed position in preparation for heel-strike and a new cycle.[4,9]

Hip

Hip motion occurs in all three planes during the gait cycle. Figure 23–8 shows the sagittal plane motion. At heel-strike, the hip is flexed about 30 degrees. The hip begins to extend during the contact phase, and this extension continues until heel-rise. The hip motion changes when propulsion begins, with flexion occurring throughout the propulsion and swing phases. At heel-strike, the hip has returned to 30 degrees of flexion.[4,12]

Motion of the hip in the frontal plane (adduction and abduction) is depicted in Figure 23–9. The position of the hip at heel-strike is dictated by the width of the walking base. Despite these variations that affect hip position, the direction of joint motion is clear. At heel-strike, the pelvis and the center of gravity are moving laterally over the limb that is accepting the body's weight. This lateral shift produces closed chain adduction during contact and the first half of the midstance phase. Once the lateral shift is decelerated, the motion of the hip changes to abduction for the rest of the stance. The path of the hip is variable during swing, but the goal is to bring the foot into proper position for heel-strike.[12]

Hip rotation in the transverse plane is depicted in Figure 23–10. Internal rotation is occurring at the hip as the leg accepts the body's weight and adapts to the ground. The motion changes to external rotation during midstance and propulsion. As swing begins, the leg initiates the internal rotation that will continue when ground contact is renewed.[4,13]

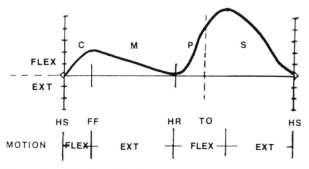

Figure 23-7. Motion of the knee joint. (For abbreviations, see Fig. 23–3.) (From Tiberio,[30] with permission.)

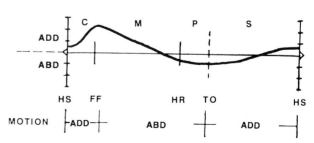

Figure 23-9. Hip abduction (ABD) and adduction (ADD) during gait. (For other abbreviations, see Fig. 23–3.) (From Tiberio,[30] with permission.)

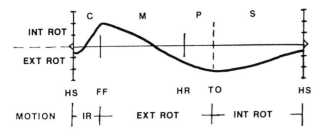

Figure 23–10. Hip internal rotation (INT ROT) and external rotation (EXT ROT) during gait cycle. (For other abbreviations, see Fig. 23–3.) (From Tiberio,[30] with permission.)

Synchronicity

The transverse plane motion of all the bone segments is consistent throughout the phases of the gait cycle.[13] Figure 23–11 shows the motions of the pelvis, femur, and tibia. It is not coincidental that the motions occur in the same direction. The bone segments exhibit an exquisite synchronicity that is essential for normal human locomotion. At the bottom of Figure 23–11, the closed chain motion of the subtalar joint during stance is shown, with the obligatory tibial rotation delineated. This rotation caused by subtalar joint motion is consistent with the rotation patterns in the proximal segments and demonstrates the importance of subtalar joint function for lower quarter mechanics.

It is clear that although the segments rotate in the same direction, the amount and rate of the motion are not the same across segments. If they were, there would be no joint motion except at the lumbosacral junction. Because the motions are not equal, a "relative rotation"

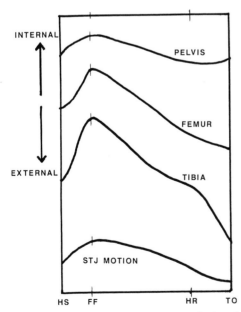

Figure 23–11. Rotation of the bone segments during the stance phase. The steepness of the slope represents the rate of rotation. The motion of the subtalar joint (STJ) as a reference appears at the bottom of the figure. (For other abbreviations, see Fig. 23–3.) (From Tiberio,[30] with permission.)

is produced at the hip and knee joints. An example of this is the fact that the femur is internally rotating faster than the pelvis during the contact phase. This produces a relative internal rotation at the hip joint. This comparison of the rate of movement between one bone and another is also critical at the knee joint.

Again referring to Figure 23–11, although both the tibia and the femur are internally rotating during the contact phase, the tibia is moving faster than the femur. This produces a relative internal rotation at the knee, which is a component motion of knee flexion during the first 15 to 20 degrees. Knee rotation facilitates the knee flexion that is vital for shock attenuation during the contact phase. During the midstance phase, all motions reverse: The subtalar joint supinates (external rotation), the knee extends (external rotation), and all the segments externally rotate while the tibia moves faster than the femur (relative external rotation). The synchronous linkage of the segments continues.

The subtalar joint continues to supinate (external rotation) during propulsion, but the knee flexes (internal rotation). The synchronicity seems to have disappeared, but actually it is still present. During the beginning of propulsion, the pelvis and the femur are externally rotating faster than the tibia. This produces relative internal rotation at the knee, which provides the component motion for knee flexion during the first 15 to 20 degrees of motion. Therefore, it is not biomechanically inconsistent that the subtalar joint can supinate while the knee flexes, as long as the rate of rotation between the femur and tibia is precise.

■ Kinetics of Locomotion

Muscle Function

The functions of muscles usually are taught on the basis of a concentric contraction when the distal segment is free to move (open chain). For example, this approach applied to the tibialis anterior muscle would describe its function as dorsiflexing the foot (concentric) or as producing the open chain action of moving the dorsum of the foot up toward the leg. Although it is certainly reasonable to learn muscle function from this perspective, it is also very limiting. Muscle function during activities in which the distal segment is fixed, thereby closing the chain, is quite different.[14]

Understanding muscle function during closed chain activities is facilitated by describing the effects of different types of muscle contractions on joint motion. A concentric contraction produces or accelerates joint motion. An eccentric contraction controls or decelerates the motion to which it is antagonistic.

Another important consideration is the function of multijoint muscles. All of the extrinsic muscles that cross the ankle joint also have functions at the subtalar joint;

many cross the midtarsal joint as well. Therefore, a muscle will have simultaneous effects on more than one joint unless a synergistic contraction of another muscle neutralizes the muscle's function at one of the joints. These synergistic functions are not well understood. Therefore, the discussion of muscle function in this chapter focuses on the acceleration and deceleration of joint movement.

Ankle

The specific function of muscles is determined when knowledge of muscle anatomy and joint motion are combined and then verified whenever possible by electromyographic research.[3,4,15–17] Figure 23–12 shows the activities of the muscles that control ankle function. During the contact phase, the ankle is plantar flexing, but the muscles that dorsiflex the foot are active. The actual motion is produced by the ground reaction force when the heel strikes the ground. The anterior tibialis works eccentrically to decelerate the foot's movement to the ground. Paralysis of this muscle produces the well-known foot slap.

Once the midstance phase begins, the calf group becomes active. These muscles decelerate the forward movement of the tibia over the foot. The activity increases to a peak at heel-rise. At this point, the calf muscles shift from an eccentric to a concentric contraction, which plantar flexes the foot. This muscle action initiates the propulsive phase. This manner of muscle function, decelerating the motion before accelerating in the opposite direction, is frequently seen in human locomotion.

As swing begins, the ankle must dorsiflex to keep the foot from dragging. This acceleration by the anterior tibialis is followed by an isometric contraction to hold the foot in position for heel-strike, when the cycle will

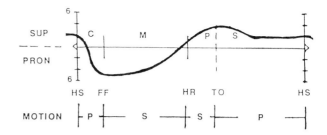

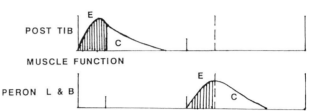

Figure 23–13. Selected muscle function at the subtalar joint. SUP, supination; PRON, pronation; POST TIB, posterior tibialis; PERON L & B, peroneus longus and brevis. (For other abbreviations, see Fig. 23–3.) (From Tiberio,[30] with permission.)

begin again. The function of these muscles at the subtalar joint cannot be overlooked. During contact, when the anterior tibialis is decelerating plantar flexion, it can also assist in the deceleration of subtalar joint pronation. The acceleration of supination during midstance and propulsion is assisted by the calf group contraction affecting ankle motion.

Subtalar Joint

It seems appropriate to consider the extrinsic muscles that function primarily at the subtalar joint. The primary decelerator of pronation during contact is the posterior tibialis (Fig. 23–13). Therefore, an eccentric contraction during contact, decelerating pronation, will transition into a concentric contraction as midstance begins with the acceleration of supination at the subtalar joint.

During propulsion, subtalar joint supination continues even though the activity of the posterior tibialis has ended. Now the lateral extrinsics need to be active to control and limit the amount of supination. Therefore, the peroneus longus and brevis work eccentrically until swing begins, and there will probably be some concentric activity to return the subtalar joint close to its neutral position before heel-strike. The peroneus longus also provides important stability to the forefoot during propulsion. It allows the forefoot to maintain ground contact during subtalar joint supination and stabilizes the first metatarsal during propulsion off the hallux.

Knee

Knee flexion for shock absorption requires the quadriceps to contract eccentrically to decelerate this motion during

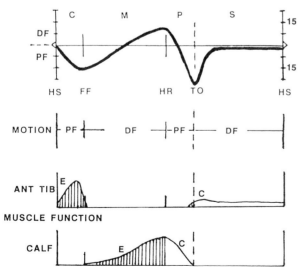

Figure 23–12. Selected muscle function at the ankle joint. The striped area represents eccentric contraction. The open area represents concentric contraction. DF, dorsiflexion; PF, plantar flexion; ANT TIB, anterior tibialis. (For other abbreviations, see Fig. 23–3.) (From Tiberio,[30] with permission.)

the contact phase. The quadriceps works concentrically during the beginning of the midstance phase as the knee extends. The quadriceps becomes active again during propulsion and early swing as the knee flexes. Because the motion is flexion, this activity of the quadriceps must be eccentric.

Figure 23–14 shows that the hamstrings are active during the contact phase at the same time the quadriceps is working. Until now, our description of muscle activity has shown that when one muscle is active, the antagonist is inactive. The hamstrings and quadriceps exhibit a different pattern. It must be remembered that the hamstrings are powerful hip extensors as well as knee flexors. Before heel-strike, the hamstrings are contracting strongly to decelerate the hip flexion and knee extension. Once the heel strikes the ground and the forward movement of the leg is slowed, the hamstring activity prevents the trunk from flexing forward at the hip. The hamstrings' ability to prevent hip flexion and then accelerate hip extension is dependent on a stable distal attachment.

Hips

As the knee flexes during contact, the hamstrings' effectiveness is lost and the activity gradually ceases. To complete hip extension, the body "substitutes" the gluteus maximus for the hamstrings because the maximus is a single-joint muscle. Figure 23–15 shows how the activity of the gluteus maximus increase correspondingly to the decrease in hamstring activity. One might logically question why the gluteus maximus is not active from the beginning of hip extension. The hamstrings, being decelerators of both knee extension and hip flexion, are already active during the end of swing. It is efficient to use the

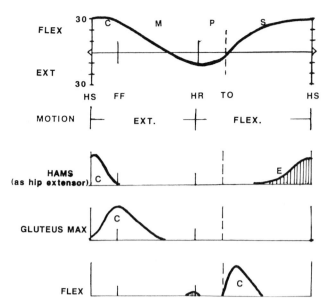

Figure 23–15. Selected muscle functions at the hip joint in the sagittal plane. FLEX, flexion; EXT, extension. (For other abbreviations, see Fig. 23–3.) (From Tiberio,[30] with permission.)

already active hamstrings as hip extensors by changing to a concentric contraction on heel-strike. This demonstrates the delicate interplay between joints and muscle that is present during efficient locomotion.

The primary role of the hip flexors is to accelerate the leg forward at toe-off. This concentric activity ceases by midswing. The hip flexors are also active just before heel-rise, apparently to limit the amount of hip extension, which peaks at this time.

The abductors of the hip begin to activate once the heel strikes the ground (Fig. 23–16), and their activity peaks during single limb support. The initial activity is eccentric, as the pelvis is shifting laterally over the stance leg. Once this lateral displacement is decelerated, the

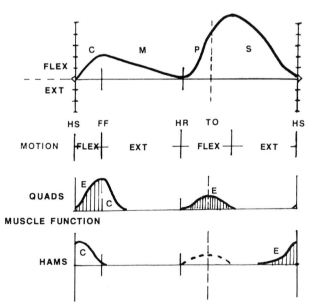

Figure 23–14. Selected muscle functions at the knee joint. FLEX, flexion; EXT, extension. (For other abbreviations, see Fig. 23–3.) (From Tiberio,[30] with permission.)

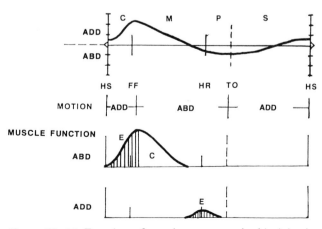

Figure 23–16. Function of muscle groups at the hip joint in the frontal plane. ADD, adduction; ABD, abduction. (For other abbreviations, see Fig. 23–3.) (From Tiberio,[30] with permission.)

abductors accelerate the pelvis back toward the opposite side. The hip adductors function at two times during the cycle. The purpose of these contractions is not clear, but the first may decelerate the abduction occurring as the body's weight shifts to the other leg. The second activity during swing may ensure proper foot placement at heel-strike. Figure 23–16 shows the activity of both groups of muscles that control the hip in the frontal plane. It may be imagined as the abductors of each hip playing "catch" with the center of gravity. One side "catches" the center of gravity eccentrically and then "throws" it back concentrically to the opposite side, which repeats the catch and throw.

Little is known about the hip rotator muscles. However, given the anatomic function of these muscles and the joint motions during gait, it would seem logical that the external rotators would work to decelerate internal limb rotation during the contact phase and to accelerate external rotation during midstance.

Ground Reaction Forces

Besides muscle forces, the ground reaction forces deserve attention. Ground reaction forces are created when gravity (and sometimes muscles) force the body against the ground, and the ground pushes back, as predicted by Newton's third law. The "collision" between the foot and the ground produces both translation (linear forces) and rotation (torques). These are measured by force plates over which subjects walk. In this section, only the translation or linear forces are presented. Most readers are familiar with the vertical ground reaction force. Figure 23–17 shows a typical ground reaction force pattern for walking.[2,3,18–20] There are two peaks to this force, one at maximum limb loading during weight acceptance and the second during propulsion. The second peak is often higher if the calf contraction at heel-rise is powerful and

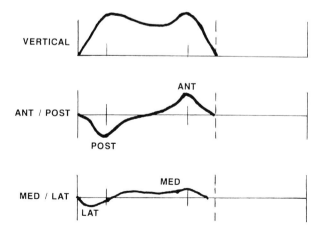

Figure 23–17. Ground reaction forces in three planes. The forces are equal in magnitude but opposite in direction to the forces applied by the body to the ground. ANT, anterior; POST, posterior; MED, medial; LAT, lateral. (From Tiberio,[30] with permission.)

if the forefoot is stable and the foot is functioning as a rigid lever.

There is also a horizontal ground reaction force that is directed anteroposteriorly (fore and aft). This reaction force (Fig. 23–17) is posterior when the heel strikes the ground and anterior during propulsion. A third ground reaction force occurs in a mediolateral direction. As the leg strikes the ground and internally rotates, the reaction force is directed laterally, but during propulsion, it shifts to a medial direction. Gravity, the ground reaction forces, and muscle contractions combine to exert large forces on the articular surfaces of the joints. This topic is beyond the scope of this chapter, but the reader should be aware that most of these joint compressive forces during dynamic activity are due to muscle contraction. The forces have been calculated to reach two to three times body weight at the hip and the tibiofemoral joint during normal walking.[20]

Running

Running is a natural form of human locomotion. As the speed of walking increases, the time during which both legs are on the ground (double leg support) decreases. As the speed of locomotion continues to increase, the stance leg will toe-off before the swinging leg contracts the surface. Double leg support is eliminated, and an airborne period is created. The locomotion is now running.

As would be expected, as the cycle time decreases, stance time decreases both absolutely and as a percentage of the cycle. The range of motion at the joints increases.[15] The increase in motion combined with the decrease in cycle time means that the speed of the joint motion increases dramatically. The muscles are required to decelerate more motion in a shorter period of time. In some cases, the mode of muscle function (eccentric or concentric) changes.

Since the advent of the running boom, running has been studied extensively. Walking was used as a reference for these studies, and emphasis was placed on the differences between walking and running. Although understanding these differences is important, just as crucial is an appreciation of the similarities between these two forms of human locomotion. During running, the primary function of the foot and lower leg remains the same. The leg must accept the body's weight, the foot must adapt to the ground, and the ground reaction force must be attenuated. Immediately thereafter, the body's weight moves forward, the knee begins to extend, and the foot propels the body forward. Joint motions consistent with these functions are present in both walking and running.[21] At ground contact, the subtalar joint pronates for surface adaptation, the knee flexes for shock absorption, and the leg internally rotates to allow synchronous motion from the pelvis down to the foot. The motions reverse during propulsion. The subtalar joint supinates to create the rigid lever, the knee extends to move the body forward, and the leg externally rotates to maintain synchronicity of the joints and to allow the pelvis to rotate with the swing of the opposite leg. The midstance or transition phase occurs rapidly as the stance phase time decreases.

The ground reaction forces are also dramatically increased. Figure 23–17 shows that the vertical ground reaction force for walking is just in excess of one body weight equivalent. Research on running has shown that this force increases as the speed of running increases and is in the range of two to three and one-half times body weight.[21–23] As in walking, there appear to be two peaks of the ground reaction force in most runners (sprinters may be the exception). The impact peak is gradual in some subjects but exhibits a sharp spike in others. Also, during running the anteroposterior shear force increases.

In 1980, Brody[24] described three different styles of running based on how the foot achieves ground contact. The foot can either (1) simulate walking with a heel-to-toe gait, (2) land simultaneously on the heel and the forefoot, or (3) land with a toe-to-heel sequence. This and other articles have associated these different styles with the speed of running. Although there is some correlation, it would be a mistake to assume that a runner uses a particular style based solely on the speed of running.

These different styles necessitate different motions at the ankle joint and therefore different muscle functions.[24] The heel-to-toe runner plantar flexes at the ankle on ground contact, putting more stress on the tibialis anterior. The other two styles dorsiflex on ground contact, placing more stress on the calf group (eccentrically). The landing pattern is also likely to alter which muscles assist the posterior tibialis in decelerating pronation. It may be that, from a biomechanical and rehabilitation standpoint, the importance of different running styles lies primarily at the ankle joint, which alters the potential for different musculotendinous units to be injured.

The Role of Clinical Analysis

Analysis of human locomotion in the clinical setting is an important evaluative procedure. Identification of gait deviations during walking or running provides information that may help the practitioner determine the cause of the patient's problem and/or decide on a particular course of treatment. Historically, gait evaluations were performed visually by the practitioner. Visual gait examinations provide valuable information when performed by the trained eye. Except for the identification of muscle contractions, visual assessments provide information on the kinematic aspects of human locomotion, information that complements other components of a physical examination.

Visual gait examinations have major limitations. Certain aspects of walking and almost all aspects of running occur too quickly for the human eye and nervous system to detect consciously. Also, the information obtained by visual assessment is very subjective, and no permanent record is available for subsequent analysis. Fortunately, with the development of video cameras and recorders, a readily available, low-cost alternative to visual examination exists. The permanent record created by the videotape combined with the slow-motion and freeze-frame capabilities of the videocassette recorder provides excellent clinical assessment of both walking and running.

Unfortunately, at present the standard videotape systems purchased for home use are not able to provide the type of kinematic data required by researchers. These data must be acquired and analyzed using equipment found only in specialized medical centers and research institutions. The data analysis is invariably performed by computer programs, whereas the acquisition systems vary greatly. High-speed film cameras, high-speed videotape, optic-electric, ultrasonic, and electromagnetic systems all provide the more exact measures necessary for scientific studies.

Information about the kinetics of human locomotion (muscle function and ground reaction force) is not commonly analyzed in the clinical environment. Electromyographic and ground reaction data from force plates or multiple transducer pads, when synchronized with kinematic data, constitute the optimal level of analysis of human locomotion. Adding to the problem are the errors inherent in two-dimensional analysis[25] and in systems with a maximum sampling rate of 60 Hz.

Motion can be abnormal if (1) its amount is too much or not enough, (2) it occurs too quickly or too slowly, or (3) it occurs at the wrong time. Too little motion may not allow proper dissipation of forces, which may increase joint compression; too much motion may generate excessive tensile forces on ligaments and muscle-tendon units. Motion that occurs too quickly may tax the ability of the muscle-tendon unit to decelerate the motion. Motion occurring at the wrong time will disrupt not only the primary functions of the foot but also the synchronous movement of the entire lower quarter.

Functional Kinematics

The importance of subtalar joint pronation and supination described previously is increased in the functional *chain reaction* concepts espoused by Gray.[26] From this perspective, the movements of individual joints must be analyzed in the context of a total body movement during a functional task. The tri-plane motion of the subtalar joint is linked to tri-plane motion in all the joints. The synchronicity described earlier becomes more important.

The contention that all joints move in three planes contradicts the classical classification of joints as uniaxial, biaxial, or triaxial. A more acceptable way to describe functional motion might be that there is significant motion and/or stress in all three planes. For example, the knee is considered biaxial, having sagittal plane (flexion/extension) and transverse plane (internal/external rotation) motion. But it is difficult to ignore the valgus and varus stresses on the collateral ligaments in the frontal plane. The motion that creates these stresses is small but observable, measurable, and important. Similarly, the bones and ligaments supplying integrity to the ankle joint are stressed by motion in the frontal and transverse planes during the uniaxial motion (dorsiflexion and plantar-flexion) in the sagittal plane.

The motions of the more proximal joints that are linked in function to the subtalar joint could be referred to as the *pronation response* and the *supination response*. Table 23–1 lists the motions in each plane that occur during the pronation and supination response of the lower extremity. The motions of the pronation response are caused by gravity and momentum in most modes of function. The motions of the supination response are the reversal of pronation. These motions are consistent with the individual joint motions described previously in this chapter. The pronation response occurs from heel-strike to just after foot-flat, when the supination response begins. During propulsion there are some exceptions to the supination response in order to minimize the vertical displacement of the body's center of mass. These exceptions are eliminated during running and jumping activities. The functional approach is an expansion of the classical concepts which allows greater insight into joint motion and, more importantly, muscle function.

Functional Muscle Actions

Also critical to an understanding of the functional approach is the link between muscle function and the prona-

tion and supination responses of the limb. If gravity and momentum accelerate the joints during the pronation response, then muscle activity would be primarily eccentric to decelerate the motion. The function of the muscle would change to concentric when the joint motions reversed during the supination response. The result is muscles working in the stretch-shorten (plyometric) mode. This again is consistent with the muscle function ascribed to individual joints previously. However, analyzing muscle function joint by joint limits our understanding of function. Should the gastrocnemius activity be assigned to the knee, ankle, or subtalar joints?

In the functional approach, all muscles are considered antigravity muscles. Their function can then be assigned by which motion needs to be decelerated. The anterior tibilias decelerates ankle plantar flexion, the quadriceps decelerate knee flexion, and the gluteus medius decelerates hip adduction. For any motion during the pronation response (in Table 23–1) the opposite muscle will be working eccentrically.

This approach may be simplistic for muscles spanning more than one joint. The hamstrings, for example, generate torques at the knee and hip. The functional assignment of the hamstrings during the pronation response would be to decelerate hip flexion (not knee extension) and then accelerate hip extension during supination. This is accurate because it focuses our attention on the hip, but it does not explain the affect of the torque at the knee joint. The hamstrings are performing an eccentric contraction at the hip, but the knee is flexing, suggesting a simultaneous concentric contraction ("econcentric"). Recently, researchers have turned their attention to this

□□□□□ □ □ □

Table 23–1. Motions for Each Joint in the Three Cardinal Planes

Joint	Pronation Response		
	Sagittal	*Frontal*	*Transverse*
STJ	Dorsiflexion	Eversion	Abduction
Ankle	DF/PF*	Eversion	Abduction
Knee	Flexion	Abduction	Internal rotation
Hip	Flexion	Adduction	Internal rotation

Joint	Supination Response		
	Sagittal	*Frontal*	*Transverse*
STJ	Plantarflexion	Inversion	Adduction
Ankle	Plantarflexion	Inversion	Adduction
Knee	Extension	Adduction	External rotation
Hip	Extension	Abduction	External rotation

* Motion depends on which part of the foot contacts the ground first.
Abbreviations: DF/PF, dorsiflexion/plantarflexion; STJ, subtalar joint.

issue,[27,28] and some have suggested that biarticular muscles can redistribute joint moments and powers.[28] The ultimate motion produced by contraction of multiarticular muscles may be dependent on the particular joint angle.

Inherent in the functional approach is the concept of the bone segments as a linked system instead of individual joints. This is not a trivial step because it then allows muscles to generate torques at joints they do not cross.[29] An important example during gait is the role of the soleus in decelerating knee flexion and accelerating knee extension. If the soleus decelerates ankle dorsiflexion, during gait it controls the forward movement of the tibia over the foot. If the femur continues to move forward at a faster rate, the resulting joint motion produced by the soleus would be knee extension. This same effect is seen with a floor reaction ankle-foot orthosis (AFO), which prevents the ankle from dorsiflexing. Similarly, the gluteus maximus can extend the knee by pulling the femur back when the foot is fixed (e.g., the method by which the transfemoral amputee extends the prosthetic knee).

Assignment of muscle function during gait has depended on whether the muscle is active and the direction of joint motion, but the locomotory system of humans is very complex. The functional approach causes us to pause when attributing a specific role to a particular muscle. Anatomic descriptions of muscle functions become insufficient. The ultimate effect of a muscle contraction depends on whether the distal segment is fixed, the position of the target and adjacent joints, the torques generated by muscles not crossing a joint, and the magnitude of external torques applied to the skeletal system.

■ Summary

Human locomotion is a sequential and synchronous activity which, when functioning properly, is a marvelous sight to behold. Its complexity becomes apparent when dysfunctions arise that present as gait deviations and when the gait deviations cause tissue symptoms. Determining the cause of the deviation, as well as the proper treatment approach to correct it, is often very difficult. Knowledge of normal human locomotion provides the template against which we compare our visual or videotape analysis. Understanding the sequential and synchronous relationships allows the clinician to find the cause of the patient's symptoms when this cause is not located in the same anatomic region as the symptoms.

Abnormal gait kinematics need to be considered from three different perspectives: the amount of motion, the speed and direction (velocity) of that motion, and the sequential timing of the motion in the gait cycle. When gait deviations are discovered, they must be analyzed in reference to (1) their effect on the primary functions of the foot and (2) the resultant tissue stresses placed on proximal structures or compensatory motions by these structures to avoid the tissue stress.

It is important for the practitioner who desires to understand and assess gait to have a comprehensive ability to assess the different segments of the lower quarter independently in both an open chain and a closed chain position. The ability to gain segmented information and then to put this information together as a whole allows the practitioner to begin to understand the causes of the gait deviations visualized and identified. There is much we do not know about human locomotion. The intricacies and the different compensations that occur in allowing an individual to walk are beyond our ability to measure, observe, or even understand. However, as we continue to strive toward a more comprehensive understanding of the biomechanics of human locomotion, we will be better equipped to offer our patients solutions to the causes of their problems with locomotion.

■ References

1. Schmidt RA: Motor Control and Learning: A Behavioral Emphasis. Human Kinetics, Champaign, IL, 1982
2. Saunders JBdeCM, Inman VT, Eberhart HD: The major determinants in normal and pathological gait. J Bone Joint Surg 35(A):543, 1953
3. Root ML, Orien WP, Week JH: Normal and Abnormal Function of the Foot. Clinical Biomechanics Corp, Los Angeles, 1977
4. Inman VT, Ralston HJ, Todd F: Human Walking. Williams & Wilkins, Baltimore, 1981
5. Inman VT: The Joints of the Ankle. Williams & Wilkins, Baltimore, 1976
6. Wright DG, Desai SM, Hengerson WH: Action of the subtalar and ankle complex during the stance phase of walking. J Bone Joint Surg 46(A):361, 1964
7. Isman RE, Inman VT: Anthropometric studies of the foot and ankle. Bull Prosthet Res 10–11:97, 1969
8. Sarrafian SK: Anatomy of the Foot and Ankle: Descriptive, Topographic, Functional. JB Lippincott, Philadelphia, 1983
9. Murray MP: Gait as a total pattern of movement. Am J Phys Med 46:290, 1967
10. McPoil T, Cornwall MW: Relationship between neutral subtalar joint position and pattern of rearfoot motion during walking. Foot Ankle Int 15:141–145, 1994
11. Pierrynowski MR, Smith SB: Rearfoot inversion/eversion during gait relative to subtalar neutral position. Foot Ankle Int 17:406–412, 1996
12. McPoil T: Invited commentary. J Orthop Sports Phys Ther 29:326–328, 1999
13. Levens AS, Inman VT, Blosser JA: Transverse rotation of the segments of the lower extremity in locomotion. J Bone Joint Surg 30(A):859, 1948
14. Gray GW: Manual: When the Foot Hits the Ground Everything Changes. Practical Programs for Applied Biomechanics, Toledo, OH, 1984
15. Mann RA, Hagy J: Biomechanics of walking, running and sprinting. Med Sci Sports Exerc 8:345, 1980
16. Ericson MO, Nisell R, Ekholm J: Quantified electromyography of lower limb muscles during level walking. Scand J Rehabil Med 18:159, 1986
17. Basmajian JV: Muscles Alive: Their Functions Revealed by Electromyography. 3rd Ed. Williams & Wilkins, Baltimore, 1974

18. Cunningham DM: Components of floor reaction during walking. Prosthetic Devices Research Project, University of California at Berkeley, Series II, Issue 14, 1950

19. Perry J: The mechanics of walking: a clinical interpretation. Phys Ther 47:778, 1967

20. Soderburg GL: Kinesiology: Application to Pathological Motion. Williams & Wilkins, Baltimore, 1986

21. Bates BT: Biomechanics of running. Presented at Medithon—A Multidisciplinary Seminar on Running Injuries, 1985

22. Frederick EC, Hagy JL: Factors influencing ground reactions forces in running. Int J Sport Biomech 2:41, 1986

23. Cavanaugh PR, LaFortune MA: Ground reaction forces in distance running. J Biomech 13:397, 1980

24. Brody DM: Running injuries. Clin Symp 32:1, 1980

25. Areblad M, Nigg BM, Ekstrand J, et al: Three-dimensional measurement of rearfoot motion during running. J Biomech 23:933–940, 1990

26. Gray GW: Rehabilitation of running injuries: biomechanical and proprioceptive considerations. Topics in Acute Care and Trauma Rehabilitation. Aspen Publishers, 1986

27. Gielen S, van Ingen Schenau GJ, Tax T, et al: The activation of mono- and bi-articular muscles in multi-joint movements. In Winters JM, Woo SL-Y (eds): Multiple Muscle Systems. Springer-Verlag, 1990

28. van Ingen Schenau GJ, Bobbert MF, van Soest AJ: The unique action of biarticular muscles in leg extensions. In Winters JM, Woo SL-Y (eds): Multiple Muscle Systems. Springer-Verlag, 1990

29. Zajac FE, Gordon ME: Determining muscle's force and action in multiarticular movement. Exerc Sport Sci Rev 17:187–230, 1989

30. Tiberio D: Course Manual: Foot Biomechanics and Orthotic Intervention. On-Site Biomechanical Education and Training, Storrs, CT, 1988

CHAPTER 24
Dysfunction, Evaluation, and Treatment of the Foot and Ankle

Ellen Wetherbee, Juan C. Garbalosa, Robert A. Donatelli, and Michael J. Wooden

This chapter briefly reviews the anatomy and normal and abnormal biomechanics of the foot and ankle. Various foot and ankle pathologies are also discussed with respect to pathomechanics, evaluation, and treatment. The pathologies include entrapment syndromes, traumatic injuries to the foot and ankle, and foot deformities. The biomechanical evaluation of the foot and ankle is also described.

■ Normal Biomechanics

Anatomy

Some 33 bones comprise the skeletal structure of the foot and ankle.[1-5] This osseous structure can be broken down into a forefoot and a rearfoot section. In the rearfoot, the osseous structures of clinical importance are the distal ends of the fibula and tibia, the talus, and the calcaneus. These four bones interact to serve as supportive structures and pulley systems for the various tendons that pass over the bones.[6] The tibia, fibula, and talus together form a hinge joint: the talocrural joint. Two types of motion occur at this joint: osteokinematic and arthrokinematic.[2-7] Osteokinematic movement is the overall movement of two bones without reference to the motion occurring between the joint surfaces (i.e., flexion and extension). Arthrokinematic movement is the motion actually occurring between the two joint surfaces (i.e., roll and spin).[5]

Plantar flexion and dorsiflexion are the osteokinematic motions occurring at the talocrural joint. Osteokinematic movement at the talocrural joint is governed and restricted primarily by the bony configuration of the joint surfaces. The primary arthrokinematic joint motions of the talocrural joint are roll and slide. Several ligaments help restrict the arthrokinematic movements found at the talocrural joint. These ligaments are the anterior tibio-

fibular, the anterior and posterior talofibular, the deltoid, and the calcaneofibular.[2-7]

A second joint found in the rearfoot, the subtalar joint, is composed of the calcaneus inferiorly and the talus superiorly.[2-8] Since the axis of the subtalar joint is located in three planes, a complex series of supination and pronation motions occurs there.[6] Supination is defined as inversion, plantar flexion, and adduction of the calcaneus on the talus in the open kinetic chain. Pronation, on the other hand, is defined as eversion, dorsiflexion, and abduction of the calcaneus on the talus.[4,6-8] These joint motions are governed by ligamentous tension and bony restraint mechanisms. The deltoid, anterior and posterior talofibular, and calcaneofibular ligaments prevent excessive motion from occurring at the subtalar joint.[3-5,7,9]

The rearfoot is separated from the forefoot by the midtarsal joint, which is composed of the cuboid, naviculus, calcaneus, and talus.[1-5] As in the subtalar joint, the triplanar motions of supination and pronation occur at the midtarsal joint. Triplanar motions at the midtarsal joint occur about two joint axes: longitudinal and oblique. The motions of eversion during pronation and inversion during supination in an open kinetic chain occur about the longitudinal axis. About the oblique midtarsal joint axis, the open kinetic chain motions of plantar flexion and abduction occur during supination and dorsiflexion, and adduction occurs during pronation.[6,7,10] Ligamentous structures restraining the motions of supination and pronation are the bifurcate, spring, short plantar, and long plantar ligaments and the plantar aponeurosis.[3-6]

The remaining osseous structures of the forefoot are the 3 cuneiforms, the 5 metatarsals, the 2 plantar sesamoids of the first metatarsal, and the 14 phalanges. These bones form several joints, of which only the metatarsophalangeal (MTP) and interphalangeal (IP) joints will be briefly discussed. The MTP joint is an ellipsoidal joint that allows the osteokinematic motions of abduction, adduction, flexion, and extension to occur. The IP joints are pure hinge joints that allow the osteokinematic motions of flexion and extension to occur. Both joints have proper joint capsules with accompanying supportive ligamentous structures.[1–5,7]

There are several muscles of clinical importance in the foot. The role many of these muscles play in the production of pathology in the foot is covered in the discussion of foot pathologies. Some of these muscles are the gastrocsoleus–tendoachilles complex, the peroneus brevis and longus, and the tibialis posterior and anterior.[2–5] These muscles are crucial in the rehabilitation of the foot and ankle.

Important neurovascular structures passing through and terminating in the foot are the posterior (which divides into the medial and lateral plantar nerves) and anterior tibial nerves, the musculocutaneous nerve, the sural nerve, the dorsalis pedis artery, and the posterior tibial artery (which divides into the medial and lateral plantar arteries).[2–5] The effect these structures have on foot pathology is further discussed in the section on entrapments.

For a more detailed discussion of the anatomy of the foot, refer to various textbooks on the subject.[3–5]

Nonweightbearing Motion

During nonweightbearing lower extremity motion at the subtalar joint, movement occurs about a fixed talus during pronation and supination, respectively.[6,11–16] The calcaneus will evert, dorsiflex, and abduct and invert, plantar flex, and adduct about the talus during pronation and supination, respectively.[6,11–16] The lack of talar motion in the nonweightbearing lower extremity is due to the absence of direct muscular attachments on the talus.[4,6,11]

During pronation, nonweightbearing lower extremity motion at the midtarsal joint consists of eversion about the longitudinal axis and abduction and dorsiflexion about the oblique axis. During supination, inversion occurs about the longitudinal axis and adduction and plantar flexion occur about the oblique axis.[6,7,10,13,14,17] The extent of permissible movement at the midtarsal joint depends upon the position of the subtalar joint. Supination of the subtalar joint causes a decrease in the available motion of the midtarsal joint; pronation at the subtalar joint causes an increase.[6,14,17–20]

MTP joint motion in the nonweightbearing lower extremity can affect the amount of joint motion seen in the forefoot and rearfoot joints. MTP joint extension will cause the forefoot and rearfoot joints to be placed in a closed-packed position. Therefore, a cinching up of the joints of the foot occurs. This cinching up is described as the "windlass effect."[4,12,21–23] It is produced by the attachments of the plantar aponeurosis onto the bases of the MTP joints and the calcaneus.[4,21] A minimum of 60 degrees of MTP extension is needed for normal MTP function during gait.[4,6,12,24]

Weightbearing Motion

There are some differences between weightbearing and nonweightbearing motion in the foot and ankle. These differences are a result of the gravitational and ground reaction forces imparted to the foot and ankle.[6,12,15,23]

One such difference between the weightbearing conditions is in the motion occurring at the subtalar joint. In the weightbearing condition, during supination, the calcaneus inverts while the talus dorsiflexes and abducts.[6,13,15,16,23] During pronation the calcaneus everts while the talus plantar flexes and adducts.[6,13,15,16,23] The chief difference between the two weightbearing conditions is the presence of talar motion in the weightbearing condition and its absence in the nonweightbearing condition.

During the gait cycle the previously cited events of lower extremity weightbearing motion can be observed. At heel-strike the subtalar joint is in a neutral to slightly supinated position, while the talocrural joint is in dorsiflexion. As the talocrural joint begins to plantar flex, the subtalar joint begins to pronate. Both of these motions occur as a result of body weight forcing the subtalar joint to pronate. Eccentric action of the evertors and dorsiflexors of the talocrural and subtalar joints controls this pronatory motion. When the gait cycle reaches the foot-flat phase, the subtalar joint is fully pronated and the talocrural joint has reached the joint's extent of plantar flexion.[4,6,8,15,23]

As the gait cycle continues, the subtalar joint begins to resupinate at midstance, reaching maximum supination at toe-off. The talocrural joint goes through a cycle of dorsiflexion-plantar flexion-dorsiflexion from midstance to the swing phase of gait. Resupination activity at the subtalar joint results from concentric muscle activity of the plantar flexors and invertors of the subtalar joint and external rotation of the lower limb. The dorsiplantar-dorsiflexion activity of the talocrural joint is due to eccentric and concentric activity of the plantar flexors of the talocrural joint.[4,6,8,15,23]

Midtarsal joint motion, as in the nonweightbearing condition, is dependent upon the position of the subtalar joint. Supination at the subtalar joint decreases the amount of available motion at the midtarsal joint. The midtarsal joint locks with subtalar joint supination. Pronation of the subtalar joint unlocks the midtarsal joint, causing the forefoot to become an unstable "loose bag of bones."[4,6,8,15,17–20]

Midtarsal joint pronation is seen from foot-flat to midstance of the gait cycle. The pronating motion consists of eversion along the longitudinal axis and dorsiflexion and abduction along the oblique axis of the midtarsal joint. Supination of the midtarsal joint is seen from just after midstance to toe-off in the gait cycle. Inversion about the longitudinal axis and plantar flexion and adduction along the oblique axis are seen during midtarsal joint supination.[4,6,8,15,23]

Eccentric muscle action of the invertors of the foot and concentric activity of the evertors cause midtarsal joint pronation. Supination is caused by concentric muscle activity of the invertors of the foot and ankle.[4,6] The extent of supination and pronation movements also depends on the subtalar joint position.

Both supination and pronation are necessary for normal function of the lower extremity. Concurrent pronation of the midtarsal and subtalar joints allows the foot to adapt to uneven surfaces and to dissipate and transmit ground reaction forces.[4,6,12,15,23] Supination transduces the foot and ankle into a rigid lever to transfer the vertical forces of propulsion to the ground from the lower extremity, thus reducing the shear forces transmitted directly to the forefoot during propulsion.[4,6,12,15,23] Supination and pronation of the subtalar joint also serve to convert the transverse plane rotations of the trunk and lower extremity into sagittal plane rotations.[8,12] During normal gait activity the trunk and lower limb rotate internally at heel-strike and externally at heel-off. The subtalar joint, in response to these transverse plane rotations, pronates during internal rotation and supinates during external rotation, thus acting as a torque convertor for the lower extremity.[6,12]

The chief activity at the MTP joints during weight-bearing activity is the dorsiflexion-plantar flexion motion of the toes. As heel-off occurs, the toes passively dorsiflex, then actively plantar flex as toe-off occurs. Passive dorsiflexion during heel-off tightens the plantar aponeurosis and cinches up the tarsal and metatarsal bones. This cinching up assists in the transduction of the foot into a rigid lever for propulsive activities. Plantar flexion of the phalanges, mainly the hallux, during toe-off acts as the chief propeller of the lower extremity.[4,6,21,23] Several sources in the literature provide in-depth discussions of the normal mechanics of the foot.[6,12,15,23]

■ Abnormal Biomechanics

Abnormal biomechanics will be discussed in reference to the weightbearing condition. The adverse effects of abnormal biomechanics are usually seen during the stance phase of gait. In the foot and ankle these adverse effects are usually the result of either excessive pronation or excessive supination.[6]

Excessive Pronation

Excessive pronation is defined as pronation that either occurs for too long a time or is excessive.[6] This excessive pronation takes place at the subtalar joint. When pronation occurs for too long a time, the subtalar joint remains pronated after the foot-flat phase of gait. If the subtalar joint exhibits more than 30 degrees of calcaneal eversion from foot-flat to the midstance phase of gait, too much pronation is present.[6]

Excessive pronation can be attributed to congenital, neuromuscular, and/or acquired factors. Only the acquired factors are discussed in this chapter. For further information on neuromuscular or congenital factors see Jahss' textbook on disorders of the foot.[25]

Acquired factors causing excessive pronation can be divided into extrinsic and intrinsic causes. Extrinsic causes are those due to events occurring outside of the foot and ankle region, in the lower leg or knee.[6] Two examples of extrinsic causes are gastrocsoleus tightness and rotational deformities of the lower extremity (e.g., femoral anteversion and tibial varus).

Intrinsic causes of excessive pronation are those that occur within the foot and ankle region.[6] These causes are usually fixed deformities of the subtalar and midtarsal joints.[6] Examples of intrinsic causes are forefoot varus and ankle joint equinus.

Both intrinsic and extrinsic causes can produce excessive compensatory subtalar joint pronation. The response to the extrinsic or intrinsic cause of excessive pronation varies from person to person, depending on the number of intrinsic and extrinsic factors present and the mobility of the subtalar, midtarsal, and other foot joints.

An alteration in the normal mechanics of the lower extremity occurs with excessive pronation at the subtalar joint. Pronation during the push-off portion of gait causes the foot to be unstable at a time when the foot needs to be a rigid lever.[4,6,15,16,23] If unstable, the foot will be unable to transmit the forces encountered during push-off.[4,6,23] This inability to transmit forces may lead to tissue breakdown within the foot (e.g., Morton's neuroma).[6] An added effect of an excessively long pronatory phase is disruption of the normal transverse rotatory cycle of the lower extremity, possibly causing pathology at the knee and hip.[4,6,18,23]

Excessive Supination

Excessive supination is much the same as excessive pronation; supination can occur for too long a time period or can be excessive.[6] As in excessive pronation, myriad causes ranging from congenital to acquired deformities may result in excessive supination.

An excessively supinated foot prevents the foot and ankle from absorbing shock.[4,6,23] The foot and ankle therefore transmit this stress up the lower extremity to the knee, hip, or back, possibly causing pathology.[6,12,16] Also, the foot remains rigid at a time when it needs to become mobile and adaptable (i.e., from heel-strike to foot-flat). Therefore, the foot is unable to adapt to uneven terrain, and the result is a loss of equilibrium (a possible perpetuating factor in repeated ankle sprains in the athlete).[6]

Excessive supination can also alter the normal transverse rotational events of the lower extremity.[6,18] This hindrance of normal rotational events may cause damage in the foot and ankle, as well as being detrimental to the remainder of the lower extremity.

■ Dysfunctions and Pathologies

Entrapments

Tarsal Tunnel Syndrome

Tarsal tunnel syndrome is an entrapment of the posterior tibial nerve and artery as they pass through a fibrous osseous tunnel located posteromedial to the medial malleolus.[26-30] The roof of the tunnel is composed of the flexor retinaculum (the laciniate ligament), and the floor is composed of the underlying bony structures. A decrease in the diameter of the tunnel may cause compression of the posterior tibial nerve and artery, resulting in symptoms.[28,29] The decrease in diameter maybe due to external or internal pathology.

Excessive pronation of the subtalar joint is an external pathology that tends to compress the tunnel. The laciniate ligament is stretched during excessive pronation, thereby decreasing the diameter of the tunnel.[27-29] Tendinitis of the posterior tibial, the flexor digitorum longus, and/or the flexor hallucis longus tendon is an example of internal pathology causing a decrease in the diameter of the tarsal tunnel.[26,28,29] Misalignment of the bony structures of the talocrural joint secondary to fracture can be considered a combination of internal and external pathologies causing a diminished tarsal tunnel diameter. All of these pathologies may compromise the tunnel either by occupying or by decreasing the space of the tunnel.[26,29]

Another purported cause of tarsal tunnel symptoms is entrapment of the posterior tibial nerve by the abductor hallucis muscle as the nerve enters the plantar aspect of the foot. The entrapment is caused by a tethering of the nerve, as the nerve enters the foot, by the abductor hallucis and the underlying bone.[30,31] This tethering stretches the posterior tibial nerve during gait activities.

Neuromas

Neuromas are fibrotic proliferations of the tissue surrounding the neurovascular bundles located between the metatarsals. The fibrotic proliferation is usually due to abnormal shearing forces between the metatarsal heads and the underlying tissues. An ischemic response of the neurovascular bundles is the end result of the tissue proliferation, ultimately leading to the symptoms felt by the patient.[6,26,30]

The pathomechanics involved in the formation of a neuroma are usually the result of abnormal pronation during the propulsive phase of gait.[6] Normally the neurovascular bundles lie plantar to and between the metatarsals. During abnormal pronation, the metatarsal heads of the first, second, and third metatarsals move in a lateroplantar direction while the fifth metatarsal head moves in a dorsomedial direction.[6,32] At the same time, ground reaction forces and the patient's shoe fix the soft tissues on the plantar surface of the foot. The metatarsal head motion establishes a shear and a compressive force. The compressive force is due to the metatarsal heads lying over the neurovascular bundles.[6] The result of these compressive and shear forces is fibrotic proliferation of the surrounding tissue in an effort to protect the neurovascular bundles.[6,26,30]

Trauma

Fractures

Talocrural fractures are the result of four basic types of abnormal force: compressive, inversion, eversion, and/or torsion.[33-35] Inversion or eversion fractures are usually accompanied by a torsional component.[34,35] An inversion or eversion fracture, with or without a torsional component, results in damage to the soft tissues and osseous structures about the talocrural and subtalar joints.[27,33-35] Depending on the severity of the injury and on whether the forefoot is in supination or pronation, a fracture of the medial and/or the lateral malleolus can be seen.[34-36] A possible concomitant injury is osteochondral fracture of the talar dome.[33-36] Disruption of the inferior tibiofibular syndesmosis may also be a consequence of an eversion or inversion fracture.[33-36]

Compression fractures of the talocrural joint are usually the result of a jumping incident.[27,33,36] In this type of fracture there is direct damage to the talus as a result of applied force. A secondary event may be disruption of the inferior tibiofibular syndesmosis as in an inversion or eversion injury.[33,36]

Metatarsal fractures generally involve either the first or the fifth metatarsal and can be a result of either trauma or excessive stress.[37] The mechanism of injury in a traumatic fracture of the first metatarsal usually involves an abduction and hyperflexion or hyperextension mechanism of injury.[27,33] In a traumatic fracture of the fifth metatarsal the mechanism of injury usually involves inversion of the foot. The peroneus brevis contracts forcefully to prevent the excessive inversion, thus avulsing the styloid process of the fifth metatarsal.[27,33]

Stress fractures are usually the result of hyperpronation of the midtarsal and subtalar joints.[6,27,38] The hyperpronation prevents the foot from locking. Instead of being transmitted up the kinetic chain, the forces of propulsion are dissipated within the foot, which is incapable of handling the extra stress of the propulsive forces.[6,38] Stress fractures can also be a result of a lack of pronation in the subtalar joint (the supinated foot). The subtalar joint is unable to pronate and therefore does not allow the forces of compression to be absorbed properly.[6]

Sprains

The mechanism of a talocrural sprain is either lateral or medial, with or without a torsional force component. In a lateral injury the mechanism of injury involves an inversion force. The injury may involve ligamentous damage occurring in the following order: the anterior talofibular, calcaneofibular, posterior talofibular, and posterior tibiofibular ligaments. As more ligaments become involved, the severity of the injury increases.[26,27,39]

Medial mechanisms of injury are the result of eversion forces. The deltoid and tibiofibular ligaments are usually torn in this type of injury.[26,27,39] An associated fracture of the fibula is the usual complication of an eversion injury.[26,27,33,36,39] Medial injuries are rare compared to lateral ligamentous injuries.

MTP sprains normally involve a hyperflexion injury to the joint. Capsular tearing, articular cartilage damage, and possible fracturing of the tibial sesamoid are seen in MTP joint sprains.[26,27] This type of injury is thought to be a causative factor in hallux limitus deformities.[6]

Tibiofibular sprains are frequently a secondary involvement of talocrural injuries or a result of a compression injury.[26] Fracture of the dome of the talus or of the distal end of the fibula is a possible complication.[26,36] The mechanism of injury often involves a rotational or compressive force with a concomitant dorsiflexion force.[26,27,36]

Pathomechanics

Hallux Abductovalgus

By definition, hallux abductovalgus is adduction of the first metatarsal with a valgus deformity of the proximal and distal phalanges of the hallux.[6,40] Hallux abductovalgus may be a result of hypermobility of the first metatarsal in a forefoot adductus, rheumatoid inflammatory disease, neuromuscular disease, or a result of postsurgical malfunction.[6,41,42] In all of these conditions a subluxation of the first MTP joint occurs initially, followed by dislocation.[6,41,42]

Classically, there are four stages in the progression of this hallux deformity. The predisposing factor is a hypermobility of the first metatarsal.[6,41,42] This hypermobility allows the hallux to abduct and the first metatarsal to adduct and invert upon the tarsus and the hallux. Abnormal pronation is usually the cause of the hypermobility of the first metatarsal.[6,40–42] Any structural or neuromuscular problem causing abnormal pronation or a laterally directed muscular force may lead to a hallux abductovalgus deformity.[6,41,42]

In stage one, a lateral subluxation of the base of the proximal phalanx is seen on the roentgenogram. Abduction of the hallux, with indentation of the soft tissues laterally, is seen once stage two is reached. Metatarsus adductus primus, an increase of the adduction angle between the first and second metatarsals, is the hallmark of stage three of the deformity. A subluxation or dislocation of the first MTP joint characterizes stage four, with the hallux riding over or under the second toe.[6]

Hallux Rigidus and Hallux Limitus

Hallux rigidus is a hypomobility of the first MTP joint. Hallux limitus is an ankylosing of the first MTP joint. A rigidus deformity may be a precursor to a limitus deformity.[6,27,40]

There are several etiologies of hallux limitus deformity. Hypermobility of the first ray associated with abnormal pronation and calcaneal eversion, immobilization of the first MTP joint, degenerative joint disease of the first MTP joint, trauma causing an inflammatory response of the joint, metatarsus primus elevatus, and an excessively long first metatarsal may all be precursors.[6,26,27] All of these precursors cause immobilization of the first MTP joint. As a result of this immobilization of a synovial joint, a limitus deformity occurs.[43–46]

The pathomechanics of a hallux limitus deformity are due to two problems: an inability of the first metatarsal to plantar flex or of the first MTP joint to dorsiflex. Abnormal pronation of the subtalar joint prevents the first metatarsal from plantar flexing because of the effect of ground reaction forces on the metatarsal. Ground reaction forces dorsiflex the first metatarsal during abnormal pronation. An excessively long first metatarsal can also prevent the metatarsal from plantar flexing.

Any trauma or inflammatory disease that causes bony deformation of the first MTP joint can prevent normal MTP joint motion. If this type of immobilization continues untreated, the end result will be a rigidus (or ankylosed) deformity of the first MTP joint.[6,26,47]

Tailor's Bunion

Tailor's bunion is the mirror image of an abductovalgus deformity of the first ray occurring at the fifth MTP joint.[6] Adduction of the fifth toe and abduction of the fifth metatarsal are seen in this deformity.[6,30] Four causes of Tailor's bunion are abnormal pronation, uncompensated forefoot varus, congenital dorsiflexed fifth metatarsal, and congenitally plantar flexed fifth metatarsal.

Abnormal pronation is reported to be a factor in the etiology of Tailor's bunion.[6] For abnormal pronation to cause a Tailor's bunion, one of the other etiologic factors noted above must also be present.[6] Abnormal pronation causes hypermobility of the fifth metatarsal. This hypermobility produces internal shearing between the metatarsal and the overlying soft tissue. As the deformity progresses, the events described in the hallux abductovalgus deformity occur.[6]

Uncompensated forefoot varus, exceeding the range of motion of pronation of the subtalar joint, causes the fifth metatarsal to bear excessive weight. This excessive weightbearing forces the fifth metatarsal to dorsiflex and evert. The dorsiflexion and eversion cause the fifth metatarsal to abduct and the proximal phalanx of the fifth toe to adduct, resulting in a Tailor's bunion.[6]

Congenital plantar flexion of the fifth metatarsal prevents the fifth metatarsal from dorsiflexing beyond the transverse plane of the other metatarsal heads. This plantar flexed attitude and abnormally pronating foot cause the fifth metatarsal to become unstable. Ground reaction forces force the fifth metatarsal to evert, abduct, and dorsiflex. Eventually the fifth metatarsal subluxates and is no longer functional.[6]

The last cause of a Tailor's bunion is a congenitally dorsiflexed fifth metatarsal. The only visual abnormality present is a dorsally located bunion. The dorsal attitude of the fifth toe causes abnormal shearing between the bone and the overlying dorsal soft tissues. This abnormal shearing is due to the firm fixation of the soft tissues by the shoe.[6]

Hammer Toes

In a hammer toe deformity, the MTP and distal interphalangeal (DIP) joints are in extension while the proximal interphalangeal joint (PIP) is in flexion.[6,30,48,49] Plantar flexed metatarsals, loss of lumbrical function, imbalance of interossei function, paralysis of the extensors of the toes, shortness of a metatarsal, forefoot valgus, hallux abductovalgus, trauma to the MTP joint causing instability, and subluxation of the fifth toe into pronation are all possible causes of a hammer toe deformity.[6,30] The common denominator among all of these pathologies is the production of a force imbalance across the MTP joint. This force imbalance may lead to a joint instability of the MTP or an imbalance of the muscles crossing the MTP joint.[4,6,30]

Claw Toes

A claw toe deformity occurs when the MTP joint is in extension and the DIP and PIP joints are in flexion.[6,30,48,49] The possible etiologic factors are forefoot adductus, congenitally plantar flexed first metatarsal, arthritis, spasm of the long and short toe flexors, weak gastrocnemius, forefoot supinatus, and pes cavus.[6,30]

Forefoot adductus, congenitally plantar flexed first ray, forefoot supinatus, and pes cavus all have the same pathomechanical effect on the toes.[6] The adduction angle of the metatarsals and the abduction angle of the phalanges increase. Instability of the MTP joints occurs as a result of this malalignment. The function of the lumbricales and flexors of the toes is altered as a result of the combined effect of instability and poor joint position. The alteration of these muscle groups instigates extension of the MTP and flexion of the DIP and PIP joints of all the digits of the foot.[6]

Arthritis of the MTPs leads to an overstretching of the restraining mechanisms of the extensor tendons of the toes, much the same as in arthritic conditions of the hand. This overstretching allows the tendons to drift laterally and alter their line of pull. Again, the alteration of the line of pull causes the toes to be abducted, and the claw toe deformity ensues.[6,30]

During heel-off and toe-off, the activity of the long toe flexors increases to compensate for the weak gastrocnemius. The increased toe flexor activity overpowers the extensors of the toes, resulting in a claw toe deformity. Spasm of the long and short toe flexors can cause a claw toe deformity in a similar fashion.[6]

Mallet Toes

The DIP joints of one or more toes are in a flexed attitude in a mallet toe deformity. The flexed attitude may be fixed or malleable. The etiology of mallet toe deformity is unknown. Some authors speculate that the condition is congenital or due to wearing shoes that are not long enough.[6,30]

Plantar Fasciitis

Plantar fasciitis involves an overstretching of the plantar fascia causing an inflammatory reaction, usually near the fascia's calcaneal attachment. The plantar fascia is overstretched, with pronation and extension of the MTP joint occurring simultaneously. Any individual who abnormally pronates during the push-off phase of gait is at risk of developing plantar fasciitis. The presence of a pes cavus foot also predisposes the individual to this condition, because in pes cavus the plantar fascia is already on stretch even when the foot is at rest.[50–53]

General Evaluation

Musculoskeletal Evaluation

A foot and ankle evaluation begins with a visual inspection of the lower extremity as a whole. Any muscular imbalances affecting structural alignment and possibly altering normal mechanics are noted. The examiner then focuses on the foot and ankle. Areas of redness, ecchymosis, effusion, edema, bony angulation, and callus formation are noted.[9,48,49] The visual inspection is followed by a palpatory examination. Any areas of tenderness and increased tissue tension are discerned.[9,48,49]

Next, a range-of-motion evaluation noting the amount of dorsiflexion and plantar flexion of the talocrural and MTP joints is performed.[9,48,49,54] For normal function of the lower extremity there should be at least 10 degrees of dorsiflexion and 30 degrees of plantar flexion of the talocrural joint.[6,9,55] There should be at least 60 degrees of dorsiflexion for normal function of the first MTP joint.[12,24,56]

A gross manual muscle test is performed next.[9,48,49] The musculature about the ankle is tested. For a more quantitative test of ankle muscle strength, an isokinetic evaluation can be performed. The examiner should expect to see normal absolute peak torque values at 30 degrees per second and at 120 degrees per second for all muscle groups tested. Peak torque values for ankle evertors and invertors should be around 21 ft-lb for men and 15 ft-lb for women at 30 degrees per second. At 120 degrees per second, the torque values should be around 15 ft-lb for men and 10 ft-lb for women.[57,58]

A general overview of the neurovascular structure ends the general screening evaluation. Areas of decreased sensation as well as areas of hyperesthesia are noted. A general circulatory examination is performed to establish circulatory integrity of the arterial supply to the foot and ankle. The dorsalis pedis and posterior tibial pulses are established.[9,48,49]

Specific Evaluative Procedures

Tarsal tunnel entrapment may be discerned by two specific manual tests: hyperpronation and Tinel's sign.[27,29,48] Hyperpronation of the subtalar joint decreases the diameter of the tarsal tunnel. During the hyperpronation test, the subtalar joint is maintained in excessive pronation for 30 to 60 seconds.[29] A positive test results in the reproduction of the patient's symptoms on a consistent basis. In Tinel's sign the examiner taps the posterior tibial nerve proximal to its entrance to the tarsal tunnel. A positive test again results in the reproduction of the patient's symptoms.

Along with these two manual tests, manual muscle and sensory testing are performed to determine the extent of nerve trunk compression. Weakness, as determined by a manual muscle test, of the muscles innervated by the medial and lateral plantar nerves may be indicative of a peripheral nerve entrapment at the tarsal tunnel.[27,29] Sensory tests are performed to determine the presence and extent of areas of hypoesthesia. These areas should correspond to the particular areas of innervation of the involved nerves.[26,27,29]

Electromyographic studies can be performed to further document the presence of tarsal tunnel entrapment. Latencies greater than 6.2 and 7.0 seconds to the abductor hallucis and the abductor digiti quinti, respectively, are indicative of entrapment of the posterior tibial nerve at the tarsal tunnel.[26]

The history obtained by the clinician will usually elicit complaints of burning, tingling, or pain in the medial arch or the plantar aspect of foot. These symptoms usually are aggravated by increased activity. The patient may complain of nocturnal pain with proximal or distal radiation of symptoms.[26,27,29]

During the general evaluation, the clinician may notice a valgus attitude of the calcaneus during static standing. This attitude of the calcaneus may be a predisposing, perpetuating, or precipitating factor in tarsal tunnel entrapment. One other evaluative procedure, a biomechanical foot evaluation, is also performed. In this evaluation other predisposing, perpetuating, or precipitating factors of tarsal tunnel may be discovered (e.g., excessive subtalar joint motion).[6,26,27,29] This portion of the evaluation is discussed in detail later in this chapter.

Patients with neuroma typically present a history of acute episodes of radiating pains and/or paresthesias into the toes. The onset of the pain is sudden and cramp-like. Initially, the symptoms occur only when the patient is wearing shoes that compress the toes; with time the pain may become intractable. The patient reports that the symptoms are or were alleviated by the removal of shoes and massaging of the toes.[6,26–30]

The chief physical therapy evaluative procedures in a patient with neuroma are a biomechanical gait analysis and a general lower kinetic chain evaluation to determine the perpetuating, predisposing, and precipitating factors for the development of a neuroma.

Fractures and sprains of the talocrural joint are evaluated in much the same manner. The major difference is that the clinician must wait until a fracture has healed sufficiently before proceeding with any evaluative tests, whereas in a patient who has sustained a sprain, the clinician may apply the evaluative tests immediately. The evaluation generally consists of obtaining a history, performing range-of-motion measurements, strength testing, noting the presence of edema or effusion, and noting the presence of any residual deformity in the foot and ankle.[27,33,36]

The osteokinematic motion of the involved joint is first assessed by range-of-motion testing. The joint itself, as well as the joints proximal and distal to it, are assessed. For example, in a talocrural fracture the range of motion of the MTP joints and the knee, as well as of the ankle, is evaluated. Once the osteokinematic movements of any joints have been assessed, the arthrokinematic movements of any restricted joints are evaluated.[27,33,36,59,60] Additionally, intermetatarsal joint play motion should be assessed to determine any lack of mobility secondary to immobilization.

Strength is evaluated using manual muscle testing techniques and/or isokinetic procedures. As in the range-of-motion testing, the joints proximal to, distal to, and at the site of injury are all tested.[27] If isokinetic tests are performed, the involved joint is tested at both slow and fast speeds.[58]

Circumferential measurements of the foot and ankle are taken to document the presence of effusion or edema. The flexibility of the heel cord is assessed to rule out heel cord tightness. A biomechanical foot evaluation may also be beneficial in assessing the impact any foot deformities may have on the patient's lower extremity.[27,33,36]

There are two added components in the evaluation of talocrural and tibiofibular sprains: ligamentous laxity and talar mobility tests. Three ligamentous laxity tests are used to evaluate the integrity of the talocrural ligaments. The first is the anterior and posterior drawer test (Fig. 24–1) to determine the integrity of the anterior and posterior talofibular ligaments.[9,27] The others are the inversion and eversion stress tests (Fig. 24–2). These tests evaluate the integrity of the calcaneofibular and deltoid ligaments.[27] Talar mobility tests consist of medial and lateral stress tests (Fig. 24–3). These tests evaluate the integrity of the inferior talofibular syndesmosis. Palpation may also be helpful in isolating the ligamentous tissues at fault.[9,27]

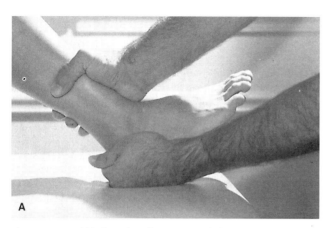
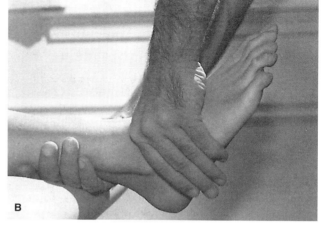

Figure 24–1. (A) Anterior drawer test; (B) posterior drawer test.

In pathomechanical conditions, the major portion of the assessment consists of a biomechanical foot and ankle evaluation and a proper medical workup. The medical workup is necessary to rule out systemic or neurologic causes for the presenting deformity.[6] Obtaining a good history from the patient may be helpful initially and later on when assessing the effects of any treatments.

One pathomechanical entity requiring a slightly different evaluative procedure is plantar fasciitis. Along with a history, medical workup, and biomechanical evaluation, the clinician needs to perform a palpatory evaluation of the calcaneal area. In the history, the patient will complain of pain and tenderness localized to the plantar aspect of the foot. The pain may radiate forward along the plantar aspect of the foot. Usually the pain is noted upon awaken-ing in the morning and worsens as the client increases the distance he or she walks or runs.

Upon visual inspection of a patient with plantar fasciitis, the clinician may note the presence of a cavus foot. Edema of the medial plantar aspect of the heel may also be seen on visual inspection. Palpation may reveal point tenderness localized to the medial aspect of the calcaneus.[27,50-52] Passive toe extension may also reproduce the patient's pain.[53]

Biomechanical Evaluation

The biomechanical assessment of the foot involves several steps. The evaluation begins with the visual inspection of the patient in a static standing posture, followed by static

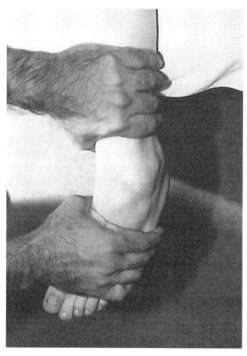

Figure 24–2. Inversion stress test.

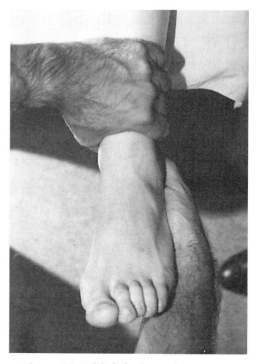

Figure 24–3. Medial talocrural stress test.

supine-lying, static prone-lying, static standing, and dynamic gait analyses.

Visual Inspection

The biomechanical evaluation begins with a visual inspection of the lower extremities while the patient is standing with the feet shoulder width apart. The clinician needs to have visual access to the patient's entire lower quarter. From the frontal view, the clinician will note the presence of tibial or genu varus or valgus disorders, toe deformities or attitudes, and the position of the forefoot. The posterior view of the client may reveal the presence of heel, tibia, or genu varus or valgus and the position of the talus (subtalar joint).

Static Supine-Lying Evaluation

During the supine-lying portion of the evaluation, the first step is to observe the foot for the presence of any callosities or deformities. Next, the range of motion of the first MTP joint is noted (Fig. 24–4). The angle of pull of the quadriceps muscle (Q angle) is discerned at this time. The angle is determined by aligning one arm of the goniometer with an imaginary line drawn from the anterosuperior iliac crest to the center of the knee joint and the other arm with the anterior border of the tibia. The axis of the goniometer will lie at the center of the knee joint. Finally, the amount of intermetatarsal mobility is evaluated by applying inferosuperior force and assessing the degree of resistance that is met by the clinician's hands. The above measurements are compared to those of the other limb for any dissimilarities.[6,27,48,60,61]

Static Prone-Lying Evaluation

The patient is positioned in a prone-lying attitude with both lower extremities over the edge of a supporting surface so that the malleoli of the ankles are even with

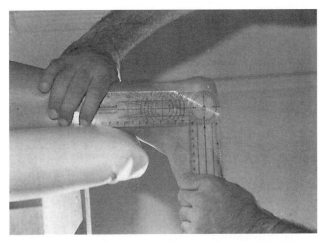

Figure 24–5. Goniometric measurement of talocrural joint dorsiflexion.

the edge of the surface. Visual inspection of the lower extremity consists of noting the presence of callosities and bony deformities of the foot and ankle.[6,27,48] Next, the range of motion of talocrural dorsiflexion and plantar flexion is evaluated with the knee in extension (Fig. 24–5).

One of the client's lower extremities is placed in slight knee flexion and abduction, with flexion and external rotation of the hip (Fig. 24–6). This posture ensures that the opposite extremity is in a plane parallel with the ground and the supporting surface, keeping the foot at a right angle to the floor. Longitudinal bisection lines are now drawn with a fine-tip marker along the posterior

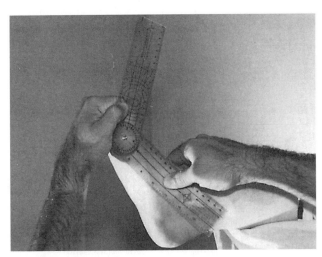

Figure 24–4. Goniometric measurement of MTP joint flexion.

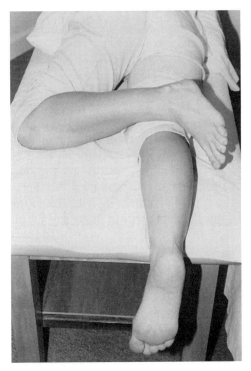

Figure 24–6. Prone-lying measurement position.

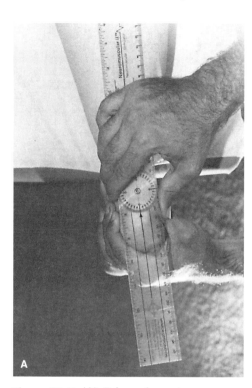 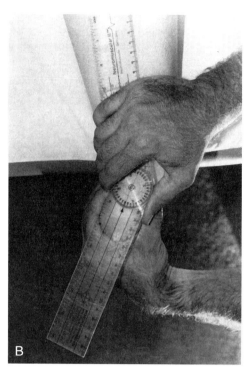

Figure 24–7. (A) Calcaneal eversion measurement; (B) calcaneal inversion measurement.

aspect of the lower third of the calf and heel of the lower extremity.[61,62] It is extremely important to draw these bisection lines accurately. The clinician should make every effort to choose the same anatomic landmarks consistently to ensure the reliability of present and future measurements. If the clinician ensures the consistency of the location and use of the appropriate anatomic landmarks, this procedure is reliable.[62]

Using the bisection lines, the clinician then measures the amount of subtalar joint range of motion. The clinician grasps the heel and the calf, as indicated in Figure 24–7. The heel is moved in one direction (into inversion or eversion) until maximal resistance is felt, and the angular displacement of the heel is recorded. The same method is repeated in the opposite direction.[61,62]

The eversion and inversion angles are summed to give the total subtalar joint range of motion. The total range of motion is divided by 3, and the quotient is subtracted from the average calcaneal eversion angle to arrive at the calculated subtalar joint neutral position (Fig. 24–8). From the subtalar neutral position, a minimum of 4 degrees of eversion and 8 degrees of inversion of the calcaneus in the frontal plane (or total subtalar joint motion) are needed for normal function of the foot.[22,61,62]

The subtalar joint is now placed in the calculated subtalar joint neutral position by grasping the distal third of the shaft of the fifth metatarsal and everting or inverting the foot. Great care must be taken to ensure that the foot is not dorsiflexed during this maneuver, as this may alter the forefoot–rearfoot frontal plane angular relationship.

Once the subtalar joint is in the neutral position, the frontal plane forefoot to rearfoot posture is determined by aligning one of the arms of a goniometer along the plane of the metatarsal heads and the other arm perpen-

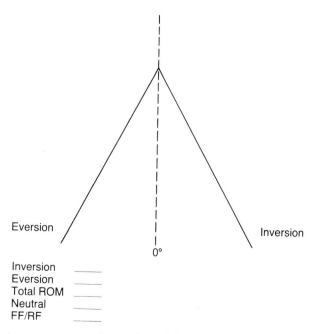

Figure 24–8. Static biomechanical foot evaluation form. "Neutral" equals eversion minus total range of motion (ROM) divided by 3; FF/RF is the frontal plane relationship.

dicular to the bisection line of the heel[61,62] (Fig. 24–9). The most prevalent forefoot to rearfoot attitude in an asymptomatic population has been reported to be a varus attitude. The least common attitude is the neutral condition. A normal forefoot varus attitude, as measured by a goniometer, is 7.8 degrees, and a normal valgus attitude is 4.7 degrees.[62]

One other instrument, cited in the literature, that can be used to measure the forefoot–rearfoot frontal plane angular relationship is the forefoot measuring device (FMD).[61–63] The preliminary measurement steps (e.g., subtalar joint positioning) are the same for the FMD as for the goniometer. The frontal plane relationship is measured with the FMD by aligning the slit on the posterior part of the FMD, with the bisection line on the posterior surface of the calcaneus. The plateau on the front part of the FMD is placed on the plantar surface of the foot, even with the fifth metatarsal[61,62] (Fig. 24–10). Two studies report the FMD to be slightly more reliable than the goniometer, but the difference is insignificant clinically.[62,63] The most prevalent frontal plane forefoot–rearfoot relationship using the FMD is also one of varus, with the average varus angle being 7.2 degrees.[62]

The possible influence of the gastrocsoleus complex on the subtalar joint can also be determined in the prone-lying position. Dorsiflexion at the talocrural joint with the knee in extension is compared to dorsiflexion with the knee in flexion. A dramatic increase in the range of motion of the talocrural joint with the knee in flexion

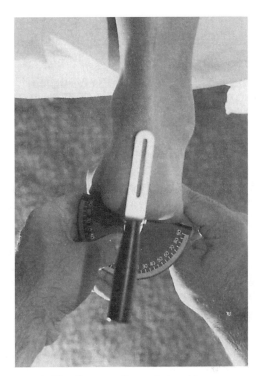

Figure 24–10. Forefoot–rearfoot relationship as measured by an FMD.

compared to extension is an indication that the gastrocsoleus complex may be affecting subtalar joint mechanics.[6]

Static Standing Evaluation

The amount of tibial and heel valgus or varus is measured with the patient in the static standing position and the feet shoulder width apart. The clinician uses a goniometer to measure the angle of the heel varus or valgus. The arms of the goniometer are aligned with the longitudinal bisection line of the heel and parallel to the ground to measure the amount of heel varus or valgus. To measure the amount of tibial varus or valgus, the arms of the goniometer are aligned with the longitudinal bisection line on the posterior aspect of the tibia and parallel to the ground.[6,27,48,61,64]

Gait Analysis

All of the above information is correlated with a dynamic gait analysis. The patient is instructed to ambulate on a treadmill or the floor, with or without shoes. The speed of the gait should be slow at first and progressively increased. The markings on the heel allow the clinician to observe the patient for variances from the normal sequence of gait. Recall that from heel-strike to foot-flat the subtalar joint pronates (the calcaneus everts). From foot-flat to heel-off, the subtalar joint resupinates (the calcaneus inverts). The relationship of the lower extremity to the body should also be noted. As the speed of the

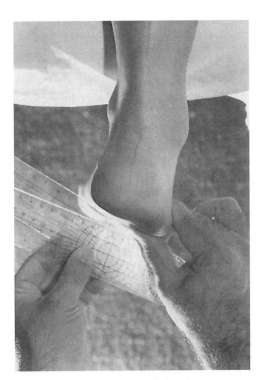

Figure 24–9. Forefoot–rearfoot relationship as measured by a goniometer.

gait increases, the extremity of the client should adduct slightly. Gait analysis is discussed further in Chapter 13.

Summary of Evaluative Procedures

The presence of a particular pathology is not based solely upon the findings from any one of the above evaluative procedures. Instead, the findings from all of the procedures should be correlated, and a decision on the particular type of or approach to treatment should then be made. For instance, the presence of a forefoot deformity (e.g., forefoot valgus or varus) by itself is not indicative of a pathology. The subtalar joint may be capable of compensating for this deformity. When the forefoot deformity is present along with some other factor (e.g., tight gastrocnemius complex), the subtalar joint may be unable to compensate for the deformity. At this time, the decision to treat the forefoot deformity by the use of biomechanical orthotics is made.[56,62,65]

■ Treatment

Entrapments

Treatment for tarsal tunnel entrapment should address the predisposing and perpetuating causes of the entrapment. Permanent biomechanical orthotics to control the perpetuating and predisposing factors of excessive pronation are an effective method of treatment. In cases where the tarsal tunnel symptoms are due to internal causes (e.g., tendonitis of the posterior tibialis tendon), an anti-inflammatory medicine may be prescribed by a physician. The physician may opt to inject the area with medication or prescribe the use of iontophoresis with an anti-inflammatory cream (such as 1 percent hydrocortisone cream).[66,67]

Conservative treatment of patients with neuromas of the foot consists of proper shoe wear. The patient is advised to wear wider shoes. Accommodative orthotics may be prescribed to relieve metatarsal head pressure on the neuroma as well as to correct the precipitating factor of abnormal pronation. Nonconservative treatment consists of surgical removal of the neuroma. For optimal results, nonconservative measures should be combined with treatments addressing the precipitating or perpetuating factors (e.g., biomechanical orthotics).[6,26,27,30]

Trauma

Treatment of traumatic injuries consists of three phases: acute, subacute, and postacute rehabilitation.

The acute phase of treatment follows the basic principles of protection from further injury, rest, ice, and compression and elevation of the injured site.[27,58,68] For the most part, the acute phase of treatment is a passive stage for the patient. This phase of treatment begins immediately after injury. Its duration is roughly the same for both fractures and sprains of the foot and ankle: 24 to 48 hours. Control and reduction of the inflammatory process are of the utmost importance during the acute stage.

The subacute phase of treatment is slightly different for fractures and sprains of the foot and ankle. Stability of the fracture site is still of paramount importance. Control and reduction of edema and effusion, prevention of muscle atrophy, and maintenance of cardiovascular fitness are key goals for the rehabilitation program during this phase of treatment of foot and ankle fractures. Elevation of the involved extremity, isometric exercises of the immobilized muscles, and the use of upper extremity ergometers are all recommended. The strengthening of uninvolved extremities to prevent disuse atrophy is also recommended.[27,58,69]

Treatment of sprains differs from that of fractures in that mobility is encouraged during the subacute phase of the rehabilitation program.[27,58] The patient is encouraged to begin sagittal plane exercises and movement. The exercises promote increased circulation as well as prevent excessive joint stiffness. Compressive supports (i.e., air splints) are used to provide stability and prevent an increase in edema when the involved lower extremity is in a dependent position. Partial weightbearing using axillary crutches is also encouraged. Isometric exercises with the peroneal muscles may also be of some benefit. As in the subacute phase of traumatic fractures, the control of effusion and edema and the maintenance of cardiovascular fitness are emphasized during the subacute phase of sprains.[27,58,68]

The postacute phase of traumatic injuries to the foot and ankle emphasizes the improvement of mobility and strength of the adjacent and involved joints and muscles. Once again, the treatment of fractures and the treatment of sprains parallel each other. The only difference between the two types of injury is in the areas of emphasis in the initial period of treatment. The initial emphasis with fractures is on the improvement of range of motion, both osteokinematic and arthrokinematic, of the involved joint, whereas the initial emphasis with sprains during the postacute phase is on improving the strength of the surrounding musculature and the proprioceptive ability of the injured joint. The strength of the invertors, evertors, dorsiflexors, and plantar flexors of the ankle is increased by the use of isokinetic exercises at high and low speeds. As previously mentioned, other involved muscle groups of the lower kinetic chain may also need strengthening. The final rehabilitation stage of both types of injury is a progression to functional activities. For the athlete, the final stage is a progression to skill and agility exercises (e.g., figure eight exercises).[27,58,70–72]

Specific treatments of talocrural fractures include mobilization of the talocrural, inferior tibiofibular, midtarsal intermetatarsal, and MTP joints. Initially, the arthrokinematic motions of roll and glide are restored through various mobilization techniques.[27,58,73] Two mobilization techniques used in treating the talocrural joint are posterior glide of the tibia and fibula on the talus and long axis distraction of the talocrural joint[59,60,73] (see Chapter 23). The glide technique is used to assist in restoring the osteokinematic motion of dorsiflexion and plantar flexion. A general capsular stretch is provided by the distractive technique. Osteokinematic motions are also performed along with the arthrokinematic motions. Usually the osteokinematic motions can be performed while the patient is in a whirlpool. The warmth of the water in the whirlpool can assist pain control and promotion of tissue plasticity. Heel cord stretching is also emphasized during treatment.[27,58,73]

Along with the improvement of movement and strength, the joint proprioceptors must also be retrained. This retraining consists of tilt board and unilateral weight-bearing exercises with the eyes shut and open.[70–72] Finally, in some cases, the prescription of a biomechanical orthotic may be of assistance in controlling any abnormal pronatory or supinatory forces that may be present. The use of orthotics may be of most use in those patients who have experienced a stress fracture of the metatarsals.

Specific treatment of MTP sprains consists of icing to reduce the inflammatory process, protective wrapping, and a nonweightbearing gait initially. Exercises that do not increase discomfort in conjunction with a graduated return to a pain-free activity program will follow. Mobilization of the MTP joint is performed when stiffness indicates this procedure to be of value.

Pathomechanical Conditions

As with entrapments, the treatments of pathomechanical conditions address the predisposing and perpetuating factors. These two factors are usually handled by the use of biomechanical orthotics, which control the abnormal pronation or supination occurring at the subtalar joint. The orthotics will also support varus or valgus deformities of the forefoot, if present.[6]

Other forms of treatment that accommodate or attempt to control the predisposing or perpetuating factors are heel lifts and accommodative shoes. For instance, decreasing the height of heels has been recommended for individuals who abnormally pronate because of intrinsic factors. Increasing the heel height has been recommended for individuals who abnormally pronate to compensate for extrinsic muscle problems (e.g., gastrocnemius tightness). Both of these heel height corrections have been recommended in the treatment of hallux abductovalgus conditions.[6,42,51]

Some pathomechanical conditions may require other forms of treatment in addition to the use of biomechanical orthotics or shoe inserts. Mobilization of any joints exhibiting limitation of movement, thereby causing abnormal pronation or supination, may be needed. Such techniques may be useful in the treatment of a plantar flexed fifth

metatarsal in a Tailor's bunion, a limitus deformity of the first MTP joint, and a mallet toe deformity. In conjunction with the mobilization techniques, the use of appropriate heating modalities has been shown to be effective in the treatment of joint hypomobility.[6,47]

Adjunctive treatments for inflammatory conditions of the foot and ankle include the use of cryotherapy to control any edema present. Iontophoresis or phonophoresis with 10 percent hydrocortisone cream can also be used to control the inflammatory reaction that is present with plantar fasciitis and to alleviate the presenting symptoms.[27,66]

Surgical correction of any deformities that are present is a promising alternative.[6,26] Surgery may also be the most effective treatment in cases where the predisposing factor is an excessively long metatarsal or elevatus condition.[6,43] Tenotomies of the flexor tendon with relocation of the tendon onto the dorsal surface of the foot are alternative forms of treatment in such conditions as mallet toes.[6]

Isokinetic strengthening of weak musculature, if present, is also advocated in pathomechanical conditions. Isokinetic exercises may also be needed in patients who have required surgery to prevent disuse atrophy from occurring during the recuperative period.

CASE STUDIES

CASE STUDY 1

MM is a 35-year-old competitive runner (masters level) with a diagnosis of plantar fasciitis of the left foot. His pain began 4 weeks earlier after a training run. The pain was centered over the medial plantar aspect of his left heel, radiating distally to the first and second metatarsal heads and proximally to the insertion of the tendoachilles (Fig. 24–11). Initially, the pain was localized to the plantar aspect of the foot. The heel pain was worse in the morning, improved by midday, and worsened by the evening. When MM trained, he was able to run approximately 6 minutes before he noticed an increase in the heel pain. He was able to continue to run for another 6 minutes before he had to stop. The pain remained elevated for approximately 30 minutes after he stopped running.

The past medical history was insignificant. Radiographs taken 2 weeks earlier were negative. MM stated that he was currently taking a prescription anti-inflammatory drug. His orthopaedist had injected a prednisone-lidocaine mixture into the plantar aspect of the left heel approximately 2 weeks earlier. The patient also stated that he was continuing to run but only for 2 miles. In the previous 2 weeks, his symptoms had remained unchanged.

Visual inspection was unremarkable except for a slight tibial varus bilaterally (calcanei are in neutral position).

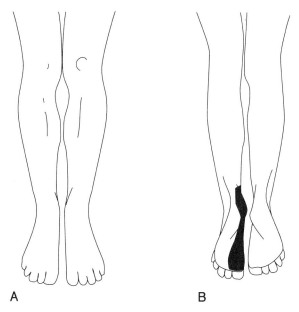

Figure 24–11. Pain drawing (see text for details).

Palpation of the left heel revealed an area of marked tenderness located over the insertion of the plantar aponeurosis. Extension of the MTPs with concomitant deep pressure applied over the insertion of the plantar aponeurosis increased MM's symptoms. A slight decrease in the intermetatarsal motion was noted during accessory joint testing of the left foot and ankle. Passive joint testing was within normal limits except for a decrease in dorsiflexion of the left ankle with the knee extended. The left ankle dorsiflexed to 0 degrees and 20 degrees with the knee

extended and flexed, respectively. Isometric break testing of the lower extremities was within normal limits.

The static biomechanical evaluation was significant for a decrease in left subtalar joint motion, bilateral forefoot varus, and bilateral tibial varum (Fig. 24–12). The dynamic biomechanical evaluation was significant for abnormal pronation of the left foot (foot pronated from midstance to toe-off). The extent of pronation (in terms of quantity, not duration) increased with the speed of gait.

Given the patient's area and behavior of pain, he appeared to be experiencing an acute inflammatory condition of a mechanical nature.[73] The source of MM's problem was not single but multiple, involving several structural and functional deficiencies that were acting conjointly to decrease his ability to adapt to the different stresses his left foot and ankle were undergoing during running. The functional factors were the limited intermetatarsal joint play, gastrocnemius tightness (limited talocrural joint dorsiflexion), and limited subtalar joint motion. The structural factors were the forefoot varus and tibial varus.

The interrelationship between the structural and functional deficiencies can best be highlighted by a hypothesized effect of tibial varus on subtalar joint mechanics of the left foot. To have the foot in contact with the ground during the foot-flat, midstance, and heel-off phases of gait, the subtalar joint must pronate to compensate for the degree of forefoot and tibial varus present. Unfortunately, there was no subtalar range of motion, which prevented the subtalar joint from compensating for the combined amount of forefoot varus and tibial varus. This lack of compensation was compounded by the inability of the metatarsals to compensate for the

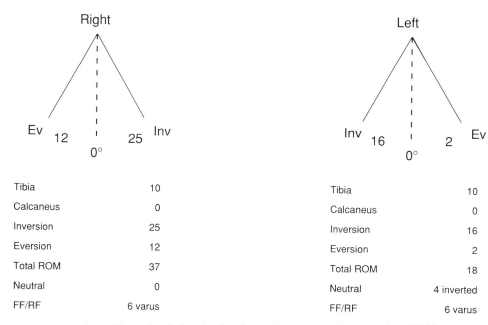

	Right			Left	
Tibia	10		Tibia	10	
Calcaneus	0		Calcaneus	0	
Inversion	25		Inversion	16	
Eversion	12		Eversion	2	
Total ROM	37		Total ROM	18	
Neutral	0		Neutral	4 inverted	
FF/RF	6 varus		FF/RF	6 varus	

Figure 24–12. Static biomechanical evaluation form. Ev; eversion; Inv, inversion; ROM, range of motion; FF, forefoot; RF, rearfoot.

forefoot varus by plantar flexing secondary to limited intermetatarsal motion. This lack of compensation on the part of the forefoot and rearfoot may place increased stress on the medial plantar structures (i.e., plantar aponeurosis), possibly causing damage to the tissues located there.[6]

Because MM's problem was multifaceted, the treatment plan that was initiated attempted to address several of the functional and structural deficiencies noted. A home exercise program was implemented, with the goal of decreasing the abnormal stress imparted to the foot, controlling any inflammatory reaction occurring in the foot, and improving the flexibility of the posterior lower leg musculature. The patient was instructed to discontinue running for 2 weeks, substituting a walking/cycling program, to apply ice packs to the left heel at night and after workouts, and to perform posterior lower leg stretches (Fig. 24–13). The walking/cycling program consisted of 30-minute pain-free workouts. If MM experienced any pain in his left foot, he was to stop the activity and apply ice to the left foot. Return to this low-level activity could begin if by the next workout there was no further increase in MM's symptoms.

An office-based treatment program was also implemented to help reduce the inflammatory reaction in the left heel, improve the mobility of the forefoot area, and reduce the abnormal biomechanical stresses in the left foot. The patient was seen three times per week for the first 2 weeks for 10-minute treatments of phonophoresis at 1.5 w/cm², using 10 percent hydrocortisone cream to the medial plantar surface of the left heel. The phonophoresis treatments were immediately followed by ice massage over the same area to which the phonophoresis was applied. At the initial office visit, a pair of temporary biomechanical orthotics was constructed using a 6 degree medial forefoot post and a 3 degree rearfoot post in an attempt to control the abnormal pronation. The patient was instructed to wear the orthotics for 1-hour periods alternating with 1-hour rest periods on the day he received the orthotics. He was to double the period of orthotics wear while keeping the rest period constant until he was able to wear the orthotics for an 8-hour period, after which he no longer needed a rest period. If at any time during this phase of treatment MM experienced any increase in his symptoms secondary to orthotics wear, he was to discontinue their use, ice the left foot, and inform the therapist.

After 2 weeks, the patient reported a significant reduction in symptoms. A return to a running program was now instituted. MM was instructed to start running approximately ¼ of a mile during his first training session and walk ¼ of a mile. He was to increase the distance by doubling his previous workout as long as he was pain-free for two consecutive workouts. Once he was able to run for 1 mile pain-free, he could continue to increase the distance of the run by half-mile increments while decreasing the walking by half-mile increments until he achieved his desired training level. Permanent semirigid orthotics were constructed with a medial 6 degree forefoot post bilaterally and a 3 degree medial rearfoot post with 2 degrees of motion. The rearfoot post incorporated 2 degrees of motion to help compensate for the decreased subtalar joint motion and tibial varus. At the 6-month follow-up exam, he stated that he was pain-free.

CASE STUDY 2

ML is a 35-year-old female who presents with primary complaints of pain posterior and superior to the medial malleolus bilaterally. The symptoms on the right are more severe than those on the left side. She is a recreational runner, who runs 5 miles four times per week. Recently, she has started experiencing pain during her runs. Initially, her symptoms commenced after running for 2 miles. Currently, they begin after running for 1 mile. The pain persists for 2 hours after she finishes running. Additionally, ML has begun experiencing pain when ascending and descending stairs and if she is on her feet for more than half an hour. Her past medical history is significant for a minor ankle sprain that she suffered approximately 1 year ago. She did not receive any medical treatment, and the sprain healed satisfactorily within a reasonable amount of time.

Visual inspection of ML was unremarkable. The patient reported tenderness to palpation along the posterior tibialis just superior to the medial malleolus. All resisted ankle movements were 5/5 in strength. Repeated resisted ankle inversion reproduced her symptoms. Goniometric assessment of the talocrural joint range of motion was unremarkable except for ankle dorsiflexion, which was limited bilaterally. ML exhibited 5 degrees and 7 degrees of dorsiflexion passively in the left and right talocrural joints, respectively. Passive ankle movements in all planes did not reproduce ML's symptoms.

A static and dynamic biomechanical foot and ankle assessment was performed. ML was positioned prone ly-

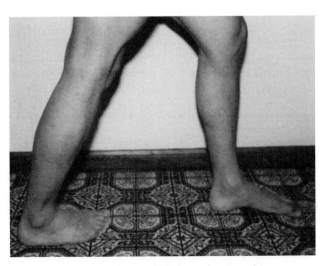

Figure 24–13. Posterior lower leg stretches.

ing, and the subtalar joint neutral position was determined. The neutral position of the subtalar joint was 10 degrees inverted for the right and 12 degrees inverted for the left lower extremity, respectively. With the rearfoot in this posture, a forefoot varus of 10 degrees was noted bilaterally. When ML was examined in weightbearing, the orientation calcaneus with respect to the floor was determined in two standing postures. With ML standing in an erect posture and the subtalar joints in a neutral position, a calcaneal position of zero degrees with respect to the floor was determined bilaterally. ML was now instructed to stand in a relaxed upright posture, and a calcaneal varum attitude of 7 degrees on the left and 4 degrees on the right was measured. ML's tibial varum was also measured with the subtalar joint in its neutral position while in double and single limb stance. Measurement of this angle during single limb stance is of special import for a runner because of the increased time in unilateral weightbearing during running gait. Tibial varum with the subtalar joint in its neutral position when in double leg stance was zero degrees bilaterally. In single leg stance, ML had 8 degrees and 6 degrees of tibial varum on the left and right lower extremities, respectively.

A visual inspection of ML's lower extremity biomechanics while walking and running was also conducted. During the initial contact to loading response phases of walking and running gaits, ML demonstrated excessive pronation of the subtalar joint bilaterally. The excessive pronation appeared to be off a greater amount during running.

Given the location of the patient's symptoms, provocation of pain with resisted inversion and palpation along the posterior tibialis, ML appeared to be experiencing tendinitis of the posterior tibialis. The excessive pronation seen during ML's walking and running gaits is an attempt by the lower extremity to compensate for the loss of ankle motion and skeletal malalignment noted during the physical evaluation. The excessive pronation has placed abnormal stress on the posterior tibialis creating the tendinitis. The control of pain and of the existing inflammatory process are the primary goals of the initial treatment program of ML. During the first week of formal treatment of ML, modalities and manual techniques were used to facilitate healing of the tendon. Ice massage followed by deep friction massage, as described by James Cyriax, were applied to the tendon during the first week of treatment.[74,75] After the massage, phonophoresis was administered at 3 MHz, 20 percent duty cycle, 0.75 W/cm² for 5 to 10 minutes to the tendon.[76] The physician was contacted to prescribe an anti-inflammatory medication to assist in the control of the inflammatory process. Additionally, ML was instructed to self-administer ice massages whenever her symptoms increased.

To address the loss of dorsiflexion noted during the passive range-of-motion examination, a mobilization program to the posterior talocrural joint capsule was instituted during the first week of treatment. In addition to the mobilization program, a home exercise program consisting of passive talocrural joint dorsiflexion stretches while in a nonweightbearing posture were instituted. The therapist must take the time to educate the patient about the correct form in which this stretch should be performed to ensure the avoidance of pronation of the subtalar joint during the stretch.

Excessive stresses must not be placed upon the tendon. Therefore, the patient was advised to discontinue running for at least 3 weeks. Alternate forms of cardiovascular training were suggested to ML, including bicycling, swimming, or running in a gravity-reduced environment (e.g., in a pool using a flotation vest).

During the second and third weeks of treatment, once ML reported less pain with walking activities, weightbearing heel cord stretching was initiated. Excessive pronation is prevented during this stretch by placing a wedge under the medial aspect of the foot. Ankle strengthening exercises using resistive tubing, weights, and isokinetics in all movement directions except for ankle inversion were initiated. Concentric and eccentric ankle inversion exercises were added to the program once ML demonstrated that she could invert her foot without provoking her symptoms. Eccentric exercises during this phase of rehabilitation were emphasized, as they have been shown to prevent the recurrence of tendinitis.[77,78]

By the third week of treatment, when ML was able to perform resistive exercises without provoking symptoms, a home exercise program was implemented that incorporated more functional demands of the lower extremity. The program included directions to discontinue these exercises if they provoked any of her symptoms. The home exercises consisted of light hopping on a compliant surface, as well as single leg balance activities to prepare the patient for increased weightbearing demands. If ML remained asymptomatic during these activities, a fast walking program with progression to running would be initiated.

The other aspect of this patient's management was the prescription of a biomechanical orthotic.[79–81] A semi-rigid orthotic with a 4 degree medial rearfoot post and a 5 degree medial forefoot post was fabricated. The instructions for use and wear of the orthotic were the same as in the previous case. The initial examination revealed that ML had excessive forefoot and calcaneal varus and diminished talocrural joint dorsiflexion. This combination of skeletal alignment and soft tissue tightness contributed to the compensatory excessive pronation that was present. Therefore, an orthotic was given to the patient to decrease the abnormal stresses that were being sustained by the posterior tibialis tendon. At the 4-month follow-up exam, ML continued to be pain-free and returned to her previous level of recreational running.

■ Summary

A review of the anatomy and biomechanics of the foot and ankle, both abnormal and normal, has been presented. Different pathologic entities, with their pathophysiology, evaluation, and treatment, have been described. A common bond between all the entities presented has been in the areas of treatment and evaluation. When treating these conditions, the clinician must be aware of adjacent areas that may require treatment. These adjacent areas are discovered through a comprehensive evaluation of the lower kinetic chain.

Much research, both demographic and cause-and-effect, needs to be performed in the area of the foot and ankle. Future research should address the effectiveness of different treatments of the pathologic entities. An attempt should also be made to establish normative data regarding the different lower extremity relationships and strength values. The foundation for a sound treatment program is sound research.

■ References

1. Bojsen-Moller F: Anatomy of the forefoot, normal and pathological. Clin Orthop 142:10, 1979
2. Jaffe WL, Laitman JT: The evolution and anatomy of the human foot. p. 1. In Jahss M (ed): Disorders of the Foot. Vol. 1. WB Saunders, Philadelphia, 1982
3. Moore KL: The lower limb. p. 491. In Clinically Oriented Anatomy. Williams & Wilkins, Baltimore, 1980
4. Sarafian SK: Anatomy of the Foot and Ankle: Descriptive Topographic Functional. JB Lippincott, Philadelphia, 1983
5. Warwick R, Williams PL: Gray's Anatomy. WB Saunders, Philadelphia, 1973
6. Root ML, Orien WP, Weed JH: Normal and Abnormal Function of the Foot: Clinical Biomechanics. Vol. 2. Clinical Biomechanics Corp., Los Angeles, 1977
7. Steindler A: The mechanics of the foot and ankle. p. 373. In Kinesiology of the Human Body Under Normal and Pathological Conditions. Charles C Thomas, Springfield, IL, 1973
8. Perry J: Anatomy and biomechanics of the hindfoot. Clin Orthop 177:9, 1983
9. Fetto JF: Anatomy and examination of the foot and ankle. p. 371. In Nicholas JA, Hershman EB (eds): The Lower Extremity and Spine in Sports Medicine. Vol. 1. CV Mosby, St. Louis, 1986
10. Elftman H: The transverse tarsal joint and its control. Clin Orthop 16:41, 1960
11. Digiovani JE, Smith SD: Normal biomechanics of the adult rearfoot: a radiographic analysis. J Am Podiatr Assoc 66: 812, 1976
12. Donatelli R: Normal biomechanics of the foot and ankle. JOSPT 7:91, 1985
13. Green DR, Whitney AK, Walters P: Subtalar joint motion: a simplified view. J Am Podiatr Assoc 69:83, 1979
14. Manter JT: Movements of the subtalar and transverse tarsal joints. Anat Rec 80:397, 1941
15. McPoil TG, Knecht HG: Biomechanics of the foot in walking: a functional approach. JOSPT 7:69, 1985
16. Subotnick SI: Biomechanics of the subtalar and midtarsal joints. J Am Podiatr Assoc 65:756, 1975
17. Hicks JH: The mechanics of the foot I: the joints. J Anat 87:345, 1953
18. Morris JM: Biomechanics of the foot and ankle. Clin Orthop 122:10, 1977
19. Inman VT: UC–BL dual axis ankle control system and UC–BL shoe insert: biomechanical considerations. Bull Prosthet Res 10–11:130, 1969
20. Phillips RD, Phillips RL: Quantitative analysis of the locking position of the midtarsal joint. J Am Podiatr Assoc 73: 518, 1983
21. Hicks JH: The mechanics of the foot II: the plantar aponeurosis and the arch. J Anat 88:25, 1954
22. Wright DG, Desai SM, Henderson WH: Action of the subtalar ankle joint complex during the stance phase of walking. J Bone Joint Surg 48(A):361, 1964
23. Mann RA: Biomechanics of the foot and ankle. p. 1. In Mann RA (ed): Surgery of the Foot. 5th Ed. CV Mosby, St. Louis, 1986
24. Bojsen-Moller F, Lamoreux L: Significance of free dorsiflexion of the toes in walking. Acta Orthop Scand 50:471, 1979
25. Jahss M (ed): Disorders of the Foot: Vols. 1 and 2. WB Saunders, Philadelphia, 1982
26. Singer KM, Jones DC: Soft tissue conditions of the ankle and foot. p. 498. In Nicholas JA, Hershman EB (eds): The Lower Extremity and Spine in Sports Medicine. Vol. 1. CV Mosby, Philadelphia, 1986
27. Roy S, Irwin R: Sports Medicine: Prevention, Evaluation, Management, and Rehabilitation. Prentice-Hall, Englewood Cliffs, NJ, 1983
28. Koppell HP, Thompson WAL: Peripheral Entrapment Neuropathies. 2nd Ed. Robert E. Krieger, Malabar, FL, 1976
29. Kushner S, Reid DC: Medial tarsal tunnel syndrome: a review. JOSPT 6:39, 1984
30. Viladot A: The metatarsals. p. 659. In Jahss M (ed): Disorders of the Foot. Vol. 1. WB Saunders, Philadelphia, 1982
31. Hendrix CL, Jolly G, Garbalosa JC, et al: Entrapment neuropathy: the etiology of intractable chronic heel pain syndrome. J Foot Ankle Surg 37(4):273, 1998
32. Oldenbrook LL, Smith CE: Metatarsal head motion secondary to rearfoot pronation and supination: an anatomical investigation. J Am Podiatr Assoc 69:24, 1979
33. Glick J, Sampson TG: Ankle and foot fractures in athletics. p. 526. In Nicholas JA, Hershman EB (eds): The Lower Extremity and Spine in Sports Medicine. Vol. 1. CV Mosby, Philadelphia, 1986
34. Segal D, Yablon IG: Bimalleolar fractures. p. 31. In Yablon IG, Segal D, Leach RE (eds): Ankle Injuries. Churchill Livingstone, New York, 1983
35. Lauge-Hansen N: Fractures of the ankle. II. Combined exploration-surgical and exploration-roentgenographic investigation. Arch Surg 60:957, 1950
36. Turco VJ, Spinella AJ: Occult trauma and unusual injuries in the foot and ankle. p. 541. In Nicholas JA, Hershman EB (eds): The Lower Extremity and Spine in Sports Medicine. Vol. 1. CV Mosby, Philadelphia, 1986
37. O'Donoghue DH: Injuries of the foot. p. 747. In Treatment of Injuries to Athletes. 3rd Ed. WB Saunders, Philadelphia, 1976
38. Hughes LY: Biomechanical analysis of the foot and ankle for predisposition to developing stress fractures. JOSPT 7:96, 1985
39. Leach RE, Schepsis A: Ligamentous injuries. p. 193. In Yablon IG, Segal D, Leach RE (eds): Ankle Injuries. Churchill Livingstone, New York, 1983

40. Mann RA, Coughlin MJ: Hallux valgus and complications of hallux valgus. p. 65. In Mann RA (ed): Surgery of the Foot. 5th Ed. CV Mosby, St. Louis, 1986

41. Greensburg GS: Relationship of hallux abductus angle and first metatarsal angle to severity of pronation. J Am Podiatr Assoc 69:29, 1979

42. Subotnick SI: Equinus deformity as it affects the forefoot. J Am Podiatr Assoc 61:423, 1971

43. Akeson WH, Amiel D, Woo S: Immobility effects of synovial joints: the pathomechanics of joint contracture. Biorheology 17:95, 1980

44. Enneking W, Horowitz M: The intra-articular effects of immobilization on the human knee. J Bone Joint Surg 54(A):973, 1972

45. Woo S, Matthews JV, Akeson WH, et al: Connective tissue response to immobility: correlative study of biomechanical and biochemical measurements of normal and immobilized rabbit knees. Arthritis Rheum 18:257, 1975

46. Donatelli R, Owens-Burkart H: Effects of immobilization on the extensibility of periarticular connective tissue. JOSPT 3:67, 1981

47. Kelikan H: The hallux. p. 539. In Mann RA (ed): Surgery of the Foot. 5th Ed. CV Mosby, St. Louis, 1986

48. Hoppenfeld S: Physical examination of the foot and ankle. p. 197. In Hoppenfeld S (ed): Physical Examination of the Spine and Extremities. Appleton-Century-Crofts, New York, 1976

49. Mann RA: Principles of examination of the foot and ankle. p. 31. In Mann RA (ed): Surgery of the Foot. 5th Ed. CV Mosby, St. Louis, 1986

50. Marshall RN: Foot mechanics and joggers' injuries. NZ Med J 88:288, 1978

51. Aronson NG, Winston L, Cohen RI, et al: Some aspects of problems in runners: treatment and prevention. J Am Podiatr Assoc 67:595, 1977

52. Leach RE, DiIorio E, Harney RA: Pathologic hindfoot conditions in the athlete. Clin Orthop 177:116, 1983

53. Turek SL: The foot and ankle. p. 1407. In Orthopaedics: Principles and Their Applications. Vol. 2. 4th Ed. JB Lippincott, Philadelphia, 1984

54. Stolov WC, Cole TM, Tobis JS: Evaluation of the patient: goniometry; muscle testing. p. 17. In Krusen FH, Kottke FJ, Ellwood PM (eds): Physical Medicine and Rehabilitation. WB Saunders, Philadelphia, 1971

55. Adelaar RS: The practical biomechanics of running. Am J Sports Med 14:497, 1986

56. Biossonault W, Donatelli R: The influence of hallux extension on the foot during ambulation. JOSPT 5:240, 1984

57. Wong DLK, Glasheen-Wray M, Andrew LF: Isokinetic evaluation of the ankle invertors and evertors. JOSPT 5:246, 1984

58. Davies GJ: Subtalar joint, ankle joint, and shin pain testing and rehabilitation. p. 123. In Davies GJ (ed): A Compendium of Isokinetics in Clinical Usage and Clinical Notes. S&S Publishers, LaCrosse, WI, 1984

59. Maitland GD: Peripheral Manipulation. 2nd Ed. Butterworths, Boston, 1977

60. Mennell JM: Joint Pain: Diagnosis and Treatment Using Manipulative Techniques. Little, Brown, Boston, 1964

61. Root ML, Orien WP, Weed JH: Biomechanical Examination of the Foot. Vol. 1. Clinical Biomechanics Corp., Los Angeles, 1971

62. Garbalosa JC, McClure M, Catlin PA, et al: Normal angular relationship of the forefoot to the rearfoot in the frontal plane. JOSPT 20(4):200, 1994

63. Lohmann KN, Rayhel HE, Schneirwind WP, et al: Static measurement of the tibia vara: reliability and effect of lower extremity position. Phys Ther 67:196, 1987

64. Murphy P: Orthoses: not the sole solution for running ailments. Phys Sportsmed 14:164, 1986

65. Harris PR: Iontophorsesis: clinical research in musculoskeletal inflammatory conditions. JOSPT 4:109, 1982

66. Boone DC: Applications of iontophoresis. p. 99. In Wolf S (ed): Clinics in Physical Therapy: Electrotherapy. Churchill Livingstone, New York, 1986

67. Sims D: Effects of positioning on ankle edema. JOSPT 8:30, 1986

68. Nicholas JA, Hershman EB (eds): The Lower Extremity and Spine in Sports Medicine. Vols. 1. and 2. CV Mosby, Philadelphia, 1986

69. DeCarlo MS, Talbot RW: Evaluation of ankle joint proprioception following injection of the anterior talofibular ligament. JOSPT 8:70, 1986

70. Rebman LW: Ankle injuries: clinical observations. JOSPT 8:153, 1986

71. Smith RW, Reischl SF: Treatment of ankle sprains in young athletes. Am J Sports Med 14:465, 1986

72. Kessler RM, Hertling D: The ankle and hindfoot. p. 448. In Kessler RM, Hertling D (eds): Management of Common Musculoskeletal Disorders: Physical Therapy Principles and Methods. Harper & Row, Philadelphia, 1983

73. Cummings GS: Orthopedic Series. Vol. 1. Stokesville Publishing Co., Atlanta, 1992

74. Davidson CJ, Ganion LR, Gehlsen GM, et al: Rat tendon morphologic and functional changes resulting from soft tissue mobilization. Med Sci Sports Exerc 29(3):313, 1997

75. Cyriax J, Coldham M: Textbook of Orthopaedic Medicine. Bailliere Tindall, London, 1984

76. Cameron MH: Physical Agents in Rehabilitation. From Research to Practice. WB Saunders, Philadelphia, 1999

77. Alfredson H, Pieteila T, Jonsson P, et al: Heavy-load eccentric calf muscle training for treatment of chronic achilles tendinosis. Am J Sports Med 26(3):360, 1998

78. Fyfe I, Stanish WD: The use of eccentric training and stretching in the treatment and prevention of tendon injuries. Clin Sports Med 11(3):601, 1992

79. McPoil TG, Hunt GC: Evaluation and management of foot and ankle disorders: present problems and future directions. JOSPT 21(6):381, 1995

80. Gross MT: Lower quarter screening for skeletal malalignment—suggestions for orthotics and shoewear. JOSPT 21(6):389, 1995

81. Johanson MA, Donatelli R., Wooden M, et al: Effects of three different posting methods on controlling abnormal subtalar pronation. Phys Ther 74(2):149, 1994

CHAPTER 25

Foot Orthotics: An Overview of Rationale, Assessment, and Fabrications

Stephanie Hoffman and Monique Ronayne Peterson

Biomechanical orthotics, also known as *functional orthotics,* are often used in the treatment of abnormal foot mechanics. As the foot hits the ground a series of abnormal compensations occur based on the mechanics and alignment of the foot and/or lower leg. A chain reaction then translates superiorly and inferiorly, depending on the ground reaction forces, weight of the body, and rotational forces. The types of orthotics are as diverse as the variety of foot types. For the clinician this diversity presents a great challenge in providing the most appropriate custom device.

This chapter includes criteria for orthotic prescriptions based on a lower extremity biomechanical evaluation and patient needs. Nonweightbearing as well as weightbearing evaluation techniques will be discussed. A brief review of gait analysis, including observational and computerized assessments, will be reviewed. Pathomechanics will also be discussed, with emphasis on compensatory pronation and supination. The use of functional orthotics to assist in reducing compensations will be reviewed. Accommodative orthotic intervention will be reviewed. Also, specialty areas such as the diabetic foot and pediatrics. Orthotic fabrication including in-office and laboratory techniques will be discussed. Finally, casting in subtalar joint neutral, corrective additions, and break-in techniques will be reviewed.

■ Criteria for Orthotics

A thorough history is an essential factor with orthotic prescription. Questions regarding symptoms and their relationship to overuse or repetitive strain from a sport or occupation should be covered. If the injury is sport related, questions regarding various terrains, training schedule, and the type of footwear should be asked. If the injury is work related, information regarding how much time one spends walking, standing, and lifting should be assessed. Any history of underlying diseases should also be obtained, including osteoarthritis, rheumatoid arthritis, or diabetes. Recent trauma or surgeries should also be discussed. Age, weight, height, and shoe types are also factors which will need to be covered when fitting a patient for orthotics.

Once the history is completed, a thorough lower extremity biomechanical evaluation should be performed prior to issuing orthotics. Muscle imbalances or soft tissue restrictions affecting the lower extremities should be addressed first. The objective evaluation begins with the patient supine, followed by prone, static, and dynamic movements and gait analysis (Fig. 25–1). Specific evaluation tests not covered in previous chapters will be described.

■ Lower Extremity Biomechanical Evaluation

Supine

Sacroiliac Joint/Leg Length Difference

The supine evaluation begins by assessing the sacroiliac (SI) joint by palpating the anterior superior iliac spines (ASIS) and checking for symmetry, followed by assessing the symmetry of the pubic tubercles. It is well documented that a posterior rotated innominate corresponds with an apparently lengthened leg, and an anterior innominate is related to an apparently shortened leg.[1] A thorough pelvic evaluation is presented in Chapter 19. Once the SI joint has been cleared of dysfunction and the pelvis is balanced with the lower limbs, the leg length can be assessed. This is measured from the ASIS to the medial or lateral malleolus and compared to the measurement of the other limb to determine if a structural leg length

Supine

Sacroiliac joint _____

Leg length difference _____ (or L _____ R _____)

    Flexibility

Hip IR/ER w/hip flex.	L _____	R _____
Hip IR/ER w/hip ext.	L _____	R _____
Hip flexors	L _____	R _____
Hamstrings	L _____	R _____
Iliotibial band	L _____	R _____
Femoral torsion	L _____	R _____
Tibial torsion	L _____	R _____

Knee

Palpation _____

Q angle	L _____	R _____

P-F tracking _____

Strength/VMO tone _____

Menicus testing	L _____	R _____
Collateral ligaments	L _____	R _____
ACL/PCL	L _____	R _____

Ankle-Foot

Palpation _____

Strength _____

Hallux valgus	L _____	R _____
Hallux dorsiflexion	L _____	R _____

Toe deviations _____

Calcaneal exostosis	L _____	R _____

Callus formation

Foot picture to mark callus

First ray

Position	L _____	R _____
Mobility	L _____	R _____

Midtarsal joint mobility

Longitudinal axis	L _____	R _____
Oblique axis	L _____	R _____

Prone

Ankle-Foot

Dorsiflex. in STJN w/knee ext.	L _____	R _____
Dorsiflex. in STJN w/knee flex.	L _____	R _____

Subtalar joint

Calcaneal inversion	L _____	R _____
Calcaneal eversion	L _____	R _____
Neutral subtalar jt.	L _____	R _____

Forefoot position

In STJN	L _____	R _____

STANDING

Genu valgus/varus	L _____	R _____
Recurvatum	L _____	R _____
Navicular height/drop	L _____	R _____
Tibial val/var in STJN	L _____	R _____
Calcaneal val/var in STJN	L _____	R _____
Calcaneal val/var wt.-bearing	L _____	R _____

GAIT

Heel-strike _____

Midstance _____

Push-off _____

Leg position ER/IR _____

Forefoot position ABD/ADD _____

Angle of gait _____

Running _____

_____

Proprioception

    Eyes open _____

    Eyes closed _____

Miscellaneous _____

_____

_____

Figure 25–1. Objective lower quarter biomechanical evaluation form.

difference is present.[2] A leg length difference of 1 to 1.5 cm is considered normal, yet even this amount can be pathologic.[2]

Muscle Flexibility

Next, hip, knee, and ankle muscle and soft tissue mobility need to be assessed. The testing is well documented in Chapter 14. Soft tissue restrictions, which can contribute to the pathomechanics, should be addressed prior to issuing an orthotic.

Femoral Torsion

Femoral torsion is measured by first palpating the lateral greater trochanter. Then passively rotate the femur medially and laterally until the most lateral prominence of the trochanter is felt under the thenar eminence. The angle

measured from the femoral condyles with respect to 90 degrees vertical will determine the amount of torsion (Fig. 25–2). This test can also be completed prone with the knee flexed to 90 degrees, followed by palpating the maximum lateral prominence of the trochanter while rotating the leg. In this position, the amount of femoral torsion is based on the goniometric measurement between the tibia and 90 degrees vertical.[3] The mean angle in adults is 8 to 15 degrees of antetorsion/anteversion.[2,4]

Tibial Torsion

To assess tibial torsion, the femoral condyles or patella are aligned in the frontal plane (parallel with the horizontal). Then the angle of the malleoli with the horizontal (representation of the tibiofemoral joint axis) is measured (Fig. 25–3). Normal adult tibial torsion ranges from 15 to 30 degrees of external torsion.[4]

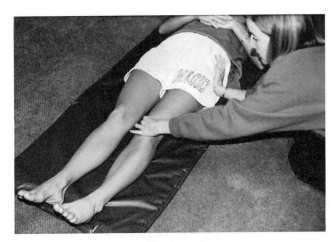

Figure 25–2. Femoral torsion.

Knee Joint

If knee symptoms exist, a full knee evaluation should be completed. See Chapter 21 for a detailed knee evaluation. If knee symptoms persist after rehabilitation and pathomechanics exist, orthotics may be a useful adjunct.

Ankle/Foot

First, a visual inspection is completed, assessing the foot for toe deviations and/or calluses which may be a result of abnormal biomechanics. This topic is covered in Chapter 24. The first metatarsophalangeal (MTP) joint should be able to dorsiflex at least 60 degrees for functional gait. A medial callus along the first toe can be related to hallux valgus. This is due to the push-off phase of gait occurring at the medial aspect of the hallux versus the plantar surface. Calluses along the plantar surface of the second, third, or fourth metatarsal heads can be related to poor

first ray stability during the push-off phase of gait. This can occur with excessive pronation.

Midtarsal Joint

To assess midtarsal or transtarsal joint mobility, the calcaneus is held with one hand and the distal region of the second through fifth metatarsals is held with the other hand. While inverting and holding the calcaneus, move the forefoot through inversion and eversion. Repeat the inversion/eversion movements of the forefoot with the calcaneus everted and compare the amount of motion in both positions (Fig. 25–4). Normally, there should be less mobility of the metatarsals with the calcaneus inverted (the subtalar joint locked in supination) due to the locking of the midtarsal joint.[5,6] If excessive movement is noted, then there is laxity along the midtarsal joint's longitudinal axis. To assess the oblique axis of the midtarsal joint, the forefoot should be moved through abduction/dorsiflexion and adduction/plantar flexion with the calcaneus inverted and then everted. Mobility is then compared. Excessive movement with the calcaneus inverted reveals oblique axis laxity. Laxity or hypermobility of the midtarsal joint can be a factor in excessive pronation, causing poor stability with the push-off phase of gait during propulsion.[7]

First Ray Position and Mobility

The first ray consists of the first metatarsal and the first or medial cuneiform. The position of the first ray is assessed by stabilizing the second through fifth metatarsal heads with one hand and grasping the first metatarsal head with the other hand. A plantar flexed first ray exists if the first metatarsal head is lower than the other metatarsal heads. If the first metatarsal head is even with the other metatarsal heads, it is neutral (Fig. 25–5). If it is above the other metatarsal heads, it is considered dorsiflexed.

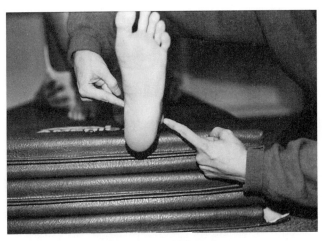

Figure 25–3. Tibial torsion.

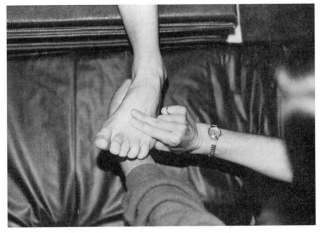

Figure 25–4. Midtarsal joint mobility.

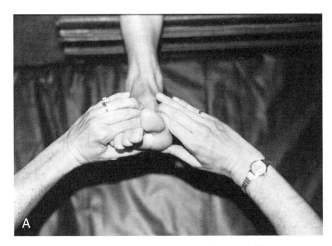
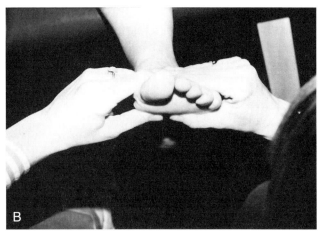

Figure 25–5. (A) Plantar flexed and (B) neutral first ray.

While maintaining the hand position described above, manually move the first metatarsal into dorsiflexion and plantar flexion while keeping the second through fifth metatarsals stable. Assess the movement of the first metatarsal and document the motion as rigid/hypomobile, semirigid (or semiflexible), or flexible/hypermobile. Normal range of motion for this joint is 20 degrees of plantar flexion and 20 degrees of dorsiflexion.[8]

Prone

Talocrural Joint Mobility

Talocrural joint mobility is assessed by measuring the amount of dorsiflexion and plantar flexion, in subtalar joint neutral, with the knee flexed and extended. See Chapter 24 for details. Ten degees of dorsiflexion to 20 degrees of plantar flexion are required for walking.[6]

Subtalar Joint Mobility and Subtalar Joint Neutral (STJN)

To assess STJN, the foot is positioned perpendicular to the ground. Subtalar joint motion is measured by the angle between the posterior longitudinal bisection of the lower one-third of the leg and the bisection of the posterior calcaneus. Manually invert the calcaneus to measure inversion with a goniometer, and evert the foot for eversion. Twenty degrees of inversion to 10 degrees of eversion are within normal limits.[9] The same bisection lines are used for STJN measurement by a palpation technique. The clinician palpates the medial aspect of the talus with the thumb and the lateral aspect of the talus with the index finger. While holding the fourth and fifth metatarsals, supinate and pronate the foot manually with the other hand. STJN is the position in which the talus is felt equally

on the medial and lateral sides (Fig. 25–6). A mathematically derived method to obtain the STJN is described in Chapter 24. Good intratester and intertester reliability is found with the mathematical method.[8,10] Using the mathematical method, one study found that the mean neutral rearfoot position was approximately 2.5 degrees of inversion in 240 asypmtomatic feet.[10] Studies have shown fair intratester reliability but poor intertester reliability with the palpation technique.[11]

Forefoot Position in STJN

Once STJN is determined, either by calculations or by palpation, the forefoot relationship is assessed. With the rearfoot maintained in STJN, the forefoot position is determined by aligning one arm of the goniometer along the plane of the metatarsal heads and aligning the other arm perpendicular to the calcaneal bisection line, as pre-

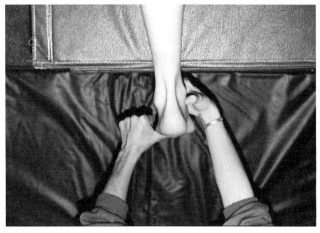

Figure 25–6. Subtalar joint neutral.

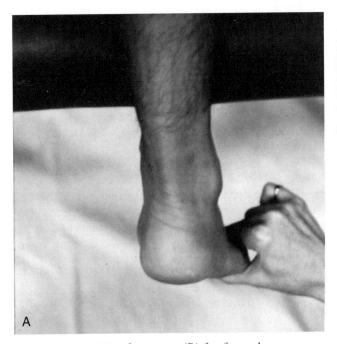

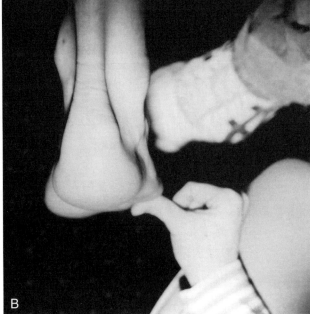

Figure 25–7. (A) Forefoot varus; (B) forefoot valgus.

viously described. The goniometer axis is held laterally for a forefoot varus measurement, and the axis is placed medially if a forefoot valgus is present (Fig. 25–7). Zero to 2 degrees of forefoot varus are within normal limits, according to one article.[4] Garbalosa et al.[10] found that the average forefoot varus angle was 7.82 degrees in 86 percent of 240 asymptomatic feet studied.[10]

Standing—Static Weightbearing

A postural assessment is completed, checking for symmetry of various bony landmarks such as the iliac crests and posterior superior iliac spines. Compensatory supination and pronation can occur due to lower limb deviations (Table 25–1). If asymmetry is noted from limb to limb, and if the SI joint is cleared with no osseous malalignment, then an apparent or functional leg length difference is present. The authors have observed that excessive supination or pronation in one limb can contribute to a functional leg length discrepancy.

Subtalar Joint Neutral (Weightbearing)

The same bisection lines discussed in the prone position for measuring STJN are used for the weightbearing STJN measurement. The neutral position is determined by using the thumb and index finger to palpate the medial and lateral talar head. The other hand passively rotates the lower leg internally and externally until the talus is felt equally under the thumb and index finger. The measurement should be identical to that found in the prone STJN position (Fig. 25–8).

Tibial Varum

While in STJN, the tibial varum/valgum position is determined by measuring the angle between the bisection of the lower leg with vertical 90 degrees. Excessive tibial

Table 25–1. Lower Quarter Deviations with Possible Compensations

Structure	Abnormality
Sacroiliac joint	
Posterior innominate	Pronation
Anterior innominate	Supination
Osseous leg length difference	
Shorter leg	Supination
Longer leg	Pronation
Femoral joint	
Anteversion	Toeing-in
Retroversion	Toeing-out
Knee	
Valgus	Pronation
Varus	Supination/pronation
Tibial joint	
Internal torsion	Toeing-in
External torsion	Toeing-out
Varum	Pronation

Note. Compensations may occur if the deviations are excessive. Not covered in the table are soft tissue restrictions or neuromuscular conditions, which can also influence compensations.

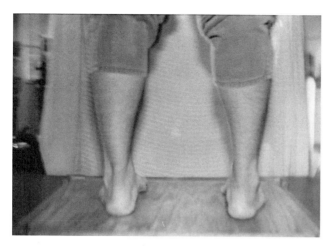

Figure 25–8. Subtalar joint neutral stance.

varum may lead to compensatory pronation at the subtalar joint.[6,8]

Calcaneal Resting Position

In a relaxed stance, the calcaneal resting position is measured by the angle of bisection of the lower one-third of the leg to the longitudinal bisection line along the calcaneus. Normal calcaneal eversion is 5 degrees.[5,12] Excessive calcaneal eversion is related to abnormal pronation. Intratester results were good for calcaneal resting position and subtalar joint neutral position using an inclinometer along the calcaneal bisection line.[11]

Navicular Drop Test

The navicular drop test (navicular height) can also be used to determine subtalar joint and midtarsal joint motion. Navicular changes relate directly to the midtarsal joint by its articulation with the talus and indirectly to the subtalar joint via the talus. The navicular tuberosity is palpated and marked. Measurements are then taken from the floor to the tuberosity in STJN (previously described) and again in a relaxed stance. The difference between the height measurements, in millimeters, is defined as the navicular height difference or navicular drop. In a recent study, high intratester and intertester reliability was found with the navicular drop test using an inclinometer. The intertester range for navicular height difference was 2.0 to 10.2 mm in 30 healthy volunteers (22 females aged 24 ± 3.6 years; 8 males aged 25 ± 5.1 years).[11] A navicular height difference greater than 10 mm is considered abnormal.[13]

Observational Gait Analysis

Once the static evaluation is completed, a gait analysis can be performed. Chapter 23 fully describes the gait

cycle. In brief, at heel-strike the calcaneus is slightly inverted and quickly everts/pronates at the talocrural and subtalar joints to unlock and adapt to the ground surfaces. Pronation continues with the unlocking of the midtarsal joint and is maximum at foot-flat. The medial longitudinal arch and the navicular bone are down during pronation with plantar flexion/adduction of the talus and eversion/abduction of the calcaneus. During early midstance, shock absorption occurs with internal rotation of the tibia and the knee.

As the tibia moves anteriorly over the foot, a reversal of pronation occurs and the subtalar joint passes through neutral and begins supinating in late midstance. Supination occurs at the midtarsal and subtalar joints to function as a rigid lever for proplusion. With the heel-off to toe-off supinatory phase, the foot is abducted no more than 10 to 15 degrees.[8] The tibia externally rotates, and the calcaneus inverts/adducts while the talus dorsiflexes/abducts. STJN occurs twice in midstance, shortly after heel-strike and prior to heel-lift.

Utilizing a treadmill can better capture gait analysis. It allows a repeated gait cycle with a consistent pattern to be viewed. In addition, a floor gait analysis should be conducted. This allows for a more natural gait without being preoccupied by the treadmill. Both forms of observational gait analysis should reveal similar findings and may assist in verifying pathomechanics.

Computerized Gait Analysis

There are several types of computerized gait analysis. One type uses a computer connected to a mat composed of more than 1600 electronic sensors. As the patient walks across the mat, the foot is scanned more than 30 times per second, taking measurements of the weight distribution and gait. An image is then produced on the computer screen, allowing the clinician to assess pressure relating to the force distribution during the gait. Another system collects and assesses information from up to four platforms simultaneously. It then analyzes parameters regarding gait, balance, and power.

Structural foot and ankle deviations can lead to abnormal lower extremity biomechanics with weightbearing. For example, excess pronation at push-off prevents a rigid lever from propelling the body forward. Abnormal mechanics such as excess supination at midstance can affect the ability of the foot to adapt to uneven terrain or to absorb shock. This could result in various lower extremity and back pathologies.[5,10] The following section covers foot and ankle pathomechanics, which can contribute to compensatory adaptations in gait.

■ Pathomechanics

Abnormal Pronation

Abnormal pronation is excessive pronation, which occurs beyond the initial 25 percent of the stance phase, that is, beyond forefoot loading.[7] This can lead to soft tissue damage of various structures along the lower extremity.[10] Abnormal pronation is a compensation for various deviations. Hypermobility of the forefoot and first ray can attribute to abnormal pronation. Here the first ray cannot overcome the ground reaction force and is thus unable to resupinate as a rigid lever for push-off. This creates increased loading at the second, third, and fourth metatarsal heads. The etiology includes congenital, neurologic, intrinsic (regarding the foot), extrinsic (regarding the lower limb), and developmental factors. This section focuses on three intrinsic factors which can lead to compensatory abnormal pronation: rearfoot varus, forefoot varus, and forefoot valgus.

Rearfoot Varus

A rearfoot varus dysfunction is excessive calcaneal inversion in subtalar joint neutral, with the forefoot parallel or neutral to the rearfoot (Fig. 25–9). Due to the inverted position of the calcaneus, the ground is farther away from the medial aspect of the foot. This requires increased calcaneal eversion to bring the medial heel to the ground with weightbearing. This compensation may cause excessive subtalar joint pronation during midstance and push-off. The abnormal pronation can cause excessive strain on soft tissue structures, leading to disorders such as anterior or posterior tibial tendinitis, tarsal tunnel syndrome, and plantar fasciitis. A chain reaction of events can then lead to pathologies at the knee, hip, and pelvic region.

Forefoot Varus

A forefoot varus is an inverted position of the forefoot on the rearfoot in subtalar joint neutral (Fig. 25–10). Compensation occurs to bring the medial aspect of the forefoot to the ground by excessively pronating at the subtalar joint. A forefoot varus has been reported as the

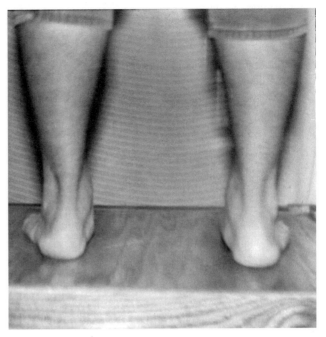

Figure 25–10. Compensated forefoot varus.

most common intrinsic deformity resulting in abnormal pronation, especially at push-off.[7,10,14] The forefoot varus deformity can also lead to pathologies mentioned with rearfoot varus. Forefoot varus can also be partially compensated or uncompensated for. This lack of compensation creates an increase in abduction of the foot from the midline of the body. This combines with eversion, leading to excess pronation at the midtarsal joint.[8]

Forefoot Valgus

Forefoot valgus is an everted forefoot position on the rearfoot in STJN.[7] Early medial forefoot loading occurs with a quick transfer to the lateral foot as the subtalar joint is supinating. Once heel-lift is completed, rapid pronation may occur in late stance, leading to instability during propulsion.[6,7] Forefoot valgus is less frequently seen.[5]

Abnormal Supination

Abnormal supination is the lack of pronation or the inability to pronate during midstance. This may cause poor shock absorption and difficulty adapting to various surfaces. Clinically, it accounts for a small proportion of the pathologies seen. Etiologic factors are neurologic, intrinsic foot deviations, or extrinsic deformities.[5] This section covers intrinsic foot deformities such as rigid forefoot valgus and rigid plantar flexed first ray. Pes cavus will be discussed under pediatric orthotics.

Rigid Forefoot Valgus

A rigid forefoot valgus is an everted forefoot position on the rearfoot in STJN[7] (Fig. 25–11). During weightbear-

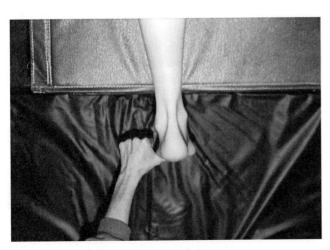

Figure 25–9. Rearfoot varus.

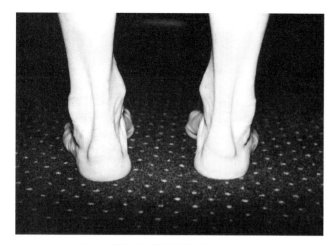

Figure 25–11. Rigid forefoot valgus.

ing, there is lack of forefoot inversion and the subtalar joint supinates to compensate during forefoot loading. Early medial forefoot loading occurs with a quick transfer to the lateral foot as the subtalar joint is supinating. Once heel-lift occurs, supination may persist through push-off, with excessive forces maintained along the lateral border of the foot.

Rigid Plantar Flexed First Ray

A rigid plantar flexed first ray is present when the first metatarsal head is plantar flexed and aligned lower then the second through fifth metatarsal heads. It is unable to return to a neutral position, aligned with the other metatarsals. There is early medial forefoot loading with a quick transfer to the lateral foot, and excessive supination occurs.

Other Foot Dysfunctions

Hallux Limitus/Hallux Rigidus

Hallux limitus is a limitation of dorsiflexion at the first MTP joint. The required 60 to 65 degrees of dorsiflexion needed during propulsion does not occur.[15] Thus, in adulthood, repeated trauma occurs at the MTP joint during gait with attempts to dorsiflex. This may lead to ankylosis of the first MTP joint, a condition referred to as *hallux rigidus*.[5] The hallux limitus and rigidus deformities have been correlated with first ray hypermobility, which occurs with abnormal pronation. They are also related to degenerative joint disease, trauma, a dorsiflexed first ray deformity, and an excessively long first metatarsal.[5] Compensation may occur with hyperextension of the first interphalangeal joint. Another compensation could be increased loads to the lateral four toes and metatarsals, which could lead to fatigue fractures.[15]

The previously described dysfunctions are some of the factors contributing to abnormal lower extremity bio-

mechanics. Other influences are trauma, congenital deformities, and neurologic pathologies, which are beyond the scope of our chapter. The next section covers correction techniques with the use of orthotics.

■ Biomechanical Orthotics

A custom, biomechanical orthotic assists in the control of excess motion of the midtarsal, subtalar joints, and talocrural joints.[14] It assists in normalizing the gait cycle with regard to heel-strike, stance phase, and push-off, thus minimizing pathomechanics. Also known as *functional* orthotics, biomechanical orthotics provide triplanar correction of the forefoot and rearfoot. They attempt to reduce compensations of the triplanar joints such as excess pronation or supination.

A semirigid orthotic provides a rigid support for biomechanical control and some flexibility for shock absorption.[6] Leather, cork, and thermoplastics are some of the materials used to fabricate these devices. Orthotic control is created primarily through a post or wedge. A forefoot and/or rearfoot post is utilized when creating a biomechanical orthotic to assist in normalizing gait. In the following subsections, additional assistive devices and other patient considerations for biomechanical orthotics will be discussed.

Posts

A post is material added to an orthotic shell. The shell can be fabricated from a patient's foot in STJN. The shell can be made at the office or sent to a custom orthotic laboratory after a negative impression cast is made at the office. Both of these situations will be discussed in the section "Orthotic Fabrication." The amount and type of correction provided as well as the type of device and the laboratories utilized, vary greatly among clinicians. An extrinsic post is a correction applied to the outside of the orthotic shell. By contrast, an intrinsic post is applied within the orthotic shell. Some clinicians and laboratories prefer to use intrinsic posting as a correction to the forefoot and extrinsic posting for the rearfoot. The authors believe that extrinsic posting may provide greater control of compensatory pronation. This may add bulk to the orthotic, which may limit the types of footwear. The intrinsic post is useful with tight footwear, such as a woman's dress shoe, but provides less control of compensatory pronation. Both types of posting are used to decrease compensatory pronation or supination at the subtalar and/or midtarsal joints. This allows the foot to function closer to neutral position.

Rearfoot Extrinsic Post

A rearfoot extrinsic post consists of material applied along the calcaneal region of an orthotic shell. If the post is for a rearfoot varus deformity, the material is higher medial and tapers down laterally. The rearfoot varus post brings the ground closer to the medial calcaneal surface, decreasing excessive subtalar joint pronation during early midstance. This improves lower extremity stability and muscle efficiency during midstance.

Forefoot Extrinsic Post

A forefoot post is material applied proximal to the metatarsal head region of an orthotic shell. A forefoot varus deformity post has more material medially and then tapers laterally to reduce excessive midtarsal joint pronation during forefoot loading. This increases stability for effective propulsion. If both a rearfoot and a forefoot varus deformity are present, a medial rearfoot and forefoot post is applied. This allows compensatory pronation at the subtalar and midtarsal joints to be reduced.

Forefoot Valgus Post

A forefoot valgus post is material built up along the lateral orthotic shell, tapering medially to reduce excessive supination. This brings the ground up to the lateral component of the foot, preventing compensatory pronation and/or supination.

Methods for Orthotic Prescription

The degree of correction determines the degree of posting needed. There is minimal research regarding the amount of orthotic posting relative to the degree of deformity and what is most effective. One study assessed the effects of various posting methods using 22 subjects with at least 8 degrees of forefoot varus deformity.[16] The subjects were required to be pain-free for at least 1 month prior to testing. A trigonometric formula was used to calculate the forefoot post height, which provided approximately 60 percent correction. The rearfoot post height was 80 percent of the height of the forefoot post. No forefoot post exceeded 7 mm, and the rearfoot post did not exceed 6 mm. The subjects were studied while walking with (1) shoes alone, (2) orthotic shells unposted, (3) orthotic shells with forefoot posts, (4) orthotic shells with rearfoot posts, and (5) shells with both rearfoot and forefoot posts. Results revealed that all types of posting and the orthotic shell alone decreased maximal pronation. Maximal control resulted with combined rearfoot and forefoot posting.[16]

Another study assessed 53 subjects with various lower extremity problems. They were fit with semirigid orthotics using the neutral casting method.[14] The casts were sent to an orthotic laboratory for fabrication, with the prescription based on the biomechanical evaluation. Patients responded to a questionnaire, and 96 percent reported relief from pain with the use of the orthotics. Tomaro and Butterfield[17] recommend various orthotics

with traumatic foot or ankle injuries after physical therapy is completed. General orthotic recommendations for subtalar joint hypomobility include a semiflexible, total contact orthotic without extrinsic posting. This allows for more shock absorption. General orthotic recommendations for excessive subtalar joint pronation include a semirigid shell with extrinsic rearfoot posting to control abnormal pronation. Excessive supination of the subtalar joint generally responds well with a lateral wedge midfoot to forefoot to assist in weight transfer to the medial forefoot. Each orthotic varies, based on the individual biomechanical evaluation. Forefoot extrinsic posts should generally not exceed 5–7 degrees. Rearfoot extrinsic posts should generally not exceed 5 degrees. The aforementioned foot mechanics with orthotic types are generally recommendations. All factors of the biomechanical orthotic must be considered.

■ Orthotic Fabrication

Many techniques exist for orthotic fabrication, such as prefabricated types or casting in STJN. Many devices are commercially available. The amount and type of correction and the terminology used vary greatly. Our focus will be on custom semirigid biomechanical (also called *functional*) orthotics. There is a wide range of semirigid orthotic devices, many of which combine control, where needed, with shock absorption. In-office fabrication and neutral casting with laboratory fabrication will be reviewed. A STJN casting technique will be described, as well as considerations during the initial use of the orthotics. Finally, a case study will be presented.

In-Office Fabrication

The advantages of fabricating an orthotic in the office is immediate delivery to the patient, as well as the ability to make the various adjustments which may be required. Patients may need an orthotic temporarily rather than a more durable laboratory device. The in-office device is typically less expensive and easier to alter due to the onsite clinician's accessibility. The in-office orthotic should still be a custom device, with posting prescribed similarly to that of the laboratory device. Criteria used to determine which in-office system to utilize should include a variety of styles and sizes of orthotics, as well as the ability to use corrective additions. Posting, heel lifts, arch pads, and relief cutouts should all be options with an in-office system. These orthotics should vary in material and consistency from rigid to semirigid to flexible. Prefabricated orthotics are typically premolded for average foot sizes and are intended for those individuals who need minimal correction.[18] The goals should be consistent: to improve lower extremity biomechanics and minimize compensatory pronation or supination.

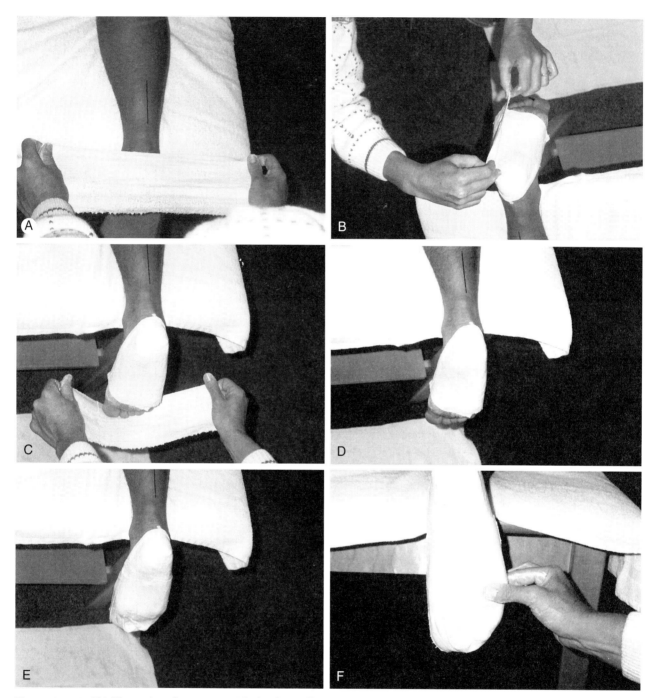

Figure 25–12. (A) The patient lies prone, with the foot off the edge of the treatment table. (B) Use two strips of quick-drying plaster doubled in length, dip the plaster in water, and ring out most of the water. (C) Lay the first strip of wet plaster down from the heel downward, create a ¼ in. edge superiorly, fold over the plaster, and smooth it down to the arch of the foot. (D) Lay the second strip of wet plaster from the toes upward, create a ¼ in. edge superiorly, fold over the plaster, and smooth it down to the arch of the foot, covering the toes. (E) Smooth out the entire arch of the foot, releasing any air bubbles and ensuring total foot contact with the plaster. (F) Align the foot in STJN and hold it in this position until the plaster is dry and hard.

Laboratory Orthotics

Many patients may need a laboratory-fabricated orthotic, which typically requires a cast imprint of the plantar surface of the foot. This type of orthotic differs from an in-office orthotic with regard to durability, choice of materials used, and the amount of rigidity required. One advantage of laboratory fabrication is a wide range of orthotics, from slim fashion to sport-specific types. The custom orthotic is based on a prescription, and, if needed, many laboratories offer technical support to assist in the orthotic preparation. A nonweightbearing neutral cast is required. Casting of the feet for this procedure will be reviewed.[19] A prescription form should accompany these casts to the laboratory, with comments on the patient's symptoms, specific anomalies of the feet, orthotic type, and posting instructions with any corrective additions.

The disadvantages of laboratory orthotics are their higher cost, slow turnaround time, and the inability of a clinician to make immediate changes if needed. The finished product can take as long as 3–4 weeks to manufacture. Further delays are added with any additions or modifications.

Neutral Casting

The neutral casting method consists of applying plaster to the foot while maintaining a STJN position. This method produces a neutral foot impression, which is sent to a laboratory for orthotic fabrication. The technique reviewed involves casting the foot in STJN while lying prone (Fig. 25–12). Upon completion and drying of the cast, the patient's name should be labeled on the cast prior to being sent for fabrication.

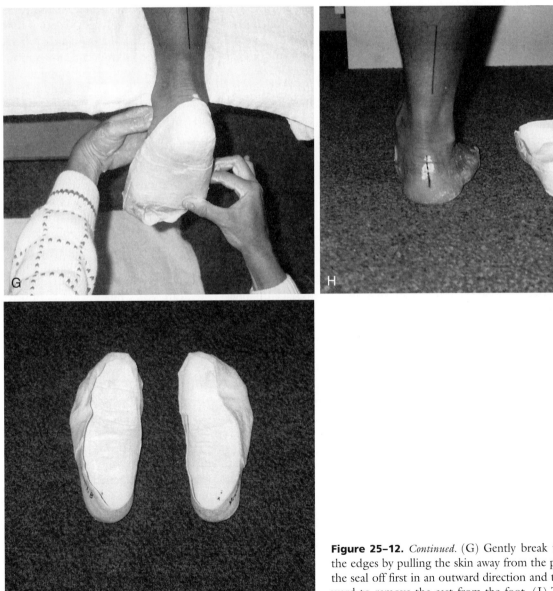

Figure 25–12. *Continued.* (G) Gently break the seal around the edges by pulling the skin away from the plaster. (H) Pop the seal off first in an outward direction and then pull downward to remove the cast from the foot. (I) The cast should resemble the deformity.

■ Corrective Additions

Heel Lifts

The function of a heel lift is to decrease the need for compensatory pronation. If an oblique ankle joint axis exists, the heel lift may assist in resupination of the foot after heel-strike, minimizing hyperpronation.[20] A heel lift provides sagittal plane correction, which may also reduce loads to the plantar fascia by elevating the heel. Heel lifts may be used independently of orthotics to provide temporary assistance in healing soft tissue strain of the gastrocnemius and soleus complex. Literature reports regarding the use of heel lifts as a significant assistance with leg length discrepancy are minimal. Changes of ⅛ to ¼ in. can generally stay in the shoe. Any changes of more than ¼ in. should be added to the heel and sole of the shoe externally. Clinically, there is evidence that lifting the entire base of the orthotic or the shoe itself may assist in reducing the strains that a leg length discrepancy may cause.

First Ray Cutout

This relief cutout allows a plantar flexed first ray to decompress the first metatarsal joint. With a rigid plantar flexed first ray, the first metatarsal hits the ground immediately after heel-strike, followed by supination to bring the lateral aspect of the foot to the floor.[20] This compensatory supination can be avoided by assisting the first ray to be more mobile.

Another method used to relieve the plantar flexed first ray consists of a metatarsal bar or pad placed proximal to the metatarsal heads. This is used to distribute the forces more evenly across the metatarsals, thus relieving metatarsalgia.

Top Covers

The purpose of a top cover is to provide additional shock absorption. A smooth transition from the orthotic to the surface of the shoe is accomplished. If reports of orthotic movement occur, a fully extended top cover may be required. If an orthotic for a women's fashion shoe is required, a narrower top cover with a streamlined shape may be indicated. Top covers come in a variety of materials with different densities and durabilities, such as leather, neoprene, poron, and vinyl.

■ Accommodative Orthotics

An accommodative orthotic is a soft insert which provides support and cushioning to the foot. Forces are mildly dissipated, giving the foot less pressure in a concentrated area. The foot is not biomechanically altered by posting material or by placing the foot in neutral position.[6] Indi-

viduals with sensitive skin, with a tendency toward skin breakdown, or with increased distal venous pressure may benefit from an accommodative orthotic to assist in pressure distribution. The accommodative orthotic should be flexible and able to adapt to a variety of terrain. It may be a thicker insole, requiring a deeper shoe. Removing the insoles of certain shoes may assist in better fitting an accommodative orthotic. Accommodative padding may also be utilized instead of a complete orthotic to provide areas of pressure relief. The foot of a diabetic patient, for example, may benefit from an accommodative device.

■ Diabetes: Epidemiology and Economics

Diabetes affects over 50 percent of adult Native Americans and Hispanics, and African Americans record it as the third leading cause of death in the United States.[19] The American Diabetes Association (ADA) reports that over 16 million Americans have diabetes, half of whom remain undiagnosed.[21] Diabetes is associated with more than 50 percent of the 120,000 lower limb amputations in this country.[19] The disease is more prevalent among the elderly population, and its incidence increases with age.[22] According to the American Physical Therapy Association (APTA), it is currently the sixth leading cause of death in the United States. Peripheral nerve disease afflicts 60–70 percent of diabetic individuals. Reports show more than 35,000 major amputations among diabetics annually, with 12,000 to 15,000 elderly individuals undergoing amputation as a result of ulcers. These ulcers may have been prevented through proper education, orthotic intervention, and medical management.[23]

Over $90 billion is spent on the complications of diabetes annually; $3 billion is spent annually on diabetic foot care alone.[21] Medicare costs range from $6000 to $30,000 per patient after hospitalization for continued medical management of the diabetic foot as a result of severe ulceration or amputation.[22] Approximately $1.2 billion is annually spent on patients undergoing amputation secondary to complications of diabetes.[24]

Pathophysiology of the Diabetic Foot

Diabetes can cause poor circulation, difficulty fighting infection, neurologic dysfunction, and associated joint pathology.[25] The diabetic foot experiences sensory loss with changes in proprioception, possible orthopedic deformity creating pressure spots, skin breakdown, and foot ulcers, often leading to amputation of the affected foot or limb. Early recognition and prophylactic intervention are imperative for the individual with diabetes. An orthotic device can assist in providing equal distribution of forces from faulty foot mechanics, thus preventing ulcer development.

Causes of Skin Breakdown

Neuropathy, ischemia, and infection are the main causes of tissue breakdown resulting in ulceration of the foot. Severe ulceration may lead to lower extremity amputation in the diabetic patient. Poor vascularity and sensory changes promote skin breakdown and predispose the foot to microtrauma.

Ischemia is a major contributor to the diabetic ulcer by delaying the process of wound repair and making infection control more difficult. A vasodilitary response may occur, although vasoconstriction is more likely. Both conditions are a result of the autonomic nerve distribution inherent in diabetes.

Another cause of skin breakdown is autonomic neuropathy, which may change hydration levels of the skin. Dry, flaky or scaly epidermal effects may be found on evaluation due to anhidrosis. Fissures may develop, which may be prone to bacterial infection secondary to decreased circulation effects. It is not unusual to witness extremely moist skin; hyperhydrosis, as well as secondary changes in vascular distribution, result from arteriovenous shunting away from the capillary bed.[26] Hyperhydrosis may result in fungus and yeast infections, also leading to skin breakdown. When motor nerves of the foot are disrupted, the intrinsic foot muscles weaken, causing changes in pressure distribution.[27] Peripheral sensation loss may coincide with this process, resulting in skin breakdown as well.

Biomechanical Factors

Proprioception, balance, and kinesthetic effectiveness are compromised in the diabetic patient. Accordingly, faulty gait mechanics may result, creating biomechanical dysfunction. Abnormal or faulty gait mechanics create high-pressure areas in prominent regions of the foot. These pressures create skin breakdown and ischemia, resulting in ulceration. The change in peripheral sensation delays the response time, preventing early recognition and treatment. Initial stages of disease in the diabetic foot are caused by trauma to the vascular system of the lower leg. The tibial and peroneal arteries are most commonly damaged. Repetitive stress to areas of decreased vascularity often begin the biomechanical process of breakdown. Peripheral vascular insufficiency often leads to poor healing due to decreased circulation. When faulty gait mechanics, increased pressure, and sensory loss occur simultaneously, a diabetic individual may not feel pain or realize that damage is being done. This creates a chronic condition and impairment. Pressure necrosis from poorly fitting shoes may also go unnoticed due to sensory loss.

Orthotic Intervention

Proper weight distribution through a normal gait cycle greatly assists the diabetic foot. When utilizing orthotics with the diabetic individual, several issues must be ad-

dressed. The primary aim when applying orthotics to the diabetic foot is to protect the plantar surface of the foot from skin breakdown, which could lead to ulcers and ultimately amputation. Additional concerns are to protect bony protuberances from excessive wear and to promote overall biomechanical efficiency. An accommodative orthotic is appropriate for this patient population. Shock-absorbing materials are recommended to assist in the equal distribution of weight. Plastazote is an easy-to-mold material which has proven to be successful in diabetic foot management. One study revealed that a total-contact insert for individuals with diabetes mellitus showed increased walking speed and higher scores on a physical performance test.[28] Another case report supports the long-term care of a neuropathic plantar ulcer with a total contact insert.[29] There is also evidence that amputations can be prevented with therapeutic footwear by protecting sensitive skin areas.[30]

Evaluation

Patient evaluation should include a diabetic foot screening in both weightbearing and nonweightbearing conditions. Weightbearing assessment may include compensations of normal gait in order to prevent further damage to sensitive skin areas. Antalgic gait and protective stance should be noted. A nonweightbearing exam should include soft tissue assessment for skin breakdown, redness, and current ulcer development. Hyperkeratosis (corns and calluses) or any skin color changes should be assessed, as well as any signs of gangrene. Palpation or popliteal, dorsal pedal, and posterior tibial pulses should be assessed. The temperature of the foot should be assessed bilaterally, with observation of redness and atrophic skin changes. Delayed venous fill time after elevation and blanching with elevation should also be examined in determining vascular compromise to the foot. Finally, sensation should be assessed, including the dermatomes of the lower extremity.

Patient Education

The key areas in educating the diabetic individual with regard to ulcer prevention are as follows. A basic understanding of foot hygiene, including drying the toes thoroughly, is required. Daily inspection of the feet for any changes in skin breakdown is imperative to early intervention. Proper footwear with a possible orthotic device should be explored. Adequate padding in a sock (such as cotton) is helpful to assist in protecting skin from breakdown. Avoidance of direct trauma to the foot should be emphasized, including exposure to hot water with changes in sensory awareness. Actions to take if problems arise and information on when to seek medical attention will also allow the diabetic individual to prevent ulcer development. Once an ulcer has developed, it will always be more vulnerable to recurring breakdown. The individual with diabetes must pay constant attention to the condition of the feet in order to stay healthy.

◼ Pediatric Orthotics

The use of orthotics with children continues to be controversial with regard to lasting effects, efficacy of treatment, and choice of orthotic devices. Practitioners who utilize orthotics with children wish to achieve functional gait throughout the growth stage.[8,31] The use of orthotics with abnormal mechanics during the early stages of walking may decrease abnormal compensations that develop later in life.[8]

A common biomechanical condition in children is hypermobile flatfeet, also known as *pes planus deformity*. This excess motion causes further stress at adjoining joints with poor musculoskeletal control to alleviate problems. One management technique for this foot type is to control the rearfoot in attempts to normalize gait mechanics.[8] A heel stabilizer will assist in providing control without the need to post the forefoot or rearfoot. A shock-absorbing insert without correction will also assist in reducing the biomechanical stress at heel-strike and further dissipate forces at push-off. If further corrections of hypermobile flatfoot are necessary, a rearfoot post is added to position the subtalar joint in neutral. Corrections can be up to 100 percent due to increased mobility of the subtalar joint and soft tissue flexibility in children.

Another pathologic foot condition in children is the pes cavus, or high-arched, foot. This is the opposite of the pes planus foot. In the pes cavus foot there is plantar flexion of the forefoot on the rearfoot.[8] This usually results in abnormal supination, which involves hypomobility of the joints in the foot. Thus, there is a lack of shock absorption in the stance phase of gait. Other terms used to classify pes cavus foot types are *clubfoot, talipes plantaris,* and *pes equinovarus.*[32] Orthotic selection for these conditions should cover neurologic as well as orthopedic issues. In general, a more flexible orthotic may be used to assist in shock absorption.

Clinicians should take into consideration the structural changes the child is going through, with recommendations to replace orthotics every 1–2 years. Orthotic material should be semirigid to promote stability of the hypermobile segments while further dissipating forces. A more rigid device may be necessary for additional control. Each child's feet should be carefully assessed to determine which orthotic is most appropriate. The main goal of utilizing an orthotic device with children is to assist in normalizing gait to decrease compensations caused by abnormal foot types.

◼ Break-In Technique

A key element in the success of a new pair of orthotics is the method the individual uses to break in the orthotics.

The abnormal foot has been accustomed to a specific faulty alignment for some time, and becoming reacquainted with normal mechanics may be a challenge. It is recommended that the individual wear new orthotics for only 1 hour on the first day, adding an hour a day until the fourth day, when 2 hours per day may be added. By the end of the first week, the individual should be able to tolerate the orthotics for 8 hours per day. For individuals who are on their feet most of the day, this break-in period may take longer. Athletes are encouraged to complete the break-in period prior to working out with their new orthotics. There is an additional break-in period for athletics after the original break-in period. Athletes should wear their orthotics for 1 hour of workout time during the first week and increase the wearing time gradually, depending on the high-impact demands of their sport. Consultation with a physical therapist is recommended on the specific break-in period for orthotics with different athletic endeavors.

It is important to educate individuals on realistic expectations of the results of wearing new orthotics. Fatigue and soft tissue strain are possible side effects; thus, more stretching may be necessary during the break-in period. Further strain to the kinetic chain as a whole may also be experienced secondary to the changes in biomechanical alignment of the body. If a patient typically is asymptomatic, regardless of abnormal foot mechanics, orthotics may not be the best intervention. Finally, it is recommended that individuals wear their orthotics during 80 percent of their weightbearing hours for the best results. No research supports the theory of permanent changes in the foot mechanics of adults from wearing orthotics. Therefore for orthotics to be effective, they must be worn. There does not appear to be any carryover of correction from an orthotic to a barefoot or nonorthotic situation.

Other Considerations with Orthotics

Patients' specific needs must also be considered in writing the orthotic prescription. The patient's activity level will play a role in determining the density of the material and the type of orthotic used. Various laboratories offer multiple sport orthotics, depending on the athletic activity. The forces loaded to the foot and the type of loading, rearfoot to forefoot or forefoot to rearfoot, vary in different sports. The athlete or the individual with a high activity level will benefit from maximum control of compensatory pronation. The sedentary individual with limited rearfoot or forefoot motion may benefit from a low-density shell. This will allow good shock absorption and minimal control. Additional devices can be added to distribute pressures evenly.

Shoe wear is also an important consideration with orthotics. Semirigid orthotics with extrinsic posting tend to be bulky, fitting mostly within larger footwear. For a dress shoe, a narrow and less dense shell is beneficial, usually with intrinsic posting to accommodate the low volume of the shoe. Top covers usually extend to the metatarsal heads or the sulcus to minimize the bulk. With a high-heeled shoe, a cobra-style orthotic can be used. The advantage is the slim design, although it provides minimal control of the foot.

Weight and height are other factors affecting orthotic fabrication. Laboratories recommend arch fills with materials such as poron or EVA if the patient weighs more than 200 lb or is more than 6 ft tall. The patient's medical history, such as osteoarthritis, rheumatoid arthritis, or diabetes, must also be considered. These factors all play a role in orthotic selection and prescription.

CASE STUDIES

Subjective Examination

The patient is a 63-year-old secretary with insidious onset of left foot and ankle swelling 2 months prior to the evaluation. The amount of swelling correlates with the duration of walking. By evening, pain is present along the medial left foot and ankle. There are no reports of parathesia and no history of lower extremity pathologies or injuries. There is a history of right "sciatic" pain for the past 6 years; however, the patient has never sought medical attention. She takes Tylenol nightly to control the sciatic symptoms. Her overall health is good.

Objective Examination

No discoloration or temperature changes are noted. There is pitting edema along the dorsal foot and the medial and lateral malleoli. Moderate pain is felt along the tendons of the tibialis posterior, flexor digitorum longus, flexor hallucis longus, and medial soleus muscle. Strength of the foot/ankle musculature is within normal limits and is asymptomatic.

Significant Findings of the LE Biomechanical Evaluation

Supine

Findings include a right anterior innominate SI joint, mild right femoral anteversion, mild restrictions of the right hip on internal and external rotation and bilateral hamstrings, moderate hallux valgus bilaterally, 50 degrees of left hallux dorsiflexion, and midtarsal joint hypermobility bilaterally. The left first ray is dorsiflexed and the right first ray is plantar flexed; both rays are flexible.

Prone

Talocrural joint mobility is within normal limits bilaterally; however, pain is present with active and passive left dorsiflexion at end-range. Mild restrictions of the left

subtalar joint occur with inversion and eversion. In STJN, there is a mild to moderate rearfoot varus bilaterally, severe left forefoot varus, and mild right forefoot varus.

Standing

There is genu varum bilaterally and excessive navicular drop. The calcaneal weightbearing position is excessive eversion, left greater than right.

Gait

Pronation is abnormal just after heel-strike through push-off. There is excessive femoral internal rotation and forefoot abduction.

Diagnosis

The patient displays a possible medial/deep compartment syndrome and a sacroiliac joint dysfunction. Abnormal pronation is also present due to lower extremity and foot/ankle dysfunctions.

Goals

The goals are to minimize the biomechanical dysfunctions, decrease the stress to the lower leg/ankle soft tissue structures, decrease the edema and pain with gait, and improve subtalar and first MTP joint mobility

Therapy

SI joint manual techniques, joint mobilization, soft tissue mobilization, and footmaxx analysis for orthotics are recommended. Because the patient wore dress shoes, an orthotic was completed with intrinsic posting and top-cover to the metatarsal heads. After the first office visit, the SI joint deviation was corrected. After two office visits and 10 days' use of the orthotics, the patient reported that she was no longer taking Tylenol due to decreased "sciatica." No pain was present with palpation of the medial left lower leg/ankle or with ankle dorsiflexion. The pitting edema resolved. The left hallux dorsiflexion was within normal limits for gait. Mild left subtalar joint inversion restrictions persisted. A follow-up exam 1 month later continued to reveal decreased left foot/ankle edema, no left foot pain during or after walking, and decreased right "sciatica."

■ References

1. Cummings G, Scholz JP, Barnes K: The effect of imposed leg length differences on pelvic bone symmetry. Spine 18(3): 368–373, 1993
2. Magee DJ: Orthopedic Physical Assessment. 2nd Ed. WB Saunders, Philadelphia, 1992

3. Ruwe PA, Gage JR, Ozonoff MB, et al: Clinical determination of femoral anteversion. A comparison with established techniques. J Bone Joint Surg 74A(6):820–830, 1992

4. Riegger-Krugh C, Keysor JJ: Skeletal malalignments of the lower quarter: correlated and compensatory motions and postures. JOSPT 23(2):164–170, 1996

5. Root ML, Orien WP, Weed JH: Clinical Biomechanics: Normal and Abnormal Function of the Foot. Vol. 2. Clinical Biomechanics Corp., Los Angeles, 1977

6. Gould JA III: Orthopaedic and Sports Physical Therapy. 2nd Ed., CV Mosby, St. Louis, 1990

7. Donatelli R: Abnormal biomechanics of the foot and ankle. JOSPT 9(1):11–16, 1987

8. Donatelli R: The Biomechanics of the Foot and Ankle. FA Davis, Philadelphia, 1990

9. Donatelli R: Normal biomechanics of the foot and ankle. JOSPT 7(3):91–95, 1985

10. Garbalosa JC, McClure MH, Catlain PA, et al: The frontal plane relationship of the forefoot to the rearfoot in an asymptomatic population. JOSPT 20(4):200–206, 1994

11. Sell KE, Verity TM, Worrell TW, et al: Two measurement techniques for assessing subtalar joint position: a reliability study. JOSPT 19(3):162–167, 1994

12. McPoil T, Cornwall MW: Relationship between neutral subtalar joint position and pattern of rearfoot motion during walking. Foot Ankle 17(3):141–145, 1994

13. Mueller M, Host J, Norton B: Navicular drop as a measure of excessive rearfoot pronation. J Am Podiatr Assoc 83:198–202, 1993

14. Donatelli R, Hurlbert C, Conaway D, et al: Biomechanical foot orthotics: a retrospective study. JOSPT 10(6):205–212, 1988

15. Boisssonault W, Donatelli R: The influence of hallux extension on the foot during ambulation. JOSPT 5(5):240–242, 1984

16. Johanson MA, Donatelli R, Wooden MJ, et al: Effects of three different posting methods on controlling abnormal subtalar pronation. Phys Ther 74(2):149–161, 1994

17. Tomaro J, Butterfield SL: Biomechanical treatment of traumatic foot and ankle injuries with the use of foot orthotics. JOSPT 21(6):373–380, 1995

18. Black E: Custom orthotics: Do you need them? Stride 1(3):21–30, 1996

19. Donatelli R: The Biomechanics of the Foot and Ankle. 2nd Ed. FA Davis, Philadelphia, 1996

20. Inman UT: The Joints of the Ankle. Williams & Wilkins, Baltimore, 1976

21. Donnelly R, Davis R, Girard S: New classification for diabetes mellitus. JAAPA 11(3):18–21, 1998

22. Gleis L: Financing the care of diabetes mellitus in the 1990's. Diab Care 13:1021–1023, 1990

23. Nemchik R: From research to practice: saving the diabetic foot. Diabetes Spectrum 1:153–155, 1990

24. Levin ME, O'Neal LW: The diabetic foot. Ann Acad Med Singapore 7:359–363, 1978

25. Edmonds M, Roberts V, Watkins P: Blood flow in the diabetic neuropathic foot. Diabetologia 22:9–15, 1982

26. Niinikoski J: Cellular and nutritional interactions in wound healing. Med Biol 58:303–309, 1980

27. Alexandria VA: Diabetic Foot Care. Am Diabetes Assoc 1990

28. Mueller MJ, Strube MJ: Therapeutic footwear: enhanced function in people with diabetes and transmetatarsal amputation. Arch Phys Med Rehabil 78(9):952–956, 1997

29. Nawoczenski DA, Birke JA, Graham SL, et al: The neuropathic foot; a management scheme: a case report. Phys Ther 69(4):287–291, 1989

30. Mueller MJ: Therapeutic footwear helps protect the diabetic foot. J Am Podiatr Med Assoc 87(8):360–364,

31. Tecklin JS: Pediatric Physical Therapy. JB Lippincott, Philadelphia, 1989

32. Jahs MH: Disorders of the Foot. Vol. 1. WB Saunders, Philadelphia, 1982

CHAPTER 26

Reconstructive Surgery of the Foot and Ankle

Leland C. McCluskey

The foot has a unique dual function, requiring the ability to convert from a flexible, shock-absorbing structure at heel-strike into a rigid lever for the push-off phase of gait. Most injuries and disabilities involving the foot can be categorized according to one of these two functions. The goal of most foot surgery is to eliminate pain and to restore normal function when possible.

The Adult Acquired Flat Foot

The most common cause of adult acquired flat foot is dysfunction of the posterior tibial tendon. Posterior tibial tendon dysfunction produces hindfoot valgus, flattening of the medial longitudinal arch, forefoot abduction, and forefoot varus. This condition is now often recognized as a precursor to the development of severe deformities or arthritis in the hindfoot. These deformities are flexible in the early stages, but they progress to become rigid in the later stages. Pes planus, obesity, and inflammatory arthritis are predisposing risks to dysfunction or rupture of the posterior tibial tendon. The normal excursion of the posterior tibial tendon is 1.5 to 2 cm. Thus, any elongation of the tendon can lead to dysfunction and disability. Positive single and double heel-rise tests are good early indicators of dysfunction as the heel fails to invert to a varus position.

Soft tissue procedures alone are adequate to treat early-stage cases with no deformity. Triple arthrodesis is required for patients with rigid hindfoot and forefoot deformities. Limited hindfoot arthrodesis is considered for those patients in Johnson and Strom's stage 2 classification in whom moderate deformities exist but flexibility remains.[1] Attempts are made to preserve subtalar motion when possible. Recent emphasis on lateral column lengthening through distraction arthrodesis of the calcaneocu-

boid joint and medial soft tissue reconstruction using flexor digitorum longus transfers have allowed good correction of moderate deformities while preserving subtalar and hindfoot function. Seventy-five percent or more of subtalar motion is maintained after fusion of the calcaneocuboid joint.[2] A medial displacement osteotomy of the body of the calcaneus can also be added in severe cases.[3]

Technique

The patient is placed in a supine position, with the iliac crest and the entire extremity prepared and draped. A lateral incision is made dorsal to the peroneal brevis tendon and plantar to the peroneus tertius tendon, extending over the calcaneocuboid joint[4] (Fig. 26–1). The superficial peroneal and sural nerves are protected. The extensor digitorum brevis muscle is split, and the entire width of the calcaneocuboid joint is exposed. The articular surfaces are removed from the joint with a 1-in. osteotome. A laminar spreader or distractors are used to distract the calcaneocuboid joint approximately 1 cm. Care is taken to avoid creating more forefoot varus. A 1-cm bicortical bone graft from the iliac crest or the posterior bursal projection of the calcaneus is harvested and placed in the osteotomy site. An AO H-plate with 3.5-mm cortical screws is used for fixation. The bony alignment and peritalar subluxation is corrected.

The flexor digitorum longus transfer to the navicular is important because it provides dynamic stability to the medial column of the foot. A medial incision is made over the posterior tibial tendon sheath from the medial malleolus to the base of the first metatarsal. The superficial fascia with the abductor hallucis is incised distally, and the muscle is retracted plantarly. The deep fascia and the medial septum are incised, and the flexor digitorum longus is identified and incised distal to the knot of Henry. Proximally, the posterior tibial tendon sheath is incised,

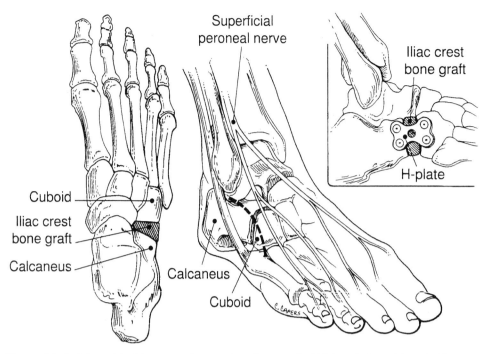

Figure 26–1. A lateral incision extends over the calcaneocuboid joint. A 1-cm bicortical bone graft from the iliac crest is placed in the osteotomy site. An AO H-plate with 3.5-mm cortical screws is used for fixation. (From McCluskey,[4] with permission.)

and the inferior one-third of the tendon is sutured into the spring ligament. The transferred flexor digitorum longus is passed plantarly to dorsally through drill holes in the navicular and then sutured back to itself with a no. 1 nonabsorbable suture. The Achilles tendon is often lengthened at this time if the foot cannot be dorsiflexed to 10 degrees with the knee in extension.

Postoperative Care

Postoperatively, patients remain in touch-down weight-bearing status in a short leg cast for 6 weeks. Next, they advance to a walking splint or cast for 4 to 6 weeks, and range-of-motion, strengthening, and proprioception exercises are initiated.

■ Ankle Instability

All first-time inversion ankle sprains, regardless of their severity, are treated with temporary immobilization followed by aggressive functional rehabilitation. The exception to this program is the acutely injured patient in whom associated ankle injuries, such as displaced fractures, displaced osteochondral lesions of the talus, and peroneal tendon ruptures or dislocations, warrant surgical intervention. Surgery is usually reserved for those patients who have chronic functional instability (episodes of giving way) and documented mechanical instability and who have not benefited from an appropriate rehabilitation program. The preferred surgical treatment for both acute and

chronic reconstructions in most patients is the Broström-Gould procedure.[5] This technique is an anatomic repair that does not sacrifice any normal structures. Subtalar instability is also addressed with this procedure by reconstructing the calcaneofibular ligament and using the extensor retinaculum to reinforce the repair.

Technique

An anterolateral incision is usually used. The surgeon makes a curvilinear incision along the anterior border of the distal fibula[6] (Fig. 26–2). The incision begins about 5 cm proximal to the fibular tip and curves posteriorly toward the peroneal tendon sheath. A posterolateral incision is considered if peroneal tendon injury is suspected. Care is taken to protect the superficial peroneal nerve and the sural nerve. Dissection is carried down to the capsule anteriorly, and the extensor retinaculum is identified distally. The capsule is incised anteriorly and extended to the distal extent of the incision, leaving a 3-mm cuff of capsule attached to the fibula. This capsular incision includes the anterior talofibular ligament. The peroneal tendons are retracted inferiorly, and the extracapsular calcaneofibular ligament is identified at the tip of the fibula and followed as it runs distal and posterior to the calcaneus. This ligament helps form the floor of the peroneal tendon sheath and is usually easily identified. A 3-mm proximal cuff is left attached to the fibula, and it is repaired first in a vest-over-pants fashion with a no. 0 nonabsorbable suture. The anterior talofibular ligament is shortened in a similar vest-over-pants fashion through drill holes in

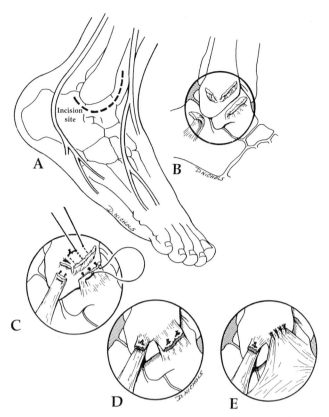

Figure 26–2. Broström-Gould procedure. (A) Anterolateral curved incision. (B) Arthrotomy leaving a 3.0-mm cuff at the distal fibula. The proximal stump of the ligament is elevated. (C) The distal stump of the ligament is sutured into the fibula. (D) The proximal stump of the ligament is sutured over the distal stump in a vest-over-pants fashion. (E) The proximal margin of the extensor retinaculum is sutured into the periosteum of the fibula. (From McCluskey,[6] with permission.)

the fibula or by using a suture-anchoring device in the fibula. The capsule is repaired with a no. 0 Vicryl suture. The Gould modification involves finding the proximal margin of the extensor retinaculum and suturing it into the periosteum of the fibula as noted in Figure 26–2E.[5,6] Subcutaneous tissue is closed with a 2-0 Vicryl suture, and the skin is closed with a subcuticular 3-0 Prolene suture.

Postoperative Care

A splint is applied for 2 weeks, followed by a short leg cast for another 2 weeks. After the cast has been removed, the patient begins range-of-motion, strengthening, and proprioception exercises. A coaptation splint is worn for approximately 4 weeks. Full activity is usually resumed within about 12 weeks.

■ Hallux Valgus

Hallux valgus deformities involve lateral deviation of the great toe and medial deviation of the first metatarsal head

(Fig. 26–3). A hereditary predisposition to these deformities is found in more than half of the people who have them. Shoe wear plays an important role in its development by initiating the lateral posturing of the great toe and, through a cam mechanism, creating the medial deviation of the metatarsal head. Overpronation of the hindfoot and instability of the medial column are also predisposing factors.

When nonoperative treatment, such as shoe wear modification, has failed, surgery can be considered for painful deformities.[7] The procedure of choice depends upon the magnitude of the deformity, the flexibility of the deformity, the amount of first tarsometatarsal instability present, and the amount of degenerative changes present. The most commonly performed procedures are the chevron osteotomy for mild to moderate deformities that are passively correctable and the basilar osteotomy with modified McBride bunionectomy for more severe deformities with incongruent metatarsophalangeal joints and significantly subluxated sesamoid bones. First metatarsophalangeal fusions are used as salvage procedures or for patients who have first metatarsophalangeal arthritis. First tarsometatarsal fusion has gained more popularity recently with the recognition of tarsometatarsal instability, but it has a higher nonunion rate and a longer recovery time.

Chevron Osteotomy

The chevron osteotomy is performed when the intermetatarsal angle is less than or equal to 15 degrees and the

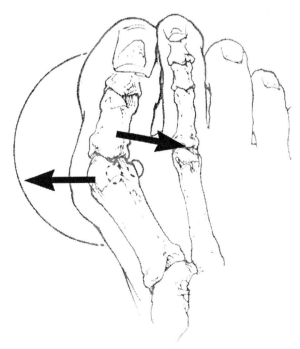

Figure 26–3. Hallux valgus. Lateral deviation of the great toe and medial deviation of the first metatarsal head describe this deformity.

metatarsophalangeal joint is passively correctable to a neutral position. The sesamoid positions are usually mildly or moderately displaced. Recently, the indications have been extended to more severe deformities by including a careful lateral release of the metatarsophalangeal joint and the adductor tendon. There is some risk of avascular necrosis to the distal fragment with a lateral release.

Technique

The chevron osteotomy is performed through a medial incision over the first metatarsophalangeal joint, taking care to protect the dorsal and plantar cutaneous nerves. A linear incision is made in the capsule, and the medial eminence is exposed and cut parallel to the medial border of the foot. The horizontal-V osteotomy is performed with the apex distal and approximately 3 mm proximal to the metatarsophalangeal joint[7] (Fig. 26–4). The angle of the osteotomy is 60 degrees. The distal fragment is then translated laterally 5 mm and is fixed with a pin or screw. The remaining medial eminence is then resected flush with the medial cortex of the metatarsal, and the capsule is repaired after excision of redundant tissue.

Postoperative Care

These reconstructions are stable, and the patient is allowed full weightbearing with a postoperative shoe immediately after surgery. Gentle range of motion of the metatarsophalangeal joint is begun early. The bunion dressing is changed at weekly intervals for 3 weeks, and then a toe separator is used for 2 weeks.

Basilar Osteotomy with Modified McBride Bunionectomy

Moderate or severe deformities can be treated surgically by performing an osteotomy at the base of the metatarsal. This technique allows correction of a greater intermeta-

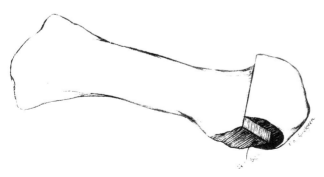

Figure 26–4. The V osteotomy subtends an angle of 50 to 60 degrees and is made parallel to the plantar aspect of the foot. If the limbs of the V osteotomy converge or diverge, it will be more difficult to displace the osteotomy and there will be less contact between the fragments. (From Johnson,[7] with permission.)

tarsal angle and simultaneous distal soft tissue reconstruction. Indications include intermetatarsal angles of more than 15 degrees, a subluxated sesamoid position, and more rigid deformities.

Technique

Two incisions are used. The first incision is a dorsal longitudinal incision over the first interspace, dissecting down through the dorsal fascia to the lateral sesamoid complex. A generous longitudinal incision is made dorsal to the lateral sesamoid through the sesamoid-metatarsal ligament. Next, the adductor hallucis tendon and the intermetatarsal ligament are incised from the attachment at the lateral sesamoid. A medial incision is made over the metatarsophalangeal joint and is extended up to the proximal metatarsal region. A capsulotomy is performed distally. The medial eminence is resected flush with the medial cortex of the metatarsal. The proximal osteotomy is performed using a crescentic osteotomy or a horizontal-V osteotomy. The intermetatarsal angle is corrected, and the proximal osteotomy is fixed with a 3.5-mm cortical screw. I prefer the proximal horizontal-V osteotomy with the apex distal and the screw placed from plantar to dorsal across the osteotomy side after correction of the intermetatarsal angle. This technique allows shortening or lengthening of the metatarsal as required and provides a more stable construct and more surface area for faster healing. Next, the distal capsule is repaired, taking care not to overtighten the capsule. Occasionally, an Akin osteotomy of the proximal phalanx is added to this procedure or to the chevron procedure to correct hallux interphalangeus.

Postoperative Care

Postoperative care for the basilar osteotomy with a modified McBride bunionectomy involves changing the dressings weekly for 4 weeks, using a toe separator for another 2 weeks, and having the patient begin range-of-motion exercises when comfortable.

■ Trauma

The foot and ankle are susceptible to trauma, and common surgical procedures are indicated for ankle fractures, calcaneal fractures, talar fractures, and Lisfranc tarsometatarsal subluxations. Some recent trends and recommendations for treatments will be discussed briefly.

Ankle Fractures

After an ankle fracture, the ankle mortise must be restored, and all intra-articular fractures must be reduced anatomically to prevent degenerative arthritis of the ankle. Medial malleolar fractures are usually fixed to prevent the

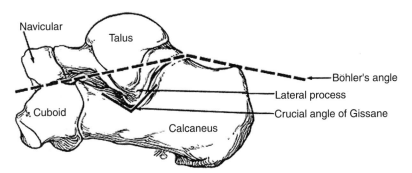

Figure 26–5. Lateral view of the calcaneus demonstrating Böhler's tuber angle (dotted line) and the crucial angle of Gissane. (From Heckman,[8] with permission.)

nonunions that occur with nonoperative treatment of even minimally displaced fractures. Lateral malleolar fractures are treated with open reduction and internal fixation if the ankle mortise is disrupted or if more than 2 mm of displacement or rotation is noted. Fractures at the level of the joint are treated with interfragmentary screws and one-third tubular plates. Care is taken to reduce these fractures anatomically and to fix the syndesmosis internally in cases where instability is noted, particularly in fracture patterns involving fibular fractures that are 3 cm or more proximal to the ankle joint.

Calcaneal Fractures

Calcaneal fractures are associated with a high risk of subtalar arthritis and disability.[8] These fractures are best treated with open reduction and internal fixation to restore the normal height, width, and articular surface at the posterior facet of the subtalar joint (Fig. 26–5). Improved results have been achievable through the use of a lateral or extensile approach and lower-profile plates and screws. Internal fixation allows early range-of-motion exercises after the incision site has healed; however, 6 weeks of nonweight-bearing is still required. For patients who have comminuted intra-articular fractures that involve more than three fracture fragments, primary subtalar arthrodeses have gained popularity. Late reconstructions usually in-

volve treatment of subtalar arthritis and require a subtalar arthrodesis.

Talar Fractures

Fractures of the neck of the talus are associated with avascular necrosis and are treated with open reduction and internal fixation to achieve anatomic reduction. The risk of avascular necrosis varies from 10 to 90 percent or more, depending on the amount of initial displacement.[9] Usually, cannulated screws are used for internal fixation from either a posterolateral or an anteromedial approach. Late reconstructive salvage procedures are used primarily to treat avascular necrosis and secondary arthritic changes. A tibial calcaneal fusion may be required if the ankle and subtalar joint are both involved. Recently, improved results from total joint ankle arthroplasty have been achieved and may be considered an alternative treatment.[10]

Lisfranc Fracture Dislocations

Subtle sprains of the Lisfranc tarsometatarsal joint are easily missed. A high index of suspicion must be present if swelling and tenderness through those midfoot joints are noted. Radiographs must include standing views and comparison views of the normal foot to recognize subtle subluxation (Fig. 26–6). The treatment for stable sprains

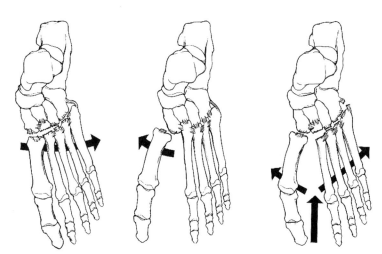

Figure 26–6. The three common patterns of tarsometatarsal joint dislocation: (left) homolateral, (center) isolated, and (right) divergent. (From Wilson FC,[11] with permission.)

is casting. Often these injuries are unstable and require closed or open reduction and internal fixation. Screws are the preferred method of fixation. Postoperative care involves casting and nonweightbearing for 6 weeks. Late reconstructive procedures include midfoot arthrodesis for patients with posttraumatic arthritis.

Summary

Thorough knowledge of the anatomy, biomechanics, and function of the foot is necessary to diagnose and treat most foot and ankle disorders. New techniques are being developed to treat these conditions—all with their recommended rehabilitation protocols. Good communication between surgeon and therapist continues to be essential for an optimal outcome in these patients.

References

1. Johnson KA, Strom DE: Tibialis posterior tendon dysfunction. Clin Orthop 239:196, 1989

2. Deland JT, Otis JC, Lee KT, et al: Lateral column lengthening with calcaneocuboid fusion: range of motion in the triple joint complex. Foot Ankle Int 16:729–735, 1994

3. Myerson MS, Corrigan J: Treatment of posterior tibial tendon dysfunction with flexor digitorum longus tendon transfer and calcaneal osteotomy. Orthopaedics 19:383–388, 1996

4. McCluskey LC: Talonavicular arthrodesis, calcaneocuboid arthrodesis, double arthrodesis, and pantalar arthrodesis. Foot Ankle Clin 2(2):329–339, 1997

5. Hamilton WG, Thompson FM, Snow SW: The modified Brostrom procedure for lateral ankle instability. Foot Ankle 14: 1–7, 1992

6. McCluskey LC: Foot and ankle injuries in sports. p. 912. In Gould JS (ed): Operative Foot Surgery. WB Saunders, Philadelphia, 1995

7. Johnson JE: Chevron osteotomy for hallux valgus: surgical indications and technique. Operative Techniques Orthopaedics 2:177–183, 1992

8. Heckman JD: Fractures and dislocations of the ankle. p. 1671. In Rockwood CA, Green DP (eds): Fractures in Adults. 2nd Ed. Lippincott, Philadelphia, 1984

9. Hawkins LG: Fractures of the neck of the talus. J Bone Joint Surg 52A:991–1002, 1970

10. Pyevich MT, Saltzman CL, Callaghan JJ, et al: Total ankle arthroplasty: a unique design. Two to twelve-year follow-up. J Bone Joint Surg 80A:1410–1420, 1998

11. Wilson FC: Fractures and dislocations of the foot. p. 1800. In Rockwood CA, Green DP (eds): Fractures in Adults. 2nd Ed. JB Lippincott, Philadelphia, 1984

CHAPTER 27
Mobilization of the Lower Extremity

Michael J. Wooden

The lower extremity mobilization techniques described in this chapter are by no means all that exist. Rather, these are the techniques that the author has found to be safe, easy to apply, and effective.

The reader is referred to Chapter 13 for a discussion of the definitions, indications, and contraindications of mobilization. Also, Chapters 21 through 26 contain descriptions of anatomy, mechanics, pathology, and evaluation of the lower limb joints.

■ Techniques

For each technique illustrated, patient position, the therapist's hand contacts, and the direction of movement are described. Table 27–1 lists each technique along with the physiologic movement it theoretically enhances.

Table 27–1. Summary of Lower Extremity Techniques

Joint	Mobilization Technique	Movement Promoted	Figure No.
Hip	Long axis distraction	General	27–1
	Distraction in flexion	Flexion	27–2
	Lateral distraction	General	27–3
	Lateral distraction in flexion	Flexion	27–4
	Posterior capsule stretch	Flexion	27–5
	Anterior capsule stretch	Extension	27–6, 27–7
	Medial capsule stretch	Abduction	
Patellofemoral	Superior glide	Extension	27–8A
	Interior glide	Flexion	27–8B
	Lateromedial glide	General	27–9
Tibiofemoral	Anterior glide	Extension	27–10, 27–12, 27–13, 27–14
	Posterior glide	Flexion	27–11, 27–13, 27–14
	Medial rotation	Medial rotation, flexion	27–15A, 27–16
	Lateral rotation	Lateral rotation, extension	27–15B, 27–16
	Long axis distraction	General	27–17
	Distraction in flexion	Flexion	27–18, 27–19
Superior tibiofibular	Anterosposterior glides	General	27–20, 27–21
	Downward glide	Downward glide of fibula	27–22
	Upward glide	Upward glide of fibula	27–23

Table continued on following page

☐☐☐☐☐ ☐ ☐ ☐

Table 27–1. Summary of Lower Extremity Techniques *Continued*

Joint	Mobilization Technique	Movement Promoted	Figure No.
Inferior tibiofibular	Tib-fib glide	Fibular movement, ankle plantar flexion and dorsiflexion	27–24
Ankle mortice	Distraction	General	27–25, 27–26, 27–27
	Anterior glide	Plantar flexion	27–28, 27–29, 27–31
	Posterior glide	Dorsiflexion	27–28, 27–30
Subtalar	Distraction	General	27–32, 27–33, 27–34
	Distraction with calcaneal rocking	Inversion, eversion	27–35
Midtarsal	Talonavicular glide	Pronation, supination	27–36
	Calcaneocuboid glide	Pronation, supination	27–37
Intermetatarsal (anterior arch)	Glides	General	27–38
Metatarsophalangeal	Distraction	General	27–39
	Dorsal glide	Dorsiflexion	27–40A, 27–42
	Plantar glide	Plantar flexion	27–40B, 27–42
	Mediolateral glide and tilt	General	27–41
Interphalangeal	Distraction	General	27–43
	Dorsoplantar glides	Dorsiflexion, plantar, flexion	27–43

■ The Hip

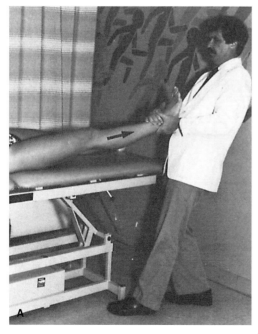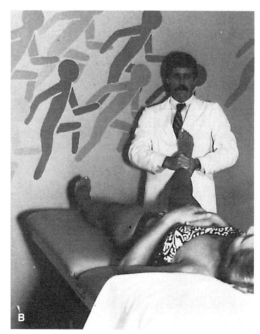

Figure 27–1. Long axis distraction.
Patient position: supine, leg extended.
Contacts: grasp the leg with both hands around the malleoli, elbows flexed: the leg is held in (A) slight flexion and (B) abduction.
Direction of movement: the therapist leans backward and pulls along the long axis of the leg.

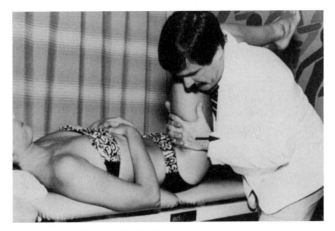

Figure 27–2. Distraction in flexion.
Patient position: Supine, hip and knee flexed to 90 degrees.
Contacts: the back of the knee rests on the therapist's shoulder; hands grasp the anterior aspect of the proximal thigh with fingers interlocked.
Direction of movement: the femoral head is pulled inferiorly.

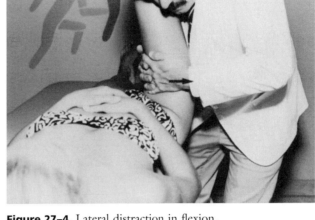

Figure 27–4. Lateral distraction in flexion.
Patient position: supine, hip and knee flexed to 90 degrees.
Contacts: the back of the knee rests on the therapist's shoulder; hands grasp the medial aspect of the proximal thigh with fingers interlocked.
Direction of movement: the femoral head is distracted laterally.

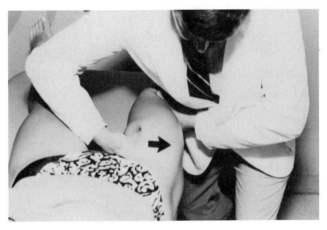

Figure 27–3. Lateral distraction.
Patient position: supine, leg extended.
Contacts: one hand stabilizes the lateral aspect of the femur above the knee; the other hand contacts the first web space against the medial aspect of the proximal femur.
Direction of movement: the femoral head is distracted laterally.

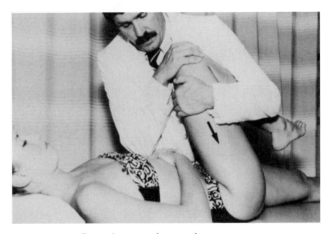

Figure 27–5. Posterior capsule stretch.
Patient position: supine, hip flexed to at least 100 degrees.
Contacts: the medial aspect of the knee rests against the therapist's chest; hands grasp the distal femur and over the patella.
Direction of movement: push downward along the long axis of the femur posteriorly, inferiorly, and slightly laterally.

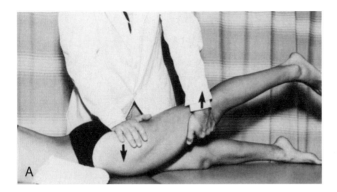

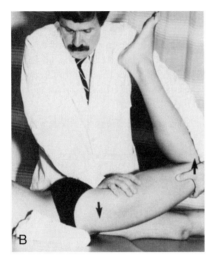

Figure 27–6. Anterior capsule stretch.

Patient position: prone, leg extended, small towel roll under the anterior superior iliac spine.

Direction of movement: (A) simultaneously lift the knee while pushing the femoral head anteriorly; (B) with the knee flexed, the same maneuver also stretches the rectus femoris.

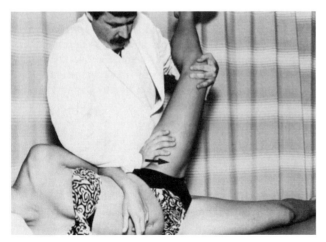

Figure 27–7. Medial capsule stretch.

Patient position: side-lying, hip at end-range abduction.

Contacts: one hand cradles the medial aspect of the knee to stabilize; the heel of the other hand contacts the lateral aspect of the hip at the greater trochanter.

Direction of movement: push the femoral head inferiorly.

■ The Knee

The Patellofemoral Joint

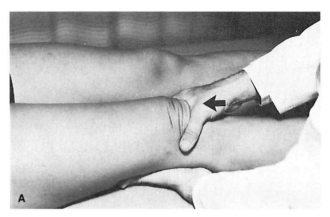

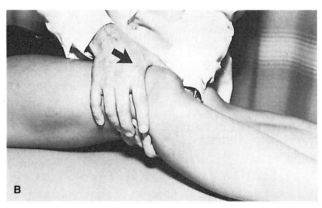

Figure 27–8. Superoinferior glide.

Patient position: supine.

Contacts: support the knee in slight flexion; contact the patella with the first web space at the base (superior) or the apex (inferior).

Direction of movement: glide (A) superiorly or (B) inferiorly.

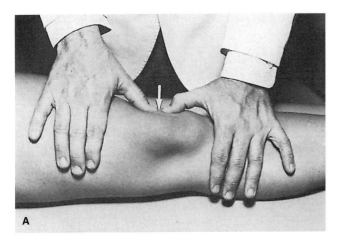

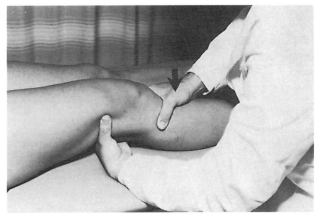

Figure 27–11. Posterior glide.
Patient position: supine, knee in slight flexion.
Contacts: stabilize the posterior aspect of the distal femur; grasp over the tibial tubercle.
Direction of movement: glide the tibia posteriorly.

Figure 27–9. Lateromedial glide.
Patient position: supine.
Contacts: use thumbtips against the medial or lateral patellar borders.
Direction of movement: glide (A) medially or (B) laterally.

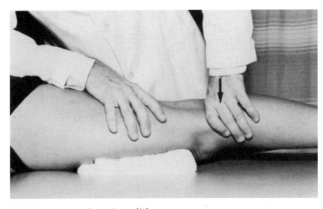

Figure 27–12. Anterior glide.
Patient position: prone, knee extended.
Contacts: the anterior aspect of the femur is stabilized with a small towel roll; the first web space contacts the posterior aspect of the proximal femur.
Direction of movement: glide the tibia anteriorly.

The Tibiofemoral Joint

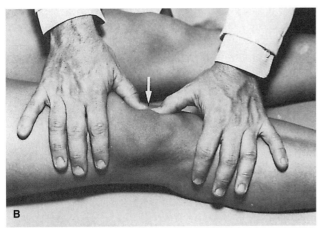

Figure 27–10. Anterior glide.
Patient position: supine, knee in slight flexion.
Contacts: stabilize the anterior aspect of the distal femur; grasp the posterior aspect of the proximal tibia.
Direction of movement: glide the tibia anteriorly on the femur.

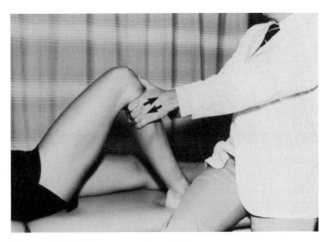

Figure 27–13. Anteroposterior glide.
Patient position: supine, knee flexed to 90 degrees.
Contacts: grasp the proximal aspect of the tibia, thumbs anterior.
Direction of movement: glide the tibia anteriorly and posteriorly.

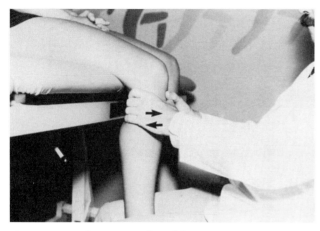

Figure 27-14. Anteroposterior glide.
Patient position: sitting, knee flexed to 90 degrees.
Contacts: grasp the proximal aspect of the tibia, thumbs anterior.
Direction of movement: glide the tibia anteriorly and posteriorly.

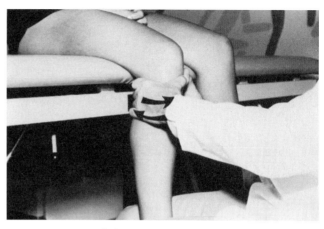

Figure 27-16. Mediolateral rotation.
Patient position: sitting, knee flexed to 90 degrees.
Contacts: grasp the proximal aspect of the tibia, thumbs anterior.
Direction of movement: combine anterior and posterior glide with medial and lateral rotation.

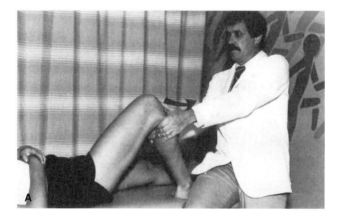

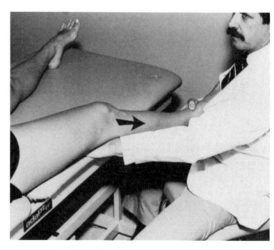

Figure 27-17. Long axis distraction.
Patient position: supine, slight flexion.
Contacts: stabilize with hand behind the knee; the other hand grasps the lower leg around the malleoli.
Direction of movement: pull along the long axis of the lower leg.

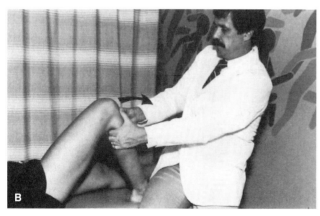

Figure 27-15. Mediolateral rotation.
Patient position: supine, knee flexed to 90 degrees.
Contacts: grasp the proximal aspect of the tibia, thumbs anterior.
Direction of movement: combine (A) anterior glide with medial and (B) lateral rotation.

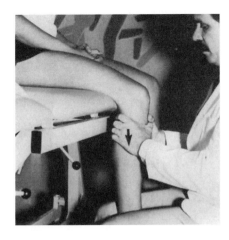

Figure 27–18. Distraction in flexion.
Patient position: sitting, knee flexed to 90 degrees.
Contacts: grasp the proximal aspect of the tibia, thumbs anterior.
Direction of movement: distract the lower leg downward; distraction can be assisted by the therapist holding the malleoli between the knees. Note: In this position, anteroposterior glides and rotations can also be applied while distracting.

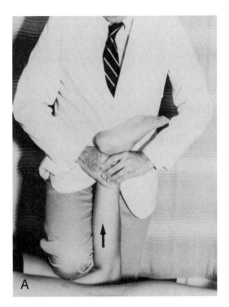

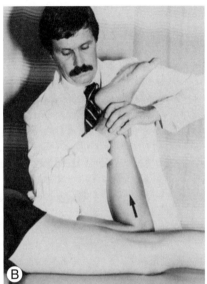

Figure 27–19. Distraction in flexion.
Patient position: prone, knee flexed to 90 degrees or more.
Contacts: grasp the distal femur with hands around the malleoli; stabilize the posterior aspect of the femur with (A) the knee or elbow and (B) a towel roll.
Direction of movement: (A) distract by pulling the leg upward; (B) distract by flexing the leg toward the stabilizing arm and simultaneously lifting the leg up.

The Superior Tibiofibular Joint

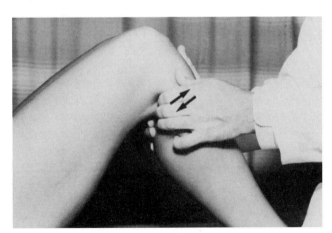

Figure 27–20. Anteroposterior glide.
Patient position: supine, knee flexed to 90 degrees.
Contacts: stabilize the medial aspect of the tibia; grasp the fibular head with thumb and forefinger.
Direction of movement: glide the fibular head anteriorly and posteriorly.

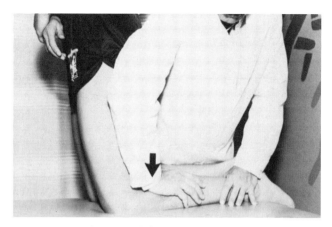

Figure 27–21. Anterior glide.
Patient position: kneeling.
Contacts: stabilize the lower leg on the table; the carpal tunnel contacts the posterior aspect of the fibular head.
Direction of movement: glide the fibular head downward (anteriorly).

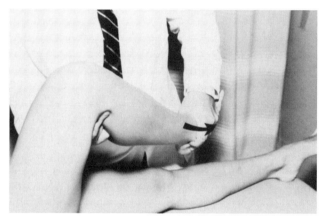

Figure 27–22. Downward glide.
Patient position: supine, hip and knee flexed to about 90 degrees.
Contacts: support the knee posteriorly while palpating the head of the fibula; the other hand grasps the leg above the ankle with the index finger hooked around the lateral malleolus.
Direction of movement: simultaneously invert the ankle and pull the lateral malleolus downward.

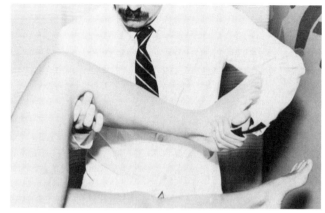

Figure 27–23. Upward glide.
Patient position: supine, hip and knee flexed to about 90 degrees.
Contacts: support the knee posteriorly while palpating the head of the fibula; the heel of other the hand contacts the lateral aspect of the plantar surface of the foot.
Direction of movement: evert the foot sharply to push the fibula upward.

■ The Foot and Ankle

The Distal Tibiofibular Joint

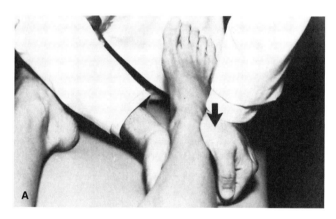

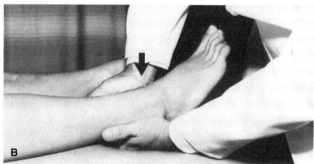

Figure 27–24. Fibular glides.
Patient position: supine.
Contacts: stabilize the medial malleolus against the carpal tunnel of the hand resting on the table; the carpal tunnel of the other hand contacts the anterior aspect of the lateral malleolus.
Direction: (A) glide the fibula posteriorly on the tibia; (B) reverse hand positions to glide the tibia posteriorly.

The Talocrural (Mortice) Joint

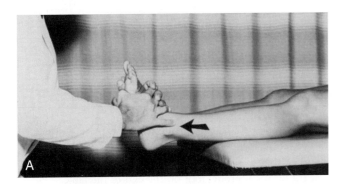

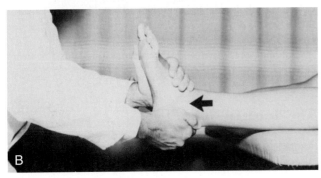

Figure 27–25. Distraction.
Patient position: supine.
Contacts: (A) grasp the foot with the second, third, and fourth fingers of both hands interlocked over the dorsum, thumbs plantar, or (B) grasp with one hand dorsomedially while the other hand holds the calcaneus laterally.
Direction of movement: distract the talus from the mortise.

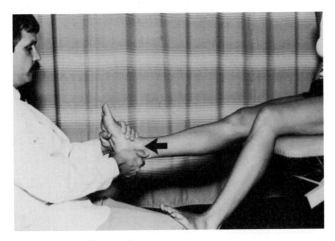

Figure 27–26. Distraction.
Patient position: sitting at the end of the table; the therapist is also sitting.
Contacts: same as in Figure 27–25; the patient adds stability by resting the opposite foot on the therapist's knee.
Direction of movement: distract the talus from the mortise.

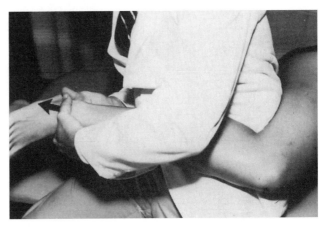

Figure 27–27. Distraction.
Patient position: side-lying.
Contacts: the posterior aspect of the femur is stabilized against the therapist's hip and iliac crest; the first web spaces grasp anterior and posterior to the talus.
Direction of movement: distract the talus from the mortise.

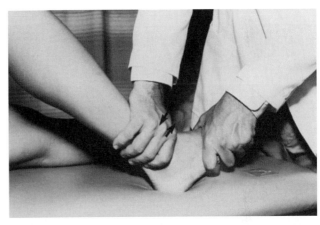

Figure 27–28. Anteroposterior glide.
Patient position: supine, knee flexed with the heel resting on the table.
Contacts: stabilize the foot by grasping dorsolaterally; the other hand grasps the anterior aspect of the lower leg above the malleoli.
Direction of movement: glide the tibia and fibula anteriorly and posteriorly on the talus.

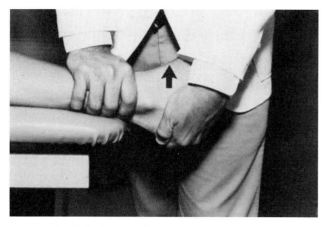

Figure 27–29. Anterior glide.
Patient position: supine, leg extended with the foot off the end of the table.
Contacts: stabilize the tibia and fibula by holding them against the table; the other hand cradles the calcaneus laterally.
Direction of movement: glide the calcaneus and talus upward (anteriorly).

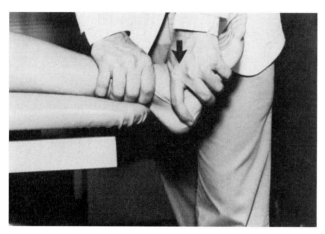

Figure 27–30. Posterior glide.
Patient position: supine, leg extended with the foot off the edge of the table.
Contacts: stabilize the tibia and fibula by holding them against the table; the other hand grasps the foot dorsolaterally with the first web space against the anterior aspect of the talus.

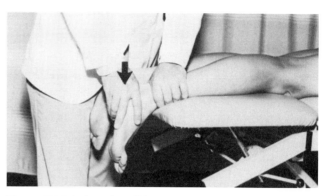

Figure 27–31. Anterior glide.
Patient position: prone, foot off the end of the table.
Contacts: stabilize the tibia and fibula by holding them against the table; the first web space of the other hand contacts the posterior aspect of the ankle.
Direction of movement: glide the calcaneus and talus downward (anteriorly) on the mortise.

The Subtalar Joint

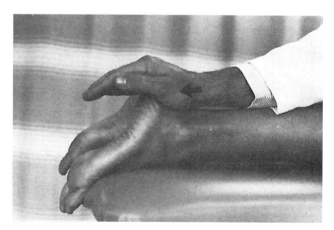

Figure 27–32. Distraction.
Patient position: prone, ankle plantar flexed, toes off the end of the table.
Contacts: the therapist's carpal tunnel contacts the posterior aspect of the calcaneus near the insertion of the Achilles tendon.
Direction of movement: distract the calcaneus from the talus by pushing caudally.

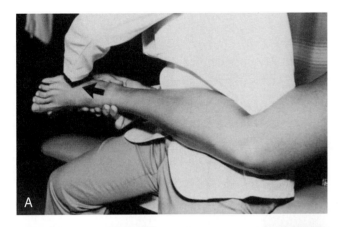

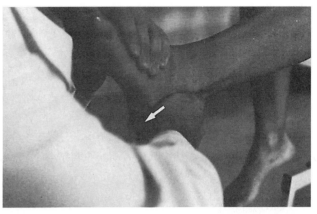

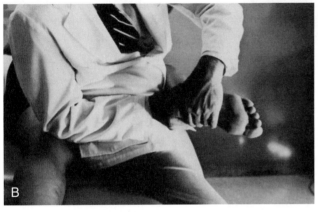

Figure 27–33. Distraction.
Patient position: side-lying.
Contacts: (A) the posterior aspect of the femur is stabilized against the therapist's hip and iliac crest; (B) first web spaces grasp the posterior and plantar aspects of the calcaneus.
Direction of movement: distract the calcaneus from the talus.

Figure 27–34. Distraction.
Patient: supine or sitting, foot off the end of the table.
Contacts: stabilize the foot by grasping it dorsomedially; the other hand grasps the calcaneus laterally.
Direction of movement: distract the calcaneus from the talus.

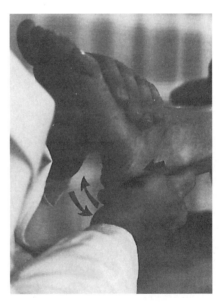

Figure 27–35. Distraction with calcaneal rocking.
Patient position: supine or sitting, foot off the edge of the table
Contacts: same as in Figure 27–34.
Direction of movement: while distracting the calcaneus, invert and evert it on the talus.

The Talonavicular Joint (Medial Aspect of the Midtarsal Joint)

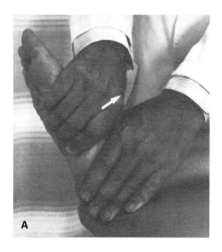

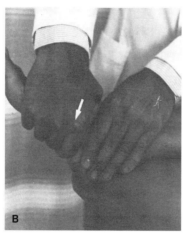

Figure 27–36. Talonavicular glide.
Patient position: supine.
Contacts: with both hands on the medial aspect of the foot, stabilize the talus and grasp the navicular with the first web space.
Direction of movement: glide the navicular in (A) dorsal and (B) plantar directions.

The Calcaneocuboid Joint (Lateral Aspect of the Midtarsal Joint)

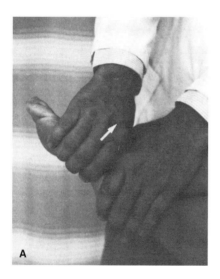

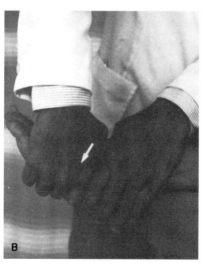

Figure 27–37. Calcaneocuboid glide.
Patient position: supine.
Contacts: with both hands on the lateral aspect of the foot, stabilize the calcaneus and grasp the cuboid with the first web space.

The Intermetatarsal Joints

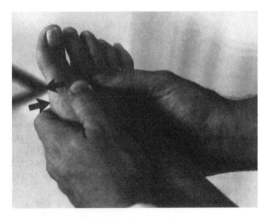

Figure 27–38. Intermetatarsal glides.
Patient position: supine.
Contacts: with the thumbs and forefingers, grasp the first and second metatarsal heads; stabilize the second metatarsal head.
Direction of movement: glide the first metatarsal head in dorsal and plantar directions; repeat at the second, third, and fourth interspaces.

The First Metatarsophalangeal (MTP) Joint

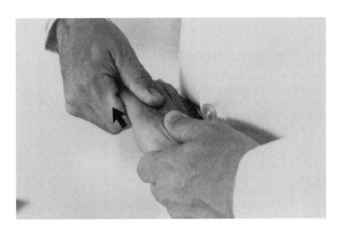

Figure 27–39. Distraction.
Patient position: supine.
Contacts: stabilize the first metatarsal head; the other hand grasps the proximal phalanx on its dorsal and plantar aspects.
Direction of movement: distract the phalanx from the metatarsal.

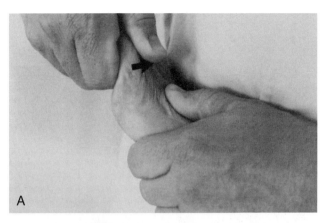

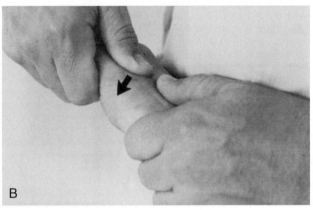

Figure 27–40. Dorsoplantar glides.
Patient position: supine.
Contacts: stabilize the first metatarsal head; the other hand grasps the dorsal and plantar aspects of the proximal phalanx.
Direction of movement: glide the phalanx in (A) dorsal and (B) plantar directions.

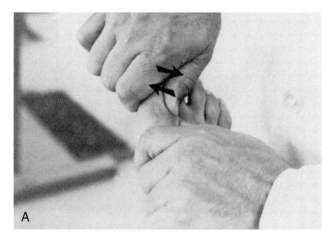

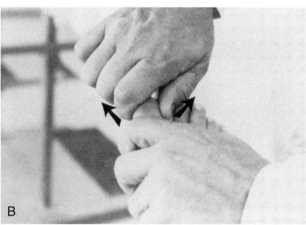

Figure 27–41. Mediolateral glide and tilt.
Patient position: supine.
Contacts: stabilize the first metatarsal head; the other hand grasps the medial and lateral aspects of the proximal phalanx.
Direction of movement: (A) glide the phalanx medially and laterally; (B) tilt the phalanx medially and laterally.

The Second to Fifth MTP Joints

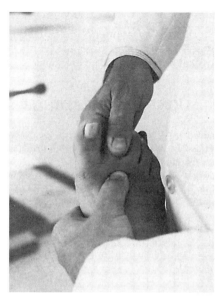

Figure 27–42. Distraction and dorsoplantar glides.
Patient position: supine.
Contacts: stabilize the second metatarsal head; the other hand grasps the dorsal and plantar aspects of the proximal phalanx.
Direction of movement: distract or glide the phalanx (as in Figs. 27–39 and 27–40); repeat at the third, fourth, and fifth MTP joints.

The Interphalangeal Joints

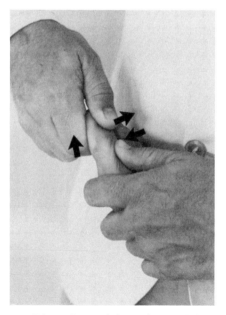

Figure 27–43. Distraction and dorsoplantar glides.
Patient position: supine.
Contacts: stabilize the proximal phalanx; grasp the dorsal and plantar aspects of the distal phalanx.
Direction of movement: distract and glide in the dorsal and plantar directions; repeat for all interphalangeal joints.

■ Acknowledgements

I thank Janie Wise, MMSc, PT (the photographer), Amelia Haselden, PT (the model), and the Physical Therapy Department at Emory University Hospital for their valuable assistance.

■ Suggested Readings

Basmajian JV, MacConail C: Arthrology. In Warwick R, Williams P (eds.): Gray's Anatomy, 35th Br. Ed. WB Saunders, Philadelphia, 1973

Brooks-Scott J: Handbook of Mobilization. In The Management of Children with Neurologic Disorders. Butterworth-Heinemann, London, 1998

Butler D: Mobilisation of the Nervous System. Churchill Livingstone, Melbourne, 1991

Corrigan B, Maitland GD: Practical Orthopaedic Medicine. Butterworths, London, 1985

Cyriax J: Textbook of Orthopaedic Medicine. Vol. 1: Diagnosis of Soft Tissue Lesions. Balliere Tindall, London, 1978

Cyriax J, Cyriax P: Illustrated Manual of Orthopaedic Medicine. Butterworths, London, 1983

D'Ambrogio KJ, Roth GB: Positional Release Therapy: Assessment and Treatment of Musculoskeletal Dysfunction. CV Mosby, St. Louis, 1997

Donatelli RA (ed): Physical Therapy of the Shoulder. 3rd Ed. Churchill Livingston, Melbourne, 1986

Glasgow EF, Twomey L (eds): Aspects of Manipulative Therapy. Churchill Livingstone, Melbourne, 1986

Hoppenfeld S: Physical Examination of the Spine and Extremities. Appleton-Century-Crofts, East Norwalk, CT, 1976

Konin JG, Wiksten DL, Isear JA: Special Tests for Orthopaedic Examination. Slack, Inc., Thorofare, NJ, 1997

Loudon J, Bell S, Johnston J: The Clinical Orthopedic Assessment Guide. Human Kinetics, Champaign, IL, 1998

Magee DJ: Orthopedic Physical Assessment. WB Saunders, Philadephia, 1987

Maitland GD: Peripheral Manipulation. Butterworths, London, 1978

Mennell JM: Joint Pain: Diagnosis and Treatment Using Manipulative Techniques. Little, Brown, Boston, 1964

■ CHAPTER 28

Measurement of Functional Status, Progress, and Outcome in Orthopaedic Clinical Practice

Jill Binkley

■ Rationale for Measuring Functional Outcome

Physical therapists are routinely challenged to determine whether a patient's condition has changed following one treatment or a series of treatments. Change may be detected as a decrease in pain measured on a pain scale or as increased range of motion. Patients may note increased ability to do an activity that they were previously unable to do, another indicator of change. We use this information regarding change and the extent of that change to make decisions about continuing, discontinuing, or changing our intervention. Information regarding the outcomes of physical therapy interventions is used to guide future clinical decision making on an informal basis and, in some cases, on a formal basis through systematic data collection, such as part of a quality assurance program. In addition, measurement of outcome is a critical component of formal clinical studies comparing interventions. Clearly, the appropriate selection of measures of patient progress and outcome is critical. While it is becoming increasingly recognized that measurement of outcome is important in physical therapy, there is little in the literature to assist clinicians in evaluating and interpreting the variety of self-report functional status scales available. The purpose of this chapter is to outline the rationale for implementing systematic functional outcome measurement in your clinical practice. Self-report functional status scales will be focused on. Criteria for selecting outcome measures will be addressed, and measures currently in the literature that meet these criteria will be reviewed.

In clinical practice, we constantly measure and remeasure patients' status through informal inquiries—"How are you doing today? Are the stairs any easier to climb?"—and through measures of impairment, such as pain, range of motion, and strength. Impairment measures are not adequate measures of outcome for four reasons. First,

there is mounting evidence that measures of impairment are not always directly related to patients' functional capacity, which is, ironically, most often the critical goal of physiotherapy intervention. We see this clinically in the lack of direct correlation between impairment and function in patients. An example is an athlete with a minor reduction in range of motion resulting in a major functional limitation such as inability to perform the sport. This lack of direct correlation between impairment and function has been documented in the literature. In patients with low back pain, only moderate correlation has been reported between impairment measures such as pain intensity, lumbar range of motion, strength, and neurologic findings and patients' functional ability.[1-3] In addition, the lack of direct correlation between knee extensor strength and functional ability has been documented.[4]

The second reason that impairment alone is not an adequate measure of patient outcome is that many measures of impairment used by orthopaedic physical therapists are diagnostic rather than evaluative. Kirshner and Guyatt[5] suggest that the three purposes of tests or measures are *discriminatory or diagnostic* (discriminating between categories of patients), *predictive* (predicting the patient's prognosis), and *evaluative* (measuring the change in a patient's status over time). With respect to the issue of categorizing patients, this refers to distinguishing between different conditions and/or between levels of severity of a particular condition. Thus, the purpose of clinical testing may be best summarized as (1) determining the diagnosis, (2) determining the prognosis, and (3) obtaining baseline measures for evaluating treatment progress and outcome. Some impairment measures, such as range of motion, may be appropriate for meeting all three goals. On the other hand, many measures of impairment, such as ligamentous testing, are not appropriate measures of physical therapy progress or outcome.

The third reason that impairment alone is not an adequate measure of patient outcome is that in many cases, a suitable measure of impairment does not exist for documenting patient change. An example of this is a patient presenting with patellofemoral pain when running for more than 5 miles. There may be no pain to measure during the assessment and no other suitable impairment measure to document the incremental change which is anticipated during the period of physical therapy intervention. An appropriate measure of function may be the only outcome measure with which to document change in this patient.

The fourth and final reason to measure function in our patients is that the goals of physical therapy are typically to increase patients' function levels (ability to sit, run, comb one's hair, or go to work). It makes sense, therefore, to measure the *functional outcome* of our patients. While impairment measures remain important in planning intervention and measuring outcome, measures of function are a critical component in documenting the patient's progress and outcome.

There are many potential benefits of incorporating standardized functional outcome measurement into practice. The first and most important one is enhancement of patient care by focusing on functional goals which are of critical importance to the patient. Patient–clinician communication is improved as patients perceive the physical therapist's interest in their functional limitations. Clinical decision making regarding continuation, change, or discontinuation of treatment is improved. Finally, there is clear communication with referral sources and payers regarding patients' functional level and the functional goals and outcomes of physical therapy. This constitutes evidence of the quality of physical therapy intervention provided to patients. In many cases, payers not only appreciate but require documentation of the patient's functional level at the initial evaluation as well as on an ongoing basis as a measure of progress and outcome.

Methods of Measuring Function in Orthopaedic Patients

Two principal types of measures are used to evaluate function in orthopaedic patients: self-report functional status scales and observed functional performance measures. Self-report functional scales vary from one page to many pages and are filled out by patients in the clinic or through a phone survey. Examples of these are the SF-36 health status scale and the Roland-Morris Back Pain Questionnaire.[6–8] Functional performance measures are obtained by the physical therapist and may consist of a simple one-task test, such as timed walking, or a more complex battery of tests, such as functional capacity evaluations for patients with low back pain. While there is an important role in physical therapy clinical practice for functional performance testing, self-report functional scales are recommended as a fundamental measure of functional progress and outcome. An increasing number of these scales are available, with documented measurement properties suited to orthopaedic physical therapy practice. Self-report functional scales are efficient and economical to implement in clinical practice and, therefore, will be the focus of this chapter.

■ Self-Report Functional Status Measures

Types of Self-Report Functional Status

Self-report functional status measures, in which patients respond verbally or in writing to questions regarding their function, are the easiest measures of function to incorporate into clinical practice. Functional status measures are classified as generic, condition-specific, and patient-specific. Generic measures are designed to be applicable across a broad spectrum of diseases, conditions, and demographic and cultural subgroups.[9] Such comparisons are of particular importance to health policy analysts. Examples of generic scales are the Sickness Impact Profile (SIP)[10] and the SF-36.[7,11] Condition-specific functional status measures are intended to assess disability and clinically important changes in disability within a specific group (e.g., patients with anterior cruciate ligament [ACL] deficiency or low back pain). Examples of condition-specific scales are the Lysholm knee scale[12] and the Roland-Morris scale[6] for use with patients with low back pain. Generic measures are referred to as *health status measures,* as they tap a variety of domains, including mental, emotional, psychosocial, and physical function. For the purposes of this chapter, all measures dealt with will be referred to as *functional status measures,* encompassing both measures of generic health status and physical function measures.

Health care policy makers and clinical researchers are interested in acquiring data on groups; clinicians are also interested in obtaining information and making decisions concerning individual patients. Both generic and condition-specific functional status measures have been conceived with the former interest in mind. More recently, there has been a growing interest in using functional status measures at the individual patient level.[13–18] In support of this position, Feinstein and colleagues have suggested that "if the index is intended to demonstrate the patient's improvement, the patient's concept of what should be improved may often be much more cogent than the particular beliefs held by the health care team."[19] In response to this need a third type of functional status measure has emerged: the patient-specific measure. The goal of patient-specific measures is to aid clinicians in making decisions about the health or functional status of individual patients. Several patient-specific measures such as the MACTAR,[14] the MacKenzie,[13] and Patient Specific Functional Scale[17,18,20] have been reported in the literature.

Criteria for Selecting Functional Status Measures for Orthopaedic Clinical Practice

The following are criteria for selecting a self-report functional status measure for use in clinical practice:

1. The measure must be developed using a systematic process of item selection and must use appropriate scaling and item weighting, where applicable.[21]
2. The measure is documented to be *reliable.*
3. The measure is documented to be *valid.*
4. The measure is documented to be *sensitive to valid change,* a form of validity.
5. The measure can be administered quickly, and is easy to score and record in the medical record.
6. The measure is appropriate for wide application to patients in the clinical practice, including patients with different initial functional levels, conditions, diseases, problems, and ages. This improves the compliance of clinicians in using the scales and simplifies the logistics of selecting scales for patients and maintaining copies of scales in the clinic.
7. The measure provides more information at a higher quality than is currently available to clinicians.

The development of a functional status measure which is scientifically sound and clinically useful is a complex process.[21] The initial step is item or question generation and is usually performed through expert clinician and patient interviews as well as literature search. The type of information included in a measure affects its measurement properties. For example, some measures combine function as well as impairment items, such as range of motion, swelling, or thigh atrophy.[12] In the Lysholm knee scoring scale, for example, data such as thigh atrophy are converted from centimeters to a 3-point scale of atrophy. The inclusion of impairment data may impact the measurement properties of the scale when the reliability of the impairment measure is lower than that of the functional items on the scale. In addition, functional change may be obscured in cases where thigh atrophy is not changing while function is improving. Finally, information is lost in converting continuous data (e.g., thigh atrophy in centimeters or range of motion in degrees) to ordinal data (e.g., a 5-point scale).

Once items are determined, the initial version of the scale is pilot tested by administering the scale to a group of appropriate patients. Items are then systematically reviewed for inclusion in or exclusion from the final scale. A critical aspect of scale development is item scaling, which includes issues such as whether responses are dichotomous (e.g., yes/no) or scaled (e.g., a 7-point scale ranging from "unable to perform the task" to "no difficulty"). The type of scale selected, number of scale points,

and labels for scale points are factors which significantly impact the reliability, validity, and sensitivity to change of a measure.

Reliability, validity, and sensitivity to valid change are termed the *measurement properties* of a test or measure. *Reliability* refers to the repeatability of the measure and reflects the error associated with a measure. For a test or measure to be reliable, it must remain stable and reflect stable differences between patients who have not truly changed over the reassessment interval.[22] Reliability is often assessed by administering a scale or test at two points in time when a change in patients' condition is not expected. *Validity* addresses the extent to which a test or measure truly measures what it is intended to measure. In the case of a functional scale, validity is the extent to which the scale captures the true functional capacity of the patients.[22] There are four types of validity: face, content, construct, and criterion validity. *Face validity* is the least rigorous form of validity and refers to the extent to which a scale *appears* to capture the concept it purports to measure.[22] For example, common sense suggests that a scale designed to measure upper extremity function which includes patients' ability to walk and run lacks face validity. *Content validity* relates to the extent to which the content included in a measure represents the attribute of interest.[22] For example, how well does a given low back functional status scale sample the overall functional ability of patients with low back pain? *Construct validity* refers to the extent to which scores or performance on a test or measure agree with a theory, or hypothesis, about the phenomenon being measured.[22] In the case of function, one theory might be that patients off work due to their back pain will be more disabled than persons with back pain who continue to work. This theory could then be used to examine the construct validity of a functional measure by determining whether, in fact, functional scores on the scale indicated that patients off work had lower levels of function than those at work. Finally, *criterion-related validity* establishes the extent to which one measure compares with another measure considered to be a direct measure of the attribute of interest.[22] An example of this would be to compare a functional scale score to a direct measure of patient function. In many cases, including the domain of functional performance, there is no gold standard, or criterion, for measurement of function. The validation process for health status and functional scales is often carried out, therefore, through a series of construct validation studies.

The capacity of a measure to detect change in an individual patient or groups of patients has been termed *sensitivity to change* or *responsiveness.*[5,21,23] The term responsiveness, however, denotes a test's capacity to measure change but does not address the validity of the change, or whether the change measured on the scale truly reflects clinically important change. The term *sensitivity to valid change* encompasses both the capacity of a measure to detect change and the validity or meaningfulness of the change.[23] Examination of the validity of the change requires the use of an external measure, such as a patient/clinician rating of change or the use of a construct in which there is evidence that one group will change at a different rate than another (e.g., comparison of patients with acute versus chronic conditions).

There are important clinical implications in selecting a tool which does not have established or acceptable measurement properties for the patient population in which it will be used clinically. For example, a clinician will be unable to determine true change in patient status versus measurement error when using a functional scale which has poor reliability. Another example is the situation in which a measure shown to be sensitive to valid change in a particular population, such as patients with knee conditions, is used for patients with other conditions, such as foot and ankle conditions. The scale may not be as sensitive to change in the foot and ankle population. The risk of incorporating a functional status measure without documented measurement properties into practice is significant. Scales not documented to be reliable, valid, and sensitive to change in the patients on which they are used may estimate patients' functional level incorrectly and fail to capture improvement in functional status.

It is critical that any scale selected for implementation in clinical practice provide information regarding patients' functional status which is germane to clinical decision making. Clinicians must be able to measure function on an ongoing basis, such as weekly, in order to evaluate incremental functional change. Ease of administration and ease of scoring are also critical. In cases where, for example, complex calculations or a computer are required to determine a score, functional scores may not be available to clinicians for day-to-day decision making. If a scale requires detailed computation of scores and/or if scoring is performed outside the clinic, clinicians should be aware that functional measures cannot be used to track the progress and outcome of individual patients.

Measurement Properties of Self-Report Scales: Application to Groups of Patients and Individual Patients

Measurement of functional status in our patients serves two important and distinct purposes: (1) documentation of physical therapy outcome in *groups* of patients for quality assurance, establishment of clinical standards, and/or research purposes and (2) documentation of functional level, setting goals, and measuring functional progress and outcome in *individual* patients.

Outcome assessment procedures to date typically focus on the process of measurement of function at initial assessment and at discharge in order to answer the question "Has the functional status of this group of patients changed during the intervention period?" This information provides clinicians, administrators, and payers with information regarding the physical therapy and clinic performance of groups of patients. Patients may be grouped by categories such as diagnosis, clinic, physical therapist, or demographic factors in order to draw conclusions regarding patient outcome in these groups. Where comparative data are available, such as in pooled databases, clinics and clinicians can compare their outcomes to those of other groups of patients and other clinics. When the goal of measuring functional outcome is to compare groups of patients within a clinic or between clinics with respect to health status and function, the critical properties required of any measure used are reliability, validity, and sensitivity to change.

There is little in the literature to assist physical therapists in the use of available functional status scales to achieve the second purpose of documenting function, setting goals and measuring the progress of individual patients. Often, self-report functional status scales are many pages in length and require detailed calculations to score. They are therefore difficult for clinicians to use on a regular basis. In order for self-report functional scales to be used to document function and change in function, the scales must be easy to administer and score on a regular basis (for example, weekly). Once these criteria related to ease of administration are met, clinicians must also be armed with information regarding the reliability, validity, and sensitivity to valid change of the tool being used. In this case, however, the information must be provided in a format that enables a clinician to answer the following questions: (1) What is the functional status of the patient at a given point in time? (2) Has the patient's functional status truly changed? and (3) Has the patient's functional status undergone a change that is clinically important?

A self-report functional scale may be used to estimate the functional status of an individual patient at a given point in time.[24] In interpreting the score on such a scale, however, one must recognize that there is inherent variability in any clinical test or measure. This variability can be attributed to the patient, examiner, instrument, and measurement process. The variability of a test or measure is its test-retest reliability and is usually expressed as a reliability coefficient, such as an intraclass correlation coefficient. A reliability coefficient of, for example, $R = .85$ can be difficult to interpret when administering a test to an individual patient. Thus, for decisions on individual patients, an alternate expression of the error associated with a measure is most helpful to the clinician. The standard error of measurement (SEM) represents the within-patient error associated with multiple measurements obtained from the same patient. The SEM is expressed in the same units as the original measure and is, therefore, easy to interpret clinically. For example, for self-report scales, the SEM will be expressed in scale points. The

SEM provides clinicians with an estimate of the potential error associated with a given measure at a single point in time for a given sample of patients. In order to apply the SEM to a patient outside of a given study, confidence intervals are calculated for the SEM. Typically, a 90 percent confidence in a measure is appropriate for physical therapy decision making. The interpretation of this estimate of error is that, given a score on a scale of, for example, 20/100, and that the error associated with a single measure (90 percent confidence interval [CI] is 5 points, one can be reasonably confident that the true score lies between 15 and 25.

The SEM assumes that error is constant over the entire range of scale scores or at all levels of disability. The conditional standard error of measurement (CSEM) differs from the SEM in that the CSEM acknowledges that the magnitude of error is dependent, or conditional, on the score or scores of interest. In the case of self-report functional measures, this is often the case, and more error is associated with scores in the middle of the range than at the extremes of the range.[24] The clinical implication of this is that, in general, less change may be required on a functional scale for patients with very high or very low levels of disability to be indicative of true functional change.

In order to determine if true change has occurred in an individual patient's functional status between the initial and follow-up assessments, one must examine the change score between these two points. In this case, however, the estimate of the error of this change score must account for potential error at both assessments. This is accomplished by calculating the minimal detectable change (MDC), a mathematical manipulation of the SEM.[24]

Finally, clinicians need to know whether the change in scale scores is an important functional change. In this case, one must be aware of the minimally clinically important difference (MCID) for the scale. The MCID is estimated for a scale from studies examining sensitivity to valid change and is defined as the minimal change in a score or measure on a scale which is indicative of a change in function which is *important* to a patient.[24,25] It is possible to measure change on a scale which is greater than the error associated with the scale (MDC), but the change may have little impact on a patient's day-to-day function. An example is an increase in knee flexion from 35 to 50 degrees. This change is probably greater than that due to error, so true change has occurred. This increase, however, may not be particularly important to the patient. On the other hand, an increase in knee flexion from 80 to 95 degrees may be functionally important in allowing sitting and stair climbing. Thus, the MCID provides an estimate of the change on a measure which is indicative of clinically important change. It is of interest that the MCID may be dependent on the starting value, as noted in the knee range of motion example.

■ Functional Status Measures Suggested for Orthopaedic Clinical Practice

The following is a review of functional status scales relevant to general orthopaedic physical therapy practice which most closely meet the criteria stated above. Many additional scales are available, such as condition-specific scales for the temporomandibular joint and arthritis scales, which may be appropriate for incorporation into practice, depending on the clinical setting. A checklist of criteria to consider when evaluating other functional scales for clinical practice is provided in Figure 28–1. The Patient-Specific Functional Scale (PSFS) will be described first. Five condition-specific scales for each of the major anatomic regions (low back, neck, upper extremity, and lower extremity) will be reviewed. In the case of low back pain, both the Roland-Morris Low Back Pain Questionnaire and the Oswestry Low Back Pain Disability Index are included, since both meet the criteria for selection.

In the PSFS patients state their own functional limitations, so the scale is equally applicable for a high-level athlete with tendinitis and a patient following total knee replacement. When the PSFS is completed weekly, the patient and the physical therapist are provided with important and immediately usable information regarding change in functional activities which are important to the patient. The main disadvantage of the PSFS is that it is impossible to compare scores between patients, since each patient reports his or her own functional limitations. For this reason, use of the PSFS in clinical practice should be considered an initial step in incorporating measurement of functional progress and outcome into clinical practice. In order to allow comparison of baseline measures of function, rate of change, and interventions, standard condition-specific functional status measures are required. For example, a lower extremity scale administered to all patients in your practice allows comparison of baseline disability in different conditions and systematic comparison of different interventions for the same conditions.

The Patient-Specific Functional Scale

Description

The PSFS was constructed by Stratford and colleagues. Its principal goals were to provide a standardized method and measure for eliciting and recording patients' disabilities.[17,18,20] The PSFS is administered at the initial assessment, during the history taking and prior to the assessment of any impairment measures. The rationale for administering it prior to the objective examination is to maximize the patient's focus on function ("I have difficulty walking down stairs") rather than impairment ("I can't flex my knee"). Patients are asked to identify up to three important activities they are having difficulty with or are unable to perform. In addition to specifying the

The following is a checklist of criteria to use when selecting a health status measure for use in clinical practice. Note that one or several papers from the literature may need to be reviewed to complete the criteria checklist for a particular health status measure.

1. **Does the measure have documented validity?**

   a. Does the scale make sense with respect to the content of questions for the intended patient group? (face validity)
      Yes _____
      No _____
   b. Does the measure compare favorably when compared directly with other scales used to document function in this patient group? (validity)
      Yes _____ (measure performs as well as or better than other measures used to document function in this group)
      No _____
   c. Does the scale measure change effectively in the patient group?
      Yes _____ (measure demonstrated to be sensitive to valid change using strongest available designs)
      In Part _____ (some indication in the literature that measure documents change)
      No _____ (no work to date or measure does not perform well with respect to measurements of change)
   d. Is the sensitivity to valid change expressed in terms to allow application to individual patients—minimal clinically important difference (MCID)?
      Yes _____, state MCID: _____ scale points
      No _____

2. **Have the reliability and error associated with the measure's use been established?**

   a. Does the scale have documented internal consistency?
      Yes _____
      No _____
   b. Does the scale have documented test-retest reliability?

3. **Is the measure appropriate for wide application to patients in the clinical practice, including patients with different initial functional levels, conditions, diseases, problems, and ages?**

   Yes _____
   No, but appropriate to wide spectrum of patients in my clinical practice _____
   No _____

Summary

Rate the health status measure with regard to *appropriateness for use in the patient population* in question:

0	1	2	3	4
Not Appropriate		**Some criteria met and/or**		**Very Appropriate**
No criteria met		best available scale		All criteria met

Figure 28–1. Criteria for selecting outcome measures.

activities, patients are asked to rate, on an 11-point scale, the current level of difficulty associated with each activity. Patients are then asked to indicate up to two activities with which they are having just a bit of difficulty. The inclusion of these minor functional limitations allows tracking of any deterioration in the patient's condition. Finally, there are two pain questions and related scales. The clinician's role is to read the script (instructions) to the patient and record the activities, the corresponding numerical difficulty ratings, and the assessment date. At subsequent reassessments, the clinician reads the follow-up script, which reminds the patient of the activities he or she identified previously. Once again, the clinician records the numerical difficulty ratings and the date.

The activities and scores are recorded on the functional goal and outcome worksheet (Fig. 28–2). The scores for the main activities indicated by the patient are averaged together to produce an average score out of 10. The scores for the additional activities with which the patient is having minimal difficulty are also averaged. The functional goal and outcome worksheet was designed to record the PSFS activities and scores, additional functional scale scores, key impairment measures, and patient goals at initial assessment and at weekly follow-up exams.

Measurement Properties

The reliability, validity, and sensitivity to change of the PSFS have been reported in three patient groups: those with knee conditions, low back dysfunction, and cervical dysfunction.[17,18,20] In these groups, the PSFS was demonstrated to be reliable (test-retest reliability based on average scores and individual activity scores: $R = 0.84–0.98$). The construct validity of the PSFS was confirmed by

PATIENT NAME:

PATIENT-SPECIFIC ACTIVITIES	Initial	DATE AND SCORE						
1.								
2.								
3.								
AVERAGE: (/10)								
ADDITIONAL ACTIVITIES:								
1.								
2.								
PSFS PAIN QUESTIONS:								
PAIN LIMITATION SCORE:								
PAIN INTENSITY SCORE:								
CONDITION-SPECIFIC MEASURE:								
IMPAIRMENT MEASURES: **(e.g., ROM, STRENGTH)**								
1.								
2.								
3.								
4.								
SHORT-TERM GOALS: 2 WEEKS								
1.								
2.								
3.								
4.								
LONG-TERM GOALS: 4 WEEKS								
1.								
2.								
3.								
4.								

Figure 28–2. Functional goal and outcome worksheet.

comparing patients' PSFS scores with existing measures: the SF-36 in the knee study,[17] the Roland-Morris Low Back Pain Questionnaire for back pain patients,[18] and the Neck Disability Index in the neck study.[20] Correlation of the PSFS with the relevant comparison scale in each study was adequate to good ($r = .49-.83$). The sensitivity to valid change of the PSFS was confirmed using a number of different constructs in each of the three studies.[17,18,20] On average, the PSFS took subjects and therapists 4 minutes 13 seconds ($s = 1.9$ minutes) to administer.[18] While further work in other conditions is desirable, it appears that the PSFS meets the criteria of established measurement properties, and it is easy and efficient to administer and incorporate into the clinical record.

With respect to individual patient decision making, the potential error associated with an average score on the PSFS at a given point in time is ±1.7 scale points (90 percent CI), the MDC is 3 scale points (90 percent CI), and the MCID is 3 scale points (90 percent CI).[17] The interpretation of this is that at a given point in time, for example initial evaluation, a clinician can be confident that a given PSFS average score out of 10 is within 1.7 scale points of the patient's true score. On follow-up, changes in the score of at least 3 scale points can be interpreted as true patient change with reasonable confidence.

Roland-Morris Back Pain Questionnaire

Description

The Roland-Morris Back Pain Questionnaire (RMQ) is a scale which meets all of the criteria for functional outcome scales above.[6,27–30] It is a one-page, 24-item self-administered scale which takes several minutes for patients to complete. The score is easily calculated as the sum of functional problems which apply to the patient. Each of the 24 items is scored either 1, if it is endorsed by a patient, or 0 if it is not endorsed. Thus, scores can vary from the most desirable health state score of 0 to the least desirable health state score of 24.

Measurement Properties

The measurement properties of the RMQ are equal to or better than those of competing measures designed to assess the functional status of persons with low back pain and are better than those of most measures obtained as part of the objective assessment.[6,26–30] Test-retest reliability coefficients of .86 to .93 have been reported.[6,31,32] The RMQ's capacity to assess valid change has been well documented.[1,28,30,33,34]

With respect to decision making concerning individual patients, the potential error associated with a score on the RMQ at a given point in time is ±3 scale points (90 percent CI), the MDC is 5 scale points (90 percent

CI), and the MCID is 5 scale points (90 percent CI).[24] The interpretation of this is that at a given point in time, for example the initial evaluation, a clinician can be reasonably confident that a given RMQ score is within 3 scale points of the patient's true score. On follow-up, changes in the score of ± 5 scale points or more can be interpreted as true patient change with reasonable confidence. In this case, the MCID is the same as the MDC, so that changes of 5 scale points or more indicate clinically important differences.

Oswestry Low Back Pain Disability Index

Description

The Oswestry Low Back Pain Disability Index (Oswestry) is a one-page, 10-item self-administered scale which takes several minutes for patients to complete.[35] Each of the 10 items, including items such as pain, personal care, lifting, sleeping, and sex life, are rated on a 6-point scale, and all the items are summed. The patient's score is easily calculated. Scores can vary from the most desirable health state score of 0 to the least desirable health state score of 100.

Measurement Properties

The measurement properties of the Oswestry are well documented in the literature.[27,28,30,35,36] The Oswestry has been found to have good test-retest reliability ($r = 0.99$[31] and $R = 0.91$[27]). With respect to construct validity, it was demonstrated to show a significant positive change over time in patients in whom a high likelihood of spontaneous recovery was predicted. In addition, the Oswestry has been shown to be sensitive to valid change.[37,38]

With respect to decision making concerning individual patients, the potential error associated with a score on the Oswestry scale at a given point in time is 11 scale points (90 percent CI), the MDC is 16 scale points (90 percent CI), and the MCID is 11 scale points (90 percent CI). These estimates of error and MDC are derived from data presented in the literature[27,28] and from unpublished data (P. Stratford, personal communication, 1997). The interpretation of this is that at a given point in time, for example the initial evaluation, a clinician can be reasonably confident that a given Oswestry score is within 11 scale points of the patient's true score. On follow-up, changes in scores of ±16 scale points or more can be interpreted as true patient change with reasonable confidence. In this case, the MCID of 11 scale points is less than the MDC, so that while changes of about 11 points may be clinically important, one cannot be sure at the 90 percent level that the change is not related to error alone unless the change is greater that the MDC of 16 points.

The Neck Disability Index

Description

The Neck Disability Index (NDI) is the only condition-specific scale reported in the literature for cervical disorders.[39] The NDI format was based on the Oswestry scale for patients with low back pain and consists of 10 items, including 5 from the original Oswestry. It is a one-page self-administered scale which takes only a few minutes to complete. Scores vary from 0 (most desirable health state) to 50 (least desirable health state).

Measurement Properties

The measurement properties of the NDI have been documented in the literature.[39,40] Test-retest reliability has been reported to be good ($r = .89$).[40] In addition, construct validity was found to be acceptable when NDI scores were compared with McGill Pain Questionnaire scores and a visual analogue pain scale score.[39] Riddle and Stratford[40] examined the validity and sensitivity to change of the NDI in a variety of cervical conditions. They found that the NDI as well as the comparison scale, the Physical Component Score and the Mental Component Score of the SF-36, were adept at measuring change over time in patients with neck conditions. The authors noted that, based on the measurement properties examined, both the NDI and component scores of the SF-36 were appropriate for use in cervical conditions, but they pointed out that from a practical point of view, the NDI is much less complex to administer and score.

With respect to decision making about individual patients, the potential error associated with a score on the NDI at a given point in time is 5 scale points (90 percent CI). The MDC is 7 scale points (90 percent CI), and the MCID is 7 scale points (90 percent CI). The error estimates and MCID were derived from the literature.[20,39] The interpretation of this is that at a given point in time, for example the initial evaluation, a clinician can be reasonably confident that a given NDI score is within 5 scale points of the patient's true score. On follow-up, changes in score of ±7 scale points or more can be interpreted as true patient change with reasonable confidence. In this case, the MCID is the same as the MDC, so that changes of 7 scale points or more indicate clinically important differences.

Disability of the Arm Shoulder and Hand Outcome Measure

The Disability of the Arm Shoulder and Hand Outcome Measure (DASH) was developed jointly by the Institute for Work and Health in Toronto and the American Academy of Orthopaedic Surgeons.[41-43] The DASH incorporates questions related to function (23 questions) and symptoms (7 questions) and includes an optional sports/performing arts section (4 questions). Each question is rated on a 5-point scale from "none"/"no difficulty" to "unable"/"extreme severity," depending on the question. It is estimated that the DASH takes about 5 minutes to complete, and it is relatively easy to score. The scores are converted to a 100-point scale for function/symptoms, and there is a separate score for sports/performing arts.

Measurement Properties

The DASH was developed through a systematic item generation and subsequent item reduction process which included extensive field testing.[41] The DASH has been demonstrated to have good internal consistency, a component of reliability.[42] Initial examination of the construct validity of the DASH suggests that it is a valid measure of upper extremity function.[43]

With respect to decision making about individual patients, the potential error associated with a score on the DASH at a given point in time and the MDC, estimated from the literature, are approximately 8 scale points on the 100-point scale (90 percent CI).[43] The MDC, also estimated from the literature, is 12 scale points (90 percent CI).[43] The MCID has not yet been reported.

The Lower Extremity Functional Scale

Description

The Lower Extremity Functional Scale (LEFS) was developed by Binkley and colleagues for measurement of function in a variety of lower extremity conditions.[44] Items were generated by sampling physical therapy orthopaedic clinicians, reviewing existing functional self-report measures, and surveying 30 patients with lower extremity musculoskeletal conditions. Systematic item analysis was performed to finalize scale items. Each of 20 activities is rated on a 5-point scale, from 0 ("extreme difficulty/unable to perform activity") to 4 ("no difficulty"). The maximum score of 80 is indicative of no disability. The 5-point rating scale, rather than a dichotomous scale, was selected to maximize the capacity of the scale to measure change. The LEFS takes about 1 minute to complete and less than 1 minute to score.

Measurement Properties

The reliability, validity, and sensitivity to change of the LEFS were examined in 105 subjects with lower extremity dysfunction.[44] Test-retest reliability was good ($R = 0.94$). The LEFS and SF-36 physical function scores were compared to investigate the construct validity of the LEFS. Correlation between the LEFS and the SF-36 physical function subscale was good ($r = 0.74$). In order to examine sensitivity to change, a prognostic rating of predicted functional change at 1 week and at 3 weeks was performed. Correlation of change on the LEFS with the prognostic rating of change was acceptable (Spearman's rho = 0.60). In summary, the LEFS appears to be reliable, valid, and sensitive to valid change in patients with lower extremity dysfunction.[44]

With respect to decision making about individual patients, the potential error associated with a score on the LEFS at a given point in time is 5 scale points on the 80-point scale (90 percent CI). The MDC is 6 scale points (90 percent CI), and the MCID is approximately 9 scale points (90 percent CI).[44] The interpretation of this is that at a given point in time, for example the initial evaluation, a clinician can be reasonably confident that a given LEFS score is within 5 scale points of the patient's true score. On follow-up, changes in a score of at least 7 scale points can be interpreted as indicating true patient change with reasonable confidence. In this case, the MCID is greater than the MDC, so that changes of 9 scale points or more are required to be reasonably confident that clinically important change has occurred.

The SF-36 Health Status Measure

Two generic scales with well documented measurement properties are the Sickness Impact Profile (SIP)[10] and the SF-36.[7,8,11] Since the SIP takes patients over 20 minutes to complete, the SF-36, which is less time-consuming, will be discussed here. The SF-36 is a multidimensional generic health status instrument that includes eight health concept scales: (1) physical functioning, (2) role limitation (physical), (3) bodily pain, (4) general health, (5) vitality, (6) social function, (7) role limitation (emotional), and (8) mental health. In total, the instrument contains 36 items that represent a broad array of health concepts. All scales are linearly transformed to a 0 to 100-point scale, with 100 indicating the most favorable health state. The SF-36 requires approximately 15 minutes to score manually or it may be computer scored. The measurement properties of the SF-36 have been well established on samples from diverse populations.[7,8,11,12,17,40,45] The physical function and pain dimensions appear to be most relevant to orthopaedic outpatients.[12,17,45] The SF-36 physical function questions appear to be most applicable to lower limb and low back problems, with little relevance to neck and upper extremity problems.

Reliability, validity, and sensitivity to change have been well documented for the SF-36.[7,8,11,12,17,45] While several of the SF-36 subscales have the capacity to measure change on patients with low back and lower extremity conditions, many of the subscales do not change in outpatient musculoskeletal conditions. For example, the mental health subscale of the SF-36 does not appear to measure important change in this patient population.[12,17,41,45] While the SF-36 taps many aspects of health in a wide variety of patient populations, this can prove to be a disadvantage when attempting to measure change in an orthopaedic outpatient with minimal overall health dysfunction. This is due to the fact that many items on generic scales may not be relevant to persons with particular orthopaedic problems. The SF-36 is an appropriate generic health scale to incorporate into orthopaedic clinical practice when the goal is to compare groups of patients on the wide variety of health attributes tapped by the SF-36, such as for a quality assurance program or for research purposes. Given the complexity of scoring the SF-36, it is not well suited to assisting clinicians in setting patient goals and in tracking progress through weekly follow-up and scoring.

■ Setting Goals and Tracking Patients' Progress Using Functional Scales

Clinicians can use a measure of patients' initial function, such as that obtained with the RMQ, to set functional goals and track patients' progress. To set short- and long-term goals based on a functional scale, the clinician must synthesize the clinical history and objective findings of the patient and the error, MDC, and MDIC of the relevant scale. These measurement properties are summarized in Table 28–1.

Consider a patient with an initial RMQ score of 15/24. Based on the error at a given point in time for the RMQ, the clinician can be confident that the actual scale score is between 12 and 18. In setting a short-term goal for this patient, one must consider the history and clinical findings as well as the MDC (5 scale points) and MCID (5 scale points) for the RMQ. If the patient is deemed to have a fairly chronic condition, to be extremely impaired, and, therefore, expected to change slowly, one might select a 2-week time frame for a change in score of 5 points. The short-term goal, then, would be: "Decrease RMQ score to less than or equal to 10/24." In setting a short-term goal for a more acutely injured patient who is predicted to change quickly, a shorter time frame of, for example, 1 week, with a greater change than the MCID, may be selected. In this case, the goal may be "Decrease RMQ score to less than or equal to 7/24." On follow-up, for example one week later, progress is determined by the amount of change on the scale. In cases where improvement greater than the MDC and MCID occurs, clinicians can be confident that true (MDC) and important (MCID) change has occurred. In cases where there is improvement that is greater than or equal to the MDC but the change falls below the MCID, clinicians can be confident that true change has occurred but that this may not be important change. Continuation of the intervention, or discharge if goals are met, would be justified in both of these scenarios. In cases where there is no change or where change is less than the MDC, clinicians may be confident that true change has not occurred. In this case, depending on the clinical picture and the interval since the previous assessment, a change in intervention or discharge may be considered. See Figure 28–1 for criteria for selecting outcome measures.

□□□□□ □ □ □

Table 28-1. Summary of Scale Properties for Decision Making Concerning Individual Patients

	Scale Range and Interpretation	Error Associated with a Single Measure (90% CI) (Scale Points)	Minimal Detectable Change MDC (90% CI) (Scale Points)	Minimal Clinically Important Difference MCID (90% CI) (Scale Points)
Patient-Specific Functional Scale	0–10 0 = no disability	1.7	3	3
Roland-Morris Back Pain Questionnaire	0–24 0 = no disability	3	5	5
Oswestry Low Back Pain Index	0–100 100 = no disability	11	16	11
Neck Disability Index	0–50 50 = no disability	5	7	7
Lower Extremity Functional Scale	0–80 0 = no disability	5	6	9
Disabilities of the Arm, Hand and Shoulder Outcome Measure	0–100 0 = no disability	10	14	Not Available

CASE STUDIES

Mrs. D is a 55-year-old woman referred to physical therapy with low back pain. She states that she has had low back pain on and off for years, which was aggravated 2 months ago when she lifted her grandchild. Mrs. D has central low back, right buttock, and right posterior thigh pain which is aggravated by sitting and bending over. Her pain is eased by a change of position and by walking. Ten minutes of sitting aggravates the pain, and it eases immediately upon changing positions. Baseline pain intensity is 3/10 (Fig. 28–2).

Mrs. D is a librarian at the local elementary school. She is active at home, with home care, gardening, and caring for her grandchildren. She walks regularly. Her RMQ score is 17/24. Her PSFS average score is 1.7/10 (Fig. 28–3).

Her general health is unremarkable. Mrs. D takes no medication. Radiographs indicate moderate degenerative changes at L5–S1 and L4–L5.

Examination

Posture: mild forward head posture, increased lumbar lordosis

Active Range of Motion (measures are the modified Shobers test[46]; the starting point is a 15-cm line measured cranially from posterior superior iliac spine)

Lumbar: Flexion 2.5 cm; pain reproduced in the right lumbar region/buttock (6/10)

Extension: 2.1 cm

Side flexion: right, full; left, three-quarter range

Special Active Movements:

Flexion-left side flexion/right rotation restricted to approximately one-half of right side; pain reproduced in right buttock and posterior thigh (8/10)

Repeated flexion negative

Segmental Mobility Testing: Posterior-anterior movements (in flexion position) at L4 and L5 are restricted and reproduce the right lumbar and buttock pain.[47] Passive intervertebral movement testing indicates restriction in flexion, left side flexion, and right rotation at L4.[47]

Neurologic Exam: negative

Other Joints

Hips: Hip extension: right, 8 degrees; left, 10 degrees; no other significant findings

Sacroiliac joint test negative.

Physical Therapy Treatment Plan: Setting Goals, Tracking Progress and Outcome

A manual therapy approach and an exercise program were implemented for Mrs. D, with the goals of increasing lumbar range of motion, particularly flexion, and decreasing pain. Impairment measures appropriate for tracking progress are identified in Figure 28–2. Goals were established considering Mrs. D's multiple previous episodes, clinical and radiographic findings, age, and active lifestyle. The physical therapy goals included correction of two

PATIENT NAME: Mrs. D

	DATE AND SCORE							
PATIENT-SPECIFIC ACTIVITIES	Initial 4/1	4/8	4/15	4/22	4/29			
1. Sitting	3	5	8	10	10			
2. Lifting/carrying grandchild	0	0	2	8	8			
3. Gardening	2	2	5	9	9			
AVERAGE: (/10)	1.7	2.3	5	9	9			
ADDITIONAL ACTIVITIES:								
1. Brushing teeth	8	9	10	10	10			
2. Panty hose/socks	7	7	10	10	10			
PSFS PAIN QUESTIONS:								
PAIN LIMITATION SCORE:	5/10	7/10	10/10	10/10	10/10			
PAIN INTENSITY SCORE:	3/10	4/10	2/10	0/10	0/10			
CONDITION-SPECIFIC MEASURE: (RMQ)	17/24	14/24	11/24	5/24	1/24			
IMPAIRMENT MEASURES: (e.g., ROM, STRENGTH)								
1. Lumbar flexion	2.5 cm	3.1	4.1	4.5	4.5			
2. Pain on flexion	6/10	5/10	2/10	0/10	0/10			
3. Pain with flexion/left side flexion/right rotation combined movement	8/10	8/10	3/10	0/10	0/10			
4.								
SHORT-TERM GOALS: 2 WEEKS								
1. Increase lumbar flexion >3.0 cm		✔						
2. Decrease pain on flexion <3/10			✔					
3. Increase PSFS average >4/10			✔					
4. Decrease RMQ score <12/24			✔					
LONG-TERM GOALS: 4 WEEKS								
1. Increase lumbar flexion >4.0 cm				✔				
2. No pain on flexion				✔				
3. Increase PSFS average >8/10				✔				
4. Decrease RMQ score <3/24					✔			

Figure 28–3. Functional goal and outcome worksheet.

measurable impairments and two functional goals based on the PSFS and RMQ scores. Goals were set to expect change greater than the MDC and MCID for each of the scales. In a patient in whom change is expected to occur more slowly, the time frame for the goals may be increased. Another option if the MCID for the scale is greater than the MCD is to set a goal just at the MDC for a scale but not as great as the MCID. In a patient in whom more rapid change is expected, the time frame may be shorter or the goals may be greater than the MDC or MCID for the scale.

Administration Issues

Three components affect the successful clinical implementation of a self-report functional measure: (1) ease of administration of the questionnaire, (2) easy interpretation of the result, and (3) efficient documentation in the medical record. To facilitate the administration of outcome measures, copies should be readily available in the clinic. To avoid excessive amounts of paper in patients' charts and to keep printing costs down, scales may be laminated or kept in a plastic sleeve. Patients respond directly on the laminated copy using a transparency marking pen. Once the scale is scored by the clinician, it can be used again. It is important that the scoring and subsequent transfer of functional scores to the medical record are efficient. The functional goal and outcome worksheet in Figure 28–1 provide an efficient method of recording (1) the PSFS activities, scores, and averages; (2) the PSFS pain limitation and intensity questions; (3) a condition-specific functional measure; (4) components of the physical assessment important to a specific patient (e.g., range-of-motion measures); and (5) short- and long-term goals. Having all of this information in one place in the medical record facilitates the use of functional scale scores for goal setting, for estimation of functional progress, and for determination of when goals have been met. In addition, this information is easily transferable to a computer spreadsheet to track patients' progress and outcome in the clinic. Regular weekly follow-up of all patients on these measures provides an efficient and comprehensive approach to documentation of patient progress and outcome.

Summary

Measurement of function is critical in documenting the outcome of physical therapy. Self-report functional status scales provide an efficient and cost-effective method of documenting function in orthopaedic physical therapy practice. The selection of scales appropriate for incorporation in practice should be based on documented measurement properties and ease of administration. If scales are to be incorporated into the clinical decision-making process,

including setting goals and measuring patient progress, regular reevaluation of function on, for example, a weekly basis is required. In this case, scales must be readily available in the clinic, and scores must be calculated and recorded with ease. The appropriate combination of patient-specific, condition-specific, and generic health status measures should be determined, depending on the patient group and the goals of outcome measurement. Clinicians can use a combination of these self-report functional measures to document the progress and outcome in individual patients, as well as to document the outcome of groups of patients for quality assurance purposes.

References

1. Deyo RA, Centor RM: Assessing the responsiveness of functional scales to clinical change: an analogy to diagnostic test performance. J Chronic Dis 39:897, 1986
2. Waddell G: Biopsychosocial analysis of low back pain. Clin Rheumatol 6:523, 1992
3. Hazard RG, Haugh LD, Green PA, et al: Chronic low back pain: the relationship between patient satisfaction and pain, impairment, and disability outcomes, abstracted. Spine 19:881, 1994
4. Buchner DM, de Lateur BJ: The importance of skeletal muscle strength to physical function in older adults. Ann Behav Med 13:91, 1991
5. Kirshner B, Guyatt G: A methodological framework for assessing health indices. J Chronic Dis 38:27, 1985
6. Roland M, Morris R: A study of the natural history of back pain. Part I: development of a reliable and sensitive measure of disability in low-back pain. Spine 8:141, 1983
7. McHorney CA, Ware JE Jr, Raczek AE: The MOS 36-item short-form health survey (SF-36): II. Psychometric and clinical tests of validity in measuring physical and mental health constructs. Med Care 31:247, 1993
8. McHorney CA, Ware JE Jr, Lu R, et al: The MOS 36-item short-form health survey (SF-36): III. Tests of data quality, scaling assumptions, and reliability across diverse patient groups. Med Care 32:40, 1994
9. Patrick DL, Deyo RA, Atlas SJ, et al: Assessing health-related quality of life in patients with sciatica. Spine 20:1899, 1995
10. Bergner M, Bobbitt RA, Carter WB, et al: The Sickness Impact Profile: development and final revision of a health status measure. Med Care 19:787, 1981
11. Ware JE Jr, Sherbourne CD: The MOS 36-item short-form health survey (SF-36) I. Conceptual framework and items selection. Med Care 30:473, 1992
12. Lysholm J, Gillquist J: Evaluation of knee ligament surgery results with special emphasis on use of a scoring scale. Am J Sports Med 10:150, 1982
13. MacKenzie C, Charlson M, DiGioia D, et al: A patient-specific measure of change in maximum function. Arch Intern Med 146:1325, 1986
14. Tugwell P, Bombardier C, Buchanan W, et al: The MACTAR patient preference disability questionnaire—an individualized functional priority approach for assessing improvement in physical disability in clinical trials in rheumatoid arthritis. J Rheumatol 14:446, 1987
15. McHorney CA, Tarlov AR: Individual-patient monitoring in clinical practice: are available health status surveys adequate? Qual Life Res 4:293, 1995

16. Ruta DA, Garratt AM, Leng M, et al: A new approach to the measurement of quality of life: the patient-generated index. Med Care 32:1109, 1994

17. Chatman AB, Hyams SP, Neel JM, et al: The Patient Specific Functional Scale: measurement properties in patients with knee dysfunction. Phys Ther 77:820, 1997

18. Stratford P, Gill C, Westaway M, et al: Assessing disability and change in individual patients: a report of a patient specific measure. Physiother Canada 47:258, 1995

19. Feinstein AR, Josephy BR, Well CK: Scientific and clinical problems in indexes of functional disability. Ann Intern Med 105:413, 1986

20. Westaway M, Stratford PW, Binkley J: The Patient Specific Functional Scale: validation of its use in persons with neck dysfunction. J Orthop Sports Phys Ther 27:331, 1998

21. Streiner DL, Norman GR: Health Measurement Scales: A Practical Guide to Their Development and Use. Oxford University Press, Oxford, 1995

22. Standards for educational and psychological testing. American Psychological Association, Washington, DC, 1985

23. Stratford PW, Binkley JM, Riddle DL: Health Status Measures: strategies and analytic methods for assessing change scores. Phys Ther 76:1109, 1996

24. Stratford PW, Binkley JM: Applying the results of self-report measures to individual patients: an example using the Roland-Morris Questionnaire. J Orthop Sports Phys Ther 29:232, 1999

25. Stratford PW, Binkley J, Solomon P, et al: Defining the minimal level of detectable change for the Roland Morris Questionnaire. Phys Ther 76:359, 1996

26. Kopec JA, Esdaile JM, Abrahamowicz M, et al: The Quebec back pain disability scale: measurement properties. Spine 20:341, 1995

27. Stratford PW, Binkley J, Solomon P, et al: Assessing change over time in patients with low back pain. Phys Ther 74:528, 1994

28. Kopec JA, Esdaile JM: Functional disability scales for back pain. Spine 20:1943, 1995

29. Beurskens AJ, de Vet HC, Koke AJ, et al: Measuring the functional status of patients with low back pain: assessment of the quality of four disease-specific questionnaires. Spine 20:1017, 1995

30. Beurskens AJHM, de Vet HCW, Koke AJA: Responsiveness of functional status in low back pain: a comparison of different instruments. Pain 65:71, 1996

31. Deyo RA: Comparative validity of the Sickness Impact Profile and shorter scales for functional assessment in low-back pain. Spine 11:951, 1986

32. Stratford PW, Finch E, Solomon P, et al: Using the Roland-Morris Questionnaire to make decisions about individual patients. Physiother Canada 48:107, 1996

33. Riddle DL, Stratford PW, Binkley JM: Sensitivity to change of the Roland-Morris back pain questionnaire: part II. Phys Ther 78:1197, 1998

34. Stratford PW, Binkley JM, Riddle DL: Sensitivity to change of the Roland-Morris back pain questionnaire: part 1. Phys Ther 78:1186, 1998

35. Fairbank JC, Couper J, Davies JB, et al: The Oswestry low back pain disability questionnaire. Physiotherapy 66:271, 1980

36. Haas M, Jacobs GH, Raphail R, et al: Low back pain outcome measurement assessment in chiropractic teaching clinics: responsiveness and applicability of two functional disability questionnaires. J Manip Physiol Ther 18:79, 1995

37. Jarvikoski A, Mellin G, Estlander A, et al: Outcome of two multimodal back treatment programs with and without intensive physical training. J Spinal Dis 6:93, 1995

38. Bombardier C, Kerr MS, Shannon HS: A guide to interpreting epidemiologic studies on the etiology of back pain. Spine 19:2047S, 1994

39. Vernon H, Mior S: The neck disability index: a study of reliability and validity. J Manip Physiol Ther 14:409, 1991

40. Riddle DL, Stratford PW: Use of generic versus region-specific functional status measures on patients with cervical spine disorders: a comparison study. Phys Ther 78:951, 1998

41. Hudak PL, Armadio P, Bombardier C, Upper Extremity Collaborative Group: Development of an upper extremity outcome measure: the DASH (Disabilities of the Arm, Shoulder, and Hand). Am J Industrial Med 29:602, 1997

42. Armadio P, Beaton D, Bombardier C, et al. Development of an upper extremity outcome measure: the "DASH" (Disabilities of the arm, shoulder and hand), abstracted. Arthritis Rheum 39:S112, 1996

43. Armadio P, Beaton D, Bombardier C, et al. Measuring disability and symptoms of the upper limb: a validation study of the DASH questionnaire, abstracted. Arthritis Rheum 39:S112, 1996

44. Binkley JM, Stratford PW, Lott S, et al: The Lower Extremity Functional Scale (LEFS): scale development, measurement properties, and clinical application. Phys Ther 79:371, 1999

45. Jette DU, Jette AM: Physical therapy and health outcomes in patients with spinal impairments. Phys Ther 76:930, 1996

46. Williams R, Binkley J, Bloch R, et al: Reliability of the modified-modified Schober and double inclinometer methods for measuring lumbar flexion and extension. Phys Ther 73:26, 1993.

47. Maitland GD: Vertebral Manipulation. 5th Ed. Butterworths, London, 1986.

CHAPTER 29
Orthopaedic Problems in the Neurologic Patient

Richard W. Bohannon

As the title indicates, this chapter addresses orthopaedic problems in the neurologic patient. In this review, the term *orthopaedic* will be considered synonymous with the term *musculoskeletal.* Therefore, only musculoskeletal problems that can be clearly related to a primary neurologic pathology are discussed. Unrelated problems such as rheumatoid arthritis in a patient with stroke are outside the scope of this chapter. Problems such as muscle weakness, which are often primarily neurologic in origin, are not covered except in relation to other musculoskeletal problems. Orthopaedic problems addressed in this chapter are those affecting bones, joints, and soft tissue. Because the problems reviewed here are not necessarily isolated to a single musculoskeletal component, they are discussed individually. The limited scope of problems addressed concerns either the pathology or impairment levels of illness[1]; such problems include heterotopic ossification, osteoporosis, range-of-motion limitations, joint malalignment, and joint pain. Five aspects of the problems are discussed: documentation/measurement, nature, determinants, implications, and treatment. The chapter concludes with a case study.

Heterotopic Ossification

Heterotopic ossification can be defined as the ossification of soft tissue in an abnormal location. Several classifications of heterotopic ossification exist; however, only neurogenic ossification is addressed in the following subsections. What distinguishes neurogenic ossification from other forms of heterotopic ossification is that it occurs in the presence of severe neurologic conditions.[2-5]

Documentation/Measurement

Once a heterotopic ossification is established, it can be documented on radiographs of the affected area (Fig.

29–1). While a heterotopic ossification is still in its formative stages, bone scans can be useful for describing the presence of the ossification process.[6-8] Even before a bone scan or a radiograph is positive, several clinical signs may herald the appearance of heterotopic ossification. The signs, which can mimic those of acute arthritis[9] and thrombophlebitis,[10] should be apparent to therapists working with the patient with neurologic symptoms. The signs include soft tissue swelling, warmth, and erythema.[2,6,7,11,12] Fever may occur.[11] With time, the swelling becomes more localized and the tissue firmer to palpation.[11] The serum level of alkaline phosphatase is increased during ectopic bone formation but apparently returns toward normal as the heterotopic ossification matures.[3,6,7,12,13] The degree of alkaline phosphatase elevation, which has been reported to range from slight to four or five times normal among patients with heterotopic ossification, does not necessarily indicate the severity of the heterotopic ossification.[6]

Nature

Heterotopic ossification is not a ubiquitous complication of neurologic pathology. Only rarely does it affect infants or individuals with congenital or progressive neurologic disorders. With some exceptions,[13-15] individuals with neurogenic ossification described in the literature are beyond early childhood and have major neurologic disorders of sudden onset. The diagnostic group in which heterotopic ossification has been reported most often is spinal cord injury.[2,3,6,11,13,16-21] Within this group, patients with cervical or thoracic lesions appear more likely to develop heterotopic ossification than patients with lumbar lesions.[16] Although the incidence of heterotopic ossification reported for spinal cord-injured individuals varies among studies, it apparently can reach 30 percent.[2] Patients with brain lesions, particularly from trauma, are also commonly

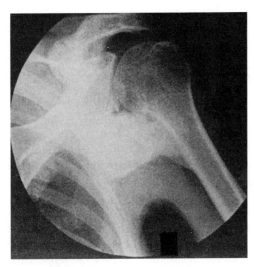

Figure 29–1. Heterotopic ossification of the shoulder. (From Greenwood et al.,[5] with permission.)

described as at risk of heterotopic ossification.[4,5,7,8,21,22] Sazbon et al.[4] reported that 36 (76.8 percent) of the 47 long-term comatose patients they examined with radiographs demonstrated heterotopic ossification. Twenty-five (22.5 percent) of 111 brain-injured patients who underwent "routine triple-phase bone scans" within 3 weeks of hospital admission were reported to demonstrate heterotopic ossification in another study.[8] Hurvitz et al.[15] reported an incidence of 14.4 percent among children and adolescents with head injuries. Greenwood et al.[5] reported an incidence of only 7 percent among head-injured patients and of only 1 percent among stroke patients, but they relied on a retrospective search of radiographs.

Heterotopic ossification, according to Stover et al.,[2] "seldom involves the muscle mass per se." Rather, it usually occurs in the connective tissue planes between muscles.[2] It can be found around a single joint or around multiple joints of an individual patient. Although more commonly found around the large proximal joints, particularly the hip,[5,8,11,13,15,19] neurogenic ossifications have also been documented at the shoulder (Fig. 29–1), elbow, knee,[2,8,15] wrist, hand, ankle, and feet.[2]

The latent period between neurologic insult and the appearance of a clearly identifiable heterotopic ossification is not fixed. Evidently, the process can begin quite early and remain active long after the onset of the neurologic pathology. Citta-Pietrolungo et al.[8] reported heterotopic ossification within 3 weeks of hospital admission among patients with traumatic brain injuries. Stover et al.[2] suggested that the most common latent period of heterotopic ossification was 1 to 4 months after injury in a sample of spinal cord-injured patients. In long-term comatose patients, Sazbon et al.[4] reported that the earliest evidence of ossification occurred 1 month after the onset of coma. In a sample of pediatric spinal cord-injured patients, the average time at which heterotopic ossification was diag-

nosed was 6½ years after injury, leading Garland et al.[13] to conclude that "pediatric patients who developed heterotopic ossification appeared to have a lower incidence, delayed onset, and fewer associated signs and symptoms compared with their adult counterparts."

Determinants

The exact determinants of heterotopic ossification remain a mystery. Clearly, in neurogenic ossification, a lesion of the nervous system is a prerequisite. However, it is probably the sudden immobility that accompanies many such lesions, rather than the lesions themselves, that contributes to the development of heterotopic ossifications. Catz et al.[21] stated that the confinement of heterotopic ossification to the region below the level of neurologic deficit in patients with spinal cord injury and to mostly the weak extremities in brain-injured patients supports a "possible causal relationship between the presence of sensorimotor disability and heterotopic ossification." All 25 patients that Citta-Pietrolungo et al.[8] identified with heterotopic ossification after traumatic brain injury had experienced a period of immobility; 24 had experienced a period of coma. Unlike the presence of coma, the actual duration of coma may not be a major determinant of the severity or extent of heterotopic ossification.[4,5] Only the findings of Hurvitz et al.[15] seem to point to coma durations as associated with a greater risk of heterotopic ossification.

Although trauma (e.g., contusions, fractures, surgery) can lead to heterotopic ossification, the evidence does not support the view that trauma or exercise are direct contributors to the formation of neurogenic ossifications.[2,15] Stover et al.[2] hypothesized that local factors such as circulatory status and tissue hypoxia may contribute to the pathogenesis of heterotopic ossification. As serum calcium is not increased during the time when heterotopic ossifications are forming, an increased amount of circulating calcium does not offer an explanation. Collagen lost from bone, however, may contribute to heterotopic ossification.[23] Galactosyl hydroxylysine, which is abundant in bone collagen, is excreted in increased amounts after spinal cord injury. The amount of the substance excreted does not return to normal until bone turnover stabilizes.[22]

Implications

Heterotopic ossification is not intrinsically problematic. It is the consequences of the ossification that are troublesome. Probably of greatest concern to therapists are the decreased range of motion[6,11,14] and pain[14] that accompany heterotopic ossification. Complete ankylosis will ultimately occur in a small percentage of cases.[7] Whether range of motion is merely reduced or impossible (as in ankylosis), impairments in range of motion can compromise therapy and function.[6,8] Other complications thought to result indirectly from heterotopic ossification are skin breakdown,[14,17] nerve and vascular compression, and lymphedema.[24]

Treatment

Three primary methods can be used to treat heterotopic ossification, either separately or together. Of greatest relevance to therapists is range-of-motion exercise. Stover et al.[2] reported no difference in the development of heterotopic ossification between patients receiving little or no physical therapy and patients receiving aggressive range-of-motion exercises. For patients with bilateral heterotopic ossification who were treated unilaterally, however, range of motion tended to improve on the side receiving "aggressive passive stretching" relative to the contralateral rested side. Greenwood et al.[5] indicated that heterotopic ossifications can be fractured by vigorous manipulation, with a resultant gain in function. What the clinician should be wary of, if providing vigorous range-of-motion exercises for a patient with heterotopic ossification, is the likelihood of concomitant osteoporosis and an increased risk of skeletal fracture.

Surgery is another possible treatment of heterotopic ossification, albeit one that Stover et al.[17] suggested should be "considered only in patients who develop limitations of function or related skin pressure areas." Although surgery can yield intraoperative increases in range of motion, postoperative recurrence of ossification[11,17] and a loss of intraoperative gains in motion are common.[6,19] According to Garland and Orwin,[19] improved postoperative range of motion is best predicted by preoperative range of motion, and recurrence of heterotopic ossification is predictable from the amount of heterotopic bone present preoperatively. Complications of surgery (other than recurrence) that have been reported include wound infections, excessive bleeding, and fractures.[19]

Pharmacologic treatment is also possible. The drug of choice is disodium etidronate, which prevents bone mineralization.[7,11,18,22] The drug has been used prophylactically to inhibit the formation of heterotopic ossification after severe head injury[22] and spinal cord injury.[18] It has also been administered after surgical removal of heterotopic ossification to prevent recurrence. Stover et al.[11] reported that as long as the drug was used, recurrence was prevented. If it was not used, recurrence could be shown on radiographs within 3 weeks. If it was used and then discontinued, recurrence was variable.

■ Osteoporosis

Osteoporosis is a disorder characterized by diminished bone mass (bone mineral density) and an increased likelihood of fractures. Osteoporosis can be classified as involutional or secondary. Involutional osteoporosis occurs naturally with age, whereas secondary osteoporosis results from a predisposing medical condition.[25]

Documentation/Measurement

Many methods of measuring bone mineral density exist and have been reviewed elsewhere.[25] Among these methods, photon absorption (single or dual) has probably had the greatest use in the recent past. According to Ostlere and Gold,[25] however, another technique, dual-energy radiography, has made dual-photon absorptiometry obsolete.

Many patients with neurologic disorders seen by physical therapists may not have undergone procedures for the documentation or measurement of bone mineral density. Nevertheless, information relevant to the presence or degree of osteoporosis may be available. Patients sometimes demonstrate overt signs that are consistent with osteoporosis and its consequences. For example, an elderly woman with a stroke may have severe thoracic kyphosis, which can result from the collapse and wedging of the osteoporotic bodies of the thoracic vertebrae. Also, radiology reports of radiographs taken for purposes other than the documentation of osteoporosis (e.g., routine chest x-rays) may allude to the presence of osteoporosis.

Nature and Determinants

Many patients with neurologic disorders, by virtue of their advanced age and female gender, are already prone to bone loss.[26] Factors such as age and gender, however, do not explain the extreme bone loss demonstrated by patients with lesions of the brain, spinal cord, and lower motor neurons.[27–42] The most likely explanation for the patients' bone loss is their impaired motor capacity, which leads to decreased stresses on bone from muscular contraction and weightbearing. Such stresses, after all, are known to retard osteoporosis and the processes (e.g., osteoclastic activity) leading to it.[43–45] Moreover, bones subject to lower muscular stresses in patients with neurologic disorders demonstrate greater reductions in density. Specifically, patients with long-standing hemiparesis, whether from stroke[29,32,33] or cerebral palsy,[38] tend to show decreased bone density on the paretic compared with the nonparetic side; patients with paraplegia show substantially reduced bone mineral content in the femur but not the lumbar vertebrae;[28,36,46] and patients with quadriplegia and paraplegia show similar bone densities at the pelvis and in the lower extremities but very different densities in the upper extremities and trunk.[47] Patients with stroke, whose paretic upper extremities are typically more impaired than their paretic lower extremities, demonstrate greater demineralization in their upper extremities.[33] Patients whose ambulatory status is more deficient also have lower bone mineral densities. A relationship between bone mineral density of the lower extremities and ambulatory status has been shown for patients with cerebral palsy[41] and myelomeningocele,[34] as has a relationship between bone mineral density of the spine and ambulatory status in patients with cerebral palsy.[37,41]

The timing and rate of bone loss following acute neurologic incidents are difficult to discern from the literature. Although many of the stresses contributing to the maintenance of bone mineral density are decreased abruptly following the incident, bone density is not lost immediately. Szollar et al.[36] concluded that for patients with spinal cord injury, "initial bone mass loss does not appear to occur prior to one year post injury." Hangartner et al.,[40] on the other hand, calculated a decrease of over 50 percent in the trabecular bone of the tibia over the first 2 years after spinal cord injury. They determined that no further bone loss occurred after 7 years. Other investigators have found that bone was lost for 2 to 3 years before stabilizing after spinal cord injury.[31,46] Hamdy et al.[33] found that among patients with stroke, demineralization of the paretic side began in the first month after onset and reached its maximum in 3 to 4 months.[33]

Implications

Concomitant with acute quadriplegia are the excretion of calcium and collagen metabolites,[48,49] both presumably from the bone matrix. These materials, however, are only signs of the underlying processes of osteoporosis. Of potentially greatest concern to therapists are fractures that occur in weakened osteoporotic bones. In a patient with paraplegia, Rafii et al.[50] reported bilateral acetabular stress fractures that were presumed to be secondary to osteoporosis and the pattern of ambulation training practiced by the patient in braces. Keating et al.[51] reported that three spinal cord-injured patients experienced fractures after only minimal trauma. Of the 14 patients with stroke described in the report by Hodkinson and Brain,[29] 10 of those with osteoporosis had also experienced a fracture of the femur. While very low spinal bone density was not associated with an increased fracture risk among children and adolescents with spastic quadriplegia, spica casting and a previous fracture were strongly related to fracture rate.[42]

Treatment

Attempts to alter the osteoporosis accompanying neurologic disorders have been made. They include both physical and pharmacologic methods. Given the known effect of exercise and weightbearing on bone density, interventions incorporating either or both would appear to have promise for patients with neurologic disorders. In reality, however, physical methods have been shown to have either no significant effect or only a limited effect. Pacy et al.[28] found no changes in the bone mineral content or density of paraplegic patients during a functional electrical stimulation exercise program consisting of 10 weeks of leg raising and 32 weeks of bicycle pedaling. Leeds et al.[52] similarly found no increase in bone mineral density in patients performing electrically stimulated cycle ergometry for 6 months. Spinal cord-injured subjects treated with functional electrical stimulation by Hangartner et al.[40] continued to lose bone density but at a slower than expected rate. Abramson[30] reported more than 40 years ago that 3 hours of standing may be required to affect the osteoporotic process among patients with paraplegia. Perhaps that explains why Kunkel et al.[39] found no alteration in the bone density of the lumbar spine or femoral neck of patients with spinal cord injury or multiple sclerosis who stood in standing frames for an average of 144 hours over a period of 135 days.

Claus-Walker and colleagues[53] administered (+)-catechin to patients with quadriplegia in an effort to stabilize body collagen content. Their pharmacologic intervention did not affect the amount of collagen degradation product or calcium noted in the urine. Thus, it is not likely that the treatment can reduce the rate of progression of osteoporosis. Pearson et al.[54] found no effect of cyclical etidronate alone on bone density loss after spinal cord injury. Patients who were given oral etidronate and were ambulatory, however, had a significantly lower rate of loss of bone mineral desity. Pearson et al. concluded, therefore, that cyclical etidronate may be a feasible treatment for patients "who eventually walk."

■ Range-of-Motion Limitations

Range-of-motion limitations are a common complication of many neurologic pathologies. Regardless of their source, they are often of concern to physical therapists who work with neurologically involved patients.

Documentation/Measurement

Although physical therapists are well acquainted with goniometry and other procedures for measuring joint range of motion, certain points relevant to such measurement merit discussion. The points relate to what is being measured, the endpoint of measurement, and the reliability of the measurements.

When range of motion is measured, the structures limiting range of motion are not identified. Thus, straight leg raising[55] or the active knee extension test[56] may give an indication of hamstring musculotendinous unit length, and the Thomas test[57] may give an indication of hip flexor musculotendinous unit length, but they are not measures of muscle length per se. Additional tests are required if the tissues responsible for decreased range of motion are to be identified.

Fortunately, many sources of information on normal range of motion exist.[58–63] Unfortunately, the sources rarely define the specific endpoint used during measurement. Range-of-motion measurements obtained at the point of first resistance,[64] where the tested individual feels maximum range has been reached,[65] at the point of pain[66,67] or at the extreme of available range where firm resistance is encountered,[65] have all been used. Presumably, the last is used most often. Nevertheless, measurements at other endpoints, for example, at first resistance[64] or at the point of pain,[66,67] have proved to be particularly appropriate for some patients with neurologic disorders.

Many studies of healthy subjects have shown range-of-motion measurements to be reliable.[68,69] Some studies of patients with neurologic disorders have reported reliable measurements as well.[66] Caution should be exercised, however, in generalizing from studies of healthy subjects. The results of several studies make this point rather clear.[70-72] Harris et al.[70] concluded that "a difference of >10–15 degrees in range of motion over time does not justify conclusions of either significant improvement or significant regression in a child with severe spastic cerebral palsy."

Nature

Nearly all, if not all, neurologic pathologies that result in muscle weakness are accompanied by limitations in range of motion. Although some joints appear to be afflicted more often than others, almost any joint can demonstrate impairments in range of motion.

For patients with stroke, the shoulder is probably the joint that shows limitations in range most often. The motions noted most frequently to be reduced are external rotation (Fig. 29–2) and elevation (flexion or abduction.[66,67,73-77] The magnitude of the limitations tends to be greater as the time since the onset of stroke increases.[66,73] Limitations in ankle dorsiflexion range of motion are also quite common among patients with stroke.[78,79]

After head injuries, particularly those that are severe, limitations in range of motion are common. Although almost any joint can be limited in range of motion, the ankle is probably most often affected. Equinus deformities are perhaps the most problematic.[80-83] Knee flexion contractures are also quite frequent.[82,84]

The range-of-motion limitations shown by patients with cerebral palsy are similar to those shown by patients with other intracranial lesions. Thus, ankle dorsiflexion is limited particularly often.[85-91] In the absence of an effec-

tive intervention, limitations in ankle dorsiflexion tend to worsen with age for many children with cerebral palsy.[85,86] Limitations at the knee and hip are also quite prevalent among patients with cerebral palsy.[92-97] Motions specifically limited in many patients are knee extension and hip extension, although hip flexion can also be deficient.[93]

Muscular dystrophy is accompanied by a host of range-of-motion limitations.[98-103] Markedly reduced ankle dorsiflexion range of motion is, however, one of the hallmark abnormalities among individuals with Duchenne muscular dystrophy. As in children with cerebral palsy, the abnormality tends to worsen with time (i.e., with increasing age).[98-100] Other joints are afflicted. Contractures at the hip, knee, wrist, and hand appear to be practically inevitable.[100-103]

Besides the diagnostic groups mentioned earlier, there are others for which limitations in range of motion are a documented problem. They include patients with spinal cord injury,[104,105] multiple sclerosis,[106] poliomyelitis,[107,108] and myelomeningocele.[109]

Determinants

Determinants of range-of-motion limitations can be described at two levels. Grossly, range limitations can be explained by other impairments. More specifically, limitations in range of motion can be explained at the tissue level.

As has been intimated before, it is the weakness that accompanies neurologic disorders and limits voluntary movement that presumably predisposes the affected individual to limitations in range of range motion. This conclusion, although deductively sound and probably true, has not been supported (to the best of my knowledge) by correlational studies.[73] Weakness that results in muscle imbalances or that increases the likelihood of prolonged times in specific positions has been blamed for range-of-motion limitations,[110] as has spasticity.[111] Statistical evidence that these impairments underlie range-of-motion limitations, however, is lacking.[109]

At the tissue level, range-of-motion limitations can arise from muscle, at the tendon, or from about the joint. Reduced muscle length, which results from a reduced number of sarcomeres in series,[86,89,112,113] can clearly reduce

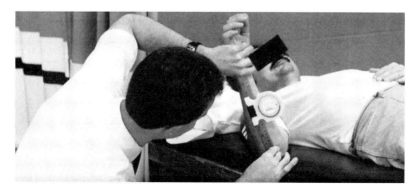

Figure 29–2. Shoulder external rotation measured to the point of pain.

joint range of motion. Whether the muscle belly is shortened (as is the case in some adult neurologic disorders)[78] or the muscle never achieves a normal length during maturation (as is apparently the case in some children with cerebral palsy),[86] the consequences for range of motion are the same. Also occurring in muscles are changes in connective tissue.[114,115] These changes can occur quite early when muscles are immobilized in a shortened position.[114] Jozsa et al.[115] indicated that the relative volume of connective tissue increases in parallel with the duration of immobilization. Although it is probably the muscle belly that is usually short when the overall length of the muscle–tendon unit is reduced, tendon length is also adaptable[116] and may contribute to length reductions. Adhesions between tendons and their sheaths and other surrounding structures can also limit movement of the tendon within the sheath.[117] The tendon, therefore, can also be responsible in some cases for range-of-motion limitations. Changes within ligaments themselves[118] and adhesions between soft tissue (e.g., capsule) and osseous tissue of a joint[119-122] can lead to extreme limitations in range of motion in patients with neurologic disorders, as well as in orthopaedic patients, in whom they have often been demonstrated.

Implications

Range-of-motion limitations have implications primarily for the normal performance of functional activities. At the shoulder, they also have a relationship with pain.

As specific joint excursions are used when functional activities are carried out in a normal manner,[123-126] the importance of critical ranges of motion is rather obvious. As "critical" ranges (e.g., knee flexion during gait) are typically less than normal end ranges, minor losses in range of motion tend not to be disabling.[127] What may be less obvious is that limitations in range of motion, even when they do not preclude the completion of functional tasks, can alter the mechanics of the task. For example, with limited knee flexion range, an increased hip extension moment is required to complete the sit-to-stand maneuver.[128] With weakness of the hip extensor muscles, this may be hard for some patients to perform. When decreased range of motion is caused by a shortened muscle–tendon unit, the angle–tension curve tends to shift to the left. At the ankle, leftward shifts have been documented during passive ankle dorsiflexion and elongation of the triceps surae muscle group.[64] Such leftward shifts involve an increased resistance to ankle dorsiflexion, which can affect ankle mechanics during both the swing and stance phases of gait.[129-131] Among the gait deviations that may occur as a result of stance phase limitations are an early heel-off on the affected side, a decreased step length on the unaffected side, and a high-velocity terminal knee extension or genu-recurvation on the affected side.

At the shoulder, particularly in patients with hemiplegia, impairments in range of motion are one of the most consistently reported correlates of pain. In practice, restricted range of motion and pain at the shoulder are so strongly associated in patients with neurologic disorders that the patients' shoulders are often described as painful and stiff, frozen, or with contracture.[74,76,104] Rizk et al.[76] indicated that the pathogenesis of shoulder pain in patients with hemiplegia is probably "similar to that of idiopathic frozen shoulder." Kumar et al.[77] reported a significant difference in the range of shoulder abduction, flexion, and internal and external rotation motion between hemiplegic patients with and without shoulder pain. In two studies that examined the relationship between multiple independent variables and shoulder pain, Bohannon and co-workers[73,75] reported range of motion to be the best predictor of pain (as measured). Joynt[132] reported corroborative findings and concluded that "pain was related most to loss of motion."

Treatment

The treatment of range-of-motion limitations can involve reduction of existing limitations, prevention of future limitations, or slowing the progression of limitations. Treatment can be categorized as surgical or nonsurgical, but in some cases it involves both options.

Surgical Treatment

Surgical interventions are directed at the tissue thought to be limiting range of motion. When the joint capsule is the site of range restrictions, the surgical lysis of adhesions there[122] or a capsulotomy[133] can be performed, with good results. In cases in which the muscle–tendon unit is of inadequate length, several options are available. Probably the most severe option is a complete muscle release by tenotomy. As the procedure totally disrupts the continuity of the muscle–tendon unit, the unit is unable postsurgically to interfere with motion. Desirable results have been reported for complete releases performed on the hamstring muscles of patients with poliomyelitis[108] and cerebral palsy,[94] on the hip abductor muscles of patients with cerebral palsy,[94] and on the subscapularis muscle of patients with stroke.[74] Less extreme methods of increasing muscle–tendon unit length to improve range of motion include aponeurosis lengthening[88,134] and tendon lengthening.[94,108,135] The latter procedure has been performed extensively on the Achilles tendons of patients with muscular dystrophy[98,99] and cerebral palsy.[85,86,91,134] Although Achilles tendon lengthening is effective in increasing ankle dorsiflexion range of motion in both types of patients, the results are not necessarily permanent.[85,86,91,98,99]

Nonsurgical Treatment

Nonsurgical approaches, although often the only ones applied to patients with neurologic disorders, can also be applied as an adjunct to surgical interventions.[106] Among the many nonsurgical options are exercise, splints and casts, and electrical stimulation.

Exercise can take many forms, but with many weak neurologically affected patients, it is passive by necessity. If passive range-of-motion exercises are to be effective, they must be applied with an adequate duration, frequency, and intensity. Although much of the research relevant to these variables has not involved neurologically affected patients per se, it is doubtless relevant. There is considerable research evidence that low-load, long-duration stretching is preferable to shorter durations of stretch (even if high loads are used).[136,137] Even though durations of stretch as short as 10 seconds have been reported to result in range-of-motion increases when applied repetitively (twice a week for 10 weeks) to sedentary women,[138] much of the research examining responses to load durations of less than 30 minutes has not provided dramatic results.[137,139,140] Durations of stretch of 30 or more minutes, however, have often been shown to be effective in increasing range of motion,[137,140,141] even in patients with neurologic disorders.[79,142] Clearly, load durations of half an hour or more cannot be applied easily or efficiently by hand. With the use of different devices, however, prolonged stretching can be achieved. Tilt tables with wedge boards for increasing ankle dorsiflexion,[79,81,143] pulley traction for increasing knee extension[108,137] and shoulder abduction,[141] screw-adjusted spreading devices for increasing hip abduction,[142,144,145] and intermittent compression devices for increasing knee extension have been used with success.[146-148] Continuous passive motion machines have also been used, but primarily as an adjunct to other interventions.[106] Good results and means of achieving them notwithstanding, clinicians should realize that many hours of stretch may be required to prevent contractures in some types of patients[90] and that, in many cases, range of motion may not increase more than a degree or so per day in response to treatment.[79,141,149] Experiments with animals provide evidence that gains realized during stretch may be augmented by heating the tissues being stretched.[150,151] Animal studies also indicate that there may be benefits to stretching (i.e., retardation of atrophy) beyond the mere maintenance or improvement in range of motion.[152-154] These potential benefits should be considered by therapists working with patients with certain neurologic pathologies.

Splints and casts are also viable devices for treating range-of-motion limitations. Although splints and other positioning devices are often used to prevent or slow losses in range of motion,[100,155,156,157] they can also be used to increase range of motion. The success of positioning devices is dependent in part on patient and caregiver compliance. Without compliance, which can be as low as 10 percent even in institutional settings (personal observations), even the best positioning devices are of little if any value. An advantage of casts is that once they are applied, compliance is ensured. Casts also have the advantage of being more restraining than splints. In patients with spasticity, spasms, and forceful posturing (e.g., traumatic brain injury), this restraining capacity may be essential to success. Serial casts can be applied to take advantage of gains in range of motion. Casting methods and their results have been described in several publications[83,158-161] and should be consulted by clinicians who are novices to the intervention.

Electrical stimulation has been described as a treatment for contractures in a few reports. Munsat et al.[162] described the effects of femoral nerve stimulation in patients with knee flexion contractures. The effects they reported, however, were related to the stimulated muscle, not to the contracture. Pandyan et al.[163] applied electrical stimulation to the wrist extensors of patients with wrist flexion contractures following stroke. The patients demonstrated increased passive wrist extension after a 2-week period of treatment, but the increase was transient.

■ Joint Malalignment

Joint malalignment, the misorientation of bones making up a joint, sometimes occurs in patients with neurologic disorders. The manner and magnitude of the malalignment can differ, as can the joints affected. In the following subsections, only hip and shoulder subluxation/dislocation are discussed, the latter far more thoroughly than the former.

Hip Malalignment

Malalignment of the femoral head relative to the acetabulum occurs in patients with neurologic disorders. It is among patients with cerebral palsy[164-167] or myelodysplasia,[168,169] however, that hip instability and subluxation/dislocation are particularly problematic.

Measurement and Nature

Although judgments about malalignment can be made by observation and palpation, radiographs are typically used to document the extent of subluxation/dislocation. Among the specific methods of quantification are migration percentage, percentage of femoral head coverage, Shenton's line, and the center edge angle.[164]

The incidence of malalignment, as documented by radiography, can be quite high in the diagnostic groups discussed earlier. Among cerebral palsy patients with "bilateral hemiplegia and severe involvement of the upper limbs," Howard et al.[165] reported a 59 percent incidence of dislocation. Huff and Ramsey[169] reported 48 subluxed and 25 dislocated hips among 130 hips of 65 patients with myelodysplasia.

Muscle weakness and imbalance have been identified as determinants of hip malalignment in patients with cerebral palsy and myelomeningocele. Howard et al.,[165] for example, stated that "it is generally agreed that spontaneous dislocation results from gluteal weakness." Regarding patients with myelodysplasia, Huff and Ramsey[169] concluded that "the hip abductors play a key role in the muscle imbalance that leads to hip instability" and that "the incidence of hip instability is much higher in patients with paralysis of this important muscle group." An inadequate amount of time walking and weightbearing through the hips has been posited to affect bone and joint architecture adversely and to contribute to the development of hip dislocation in children with cerebral palsy.[165] In patients with cerebral palsy and pelvic obliquity, hip dislocations and subluxations occur predominantly on the high side.[167,170]

Implications and Treatment

Just as a limited amount of walking is thought to affect hip alignment, hip alignment is considered to influence walking. In both cerebral palsy and myelodysplasia, walking has been described as enhanced by hip stability.[168,169] Both dislocation and subluxation predispose the hips to degenerative arthritis.[166] Hip dislocation is accompanied by hip pain and may also have a causal relationship with back pain.[169]

The treatment of hip malalignment can involve nonoperative options, operative interventions, or both. Although favorable results have been reported for splints alone,[171] Huff and Ramsey[169] stated that "a lasting reduction was seldom achieved by closed means alone." Surgical corrections, which are seldom indicated in the absence of quadriceps femoris function,[169] typically involve a release of the hip adductors, a posterior transfer of the psoas, and one or more bony procedures (e.g., derotation or varus osteotomy, acetabuloplasty).[164,166,168,169] Surgery is often followed by the application of a splint that holds the hips in abduction and internal rotation.[164,169] The results of surgery followed by splinting are generally quite favorable, but hip flexion tends to be weakened by the psoas transfer,[168] and hip abduction contractures sometimes occur.[164]

Shoulder Malalignment

Malalignment of the humeral head relative to the glenoid occurs in patients with a variety of neurologic disorders. The malalignment, which typically takes the form of an inferior subluxation, is particularly prevalent among patients with stroke.[67,75,77,132,172–178] Thus, shoulder subluxation in such patients is the focus of this section.

Measurement

Clinically, inferior subluxation of the shoulder is typically measured by palpation (Fig. 29–3). Subluxation so measured has been categorized as "clearly subluxed" versus "not clearly subluxed,"[75] or as "none," "minimal," or "substantial,"[67] or has been described by the number of

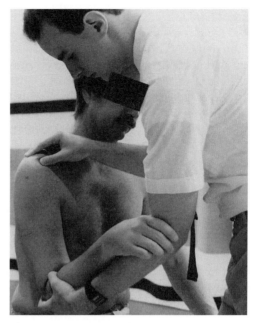

Figure 29–3. Measurement of shoulder subluxation by palpation.

finger breadths separating the acromial process and the humeral head.[172,179,180] Although subjective, judgments of subluxation based on palpation have been shown to be reliable[67] and have correlated significantly (r = .69–.76) with a radiologic measure of subluxation.[172,179,180]

Quantitative methods of measuring subluxation without radiographs have also been reported. The methods involve measuring with calipers[172,180] or a jig.[179,180] Both of these instruments provide measurements that correlate significantly, but not always strongly, with radiographically obtained measurements.[172,179,180]

In many studies, the presence or degree of subluxation has been documented radiographically.[172,175,177] Clearly, radiographs obtained with the upper extremity dependent (e.g., unsupported in sitting) are more likely than radiographs taken with the patient recumbent to reveal the full extent of malalignment.[177] Several methods of quantifying the magnitude of subluxation from radiographs have been described in sufficient detail to allow replication.[172,174,175,179–182] The specifics of the methods will not be outlined here. What should be of interest to the reader, however, is that different measurements tend to correlate strongly.[172]

Nature and Determinants

The subluxation accompanying hemiplegia is primarily inferior but also has anterior[183] and lateral components.[172,174,175,180] Even before a frank inferior subluxation occurs, a "V-shaped space between [the] humeral head and glenoid cavity" can be noted on radiographs.[174] As subluxation progresses, the position of the humeral head becomes increasingly inferior relative to the glenoid. In severe cases (dislocation), "the most superior margin of the humeral head is level with or below the most inferior margin of the glenoid fossa."[175]

Although there may be multiple determinants of subluxation, weakness of the shoulder elevation muscles is definitely foremost. Secondary analysis of contingency table data by Miglietta et al.[177] and by Najenson and Pikielny[173] shows a very strong relationship between paresis and the presence of malalignment/subluxation. Chaco and Wolf[178] reported that, among all the hemiplegic patients they studied, subluxation occurred in the shoulders of all of those whose affected supraspinatus did not respond to loading. Although downward rotation of the scapula has been proposed as a factor predisposing the shoulder to subluxation, objective documentation of the scapular position in patients with hemiplegia has refuted this idea.[184] Culham et al.[185] concluded, as a consequence of their research, that there is "no support for the concept of a relationship between scapular and humeral orientation and glenohumeral subluxation."

Implications

No doubt, the mechanics of a shoulder that is malaligned are altered. The chief consequence attributed to shoulder subluxation, however, is pain. That attribution, needless to say, is not much supported by statistical evidence. At least five studies addressing the issue have failed to show a significant relationship between shoulder subluxation and pain in patients with hemiplegia.[67,75,77,132,175] Of studies indicating a possible connection between shoulder malalignment and shoulder pain, two have methods that are described scantily[183,186] and one reports only that an early V-shaped widening is predictive of future shoulder pain.[174]

Treatment

To prevent shoulder subluxation, Chaco and Wolf[178] suggested that loading of the glenohumeral joint "should be avoided as long as the affected limb is flaccid." The sound logic of their recommendation notwithstanding, I am not aware of any published clinical report or research that documents the successful prevention of shoulder subluxation by the avoidance of joint traction. What research has addressed is the adequacy of alternative methods for reducing the inferior displacement of the humerus of shoulders that are already subluxed. Most of this research focuses on the ability of passive supports to reduce subluxation while they are applied. A survey of Canadian therapists revealed that the supports they used most often were the lap board, the cuff-type arm sling, the arm trough support, and the Bobath axial roll.[187] These and other devices have been described by others in the literature.[181,182,188–194] While applied, all supports are not equally effective. Williams et al.[182] found that the Henderson shoulder ring and the Bobath shoulder roll both provided comparable, albeit incomplete, corrections of subluxa-

tion. Brooke et al.[181] reported that the Harris hemisling provided greater reduction of subluxation than the Bobath sling. Zorowitz et al.[193] found that the single-strap hemisling was best overall for reducing vertical subluxation and that neither the single-strap hemisling nor any of the other three supports they examined was most effective for all subjects. Several studies have demonstrated that the Bobath sling tends to distract the humerus laterally.[181,193] Brooke et al.[181] also noted that the arm trough or lap board tended to overcorrect subluxation. A different type of support has been described by Morin and Bravo.[194] That support, which is provided by tape strapping, significantly reduced subluxation when used in combination with a conventional sling. Faghri et al.[195] provided active support to subluxed shoulders by applying up to 6 hours of functional electrical stimulation daily to the supraspinatus and posterior deltoid muscles. Compared to patients in a control group, patients receiving the stimulation achieved a reduction in shoulder subluxation.

Much debate has centered on whether supports, particularly slings, should be used. The intention of this section is not to resolve the debate. In contemplating the use of supports, however, clinicians should consider three issues. First, many supports restrict the use of an already hypomobile extremity; second, some supports (e.g., the Bobath roll) may actually do harm; and third, the provision of a support does not ensure that it can or will be used as intended.[196]

■ Joint Pain

Joint pain is a relatively common problem accompanying neurologic disorders, particularly stroke and spinal cord injury. Sie et al.,[197] who monitored upper extremity pain in patients with spinal cord injury, found that 55 percent of those with quadriplegia and 64 percent of those with paraplegia had pain. In these patients[197–200] and in patients with stroke[76,77,104,105,174,183,186,199,200,203–206] it is the shoulder that is most often painful. Hence, this section focuses on pain in or around that joint.

Measurement

Although in many publications focusing on shoulder pain the magnitude of the pain is either not described or the pain is described merely as existing or present,[76,77,104,105,174,183,186,199,200,203] several means of quantification are available to the clinician. Categorically, methods of quantifying pain deal with pain on movement of the shoulder, pain in the absence of movement, and pain as a factor affecting activities of daily living.

Research studies of shoulder pain in patients with stroke or spinal cord injury are sometimes not specific as to the conditions under which pain is experienced and indicate merely that it is absent or present.[201,206] Most often, however, pain is described during movement. Most simply, researchers have reported looking for a patient's reaction to movement—for example, when the shoulder is passively flexed to 90 degrees.[207] Inaba and Piorkowski[208] judged increased mobility of the shoulder to be an indirect indicator of a decrease in pain. Other investigators have used ordinal scales to describe pain with movement. Joynt[132] categorized pain as none or mild, moderate, or severe. Bohannon et al.[73] used the scale of Fugl-Meyer and coworkers (pronounced pain during all of the movement or marked pain at the end of movement, some pain, and no pain). The scale of the Ritchie articular index has been used to quantify the response of stroke patients to shoulder external rotation of the shoulder.[67,75,209] On that scale, 0 represents no pain, 1 represents complaint of pain, 2 represents complaint of pain and wince, and 3 represents complaint of pain, wince, and withdrawal. Two studies have described the reliability of measurements assigned using the scale. In one case, raters agreed on 85.3 percent of their ratings ($K = .759$); in the other; raters agreed on 70.8 percent of their ratings ($K = .677$). A 6-point ordinal scale has been used in two studies to describe the pain generally felt during the preceding 7 days (none, mild, moderate, severe, very severe, intense).[175,210] Probably the most precise method of measuring shoulder pain is to move the shoulder until pain is first reported and to record the range of motion at that point.[66,67,195] Measurements so obtained are reliable and correlate significantly ($r = -.776$; $P < .001$) with Ritchie scale grades assigned during the same movement (external rotation).[67]

The number of alternatives reported in the literature for measuring pain at rest are few. One of the ordinal scales used to describe pain at rest is the same as that used to measure pain on movement.[175,210] Secondary analysis of shoulder pain so measured,[175] however, shows it to be significantly less ($P < .001$) than pain during movement. Secondary analysis of the data of Peszczynski and Rardin,[207] however, showed a strong relationship (Yules $Q = .859$) between pain responses to palpation of the supraspinatus and biceps (long head) tendons and passive shoulder flexion. Savage and Robertson[211] and Sindou et al.[212] described a three-level ordinal scale for pain.

At least three investigators have described pain in terms of its effects on daily activities among patients with spinal cord injury. Sie et al.[197] defined significant pain as that requiring analgesics, associated with two or more activities of daily living, and severe enough to result in cessation of an activity. Silfverskiold and Waters[198] rated pain on a three-level scale (mild, moderate, severe). "Mild" pain represented discomfort, during activities of daily living, that did not limit the activities. "Severe" pain prevented the performance of two or more functional activities. Curtis et al. described a 15-item index for assessing shoulder pain during self-care,[213] transfers, wheelchair mobility, and general activities. They found the index to be both reliable and valid.[214]

Nature

Shoulder pain in patients with stroke and patients with spinal cord injury may have some common characteristics. There are enough dissimilarities, however, that the two groups of patients will be discussed separately below.

The incidence of shoulder pain in patients with stroke has been reported to be anywhere from 22 to 100 percent, depending on the study and on how pain was measured.[67,73,75,77,132,175,183,186,204,205,207,209,210] Higher incidences are noted when pain is measured with movement of the affected shoulder.[132,175] VanLangenberghe and Hogan,[175] for example, found pain among 45.4 percent of their patients under a condition of rest but among 100 percent of their patients under a condition of movement. Stress to the shoulder at the limit of motion can be particularly painful.[76] Apparently, the pain begins within 2 months of the stroke for most patients who have shoulder pain.[132,205] The likelihood of pain and the severity of pain, however, tend to increase with the time since onset.[73,75,76,209] Joynt[132] reported, for the cases he examined, that the pain was located in the lateral shoulder in 25 percent of cases, the shoulder in general in 22 percent, and the top of the shoulder in 19 percent. The pain was characterized as vague (37 percent), sharp (31 percent), and achy (19 percent). It radiated into the neck or arm in 49 percent of the cases.

The incidence of shoulder pain in patients with spinal cord injury can surpass 50 percent[199] but varies, depending on the level of the lesion and the time since the injury. Patients with quadriplegia tend to have a higher incidence of shoulder pain. In three studies, more than 70 percent of the patients with quadriplegia were found to have shoulder pain.[198,200,201] Among these patients, the incidence decreased with the time since onset.[198,200] Reports describing separately the proportion of patients with quadriplegia and paraplegia with shoulder pain indicate a lower incidence of pain among the latter. Sie et al.[197] indicated an incidence of 36 percent for patients with paraplegia compared with 46 percent for patients with quadriplegia. Silfverskiold and Waters[198] described the incidence of shoulder pain by 6 months of injury to be 87 percent and 35 percent for patients with quadriplegia and paraplegia, respectively. In patients with shoulder pain, Waring and Maynard[200] found that 61 percent had bilateral pain. The pain experienced by patients with spinal cord injury was characterized by Silfverskiold and Waters[198] as localized around the acromioclavicular and glenohumeral joints. The patients' subdeltoid bursas, rotator cuffs, and biceps tendons were tender to palpation.

Determinants

Only one variable has been shown consistently to correlate with shoulder pain—range of motion. In patients with either spinal cord injuries or stroke, shoulder pain is associated with range-of-motion limitations. Contracture and/or capsulitis was found by Campbell and Koris[202] to be the most common etiology of shoulder pain in patients with acute cervical spinal cord injuries. Range-of-motion limitations themselves have been attributed to improper positioning,[104] inadequate or inappropriate exercises,[77,200] and weakness.[75,200] Regarding the last factor, Bohannon[75] stated that "patients with greater weakness may be more prone to the development of pain because their muscles lack adequate strength to move the joint enough to prevent the development of adhesive capsulitis." Nevertheless, all studies examining the relationship between upper extremity strength and shoulder pain have not reported significant findings. Joynt,[132] Kumar et al.,[77] and Bohannon et al.,[73] in three separate studies of patients with stroke, showed no significant relationship between the variables. In another study, however, Bohannon[75] did find significant correlations between shoulder pain and muscle weakness among patients with stroke. Ring et al.[206] and Jespersen et al.[205] have also reported the development of shoulder pain to be significantly related to the degree of paralysis of the shoulder muscles. Chalsen et al.[215] provided perhaps the best summary of the importance of muscle weakness when discussing shoulder hand syndrome. They stated that "weakness is a necessary but not sufficient cause."

The possible role of shoulder subluxation in shoulder pain was discussed earlier in this chapter. In the same way that subluxation was shown to be an unlikely determinant of shoulder pain, the role of several other variables in determining shoulder pain is either unlikely or equivocal. An age of more than 50 years has been reported as predictive of shoulder pain in patients with spinal cord injury,[200] but age has not been reported to correlate positively with pain in patients with stroke.[73,209] In fact, Jespersen et al.[205] found that younger patients were more likely than older patients to have shoulder pain following stroke. One study has[186] but two studies have not[73,132] shown a significant relationship between spasticity and shoulder pain after stroke. Two studies examining the association of sensory status and shoulder pain have presented differing results.[132,186] DeCourval et al.[186] reported no relationship between shoulder pain and unilateral neglect in patients with stroke.

Implications and Treatment

Although pain itself might be considered a problem, it has further implications. As was intimated earlier in the section on the measurement of shoulder pain, pain can interfere with the performance of functional activities by patients with spinal cord injuries.[197,198] Ohry et al.[105] reported a specific example of pain's interference with wheelchair propulsion. In patients with stroke, shoulder pain has been shown to have a significant influence on

arm function and length of the hospital stay.[216] Nichols et al.[199] found that 36.1 percent of the wheelchair users they surveyed had a slight loss of sleep secondary to shoulder pain. A severe loss of sleep was experienced by 7.5 percent. Patients with stroke who have shoulder pain have significantly more sleep disturbances than patients without shoulder pain. They also show less general well-being.[217]

Like other types of pain, shoulder pain can be treated using a wide variety of pharmacologic, surgical, and physical means. Only physical means are addressed hereafter. Among such means, the effectiveness of exercise, positioning and handling advice, cryotherapy, ultrasound, and electrical nerve stimulation have been examined. Given the unequivocal relationship between range-of-motion impairments and pain of the shoulder, exercises and positioning focused on preventing or reducing limitations in range of motion would appear to be in order. Unfortunately, there is little research evidence of the effectiveness of any specific approach. What research has shown is that (1) patients with stroke whose shoulders are ranged by a therapist or who use a skateboard for exercise are less likely than patients using pulleys to develop shoulder pain;[77] (2) consistent and meticulous positioning may be able to prevent the onset of shoulder pain and contracture among spinal cord-injured patients;[104] and (3) an approach involving advice and instruction regarding positioning, handling, and exercise resulted in a higher incidence of no pain or only occasional pain than cryotherapy.[210] The study by Partridge et al.[210] also showed, however, that whether given advice and instruction or cryotherapy, patients with stroke tended to have a reduction in pain and that patient distress did not vary with the type of treatment. Inaba and Piorkowski,[208] who treated three groups of stroke patients with painful shoulders with exercise and positioning, found no significant difference in the outcome of these groups based on whether no ultrasound, ultrasound, or mock ultrasound was added. Using range of motion as an indicator of shoulder pain, Leandri et al.[218] found significant improvements among patients receiving high-intensity transcutaneous electrical nerve stimulation but not among patients treated with low-intensity or placebo stimulation. Patients with shoulder muscle flaccidity secondary to stroke who received functional electrical stimulation to their supraspinatus and posterior deltoid for up to 6 hours per day for 6 weeks fared much better than patients who did not. They demonstrated less subluxation and greater pain-free range of motion and arm function. This treatment appears particularly promising.

CASE STUDIES

This case study describes the response of a patient with a painful, stiff shoulder following stroke to a regimen of strengthening and range-of-motion exercises. Given the relationships between pain, range of motion, strength, and function, an intervention aimed at increasing both muscle strength and joint range of motion seemed appropriate.

The patient was a 63-year-old right-handed man who was hemiparetic on the left side after an ischemic stroke in the distribution of the right middle cerebral artery 50 weeks before the initiation of this study. When this study began, he was still working as the pastor of a small church and living at home. Although he had not received any formal physical therapy in 4 months, he still was occasionally performing a few exercises from an old home program.

The patient was able to follow complex verbal instructions. He had no discernible sensory loss or visual neglect. No subluxation was apparent by palpation of his left shoulder. That shoulder, however, was painful at the extreme of the patient's available abduction and external rotation range of motion. The patient was independent in all mobility and with most aspects of dressing and grooming.

Measurements

The status of the patient's paretic upper extremity was determined initially and on a weekly basis thereafter. The impairments measured were shoulder range of motion and muscle strength. Disability was characterized by the Frenchay arm test.

Two shoulder motions were measured in the paretic upper extremity: abduction and external rotation. Both were measured twice passively to the point of pain while the subject was supine. The mean of the two measurements was recorded.

The strength of the upper extremity was described using dynamometer scores. A Jamar hand grip dynamometer (TEC, Clifton, NJ)—with the handle in the second position—and the technique described by Mathiowetz et al.[219] were used to quantify grip strength. An Ametek Accuforce II hand-held dynamometer and the technique described by Bohannon[220] were used to describe quantitatively the isometric strength of the elbow flexor and extensor muscles and the shoulder abductor, external rotator, and internal rotator muscles. Each of the six dynamometer measurements was taken twice and averaged. Thereafter, the average measurements were added together to obtain a sum score.

The Frenchay arm test, which has been described extensively elsewhere, requires the performance of five activities with the paretic upper extremity.[221] The five activities are stabilizing a ruler for drawing a line, picking up a dowel, drinking from a cup, combing the hair, and removing or replacing a clothespin on a dowel. For each activity passed, the patient is given 1 point, for a maximum score of 5 points.

Treatments

The patient was treated two sessions per week, with session durations of about 40 minutes. Treatments focused on increasing the range of motion of the paretic shoulder and increasing the strength of the main muscle groups of the paretic upper extremity. More specifically, treatment consisted of three primary components: a home program, passive shoulder range-of-motion exercises, and manually resisted strengthening exercises.

The home program consisted of three parts. First, the patient was counseled to avoid placing the involved upper extremity in a position of adduction and internal rotation when sitting or recumbent. He was given specific suggestions for positioning. Second, the patient was instructed to practice weightbearing, for at least 10 minutes per day, on the paretic hand while the fingers were outstretched. Third, the patient was to practice grasping his cane in his paretic hand while slowly pronating and supinating his paretic forearm.

Passive range-of-motion exercise involved five repetitions of shoulder external rotation just past the point of pain. Each repetition was of 2 minutes' duration. Thus, a total of 10 minutes of stretch was provided.

Three sets of 10 repetitions of manually resisted concentric/eccentric exercises were applied to the finger flexor, wrist extensor, forearm pronator and supinator, elbow flexor and extensor, and shoulder internal and external rotator and abductor muscles. Verbal encouragement and occasional quick stretches were used to reinforce the patient's efforts.

Data Analysis

An AB single-subject design was used to investigate the outcome of the interventions. The A period was a 6-week baseline. The B period was 6 weeks of treatment. The treatment began immediately after the 6-week baseline measurements were obtained. Mean range of motion for shoulder external rotation and abduction and the sum of the six muscle group strengths (obtained by dynamometer) were plotted. Analysis of variance was performed to determine whether the patient's impairments in range of motion and strength were affected by the interventions.

Results

Figure 29–4 is a line graph comparing shoulder abduction and external rotation across the A and B periods. Neither motion was significantly different between the two periods (external rotation: $F = .813$, $P = .409$; abduction: $F = 2.841$, $P = .153$). Figure 29–5 is a line graph comparing the muscle group strength sums across the two periods. It is apparent from the graph that strength changed abruptly within 1 week of the initiation of the intervention. The analysis of variance showed the difference in strength between the two periods to be significant ($F = 41.8$; $P = .001$). The total Frenchay arm test score was 3 during the first eight measurement sessions and 4 thereafter. The improvement resulted from the patient's passing the clothespin task. He remained unable to pass the hair-combing tasks throughout the study period.

Discussion

The range-of-motion and strength regimens applied to the patient in this study were designed to improve pain-free range of motion, strength, and function. They did not have a significant affect on range of motion. The interventions, however, did result in a significant increase in strength, as measured by dynamometry. That the largest improvement in strength occurred soon after the initiation of therapy suggests that the strengthening component may have had a motor learning effect. That is, the intervention may have provided the patient with a sense of how to use the paretic muscles more effectively, knowledge which he was then able to generalize beyond the exercise situation. The interventions were accompanied by an improvement in only one functional activity of the Frenchay arm test. In the view of third-party payers, such limited improvement in function may not justify the usual cost of the treatments provided to the patient. As the patient in this study was not billed for treatment, such justification was not required.

Whether other patients will respond similarly to the patient in this study is uncertain. Perhaps an increased frequency or duration of treatment would have resulted in a more dramatic effect. That, however, would normally result in greater costs. Regardless, before intensive and potentially expensive interventions are applied, it makes

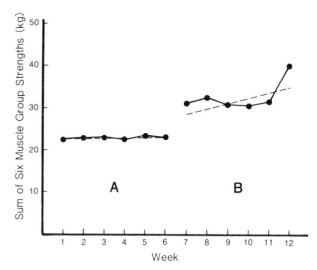

Figure 29–5. Sum of the strengths of six muscle groups measured during a baseling period of no intervention (A) and a period of intervention (B). The broken lines are the linear regression lines for the 6 data points of each period.

sense to establish a baseline of objective measures against which the outcome can be measured.

■ References

1. World Health Organization: International Classification of Impairments, Disabilities, and Handicaps. WHO, Geneva, 1980
2. Stover SL, Hataway CJ, Zeiger HE: Heterotopic ossification in spinal cord-injured patients. Arch Phys Med Rehabil 56:199, 1975
3. Furman R, Nicholas JJ, Jivoff L: Elevation of the serum alkaline phosphatase coincident with ectopic-bone formation in paraplegic patients. J Bone Joint Surg 52(A):1131, 1970
4. Sazbon L, Najenson T, Tartakovsky M, et al: Widespread periarticular new-bone formation in long-term comatose patients. J Bone Joint Surg 63(B):120, 1981
5. Greenwood R, Luder R, Gilchrist E: Neurogenic para-articular ossification: a retrospective survey of 48 cases occurring after brain damage. Clin Rehabil 3:281, 1989
6. Hsu JD, Sakimura I, Stauffer ES: Heterotopic ossification around the hip joint in spinal cord injured patients. Clin Orthop 112:165, 1975
7. Baron M, Stern J, Lander P: Heterotopic ossification heralded by a knee effusion. J Rheumatol 10:961, 1983
8. Citta-Pietrolungo TJ, Alexander MA, Steg NL: Early detection of heterotopic ossification in young patients with traumatic brain injury. Arch Phys Med Rehabil 73:258, 1992
9. Goldberg MA, Schumacher R: Heterotopic ossification mimicking acute arthritis after neurologic catastrophes. Arch Intern Med 137:619, 1977
10. Venier LH, Ditunno JF: Heterotopic ossification in the paraplegic patients. Arch Phys Med Rehabil 52:475, 1971
11. Stover SL, Niemann KMW, Miller JM: Disodium etidronate in the prevention of postoperative recurrence of heterotopic ossification in spinal-cord injury patients. J Bone Joint Surg 58(A):683, 1976

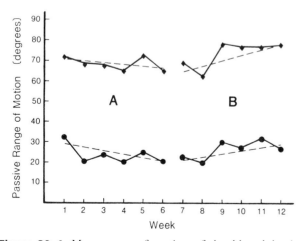

Figure 29–4. Mean range of motion of shoulder abduction (diamonds) and external rotation (circles) of the paretic side measured during a baseline period of no intervention (A) and a period of intervention (B). Broken lines are the linear regression lines for the 6 data points of each period.

12. Nicholas JJ: Ectopic bone formation in patients with spinal cord injury. Arch Phys Med Rehabil 54:354, 1973

13. Garland DE, Shimoyama ST, Lugo C, et al: Spinal cord insults and heterotopic ossification in the pediatric population. Clin Orthop 245:303, 1989

14. Lee M, Alexander MA, Miller F, et al: Postoperative heterotopic ossification in the child with cerebral palsy. Three case reports. Arch Phys Med Rehabil 73:289, 1992

15. Hurvitz EA, Mandac BR, Davidoff G, et al: Risk factors for heterotopic ossification in children and adolescents with severe traumatic brain injury. Arch Phys Med Rehabil 73:459, 1992

16. Wittenberg RH, Peschke V, Botel U: Heterotopic ossification after spinal cord injury. Epidemiology and risk factors. J Bone Joint Surg 74(B):215, 1992

17. Stover SL, Niemann KM, Tulloss JR: Experience with surgical resection of heterotopic bone in spinal cord injury patients. Clin Orthop 263:71, 1991

18. Stover SL, Hahn HR, Miller JM: Disodium etidronate in the prevention of heterotopic ossification following spinal cord injury (preliminary report). Paraplegia 14:146, 1976

19. Garland DE, Orwin JF: Resection of heterotopic ossification in patients with spinal cord injuries. Clin Orthop 242:169, 1989

20. Kiwerski J: Prevention of long-term immobilization in treatment of cervical spinal cord injuries. Clin Rehabil 6:49, 1992

21. Catz A, Snir D, Groswasser Z, et al: Is the appearance of periarticular new bone formation related to neurological disability? Paraplegia 30:361, 1992

22. Spielman G, Gennarelli TA, Rogers CR: Disodium etidronate: its role in preventing heterotopic ossification in severe head injury. Arch Phys Med Rehabil 64:539, 1983

23. Rodriguez GP, Claus-Walker J, Kent MC, et al: Collagen metabolite excretion as a predictor of bone- and skin-related complications in spinal cord injury. Arch Phys Med Rehabil 70:442, 1989

24. Varghese G, Williams K, Desmet A, et al: Nonarticular complication of heterotopic ossification: a clinical review. Arch Phys Med Rehabil 72:1009, 1991

25. Ostlere SJ, Gold RH: Osteoporosis and bone density measurement methods. Clin Orthop 271:149, 1991

26. Thomsen K, Gotfredsen A, Christiansen C: Is postmenopausal bone loss an age-related phenomenon? Calcif Tissue Int 39:123, 1986

27. Gross M, Roberts JG, Foster J, et al: Calcaneal bone density reduction in patients with restricted mobility. Arch Phys Med Rehabil 68:158, 1987

28. Pacy PJ, Hesp R, Halliday DA, et al: Muscle and bone in paraplegic patients and the effect of functional electrical stimulation. Clin Sci 75:481, 1988

29. Hodkinson HM, Brain AT: Unilateral osteoporosis in long standing hemiplegia in the elderly. J Am Geriatr Soc 15:59, 1967

30. Abramson AS: Bone disturbances in injuries to the spinal cord and cauda equina (paraplegia). J Bone Joint Surg 30(A):982, 1948

31. Griffiths HJ, D'Orsi CJ, Zimmerman RE: Use of 125 I photon scanning in the evaluation of bone density in a group of patients with spinal cord injury. Invest Radiol 7:107, 1972

32. Hamby RC, Krishnaswamy G, Cancellaro V, et al: Changes in bone mineral density after stroke. Am J Phys Med Rehabil 72:188, 1993

33. Hamdy RC, Moore SW, Cancellaro VA, et al: Long-term effects of strokes on bone mass. Am J Phys Med Rehabil 74:351, 1995

34. Rosenstein BD, Greene WB, Herrington RT, et al: Bone density in myelomeningocele: the effects of ambulatory status and other factors. Dev Med Child Neurol 29:486, 1987

35. Taggart H, Crawford V: Reduced bone density of the hip in elderly patients with Parkinson's disease. Age Ageing 24:326, 1995

36. Szollar SM, Martin EME, Parthemore JG, et al: Demineralization in the tetraplegic and paraplegic man over time. Spinal Cord 35:223, 1997

37. Wilmshurst S, Ward K, Adams JE, et al: Mobility status and bone density in cerebral palsy. Arch Dis Child 75:164, 1996

38. Lin PP, Henderson RC: Bone mineralization in the affected extremities of children with spastic hemiplegia. Dev Med Child Neurol 38:782, 1996

39. Kunkel CF, Scremin AME, Eisenberg B, et al: Effect of "standing" on spasticity, contractures, and osteoporosis in paralyzed males. Arch Phys Med Rehabil 74:73, 1993

40. Hangartner TN, Rogers MM, Glaser RM, et al: Tibial bone density loss in spinal cord injured patients: effects of FES exercise. J Rehabil Res 31:50, 1994

41. Henderson RC, Lin PP, Greene WB: Bone-mineral density in children and adolescents who have spastic cerebral palsy. J Bone Joint Surg 77A:1671, 1995

42. Henderson RC: Bone density and other possible predictors of fracture risk in children and adolescents with spastic quadriplegia. Dev Med Child Neurol 30:224, 1997

43. Oyster N, Morton M, Linnell S: Physical activity and osteoporosis in post-menopausal women. Med Sci Sports Exerc 16:44, 1984

44. Chappard D, Petitjean M, Alexandre C, et al: Cortical osteoclasts are less sensitive to etidronate than trabecular osteoclasts. J Bone Mineral Res 6:673, 1991

45. Lips P, van Ginkel FC, Netelenbos JC, et al: Lower mobility and markers of bone resorption in the elderly. Bone Mineral 9:49, 1990

46. Biering-Sorensen F, Bohr HH, Schaadt OP: Longitudinal study of bone mineral content in the lumbar spine, the forearm and the lower extremities after spinal cord injury. Eur J Clin Invest 20:330, 1990

47. Garland DE, Stewart CA, Adkins RH, et al: Osteoporosis after spinal cord injury. J Orthop Res 10:371, 1992

48. Claus-Walker JL, Campos RJ, Carter RE, et al: Calcium excretion in quadriplegia. Arch Phys Med Rehabil 53:14, 1972

49. Claus-Walker JL, Carter RE, Campos RJ, et al: Sitting, muscular exercises, and collagen metabolism in tetraplegia. Am J Phys Med 58:285, 1979

50. Rafii M, Firooznia H, Golimbu C, et al: Bilateral acetabular stress fractures in a paraplegic patient. Arch Phys Med Rehabil 63:240, 1982

51. Keating JF, Kerr M, Delargy M: Minimal trauma causing fractures in patients with spinal cord injury. Disabil Rehabil 14:108, 1992

52. Leeds EM, Klose KJ, Ganz W, et al: Bone mineral density after bicycle ergometry training. Arch Phys Med Rehabil 71:207, 1990

53. Claus-Walker J, DiFerrante N, Halstead LS, et al: Connective tissue turnover in quadriplegia. Am J Phys Med 61:130, 1982

54. Pearson EG, Nance PW, Leslie WD, et al: Cyclical etidronate: its effect on bone density in patients with acute spinal cord injury. Arch Phys Med Rehabil 78:267, 1997

55. Bohannon RW: Cinematographic analysis of the passive straight-leg-raising test for hamstring muscle length. Phys Ther 62:1269, 1982

56. Gajdosik R, Lusin G: Hamstring muscle tightness: reliability of an active-knee-extension test. Phys Ther 63:1085, 1983

57. Milch H: The measurement of hip motion in the sagittal and coronal planes. J Bone Joint Surg 41(A):731, 1959

58. Walker JM, Sue D, Miles-Elkousy N, et al: Active mobility of the extremities in older subjects. Phys Ther 64:919, 1984

59. James B, Parker AW: Active and passive mobility of lower limb joints in elderly men and women. Am J Phys Med Rehabil 68:162, 1989

60. Boone DC, Azen SP: Normal range of motion of joints in male subjects. J Bone Joint Surg 61(A):756, 1979

61. Svenningsen S, Terjesen T, Auflem M, et al: Hip motion related to age and sex. Acta Orthop Scand 60:97, 1989

62. Bassey EJ, Morgan K, Dallosso HM, et al: Flexibility of the shoulder joint measured as range of abduction in a large representative sample of men and women over 65 years of age. Eur J Appl Physiol 58:353, 1989

63. Rooas A, Andersson GBJ: Normal range of motion of the hip, knee, and ankle joints in male subjects, 30–40 years of age. Acta Orthop Scand 53:205, 1982

64. Tardieu G, Tardieu C: Cerebral palsy. Mechanical evaluation and conservative correction of limb joint contractures. Clin Orthop 219:63, 1987

65. Gajdosik RL, LeVeau BF, Bohannon RW: Effects of ankle dorsiflexion on active and passive unilateral straight leg raising. Phys Ther 65:1478, 1985

66. Andrews AW, Bohannon RW: Decreased shoulder range of motion on paretic side after stroke. Phys Ther 69:768, 1989

67. Bohannon RW, Andrews AW: Shoulder subluxation and pain in stroke patients. Am J Occup Ther 44:507, 1990

68. Boone DC, Azen SP, Lin C-M, et al: Reliability of goniometric measurements. Phys Ther 58:1355, 1978

69. Gogia PD, Braatz JH, Rose SJ, et al: Reliability and validity of goniometric measurements at the knee. Phys Ther 67:192, 1987

70. Harris SR, Smith LH, Krukowski L: Goniometric reliability for a child with spastic quadriplegia. J Pediatr Orthop 5:348, 1985

71. Stuberg WA, Fuchs RH, Miedaner JA: Reliability of goniometric measurements of children with cerebral palsy. Dev Med Child Neurol 30:657, 1988

72. Pandya S, Florence JM, King WM, et al: Reliability of goniometric measurements in patients with Duchenne muscular dystrophy. Phys Ther 65:1339, 1985

73. Bohannon RW, Larkin PA, Smith MB, et al: Shoulder pain in hemiplegia: statistical relationship with five variables. Arch Phys Med Rehabil 67:514, 1986

74. Braun RM, Mooney V, Nickel VL et al: Surgical treatment of the painful shoulder contracture in the stroke patient. J Bone Joint Surg 53(A):1307, 1971

75. Bohannon RW: Relationship between shoulder pain and selected variables in patients with hemiplegia. Clin Rehabil 2:111, 1988

76. Rizk TE, Christopher RP, Pinals RS et al: Arthrographic studies in painful hemiplegic shoulders. Arch Phys Med Rehabil 65:254, 1984

77. Kumar R, Metter EJ, Mehta AJ, et al: Shoulder pain in hemiplegia. The role of exercise. Am J Phys Med Rehabil 69:205, 1990

78. Halar EM, Stolov WC, Venkatesh B, et al: Gastrocnemius muscle belly and tendon length in stroke patients and able-bodied persons. Arch Phys Med Rehabil 59:476, 1978

79. Bohannon RW, Larkin PA: Passive ankle dorsiflexion increases in patients after a regimen of tilt table–wedge board standing. Phys Ther 65:1676, 1985

80. Conine TA, Sullivan T, Mackie T, Goodman M: Effect of serial casting for the prevention of equinus in patients with acute head injury. Arch Phys Med Rehabil 71:310, 1990

81. Richardson DLA: The use of the tilt-table to effect passive tendo Achillis stretch in a patient with head injury. Physiother Theory Pract 7:45, 1991

82. Booth BJ, Doyle M, Montgomery J: Serial casting for the management of spasticity in the head-injured adult. Phys Ther 63:1960, 1983

83. Moseley AM: The effect of casting combined with stretching on passive ankle dorsiflexion in adults with traumatic head injuries. Phys Ther 77:240, 1997

84. Cherry DB, Weigand GM: Plaster drop-out casts as a dynamic means to reduce muscle contracture. Phys Ther 61:1601, 1981

85. Truscelli D, Lespargot A, Tardieu G: Variation in the long-term results of elongation of the tendo Achillis in children with cerebral palsy. J Bone Joint Surg 61(B):466, 1979

86. Tardieu G, Tardieu C, Colbeau-Justin P, et al: Muscle hypo-extensibility in children with cerebral palsy: II. Therapeutic implications. Arch Phys Med Rehabil 63:103, 1982

87. Watt J, Sims D, Harckham F, et al: A prospective study of inhibitive casting as an adjunct to physiotherapy for cerebral-palsied children. Dev Med Child Neurol 28:480, 1986

88. Olney BW, Williams PF, Menelaus MB: Treatment of spastic equinus by aponeurosis lengthening. J Pediatr Orthop 8:422, 1988

89. Tardieu C, Huet de la Tour E, Bret MD, et al: Muscle hypoextensibility in children with cerebral palsy: I. Clinical and experimental observations. Arch Phys Med Rehabil 63:97, 1982

90. Tardieu C, Lespargot A, Tabary C, et al: For how long must the soleus muscle be stretched each day to prevent contracture? Dev Med Child Neurol 30:3, 1988

91. Sala DA, Grant AD, Kummer FJ: Equinus deformity in cerebral palsy: recurrence after tendo Achillis lengthening. Dev Med Child Neurol 39:45, 1997

92. Anderson JP, Snow B, Dorey FJ, et al: Efficacy of soft splints in reducing severe knee-flexion contractures. Dev Med Child Neurol 30:502, 1988

93. Thometz J, Rosenthal R: The effect on gait of lengthening of the medial hamstrings in cerebral palsy. J Bone Joint Surg 71(A):345, 1989

94. Matsoo T, Hara H, Tada S: Selective lengthening of psoas and rectus femoris and preservation of the iliacus for flexion deformity of the hip in cerebral palsy patients. J Pediatr Orthop 7:690, 1987

95. Hiroshima K, Ono K: Correlation between muscle shortening and derangement of the hip joint in children with spastic cerebral palsy. Clin Orthop 144:186, 1979

96. Bowen JR, MacEwen GD, Mathews PA: Treatment of extension contracture of the hip in cerebral palsy. Dev Med Child Neurol 23:23, 1981

97. Bar-On E, Malkin C, Eilert RE, et al: Hip flexion contracture in cerebral palsy. Clin Orthop 281:97, 1992

98. Seeger BR, Caudrey DJ, Little JD: Progression of equinus deformity in Duchenne muscular dystrophy. Arch Phys Med Rehabil 66:286, 1985

99. Williams EA, Read L, Ellis A, et al: The management of equinus deformity in Duchenne muscular dystrophy. J Bone Joint Surg 66(B):546, 1984

100. Scott OM, Hyde SA, Goddard C, et al: Prevention of deformity in Duchenne muscular dystrophy. Physiotherapy 67:177, 1981

101. Archibald KC, Vignos PJ: A study of contractures in muscular dystrophy. Arch Phys Med Rehabil 40:150, 1959

102. Siegel IM: Pathomechanics of stance in Duchenne muscular dystrophy. Arch Phys Med Rehabil 53:403, 1972

103. Wagner MB, Vignos PJ, Carlozzi C: Duchenne muscular dystrophy: a study of wrist and hand function. Muscle Nerve 12:236, 1989

104. Scott JA, Donovan WH: The prevention of shoulder pain and contracture in the acute tetraplegia patient. Paraplegia 19:313, 1981

105. Ohry A, Brooks ME, Steinbach TV, et al: Shoulder complications as a cause of delay in rehabilitation of spinal cord injured patients. Paraplegia 16:310, 1978–1979

106. Pope PM, Bowes CE, Tudor M, et al: Surgery combined with continuing post-operative stretching and management for knee flexion contractures in cases of multiple sclerosis—a report of six cases. Clin Rehabil 5:15, 1991

107. Sharma JC, Gupta SP, Sankhala SS, et al: Residual poliomyelitis of lower limb—pattern and deformities. Indian J Pediatr 58:233, 1991

108. Parekh PK: Flexion contractures of the knee following poliomyelitis. Int Orthop 7:165, 1983

109. Wright JG, Manelaus MB, Broughton NS, et al: Natural history of knee contractures in myelomeningocele. J Pediatr Orthop 11:725, 1991

110. Sharrard WJW: Paralytic deformity in the lower limb. J Bone Joint Surg 49(B):731, 1967

111. Botte MJ, Nickel VL, Akeson WH: Spasticity and contracture. Physiologic aspects of formation. Clin Orthop 233:7, 1988

112. Tabary JC, Tabary C, Tardieu C, et al: Physiological and structural changes in the cat's soleus muscles due to immobilization at different lengths by plaster casts. J Physiol 224:231, 1972

113. Goldspink G, Tabary C, Tabary JC, et al: Effect of denervation on the adaptation of sarcomere number and muscle extensibility to the functional length of the muscle. J Physiol 236:733, 1974

114. Williams PE, Goldspink G: Connective tissue changes in immobilized muscle. J Anat 138:343, 1984

115. Jozsa L, Kannus P, Thoring J, et al: The effect of tenotomy and immobilization on intramuscular connective tissue. J Bone Joint Surg 72(B):293, 1990

116. Tardieu C, Blanchard O, Tabary JC, et al: Tendon adaptation to bone shortening. Conn Tissue Res 11:35, 1983

117. Hagberg L, Wik O, Gerdin B: Determination of biomechanical characteristics of restrictive adhesions and functional impairment after flexor tendon surgery: a methodological study of rabbits. J Biomech 24:935, 1991

118. Wilson CJ, Dahners LE: An examination of the mechanism of ligament contracture. Clin Orthop 227:286, 1988

119. Thorpe CD, Bocell JR, Tullos HS: Intra-articular fibrous bands. J Bone Joint Surg 72(A):811, 1990

120. Enneking WF, Horowitz M: The intra-articular effects of immobilization on the knee. J Bone Joint Surg 54(A):973, 1972

121. Benum P: Operative mobilization of stiff knees after surgical treatment of knee injuries and posttraumatic conditions. Acta Orthop Scand 53:625, 1982

122. Langeland N, Carlsen B: Release surgery in stiffness of the knee. Acta Orthop Scand 54:252, 1983

123. Laubenthal KN, Smidt GL, Kellelkamp DB: A quantitative analysis of knee motion during activities of daily living. Phys Ther 52:34, 1972

124. Andriacchi TP, Andersson GBJ, Fermier RW, et al: A study of lower-limb mechanics during stair climbing. J Bone Joint Surg 62(A):749, 1980

125. Ryu J, Cooney WP, Askew LJ, et al: Functional ranges of motion of the wrist joint. J Hand Surg 16(A):409, 1991

126. Morrey BF, Askew LJ, An KN, et al: A biomechanical study of normal functional elbow motion. J Bone Joint Surg 63(A):872, 1981

127. Bergstrom G, Aniansson A, Bjelle A, et al: Functional consequences of joint impairment at age 79. Scand J Rehabil Med 17:183, 1985

128. Fleckenstein SJ, Kirby RL, MacLeod DA: Effect of limited knee-flexion range on peak hip moments of force while transferring from sitting to standing. J Biomech 21:915, 1988

129. Maurer BT, Siegler S, Hillstrom HJ, et al: Quantitative identification of ankle equinus with applications for treatment assessment. Gait Posture 3:19, 1995

130. Siegler S, Moskowitz GD, Freedman W: Passive and active components of the internal moment developed about the ankle joint during human locomotion. J Biomech 17:647, 1984

131. Eames NWA, Baker RJ, Cosgrove AP: Defining gastrocnemius length in ambulant children. Gait Posture 6:9, 1997

132. Joynt RL: The source of shoulder pain hemiplegia. Arch Phys Med Rehabil 73:409, 1992

133. Heydarian K, Akbarmia BA, Jabalameli M, et al: Posterior capsulotomy for the treatment of severe flexion contractures of the knee. J Pediatr Orthop 4:700, 1984

134. Reimers J: Functional changes in the antagonists after lengthening the agonists in cerebral palsy. I. Triceps surae lengthening. Clin Orthop 253:30, 1990

135. Reimers J: Contracture of the hamstrings in spastic cerebral palsy. J Bone Joint Surg 56(B):102, 1974

136. Kottke FJ, Pauley DL, Ptak RA: The rationale for prolonged stretching for correction of shortening of connective tissue. Arch Phys Med Rehabil 47:345, 1966

137. Light KE, Nuzik S, Personius W, et al: Low-load prolonged stretch versus high-load brief stretch in treating knee contractures. Phys Ther 64:330, 1984

138. Borms JB, Roy PV, Santens J-P, et al: Optimal duration of static stretching exercises for improvement of coxo-femoral flexibility. J Sport Sci 5:39, 1987

139. Bohannon RW: Effect of repeated eight-minute muscle loading on the angle of straight leg raising. Phys Ther 64:491, 1984

140. Williams PE: Effect of intermittent stretch on immobilized muscle. Ann Rheum Dis 47:1014, 1988

141. Rizk TE, Christopher RP, Pinals RS, et al: Adhesive capsulitis (frozen shoulder): a new approach. Arch Phys Med Rehabil 64:29, 1983

142. Odeen I: Reduction of muscular hypertonus by long-term muscle stretch. Scand J Rehabil Med 13:93, 1981

143. Guccione AA, Peteel JO: Standing wedge for increasing ankle dorsiflexion. Phys Ther 59:766, 1979

144. Rankin J, Greninger L, Ingersoll C: The effects of the power stretch device on flexibility of normal hip joints. Clin Kinesiol 45:23, 1992

145. Bohannon RW: Device for stretching spastic hip adductor muscles. Phys Ther 63:343, 1983

146. Allen AL: Use of "Flowtron" in hemophiliac patients and others with fixed flexion deformity problems. Physiotherapy 74:581, 1988

147. Nelson IW, Atkins RM, Allen AL: The management of knee flexion contractures in hemophilia: brief report. J Bone Joint Surg 71(B):327, 1989

148. Majkowski RS, Atkins RM: Treatment of fixed flexion deformities of the knee in rheumatoid arthritis using the Flowtron intermittent compression stocking. Br J Rheumatol 31:41, 1992

149. Bohannon RW, Chavis D, Larkin P, et al: Effectiveness of repeated prolonged loading for increasing flexion in knees demonstrating postoperative stiffness. Phys Ther 65:494, 1985

150. Lehmann JF, Masok AJ, Warren CG, et al: Effect of therapeutic temperatures on tendon extensibility. Arch Phys Med Rehabil 51:481, 1970

151. Warren CG, Lehmann JF, Koblanski JN: Heat and stretch procedures: an evaluation using rat tail tendon. Arch Phys Med Rehabil 57:122, 1976

152. Frankeny JR, Holly RG, Ashmore CR: Effects of graded duration of stretch on normal and dystrophic skeletal muscle. Muscle Nerve 6:269, 1983

153. Patejan JH, Songster G, McNeil D: Effects of passive movement on neurogenic atrophy in rabbit limb muscles. Exp Neurol 71:92, 1981

154. Pachter BR, Eberstein A: Effects of passive exercise on neurogenic atrophy in rat skeletal muscle. Exp Neurol 90:467, 1985

155. Bell E, Watson A: The prevention of positional deformity in cerebral palsy. Physiother Pract 1:86, 1985

156. Bohannon RW, Thorne M, Mieres AC: Shoulder positioning device for patients with hemiplegia. Phys Ther 63:49, 1983

157. Anderson JP, Snow B, Dorey FJ, et al: Efficacy of soft splints in reducing severe knee-flexion contractures. Dev Med Child Neurol 30:502, 1988

158. Cherry DB, Weigand GM: Plaster drop-out casts as a dynamic means to reduce muscle contracture. Phys Ther 61:1601, 1981

159. Sullivan T, Conine TA, Goodman M, et al: Serial casting to prevent equinas in acute traumatic head injury. Physiother Can 40:346, 1988

160. Booth BJ, Doyle M, Montgomery J: Serial casting for the management of spasticity in the head-injured adult. Phys Ther 63:1960, 1983

161. Conine TA, Sullivan T, Mackie T, et al: Effect of serial casting for the prevention of equinas in patients with acute head injury. Arch Phys Med Rehabil 71:310, 1990

162. Munsat TL, McNeal D, Waters R: Effects of nerve stimulation on human muscle. Arch Neurol 33:608, 1976

163. Pandyan AD, Granat MH, Stott DJ: Effects of electrical stimulation of flexion contractures in hemiplegic wrist. Clin Rehabil 11:123, 1997

164. Houkom JA, Roach JW, Wenger DR, et al: Treatment of acquired hip subluxation in cerebral palsy. J Pediatr Orthop 6:285, 1986

165. Howard CB, McKibbin B, Williams LA, et al: Factors affecting the incidence of hip dislocation in cerebral palsy. J Bone Joint Surg 67(B):510, 1985

166. Bagg MR, Farber J, Miller F: Long-term follow-up of hip subluxation in cerebral palsy patients. J Pediatr Orthop 13:32, 1993

167. Black BE, Griffin PP: The cerebral palsied hip. Clin Orthop 338:42, 1997

168. Lee EH, Carroll NC: Hip stability and ambulatory status in myelomeningocele. J Pediatr Orthop 5:522, 1985

169. Huff CW, Ramsey PL: Myelodysplasia. The influence of the quadriceps and hip abductor muscles on ambulatory function and stability of the hip. J Bone Joint Surg 60(A):432, 1978

170. Letts M, Shapiro L, Mulder K, et al: The windblown hip syndrome in total body cerebral palsy. J Pediatr Orthop 4:55, 1984

171. McKibbin B: The use of splintage in the management of paralytic dislocation of the hip in spina bifida cystica. J Bone Joint Surg 55(B):163, 1973

172. Prévost R, Arsenault AB, Dutil E, et al: Shoulder subluxation in hemiplegia: a radiologic correlational study. Arch Phys Med Rehabil 68:782, 1987

173. Najenson T, Pikielny SS: Malalignment of the gleno-humeral joint following hemiplegia. Ann Phys Med 8:96, 1965

174. Shai G, Ring H, Costeff H, et al: Glenohumeral malalignment in the hemiplegia shoulder. Scand J Rehabil Med 16:133, 1984

175. VanLangenberghe HVK, Hogan BM: Degree of pain and grade of subluxation in the painful hemiplegic shoulder. Scand J Rehabil Med 20:161, 1988

176. Taketomi Y: Observations on subluxation of the shoulder joint in hemiplegia. Phys Ther 55:39, 1975

177. Miglietta O, Lewitan A, Rogoff JB: Subluxation of the shoulder in hemiplegia patients. NY State Med J 59:457, 1959

178. Chaco J, Wolf E: Subluxation of the glenohumeral joint in hemiplegia. Am J Phys Med 50:139, 1971

179. Hall J, Dudgeon B, Guthrie M: Validity of clinical measures of shoulder subluxation in adults with poststroke hemiplegia. Am J Occup Ther 49:526, 1995

180. Boyd EA, Goudreau L, O'Riain MD, et al: A radiological measure of shoulder subluxation in hemiplegia: its reliability and validity. Arch Phys Med Rehabil 74:188, 1993

181. Brooke MM, deLateur BJ, Diana-Rigby GC, et al: Shoulder subluxation in hemiplegia: effects of three different supports. Arch Phys Med Rehabil 72:582, 1991

182. Williams R, Raffs L, Minuk T: Evaluation of two support methods for the subluxated shoulder of hemiplegic patients. Phys Ther 68:1209, 1988

183. VanOuwenaller C, Laplace PM, Chatraine A: Painful shoulder in hemiplegia. Arch Phys Med Rehabil 6:23, 1986

184. Prévost R, Arsenault AB, Dutil E, et al: Rotation of the scapula and shoulder subluxation in hemiplegia. Arch Phys Med Rehabil 68:786, 1987

185. Culham EG, Noce RR, Bagg SD: Shoulder complex position and glenohumeral subluxation in hemiplegia. Arch Phys Med Rehabil 76:857, 1995

186. deCourval LP, Barsauskas A, Berenbaum B, et al: Painful shoulder in the hemiplegic and unilateral neglect. Arch Phys Med Rehabil 71:673, 1990

187. Boyd E, Gaylord A: Shoulder supports with stroke patients: a Canadian survey. Can J Occup Ther 53:61, 1986

188. Walsh M: Half-lapboard for hemiplegic patients. Am J Occup Ther 41:533, 1987

189. Brudny J: New orthosis for treatment of hemiplegic shoulder subluxation. Orthot Prosthet 39:14, 1985

190. Sodring KM: Upper extremity orthoses for stroke patients. Int J Rehabil Med 3:33, 1980

191. DeVore J, Denny E: A sling to prevent a subluxed shoulder. Am J Occup Ther 24:580, 1970

192. Moodie NB, Brisbin J, Morgan AMG: Subluxation of the glenohumeral joint in hemiplegia: evaluation of supportive devices. Physiother Can 38:151, 1986

193. Zorowitz RD, Idank D, Ikai T, et al: Shoulder subluxation after stroke: a comparison of four supports. Arch Phys Med Rehabil 76:963, 1995

194. Morin L, Bravo G: Strapping the hemiplegic shoulder: a radiographic evaluation of its efficacy to reduce subluxation. Physiother Canada 49:103, 1997

195. Faghri PD, Rodgers MM, Glaser RM, et al: The effects of functional electrical stimulation on shoulder subluxation,

arm function recovery, and shoulder pain in hemiplegic stroke patients. Arch Phys Med Rehabil 75:73, 1994

196. Miller J: Shoulder pain from subluxation in the hemiplegic. Br Med J 4:345, 1975

197. Sie IH, Waters RL, Adkins RH, et al: Upper extremity pain in the post rehabilitation spinal injured patients. Arch Phys Med Rehabil 73:44, 1992

198. Silfverskiold J, Waters RL: Should pain and functional disability in spinal cord injury patients. Clin Orthop 272:141, 1991

199. Nichols PJR, Norman PA, Ennis JR: Wheelchair user's shoulder? Scand J Rehabil Med 11:29, 1979

200. Waring WP, Maynard FM: Shoulder pain in acute traumatic quadriplegia. Paraplegia 29:37, 1991

201. MacKay-Lyons M: Shoulder pain in patients with acute quadriplegia: a retrospective study. Physiother Canada 46:255, 1994

202. Campbell CC, Koris MJ: Etiologies of shoulder pain in cervical spinal cord injury. Clin Orthop 322:140, 1996

203. Hakuno A, Sashika H, Ohkawa T, et al: Arthrographic findings in hemiplegic shoulders. Arch Phys Med Rehabil 65: 706, 1984

204. Poduri KR: Shoulder pain in stroke patients and its effects on rehabilitation. J Stroke Cerebrovasc Dis 3:261, 1993

205. Jespersen HF, Jorgensen HS, Nakayama H, et al: Shoulder pain after stroke. Int J Rehabil Res 18:273, 1995

206. Ring H, Feder M, Berchadsky R, et al: Prevalence of pain and malalignment in the hemiplegic's shoulder at admission for rehabilitation. Eur J Phys Med Rehab 3:199, 1993

207. Peszczynski M, Rardin TE: The incidence of painful shoulder in hemilegia. Bull Polish Med Sci Hist 8:21, 1965

208. Inaba MK, Piorkowski M: Ultrasound in treatment of painful shoulders in patients with hemiplegia. Phys Ther 52:737, 1972

209. Bohannon RW, LeFort A: Hemiplegic shoulder pain measured with the Ritchie articular index. Int J Rehabil Res 9:379, 1986

210. Partridge CJ, Edwards SM, Mee R, et al: Hemiplegic shoulder pain: a study of two methods of physiotherapy treatment. Clin Rehabil 4:43, 1990

211. Savage R, Robertson L: The relationship between adult hemiplegic shoulder pain and depression. Physiother Canada 34:86, 1982

212. Sindou M, Mifsud JJ, Boisson D, et al: Selective posterior rhizotomy in the dorsal root entry zone for treatment of hyperspasticity and pain in the hemiplegic upper limb. Neurosurgery 18:587, 1986

213. Curtis KA, Roach KE, Brooks E, et al: Development of the Wheelchair User's Shoulder Pain Index (WUSPI). Paraplegia 33:290, 1995

214. Curtis KA, Roach KE, Applegate EB, et al: Reliability and validity of Wheelchair User's Shoulder Pain Index (WUSPI). Paraplegia 33:595, 1995

215. Chalsen GG, Fitzpatrick KA, Navia RA, et al: Prevalence of the shoulder-hand pain syndrome in an inpatient stroke rehabilitation population: a quantitative cross-sectional study. J Neurol Rehabil 1:137, 1987

216. Roy CW, Sands MR, Hill LD, et al: The effect of shoulder pain on outcome of acute hemiplegia. Clin Rehabil 9:21, 1995

217. Kücükdeveci AA, Tennant A, Hardo P, et al: Sleep problems in stroke patients: relationship with shoulder pain. Clin Rehabil 10:166, 1996

218. Leandri M, Parodi CI, Corrieri N, et al: Comparison of TENS treatments in hemiplegic shoulder pain. Scand J Rehabil Med 22:69, 1990

219. Mathiowetz V, Weimer DM, Federman SM: Grip and pinch strength: norms for 6 to 19 year olds. Am J Occup Ther 40: 705, 1986

220. Bohannon RW: Hand-held dynamometry. p. 69. In Amundsen L (ed): Muscle Strength Testing. Churchill-Livingstone, New York, 1990

221. Wade DT, Langton-Hewer R, Wood VA, et al: The hemiplegic arm after stroke: measurement and recovery. J Neurol Neurosurg Psychiatry 46:521, 1983

CHAPTER 30
Soft Tissue Mobilization

Gregory S. Johnson

Manual treatment of the soft tissues has existed since the beginning of recorded history in the form of massage and manipulation.[1] The primary purpose of these approaches was apparently to treat symptomatic soft tissues. The functional orthopaedics approach to soft tissue mobilization (STM) has been developed not only to evaluate and treat soft tissue dysfunctions that precipitate myofascial pain, but also to evaluate and treat those dysfunctions that alter structure and function and produce mechanical strains upon symptomatic structures.[2] In addition, STM offers a functional approach for evaluating and improving the patient's capacity to achieve and maintain a balanced posture, which enhances the ability to learn and perform efficient body mechanics. This approach is integrated into a broader treatment strategy of joint mobilization and neuromuscular reeducation and is coupled with a specific training, conditioning, and flexibility program.

STM is intended to be used as a component of a complete manual therapy program that includes evaluation and treatment of articular, neurovascular, and neuromuscular dysfunctions. The approach encompasses evaluation of the soft tissue system and application of specifically directed manual therapy techniques to facilitate normalization of soft tissue dysfunctions.[2,3] We have termed this integrated treatment approach *functional mobilization.*[4]

This chapter defines STM and describes its contribution to the conservative care of musculoskeletal dysfunction. This will be achieved by (1) defining the relevant soft tissue structures, (2) outlining a specific system of subjective, objective, and palpatory evaluations, (3) presenting basic treatment techniques, and (4) providing clinical correlations and case studies to develop an anatomic, biomechanical, and conceptual rationale for the use of STM.

■ Soft Tissue Components

The four primary soft tissues of the body are epithelial, muscular, nervous, and connective.[5,6] All soft tissue structures have individual and unique functions, integrated together into a dynamic biomechanical unit.[7,8] Grieve[7] emphasized this by stating that "the nerve, connective tissue, muscle, and articular complex produces multiple and varied arthrokinetic systems which are functionally interdependent upon each other."

Many authorities have stated that dysfunctions of the soft tissue system play a primary role in the onset and perpetuation of musculoskeletal symptoms.[7,9–13] Grieve[7] stated: "An explanation of the incidence of vertebral joint syndromes, and of some unsatisfactory long-term therapeutic results, might be assisted by regarding joint problems in a wider context than that of the joint alone. Much abnormality presenting, apparently simply, as joint pain may be the expression of a comprehensive underlying imbalance of the whole musculoskeletal system, i.e., articulation, ligaments, muscles, fascial planes and intermuscular septa, tendons and aponeuroses. . . ."

The human system can develop to be efficient, strong, and flexible by responding appropriately to the various types of controlled physical, mental, and emotional stress.[14–16] When the system is unable to adapt appropriately, physical compensations occur (Fig. 30–1).

The most common factor that precipitates soft tissue pain and functional impairment is trauma.[17,18] Trauma, whether from a significant external force or from repetitive internal or external microtraumas, can produce long-standing soft tissue changes[19,20] (Table 30–1). These soft

Portions of this chapter have been adapted from Johnson GS, Saliba V: Soft tissue mobilization. p. 169. In White AH, Anderson R (eds): Conservative Care of Low Back Pain. Williams & Wilkins, Baltimore, 1991, with permission.

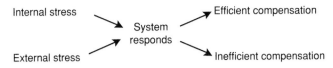

Figure 30–1. Internal and external stresses that impact upon the health of the system.

tissue dysfunctions may be the primary source of symptoms or the secondary source through impeded structural and functional capacity. Structurally, a balanced posture is no longer available due to the lack of flexibility of the soft tissue structures. This affects the efficient distribution of weight into the base of support and alters articular range of motion (ROM). These changes in soft tissue extensibility and mobility can cause abnormal forces and compressions to articular structures and can be a factor in precipitating and perpetuating pathology and symptomatology.[7,9,11,21,22]

Soft tissue dysfunctions can be specifically identified through an organized and precise subjective, objective, and palpatory evaluation. The therapist should have a working knowledge of the body's normal functional anatomy, biomechanics, and neuromuscular control to conduct and interpret this evaluation and to provide effective treatment. An understanding of soft tissue pathokinetics is essential to correlate the objective findings with possible soft tissue dysfunction. STM primarily addresses the evaluation and treatment of four soft tissue structures: (1) irregular and regular connective tissues, (2) skin, (3) skeletal muscle, and (4) neurovascular components.[5,23–25] For an in-depth description of the connective tissue structures, see Chapter 1.

Connective Tissue Structures

The primary connective tissue structures evaluated and treated by STM are the regular or dense tissues such as tendons and ligaments and the irregular or loose tissues such as fascia, intrinsic elements of muscle, articular capsules, and aponeuroses.

The fascial system is one of the primary soft tissues treated by STM. The fascial system ensheathes and permeates all tissues and structures; supplies the mechanical supportive framework that holds and integrates the body together and gives it form; provides passive support during lifting activities;[26] provides for the space and lubrication between all bodily structures; and creates pathways for nerves, blood, and lymphatic vessels.

Hollingshead[8] states, "If it were possible to dissolve out all the tissues of the body so as to leave only the fibrous (irregular) connective tissues, the essential organization of the body would still be represented and recognizable."

The fascial system is composed of laminated sheathes of connective tissues of varying thickness and density. These sheathes extend from the periosteum of bone to the basement membrane of the dermis. They are continuous throughout the body and are interconnected with the connective tissue structures of muscle (intrinsic elements, tendons, and aponeuroses), the articular structures (ligaments and capsules), and the intrinsic elements of peripheral nerves (endoneurium, perineurium, and epineurium).[5,6,8,23] This ensheathing organization of fascia allows structures to have independent three-dimensional mobility while connecting the system together into an integrated functional unit.[5,17]

Any system designed for function must have interfaces that allow motion. For the skeletal structures these interfaces are termed *joints*, while in the soft tissue system these interfaces are termed *functional joints*.

Functional Joint Concept

Gratz[27] defined the normal spaces that are maintained between all structures by fascia as functional joints. He defined a functional joint as "a space built for motion." Each functional joint creates a mechanical interface that allows the adjoining structures to move three-dimensionally in relation to each other.[2,13,17,27] In myofacial structures, the functional joints maintained by facial tissues include the spaces between individual muscle fibers on the micro level as well as the spaces that exist between a muscle and the surrounding structures. All these spaces are maintained and lubricated by the amorphous ground substance. The amorphous ground substance is a viscous gel containing a high proportion of water (60 to 70 percent) and long chains of carbohydrate molecules called *mucopolysaccharides*, principally glycosaminoglycans (GAGs).[6,23,28]

In an optimal state, the three-dimensional mobility that exists at functional joints is termed *normal play*.[2,28,29]

Table 30–1. Macrotraumas and Microtraumas

External Macrotraumas	Internal or External Microtraumas
Blows	Faulty posture
Falls	Improper neuromuscular mechanisms
Improper heavy lifting	Poor body mechanics
Surgery	Muscular imbalance
Whiplash	Improper foot wear
	Repetitive stressful activities
	Poorly organized work surfaces
	Nonsupportive sitting and sleeping surfaces
	Chronic anxiety or depression
	Overweight

The degree of normal play varies according to the functional demands and requirements of the individual structures and their mechanical interface. When the normal extensibility, accessory mobility, and biomechanical function of the tissues and surrounding structures are restricted, this dysfunctional state is called *restricted* or *decreased play*. These dysfunctions are clinically identifiable through skilled palpation, ROM testing, and observable alteration in function.[2,29]

Mennell[30] stated: "It is very remarkable how widespread may be the symptoms caused by unduly taut fascial planes. Though it is true that the fascial bands play a principal part in the mobility of the human body, they are often conducive to binding between two joint surfaces."

Dysfunctional Factors

There is no exact scientific explanation for restricted play and decreased extensibility of tissues, and further research is needed to provide more in-depth physiologic understanding. However, some possible physiologic explanations include the following.

Scar Tissue Adhesions

Following an injury, laceration, or surgery, fibroblastic activity forms new connective tissue fibers to reunite the wound as part of the postinflammatory fibroplastic phase.[31,32] These fibers are formed through random fibroblastic activity. If the appropriate remodeling stimuli are not applied during the healing process, the scar will become inextensible, with poor functional capacity.[10,14,33–36] Localized adhesions are generally produced as scar tissue forms.[10] In addition, there is often a restrictive matrix that has spider-web-like tentacles attached to surrounding structures that can alter and limit their normal mobility.[37,38] For example, the restrictive matrix of the scar tissue that is formed after abdominal surgery can often be palpated in other regions of the abdominal cavity.

Hollingshead[8] states that scar tissue "may be a major factor in altering the biomechanics of the whole kinematic chain, placing strain on all related structures." The abnormal strain caused by adherent and inextensible scar tissue may contribute to a chronic inflammatory process and further perpetuate symptoms.[10,37,39] The scar tissue matrix may also compromise neurovascular and lymphatic structures affecting the nerve conduction, the fluid balance, the exchange of metabolites, and the removal of waste products from the region.

Lymphatic Stasis and Interstitial Swelling

An increase in interstitial fluids alters the mechanical behavior of the adjacent structures and restricts normal mobility of the functional joints. This fluid imbalance may be related to immobility, poor lymphatic drainage, scar tissue blockage, or inflammation.[40,41]

Ground Substance Dehydration and Intermolecular Cross-Linking

Research has been conducted to determine the effects of forced immobilization on the periarticular tissues of various mammalian populations. This research has revealed that such immobilization contributes to soft tissue changes and development of restricted mobility of joints.[42–45] Researchers have identified biochemical and biomechanical compensations within the ligaments, tendons, capsule, and fascia of these restricted regions.[28,46] A primary component of these dysfunctions is ground substance dehydration.[28,42,43,47–49] Two results of this dehydration are thixotrophy and loss of critical fiber distance.

Thixotrophy is a state in which the ground substance becomes more viscous, resulting in increased tissue rigidity and stiffness. This increased viscosity of the ground substance requires more force to elongate and compress the tissues.[38,49]

With the loss of water from the ground substance, the critical distance that is required between fibers and structures is diminished. In this state there is a higher potential for and a significant increase in formation of restrictive intermolecular cross-link fibers[35,42–44,49] (Fig. 30–2). These intermolecular cross-links restrict interfiber mobility and extensibility, and may be partially responsible for restricted soft tissue mobility and play. Furthermore, it has been shown that this reduced mobility affects the synthesis and orientation of new collagen fibrils, which further contributes to the pathogenesis of restricted fascial mobility.[49] (See Chapter 1 for a description of the effects of immobilization on connective tissue for biomechanical changes and intermolecular cross-linking.)

Response to Treatment

It is reasonable to postulate a correlation between these research findings and the clinically identifiable decreased mobility and play found in dysfunctional soft tissues. Clinically, through the application of STM, the mobility of

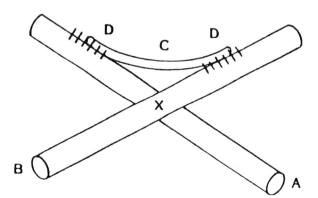

Figure 30–2. Idealized model of a collagen cross-link at the molecular level. (*A,B*) preexisting fibers; (*C*) newly synthesized fibril; (*D*) cross-link as the fibril joins the fiber; (*X*) nodal point where the fibers normally slide freely past one another. (From Akeson et al.,[49] with permission.)

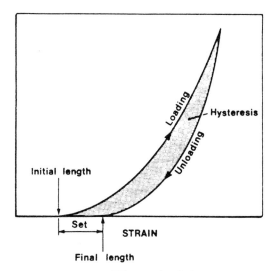

Figure 30–3. Hysteresis. When unloaded, a structure regains its shape at a rate different from that at which it deformed. Any difference between the initial and final shapes is the "set." (From Bogduk and Twomey,[51] with permission.)

these dysfunctional soft tissues can be improved. These results may be a result of one or more of the following factors:

1. An alteration of the scar tissue matrix[37,45]
2. A redistribution of interstitial fluids[7]
3. The stimulation of GAG synthesis, restoring normal or improved lubrication and hydration
4. The breaking of restrictive intermolecular cross-links[38,49]
5. The mechanical and viscoelastic elongation of existing collagenous tissues through the phenomena of creep and hysteresis, as demonstrated by the stress–strain curve[50-52] (Fig. 30–3)
6. A neuroreflexive response that may alter vascular, muscular, and biochemical factors related to immobility[53-58]

Skin

The skin is composed of two layers, an outer epidermis of ectodermal origin and the deeper dermix of mesodermal origin.[59] The skin is continuous with the deep fascia and underlying structures through the attachment of the superficial fascia to the basement membrane of the dermis.[6]

Due to the orientation and weave of the collagen and elastin fibers, the skin demonstrates considerable mechanical strength and a high degree of intrinsic flexibility and mobility. This intrinsic mobility allows the skin to have considerable extensibility and, due to its elastin content, the ability to recoil to its original configuration.[35,50] Because of the pliability of the superficial fascia, the skin also has extensive extrinsic mobility in all directions along the interface with deeper structures.[8,23] The skin in regions superficial to joints allows motion through its ability to

fold and stretch in response to the underlying movements.[10,35]

The skin can lose normal mobility secondary to trauma, scar tissue formation, and immobility. With the loss of this mobility, the underlying structures can be impeded in their functional capacity and the normal coordinated movement patterns of the kinetic chain altered.

Response to Treatment

Dysfunctions of the intrinsic and extrinsic mobility of the skin can be assessed and specific foci of restrictions identified. The mobility of these dysfunctions can be improved through the application of specific soft tissue techniques. These structural improvements are often clinically associated with dramatic reduction in pain and improved musculoskeletal function. These improvements may be related to the following possibilities:

1. More efficient biomechanical function due to release of fascial tension.
2. Local and general changes in the vascular and lymphatic circulation.[40,56]
3. A neuroreflexive inhibition of muscle tone and pain, which may be a response to the existing pathology in deeper structures,[54,56] including that of underlying spinal dysfunctions.[7,60,61] These are passed through both afferent and autonomic pathways.[62]

Skeletal Muscle

The two basic components of skeletal muscle are the muscle fibers (the contractile components) and the surrounding connective tissue sheaths (the noncontractile components). The connective tissue components are the endomysium, perimysium, and epimysium (Fig. 30–4). They envelop each muscle fiber, fascicle, and muscle belly, respectively, and invest at the muscle's terminus to form

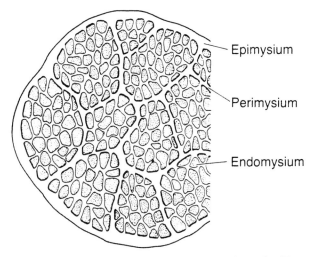

Figure 30–4. Connective tissue components of muscle. (From Ham and Cormack,[6] with permission.)

tendon, fascia, and aponeurosis.[6,23] These connective tissues provide for the following:

1. The mechanical and elastic characteristics of muscle for broadening during contraction and lengthening during passive elongation (functional excursion).[37,63] They may be the major component affected by passive muscle stretching.[64]
2. The elastic property of muscle, possibly due to the parallel arrangement of these sheaths with the contractile components.[65]
3. The tension regulation of the muscle, which influences contractile strength,[64] ability to withstand high-impact loads, and adaptive and recoil capability.[66]
4. The support, cohesion, and protective restraint of the muscle.[67]
5. The space and lubrication for normal extensibility and play of (a) the intrinsic contractile elements and (b) the muscle belly (through the epimysium) in relation to surrounding structures.[8,10]
6. A soft tissue continuum (the myofascial unit) as they interconnect with each other, as well as the loose connective tissue and fascia surrounding the muscle through the superficial epimysium.[13]
7. A conduit for blood vessels and nerve fibers[6,23] (see Chapter 1).

Dysfunctions of the Myofascial Unit

Several authors believe that the myofascial unit is often the primary precipitator of pathology and symptoms (refs. 9, 12,[68]; Sahrmann SA: course notes, 1988). The primary structural and functional dysfunctions of the myofascial unit include the following:

Restrictive scar tissue[18]

Restricted muscle play[69]

Weakness or increased tone through impaired peripheral and central innervation

Restricted extensibility and play of the connective tissue elements (fibrosis)

Adaptive muscle shortening, possibly through the loss of sarcomeres[10,13,41,70,71]

Injury of the musculotendinous structures[64]

Generalized hypertonus[1] and localized myofascial trigger points[12]

Alteration in motor control and recruitment[9,72–74]

The Myofascial Cycle

Dysfunctions of the myofascial cycle can be attributed to a variety of factors. Kirkaldy-Willis[9] has proposed a model for the evolution of spinal pathology termed the *myofascial cycle*. This model presents possible courses of degeneration termed the *degenerative cascade*, which leads to

spinal pathology and symptomatology (Fig. 30–5). This cycle begins with a minor trauma or emotional disturbance that facilitates a chronic neuromuscular response. This response facilitates chronic muscular changes such as fibrosis, weakness, limited extensibility, and altered recruitment patterns. Specifically, when the multifidi become dysfunctional, significant alteration of the arthrokinematics of the spinal segment occurs, leading to possible facet and disk deterioration.[75] Grieve,[7] in discussing tone, which Kirkaldy-Willis[9] refers to as the *chronic neuromuscular response*, states that tone in striated muscle is due to three sets of influences:

The elastic tension of the connective tissue elements

The degree or extent of interdigitation overlap of the actin and myosin elements

The number of active motor units

Myofascial Trigger Points

The number of active motor units can be influenced by multiple factors, such as trauma,[7,13] scarring from disease or injury,[13] supraspinal influences,[7] protective spasm, chronic reaction to situational stress, and repetitive habitual holding and movement patterns.[2,76] In a pathologic

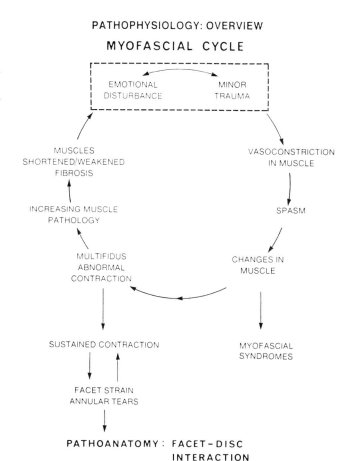

Figure 30–5. Myofascial cycle. (From Kirkaldy-Willis and Hill,[78] with permission.)

state these foci of increased tone have been termed *myofascial trigger points* by Travell and Simons.[12]

Myofascial trigger points are defined as "hyperirritable spots, usually within a taut band of skeletal muscle or in the muscle's fascia, that are painful on compression and that can give rise to characteristic referred pain, tenderness, and autonomic phenomena."[12] Travell and Simons report that the palpable hardness identified with myofascial trigger points may be caused by increased fibrous connective tissue, edema, altered viscosity of muscle, ground substance infiltrate, contracture of muscle fibers, vascular engorgement, and fatty infiltration.[12] Within the STM system, myofascial trigger points are included in the category of specific or general muscle hypertonus.

A state of increased tone may be the primary source of symptoms[12] or a secondary one through a reflex response to underlying or related pathology. In addition to local and referred pain, increased muscle tonus and myofascial trigger points may also precipitate altered movement patterns[77] and restricted ROM.[9,12,37,72] Due to the individual variability of response to pain and the possibility that referred pain or protective spasm may be caused by the hypertonic state, the location of muscle tone or tenderness is often not a reliable indicator of the location of the source of pathology.[7] Both muscular hypertonus and myofascial trigger points usually normalize in response to a treatment program of STM. However, if the hypertonus or trigger points are in protective or secondary spasm due to a primary dysfunction elsewhere, the objective signs and symptoms often return, partially or completely, within a short period of time.[2]

Neuromuscular Control

Another factor that must be taken into consideration when addressing the myofascial system is neuromuscular control. The movement control of the neuromuscular system must be precise and allow for few deviations to protect the articular and soft tissue structures.[17,68,78] Many authors report that dysfunctions of the myofascial unit are often preceded by faulty posture, poor neuromuscular control, and altered recruitment patterns.[17,68,73,74,79,80] These conditions often lead to length-associated muscle imbalances between antagonistic muscle groups and affect the balanced force production, coordination, fine motor control, and distribution of forces necessary to protect the spinal segment during movement and static postures.[7,17,68]

For efficient neuromusculoskeletal function to occur, there must be normal joint and soft tissue mechanics. Normal voluntary and involuntary neuromuscular control is developed primarily through learned activities. Various factors may precipitate a state of altered recruitment patterns.[17,68] Janda[68] has observed that there are consistent neuromuscular patterns when altered recruitment exists. Muscles composed primarily of tonic (slow twitch) fibers become chronically facilitated and respond to stressful situations and pain by increased tone and tightness. Those that are primarily composed of phasic (fast twitch) fibers are inhibited, becoming weak, atrophied, and overstretched, thus creating length-associated muscle imbalances[68,77] (Figs. 30–6 and 30–7).

Recent research[81,82] has confirmed the long-held proprioceptive neuromuscular facilitation (PNF) concept regarding the importance of the multifidus in stabilization of individual spinal segments and in controlling motion between those segments. In conjunction with the multifidus, researchers have found that the transversus abdominis contracted prior to the other abdominal muscles and in conjunction with the multifidus to produce stability.[83–85] Other researchers have also found that the multifidus is inhibited in individuals with low back pain.[86–89] Even in individuals with first-time acute episodes, the multifidi will frequently be inhibited and will not demonstrate the normal recrutment patterns. Research has found that the multifidus does not recover normal function after the episode has resolved. Therefore, through the functional mobilization approach to rehabilitation, the following treatment strategy would be followed. Initially, manual therapy would be applied to normalize the condition of the myofascial and articular structures. Then specific training would be used to facilitate contractions of the deep stabilizing muscles (multifidus, transverse abdominus,

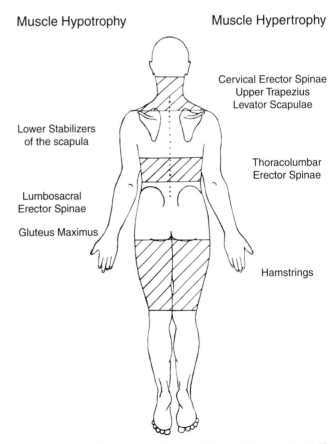

Figure 30–6. The layer syndrome. (From Jull and Janda,[93] with permission.)

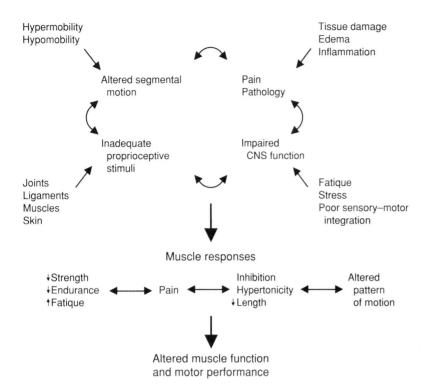

Figure 30–7. Sources of adverse stimuli and muscular responses. (From Jull and Janda,[93] with permission.)

deep fibers of the psoas and quadratus lumborum) through PNF trunk patterns and functional movement patterns (described later). This would be followed by specific body mechanic training to utilize proper biomechanics and motor sequencing.

An example of an altered recruitment pattern is excessive activation and tightness of the trunk extensors during a poorly performed sit-up. In an individual who exhibits such an altered movement pattern, one can palpate the extensors while the sit-up is being performed and note substantial activation. This unnecessary activation of the extensors creates a state of neuromuscular imbalance that decreases the facilitation of the lower abdominals. This motor recruitment dysfunction is carried over to the performance of daily activities and alters the normal neuromuscular, postural, and mechanical dynamics of the lumbar spine. The treatment strategy for this condition would include STM and stretching of the shortened extensors,[2,11,68,77] strengthening of the weakened flexors,[11,70,89] neuromuscular reeducation to restore proper movement and recruitment patterns,[17,73,74,79,90] and body mechanics training to change stressful activities of daily living (ADL) patterns.[89]

Patients who are forced into inefficient postures due to soft tissue dysfunctions often have difficulty performing dynamic, coordinated, and balanced motions while simultaneously maintaining trunk stability and controlled mobility. STM directed toward improving posture often elicits an almost immediate improvement in neuromuscular control, recruitment patterns, and stabilization abilities.[2,89]

■ Evaluation

A specific, organized evaluation system is an integral part of a rehabilitation and manual therapy program. The subjective and objective evaluation process is systematic and specific, providing baseline data from which to develop and perform a treatment program and to assess the effectiveness of treatment. The following components of evaluation can assist the therapist in identifying musculoskeletal dysfunction and determining the vigor of the treatment process:

Patient's subjective report

Structural analysis

Motion analysis

Palpation

Subjective Evaluation

Through a careful subjective evaluation, a therapist can identify many of the factors that cause and precipitate musculoskeletal symptoms. The subjective evaluation is the critical link between the patient's symptomatic and historical report and the objective findings. Cyriax and Cyriax[91] stated that most soft tissue dysfunctions have "distinctive histories."

The four primary goals of the initial subjective evaluation are as follows:

1. To develop rapport with the patient
2. To gather detailed historical information

3. To understand the specific symptoms and their irritability
4. To make the patient aware of his or her condition and of the need to take responsibility for his or her own care

Within the framework of a normal subjective evaluation, there are certain questions that are important in determining soft tissue involvement. These questions (refs. 14, 84, and Paris S, Loubert P: course notes, 1990) are designed to identify the following:

Location and type of symptoms. The patient is guided in listing each symptom, beginning with the most bothersome and proceeding to the least bothersome. Each symptom is analyzed for its precise location, type, quality, and intensity.

Course of symptoms and irritability. Identifying the general or average course of symptoms assists in determining the degree of irritability and identifying the symptom-generating structures. The patient is asked to identify the postures and motions that exacerbate or ease the symptoms, and the therapist attempts to secure quantifiable measures of irritability.

Duration of symptoms. The therapist should inquire primarily about those symptoms related to the chronic protective spasm and inactivity that could precipitate fibrotic changes within muscles and a remodeling of soft tissues.

Precipitating trauma or activity. It is important to carefully identify the direction of trauma and the movement pattern that occurred. This information is helpful in understanding the presenting symptoms, in analyzing the structural deviations, and in identifying which soft tissues should be evaluated. It is often important to know the patient's emotional state at the time of injury.[17]

Previous traumas. One should look for earlier traumas that may have precipitated soft tissue changes, altered the biomechanics of the kinematic chain, or affected the performance of normal motor function. These alterations contribute to the presenting symptoms.

Previous surgeries. It is important to inquire about previous surgeries, since scar tissue can dramatically affect efficient function in the whole kinematic chain. We have seen several cases in which restriction of scar tissue from abdominal surgery was a primary factor in the onset of shoulder symptoms. This was due to the restricted extensibility of the anterior region that altered the kinetics of throwing a ball and serving in tennis.

Stressful employment, leisure and recreational activities. It is important to identify repeated patterns of postural dysfunction and aberrant movement patterns that may create dysfunctional soft tissue and

muscular changes related to the presenting complaint.

Postural and sleeping habits. One should identify prolonged and habitual positions that may cause adaptive shortening of soft tissues and perpetuate symptoms.

Objective Evaluation

In clinical practice, we must make many choices every day in providing effective patient care. Some of these decisions are minor and obvious, while others are difficult and require careful analysis. Informed decision making is most effectively accomplished when all of the pertinent facts are gathered and analyzed. However, facts alone are not enough. Once the information is compiled, one must use discernment to sift through it. Discernment is drawn from previous experience, knowledge of anatomy, pathology, and kinesiology, and a flexible scientific and intuitive decision-making process. This process requires a consistent and organized objective evaluation system.

A carefully performed objective evaluation provides a means to assess the physical and functional status of the whole patient. The objective evaluation assists in identifying abnormal postural and functional factors in both the symptomatic and related asymptomatic regions. The organization and vigor of the objective evaluation are determined by data gained from the subjective evaluation (location, type, irritability, and nature of the symptoms). The components of an objective evaluation are observation (structural, movement, and functional analysis), palpation, neuromuscular control, and neurologic and special needs testing.

Data gathered through the objective evaluation will assist in developing a treatment plan, setting realistic goals, and objectifying the effectiveness of treatment.[77,92] Objective evaluation includes three components: structural evaluation, movement analysis, and palpation assessment.

Structural Evaluation

Through careful observation, the postural and soft tissue components are analyzed for patterns of dysfunction that are directly or indirectly related to the symptomatology. They are observed through structural and postural analysis and through soft tissue contours and proportions.

Structural and Postural Analysis

The structural and postural analysis is the building block of an objective evaluation and is based upon the interrelationship that exists between structure and function. A system's inherent functional capacity is dependent upon its structural integrity. Functionally, the body utilizes both static and dynamic postures. Static postures are primarily used for rest, which dynamic ones provide support for all functional activities.

Taking into account the natural asymmetric state of each individual, *efficient posture* can be defined as the balanced three-dimensional alignment of the body's skeletal and soft tissue structures in an arrangement that provides for optimal weight attenuation, shock absorption, and functional capacity. This balanced posture is termed *neutral alignment*. This optimal skeletal arrangement provides for minimal energy expenditure and efficient neuromuscular control. In the neutral alignment, *articulations* are inherently protected in their midrange position; *muscles* are at an optimal length for function; and *biomechanical potential* is established for optimal coordinated function.

I do not intend to imply that all functional activities occur in this neutral structural alignment. However, the capacity to assume this structural arrangement gives the neuromuscular system a flexible supportive structure and provides optimal function and protection for the articular and myofascial components.

Inefficient posture is often a major factor in the pathogenesis and perpetuation of symptoms.[17,93] Improper postural alignment places abnormal stress upon sensitive structures and affects normal weight distribution, shock absorption, segmental biomechanics, and energy expenditure. These alterations can precipitate pathology and symptoms in the articular and soft tissue structures. Poor skeletal alignment is especially significant clinically when symptom-producing postures are sustained and repeated for extended periods of time.

Inefficient alignment is usually a result of two closely interrelated factors:

Structural and mechanical dysfunctions. Hyper- or hypomobility of articular and soft tissue structures that alter normal functional capacity.

Functional compensations. Chronic or habitually held postures that alter the system's structural and functional capacity. Functional compensations develop because of either habitual use of stressful postures and motions or chronic unresolved emotional or mental physical responses.[77] The neuromuscular skeletal system compensates for these habitual or unresolved responses through unnecessary muscular effort, inefficient postural alignment, aberrant movement patterns, and reduced kinesthetic awareness. These functional compensations, when unidentified, may be primary factors in causing and perpetuating unresolved symptoms.

Observational evaluation begins with a *global view* of the patient that guides the therapist to regions in need of specific assessment. One should generally assess the overall body type,[14] contour, integrity, and balance of the patient's posture. The structural vertical and horizontal alignment should be evaluated for general patterns of imbalance and poor alignment, which may precipitate excessive stress on symptomatic structures.

Once regions and patterns of dysfunction are identified, a regional evaluation is conducted. A systematic *regional structural evaluation* begins with the analysis of the base of support and then progresses superiorly to scan each movement segment. (See Fig. 30–8 for a block representation of the movement segments.) It is at the transitional zones between these general movement segments that many dysfunctions and symptoms occur. Each segment is assessed for position, relationship of the structural and soft tissue components, and relative structural proportions of each movement segment.[2,76,94–96] Special attention is given to the evaluation of the symptomatic region or regions, with a focus on the patient's capacity to assume a neutral posture.[2,77,93]

The regional assessment is followed by a specific evaluation to closely assess the dysfunctional regions for specific structural and movement dysfunctions. This evaluation is most effectively conducted in conjunction with exploratory palpation. Combining observation with palpation provides a valuable learning experience and an opportunity to correlate the observed structural changes and palpable findings. The specific evaluation can progress to the *vertical compression test*.[89,97]

The vertical compression test assesses the integrity and force attenuation capacity of the spine and extremities in weightbearing positions. The test evaluates for the quality of weight distribution, the compliance of the structural components, and the symptoms produced by habitual postures.[69]

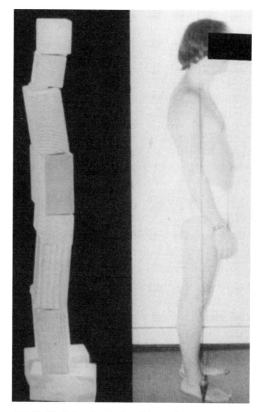

Figure 30–8. Positional relationships of movement segments.

The vertical compression test is performed in weightbearing postures such as standing, sitting, and on the hands and knees by applying a gentle vertical pressure to the head, shoulders, pelvis, or knees (Fig. 30–9). During the application of vertical compression, the therapist evaluates the inherent stability of the weightbearing structures.

When the test is applied in an optimal state, the structure will be stable, with the force felt and seen to be transmitted directly through each movement segment into the base of support. However, if a segment or a combination of segments is malpositioned, vertical compression will produce noticeable buckling or pivoting at the transitional zones. These unstable transitional zones are often the regions of presenting symptoms, and they will be increased by the test if there is a postural component to the symptoms. These zones will often be used as primary fulcrums during functional activities. This excessive overutilization of individual segments often alters neuromuscular patterns, precipitates degeneration, develops a low-grade inflammatory response, creates hypermobility, facilitates chronic muscular activity, and produces associated soft tissue adaptations (Paris S: course notes, 1977).

The therapist, while applying the vertical compression test, questions the patient about the status of the symptoms. Caution must be used with the force and number of retests applied, especially with highly irritable patients or those suspected of being load sensitive. The test can help patients recognize existing postural deviations and their functional and symptomatic effects.

Treatment Strategy. Once the dysfunctional segments are identified and symptoms assessed, the next goal is to improve the patient's posture. Utilizing both manual and verbal cues, the therapist guides each segment to a more balanced neutral position. When a more efficient alignment is achieved, vertical compression is again applied to reevaluate the vertical integrity and associated symptoms. Several postural corrections may be needed to achieve an optimal stable position. The retest also provides the patient with further kinesthetic feedback on the more stable and balanced alignment.

Those segments that cannot be repositioned due to structural limitations are identified for more in-depth soft tissue evaluation and treatment. For example, in the lumbar spine the most important and most frequently identified alignment problem is backward bending of the thoracic cage in relation to the pelvis.[2,91] The myofascial structures that are most often found to be dysfunctional are the deep fibers of the psoas, the lumbar extensors, and the anterior cervical muscles. When these and associated articular dysfunctions are normalized, the patient can assume a more balanced alignment with greater ease. Evaluation should progress to testing for the lumbar protective mechanism; balancing reactions and functional training should be emphasized.[89,97]

Except in cases where a forced posture controls pain (such as maintaining a pelvic tilt to open the intervertebral foramens in cases of advanced foraminal stenosis), increased muscular effort should not be used to assume an improved posture against underlying soft tissue tension. The effort of forcing a fixed posture often causes secondary compensations, biomechanical stresses, and structural shortening.[2,74] Therefore, restrictive soft tissues should be normalized through STM and stretching so that an improved alignment can be assumed with greater ease. This decreased effort enhances patient compliance and comfort.

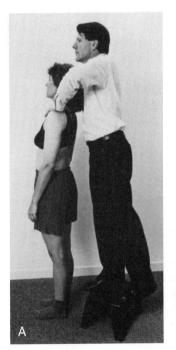
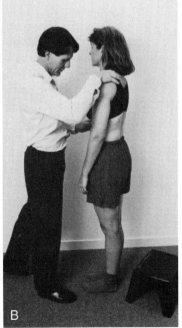
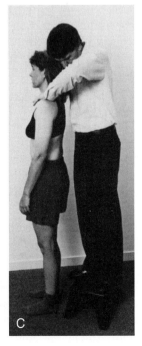

Figure 30–9. Vertical compression. (A) Test. (B) Correction. (C) Retest.

With improved postural alignment, increased emphasis should be placed on body mechanics training and a conditioning exercise program to strengthen weak muscles, stretch shortened structures, develop the lumbar protective mechanism, reestablish proper movement patterns, and improve kinesthetic awareness and balancing reactions.

Soft Tissue Observation

There is a symbiotic relationship between the soft tissues and the underlying supportive bony structure. The following soft tissue components should be assessed for dysfunctional states:

The *surface condition* for changes in texture, color, moisture, and scars.

The *surface contours* by assessing the body's outline for circumferential and segmental bands, regions of bulges or protrusions, and areas that appear flattened or tightened.

The *soft tissue proportions* by comparing the bulk of soft tissues between the front and back, right and left, and inferior and superior. Areas of imbalance can lead to the identification of regions of overdevelopment or a general deconditioned state or atrophy. Any proportional imbalances in soft tissue development require further evaluation and the initiation of an appropriate muscle conditioning program.[2,76,95,96]

The *inherent patterns of dysfunction*. The full structure is assessed using a global view to note any patterns in the organization of the soft tissue dysfunctions. These patterns often exist in observable and palpable zigzag and spiral patterns away from the central dysfunction. If a pattern is identified, one should try to determine where the primary restrictions exist and if they are due primarily to underlying mechanical dysfunctions or to functional compensations (Fig. 30–10). Frequently, normalization of these primary restrictions enhances the rehabilitation program by reducing the inherent stress placed on symptomatic structures.

The *three-dimensional structural proportions*. In the efficient state, each individual has an inherent proportional balance between the length, width, and depth of his or her structural components (skeletal and soft tissue systems). Dysfunctions often diminish one dimension and restrict functional capacity and weight distribution.[76,95,96] The treatment strategy is to increase the diminished dimension through manual therapy and reeducation.

Movement and Functional Analysis

Once postural abnormalities and soft tissue changes are identified, it is important to evaluate the mobility of these regions while the patient performs physiologic and func-

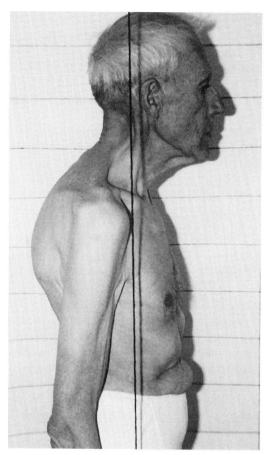

Figure 30–10. Evaluation of patterns of spiral and zigzag soft tissue compensations.

tional movements. An important and often overlooked assessment of the soft tissue system is the observation and palpation of these regions during the performance of guided motions and functional activities. Since the soft tissue system is continuous, movement that occurs in one region precipitates normal adjustments throughout the soft tissue and skeletal systems. However, dysfunctions in one region can affect the mobility and quality of movement in related regions, possibly altering the efficient function and overall adaptive potential of the entire kinematic chain.

Dysfunctional soft tissues impede efficient movement by limiting the ability of structures to elongate, fold, conform, and/or slide in relation to each other. Increased strain occurs as the motion transfers from regions of relative immobility to regions of relative hypermobility or vice versa, resulting in alterations in the function of the underlying articulations.

Through careful observation of the patient's ability to perform physiologic movement patterns, normal functional activities, functional movement patterns, and the adverse neural tension test, the therapist can identify soft tissue dysfunctions and grade the effects of those dysfunctions on movement performance.

Physiologic Movement Patterns

The conventional active ROM evalution yields significant information about the mobility of articular and soft tissue structures. Movement evaluation is performed in weight-bearing postures such as standing, sitting, and quadruped. The evaluator should look and palpate for the following:

Quality and sequencing of motion

Range of movement (delineating structural and symptomatic limitations)

Effect of movement on the intensity, location, and type of pain

Mobility of individual segments

Mobility of soft tissues in relation to each other

Freedom of soft tissues to move in relation to underlying structures

Ability of soft tissues to elongate and fold

Proper utilization of the base of support

Careful assessment and recording of specific limitations of physiologic motions provide the therapist with parameters for reevaluation and thus the ability to correlate the effects of soft tissue treatment.

Normal Functional Activities

Observation of an individual performing normal ADL, particularly those that produce symptoms, often reveals soft tissue dysfunctions associated with the presenting complaint and exacerbations. Many of the patients who present with nontraumatic muscular skeletal symptoms have what we describe as the *self-inflicted pain syndrome*. In any patient whose symptoms are perpetuated through stressful usage, the aim of therapy is to assist them in becoming aware of the relationship between their actions and their pain and educating them in the use of less stressful body mechanics.

A functional evaluation should include all functional activities frequently performed by the patient that may stress the symptomatic region, including the following:[76,89]

Coming to sitting

Sitting

Rising to standing

Walking

Bending

Reaching

Pushing

Pulling

Lifting

Functional limitations such as a tight calf compartment, limitations in hip ROM, and restrictions in shoulder girdle mobility are frequently identified through careful analysis.

Another critical component of a functional evaluation is the assessment of dynamic balance and balancing reactions. As anyone who has studied ballet, gymnastics, martial arts, or any athletic endeavor discovers, performance is often dependent upon proper structural alignment, neuromuscular coordination, muscular strength, soft tissue compliance, and balancing capacity.

When a functional approach is used, the success of treatment can be gauged through documented improvements in the tested functional activities and abilities.[89]

Functional Movement Patterns

Functional movement patterns[3] were adapted primarily from the proprioceptive neuromuscular facilitation (PNF) diagonal movement patterns[79,90] and Awareness Through Movement lessons developed by Moshe Feldenkrais.[74] These movement patterns provide a means to quickly and effectively assess motor control, muscle recruitment patterns, soft tissue compliance, and articular mobility of specific body segments, regions, and/or the body as a whole. Functional movement patterns offer additional tools for evaluating specific limitations in dynamic range and sequencing of motion. For example, lower quadrant movement patterns such as the pelvic clock, lower trunk rotation, unilateral hip rotation, and pelvic diagonals can provide information about three-dimensional active compliance of the soft tissues, mobility of the underlying articulations, and quality of neuromuscular control. Also, movement patterns such as side-lying shoulder girdle circles and arm circles reveal the mobility and compliance of the rib cage and upper extremity soft tissues.

Treatment is applied through sustained pressure on the dysfunctional tissue or joint while the patient actively performs the functional movement pattern. The motion can vary from large excursions to very small ones. The purpose is to produce intermittent pressure and relaxation upon the dysfunctions. Following the resolution of these dysfunctions, the therapist performs neuromuscular reeducation by having the patient integrate the functional movement pattern into the new range in slow, controlled motions. The movement pattern can then be transferred to a home program for further training and strengthening.

Adverse Neural Tension Test

Adverse neural tension tests, as described by Maitland,[92] Elvey,[25] and Butler,[24] test the extensibility of the neural components from the dural tube through the peripheral aspects. Restricted motion and symptom production indicate a dysfunction through possible compression, adherence, or contractile and noncontractile restriction.[98]

Evaluations for both upper and lower limb neurovascular structures are performed by placing the individual nerves on selective tension through movement of the trunk and extremity. In the efficient state, when the neurovascular structures are placed at their lengthened range, there is a springy end-fell and the patient does not experience any discomfort. In a dysfunctional state, the range is restricted, there is palpable tension, and the patient reports reproduction of symptoms or discomfort. The most efficient procedure for evaluation of the peripheral nerve in all regions where it is accessible for palpation is to have the patient perform oscillatory motions of the distal component (using the wrist for the upper extremity and the ankle for the lower one). The therapist palpates the nerve along its course, assessing for free motion and efficient play. When restricted mobility is identified, sustained pressure is placed on the dysfunctional tissues while the oscillations continue to be performed at the distal and/or proximal components.[4]

Palpatory Evaluation

Palpatory evaluation is performed by placing selective tension upon the tissues to be assessed. Through palpation, mechanical dysfunctions that restrict structures from their efficient functional excursion and independent play are identified.

Palpation evaluation is guided by the data gained through the subjective, postural, and movement evaluations and includes the specific assessment of the condition and the three-dimensional mobility of the individual layers of tissues. The soft tissues are initially evaluated in their resting positions; however, the associated functional deficits may be appreciated better by palpating the tissues during the performance of passive, active, or resisted motions.[3] The assessment is organized to evaluate the condition and the three-dimensional mobility of each layer, beginning superficially and progressing deeper. The individual layers are defined by the individual strata of muscles. This is important because skin, muscles, and neurovascular elements all exist in individual layers and compartments and are separated by loose connective tissue.[2,99]

Through proper layer palpation, most dysfunctional soft tissues can be identified. These dysfunctions exist within a specific layer or extend through several distinct layers. Such restricted regions have a single or several central epicenters of maximal restriction. Epicenters vary from the size of a pea to the size of a grain of sand. Most restrictions have spiral patterns of adherence that should be identified. A strong indicator of soft tissue dysfunction is *tenderness* to normal palpation. Therefore, patients can assist in locating the epicenter of tenderness. It should be noted that some tissues without any identifiable dysfunction will be tender to normal palpation. These tissues may be in a state of low-grade inflammation, resulting in dysfunction of soft tissue structures.[2]

Referred pain is another clinical aspect of dysfunctional soft tissues. Referred pain patterns are elicited and assessed through normal palpation to epicenter restriction. By assessing these referred pain patterns, the therapist can discern whether the dysfunction is a primary or secondary source of symptoms or dysfunction.[54,91]

While performing a palpatory evaluation, the therapist must remember that proper and sensitive palpation is a critical means of communication. One of the fastest ways to develop the patient's confidence is through a caring and competent touch. Often the difference between successful and unsuccessful manual treatment is the development of patient confidence, which influences the patient's ability to relax. It is recommended that the therapist strive to develop skills of touching and to assist this process by frequently asking patients for feedback and assistance.[100,101]

Soft tissue dysfunctions are identified through palpable changes in tissue extensibility, recoil, end-feel, and independent play.[2]

Extensibility and Recoil

Tissue extensibility is the ability of tissues to elongate to an optimal range and still have a springy end-feel. Tissue extensibility is evaluated through precise direct pressure upon the tissues or through elongation of those tissues by joint motion. Recoil is evaluated by how the tissue returns to its normal resting length.

As soft tissues are deformed through their functional excursion, points of increased resistance may be palpated. These restrictions or changes in density may exist through all or part of the tissue excursion. The specific restrictive points, epicenters, and direction of greatest restriction must be identified since the treatment technique is applied to the adherent tissues at the point and direction of greatest restriction.

End-Feel

Tissue end-feel[37] is the quality of tension felt when a tissue is manually deformed to the limit of its physiologic or accessory range. In a healthy state, tissues have a springy end-feel that can be compared to the quality of elasticity and recoil felt when a new rubber band is taken to end-range. The excursion (range of deformation) of soft tissues varies throughout the body, but in a healthy state the end-feel is consistently springy.

Dysfunctional tissues have varying degrees of hard end-feel and motion loss. These limitations are defined by their specific three-dimensional limitation of precise depth, direction, and angle of maximal restriction. The goal of this evaluation process is to localize the dysfunction so that treatment can be more specific, more effective, and less invasive.[2]

Independent Play

All soft tissue structures in their efficient state have *independent accessory mobility* in relation to surrounding structures. The degree and extent of mobility vary from structure to structure. In a healthy state this is described as *normal play*. In a dysfunctional state there is *reduced play* between adjoining tissues. In myofascial tissue this is termed *restricted muscle play*. Dysfunctional tissues and structures can be evaluated most effectively by conducting

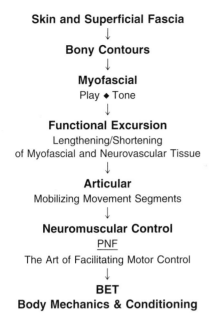

Skin and Superficial Fascia

↓

Bony Contours

↓

Myofascial

Play ◆ Tone

↓

Functional Excursion

Lengthening/Shortening
of Myofascial and Neurovascular Tissue

↓

Articular

Mobilizing Movement Segments

↓

Neuromuscular Control

<u>PNF</u>

The Art of Facilitating Motor Control

↓

BET

Body Mechanics & Conditioning

Figure 30–11. Selective and layer treatment progression. (© 11/97 The Institute of Physical Art.)

palpation during passive and active movements that reveal associated functional limitations.

Evaluation Procedures for Soft Tissue Structures

The following are the individual structures specifically assessed through layer palpation: skin and superficial fascia, bony contours, and myofascial tissues (Fig. 30–11).

Skin and Superficial Fascia Assessment

The skin is assessed for changes in tissue texture, temperature, and moisture by running the fingers or the back of the hand lightly over the surface of the skin. Changes in any of these parameters can guide the evaluation to underlying acute or chronic conditions.

The skin is evaluated for intrinsic and extrinsic mobility by fingertip palpation. The intrinsic mobility (within the skin) is assessed for extensibility, end-feel, and recoil. The extrinsic mobility is assessed for independent play of the skin in relation to underlying structures.

Techniques for evaluation of the skin and superficial fascia include skin gliding, finger sliding, and skin rolling.

Skin Gliding

Skin gliding is performed by using either general (forearm, palm, elbow, knuckles) or specific (fingertips and thumbs) contacts. The skin's two-dimensional mobility is evaluated for its ability to slide in relation to underlying structures (extrinsic mobility).

To evaluate, the manual contact point is fixed to the skin over the region to be assessed. The skin is pulled to the end-range, evaluating the functional excursion, quality of extensibility, and end-feel. The exact location of the adherence that is limiting its mobility is found through tracing and isolating along the direction of restriction. Restrictions are assessed utilizing the clock face concept. Through this approach of evaluating the 360 degrees of two-dimensional motion around a single contact point, restrictions are localized.

Finger Sliding

Finger sliding evaluates the ease with which the fingertips slide across the skin (Fig. 30–12). In normal tissue the finger slides with ease, creating a wave of skin in front. In restricted regions, the ability of the finger to slide across the skin is diminished. The goal is to isolate the specific location and direction of maximal restriction. Skin sliding is often used initially to trace and isolate regions of restriction and finger sliding provides a means to localize the precise location and direction of restriction.

Skin Rolling

Skin rolling is performed by lifting the skin between the thumb and the index and middle fingers to evaluate its ability to lift from underlying structures. Skin rolling is

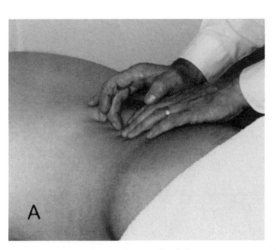

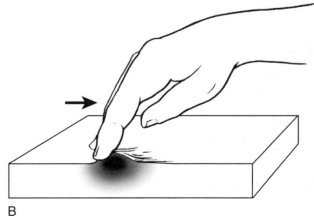

Figure 30–12. Skin and superficial fascia assessment: finger sliding.

accomplished by keeping a wave of skin in front of the thumb while the finger feeds tissue toward the thumb. This procedure is especially effective over bony prominences.

Bony Contours Assessment

Scott-Charlton and Roebuck[102] state that "a great deal of spinal pain may well be pain felt where muscle, tendon, ligament and capsule are attached to sensitive periosteum of the spine." Therefore, evaluation of the soft tissues along bony contours (i.e., iliac crest, vertebral bodies, scapula, tibia) may provide valuable information related to the overall condition of the multiple layers of soft tissues that attach to the bony contour. In addition, the bony contours are often the primary avenue for lymphatic drainage. If lymphatic drainage is impeded by restricted soft tissues, further immobility may result.

A bony contour evaluation is performed by sliding the fingers parallel (longitudinally) at progressively deeper depths along the edges of the bone, noting any points of adherence and restricted mobility. The restrictions are defined by depth and direction, utilizing the clock face concept (Fig. 30–13). Corrective treatment often facilitates functional and symptomatic improvements, possibly due to enhancement of the normal dynamic soft tissue tension and mobility altering the stress on affected structures.

Myofascial Assessment

Evaluation of the myofascial structures should include assessment of the four conditions of muscle tone, muscle play, muscle functional excursion, and neuromuscular control.

Muscle Tone

Muscles in a state of increased tone feel harder, denser, and often tender to normal palpation.[27,103] When in a state of increased tone, myofascial tissue always has specific points or epicenters of maximal density. These points exist whether the entire muscle belly is involved or the dysfunction is localized to the individual foci of hypertonia. More specifically, the exact location, depth, and direction of the increased tone should be located and treated.

Muscle Play

Concepts of muscle play have been discussed above in the section on the concepts of functional joints. The assessment of muscle play includes the following:

> The quality of accessory mobility of a muscle in relation to the surrounding structures, which allows full functional excursion and efficient biomechanical function during muscular contraction
>
> The ability of the muscle belly to expand during contraction, which allows full muscular shortening
>
> The ability of the muscle cell bundles to slide in relation to each other, which allows full passive and active functional excursion of that muscle

Muscle play is evaluated through perpendicular (transverse) deformation and parallel (longitudinal) separation of the muscle belly from surrounding structures. Each restriction is noted for its specific depth and direction. Due to the functional limitations caused by restricted muscle play, evaluation should also be conducted during passive and active motions.

Muscle Functional Excursion

Muscle functional excursion is defined as the muscle's capacity both to lengthen and narrow and to shorten and broaden. A muscle's ability to lengthen and narrow is evaluated by stretching the origin of the muscle from its insertion, identifying the specific direction of maximal restriction, and treating with STM in conjunction with contract or hold-relax techniques[73,79,104] (Fig. 30–14). The patient can assist in the evaluation process by identify-

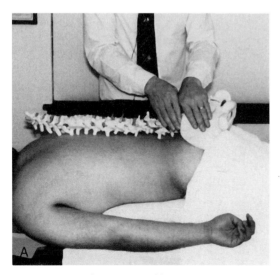
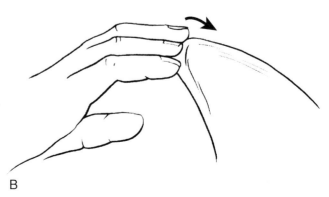

Figure 30–13. Assessment of bony contours.

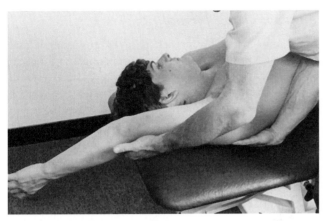

Figure 30–14. Evaluation of muscle functional excursion of the shoulder extensors.

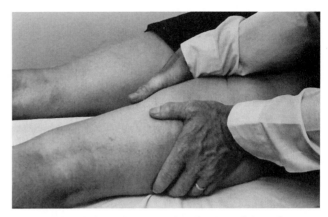

Figure 30–16. Three-dimensional evaluation of the soft tissues of the thigh.

ing where the stretch is felt when the muscle is positioned in a lengthened range.

The ability of a muscle to shorten and broaden can be evaluated through passive and active methods. Passive evaluation is performed through transverse fiber palpation to assess the play of the intrinsic fiber components. Active evaluation is similar except that active or active-resisted movements may be performed during the evaluation, which offers additional information on the dynamic capacity of the muscle.

Neuromuscular Control

Neuromuscular control is effectively evaluated and treated by using the principles and techniques of PNF[79,90] (Fig. 30–15). Inefficient coordination, recruitment, and sequencing of normal patterns of movement often lead to strain upon the soft tissues. Improvement in neuromuscular control decreases the stress on articular structures and ensures long-term maintenance of improvement in posture, available movement, and symptoms.[75,89,92]

General Three-Dimensional Evaluation

Three-dimensional palpation is a means of evaluating the general ease or difficulty with which soft tissues surround-

ing a segment of the body move. An example is evaluation of the mobility of the circumferential soft tissues of the upper thigh, in which one hand is placed over the region of the quadriceps while the other hand is placed over the hamstrings (Fig. 30–16). The therapist can evaluate the mobility of each layer circumferentially around the leg by moving the tissues in congruent motions of superior or inferior, internal or external circumferential rotation, or in a motion combining diagonal and spiral directions. Through this evaluation, one can identify those patterns in which the tissues are restricted and those in which they move freely. This distinction helps identify movement patterns that are frequently used to produce tissue mobility and those that are not used to create tissue immobility.[3,55,76]

PNF Patterns

Through the use of PNF patterns, one can identify inherent tissue tension patterns that limit the normal execution of the pattern. Because of the dynamic spiral nature of PNF patterns, many of the soft tissue restrictions that limit function can be identified (Fig. 30–17). When those

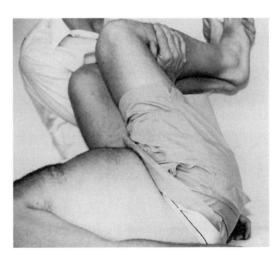

Figure 30–17. PNF lower trunk extension pattern with emphasis on the spinal intersegmental muscles and the quadratus lumborum.

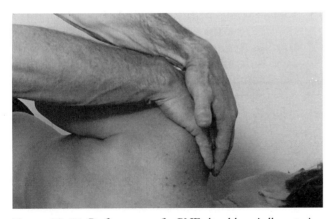

Figure 30–15. Performance of a PNF shoulder girdle anterior elevation pattern.

patterns of restriction are corrected, the PNF patterns that were previously restricted should be performed to reeducate movement within the new available range.[73,79,90]

Associated Oscillations

Associated oscillations are rhythmic oscillatory motions that are manually applied to a body part. They are executed at a rate and excursion that will create wave-like motion in the soft tissues under evaluation. Associated oscillations are used to assess the patient's ability to relax, the mobility of the soft tissues, the play of muscles, and the ease of segmental motion.[2,3] Through the application of associated oscillations the therapist can quickly identify general and specific sites of soft tissue restriction. These region are identified due to the fact that dysfunctional tissues oscillate at a slower and impeded rate or are completely restricted and appear not to move. These restricted regions are termed *still points*.

■ Treatment Approach

Physical therapy is based on the ability to touch in a knowledgeable, conscious, therapeutic, and sensitive manner. The primary tools of the profession are based on the manual art of skilled palpation. This is an art that all therapists should develop. Initially, some students possess more enhanced natural palpation perception, but the ultimate mastery of the skill in all cases is achieved through experience and extensive directed practice. Because the ability to palpate is a foundational component of our profession, students should practice the art of palpation from the first day and continue throughout their undergraduate and postgraduate training.

Evaluation and treatment must be interrelated for the application of STM to be effective. Treatment is based on subjective and objective measures such as signs, symptoms, and the mechanical behavior of the symptomatic region.[92,105] The success of treatment is also dependent on the active involvement of the patient with the process through conscious relaxation and appropriate feedback.

Treatment Strategies

There are two interrelated but distinct treatment strategies: *localized* and *biomechanical*.[3]

Localized Approach

The localized approach focuses primarily upon evaluation of the painful or dysfunctional region, providing treatment of the localized symptomatic and dysfunctional structures. This treatment strategy is guided by changes in the presenting signs and symptoms.

Biomechanical Approach

The biomechanical approach is a systems analysis and treatment approach directed at optimizing the function of the kinematic chain. Through this approach, dysfunctions of posture, mobility, and neuromuscular control affecting the symptomatic region are identified and treated. These dysfunctions are often asymptomatic, but they precipitate perpetuation of symptoms and slowing of the healing processes through repeated irritation and reinjury. The primary evaluation tools used are analysis of the positional relationship of segments, vertical compression, three-dimensional proportions analysis, functional movement patterns, PNF, and functional activity evaluations.

The following example is provided to illustrate the use of the biomechanical approach. A load-sensitive right lumbar problem that was not resolving with a localized treatment approach was assessed biomechanically.[106] It was noted that the patient's right shoulder girdle was positioned anterior and limited in its ability to be seated (like a yoke) and centered on the convexity of the rib cage. It appeared that the primary factor contributing to the patient's position was limited functional excursion of the right pectoralis minor. This dysfunctional position affected the shoulder girdle's normal arthrokinematics and force distribution capacity. Two primary biomechanical compensations were potentially affecting the lumbar spine.

1. *Thoracic spine.* The shoulder girdle and arm were forced into an anterior position to the frontal plane, shifting the center of gravity of the upper body asymmetrically anterior of the vertical axis. The patient compensated for this imbalance by bending the thoracic cage backward from the midlumbar spine. This backward-bent position altered the vertical alignment, accentuated the lumbar lordosis, and increased the strain upon the posterior elements of the symptomatic movement segments. There was reproduction of symptoms and noticeable instability of the lumbar spine during application of the vertical compression test.

2. *Cervical spine.* When optimally positioned upon the rib cage, the shoulder girdle distributes the weight and force of upper extremity loading into the rib cage, the trunk, and the base of support. However, due to the protracted position of the patient's shoulder girdle, the primary mechanism of shoulder girdle support and force distribution was assumed by the shoulder girdle muscles attached to the cervical spine. This alteration in cervical muscular function placed abnormal strain upon the cervical spine and precipitated myofascial adaptive shortening. The primary muscles affected were the longus coli, anterior scalenes, levator scapulae, upper trapezius, sternocleidomastoids, and suboccipitals. These myofascial restrictions precipitated a forward head position with

an accentuated cervical lordosis. This further altered the weight distribution and postural balance, increasing the strain on both the cervical and lumbar spines.

As the patient's ability to position her shoulder girdle and assume a balanced alignment improved, she noted that she was able to be upright for longer periods of time without exacerbating her symptoms. This enhanced both her rehabilitative program and her functional capacity.

Principles of Technique Application

Patient Preparation

Prior to providing any manual treatment, the therapist should describe to the patient the treatment that will be performed. The patient should also understand his or her responsibilities during the treatment process. Treatment is most effective when the patient is placed in a comfortable position that also allows for the greatest accessibility of the affected tissues. The patient is instructed to attempt to soften and relax the region being treated. Breathing is one of the most important adjuncts that can assist a patient in relaxation. In addition, the patient can be instructed to perform small, active oscillatory, physiologic, or functional movement patterns.

Soft Tissue Layer Concept

A foundational concept of this treatment method is to respect and treat according to the specific layer of tissue restriction or motion barrier. The superficial layers are evaluated and treated before attempting to correct the restrictions of deeper layers. By following this rule, the therapist will require the least amount of force to access the deeper restrictions. In addition, correction of superficial dysfunctions often improve the condition of restrictions of deeper layers. Dysfunctions are identified by specific depth, direction, and angle of restriction.

Technique Application

After assessing and localizing a soft tissue dysfunction, the therapist selects a specific STM technique and applies the appropriate amount of force in the direction of maximum density/restriction. The goal in applying soft tissue techniques is to achieve the desired results while using the least amount of force. It is important for the therapist to be patient and give the tissues time to respond and to allow both the mechanical and viscoelastic effects to occur.

Degree of Force

Increased force is only used as a last resort when all other options for release have been attempted or when less mobile tissues such as scar adhesions and contractures are present. These tissues may require more force. The exact amount of force is dependent upon the extent of restriction, the amount of discomfort, and the degree of irritability. The general rule is to place sufficient force upon the restriction, in the precise depth, direction, and angle, to take and maintain the dysfunctional tissues to their end range. As the restriction begins to release, the therapist should continue to maintain pressure on the dysfunctional tissues and follow the path of the tissues that are letting go.

Progression of Technique

During application of a soft tissue technique, improvement in the dysfunction should be noted through a palpable normalization in tissue mobility or density. If there is a palpable improvement in the restriction, the subjective and objective signs should be reevaluated. If the restriction does not begin to improve within a short period of time (i.e., 10 seconds), the therapist should alter or choose another technique. If after the application of two to three separate techniques there is no change, as a general rule the therapist should do the following:

Reevaluate the region for underlying or more remote dysfunctions

Treat other dysfunctions and return to the unresponsive dysfunction later during the treatment session

Reassess and treat the dysfunction during subsequent treatment sessions

Dysfunctions related to scar tissue, decreased muscle play, or fascial tightness generally maintain the improvements gained during treatment. However, dysfunctions related to hypertonus or swelling and those of a neuroreflexive nature may return with time. Gains are more likely to be maintained if improved postures and ROM are reinforced through application of resisted neuromuscular reeducation techniques, if the patient is trained in efficient body mechanics, and if a specific conditioning and rehabilitation program is designed to address the soft tissue dysfunction.

Treatment Techniques

Techniques are applied by using one hand to apply pressure upon the restriction while the other hand assists to facilitate a release. The treatment hand can apply pressure through specific (fingers or thumb) or general (heel of the hand, elbow, forearm) contacts. The multiple options of manual contacts provide the therapist with a mosaic of treatment options. The selection of a general or specific contact surface depends on the type and size of dysfunctional tissue(s) and the degree of irritability caused by the presenting symptoms.

Treatment pressure is applied in the direction of the restriction, and as it releases, the slack is taken up to keep a consistent pressure upon the resolving restriction. The direction of the restriction often changes as the release occurs, and appropriate adjustments in the direction of force are needed to maintain the pattern of release. *An inherent aspect of effective application of soft tissue mobilization techniques is the therapist's use of proper body position and mechanics.*

There is a natural progression of technique application. This progression generally begins with sustained pressure. If the restriction does not release, the therapist should add or progress to additional techniques until the restriction begins to disappear (Fig. 30–18).

Treatment Hand Techniques

Sustained Pressure

Pressure should be applied directly to the epicenter of the restricted tissue at the exact depth, direction, and angle of maximal restriction. The therapist should be positioned so that the technique can be applied either away from (pushing) or toward (pulling) his or her body. The pressure is sustained, and as the restriction resolves, the slack is taken up (Fig. 30–19).

When applied to bony contours or myofascial tissues, sustained pressure is further defined according to the direction of motion in relation to the boundary of the structure.

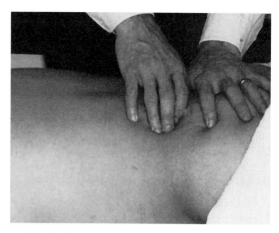

Figure 30–19. Sustained pressure with surrounding tissues placed on tension.

Unlocking Spiral

If a restriction does not resolve, the therapist can use an unlocking spiral to initiate a release. While maintaining a sustained pressure technique, the therapist assesses for the degree of tissue tension caused by clockwise and counterclockwise rotary motions. These motions are accomplished by moving the elbow away from or toward the body, spiraling the finger on the restriction as a screwdriver turns a screw. One motion creates greater tension in the tissues, while the other creates an easing of tension. When the direction of ease is identified, the therapist, while maintaining sustained pressure on the restriction, rotates in the direction of ease until the restriction begins to soften. At that point, the spiral motion is eased and the sustained pressure is continued following the pattern of release. Upon reassessment, the direction of tissue spiral that was of greater restriction (the opposite of the direction of ease) is evaluated for any remaining dysfunction and treated (Fig. 30–20).

Direct Oscillations

The technique of direct oscillations involves an extension of the sustained pressure technique, but with repeated, rhythmic, end-range deformation at the point of maxim dysfunction (grade III or IV of the Maitland system). These gentle oscillations places rhythmic pressure on and off a restriction (motion barrier). As the restriction resolves, the tissue slack is taken up.[92]

Perpendicular Mobilization

Perpendicular mobilization involves sustained pressure applied at right angles or transverse to a bony contour or myofascial tissue to improve muscle and soft tissue play (Fig. 30–21). Direct oscillation and unlocking spiral techniques can be used.

Parallel Mobilization

Parallel mobilization involves applying pressure longitudinally to restrictions along the edge of the muscle belly,

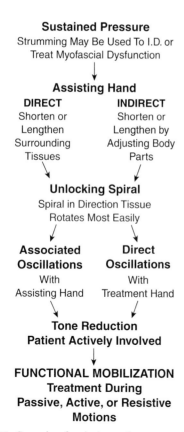

Sustained Pressure
Strumming May Be Used To I.D. or
Treat Myofascial Dysfunction
↓
Assisting Hand

DIRECT	INDIRECT
Shorten or Lengthen Surrounding Tissues	Shorten or Lengthen by Adjusting Body Parts

Unlocking Spiral
Spiral in Direction Tissue
Rotates Most Easily

Associated Oscillations	**Direct Oscillations**
With Assisting Hand	With Treatment Hand

Tone Reduction
Patient Actively Involved
↓
FUNCTIONAL MOBILIZATION
Treatment During
Passive, Active, or Resistive
Motions

Figure 30–18. Cascade of techniques for progressive treatment of specific soft tissue restrictions. (© 11/97 The Institute of Physical Art.)

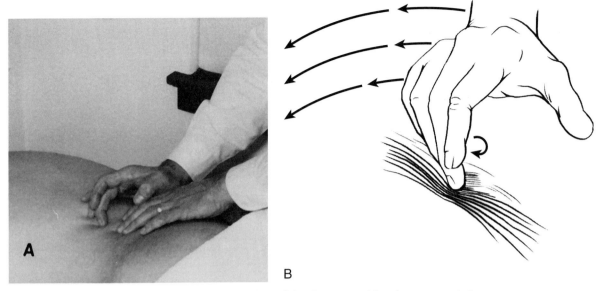

Figure 30–20. Unlocking spiral. The twisting action of the forearm and hand causes a spiral motion of fingers upon restriction.

to the seam between two muscles, or along bony contours. The purpose is to normalize the restriction and to improve muscle play and soft tissue mobility. Direct oscillations and unlocking spiral techniques can be used (Fig. 30–22).

Perpendicular (Transverse) Strumming

Perpendicular strumming is used to evaluate for and treat increased tone and the loss of myofascial play. The technique is applied through repeated, rhythmic deformation of a muscle belly, as one would strum the string of a guitar. Perpendicular pressure is applied to the border of a muscle belly, deforming it until the end-range is attained. The fingers are then allowed to slide over the top of the belly of the muscle as it springs back into position.

This technique produces rhythmic oscillations throughout the body. It allows the therapist to know if the patient is relaxing, and it provides the relaxation qualities of oscillatory motions (mechanoreceptors) (Fig. 30–23).

Friction Massage

Friction massage is a technique defined by Cyriax[37] involving repeated cross-grain manipulation of lesions of tendinous and ligamentous tissues.[39,91]

Assisting Hand Techniques

The following procedures applied by the assisting hand can be used with any of the above-mentioned treatment hand procedures to hasten or facilitate resolution of tissues being treated.

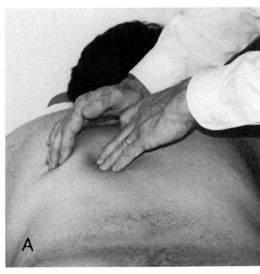

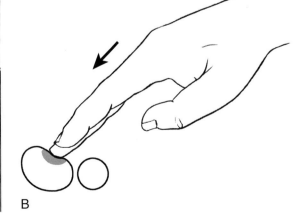

Figure 30–21. Perpendicular mobilization.

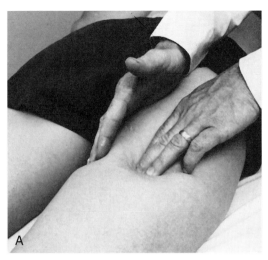
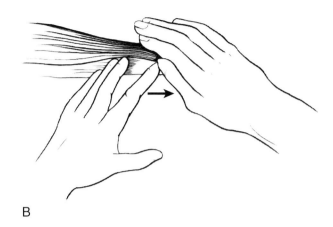

Figure 30–22. Parallel mobilization.

Placing Tissues on Slack

Placing tissues on slack involves adjusting the tissues surrounding the restriction in a shortened range to ease the tension on the restriction. This can occur from any direction in relation to the restriction (360 degrees). The tissues are shortened at the same tissue depth as the restriction.

Placing tissues on slack is generally the first assisting tool to be used, especially if the symptoms are acute or easily exacerbated. If a release does not begin within 10 seconds, the therapist should choose another direction

of shortening for the tissues or choose another assisting technique (Fig. 30–24).

Placing Tissues on Tension

Placing tissues on tension involves adjusting the surrounding tissues in a lengthened range to place tension on the restriction. This technique is applied in the same manner as placing tissues on slack, with the exact depth and direction of tensing the surrounding tissues depending on the restriction. It is used more often in chronic conditions and as a means to place more demand upon

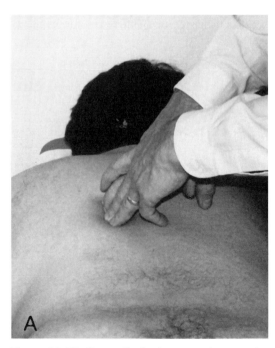
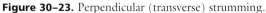
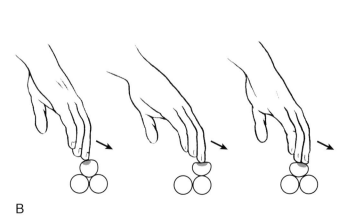

Figure 30–23. Perpendicular (transverse) strumming.

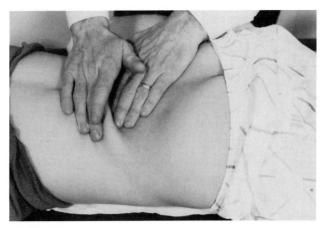

Figure 30–24. Placing tissues on slack with the assisting hand.

a restriction. All tissues should ultimately be checked in a lengthened position for the complete resolution of a restriction (Fig. 30–25).

Using Both Hands

There are conditions in which both hands are used together and no distinction is made between the treatment and assisting hands. For example, when performing a three-dimensional technique (which evolves from the three-dimensional evaluation covered in the section on palpatory evaluation above), the two hands function together to improve the mobility of the tissues as an extension of the evaluation process.[3,55,76]

Passive Associated Oscillations

Passive associated oscillations of a body part create a whole body oscillation, but with focal oscillations upon the restricted region. These oscillations are applied while sustained pressure is placed upon the restriction. When used appropriately, these oscillations help the patient relax, decrease the discomfort of the pressure on the restriction, and promote normalization of the tissues. It is important to sense the degree to which the patient is able to relax and how well the oscillations translate through the body. The frequency of the oscillations varies according to the patient's body type and the type of dysfunction.[94]

Manual Resistance

While the treatment hand is maintaining pressure upon restricted tissues, the assisting hand applies resistance to produce an isometric or isotonic contraction of the dysfunctional myofascial tissues. There are many creative ways to use this assisting hand tool. For example, in the side-lying position, treatment of dysfunctions of the soft tissues of the cervical spine can be enhanced by applying resistance to scapula patterns. These concepts are basic to the functional mobilization approach.[4,73]

Cascade of Techniques

The cascade of techniques flow chart can be used to better visualize and understand the options the therapist has for treating specific dysfunctions. This provides a mechanism for altering the treatment tools being utilized to meet the requirements of a specific restriction (Fig. 30–26).

General Techniques

General techniques provide a larger contact surface to evaluate and treat larger regions of the body. They are often used when a general evaluation and treatment is desired, such as when a large region of restrictions is present and as an initial or completion stroke. General techniques are also useful to protect or reduce the use of fingertips and thumbs, which are stressed by the use of specific techniques[107] (Fig. 30–27).

Functional Mobilization

Functional mobilization is the integrated use of soft tissue and joint mobilization combined with the dynamic principles and procedures of PNF. This is a step-by-step evaluation and treatment approach which combines mobilization or stabilization with neuromuscular reeducation. With the combined tools of PNF and STM, the therapist is able to combine the evaluation of the condition of the soft tissues, articulations, and neuromuscular control of multiple movement segments. (Fig 30–28).

Progression of Care

As noncontractile and contractile soft tissues regain their normal state of free and independent mobility, decreased tone, and normal physiologic length, the patient can assume a more efficient alignment and move with greater ease and coordination (Fig. 30–28). New postures and ROM should be reinforced through application of resisted neuromuscular reeducation techniques,[79,90] and em-

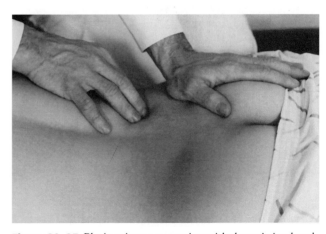

Figure 30–25. Placing tissues on tension with the assisting hand.

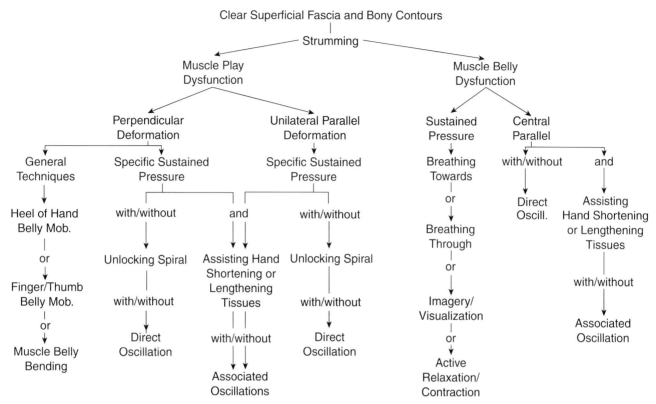

Figure 30–26. Myofascial cascade of techniques. (© 9/92 Revised 9/96: The Institute of Physical Art.)

phasis should be placed upon a specific body mechanics training and rehabilitation program.[89,105]

Precautions and Contraindications

As with any manual therapy approach, the application of any treatment technique needs to be done in a judicious manner, with recognition of the known pathologies and irritabilities and with common sense. The following list of contraindications and precautions is provided as a guide. Therapists with extensive experience and training in man-

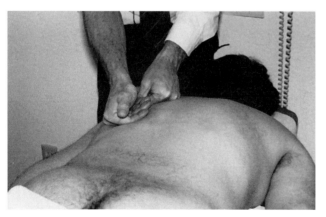

Figure 30–27. General techniques for the paraspinals.

ual therapy may judiciously treat a condition that less experienced therapists should avoid.

Malignancy

Inflammatory skin condition

Fracture

Sites of active hemorrhage

Obstructive edema

Localized infections

Aneurysm

Acute rheumatoid arthritis

Osteomyelitis

Osteoporosis

Advanced diabetes

Fibromyalgia (while in an inflammatory state)

Any symptoms that have previously been exacerbated by appropriately applied STM

■ Clinical Correlations

This overview of clinical correlations is intended to assist the reader in understanding the relevance of STM to the overall management of a patient and to illuminate the

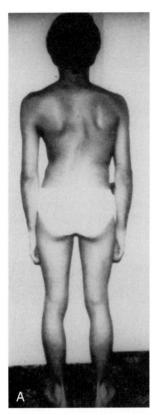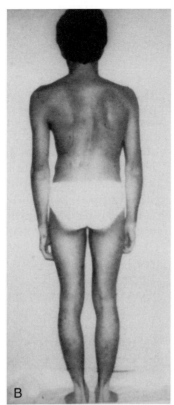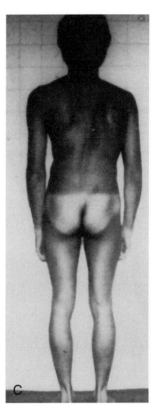

Figure 30–28. Postural changes following treatment. (A) Initial. (B) After 10 treatments. (C) One year after discharge.

possible interaction of specific soft tissue restrictions with lumbar pathology. The lumbar spine has been chosen to illustrate the soft tissue dysfunctions associated with spinal dysfunction. Most of the functional changes reported are correlations made from observations following normalization of soft tissue dysfunctions.

Skin and Superficial Fascia

Improvements achieved through correction of skin restrictions are often dramatic in comparison with the subtleness of the restriction. The most frequently noted functional improvements (increased range of physiologic and functional motions; improvements in alignment and segmental spinal mobility; and reduced symptoms) are often noted following the treatment of abdominal or posterior surgical scars.[2,54]

Lumbar Muscles and Thoracolumbar Fascia

The lumbar muscles (Fig. 30–29) can be divided into three groups and layers:[51] (1) the short intersegmental muscles—the interspinales and the intertransversarii; (2) the polysegmental muscles—the multifidus, the rotories, and the lumbar components of the longissimus, spinalis, and iliocostalis; and (3) the long polysegmental mus-

cles—represented by the thoracic components of the longissimus and iliocostalis lumborum that span the lumbar region from thoracic levels to the ilium and sacrum.

The deeper intersegmental and polysegmental muscles, particularly the multifidi, are primarily stabilizers controlling posture and assisting in fine adjustments and segmental movement.[8,9,23,108] The multifidus is also believed to protect against impingement of the facet capsule during joint movements because of its attachments to the joint capsule.[51] Kirkaldy-Willis[9] reports that uncontrolled contraction of the multifidus may be a primary factor in the production of torsional injury to the facet joints and disk. The more superficial and polysegmental muscles (erector spinae), the longissimus, spinalis, and iliocostalis, produce the grosser motions of thoracic and pelvic backward bending, sidebending, and rotation that increase lumbar lordosis.[9,23,109] Some authors have reported that the erector spinae are active in maintaining upright posture.[109]

The extensive thoracolumbar fascia attaches to the transverse processes of the lumbar vertebrae, the iliac crest and iliolumbar ligament, the 12th rib, the quadratus lumborum, the lateral portion of the psoas major, and the aponeurotic origin of the transversus abdominis.[23,110] Each layer of lumbar musculature is separated and compartmentalized by the thoracolumbar fascia, and in an efficient state can be palpated for having independent

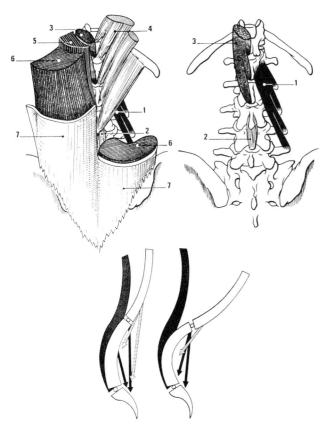

Figure 30–29. Lumbar musculature. (1) Transversospinalis; (2) interspinalis muscles; (3) spinalis muscle; (4) serratus posterior inferior; (5) longissimus; (6) iliocostalis; (7) aponeurosis of the latissimus dorsi. (From Dupuis and Kirkaldy-Willis,[112] with permission.)

mobility from surrounding structures. The lumbar musculature is most effectively assessed in the side-lying and prone positions. Its extensibility is most effectively appraised through evaluation of end-ranges of PNF trunk patterns.

Restricted play of the erector spinae can limit ROM of the lumbar spine due to the inability of the muscles to slide normally upon each other. This is noted especially with the motions of sidegliding (lateral shear), forward bending, and rotation. When muscles are in a state of increased tone or restricted play, they may have difficulty folding on each other and will restrict motions such as sidebending to the same side and backward bending.

Increased tone of the deeper musculature can be the primary source of symptoms and can limit the mobility of individual segments. With unilateral soft tissue dysfunction, there will often be a deviation to the affected side during forward bending. In conjunction with the improvement of alignment, ROM, and pain, improvement in the patient's ability to control active movement is often observed following treatment.

When the more lateral intertransversarii lateralis and quadratus lumborum have limited extensibility, the region often appears shortened and restricted in motions such as sidebending and pelvic lateral shear (sidegliding).

The quadratus lumborum will often have restricted normal play in relation to the erector spinae and psoas, affecting most spinal motions.

Abdominal Scar

Scar tissue in the abdominal region often produces marked pathomechanics of the soft tissues and the articulations of the lumbopelvic girdle region. These scar tissue dysfunctions can alter efficient function from the superficial fascia to the deep abdominal region. Through careful palpation, spider-web-like tentacles of restricted tissue can be traced extending away from the central scar, possibly extending throughout the abdominal cavity and to the posterior wall. If the palpation is performed with superimposed movement (such as a functional movement or PNF pattern), the effects of these limitations and the altered biomechanics can be noted. This restricted matrix can affect proper alignment and functional movements such as forward bending (possibly due to the inability of the abdominal tissues to fold upon themselves) and backward bending secondary to decreased extensibility of the anterior section.

In individuals with hypermobilities or spondylolisthesis, dramatic improvement in functional abilities has been observed through normalization of the abdominal scar. Improvement is often noted in static postures and in the performance of functional movement patterns such as the pelvic clock and lower trunk rotation. Through appropriate soft tissue mobilization the scar tissue may become more pliable, but the primary effect appears to be improved mobility of the surrounding structures and of the restricted spider-web-like matrix. This probably facilitates a more neutral position of the lumbar spine and allows movement to be distributed through the spine into the pelvis more efficiently.

Rectus Abdominus

The rectus abdominus originates primarily from the costal cartilage of the fifth, sixth, and seventh ribs and inserts on the crest of the pubis. It is enclosed between the aponeuroses of the oblique and transversus forming the rectus sheath, which separates it from the other abdominals.[23] If the rectus is adhered to the underlying structures, motions such as rotation and pelvic lateral shearing are restricted due to the inability of the rectus abdominus to slide over the underlying abdominals. The umbilicus should also be evaluated for free three-dimensional mobility, as restrictions will also affect the mobility of the rectus abdominus.

The rectus abdominus will often be found to be in a shortened state that holds the rib cage down, increasing a forward head posture and thoracic kyphosis. There is often a compensatory backward bending of the thoracic cage, increasing thoracolumbar or midlumbar lordosis.

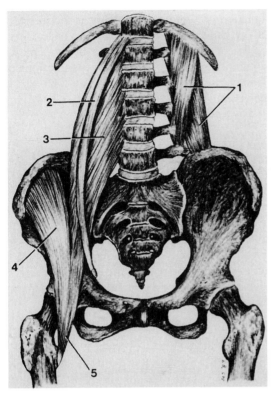

Figure 30–30. Muscles of the anterior spinal column. The intrinsic flexors of the lumbar spine: (1) two layers of the quadratus lumborum; (2) psoas minor; (3) psoas major; (4) iliacus; (5) conjoined attachment of the psoas and iliacus of and around the lesser femoral trochanter. (From Dupuis and Kirkaldy-Willis,[112] with permission.)

We often find shortened rectus abdominus muscles in individuals who do many sit-ups in a flexed position.

One of the myofascial complications of pregnancy is diastasis of the rectus abdominus. This is the separation of the two sections along the midline, the linea alba. Clinically, it has been observed that this separation occurs mostly in women who have restrictions of the lateral borders of the rectus abdominus, which prevent the muscle from stretching forward as a unit. This lack of mobility of the lateral aspect places excess stress on the central linea alba and produces separation.

Psoas and Iliacus Muscles

The psoas arises from the anterior surfaces and lower borders of the transverse processes of the 12th thoracic vertebra and all of the lumbar vertebrae, creating a muscle with multiple distinct layers (Fig. 30–30). At each segmental level it is attached to the margin of each vertebral body, the adjacent disk, and the fibrous arch that connects the upper and lower aspects of the lumbar vertebral body.[23,51] The iliacus originates primarily from the superior two-thirds of the concavity of the iliac fossa and the upper surface of the lateral part of the sacrum, and most of the fibers converge into the lateral side of the psoas

tendon.[23] The psoas and iliacus are covered with the iliac fascia, which attaches to the intervertebral disks, the margins of the vertebral bodies, and the upper part of the sacrum, and are continuous with the inguinal ligament and the transversalis fascia. The iliopsoas flexes the femur upon the pelvis or flexes the trunk and pelvis upon the lower extremities. Some authors attribute a distinct postural component to the deeper spinal fibers of the psoas.[14,109]

The iliopsoas muscles are often found to have limited extensibility, play, or increased tone at the level of spinal pathology.[7,30,68,110] Due to the psoas' centralized biomechanical position, minor dysfunction of the psoas can have a dramatic effect upon posture and the length of the lumbar region, and can place excessive stress upon the intervertebral disks and the performance of functional motions.[26,110] Restricted extensibility limits the posterior tilt of the pelvis, which increases lumbar lordosis. Such restrictions can decrease movement in all directions, especially limiting backward and forward bending. The function of the psoas is often altered by dysfunctions in the lower extremities, especially if the dysfunction is unilateral, thus altering the dynamics and the capacity for the two psoas muscles to act symmetrically during spinal function.

Through clinical experience, it has been observed that with improved length, play, and normalized tone of the psoas, an increase in forward bending of the lumbar spine often occurs. This improved mobility may be due to the ability of the psoas to fold upon itself and the ability of the transverse processes, which are posterior to the central axis of motion, to separate from each other and allow the spine to bow convexly posteriorly. It has also been noticed that restricted play of a psoas at a specific level can limit mobility of that segment, specifically affecting rotation and bending to the opposite side. Often pressure applied to the localized foci of tone will cause referred pain that duplicates the reported symptoms (Fig. 30–31). In many cases, normalization of psoas mobility and improved neuromuscular control have facilitated dramatic improvements in symptoms and function.

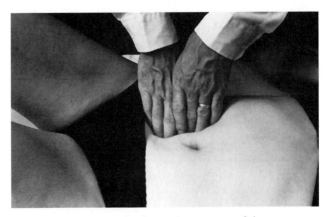

Figure 30–31. Evaluation and treatment of the psoas.

Lower Extremities and Hip

Limited mobility of the myofascial structures of the lower extremities is a primary contributing factor that forces the individual to utilize the lumbar spine instead of the lower extremities as a primary axis of motion. Several authors have suggested a correlation between poor flexibility of the lower extremities and lumbar symptoms.[26,110] Also, myofascial tightness of the lower extremities may cause a decrease in blood and lymph flow, which contributes to restricted mobility, fluid stasis, and greater muscular fatigability.

Of primary importance are dysfunctions that affect extensibility and normal play of the hip rotators, hamstrings, rectus femoris, iliotibial band, adductors, and gastrocsoleus (triceps surae).

Hip Rotators

Restricted play and decreased extensibility of these closely interrelated muscles limit hip mobility and affect pelvic motion and coordination for performance of forward-oriented tasks. The ability to rotate the body through the hips over a fixed base of support while maintaining a stable lumbar spine is affected when there is limited extensibility and play of the hip rotators (Fig. 30–32).

Hamstrings

Shortened hamstrings limit pelvic anterior tilt and therefore restrict a patient's ability to maintain a neutral spine while bending forward in standing and sitting. Restricted play between the three bellies can cause abnormal torsion on the ilium and affect the eccentric control of lower extremity and pelvic motions.

In the efficient state, the hamstrings fold around the femur during forward bending and rotational activities. This folding action provides additional range to the motions. However, the bellies of the hamstrings frequently become restricted together, preventing normal play. One of the most effective means to increase hamstrings range

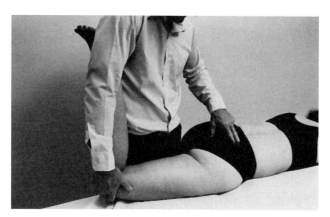

Figure 30–32. Function mobilization of the external rotators of the hip.

and function is to improve mobility at the interface between the hamstring bellies. The sciatic nerve between the bellies of the long head of the biceps femoris and the semitendinosus can be assessed. Restrictions of the hamstrings can be felt to restrict the mobility of the sciatic nerve.

Rectus Femoris

Decreased flexibility of the rectus femoris restricts the ability of the pelvis to tilt posteriorly upon the head of the femur, often limiting the individual's ability to assume a neutral lumbar position in standing. Restricted mobility of the rectus femoris in relation to the sartorius, the tensor fascia lata, and the underlying quadriceps affects performance of each muscle's independent actions. Soft tissue restrictions within and around the rectus femoris can also limit hip extension during gait and result in compensatory backward bending of the lumbar spine.

Iliotibial Band

The iliotibial band is a lateral stabilizer and is important for maintaining posture during gait. Limited mobility and play of the iliotibial band is probably a major contributor to lumbar immobility and pain.[30] Tightness often reduces the individual's ability to shift weight over the base of support (due to lateral tightness) and to perform any lateral motion. In cases of sacroiliac hypermobility, limited extensibility of the iliotibial band is often seen on the side of hypermobility.

Adductors

As with the iliotibial band, adductor tightness and limited play affect pelvic position, mobility, and the dynamics of lateral movements.

Gastrocsoleus

When the soleus is shortened, the heel lifts off the ground, decreasing the base of support and impairing balance during bending and lifting activities. This may further contribute to rearfoot deformities such as calcaneal valgus, which may cause aberrant lower quadrant function. Ankle coordination can be affected by restricted play between the bellies of the gastroc and soleus and also between the soleus and the deeper toe flexors and posterior tibialis.

CASE STUDIES

CASE STUDY 1

The following case study of a 38-year-old woman with right upper quadrant symptoms illustrates the merging of STM in an integrated manual therapy program. We have termed this approach *functional mobilization*.[4]

Presenting Symptoms

The patient presented with a 9-month duration of cervical and right upper extremity pain with limited range secondary to involvement in a rear-end automobile accident. She denied experiencing any numbness, tingling, or weakness.

Mechanics of Injury

The patient was stopped at a traffic signal when another vehicle hit her from behind at approximately 40 mph. At the time of impact her head was turned right, looking in the rear-view mirror, her right hand was on the steering wheel, and her right foot was on the brake. This information is presented because the mechanical dysfunctions of the cervical spine, right shoulder, and pelvic girdle appear to have a bearing on the patient's posture and motion during the trauma.

Symptom Onset and Progression

The patient reported an immediate onset of headache and cervical symptoms. Over the next 2 to 3 weeks, she developed right upper extremity symptoms.

Test Results

Magnetic resonance imaging revealed a minor disk bulging at the right C4–C5 level without thecal sac impingement.

Therapeutic Intervention and Symptomatic Progression

Initial therapeutic intervention consisted of anti-inflammatory and muscle relaxant medications, which controlled the patient's symptoms so that she could return to her secretarial position within 1 week. One month after the trauma she continued to experience substantial symptoms, and her physician referred her for 6 weeks of physical therapy, three times per week, at another clinic. Following 6 weeks of hot packs, ultrasound, cervical traction, and massage, the patient reported that she was experiencing increased symptoms, most notably in her right hand and wrist. Upon return to her physician, she was diagnosed as having carpal tunnel syndrome secondary to her frequent computer usage and was given workman's compensation.

Six months later, she was referred to our clinic at the suggestion of a friend. She was still unable to return to work. Her presenting problems now included right shoulder limitation and pain. During the preceding 6-month period, she had received further physical therapy in addition to chiropractic care and acupuncture.

Symptom Analysis

The following presenting symptoms are listed in the order of the patient's perceived intensity:

1. Right C7–T1 region: Pain at the approximate location of the first rib costovertebral articulation, described as a deep, boring aching pain.
2. Right C4–C5: Deep, sharp pain, especially with right rotation, sidebending, and quadrant motions.
3. Right anterior and lateral shoulder pain. In addition to the range limitations, symptoms increased with flexion and abduction.
4. Right hand and wrist pain: Primarily the medial aspect of the hand, which increased with hand usage.
5. Right medial scapula pain: Associated with forward-oriented tasks.
6. Periodic right suboccipital and temporal headaches: Often precipitated with prolonged forward-oriented tasks or poor sleeping postures.

Significant Objective Findings

1. Cervical ROM
   Right rotation: 50 percent with pain increasing at the right C4–C5
   Right extension quadrant: 30 percent with pain radiating into the right upper extremity to the hand
   Right sidebending: 30 percent with pain radiating into the right side neck and shoulder
2. Right first rib: Elevated with restricted caudal mobility, especially the posterior articulation
3. Right glenohumeral articulation ROM
   Flexion: 140 degrees with the scapula stabilized
   Abduction: 80 degrees with pain in the subdeltoid region
   External rotation: 45 degrees
   Resisted test: Positive pain elicited with resisted abduction (superspinatus) and external rotation (infraspinatus)
   Accessory mobility: Marked restriction of glenohumeral downward glide and acromioclavicular anterior mobility
4. Upper limb nerve tension test: Tested according to the procedures of Elvey and Butler;[24,25] positive with scapula depression, with radiation of symptoms into the hand; positive for the median nerve involvement
5. Right wrist: 70 percent extension
6. Pelvic girdle: Right innominate restricted in ability to extend and internally rotate (fixated in posterior torsion and outflare); region asymptomatic but functionally affecting the base of support, balance of the spine over the pelvis, and gait

Treatment Strategies

Treatment strategies for a patient presenting with such complicated and systemwide problems require a multi-

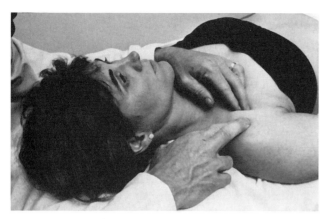

Figure 30–33. Mobilization of soft tissues of bony contours of the right clavicle and mobilization of the acromioclavicular joint.

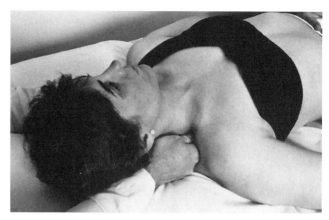

Figure 30–35. Mobilization of the right first rib with soft tissues on slack.

level and integrated approach. The following presentation emphasizes the progression and principles of treatment utilized for each dysfunctional region. Presented are the major components of the integrated treatment program:

1. Self-care was the initial emphasis of care. Training the patient to utilize more efficient postures and body mechanics to reduce the self-perpetuated exacerbations. Education and training was the basic component of the treatment program and was addressed at each visit as symptoms and functional level improved.
2. During each visit a progressive and specific stretching, strengthening, and stabilization program was addressed. This program initially focused on the positive upper limb tension sign, elevated first rib, limited cervical ROM, self-resisted dorsal glide, and pivot prone for postural training.
3. In conjunction with education and training is the manual therapy treatment of the most obvious mechanical dysfunctions. This *functional mobilization* approach includes STM, joint mobilization, and neu-

romuscular reeducation. The concept is to treat the soft tissue dysfunctions prior to treatment of articular dysfunctions, combining each with neuromuscular reeducation.

The following is an overview of the treatment rendered to each dysfunctional region.

1. *Thoracic girdle.* The basic philosophy of functional mobilization is that dysfunctions of the base of support of a symptomatic segment should generally be normalized prior to treatment of the symptomatic structures. The thoracic girdle consists of the manubrium, the first ribs, and the first thoracic vertebra. The primary dysfunction of the thoracic girdle was the posterior aspect of the right first rib restricted in caudal glide.

   Treatment strategy: The initial strategy was to normalize the superficial fascia, bony contours, and mobilization of the acromioclavicular articulation (Fig. 30–33). In addition, STM was applied to the

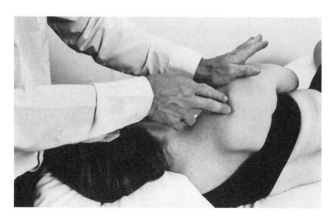

Figure 30–34. Mobilization of soft tissues of the superior right scapular border.

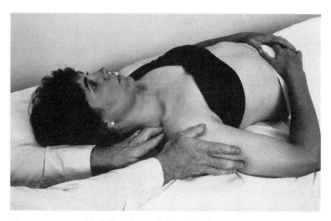

Figure 30–36. Mobilization of the right first rib with soft tissues on stretch.

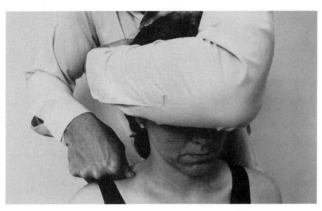

Figure 30–37. Mobilization of the right first rib in the sitting position coupled with cervical contraction/relaxation.

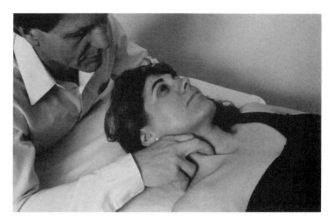

Figure 30–39. Strumming of the right longus coli.

superior border of the scapula (Fig. 30–34). There were significant restrictions of play and increased tone of the right anterior and medial scaleni that, when reduced, improved the mobility of the first rib.

Mobilization of the first rib was performed in the supine position, with the soft tissues placed on slack through cervical right sidebending. Sustained pressure was applied with the thumbs, the fingers, or the lateral first metacarpophalangeal to the most restricted portion and direction of the posterior first rib. Coupled with the sustained pressure was the use of directed breathing and contract relaxation (Figs. 30–35 and 30–36).

Treatment progressed to sitting once the rib's mobility was returned to normal. The surrounding soft tissues were treated with the cervical spine in neutral and in left sidebending to increase their functional excursion (Fig. 30–37).

Home program: The patient was instructed to use a towel or strap to maintain the downward and posterior mobility of the first rib.

2. *Cervical spine.* Once the first rib was normalized, the amount of muscle spasm in the deep cervical musculature was reduced. Noted dysfunctions included the following:
   a. Marked superficial fascia tightness posterior along the spinous processes and in the right occipital and suboccipital region
   b. Adherence between the right semispinalis capitis and the splenius muscles, especially in the lower cervical spine (Fig. 30–38)
   c. Dysfunctions of play and tone of the right longus coli, anterior and medial scaleni, sternocleidomastoid, and upper trapezius (Figs. 30–39 to 30–41)
   d. Marked tenderness and swelling of the right C4–C5 articular facet
   e. Limitation of C4 in left diagonal anterior glide and right rotation and sidebending
   f. General restriction of posterior longitudinal and interspinous ligaments, with most restriction at the C5–C6 level

   Treatment strategy: The initial strategy was to treat the soft tissues to increase play and decrease tone. The

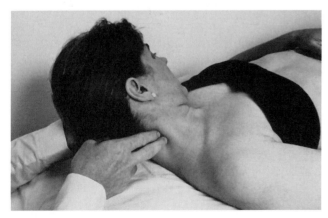

Figure 30–38. Parallel technique to improve play between the right semispinalis capitus and the spenius.

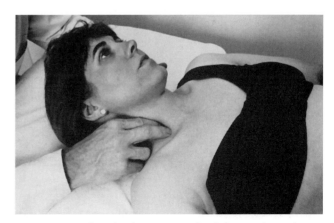

Figure 30–40. Sustained pressure to the right anterior scalenus.

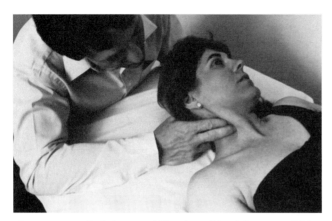

Figure 30–41. Soft tissue mobilization of the right sternocleido-mastoid.

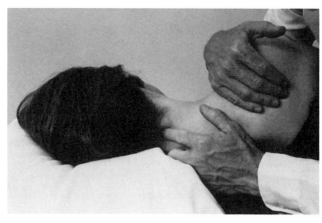

Figure 30–43. Mobilization of the interspinous ligament between C5 and C6 to increase extensibility.

tone of the muscles in the region of the right C4–C5 articular facet did not respond to tone-reducing techniques; therefore, treatment progressed to improving mobility of that intervertebral segment. Using functional mobilization techniques to localize the C4 restriction to the specific diagonal direction and using hold relax procedures improved mobility and decreased the surrounding tone (Fig. 30–42).

Additional treatment was used to reduce the tightness of the C5–C6 interspinous ligament by applying gentle fingertip traction to the C5 spinous process while the patient performed active axial extension. During the procedure the other hand performed STM to reduce anterior and posterior restrictions (Fig. 30–43). To promote the ability of the cervical spine to balance on the rib cage, the O-1 and T1–T2 segments were mobilized (Fig. 30–44).

Home program: The home program consisted of resisted axial extension, short neck and long neck flexor strengthening, and resisted pivot prone.

3. *Right shoulder.* There were both subjective and objective gains in the shoulder following treatment of the first rib and cervical spine. Treatment was directed to the following primary dysfunctions:

a. STM, primarily strumming of the bodies of the infra- and supraspinatus muscles (Fig. 30–45)
b. Friction massage to the supraspinatus and infraspinatus tendons (Fig. 30–46)
c. In the left sidelying position, selected PNF patterns to the right shoulder girdle in conjunction with STM (Fig. 30–47)
d. Mobilization of the scapular thoracic articulation by lifting the scapula from the rib cage (Fig. 30–48)

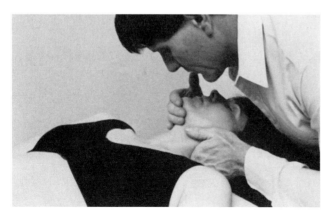

Figure 30–42. Functional mobilization to improve left anterior diagonal mobility of C4.

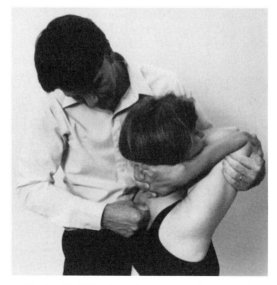

Figure 30–44. Mobilization of the upper thoracic spine to increase backward bending of T1–T2.

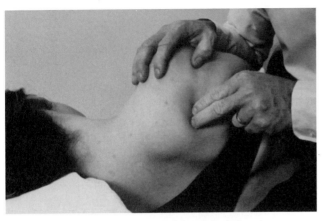

Figure 30–45. Strumming of the right infraspinatus.

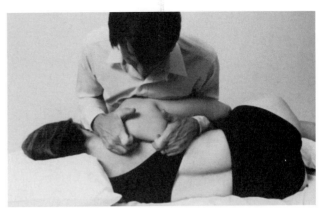

Figure 30–48. Mobilization of the right scapulothoracic articulation.

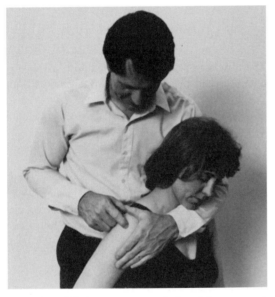

Figure 30–46. Friction massage of the right superspinatus tendon.

e. STM to the subscapularis and pectoralis minor muscles in the supine position (Figs. 30–49 and 30–50)

f. Distraction of the humeral head with STM and contract relaxation (Fig. 30–51)

g. Mobilization of the head of the humerus caudally, performed with the patient sitting and resting her right elbow on the table while the therapist placed downward pressure on the humerus (Fig. 30–52)

h. Neuromuscular reeducation of the rotator cuff through manual resistance applied in the same position, with emphasis on the humeral depressors

i. Increasing ROM of the right upper extremity by placing the arm at restricted ranges and performing STM and contract relaxation on the restricted tissues (Fig. 30–53)

j. Using upper extremity PNF patterns to identify and treat weaknesses and motor recruitment problems (Figs. 30–54 and 30–55)

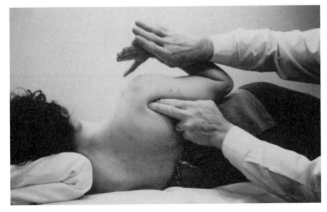

Figure 30–47. PNF for posterior depression, scapular pattern, with soft tissue mobilization.

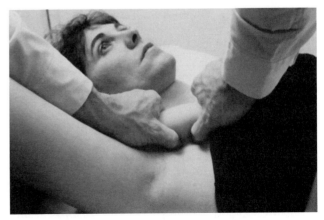

Figure 30–49. Soft tissue mobilization of the right pectoralis minor.

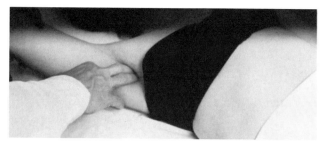

Figure 30–50. Soft tissue mobilization of the right subscapularis.

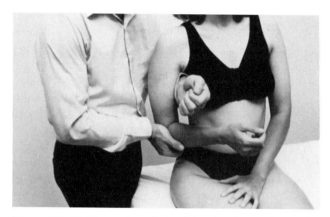

Figure 30–51. Distraction of the right glenohumeral articulation with contract relaxation.

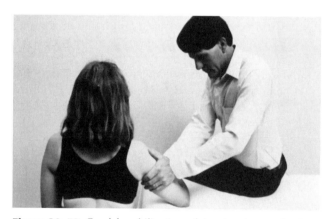

Figure 30–52. Caudal mobilization of the glenohumeral articulation with contract relaxation. Not shown is resistance to the depressors of the humeral head.

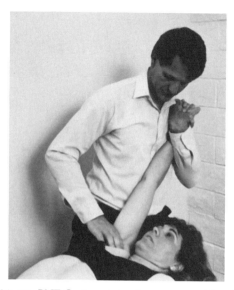

Figure 30–53. PNF flexion abduction pattern with soft tissue mobilization.

Home program: This consists of rotator cuff and upper extremity diagonal resistance using a sports cord, arm circles, and stretching to assist in maintaining and gaining ROM (Fig. 30–56)

4. *Upper limb nerve tension.* Following improvements in the mobility of the right first rib, C4–C5, and glenohumeral function, the upper limb nerve tension test was negative with shoulder girdle depression.

When the test was expanded to include a combination of shoulder girdle depression, 30 degrees of shoulder abduction, elbow extension, and wrist extension to 50 percent, the symptoms to the hand were elicited[24,25] (Fig. 30–57).

Treatment for these symptoms was addressed over several visits with three different protocols:

a. Evaluation and treatment of structures that may have been contributing to the adherent nerve (i.e., cervical spine, anterior and medial scaleni, clavical, subclavious, first rib [also ribs two to four], clavicle, coracoid process, pectoralis minor, lateral boarder of the scapula, soft tissues of the axilla arm, and forearm region, and the nerves themselves) (Fig. 30–58).

b. Performance of the upper limb nerve tension test, with the therapist moving the extremity until the patient or therapist first felt restriction; through tracing and isolation, the therapist and patient identified restricted tissues and applied appropriate treatment techniques (Fig. 30–59).

c. In the test position, the patient performed mid-range wrist flexion and extension or cervical rotation and sidebending while the therapist palpated the nerve to determine the locations of restrictions. This approach should not be used with irritable patients, as excessive motion will generally exacerbate symptoms.

Home program: The program was designed according to the protocol developed by Peter Edgelow.[111] This program includes diaphragmatic breathing, stretching of the upper thoracic spine and ribs over a fulcrum, and midrange oscillations of the wrist in a position short of beginning resistance.

5. *Right wrist.* Treatment was performed to increase wrist extension and improve the mobility of the liga-

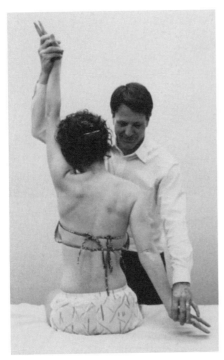

Figure 30–54. Extension adduction PNF pattern.

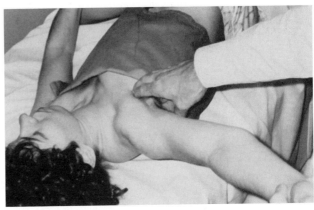

Figure 30–56. Functional movement pattern: arm circles with soft tissue mobilization.

ments. The primary mechanical dysfunctions limiting wrist extension were a restriction of the ability of the distal ends of the radius and ulna to separate and volar mobility of the lunate. It is possible that these dysfunctions occurred at the time of the accident and were a factor in the onset of wrist and hand pain secondary to computer keyboard usage.

The initial purpose of treatment was to mobilize the soft tissues and articulations of the wrist. As mobil-

ity improved, the extremity was placed at the end of the flexion abduction and extension abduction patterns to further treat the mechanical limitations of wrist extension and to initiate selective neuromuscular reeducation (Figs. 30–60 and 30–61). Treatment of the wrist in weightbearing was the final phase of functional mobilization (Fig. 30–62). The patient was sitting on the table and bearing weight on her hand, which was placed at the side in varying degrees of rotation. Weightbearing mobilization was applied while the patient actively moved over the fixed base of support.

Home program: This consisted of stretching in weightbearing and resisted PNF wrist pivots with a sports cord.

6. *Pelvic girdle.* During the patient's second visit, the pelvic girdle dysfunctions were normalized. The right innominate fixation in flexion and external rotation was probably precipitated during the accident secondary to the foot's position on the brake pedal. Pelvic girdle dysfunctions alter the normal weight distribution, base of support, and motor recruitment of the upper quadrant. It is our belief that the pelvic girdle

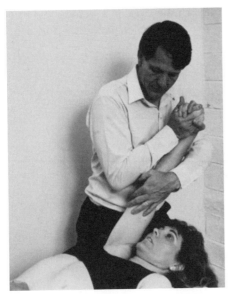

Figure 30–55. Bilateral asymmetric reciprocal pattern for trunk and shoulder girdle stability while sitting.

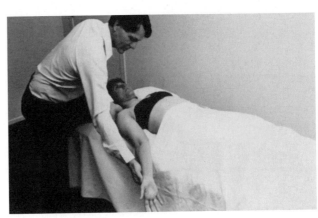

Figure 30–57. Position for the upper limb nerve tension test.

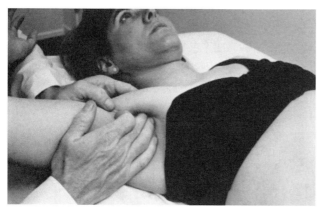

Figure 30–58. Mobilization of soft tissue around the axillary nerve track.

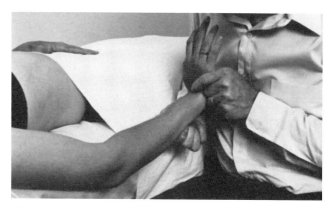

Figure 30–60. Wrist soft tissue and joint mobilization in the extension abduction pattern.

should be evaluated for dysfunctions whenever the present problem involves a weightbearing structure.

The following soft tissue structures were evaluated and treated: the right psoas, iliacus, and piriformis (Figs. 30–63 to 30–65). The following articulations were mobilized: the right sacral base with a fulcrum technique (Fig. 30–66) and extension and internal rotation mobilization of the right innominate (Fig. 30–67). Mobilization of the innominate was performed in a prone position, with the patient's left leg off the table to stabilize the lumbar spine. The right lower extremity was placed at the end-range of the extension abduction pattern, and contract relaxation was performed toward flexion adduction. During performance of the contract relaxation technique, pressure was applied on the upper lateral iliac crest to mobilize the superior innominate anterior and medially.

Treatment Progression and Results

The patient was seen initially for 7 visits over a 3-week period, with emphasis placed on education and training and manual therapy applied to the primary dysfunctions. Following this period, the subjective and objective signs of the cervical spine and shoulder improved 70 to 80 percent. The upper limb nerve tension improved 40 to 50 percent and became the primary emphasis of treatment. The patient was then seen once a week for the next 5 weeks for further training and treatment of the remaining dysfunctions. The emphasis of this component of treatment was on having the patient perform and progress in her exercise program and increase her level of daily activities.

At the end of this 5-week period the patient returned to work. Following 3 days of work she experienced increased cervical and peripheral symptoms, and we initiated treatment twice a week for the next 3 weeks to assist her transition to full-time employment. She was then seen for follow-up appointments every 3 to 4 weeks for 3 months.

At the end of 3 months she was discharged, with occasional peripheral symptoms secondary to excessive activity, but with the capacity to resolve and control these symptoms through self-management and a home program.

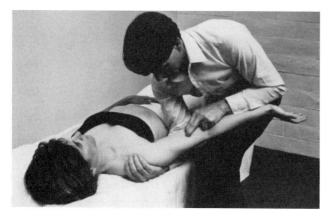

Figure 30–59. Position for the upper limb nerve tension test with tracing and isolating for soft tissue mobilization.

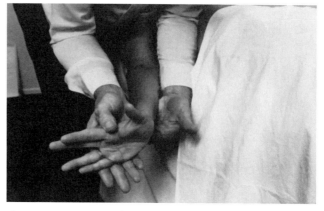

Figure 30–61. Resisted reeducation of a tight wrist in extension abduction.

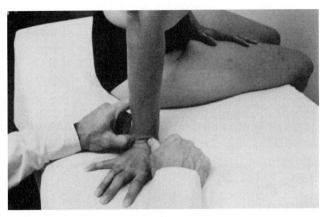

Figure 30–62. Mobilization of the wrist in weightbearing.

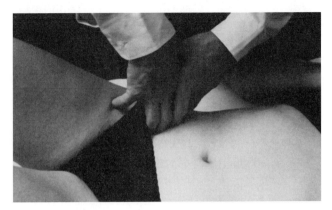

Figure 30–64. Soft tissue mobilization of the right iliacus.

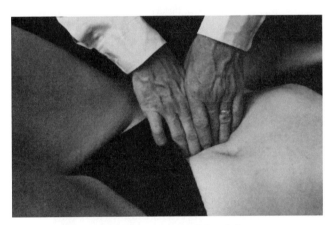

Figure 30–63. Strumming of the right psoas.

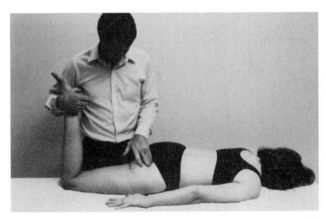

Figure 30–65. Sustained pressure to the right piriformis with associated oscillations.

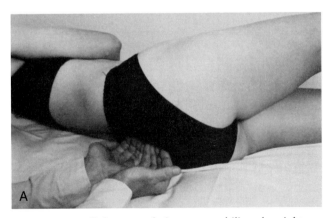

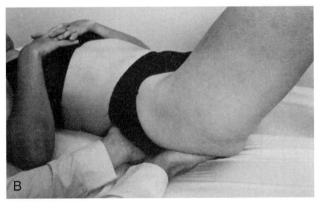

Figure 30–66. Fulcrum technique to mobilize the right sacral base. (A) Finger position. (B) Technique.

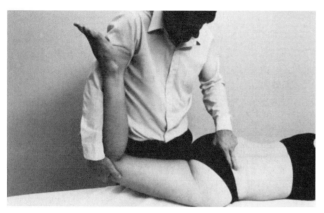

Figure 30–67. Functional mobilization of the right innominate into anterior torsion and in-flare.

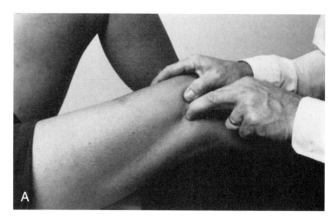

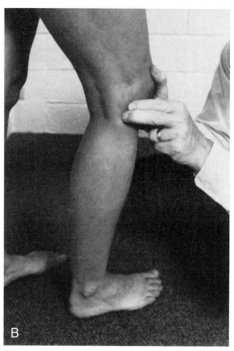

Figure 30–68. Scar tissue mobilization. (A) Nonweightbearing. (B) Weightbearing.

CASE STUDY 2

The following case study illustrates the role that dysfunctional scar tissue can play in altering normal biomechanics and the results achieved with normalization.

The patient presented with right knee pain and dysfunction 1 year after anterior cruciate reconstructive surgery. She complained of lateral joint line and medial infrapatella pain after extended use. She also stated that she was having difficulty developing strength and muscular bulk in the quadriceps, especially the vastus medialis obliques. The functional evaluation revealed that she was tracking medially, with difficulty moving her knee over the lateral aspect of her foot. It was noted that the lateral scar tissue developed significant tightness during knee tracking, with restricted posterior mobility.

Treatment of the scar was initially applied in nonweightbearing and progressed to weightbearing, with the patient attempting to track over the middle toe. The primary treatment technique used was unlocking spirals (Fig. 30–68).

Following normalization of the scar tissue, there was a natural tendency to track over the second toe. In addition, the patient was able to perform dynamic quad setting exercises of the vastus medialis. This confirmed the limitations on lower extremity function produced by the scar tissue.

■ Summary

The soft tissues of the body are often found to have inefficient mobility and tone, which precipitates and perpetuates many musculoskeletal symptoms. STM can play a valuable role in the treatment of these soft tissue dysfunctions. This treatment approach will achieve optimal results when used in conjunction with patient education, body mechanics training, a musculoskeletal conditioning program, and other manual therapy approaches (joint mobilization and neuromuscular education). A well-rounded and comprehensive conservative care program is required to return an individual to optimal function while avoiding nonconservative methods of management such as surgical intervention.

■ References

1. Harris J: History and development of manipulation and mobilization. p. 7. In Basmajian J, Nyberg R (eds): Rational Manual Therapies. Williams & Wilkins, Baltimore, 1933
2. Johnson GS, Saliba-Johnson VL: Functional Orthopedics I: Course Outline. The Institute of Physical Art, San Anselmo, CA, 1993
3. Johnson GS, Saliba-Johnson VL: Functional Orthopedics II: Course Outline. The Institute of Physical Art, San Anselmo, CA, 1992

4. Johnson GS, Saliba-Johnson VL: Functional Mobilization UQ and LQ: Course Outlines. Institute of Physical Art, San Anselmo, CA, 1992

5. Gray H: Anatomy of the Human Body. Lea & Febiger, Philadelphia, 1966

6. Ham A, Cormack D: Histology. 8th Ed. JB Lippincott, Philadelphia, 1979

7. Grieve GP: Common Vertebral Joint Problems. 2nd Ed. Churchill Livingstone, London, 1988

8. Hollingshead WH: Functional Anatomy of the Limbs and Back: A Text for Students of the Locomotor Apparatus. WB Saunders, Philadelphia, 1976

9. Kirkaldy-Willis WH: Managing Low Back Pain. 2nd Ed. Churchill Livingstone, New York, 1988

10. Cummings GS, Crutchfield CA, Barnes MR: Orthopedic Physical Therapy. Vol. 1. Soft Tissue Changes in Contractures. Strokesville, Atlanta, 1983

11. Kendall HO, Kendall FP, Boynton DA: Posture and Pain. Robert E. Krieger, Huntington, NY, 1977

12. Travell JG, Simons DG: Myofascial Pain and Dysfunction: The Trigger Point Manual. Vols. I and II. Williams & Wilkins, Baltimore, 1983, 1992

13. Woo S, Buckwalter JA: Injury and Repair of the Musculoskeletal Soft Tissues. American Academy of Orthopedic Surgeons, Park Ridge, IL, 1988

14. Porterfield J, DeRosa C: Mechanical Low Back Pain. WB Saunders, Philadelphia, 1991

15. Adams A: Effect of exercise upon ligament strength. Res Q 37:163, 1966

16. Faulkner JA: New perspectives in training for maximum performance. JAMA 205:741, 1986

17. Cailliet R: Soft Tissue Pain and Disability. FA Davis, Philadelphia, 1977

18. Woo S, Ritter MA, Amiel D, et al: The effects of exercise on the biomechanical and biochemical properties of swine digital flexor tendons. J Biomech Eng 103:51, 1981

19. Ames DL: Overuse syndrome. J Fla Med Assoc 73:607, 1986

20. Sikorski JM: The orthopaedic basis for repetitive strain injury. Aust Fam Physician 17:81, 1988

21. Farfan HF: Mechanical factors in the genesis of low back pain. In Bonica JJ (ed): Advances in Pain Research and Therapy. Vol 3. Raven Press, New York, 1979

22. Wadsworth CT: Manual Examination and Treatment of the Spine and Extremities. William & Wilkins, Baltimore, 1988

23. Warwick R, Williams PL (eds): Gray's Anatomy. 37th Ed. Churchill Livingstone, Edinburgh, 1989

24. Butler D: Mobilization of the Nervous System. Churchill Livingstone, New York, 1991

25. Elvey RL: Treatment of arm pain associated with abnormal brachial plexus tension. Aust J Physiother 32:224, 1986

26. Farfan H, Gracovetsky S: The optimum spine. Spine 11:543, 1986

27. Gratz CM: Air injection of the fascial spaces. Am J Roentgenol 35:750, 1936

28. Donatelli R, Owens-Burkart H: Effects of immobilization on the extensibility of periarticular connective tissue. J Soc Phys Ther 3:67, 1981

29. Mennell JM: Joint Pain. Little, Brown, Boston, 1964, p. 6

30. Mennell JB: The Science and Art of Joint Manipulation. Vol. 2. Churchill Livingstone, London, 1952

31. Forrest L: Current concepts in soft tissue wound healing. Br J Surg 70:133, 1983

32. Woo S, Mathews JV, Akeson WH, et al: Connective tissue response to immobility: correlative study of biomechanical and biochemical measurements of normal and immobilized rabbit knees. Arthritis Rheum 18:257, 1975

33. Nikolaou PK, MacDonald BL, Glisson RR, et al: Biomechanical and histological evaluation of muscle after controlled strain injury. Am J Sports Med 15:9, 1987

34. Arem JA, Madden JW: Effects of stress on healing wounds. I. Intermittent noncyclical tension. J Surg Res 20:93, 1976

35. Peacock E, VanWinkle W: Wound Repair. 2nd Ed. WB Saunders, Philadelphia, 1976

36. Van der Muelen JCH: Present state of knowledge on processes of healing in collagen structures. Int J Sports Med 3:4, 1982

37. Cyriax J: Textbook of Orthopedic Medicine: Diagnosis of Soft Tissue Lesions. 8th Ed. Williams & Wilkins, Baltimore, 1984

38. Noyes F: Functional properties of knee ligaments and alteration induced by immobilization: a correlative biomechanical and histological study in primates. Clin Orthop 123:210, 1977

39. Palastanga N: The use of transverse frictions for soft tissue lesions. p. 819. In Grieve G (ed): Modern Manual Therapy of the Vertebral Column. Churchill Livingstone, London, 1986

40. Ganong A: Textbook of Medical Physiology. 3rd Ed. WB Saunders, Philadelphia, 1968, p. 833

41. Lowenthal M, Tobis JS: Contracture in chronic neurological disease. Arch Phys Med 38:640, 1957

42. Amiel D, Frey C, Woo S, et al: Value of hyaluronic acid in the prevention of contracture formation. Clin Orthop 196:306, 1985

43. Woo S, Gomez MA, Woo YK, et al: The relationship of immobilization and exercise on tissue remodeling. Biorheology 19:397, 1982

44. Meyer K: Nature and function of mucopolysaccharides of connective tissue. Mol Biol 69, 1960

45. Enneking W, Horowitz M: The intra-articular effects of immobilization on the human knee. J Bone Joint Surg 54A:973, 1972

46. Amiel D, Akeson W, Woo S: Effects of nine weeks immobilization of the types of collagen synthesized in periarticular connective tissue from rabbit knees. Trans Orth Res Soc 5:162, 1980

47. Akeson W: Wolff's law of connective tissue: the effects of stress deprivation on synovial joints. Arthritis Rheum 18(Suppl 2):1, 1989

48. Akeson W: Value of 17-β-oestradial in prevention of contracture formation. Ann Them Dis 35:429, 1976

49. Akeson WH, Amiel D, Woo S: Immobility effects on synovial joint: the pathomechanics of joint contracture. Biorheology 17:95, 1980

50. Frankle VH, Nordin M: Basic Biomechanics of the Skeletal System. Lea & Febiger, Philadelphia, 1980

51. Bogduk N, Twomey LT: Clinical Anatomy of the Lumbar Spine. Churchill Livingstone, New York, 1987

52. Frank C, Amiel D, Woo S, et al: Pain complaint–exercise performance relationship in chronic pain. Pain 10:311, 1981

53. Cottingham JT, Porges SW, Richmond K: Shifts in pelvic inclination angle and parasympathetic tone produced by rolfing soft tissue manipulation. Phys Ther 68:1364, 1988

54. Dicke E, Shliack H, Wolff A: A Manual of Reflexive Therapy of the Connective Tissue (Connective Tissue Massage) "Bindegewebsmassage." Sidney S. Simone, Scarsdale, NY, 1978

55. Fabian P: Myofascial Strategies I: Course Outline. Institute of Physical Art, San Anselmo, CA, 1988, p. 8

56. Korr IM: The Collected Papers. American Academy of Osteopathy, Colorado Springs, CO, 1979

57. Levine P: Stress. p. 331. In Coles MGH, et al (eds): Psychophysiology: Systems, Processes, and Applications. Guilford Press, New York, 1986

58. Ward RC: The myofascial release concept. Course Manual: Tutorial on Level 1 Myofascial Release Technique. Michigan State University, College of Osteopathic Medicine, 1987

59. Basmajian JV: Grant's Method of Anatomy. 9th Ed. Williams & Wilkins, Baltimore, 1975

60. Korr IM: The neurobiologic mechanisms in manipulative therapy. Plenum Press, New York, 1978

61. Stoddard A: Manual of Osteopathic Practice. Hutchinson & Co, London, 1959

62. Tappan F: Healing Massage Techniques: A Study of Eastern and Western Methods. Prentice-Hall, Reston, VA, 1975

63. Sapega A, Quedenfeld T, Moyer R, et al: Biophysical factors in range-of-motion exercise. Physician Sportmed 9:57, 1981

64. Malone TR: Muscle injury and rehabilitation. Williams & Wilkins, Baltimore, 1988

65. Hill A: The mechanics of active muscle. Proc R Soc Lond 141:104, 1953

66. Komi PV: Training of muscle strength and power: interaction of neuromotoric, hypertrophic and mechanical factors. Int J Sports Med 7:10, 1986

67. Locker LH, League NG: Histology of highly-stretched beef muscle: the fine structure of grossly stretched single fibers. J Ultrastruct 52:64, 1975

68. Janda V: Muscle weakness and inhibition (pseudoparesis) in back pain syndromes. p. 198. In Grieve G (ed): Modern Manual Therapy of the Vertebral Column. Churchill Livingstone, London, 1986

69. Saliba V, Johnson G: Lumbar protective mechanism. p. 112. In White AH, Anderson R (eds): The Conservative Care of Low Back Pain. Williams & Wilkins, Baltimore, 1991

70. Grossmand MR, Sahrmann SA, Rose SJ: Review of length-associated changes in muscle. Phys Ther 62:1799, 1982

71. Tardieu C, Tarbary J, Tardieu G, et al: Adaptation of sarcomere numbers to the length imposed on muscle. p. 103. In Gubba F, Marecahl G, Takacs O (eds): Mechanism of Muscle Adaptation to Functional Requirements. Pergamon Press, Elmsford, NY, 1981

72. Dvorak J, Dvorak V: Manual Medicine: Diagnostics. Georg Thieme Verlag, Stuttgart, 1984

73. Saliba V, Johnson G, Wardlaw C: Proprioceptive neuromuscular facilitation. p. 243. In Basmajian J, Nyberg R (eds): Rational Manual Therapies. Williams & Wilkins, Baltimore, 1993

74. Feldenkrais M: Awareness Through Movement. Harper & Row, New York, 1977

75. Jowett RL, Fidler MW: Histochemical changes in the multifidus in the mechanical derangements of the spine. Orth Clin North Am 6:145, 1975

76. Aston J: Aston Patterning. Aston Training Center. Incline Valley, NV, 1989

77. Jull GA: Examination of the lumbar spine. p. 547. In Grieve G (ed): Modern Manual Therapy of the Vertebral Column. Churchill Livingstone, London, 1986

78. Kirkaldy-Willis WH, Hill RJ: A more precise diagnosis for low back pain. Spine 4:102, 1979

79. Knott M, Voss DE: Proprioceptive neuromuscular facilitation. 2nd Ed. Harper & Row, New York, 1968

80. Lewit K: The contribution of clinical observation to neurological mechanisms in manipulative therapy. p. 3. In Korr I (ed): The Neurobiologic Mechanisms in Manipulative Therapy. Plenum Press, London, 1978

81. Hodges PW, Richardson CA: Contraction of the abdominal muscles associated with movement of the lower limb. Phys Ther 77:2, 1997

82. Wilke HJ, Wolf S, Dlaes LE, et al: Stability of the lumbar spine with muscle groups—a biomechanical in vitro study. Spine 20:2, 1995

83. Hodges PW, Richardson CA: Inefficient muscular stabilization of the lumbar spine associated with low back pain—a motor control evaluation of transversus abdominis. Spine 21:22, 1996

84. Hodges PW, Richardson CA: Feedforward contraction of transversus abdominis is not influenced by the direction of arm movement. Exp Brain Res 114:362, 1997

85. Hides JA, Richardson CA, Jull GA: Multifidus muscle recovery is not automatic after resolution of acute, first-episode low back pain. Spine 21:23, 1996

86. Hides JA, Stokes MJ, Saide M, et al: Evidence of lumbar multifidus muscle wasting ipsilateral to symptoms in patients with acute/subacute low back pain: Spine 19:2, 1994

87. Hides JA, Richardson CA, Jull GA: Magnetic resonance imaging and ultrasonography of the lumbar multifidus muscle. Spine 20:1, 1995

88. Kong WK, Goel VK, Gilbertson LG, et al: Effects of muscle dysfunction on lumbar spine mechanics: Spine 21:19, 1996

89. Johnson GS, Saliba-Johnson VL: Back Education and Training: Course Outline. Institute of Physical Art, San Anselmo, CA, 1988

90. Johnson GS, Saliba-Johnson VL: PNFI: The Functional Approach to Movement Reeducation. Institute of Physical Art, San Anselmo, CA, 1987

91. Cyriax J, Cyriax P: Illustrated Manual of Orthopaedic Medicine. Butterworths, Bourough Green, England, 1983

92. Maitland GD: Vertebral Manipulation. 5th Ed. Butterworths, London, 1986

93. Jull G, Janda V: Muscles and motor control in low back pain: assessment and management. p. 253. In Twomey LT, Taylor JR (eds): Physical Therapy of the Low Back. Churchill Livingstone, New York, 1987

94. Todd ME: The Thinking Body: A Study of the Balancing Forces of Dynamic Man. Dance Horizons, Brooklyn, NY, 1937

95. Klein-Vogelback S: Functional Kinetics. English Ed. Springer-Verlag, London, 1990

96. Carriere B, Felix L: In consideration of proportions. Clin Manage 4:93, 1993

97. Johnson G, Saliba VA: Lumbar Protective Mechanism. p. 113. In White A, Anderson R (eds): The Conservative Care of Low Back Pain. Williams & Wilkins, Baltimore, 1991

98. Pacina M, Krmpotic-Nemanic J, Markiewitz A: Tunnel Syndromes. CRC Press, Boca Raton, FL, 1991

99. Greenman P: Principles of Manual Medicine. Williams & Wilkins, Baltimore, 1989

100. Miller B: Learning the touch. p. 3. In Physical Therapy Forum (Western ed.) Vol. 6. Forum Publishing, King of Prussia, PA, 1987

101. Montagu A: Touching: The Human Significance of Skin. 2nd. Ed. Harper & Row, New York, 1978

102. Scott-Charlton W, Roebuck DJ: The significance of posterior primary divisions of spinal nerves in pain syndromes. Med J Aust 2:945, 1972

103. O'Brien J: Anterior spinal tenderness in low back pain syndromes. Spine 4:85, 1979

104. Evjenth O, Hamberg J: Muscle Stretching in Manual Therapy: A Clinical Manual. Alfta Rehab Forlag, Alfta, Sweden, 1985

105. Morgan D: Concepts in functional training and postural stabilization for the low-back-injured. Top Acute Care Trauma Rehabil 2:8, 1988

106. Vollowitz E: Furniture prescription for the conservative management of low back pain. Top Acute Care Trauma Rehabil 2:18, 1988

107. Rolf R: Rolfing. Dennis-Landman, Santa Monica, CA, 1977

108. Wyke B: The neurology of joints. Ann R Coll Sur 41:25, 1967

109. Basmajian JV: Muscles Alive: Their Functions Revealed by Electromyography. Williams & Wilkins, Baltimore, 1978

110. Saal JS: Flexibility training. Phys Med Rehab 1:537, 1987

111. Edgelow P: Adverse Neural Tension Course Notes. Vol. 26, p. 716. Hayward, CA, 1969

112. Dupuis PR, Kirkaldy-Willis WH: The spine: integrated function and pathophysiology. p. 673. In Cruess RL, Rennie WRJ (eds): Adult Orthopaedics. Churchill Livingstone, New York, 1984

CHAPTER 31

Evaluation and Treatment of Neural Tissue Pain Disorders

Toby M. Hall and Robert L. Elvey

When considering injury to or disorders of the peripheral nervous system, musculoskeletal medicine generally considers altered axonal conduction. Axonal conduction loss occurs with readily diagnosable forms of peripheral neuropathy such as nerve root compression, peripheral nerve entrapments, transections, and stretch injuries, but these are relatively rare in comparison to the multitude of other disorders to which physiotherapists must attend.[1,2]

By contrast, pain in the upper or lower quarter in the absence of any neurologic deficit of the peripheral nervous system and in the absence of clinically relevant information from diagnostic tests such as radiologic imaging exams is a common clinical presentation.[3] In recent years there has been considerable interest in the role neural tissue may play in this type of pain disorder.[4-8] Of particular interest is the possible involvement of the nervi nervorum[4] and the presence of abnormal nerve trunk mechanosensitivity in neurogenic pain.

There is very little information with respect to the proportion of pain disorders that have abnormal neural tissue mechanosensitivity as the primary source of symptoms. Hall et al.[5] investigated subjects with neck and shoulder pain and found, through manual examination, that approximately one-third of them had abnormal neural tissue mechanosensitivity with no neurologic deficit. This evidence alone indicates that an important aspect of management of the patient with upper or lower quarter pain is a thorough investigation of the mechanosensitivity of neural tissue. In neuromusculoskeletal disorders, identification of the source of pain is essential prior to administration of physical treatment or the prescription of exercise programs.

Although the concept of neurogenic pain in disorders of the neuromusculoskeletal system is not new,[9,10] the development in recent years of neural tissue physical examination and manual treatment techniques can be attributed to Elvey[11-13] and Butler.[6] Contemporary understanding of pain physiology and how this might relate to neural tissue involvement in pain disorders has enhanced the physical examination and treatment of neurogenic pain.[7,14] This knowledge requires careful consideration in the management of neural tissue disorders and has necessitated a change in the understanding of the physical treatment of pain,[15] particularly neurogenic pain.[16]

This chapter presents a brief overview of peripheral neurogenic pain together with a scheme for the clinical examination necessary to evaluate the involvement of neural tissue in a disorder of pain and dysfunction unaccompanied by a neurologic deficit. In addition, a treatment approach is outlined which is suitable only when there is a reversible cause of the neurogenic pain disorder.

Pain

In the evaluation of pain and the various types of pain patterns that may accompany disorders of the upper and lower quarters, it is essential for the clinician to keep an open mind with respect to any judgment of the tissue of origin of pain. Although symptoms such as tingling, burning, pins and needles, and numbness are generally accepted as an indication of pathology affecting the nerve root or peripheral nerve trunk, pain unaccompanied by paresthesia may be very difficult to analyze in terms of tissue of origin.

Pain can be of two types, nociceptive or neuropathic, or a combination of both.[17] Nociceptive pain arises from chemically or mechanically induced impulses from nonneural tissues and can be further classified as follows:[1,17]

1. Local pain, which may be an indication of pathology of somatic tissues immediately underlying the cutaneous area of perceived pain

2. Visceral referred pain, in which a visceral disorder may cause a perception of pain in cutaneous tissues distant from the viscera involved
3. Somatic referred pain giving rise to perceived pain in cutaneous tissues distant from the somatic tissue

Neuropathic pain arises from neural structures.[17] This type of pain is perceived in cutaneous tissues that may be distant from the pathologic neural tissue. The nervi nervorum is the sensory supply of the peripheral neural system. Pain arising from noxious stimulation of the nervi nervorum does not appear to have been classified as either nociceptive or neuropathic. Although physiologically it is nociceptive, we consider pain resulting from stimulation of the nervi nervorum to be included in the neuropathic category.

In the clinical setting there may be any combination of nociceptive and neuropathic pain, either local or referred. Pain disorders rarely fit into one category.

Although detailed descriptions of nociception—the physiology of pain and the mechanism of somatic referral, visceral referral, and neuropathic pain—are beyond the scope of this chapter, an outline will be given of peripheral neuropathic pain to help provide an understanding of the topic.

■ Peripheral Neuropathic Pain

The term *peripheral neuropathic pain* has been suggested to embrace the combination of positive and negative symptoms in patients in whom pain is due to pathologic changes or dysfunction in neural tissues distal to the dorsal horn.[18] These structures include peripheral nerve trunks, plexuses, dorsal and ventral rami, nerve roots, and dorsal root ganglion.

Two types of neuropathic pain following peripheral nerve injury have been recognized: *dysesthetic pain* and *nerve trunk pain*.[19] Dysesthetic pain results from volleys of impulses arising in damaged or regenerating nociceptive afferent fibers. Characteristically, dysesthetic pain is felt in the peripheral sensory distribution of a sensory or mixed nerve. This pain has features that are not found in deep pain arising from either somatic or visceral tissues. These features include abnormal or unfamiliar sensations, frequently having a burning or electrical quality; pain felt in the region of the sensory deficit; pain with a paroxysmal brief shooting or stabbing component; and the presence of allodynia.[20,21]

In contrast, nerve trunk pain has been attributed to increased activity in mechanically or chemically sensitized nociceptors within the nerve sheaths.[19] This kind or pain is said to follow the course of the nerve trunk. It is commonly described as deep and aching, familiar like a toothache, and worsened with movement, nerve stretch, or palpation.[19]

Peripheral nerve trunks are known to be mechanosensitive, for their connective tissues possess afferents normally capable of mechanoreception.[22,23] These afferents are known as the *nervi nervorum*. Many of them are unmyelinated, forming a sporadic plexus in all the connective tissues of a peripheral nerve, and have predominantly free endings.[22]

Electrophysiologic studies have demonstrated that at least some of the nervi nervorum have a nociceptive function, for they respond to noxious mechanical, chemical, and thermal stimuli.[24] Most nervi nervorum studied by Bove and Light were sensitive to excess longitudinal stretch of the entire nerve they innervated, as well as to local stretch in any direction and to focal pressure.[4] They did not respond to stretch within normal ranges of motion. This evidence is supported by clinical studies showing that under normal circumstances nerve trunks are insensitive to nonnoxious mechanical stimuli.[25,26]

Recent evidence has shown that the nervi nervorum contain neuropeptides including substance P and calcitonin gene-related peptide, indicating a role in neurogenic vasodilation.[4,27] It has been suggested that local nerve inflammation is mediated by the nervi nervorum, especially in cases with no intrafascicular axonal damage.[4] In keeping with this suggestion, it has been postulated that the spread of mechanosensitivity along the length of the nerve trunk distant from the local area of pathology seen in nerve trunk pain is mediated through neurogenic inflammation via the nervi nervorum.[28] The entire nerve trunk then behaves as a sensitized nociceptor, generating impulses in response to minor mechanical stimuli.[29]

The mechanism of neurogenic inflammation may help to explain mechanical allodynia of structurally normal nerve trunks, where the pathology is more proximal in the nerve root. An alternative explanation is that nonnociceptive input from the presumed nerve trunk mechanoreceptors is being processed abnormally within the central nervous system.[25] This is probably the result of a sustained afferent nociceptive barrage from the site of the nerve,[30] a pathologic process termed *central sensitization*.[31]

In the lumbar spine, the most commonly cited form of neural pathology is nerve root compression, which usually results from intervertebral disc herniation but also is commonly caused by age-related changes.[1] Slow-growing osteophytes from lumbar zygapophyseal joints can compress the nerve root in the intervertebral foramen, leading to radicular symptoms and neurologic signs.[32]

Although pain is not a necessary feature of nerve root compression,[33–35] radicular pain in the absence of nerve root inflammatory changes is presumably due to chronic compression of axons within the nerve root.[1] Under these circumstances, there may be minimal sensitization of the nervi nervorum and little evidence of neural tissue mechanosensitivity on neural tissue provocation tests such as the straight leg raise.[33,36] However, unless the condition is minor, there should be clinical, radiologic, and probably electrodiagnostic evidence of compressive neurologic compromise. Clinical neurologic tests should include deep tendon reflexes, muscle power, and skin sensation tests.

Alternatively, radicular pain, even when severe, may occur in an area where axonal conduction is normal but the nerve trunk is highly sensitized mechanically. In this case, clinical neurologic and electrodiagnostic test findings may be normal, suggesting a lack of nerve root compression. What appears to be the significant factors are chemical or inflammatory[37] sensitization of the nervi nervorum and mechanical allodynia of peripheral nerve trunks.

In a patient with nerve injury, dysesthetic pain and nerve trunk pain may exist in isolation; however it is more common for both to be present.[19,33] For this reason, it may be difficult to distinguish, from the subjective descriptive term *pain*, between referred pain arising from somatic tissues and referred pain arising from neural tissues.[38,39]

The pain and paresthesia that occur in cervical and lumbar radiculopathy may not be well localized anatomically because different nerve roots have similar dermatomal distributions. In a series of 841 patients with cervical radiculopathy, only 55 percent presented with pain following a typical discrete dermatomal pattern.[40] The remainder presented with diffuse nondermatomally distributed pain. Rankine et al.[39] found that the location of pain and paresthesia was not a good predictor of the presence of lumbar nerve root compression. As is always the case, information from the subjective examination should be interpreted with caution and within the context of the complete clinical evaluation.

■ Clinical Examination

In disorders evaluated for physical therapy intervention, the combinations of local pain of somatic origin, somatic referred pain, and neurogenic pain can create a dilemma for the physical therapist who must evaluate the disorder.

The purpose of the clinical examination and evaluation is to determine the source of the patient's subjective pain complaint in order to make a diagnosis and to prescribe appropriate treatment options. To effectively evaluate a particular disorder for manual therapy, the clinician must first carry out a thorough subjective examination. An intimate knowledge of the subjective complaint will allow the clinician to plan the scope and range of physical examination tests to elicit a sufficient number of consistent signs in order to make a diagnosis. It is also particularly important that the nature of those signs on physical examination is consistent with the severity, degree of trauma, and history of the subjective complaint. Minor signs of increased upper quarter neural tissue mechanosensitivity in a clinical presentation of severe neck, scapula, and arm pain would not be consistent with a neuropathy.

The primary source of the pain should be sought elsewhere.

Physical evaluation of neural tissue follows the same principles used in examination of any other structure in the body. For example, a clinical presentation of hamstring pain following an injury such as a "pulled muscle" requires a number of physical examination tests whose findings correlate with each other before a diagnosis of muscle strain can be supported. Such tests would include static isometric muscle contraction, hamstring muscle stretch, and palpation of the muscle. These physical tests provide mechanical stimuli to the injured muscle tissue and so are provocative tests seeking a subjective pain response. It is therefore apparent that no test in isolation is sufficient to provide a consistently accurate diagnosis.

In pain disorders, multiple tissues are frequently involved. A very careful physical examination is required to ascertain from which tissue pain predominates.

To determine the level of involvement of neural tissue, a process of clinical reasoning must be employed. Although similar, the examination and clinical reasoning are more sophisticated than the example given for hamstring pain, and a number of specific correlating signs must be present. For instance, it is not possible to say that a straight leg raise (SLR) test alone is positive or negative in the diagnosis of lumbosacral nerve root pathology. The mechanical stress of SLR is not isolated to the neural structures.[41] SLR induces posterior pelvic rotation within a few degrees of lifting the leg from the horizontal.[42] Structures in the posterior thigh, pelvis, and lumbar spine are mechanically provoked. The findings of the SLR test must be interpreted within the clinical context of a number of other procedures before a diagnosis of nerve root pathology can be made.

Physical Signs of Neural Tissue Involvement

According to Elvey and Hall,[13] the physical signs of neural tissue involvement should include the following:

1. Antalgic posture
2. Active movement dysfunction
3. Passive movement dysfunction which correlates with the degree of active movement dysfunction
4. Adverse responses to neural tissue provocation tests, which must relate specifically and anatomically to tests 2 and 3
5. Mechanical allodynia in response to palpation of specific nerve trunks, which relates specifically and anatomically to tests 2 and 4
6. Evidence from the physical examination of a local cause of the neurogenic pain, which involves the neural tissue showing the responses in tests 4 and 5

The peripheral nervous system is well adapted to movement, as well as being a conductive system relaying impulses from the central nervous system to the periphery.

Under normal circumstances peripheral nerve trunks slide and glide with movement, relative to the associated movement of surrounding structures, adapting to positional changes of the trunk and limbs.[11,43,44,45] In addition, the spinal cord, nerve roots, and spinal meninges can readily adapt to normal movements of the spinal column with changes in length and tension.[46,47] With a sound knowledge of applied anatomy, it becomes clearly evident that different anatomic positions of the peripheral joints influence the peripheral nerve trunks in different ways. The clinician can utilize this knowledge to stress individual nerve trunks as part of the physical examination.

When neural tissue is sensitized or inflamed, limb movement and positional change cause a provocative mechanical stimulus resulting in pain and therefore noncompliance of the neural tissue to movement or postural change. This lack of compliance is demonstrated by painful limitation of movement caused by muscles antagonistic to the direction of movement acting to prevent further pain. Muscle contraction, as measured by electromyography, in response to provocation of neural tissue has been demonstrated in both animal and in vivo human experiments.[25,48–51] In patients with a neuropathic pain disorder in which there is evidence of heightened neural tissue mechanosensitivity, muscle activity occurs at the onset of pain provocation, whereas in normal subjects muscle activity occurs according to the level of the subject's pain tolerance.[49] It appears that muscles are recruited via central nervous system processes to prevent pain associated with the provocation of neural tissue.[25,52]

Posture

The initial observation and inspection of the static posture of the cervicobrachial and lumbopelvic regions is particularly important in the evaluation of disorders of the upper and lower quarters. However, it is important to remember

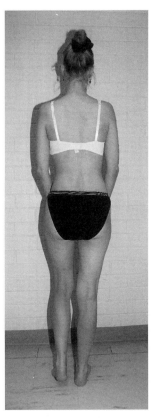

Figure 31–2. Antalgic posture associated with severe left lower quarter neural tissue sensitization.

not to diagnose a problem solely on the basis of a person's posture in a given area. The real importance of posture lies in its relationship to function. An antalgic posture that shortens the anatomic distance over which a peripheral nerve trunk courses may be the first clinical consideration in diagnosing neuropathic pain. Two examples of antalgic posture assumed in response to sensitization of upper and lower quarter neural tissue are presented in Figures 31–1 and 31–2.

In the first example (Fig. 31–1) of a patient with neck, shoulder, and arm pain related to a brachial plexopathy, the posture adopted to relieve provocation of the sensitized neural tissue is a combination of shoulder girdle elevation, cervical spine ipsilateral lateral flexion, and elbow flexion. In the second example (Fig. 31–2) of a patient with buttock and leg pain, the posture adopted to relieve provocation of the sensitized S1 nerve root is a combination of knee flexion, ankle plantar flexion, and lumbar spine ipsilateral lateral flexion.

When sensitization of a lumbar nerve root is associated with an acute, painful intervertebral disc prolapse, there is the added problem of minimizing the stress on the disc. The bulge is greatest on extension or on ipsilateral flexion.[47] The conflict between minimizing the disc bulge and reducing the provocation of neural tissue is resolved in a variety of postures, one of which, seen commonly, is a list toward the painful side together with a flattened lumbar lordosis.

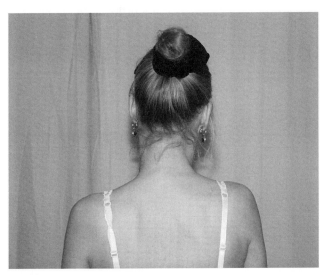

Figure 31–1. Antalgic posture associated with severe right upper quarter neural tissue sensitization.

Guarded postures to avoid movement of the sensitized nerve site have been demonstrated in an animal model.[53] In animal experiments, Hu et al.[50,51] showed that the application of a small-fiber irritant to cervical neuromeningeal tissues resulted in increased electromyographic activity in the upper trapezius and jaw muscles. It appears that the most likely mechanism for altered posture is protective muscle contraction or spasm.

It is important to remember that the magnitude of an antalgic posture will vary with the severity of pain. In the authors' experience, it is the more severe forms of pain disorder that present with antalgic postures. Minor pain problems usually present with no postural change related to abnormal neural tissue mechanosensitivity.

Active Movement

In the majority of less painful disorders, active movement dysfunction may be the first aspect of the physical examination that provides evidence of involvement of the neural system. As with active movement at any joint complex, the clinician should inquire about symptom reproduction, as well as observe the quantity and quality of movement. Poor-quality movement may present as excessive concurrent movement in the joints proximal and distal to the joint being analyzed.

Figure 31–3 demonstrates active shoulder abduction. In this example, the patient has compensated for the lack of compliance of neural tissue in the upper quarter by adopting ipsilateral cervical spine lateral flexion, shoulder girdle elevation, and elbow flexion. This movement dysfunction can be observed in many other types of disorders involving the shoulder girdle, and a hypothesis of abnormal neural tissue mechanosensitivity must be supported by a series of other specific examination procedures.

With an understanding of applied anatomy, the clinician can examine active movements in various ways to support the clinical hypotheses of a neuropathic pain dis-

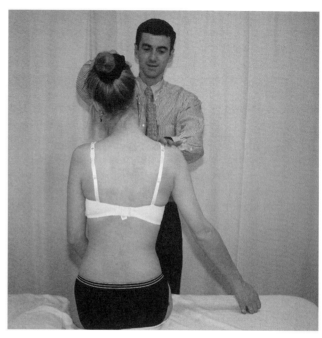

Figure 31–4. Active shoulder abuduction with cervical spine contralateral lateral flexion and the shoulder girdle lightly stabilized.

order. In the upper quarter various active movements will be affected, depending on the particular nerve tract involved. Shoulder abduction and contralateral lateral flexion of the cervical spine will increase the mechanical stress on the brachial plexus and associated tracts of neural tissue.[11,54,55] Therefore, these are the movements most likely to be affected by increased mechanosensitivity of the neural tissues forming the brachial plexus.

If active shoulder abduction or cervical spine contralateral lateral flexion is painful or limited in range, the clinician can differentiate between local pathology and neural tissue pathology by repeating the movement with neural sensitizing maneuvers such as wrist extension. Wrist extension will place greater provocation on the neural tissue of the upper quarter via the median nerve trunk.[56,57]

Figure 31–4 demonstrates shoulder abduction with the cervical spine positioned in contralateral lateral flexion and the wrist extended. Great care must be taken to avoid changing the position of the shoulder girdle complex. A typical response to cervical spine contralateral lateral flexion when upper quarter neural tissue is sensitized is for the patient to elevate the shoulder girdle in an attempt to compensate for the additional mechanical stress of side flexion. The clinician can maintain a consistent shoulder girdle position through the range of abduction with light fixation over the acromion. Using this hand position, the clinician is able to detect compensatory involuntary upper trapezius muscle activity, which can be associated with upper limb neural tissue provocative maneuvers.[58] Without this careful handling, the clinician may misinterpret the outcome of this examination procedure.

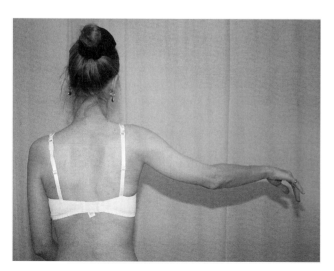

Figure 31–3. Active shoulder abduction with compensatory mechanisms.

In lower quarter lumbar flexion with hip flexion, knee extension and ankle dorsiflexion are provocative to the sciatic nerve, its terminal branches, and the L4–S3 nerve roots.[44,59,60] If pain is provoked or range of movement is limited on active lumbar flexion in standing, the clinician may consider using a process to differentiate between pathology in the lumbar somatic structures and neural tissues. The ankle is positioned in dorsiflexion or the cervical spine in flexion, and the movement is repeated (Fig. 31–5). If neural tissue is involved, the response to active lumbar flexion is more painful and the range of movement is further limited. Again, the clinician must take great care to prevent compensatory involuntary movement of knee flexion, which is presumably a protective hamstring muscle response.

In contrast to the sciatic nerve, the femoral nerve arises from the L2–L4 nerve roots and lies anterior to the coronal axis for sagittal plane movements of the hip and knee. As a consequence, the femoral and the L2–L4 nerve roots are mechanically stressed by a combination of, among other movements, lumbar contralateral lateral flexion, hip extension, and knee flexion.[43,61,62] Differentiation of somatic and neural structures as the source of pain can be considered by using a combination of remote movements sensitizing the neural structures, as previously outlined. Figure 31–6 demonstrates assessment during standing of active lumbar lateral flexion with the knee positioned in flexion. It is essential that the position of

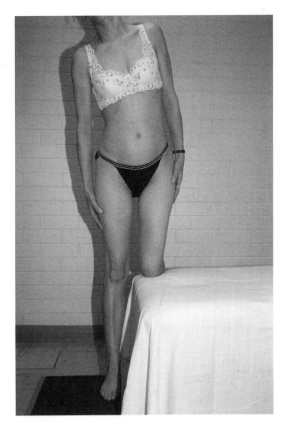

Figure 31–6. Active lumbar lateral flexion with the knee flexed.

the femur and the lumbopelvic posture not be changed between trials; otherwise, the test is invalidated. If there is significant sensitization of the neural tissue associated with the femoral nerve and the L2–L4 nerve roots, range of lumbar lateral flexion will be diminished or more painful with the knee in greater range of flexion.

This is a basic approach to analysis of active movement in the physical evaluation of neural tissue. With some thought to applied anatomy, the clinician can examine active movements in different directions and in various ways to support a clinical hypothesis formed at this early stage of evaluation. For example, a disorder of the C4–C5 motion segment may involve the C5 nerve root or the spinal nerve, which may cause an observable dysfunction of shoulder abduction and movement of the hand behind the back due to the mechanically induced stimulus produced by these movements on the suprascapular and axillary nerve trunks. Contralateral flexion of the head and neck would increase the dysfunction of shoulder abduction in this example.[13]

Passive Movement Dysfunction

It is obvious that both active and passive movement has the same or a similar mechanical stimulus effect on neural tissues. Therefore, in neuropathic pain disorders, there should be consistent limitation of range of passive movement of articulations by pain in the same direction as active movement limitation. However, in addition to as-

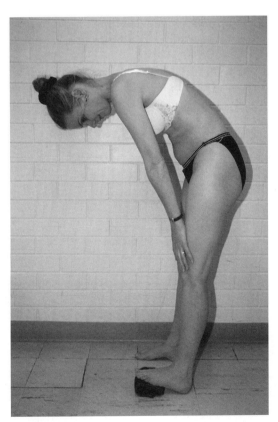

Figure 31–5. Lumbar active flexion with the ankle in end-range dorsiflexion.

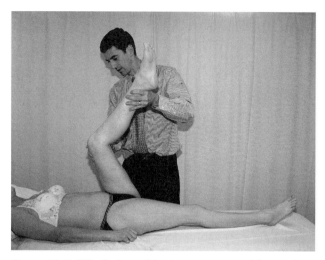

Figure 31–7. Hip flexion adduction maneuver with neural tissue provocation.

sessment of the quantity and quality of range, the clinician must evaluate any change in the feel of articular passive movement which is perceived as a change in the nature and quality of resistance.[63]

The flexion/adduction maneuver of the hip and the quadrant position of the shoulder[64] are two important passive movement tests of those joints. These movements stress not only the hip joint and shoulder complex but also certain peripheral nerve trunks.[13,59]

For example, the sciatic nerve lies posterior and lateral to the axis of motion of hip flexion adduction, so this movement will be provocative to the sciatic nerve and hence to the L4–S2 nerve roots. Possible neural tissue involvement where flexion adduction of the hip is painful and limited in range can be determined by performing the same movement with the knee more extended (Fig. 31–7). A significant decrease in range of movement should be seen if neural tissue is involved in the condition.

In the quadrant position of the shoulder,[64] the humeral head has an upward fulcrum effect on the overlying neurovascular bundle in the region of the axilla.[11] Therefore, it is possible to use this test not only for the shoulder but also for the compliance of the neurovascular tissues to the quadrant position. In the context of this chapter, this test specifically includes the neural tissues of the brachial plexus and its proximal and distal extensions. To differentiate between pain evoked from somatic structures and pain from neural tissue, the test can be performed with the shoulder girdle in elevation and depression and with the head and neck in ipsilateral and contralateral lateral flexion.[13] If the source of pain is somatic structures, there should be little change in response between these positions. By contrast, there should be a predictably increased or decreased response if pain is arising from mechanosensitive neural tissues of the upper quarter.

Adverse Responses to Neural Tissue Provocation Tests

Provocation tests are passive tests that are applied to selectively stress different neural tissues in order to assess their sensitivity to mechanical provocation. A variety of tests have been shown to mechanically provoke various components of the neural system. The most common of these provocative tests is the SLR test.[44] Other tests provocative to neural tissue are the slump test,[46] the femoral nerve stress test,[62] the passive neck flexion test,[65] the median nerve stress test,[56] and the brachial plexus tension test.[66]

Provocation tests can be carried out only within the available ranges of passive movement, which are governed by the severity of pain associated with the disorder being evaluated. For instance, in severe cervicobrachial pain conditions, only limited range of shoulder abduction can be achieved. Therefore, it is unrealistic to use a standard provocation test. The clinician is required to formulate a test according to each patient's signs and symptoms.

A methodologic approach to neural tissue provocation tests for the upper quarter has been documented.[3,13] This approach offers guidelines for examination that allow the test technique to be tailored to the severity of the neurogenic pain disorder. The suggested approach incorporates provocative maneuvers directed to the median, radial, and ulnar nerve trunks from a proximal to a distal direction and vice versa.

Figures 31–8 to 31–10 illustrate the test technique from distal to proximal. For confirmation, to verify the responses to the tests just described, it is important to apply provocative maneuvers from proximal to distal. Figures 31–11 to 31–13 illustrate these maneuvers.

A similar flexible approach is recommended for the lower quarter, although it is not feasible to undertake passive tests from proximal to distal. For a disorder involv-

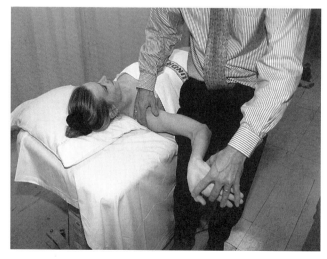

Figure 31–8. Neural tissue provocation test biased to the median nerve trunk (distal to proximal).

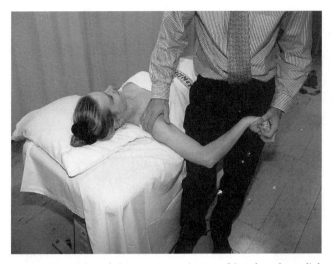

Figure 31–9. Neural tissue provocation test biased to the radial nerve trunk (distal to proximal).

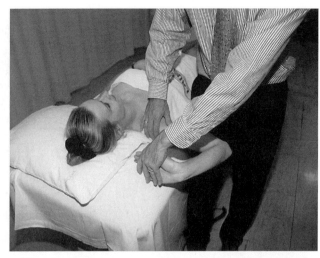

Figure 31–10. Neural tissue provocation test biased to the ulnar nerve trunk (distal to proximal).

ing the lumbar spine, provocative maneuvers directed to the sciatic, femoral, and obturator nerve trunks are required. The use of sensitizing maneuvers is a necessary part of each test. For the SLR test (Fig. 31–14) these include, among others, ankle dorsiflexion, medial hip rotation, and hip adduction, which have all been shown to increase mechanical provocation on the sciatic nerve tract.[59,61] Although cervical spine flexion has also been shown to move and tension lumbar nerve roots,[56,61] the clinical use of cervical spine flexion as a sensitizing maneuver for SLR has been shown to be questionable.[49]

Neural tissue provocative maneuvers directed to the femoral and obturator nerve trunks are shown in Figures 31–15 and 31–16. Lumbar spine lateral flexion can be used as a sensitizing maneuver. The slump test[67] is an important procedure when determining the involvement of neural tissue mechanosensitivity in lower quarter pain disorders. This test may be performed as described by Maitland,[67] with the patient sitting on the edge of the examination table (Fig. 31–17), or, if the patient cannot tolerate this position, in the side-lying position.[68] Hall et al.[68] demonstrated that, in the side-lying position, changing the lumbosacral (L5–S1) spine postures from flexion to extension has a significant sensitizing effect on SLR, presumably by increasing provocation on the lumbosacral trunk and the L4 and L5 nerve roots.[68] This procedure can be used in the differential diagnosis of lower lumbar and sacral nerve root disorders.

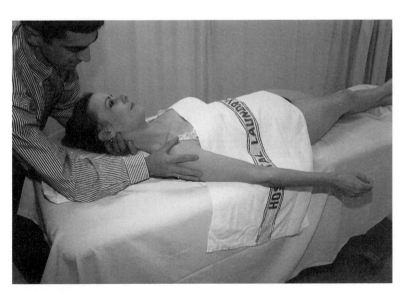

Figure 31–11. Neural tissue provocation test biased to the median nerve trunk (proximal to distal).

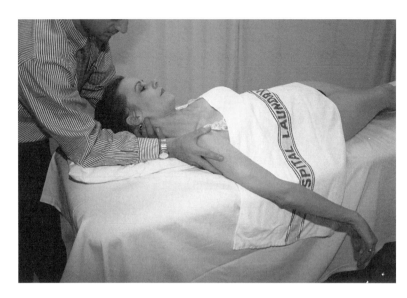

Figure 31–12. Neural tissue provocation test biased to the radial nerve trunk (proximal to distal).

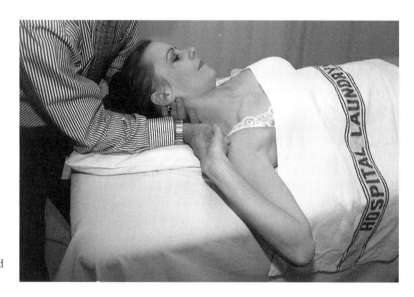

Figure 31–13. Neural tissue provocation test biased to the ulnar nerve trunk (proximal to distal).

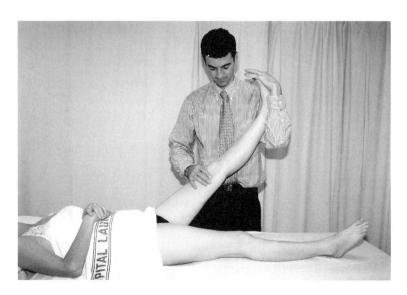

Figure 31–14. SLR with ankle dorsiflexion.

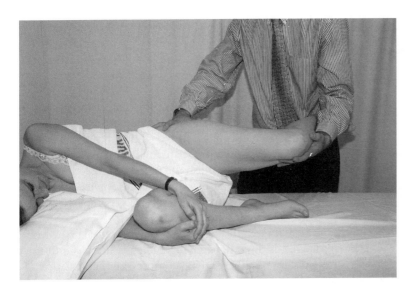

Figure 31–15. Femoral nerve provocation test in the side-lying position.

Neural tissue provocation tests are passive movement tests. The examiner must appreciate changes in muscle tone or activity in addition to a subjective pain response. Increased muscle activity is a reflection of increased mechanosensitivity of the neural tissue being tested and is indicated by an increase in resistance to movement.[69] This increase in resistance, due to onset of protective muscle activity, should coincide with the patient's report of onset of pain[49] and reproduction of the pain complaint. Symptom reproduction is the second important response. *Moments* are a more appropriate biomechanical term to describe angular forces during limb movement. Figure 31–18 is typical of the subjects in this study and represents the moment of stretched tissue, measured objectively by a load cell, during SLR (in the clinical context, moment of stretched tissue is perceived by the examiner as resistance).[69] In this example, the subject tested had significant evidence of lumbosacral neural tissue mechanosensitivity. A change in moment of tissue stretch (increased resistance) occurs only at the onset of muscle activity. The change in resistance associated with the onset of muscle activity is readily appreciable to the clinician during all passive neural tissue provocation procedures.

Mechanical Allodynia in Response to Palpation of Specific Nerve Trunks

An example has been given of an acute muscle tear, where pain on palpation is an important factor in diagnosis. Likewise, if the nervi nervorum is sensitized and pain is provoked by stress applied through the length of the nerve, focal pressure directly over the nerve trunk should also be painful.

It is well known that normal peripheral nerve trunks and nerve roots do not evoke pain in response to nonnoxious mechanical stimuli.[25,26,70,71] By contrast, inflamed nerve roots are exquisitely sensitive to even mild mechanical provocation.[26,71] Similarly, Dyck[72] reported that the entire extent of the sciatic nerve trunk is invariably tender when a lumbosacral nerve root is traumatized. Compara-

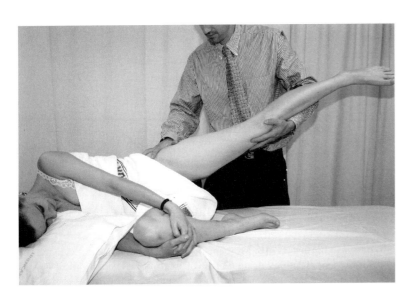

Figure 31–16. Obturator nerve provocation test in the side-lying position.

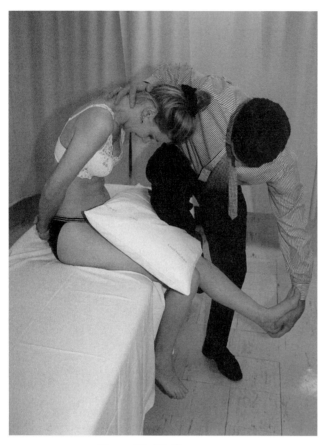

Figure 31–17. Slump test.

ble findings have been reported in cervical radiculopathy.[25]

The spread of mechanosensitivity along the length of the nerve trunk following proximal nerve trauma has been reported elsewhere[18] and has been interpreted as reflecting mechanosensitivity of regenerating axon sprouts either freely growing or arrested in disseminated microneuromas. An alternative interpretation suggests that abnormal responses to mechanical provocation of neural tissue in radiculopathy arise from the nervi nervorum.[4] The spread of sensitization of the nervi nervorum has been attributed to neurogenic inflammation.[28] Activation of the nervi nervorum in response to nerve insult is likely to result in neuropeptide release leading to intraneural edema. This edema, particularly within the epineurium, is likely to spread longitudinally, as peripheral nerves and spinal nerve roots at the level of the intervertebral foramen have very poor lymphatic drainage.[73] The endoneurium and epineurium act as closed compartments[74] that become distorted by fluid pressure[75] and so cause further sensitization of the nervi nervorum. The spread of inflammatory mediators within the edema along the course of the nerve may also sensitize the nervi nervorum.

Palpation of neural tissue must be undertaken with care. When sensitized, peripheral nerve trunks can be exquisitely tender to even very gentle palpation. In addi-

tion to assessing the pain, the clinician should be watching and palpating for associated reflex muscle responses.[25]

Mild nonnoxious pressure should be applied to the nerve trunks on the uninvolved side first in order to allow the patient to make a comparison. In some instances, palpation can be made directly over the nerve trunk, which can be identified as a distinct structure. In other locations, nerve trunks must be palpated through muscle or they are so closely associated with vascular tissues that it is difficult to distinguish the nerve as a structure. When this is the case, broad-based pressure is applied in the area of the nerve trunk and the response is compared to that on the uninvolved side.

Great care must be taken when the neural tissue being palpated is directly overlying bone, as there is a distinct possibility of an iatrogenic compression neuropathy.

Many nerves can be readily palpated, but in the clinical context of upper and lower quarter pain syndromes, the most relevant and commonly palpated nerves include the following:

> Spinal nerves as they exit from the gutters of the transverse processes of C4–C6
>
> Upper and middle trunks of the brachial plexus
>
> Neurovascular bundle of the brachial plexus underlying the tendon of the pectoralis minor
>
> Neurovascular bundle in the axilla incorporating the axillary artery and vein together with the median, radial, and ulnar nerves
>
> Median, radial, ulnar, axillary, suprascapular, and dorsal scapular nerves

Figure 31–19 demonstrates landmarks for palpation of the upper and middle trunks of the brachial plexus, which lie posterior to the sternocleidomastoid and between the belly of the scalenus anterior and scalenus medius. Figures 31–20 and 31–21 demonstrates palpation

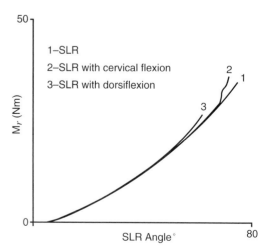

Figure 31–18. Moment of stretched tissue plotted against the SLR angle during SLR, SLR with dorsiflexion, and SLR with cervical spine flexion. (From Hall et al.,[69] with permission.)

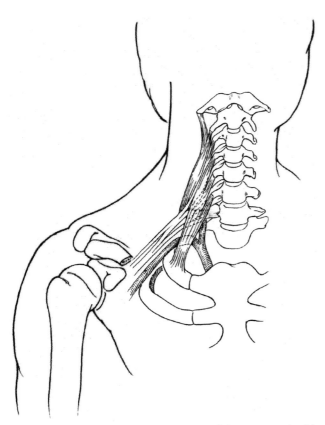

Figure 31–19. Landmarks for palpation of the upper and middle trunk.

of the median nerve in the upper arm and the neurovascular bundle in the axilla.

In the lower quarter, the following neural structures can be examined:

Ventral rami within the belly of the psoas

Sciatic nerve in the gluteal region

Tibial, common peroneal (fibular), and femoral nerves

Figures 31–22 and 31–23 demonstrate palpation of the femoral and common peroneal (fibular) nerves. To verify that a particular nerve trunk is sensitized, the clinician is advised to examine a number of different sites along the course of the nerve trunk. For example, the median nerve can be palpated within the neurovascular bundle in the axilla as well as the upper arm (Figs. 31–20 and 31–21), medial to the biceps tendon in the cubital fossa, and deep within the carpal tunnel. If the median nerve trunk is sensitized, there should be a consistent pain response throughout.

Evidence of a Local Area of Pathology

The examination procedures presented so far have focused on identification of the presence or absence of increased neural tissue sensitization. Once this has been established, it is important to identify a local cause for the neurogenic state. Many peripheral neurogenic pain disorders present to physical examination with all the features discussed. This does not mean that they are amenable to manual therapy treatment. It is quite possible for other conditions, such as painful diabetic neuropathy or a painful neuropathy caused by tumor infiltration, to cause all of the features discussed so far, including limitation of active and passive movement.[13] Therefore, the clinician must determine a cause for the neurogenic pain disorder.

For example, in the upper quarter, intervertebral disc pathology will often result in radicular arm pain and a specific cervical spine motion segment dysfunction. Examination procedures for a local cause of pathology in the cervical spine include palpation and passive segmental mobility tests.[76] Abnormal findings are aberrant spinal segmental mobility associated with pain. One example is a C7 radiculopathy, which may have all the features previously discussed together with a C6–C7 motion segment dysfunction. This would suggest a spinal cause of

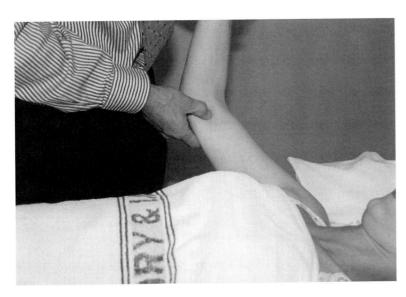

Figure 31–20. Palpation of the median nerve in the upper arm.

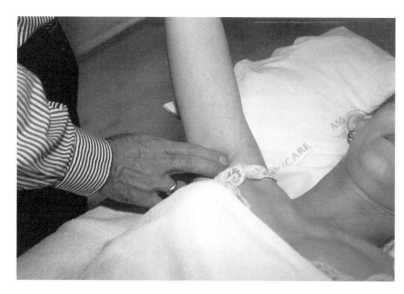

Figure 31–21. Palpation of the neurovascular bundle in the axilla.

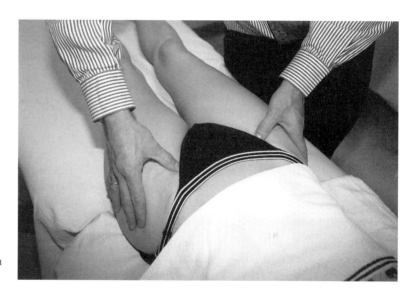

Figure 31–22. Palpation of the femoral nerve in the inguinal region.

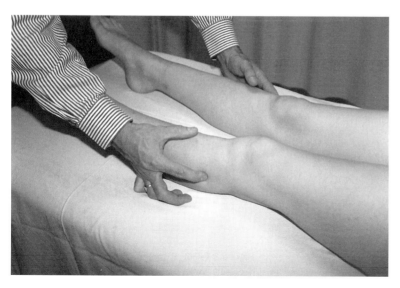

Figure 31–23. Palpation of the common peroneal (fibular) nerve at the neck of the fibula.

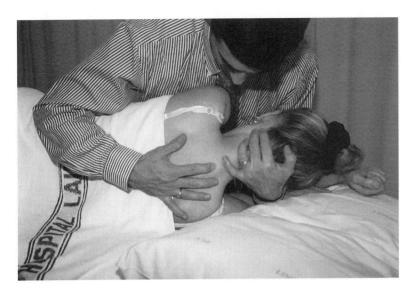

Figure 31–24. Passive segmental mobility test of flexion/extension at C6–C7.

the arm pain. Without the palpation findings it may not be possible to determine such a cause, and further medical investigation would be necessary to exclude nonneuromusculoskeletal causes.

Figure 31–24 shows a typical test technique for the determination of a local area of pathology. In this example, passive intervertebral segmental mobility tests should reveal dysfunction at the C6–C7 level.

An important aspect of the evaluation of neural tissue disorders is the assessment of neurologic function. In the clinical setting, the neurologic examination is the only means of determining whether abnormal axonal conduction exists. The neurologic examination incorporates both subjective inquiry and physical tests of nerve function.

The subjective neurologic examination must delineate the specific type and area of symptoms, including paresthesias and sensory loss. These areas can then be compared with typical dermatomal, sclerotomal, and myotomal maps. However, it is important to remember that this information alone is insufficient to determine the specific spinal segmental level of involvement. Physical neurologic examination procedures must include sensory, reflex, and muscle strength testing. For a true measure of muscle strength, the muscle must be tested to maximum voluntary contraction, which is determined by maximal resistance to the breaking point. However, in many neurogenic pain disorders, evaluation of neurogenic muscle weakness is not possible because of pain inhibition.

There is little information in the literature on the sensitivity or reliability of the neurologic examination. Other tests of nerve function include electrodiagnostic tests such as electromyography. These are invasive procedures that are more specific in the evaluation of motor or sensory conduction loss,[77] but they are not helpful if the problem is related to increased mechanosensitivity of the nerve trunk. Other diagnostic tests such as magnetic resonance imaging, x-ray tests, and other radiologic investigations have, in the past, been largely unhelpful in visual-

izing pathologic peripheral neural tissue and have been particularly unhelpful when the disorder is one of sensitization rather than mechanical compression and conduction loss. Recent advances in magnetic resonance imaging technology have enabled the visualization of peripheral neural tissues including spinal nerves, the brachial plexus, and peripheral nerve trunks.[78–80] There has been no correlation of abnormal neural tissue radiologic findings with symptoms, physical signs on neurologic examination, and neural tissue provocation tests.

We believe that the above examination scheme is effective in determining the presence of abnormal nerve trunk mechanosensitivity and the presence of nerve trunk pain. One study has used this examination protocol to determine the incidence of nerve trunk pain in a particular disorder.[5] In this study, one-third of the subjects with chronic cervicobrachial pain syndrome were found to have neural tissue mechanosensitization as the dominant source of the subjective complaint of pain. The finding of this study had some validity, as all subjects found to have nerve trunk pain responded positively to a prescribed treatment program specifically aimed at addressing nerve trunk mechanosensitivity.

■ Treatment

The most difficult aspect of the management of chronic and acute pain disorders is determining from which structure pain predominates. "Generally speaking, the more evidence there is, the greater the likelihood of focusing on the precise spot."[47] These words are particularly significant in the assessment of neural tissue pain disorders.[47]

In this chapter, a distinction has been made between two types of peripheral neurogenic pain disorder: dysesthetic pain and nerve trunk pain. This distinction is important in regard to manual therapy treatment options, which must be different for each disorder. A problem arises when a particular pain disorder presents elements of both types of pain. Under these circumstances, the clinician must judge whether it is appropriate to apply manual therapy techniques directed at reducing nerve trunk sensitization. In our opinion, if there were signs of reduced axonal conduction on the neurologic examination, neural tissue mobilization techniques would be contraindicated at that time. In the authors' clinical experience, the majority of disorders seen in clinical practice relate to increased sensitization of neural tissue rather than altered axonal conduction.

Under normal circumstances, peripheral nerve trunks are protected from the effects of nerve stretch and compression.[81] However, severe conduction loss may occur at strains as low as 6 percent.[82] As the fasciculi are stretched, their cross-sectional area is reduced, the intrafascicular pressure is increased, nerve fibers are compressed, and the intrafascicular microcirculation is compromised.[81] Even slight pressure on the outside of a nerve will lead to external hyperemia, edema, and demyelination of some axons lasting for up to 28 days.[4] Elsewhere it has been observed that 8 percent elongation of a defined nerve segment may result in impaired venular flow. At elongation of approximately 10 to 15 percent, an upper stretch limit is reached where there is complete arrest of all blood flow in the nerve.[83,84]

In a neurogenic pain disorder, it is likely that the microcirculation within the nerve is abnormal. Therefore, minimal nerve stretch will lead to further circulatory compromise and reduced nerve function. For these reasons, it is unwise to treat a damaged, compressed, or edematous nerve trunk with stretching or lengthening techniques.

The treatment of nerve trunk pain can involve the use of passive movement techniques, but we believe that nerve "lengthening" or stretching techniques are contraindicated. We advocate the use of gentle, controlled oscillatory passive movements of the anatomic structures surrounding the affected neural tissues at the site of involvement. At no time should pain be evoked by the technique. Treatment can be progressed by using passive movement techniques in a similar manner but involving movement of the surrounding anatomic tissues or structures and the affected neural tissues together in an oscillatory movement.[12]

Cervical Lateral Glide

A cervical lateral glide technique described by Elvey[12] is an example of a treatment approach that has been found to be most useful.[5,85] In C6 nerve root involvement, the arm should be positioned in some degree of abduction, with the elbow flexed and the hand resting on the abdomen. The technique involves a gentle glide of the C5–C6 motion segment to the contralateral side in a slow, oscillating manner.

During the technique, the treating clinician will be aware of the onset of protective muscle activity that represents the limit in range of the oscillatory movement or the treatment barrier.[13] If this barrier is not reached, the patient's arm is positioned in greater range of abduction or elbow extension (Fig. 31–25).

Progression of the technique on subsequent days is made by performing the technique with the shoulder in gradually increasing range of abduction.

Shoulder Girdle Oscillation

A logical development of the cervical lateral glide technique would be to add a movement of the surrounding anatomic tissues or structures and the affected neural tissues together. Shoulder girdle oscillation can be performed in a caudad-cephalad direction in the prone position while the patients symptomatic arm is supported with the hand behind the back. The range of oscillation is governed by the onset of muscle activity or the treatment barrier. The technique can be progressed at subsequent

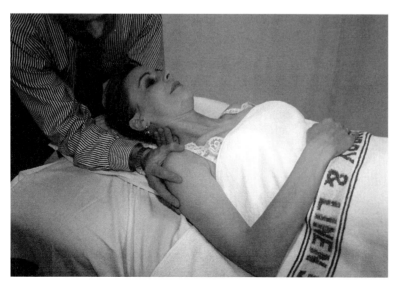

Figure 31–25. Cervical lateral glide technique.

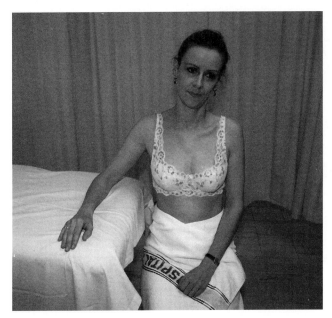

Figure 31–26. Home exercise—upper quarter neural tissue mobilization.

sessions, when indicated, by performing the oscillation while gradually extending the duration of the hand-behind-the-back position.

At some point in the treatment, a home exercise program which is an adjunct to the treatment provided by the clinician should be incorporated. Home exercise should be introduced only when consistent beneficial effects of manual therapy have been demonstrated. An example of a home exercise found to be frequently useful is shown in Figure 31–26. The patient is instructed that there should be no pain during the movement; the exercise should *not stretch* the neural tissues. Three movements of lateral flexion with the arm against the wall are performed once per day.

Evidence of the efficacy of this approach has been demonstrated in subjects with lateral elbow pain[85] and

chronic cervicobrachial pain.[5] Hall et al.[5] showed significant improvements in pain and functional capacity, as well as cervical spine and shoulder girdle mobility, after a 4-week treatment period utilizing this concept of management. Improvements were maintained at follow-up 3 months later.[5]

In the lower quarter, a similar approach can be utilized. Lateral glide is not possible; instead, a modified lateral flexion maneuver has been found to be most effective (Fig. 31–27). The example seen in Figure 31–27 is for the treatment of a left L5 nerve root involvement. The symptomatic leg is positioned in approximately 50 degrees of hip flexion, with the knee flexed to at least 30 degrees of flexion. The leg is supported to prevent adduction, medial rotation, and further provocation of the neural tissue. The range of hip and knee flexion is dependent on the severity and irritability of the disorder. The motion segment to be mobilized is positioned in flexion. The clinician localizes the movement to the L5–S1 segment by transverse pressure to the right via the L5 spinous process, with an attempt to restrict movement above this level. The clinician applies gentle force through the pelvis to create contralateral lateral flexion in a slow, oscillating manner.

As with the cervical lateral glide, the treating clinician will be aware of the onset of protective muscle activity that represents the treatment barrier while using the technique. If this barrier is not reached, the patient's leg is positioned in a greater range of hip flexion and thereby greater neural tissue provocation.

The therapy is progressed on subsequent days by performing the technique with the hip in a gradually increasing range of flexion. A logical development would be to add a movement of the surrounding anatomic tissues or structures and the affected neural tissues together in an oscillatory movement. In the side-lying position, hip flexion is performed with the knee in 50 degrees of flexion. At no time should the patient's symptoms or any paresthesias be evoked.

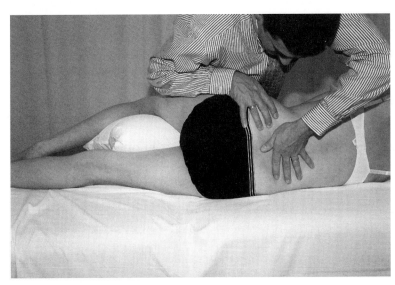

Figure 31–27. Right lateral flexion at L5–S1 for left leg pain.

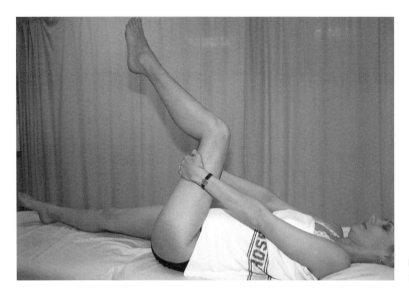

Figure 31–28. Home exercise: lower quarter neural tissue mobilization.

As a home exercise, the patient can perform hip flexion while lying supine (Fig. 31–28). The knee must be flexed to prevent stretching of the neural elements. Again, the patient must understand that the exercise should not cause pain or paresthesias.

CASE STUDIES

CASE STUDY 1

History

A 36-year-old female presented with pain as per the body chart (Fig. 31–29). The problem evolved 18 months previously after a particularly vigorous 3-hour dinghy sailing session. There was no specific incident, but midthoracic, shoulder, and arm pain developed gradually during the evening after sailing and worsened over subsequent days. The patient sought advice from her medical practitioner, who prescribed nonsteroidal anti-inflammatories, rest, and a shoulder x-ray, which was normal. Feeling no improvement over the next 2 weeks, she sought treatment from an osteopath, who manipulated her neck and back, which relieved the thoracic pain. Subsequent treatment gave no relief from the shoulder or arm pain. Since this time, the patient has "learned to live with it." The disorder did not progress, but it worsened temporarily if she tried to perform any physical activity such as sailing. Subsequent investigations by the medical practitioner revealed no abnormality on cervical spine x-ray or ultrasound imaging of the shoulder.

Physical Evaluation

At the initial evaluation, active right shoulder function was recorded as 70 degrees of abduction, 30 degrees of external rotation, and 120 degrees of flexion. A poor pattern of scapulohumeral rhythm was recorded for both flexion and abduction, with excessive scapula movement. Active cervical mobility was restricted in left lateral flexion compared to lateral flexion to the right. Of further interest was the fact that active shoulder mobility was more painful and more restricted in range when the head and neck were positioned in left lateral flexion and when the right wrist was extended.

Shoulder passive mobility was restricted in a fashion consistent with active movements. Again of interest was the fact that passive shoulder abduction was more painful and more restricted in range when the head and neck were positioned in left lateral flexion.

Neural tissue provocation tests were carried out from central to peripheral and vice versa for the median, radial, and ulnar nerve trunks. With the arm positioned in 60 degrees of abduction and the cervical spine in contralateral lateral flexion, wrist and finger extension reproduced the arm pain. Cervical left lateral flexion with the arm positioned in 60 degrees of abduction and shoulder girdle depression reproduced the arm and shoulder pain. Provocative maneuvers of the ulnar nerve were not symptomatic.

Mild pressure over the median, radial, axillary, and suprascapular nerve trunks of the right upper quarter, as well as over the upper trunk of the brachial plexus and the neurovascular bundle in the axilla, produced painful responses that were not present on the left side.

Passive segmental mobility tests of the cervical spine revealed restricted motion at C5–C6. Accessory motion palpation indicated pain and stiffness at the same level. Accessory motion palpation of the glenohumeral joint revealed restriction in range, but with only mild pain.

There was no evidence of a neurologic deficit, and other tests for the shoulder girdle and cervical regions were unremarkable.

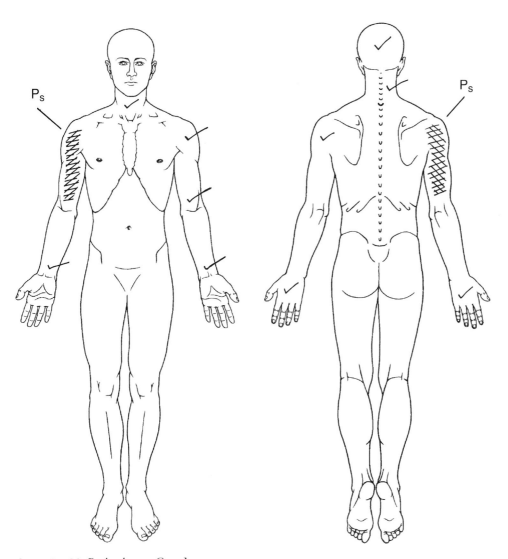

Figure 31–29. Body chart—Case 1.

The physical findings correlated accurately with the subjective complaint and supported a diagnosis of cervicobrachial pain syndrome, in which there was strong evidence of neural tissue involvement and of its being the major source of the pain. There was evidence of glenohumeral joint dysfunction that was contributing to the disorder, but it was felt that the principal problem related to sensitization of neural tissue originating at the C6 nerve root.

Treatment

Treatment commenced with a gentle, controlled oscillation of left lateral glide from the midline of C5 on C6. The right arm was positioned in 20 degrees of abduction, with the elbow flexed to 90 degrees and the hand resting on the abdomen. Treatment was initially carried out three times per week. The patient was asked to refrain from any activity involving shoulder abduction or shoulder girdle depression. In the authors' experience, a significant part

of treatment is the advice that is given to the patient about avoiding activities that provoke symptoms, thereby preventing prolongation of the disorder.

Subjective improvement occurred within the first few treatments; concomitant improvement occurred in active and passive shoulder mobility. After 2 weeks of treatment, active shoulder abduction was 120 degrees and flexion was 160 degrees. Cervical lateral glide was continued with the arm in a progressively greater range of abduction but with the elbow maintained at 90 degrees of flexion. A home exercise program was also introduced which involved sitting sideways at a table with the right arm supported on a pillow to achieve 30 degrees of abduction. Active cervical left lateral flexion was performed without pain five times once per day. Further progress was made and the severity of pain was reduced together with an increase in the range of right shoulder mobility.

After 4 weeks of treatment, manual therapy techniques directed at restoring normal accessory glide of the glenohumeral joint were introduced in conjunction with the cervical lateral glide. At the end of the treatment, the patient had regained 90 percent of shoulder mobility and was able to undertake daily tasks without discomfort.

This case is an example of the situation in which treatment is initially directed at the sensitized neural tissue as the primary source of symptoms, but it was also necessary to address the dysfunctional glenohumeral joint as a secondary contributing factor. In the authors' experience, if the treatment approach had been reversed and the glenohumeral joint treated first, the outcome would have been poor.

CASE STUDY 2

History

A 43-year-old male presented with pain as per the body chart (Fig. 31–30). The problem developed 3 months prior to assessment as a result of unloading a pallet stackedwith boxes of photocopy paper. The patient was aware of pain in the low back that gradually worsened overnight and spread to his left leg. The patient saw the company doctor, who sent him home with muscle relaxants, painkillers, and nonsteroidal anti-inflammatory medication. The doctor also ordered a plane lumbar x-ray and a computed tomography (CT) scan. According to the radiologist's report, the CT scans revealed evidence of an L4–L5 broad-based posterior disc bulge which did not impinge on the thecal sac, and there was no evidence of nerve root impingement. The patient had a history of previous low back pain associated with lifting injuries at work. There was no history of leg pain. The previous low back episode occurred 3 years previously, at which time a CT scan revealed the same findings. There had been no change in the radiologic findings between the two scans. No other abnormality was detected apart from a

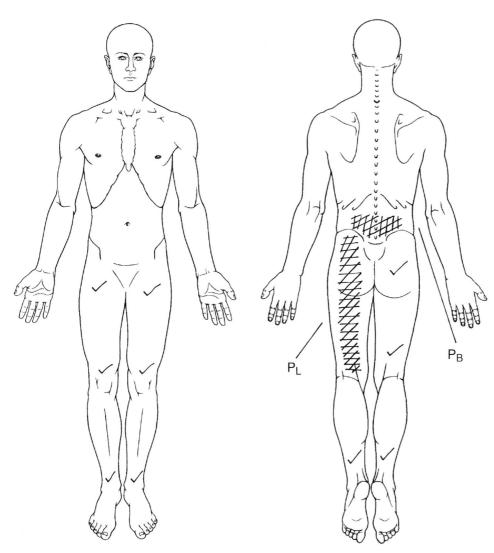

Figure 31–30. Body chart—Case 2.

mild scoliosis. The patient had attempted to return to work with light duties, working in the company office, but this had been unsuccessful.

As a result of the work trial, the patient was referred to a pain specialist, who requested physiotherapy management.

Physical Evaluation

At the initial examination, the patient presented with an antalgic posture, the left hip and knee were flexed, and the left iliac crest was elevated with respect to the right. The lumbar spine was laterally flexed to the left. Correction of the deformity increased the leg pain.

Active lumbar mobility was recorded as: flexion—finger tips to the knee joint line limited by left leg pain; side flexion to the right—finger tips 6 cm above the knee joint line limited by back pain; side flexion to the left and extension were both pain-free. Of further interest was the fact that active lumbar flexion and right lateral flexion mobility were more painful and more restricted in range when the left ankle and foot were positioned in dorsiflexion and when the left hip was flexed.

Hip passive mobility was restricted in flexion and flexion/adduction. Again of interest was the fact that passive hip flexion/adduction was more painful and more restricted in range when the knee was positioned in greater range of extension.

Neural tissue provocation tests were carried out for the sciatic, femoral, and obturator nerve trunks. SLR was limited to 40 degrees and reproduced the leg pain. With the ankle/foot in dorsiflexion, SLR was more painful and limited in range. SLR was limited to 80 degrees, without pain on the right side. Provocative maneuvers to the femoral and obturator nerve trunks did not produce symptoms. Left knee extension with the left hip in 90 degrees of flexion, tested in the right side-lying position, was more painful and restricted in range when the lumbosacral spine was positioned in extension compared to flexion.

Mild pressure over the sciatic and common peroneal (fibular) nerve trunks of the lower quarter produced painful responses that were not present on the right side. There were no responses to pressure over the femoral nerve trunk or the tibial nerve on either side.

Passive segmental mobility tests of the lumbar spine revealed restricted motion at L4–L5 and L5–S1. Accessory motion palpation produced pain and stiffness that were greater at the L4–L5 level than at the L5–S1 level. Sacroiliac joint stress tests produced no symptoms.

There was no evidence of a neurologic deficit, and other physical examination tests for the lumbar region were unremarkable.

Treatment

Treatment commenced with a gentle, controlled oscillation of right lateral flexion at L4–L5. The left leg was positioned in 50 degrees of hip and knee flexion. Treatment was initially carried out three times per week. The patient was asked to avoid a slumped spinal posture while sitting and to refrain from any activity involving lumbar flexion with the knee in extension.

Subjective improvement occurred gradually over 3 weeks. Significant improvement occurred in active and passive lumbar and hip mobility. After 3 weeks of treatment, active lumbar flexion was to mid shin and SLR was 70 degrees. Localized L4–L5 lateral flexion was continued with the leg positioned in a progressively greater range of hip flexion and with the knee flexed to 30 degrees.

A home exercise program was also introduced, which involved sitting sideways at a low table with the left leg supported on the table and with the left knee flexed to 30 degrees. Active lumbar right lateral flexion was performed without pain five times once per day. A further addition to treatment was a right side-lying technique involving passive left hip flexion with the left knee maintained at 30 degrees of flexion. The endpoint of hip flexion was always short of symptom reproduction.

The patient continued to experience a reduction in pain and increased lumbar and hip mobility.

After 4 weeks of treatment, the patient returned to light duties in an office environment. After 6 weeks of treatment, he was introduced to a gradual work-hardening program that involved a gym program. After a period of reconditioning, the patient returned to his original duties.

■ Summary

This chapter has provided a management protocol for upper and lower extremity neurogenic pain disorders which have as an essential element increased mechanical sensitization of the nerve trunk. A distinction has been made between neurogenic pain disorders involving mechanical sensitization and those with reduced axonal conduction. A description of peripheral neuropathic pain has also been presented. This subject is fundamental to the presented approach; it is recommended that the individual study this topic in greater detail. Finally, in the application of this approach, the role of the central nervous system in pain disorders must never be underestimated.

■ References

1. Bogduk N: Clinical Anatomy of the Lumbar Spine and Sacrum. 3rd Ed. Churchill Livingstone, Melbourne, 1997
2. Drye C, Zachazewski J: Peripheral nerve injuries. pp. 441–462. In Zachazewski J, Magee D, Quillen W (eds): Athletic Injuries and Rehabilitation. WB Saunders, Philadelphia, 1996
3. Hall T, Elvey R: Nerve trunk pain: physical diagnosis and treatment. Manual Ther 4(2):63–73, 1999

4. Bove G, Light A: The nervi nervorum: missing link for neuropathic pain? Pain Forum 6(3):181–190, 1997

5. Hall T, Elvey R, Davies N, et al: Efficacy of manipulative physiotherapy for the treatment of cervicobrachial pain. pp. 73–74. In Tenth Biennial Conference of the MPAA. Manipulative Physiotherapists Association of Australia, Melbourne, 1997

6. Butler D: Mobilisation of the Nervous System. Churchill Livingstone, Melbourne, 1991

7. Greening J, Lynn B: Minor peripheral nerve injuries: an underestimated source of pain. Manual Ther 3(4):187–194, 1998

8. Quintner J, Cohen M: Referred pain of peripheral nerve origin: an alternative to the "myofascial pain" construct. Clin J Pain 10:243–251, 1994

9. Madison Taylor J: Treatment of occupation neuroses and neuritis in the arms. JAMA 53(3):198–200, 1909

10. Marshall J: Nerve stretching for the relief or cure of pain. Br Med J 15:1173–1179, 1883

11. Elvey R: Brachial plexus tension tests and the pathoanatomical origin of arm pain. pp. 105–110. In Idczak R (ed): Aspects of manipulative therapy. Lincoln Institute of Health Sciences, Melbourne, 1979

12. Elvey R: Treatment of arm pain associated with abnormal brachial plexus tension. Aust J Physiother 32:225–230, 1986

13. Elvey R, Hall T: Neural tissue evaluation and treatment. pp. 131–152. In Donatelli R (ed): Physical Therapy of the Shoulder. 3rd Ed. Churchill Livingstone, New York, 1997

14. Zusman M: Irritability. Manual Ther 3(4):195–202, 1998

15. Butler D: Commentary: Adverse mechanical tension in the nervous system: a model for assessment and treatment. pp. 33–35. In Maher C (ed): Adverse Neural Tension Revisited. Australian Physiotherapy Association, Melbourne, 1998

16. Elvey R: Commentary: Treatment of arm pain associated with abnormal brachial plexus tension. pp. 13–17. In Maher C (ed): Adverse neural tension revisited. Australian Physiotherapy Association, Melbourne, 1998

17. Elliot K: Taxonomy and mechanisms of neuropathic pain. Semin Neurol 14(3):195–205, 1994

18. Devor M, Rappaport H: Pain and pathophysiology of damaged nerve. pp. 47–83. In Fields HL (ed): Pain Syndromes in Neurology. Butterworth Heinemann, Oxford, 1990

19. Asbury A, Fields H: Pain due to peripheral nerve damage: an hypothesis. Neurology 34:1587–1590, 1984

20. Devor M: Neuropathic pain and injured nerve: Peripheral mechanisms. Bri Med Bull 47(3):619–630, 1991

21. Fields H: Pain. McGraw-Hill, New York, 1987

22. Hromada J: On the nerve supply of the connective tissue of some peripheral nervous system components. Acta Anat 55:343–351, 1963

23. Thomas P, Berthold C, Ochoa J: Microscopic anatomy of the peripheral nervous system. pp. 28–91. In Dyck P, Thomas P (eds): Peripheral Neuropathy. 3rd Ed. Vol. 1. WB Saunders, Philadelphia, 1993

24. Bove G, Light A: Unmyelinated nociceptors of rat paraspinal tissues. J Neurophysiol 73:1752–1762, 1995

25. Hall T, Quintner J: Responses to mechanical stimulation of the upper limb in painful cervical radiculopathy. Aust J Physiother 42(4):277–285, 1996

26. Kuslich S, Ulstrom C, Cam J: The tissue origin of low back pain and sciatica: A report of pain responses to tissue stimulation during operations on the lumbar spine using local anaesthesia. Orthop Clin North Am 22(2):181–187, 1991

27. Zochodne D: Epineural peptides: a role in neuropathic pain. Can J Neurol Sci 20:69–72, 1993

28. Quintner J: Peripheral neuropathic pain: A rediscovered clinical entity. In Abstracts of the 19th annual general meeting of the Australian Pain Society. Australian Pain Society, Hobart, April, 1998

29. Devor M: The pathophysiology of damaged peripheral nerves. pp. 63–81. In Wall P, Melzack R (eds): Textbook of Pain. Churchill Livingstone, Edinburgh, 1989

30. Sugimoto T, Bennett G, Kajanda K: Strychnine-induced transynaptic degeneration of dorsal horn neurons in rats with an experimental neuropathy. Neurosci Lett 98:139–143, 1989

31. Woolf C: Generation of acute pain: central mechanisms. Br Med Bull 47:523–533, 1991

32. Epstein J, Epstein B, Levine L, et al: Lumbar nerve root compression at the intervertebral foramina caused by arthritis of the posterior facet. J Neurosurg 39:362–369, 1973

33. Rydevik B, Garfin S: Spinal nerve root compression. pp. 247–261. In Szabo R (ed): Nerve Root Compression Syndromes: Diagnosis and Treatment, Slack, Thorofare, NJ, 1989

34. MacNab I: The mechanism of spondylogenic pain. pp. 89–95. In Hirsch C, Zotterman Y (eds): Cervical Pain. Pergammon Press, New York, 1972

35. Wiesel S, Tsourmas N, Feffer H, et al: A study of computer-assisted tomography: 1. The incidence of positive CAT scans in an asymptomatic group of patients. Spine 9:549–551, 1984

36. Amundsen T, Weber H, Lilleas F, et al: Lumbar spinal stenosis: clinical and radiologic features. Spine 20(10):1178–1186, 1995

37. Olmarker K, Rydevik B: Pathophysiology of sciatica. Orthop Clin North Am 22(2):223–234, 1991

38. Dalton PA, Jull GA: The distribution and characteristics of neck-arm pain in patients with and without a neurological deficit. Aust J Physiother 35:3–8, 1989

39. Rankine J, Fortune D, Hutchinson C, et al: Pain drawings in the assessment of nerve root compression: a comparative study with lumbar spine magnetic resonance imaging. Spine 23(15):1668–1676, 1998

40. Henderson C, Hennessy R, Shuey H: Posterior lateral foraminotomy for an exclusive operative technique for cervical radiculopathy: a review of 846 consecutively operated cases. J Neurosurg 13:504–512, 1983

41. Kleynhans A, Terrett A: The prevention of complications from spinal manipulative therapy. pp. 171–174. In Glasgow EF Twomey LT (eds): Aspects of Manipulative Therapy. Churchill Livingstone, Melbourne, 1986

42. Fahlgren Grampo J, Reynolds H, Vorro J, et al: 3-D motion of the pelvis during passive leg lifting. pp. 119–122. In Anderson P, Hobart D, Danoff J (eds): Electromyographical Kinesiology. Elsevier, Stockholm, 1991

43. Breig A: Adverse Mechanical Tension in the Central Nervous System: Relief by Functional Neurosurgery. Almquist and Wiksell, Stockholm, 1978

44. Goddard M, Reid J: Movements induced by straight leg raising in the lumbo-sacral roots, nerves and plexus and in the intrapelvic section of the sciatic nerve. J Neurol Neurosurg Psychiatry 28:12–18, 1965

45. McLellan D, Swash M: Longitudinal sliding of the median nerve during movements of the upper limb. J Neurol Neurosurg Psychiatry 39:566–570, 1976

46. Louis R: Vertebroradicular and vertebromedullar dynamics. Anat Clin 3:1–11, 1981

47. Troup J: Biomechanics of the lumbar spinal canal. Clin Biomech 1:31–43, 1986

48. Balster S, Jull G: Upper trapezius muscle activity during the brachial plexus tension test in asymptomatic subjects. Manual Ther 2(3):144–149, 1997

49. Hall T, Zusman M, Elvey R: Manually detected impediments during the SLR test. pp. 48–53. In Jull G (ed): Manipulative Physiotherapists Association of Australia: Ninth Biennial Conference. Manipulative Physiotherapists Association of Australia, Gold Coast Queensland, 1995

50. Hu J, Yu X, Vernon H, et al: Excitatory effects on neck and jaw muscle activity of inflammatory irritant applied to cervical paraspinal tissues. Pain 55:243–250, 1993

51. Hu J, Vernon H, Tatourian I: Changes in neck electromyography associated with meningeal noxious stimulation. J Manip Physiol Ther 18:577–581, 1995

52. Elvey R: Nerve tension signs. p. 85. In Paris S (ed): Proceedings of the Fifth International Conference of the International Federation of Manipulative Therapists. International Federation of Manipulative Therapists, Vail, CO, 1992

53. Laird J, Bennett G: An electrophysiological study of dorsal horn neurons in the spinal cord of rats with an experimental peripheral neuropathy. J Neurophysiol 69(6):2072–2085, 1993

54. Ginn K: An investigation of tension development in upper limb soft tissues during the upper limb tension test. pp. 25–26. In Proceedings of the International Federation of Orthopaedic Manipulative Therapist's Conference, Cambridge, 1988

55. Reid S: The measurement of tension changes in the brachial plexus. pp. 79–90. In Dalziel B, Snowsill J (eds): Proceedings of the Fifth Biennial Conference of the Manipulative Therapists Association of Australia, Melbourne, 1987

56. Kleinrensink G, Stoeckart R, Vleeming A, et al: Mechanical tension in the median nerve. The effects of joint positions. Clin Biomech 10(5):240–244, 1995

57. Lewis J, Ramot R, Green A: Changes in mechanical tension in the median nerve: possible implications for the upper limb tension test. Physiotherapy 84(6):254–261, 1998

58. Van der Heide B: Muscle activity as a response to neural tissue testing in the upper limb. pp. 207–209. In Tenth Biennial Conference of the MPAA. Manipulative Physiotherapists Association of Australia, Melbourne, 1997

59. Breig A, Troup J: Biomechanical considerations of the straight-leg-raising test. Spine 4(3):242–250, 1979

60. Lew P, Morrow C, Lew A: The effect of neck and leg flexion and their sequence on the lumbar spinal cord: implications in low back pain and sciatica. Spine 19(21):2421–2425, 1994

61. O'Connell JEA: Protrusions of the lumbar intervertebral disc. J Bone Joint Surg 33B(1):8–17, 1951

62. Sugiura K, Yoshida T, Katoh S, et al: A study on tension signs in lumbar disc hernia. Int Orthop 3:225–228, 1979

63. Jull G, Bullock M: A motion profile of the lumbar spine in an ageing population assessed by manual examination. Physiother Pract 3:70–81, 1987

64. Maitland G: Peripheral Manipulation. 3rd Ed. Butterworth-Heinemann, London, 1991

65. Yuan Q, Dougherty L, Margulies S: In vivo human cervical spinal cord deformation and displacement in flexion. Spine 23(15):1677–1683, 1998

66. Elvey R: Brachial plexus tension tests and the pathoanatomical origin of arm pain. pp. 116–122. In Glasgow EF, Twomey LT, Scull ER, et al (eds): Aspects of Manipulative Therapy. 2nd Ed. Churchill Livingstone, Melbourne, 1985

67. Maitland G: Negative disc exploration: positive canal signs. Aust J Physiother 25(3):129–133, 1979

68. Hall T, Hepburn M, Elvey R: The effect of lumbosacral postures on the modified SLR test. Physiotherapy 79:566–570, 1993

69. Hall T, Zusman M, Elvey RL: Adverse mechanical tension in the nervous system? Analysis of straight leg raise. Manual Ther 3(3):140–146, 1998

70. Howe J, Loeser J, Calvin W: Mechanosensitivity of dorsal root ganglia and chronically injured axons: a physiological basis for the radicular pain of nerve root compression. Pain 3:25–41, 1977

71. Smyth M, Wright V: Sciatica and the intervertebral disc. An experimental study. J Bone Joint Surg 40A:1401–1418, 1958

72. Dyck P: Sciatic Pain: Lumbar Discectomy and Laminectomy. Aspen, Rockville, MD, 1987

73. Sunderland S: Nerve Injuries and Their Repair. Churchill Livingstone, Edinburgh, 1991

74. Rydevik B, Brown M, Lundborg G: Pathoanatomy and pathophysiology of nerve root compression. Spine 9(1):7–15, 1984

75. Lundborg G, Myers R, Powell H: Nerve compression injury and increased endoneurial fluid pressure: a "miniature compartment syndrome." J Neurol Neurosurg Psychiatry 46:1119–1124, 1983

76. Maitland G: Vertebral Manipulation. 5th Ed. Butterworths, London, 1986

77. Haldeman S: The electrodiagnostic evaluation of nerve root function. Spine 9:42–47, 1984

78. Dailey T, Goodkin R, Filler A, et al: Magnetic resonance neurography for cervical radiculopathy: a preliminary report. Neurosurgery 38(30):488–492, 1996

79. Filler A, Hayes C, Bell B, et al: Application of magnetic resonance neurography in the evaluation of patients with peripheral nerve pathology. J Neurosurg 85:299–309, 1996

80. Panasci D, Holliday R, Shpizner B: Advanced imaging techniques of the brachial plexus. Hand Clin 11(4):545–553, 1995

81. Sunderland S: The anatomy and physiology of nerve injury. Muscle Nerve 13:771–784, 1990

82. Kwan M, Wall E, Massie J, et al: Strain, stress and stretch of peripheral nerve: rabbit experiments in vitro and in vivo. Acta Orthop Scand 63(3):267–272, 1992

83. Lundborg G, Rydevik B: Effects of stretching the tibial nerve of the rabbit: a preliminary study of the intraneural circulation and the barrier function of the perineurium. J Bone Joint Surg 55B(2):390–401, 1973

84. Ogato K, Naito M: Blood flow of peripheral nerves: effects of dissection, stretching and compression. J Hand Surg 11:10, 1986

85. Vicenzino B, Collins D, Wright A: Cervical mobilisation: immediate effects on neural tissue mobility, mechanical hyperalgesia and pain free grip strength in lateral epicondylitis. pp. 155–156. In Jull G (ed): Clinical Solutions. Manipulative Physiotherapists Association of Australia, Gold Coast Queensland, 1995

Index